SAUER'S MANUAL OF SKIN DISEASES

ELEVENTH EDITION

Brian J. Hall, MD
Department of Pathology
University of Utah
Salt Lake City, Utah

John C. Hall, MD
Primary Staff
St. Luke's Hospital
Lecturer of Medicine
University of Missouri-Kansas
City School of Medicine
Clinician
Kansas City Free Health Clinic
Kansas City, Missouri

With 88 Contributing Authors

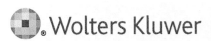

. Wolters Kluwer

Philadelphia • Baltimore • New York • London
Buenos Aires • Hong Kong • Sydney • Tokyo

Executive Editor: Rebecca Gaertner
Senior Developmental Editor: Kristina Oberle
Editorial Coordinator: Maria M. McAvey
Marketing Manager: Rachel Mante Leung
Production Project Manager: David Saltzberg
Design Coordinator: Teresa Mallon
Manufacturing Coordinator: Beth Welsh
Prepress Vendor: S4Carlisle Publishing Services

9 8 7 6 5 4

Eleventh Edition

Printed in the United States of America

Library of Congress Cataloging-in-Publication Data

Names: Hall, Brian J. (Brian John), 1981- editor. | Hall, John C., 1947- editor.
Title: Sauer's manual of skin diseases / [edited by] Brian J. Hall, John C. Hall.
Other titles: Manual of skin diseases
Description: Eleventh edition. | Philadelphia: Wolters Kluwer Health, [2017]
 | Includes bibliographical references and index.
Identifiers: LCCN 2017004087 | ISBN 9781496329936
Subjects: | MESH: Skin Diseases
Classification: LCC RL74 | NLM WR 140 | DDC 616.5—dc23 LC record available at https://lccn.loc.gov/2017004087

LWW.com

DEDICATION

To Charlotte and Jamie; and to Gordon Sauer, whose book this will always be.

Contributing Authors

Saquib R. Ahmed, MD
Division of Dermatology
University of Kansas Medical Center
Kansas City, Kansas
Chapter 19: Urticaria

Daniel Aires, MD, JD
Stiefel Professor and Division Director
Division of Dermatology
University of Kansas School of Medicine
Kansas City, Kansas
Chapter 46: General Principles of Skin Aging

Mackenzie C. Asel, MD
Dermatology Resident
Dartmouth-Hitchcock Medical Center
Lebanon, New Hampshire
Chapter 53: Dermatoses of Pregnancy

Rodney S. W. Basler, MD
Founding Chair
Taskforce on Sports Medicine
American Academy of Dermatology
Adjunct Associate Professor
Department Internal Medicine (Dermatology)
University of Nebraska Medical Center
Omaha, Nebraska
Chapter 51: Sports Medicine Dermatology

Cheryl B. Bayart, MD, MPH
Department of Dermatology
Cleveland Clinic Foundation
Cleveland, Ohio
Chapter 35: Diseases Affecting the Hair

Wilma F. Bergfeld, MD
Professor, Dermatology and Pathology
Cleveland Clinic Foundation
Cleveland, Ohio
Chapter 35: Diseases Affecting the Hair

Francisco G. Bravo, MD
Associate Professor
Pathology
Universidad Peruana Cayetano Heredia
Lima, Peru
Chapter 50: Tropical Diseases of the Skin

Cheryl M. Burgess, MD
Assistant Clinical Professor
Department of Dermatology
Georgetown University Medical Center
George Washington University Hospital
Washington, DC
Chapter 38: Skin Diseases in Ethnic Skin

Antoanella Calame, MD
Medical Director
Poway Dermatology
Poway, California
Chapter 27: Cutaneous Diseases Associated With Human Immunodeficiency Virus

Nicole M. Candelario, MD
Department of Dermatology
University of Puerto Rico
San Juan, Puerto Rico
Chapter 27: Cutaneous Diseases Associated With Human Immunodeficiency Virus

Chia-Yu Chu, MD, PhD
Associate Professor
Department of Dermatology
National Taiwan University Hospital and National Taiwan University College of Medicine
Taipei, Taiwan
Chapter 9: Drug Eruptions

Clay J. Cockerell, MD
Professor
Dermatology and Pathology
University of Texas Southwestern
Dallas, Texas
Chapter 27: Cutaneous Diseases Associated With Human Immunodeficiency Virus

Matthew Dacunha, BS
Division of Dermatology
University of Kansas Medical Center
Kansas City, Kansas
Chapter 19: Urticaria

Dayna G. Diven, MD
Professor
University of Texas Dell Medical School
Austin, Texas
Chapter 29: Sexually Transmitted Infections

Zoe D. Draelos, MD
Consulting Professor
Department of Dermatology
Duke University School of Medicine
Durham, North Carolina
President
Dermatology Consulting Services
High Point, North Carolina
Chapter 7: Cosmetics for the Physician

Steven E. Eilers, MD
Dermatology Resident
Rutgers New Jersey Medical School
Newark, New Jersey
Chapter 34: Cutaneous T-cell Lymphoma

Carly Elston, MD
Dermatology Resident
Cleveland Clinic
Cleveland, Ohio
Chapter 8: Dermatologic Allergy

Dirk M. Elston, MD
Professor
Kathleen A. Riley Chair of Dermatology
Chair, Department of Dermatology and Dermatologic
  Surgery
Medical University of South Carolina
Charleston, South Carolina
Chapter 8: Dermatologic Allergy

Steven R. Feldman, MD, PhD
Director
Center for Dermatology Research
Professor
Department of Dermatology
Department of Pathology
Department of Public Health Sciences
Wake Forest School of Medicine
Winston-Salem, North Carolina
Chapter 52: Cutaneous Signs of Bioterrorism

Kristen H. Fernandez, MD
Assistant Professor
University of Missouri
Chief of Dermatology
Harry S Truman VA
Columbia, Missouri
Chapter 14: Vasculitis

Nicholas Golda, MD
Assistant Professor of Dermatology
Director of Dermatology Surgery
University of Missouri Health
School of Medicine
Columbia, Missouri
Chapter 31: Common Nonmelanoma Skin Cancers

James L. Griffith, MD
Clarence S. Livingood Clinical Research Fellow
Department of Dermatology
Henry Ford Health System
Detroit, Michigan
**Chapter 43: Dermatologic Reactions to Ultraviolet,
  Visible Light, and Infrared Radiation**

Deepti Gupta, MD
Assistant Professor
Department of Pediatrics/Division of Dermatology
Seattle Children's Hospital/University of Washington
Seattle, Washington
Chapter 44: Genodermatoses

John C. Hall, MD
Primary Staff
St. Luke's Hospital
Lecturer of Medicine
University of Missouri-Kansas City School of
  Medicine
Clinician
Kansas City Free Health Clinic
Kansas City, Missouri
**Chapters 3, 4, 12, 13, 15, 17, 18, 20, 21, 22, 24, 25, 28,
  30, 37, 40, 55, and Index: Dermatologic Diagnosis,
  Dermatologic Therapy, Pruritic Dermatoses, Vascular
  Dermatoses, Seborrheic Dermatitis, Acne, and Rosacea,
  Other Papulosquamous Dermatoses, Granulomatous
  Dermatoses, Dermatologic Parasitology, Bullous
  Dermatoses, Exfoliative Dermatitis, Dermatologic
  Bacteriology, Spirochetal Infections, Dermatologic
  Mycology, Tumors of the Skin, Diseases of the Mucous
  Membranes, Pigmentary Dermatoses, Where to Look
  for More Information About a Skin Disease, and
  Dictionary–Index**

Suzana L. Hadžavdić, MD, PhD
Associate Professor
Department of Dermatology and Venerology
University Hospital Center Zagreb
Zagreb, Croatia
Chapter 11: Atopic Dermatitis

Tiffany J. Herd, MD
University of Kansas Medical Center
Kansas City, Kansas
Chapter 46: General Principles of Skin Aging

Ingrid Herskovitz, MD
Wound Research Fellow
Dermatology and Cutaneous Surgery Department
University of Miami
Miami, Florida
**Chapter 10: Ulcer Management: Evaluation and
  Care**

Warren R. Heymann, MD
Head, Division of Dermatology
Professor of Medicine and Pediatrics
Cooper Medical School of Rowan University
Camden, New Jersey
Clinical Professor of Dermatology
Perelman School of Medicine at the University of
  Pennsylvania
Philadelphia, Pennsylvania
Chapter 42: The Skin and Internal Disease

Dane Hill, MD
Center for Dermatology Research
Department of Dermatology
Wake Forest School of Medicine
Winston-Salem, North Carolina
Chapter 52: Cutaneous Signs of Bioterrorism

Kimberly A. Horii, MD
Division of Dermatology
Children's Mercy Hospital & Clinics
Associate Professor of Pediatrics
University of Missouri-Kansas City School of Medicine
Kansas City, Missouri
Chapter 45: Pediatric Dermatology

Olivia Hughes, BS
Clinical Researcher
Department of Dermatology and Cutaneous Surgery
University of Miami Miller School of Medicine
Miami, Florida
**Chapter 10: Ulcer Management: Evaluation and
  Care**

Tracy T. Hung, BS
Medical Student
Drexel University College of Medicine
Philadelphia, Pennsylvania
Chapter 42: The Skin and Internal Disease

Beverly A. Johnson MD
Dermatology Attending
Department of Medicine
Howard University Hospital
Private Practice
Silver Spring, Maryland
Chapter 38: Skin Diseases in Ethnic Skin

Joseph L. Jorizzo, MD
Professor, Former (Founding) Chair
Department of Dermatology
Wake Forest University School of Medicine
Winstm-Salem, North Carolina
Chapter 41: Autoimmune Connective Tissue Diseases

Kevin C. Kin, DO
Center for Dermatology Research
Department of Dermatology
Wake Forest School of Medicine
Winston-Salem, North Carolina
Chapter 52: Cutaneous Signs of Bioterrorism

Robert S Kirsner, MD, PhD
Chairman and Harvey Blank Professor
Department of Dermatology and Cutaneous Surgery
Professor of Epidemiology and Public Health
Director, University of Miami Hospital Wound Center
University of Miami Miller School of Medicine
Miami, Florida
Chapter 10: Ulcer Management: Evaluation and Care

Christopher J. Kligora, MD
Partner
Southeastern Pathology Associates
Rome, Georgia
Chapter 2: Laboratory Procedures and Tests

Laurie L. Kohen, MD
Chief Resident
Dermatology
Henry Ford Hospital
Detroit, Michigan
**Chapter 43: Dermatologic Reactions to Ultraviolet,
  Visible Light, and Infrared Radiation**

Nita Kohli, MD
Fellow, Micrographic Surgery and Dermatologic Oncology
Department of Dermatology
University of Missouri Health
School of Medicine
Columbia, Missouri
Chapter 31: Common Nonmelanoma Skin Cancers

John Koo, MD
Phototherapy Unit
Clinical Research Unit and Psychodermatology Clinic
UCSF Psoriasis and Skin Treatment Center
Department of Dermatology
University of California, San Francisco
San Francisco, California
Chapter 23: Psychodermatology

Frank C. Koranda, MD, MBA
Associate Clinical Professor
Otolaryngology—Head and Neck Surgery
Dermatology
University of Kansas Medical Center
Kansas City, Kansas
**Chapters 5 and 6: Technologic Applications in
  Dermatology and Fundamentals of Cutaneous Surgery**

Rachel L. Laarman, MD
Pediatric Dermatology Fellow
Children's Mercy Hospitals and Clinics
Kansas City, Missouri
Chapter 45: Pediatric Dermatology

W. Clark Lambert, MD, PhD
Professor and Associate Head, Dermatology
Director, Dermatopathology
New Jersey Medical School
Rutgers University
Newark, New Jersey
Chapter 34: Cutaneous T-cell Lymphoma

Walter F. Lambert, MD
Associate Professor of Clinical Pediatrics
Medical Director, UM Child Protection Team
Department of Dermatology and Cutaneous Surgery
University of Miami Miller School of Medicine
Miami, Florida
Chapter 49: Cutaneous Manifestations of Child Abuse

Robin S. Lewallen, MD
Resident
Wake Forest University School of Medicine
Winston-Salem, North Carolina
Chapter 41: Autoimmune Connective Tissue Diseases

Marilyn G. Liang, MD
Associate Professor in Dermatology
Harvard Medical School
Boston Children's Hospital
Boston, Massachusetts
Chapter 33: Vascular Tumors

Maryam Liaqat, MD
Resident
Department of Dermatology
Cooper University Hospital
Camden, New Jersey
Chapter 42: The Skin and Internal Disease

Henry W. Lim, MD
Chairman and C.S. Livingood Chair
Department of Dermatology
Henry Ford Hospital
Detroit, Michigan
**Chapter 43: Dermatologic Reactions to Ultraviolet,
    Visible Light, and Infrared Radiation**

Jasna Lipozenčić, MD, PhD
Professor, Acting Head
Department of Dermatology and Venerology
University Hospital Center Zagreb, School of Medicine
Zagreb, Croatia
Chapter 11: Atopic Dermatitis

Alex Lombardi, MD
MS Human Biology
North Carolina State University
Raleigh, North California
Chapter 36: Diseases Affecting the Nail Unit

Tracy V. Love, MD
CPT, MC, USA
PGY-4, Dermatology
Walter Reed National Military Medical Center
Bethesda, Maryland
Chapter 39: Military Dermatology

Flor MacQuhae, MD
Clinical Researcher
Department of Dermatology and Cutaneous Surgery
University of Miami Miller School of Medicine
Miami, Florida
Chapter 10: Ulcer Management: Evaluation and Care

Andrew M. Margileth, MD
Department of Pediatric Dermatology
University of Miami Health System
Miami, Florida
Chapter 49: Cutaneous Manifestations of Child Abuse

Kari L. Martin, MD
Assistant Professor of Dermatology and Child Health
Residency Program Director of Dermatology
Department of Dermatology
University of Missouri
Columbia, Missouri
Chapter 14: Vasculitis

Margaret L. McKinnon, MD, BSc
Investigator, BC Children's Hospital
Assistant Professor, Department of Medical Genetics
Faculty of Medicine
University of British Columbia
Program Director, UBC Medical Genetics Residency
    Program
BC Children's Hospital
Vancouver, British Columbia
Chapter 44: Genodermatoses

Bradley Merritt, MD, FACMS
Director of Mohs Surgery
Department of Dermatology
The University of North Carolina at Chapel Hill
Chapel Hill, North California
Chapter 36: Diseases Affecting the Nail Unit

Jon H. Meyerle, MD
Assistant Professor, Dermatology
Uniformed Services University of the Health Sciences
Bethesda, Maryland
Chapter 39: Military Dermatology

Salim Mohanna, MD
Clinical Research Associate
Instituto de Medicina Tropical "Alexander von Humboldt"
Universidad Peruana Cayetano Heredia
Lima, Peru
Chapter 50: Tropical Diseases of the Skin

Annie O. Morrison, MD
Dermatopathology Fellow
University of Texas Southwestern
Cockerell Dermatopathology
Dallas, Texas
**Chapter 27: Cutaneous Diseases Associated With Human
    Immunodeficiency Virus**

Mio Nakamura, MD
Clinical Research Fellow
UCSF Psoriasis and Skin Treatment Center
Department of Dermatology
University of California
San Francisco, California
Chapter 23: Psychodermatology

Zeena Y. Nawas, MD
Internal Medicine Chief Resident
The University of Texas Health Science Center
Houston, Texas
Chapter 26: Dermatologic Virology

Marcy Neuburg, MD
Professor
Departments of Dermatology, Plastic and reconstructive
    surgery and otolaryngology
Medical College of Wisconsin
Milwaukee, Wisconsin
Chapter 48: Skin Disease in Transplant Patients

Kate E. Oberlin, MD
Dermatology Resident
Department of Dermatology and Cutaneous Surgery
University of Miami
Miami, Florida
Chapter 49: Cutaneous Manifestations of Child Abuse

Marianne N. O'Donoghue, MD
Associate Professor
Department of Dermatology
Rush Presbyterian—St. Luke's Medical Center
Chicago, Illinois
Chapter 7: Cosmetics for the Physician

Edit B. Olasz, MD, PhD
Associate Professor
Department of Dermatology
Medical College of Wisconsin
Milwaukee, Wisconsin
Chapter 48: Skin Disease in Transplant Patients

Yetunde M. Olumide, MD
Professor Emeritus of Medicine
Consultant Physician and Dermatologist
Department of Medicine
College of Medicine of the University of Lagos
Surulere, Lagos
Chapter 54: Nutritional and Metabolic Diseases and the Skin

Andrew J. Peranteau, MD
Center for Clinical Studies
Houston, Texas
Chapter 26: Dermatologic Virology

Rachel T. Pflederer, MD
Dermatology Resident
University of Kansas Medical Center
Kansas City, Missouri
Chapter 46: General Principles of Skin Aging

Anand Rajpara, MD
Assistant Professor
Department of Dermatology
University of Kansas Medical Center
Kansas City, Missouri
Chapter 46: General Principles of Skin Aging

Kellie E. Reed, MD
Dermatology
The University of Texas Dell Medical School
Austin, Texas
Chapter 29: Sexually Transmitted Infections

Patrick Retterbush, MD
Lockman Dermatology
Athens, Georgia
Chapter 36: Diseases Affecting the Nail Unit

Christie Riemer, BS
Medical Student, Class of 2016
Michigan State University College of Human Medicine
Grand Rapids, Michigan
**Chapter 27: Cutaneous Diseases Associated With Human
    Immunodeficiency Virus**

David J. Rosenfeld, MA, BS
University Hospital MS3
Medical Student
University of Missouri School of Medicine
Columbia, Missouri
Chapter 47: Obesity and Dermatology

Lawrence A. Schachner, MD
Director of Pediatric Dermatology
Department of Dermatology and Cutaneous Surgery
University of Miami Miller School of Medicine
Miami, Florida
Chapter 49: Cutaneous Manifestations of Child Abuse

Richard K. Scher, MD, FACP
Clinical Professor of Dermatology
Weil Cornell Medical College
New York, New York
Chapter 36: Diseases Affecting the Nail Unit

Robert A. Schwartz, MD, MPH, DSc (Hon), FAAD, FRCP (Edin)
Professor and Head, Dermatology
Professor of Medicine
Professor of Pediatrics
Professor of Pathology
Rutgers New Jersey Medical School
Visiting Professor
Rutgers School of Public Affairs and Administration
Newark, New Jersey
Chapter 34: Cutaneous T-cell Lymphoma

Jeff K. Shornick, MD, MHA
Private Practice
Groton, Connecticut
Chapter 53: Dermatoses of Pregnancy

Nora K. Shumway, MD
Dermatology Resident
PGY-4
University of Missouri
Kansas City, Missouri
Chapter 47: Obesity and Dermatology

Johanna S. Song, MD MS
Resident Physician
Department of Pediatrics
Massachusetts General Hospital
Harvard Medical School
Boston, Massachusetts
Chapter 33: Vascular Tumors

Gabriela M. Soza, MD
Texas A&M College of Medicine
Bryan, Texas
Chapter 29: Sexually Transmitted Infections

Lindsay C. Strowd, MD
Assistant Professor of Dermatology
Wake Forest University School of Medicine
Winston-Salem, North California
Chapter 41: Autoimmune Connective Tissue Diseases

Yun Tong, MD
Center for Clinical Studies
Houston, Texas
Chapter 26: Dermatologic Virology

Stephen K. Tyring, MD, PhD
Clinical Professor
Dermatology
University of Texas Health Science Center
Houston, Texas
Chapter 26: Dermatologic Virology

Ting Wang, MD, PhD
Assistant Professor
Division of Dermatology
Department of Internal Medicine
University of Kansas Medical Center
Kansas City, Kansas
Chapter 32: Melanoma

Kenneth R. Watson, DO
Pathologist
MAWD Pathology Group, PA
Kansas City, Missouri
Chapters 1 and 2: Structure of the Skin and Laboratory Procedures and Tests

Jeffrey M. Weinberg, MD
Department of Dermatology
Mount Sinai St. Luke's
Mount Sinai Beth Israel
Associate Clinical Professor of Dermatology
Icahn School of Medicine at Mt Sinai
New York, New York
Chapter 16: Psoriasis

Robin S. Weiner, MD
Sanford Dermatology Clinic
Sioux Falls, South Dakota
Chapter 32: Melanoma

Christopher L. Wilson, MD
M.D. Candidate, Class of 2018
University of Missouri School of Medicine
Columbia, Missouri
Chapter 31: Common Nonmelanoma Skin Cancers

Jaeyoung Yoon, MD, PhD
Forefront Dermatology;
Mercy Hospital St. Louis
St. Louis, Missouri
Chapter 32: Melanoma

Preface

This is by far the most complete edition of this book.

All chapters, figures, and Dictionary–Index have been supplemented and updated. New chapters are **Contact Dermatitis, Cutaneous Drug Reactions, Ulcer Management: Evaluation and Care, Vasculitis, Skin Diseases in the Military,** and **Skin Disease in the Abused Patient.**

We will be forever grateful to all the outstanding authors.

We appreciate that the trust put in all of us by our patients is the true measure of success, and we thank them for that trust. The patients are the heroes, and their hopes and fears are always what is in the forefront of our efforts as physicians.

—**John C. Hall, MD**

Preface to the First Edition

(Abridged)

Approximately 15% of all patients who walk into the general practitioner's office do so for the care of some skin disease or skin lesion. It may be for such a simple treatment as the removal of a wart, for the treatment of athlete's foot, or for something as complicated as severe cystic acne. There have been so many recent advances in the various fields of medicine that the medical school instructor can expect his or her students to learn and retain only a small percentage of the material that is taught. I believe that the courses in all phases of medicine, and particularly the courses of the various specialties, should be made as simple, basic, and concise as possible. If the student retains only a small percentage of what is presented, he or she will be able to handle an amazing number of walk-in patients. I am presenting in this book only the material that medical students and general practitioners must know for the diagnosis and the treatment of patients with common skin diseases. In condensing the material, many generalities are stated, and the reader must remember that there are exceptions to every rule. The inclusion of these exceptions would defeat the intended purpose of this book. More complicated diagnostic procedures or treatments for interesting problem cases are merely frosting on the cake. This information can be obtained by the interested student from any of several more comprehensive dermatologic texts.

This book consists of two distinct but complementary parts. The first part contains the chapters devoted to the diagnosis and the management of the important common skin diseases. In discussing the common skin diseases, a short introductory sentence is followed by a listing of the salient points of each disease in outline form. All diseases of the skin have primary lesions, secondary lesions, a rather specific distribution, a general course that includes the prognosis and the recurrence rate of the diseases, varying subjective complaints, and a known or unknown cause. Where indicated, a statement follows concerning seasonal incidence, age groups affected, family and sex incidence, contagiousness, relationship to employment, and laboratory findings. The discussion ends with a paragraph on differential diagnosis and treatment. Treatment, to be effective, has to be thought of as a chain of events. The therapy outlined on the first visit is usually different from the one given on subsequent visits or for cases that are very severe. The treatment is discussed with these variations in mind.

The second part consists of a very complete Dictionary–Index to the entire field of dermatology, defining the majority of rare diseases and the unusual dermatologic terms. The inclusion of this Dictionary–Index has a dual purpose. First, it enables me to present a concise first section on common skin diseases unencumbered by the inclusion of the rare diseases. Second, it provides rather complete coverage of all of dermatology for the more interested student. In reality, two books are contained in one.

Dermatologic nomenclature has always been a bugaboo for the new student. I heartily agree with many dermatologists that we should simplify the terminology, and that has been attempted in this text. Some of the changes are mine, but many have been suggested by others. However, after a diligent effort to simplify the names of skin diseases, one is left with the appalling fact that some of the complicated terms defy change. One of the main reasons for this is that all of our field, the skin, is visible to the naked eye. As a result, any minor alteration from normal has been scrutinized by countless physicians through the years and given countless names. The liver or heart counterpart of folliculitis ulerythematosa reticulata (ulerythema acneiform, atrophoderma reticulatum symmetricum faciei, atrophoderma vermiculatum) is yet to be discovered.

What I am presenting in this book is not specialty dermatology but general practice dermatology. Some of my medical educator friends say that only internal medicine, pediatrics, and obstetrics should be taught to medical students. They state that the specialized fields of medicine should be taught only at the internship, residency, or postgraduate level. That idea misses the very important fact that cases from all of the so-called specialty fields wander into the general practitioner's office. The general practitioner must have some basic knowledge of the varied aspects of all of medicine so that he or she can properly take care of his or her general everyday practice. This basic knowledge must be taught in the undergraduate years. The purpose of this book is to complement such teaching.

—**Gordon C. Sauer, MD**

Acknowledgments

Special thanks to all of our excellent contributors and, to our editor, Kristina Oberle.

Charlotte is more than a wife. She is an inspiration, cheerleader, and friend.

Kim and Shelly, my daughters, and Tony and Tori, my grandchildren, give me my grounding and reasons for pursuit of scholarship.

My office staff kept my practice afloat while I was having fun writing. They are Kelly Howell, office manager; Lori Winters, office administrator; Larene Larson, receptionist; and Kelly Hudgens, nurse.

As brevity is the soul of wit, it is also the soul of understanding a complex subject. An overview is more priceless at the onset of learning than a mountain of detail. To stir one's interest and curiosity about a field of scientific endeavor, one needs to see that field as a whole. Therein lies the true genius of Gordon Sauer.

I frequently hear from dermatologists and nondermatologists alike that this book is their first exposure to the study of skin diseases. The tenth edition and all preceding editions are a tribute to Dr. Sauer's ability to open up the specialty of dermatology to those who wish to use its magic to help in the care of their patients.

Contents

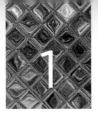

Structure of the Skin

Kenneth R. Watson, DO

The skin is the largest organ of the human body. It is composed of tissue that grows, differentiates, and renews itself constantly. Because the skin is a barrier between the internal organs and the external environment, it is uniquely subjected to noxious external agents and is also a sensitive reflection of internal disease. An understanding of the cause and effect of this complex interplay in the skin begins with knowledge of the basic structure of this organ.

LAYERS OF THE SKIN

The skin is divided into three distinct layers. From the external surface inward, they are the epidermis, dermis, and subcutaneous tissue (Fig. 1-1). There are regional variations of these layers that probably represent adaptations to different functions, such as:

1. a thickened keratin layer of the epidermis on the palms and soles,
2. numerous nerve fibers within the fingertips for improved tactile function,
3. increased numbers of sebaceous glands on the face, and
4. thickened dermis on the back.

Epidermis

The epidermis is the most superficial of the three layers of the skin and averages in thickness about the width of the mark of a sharp pencil (<1 mm). It contains several types of cells including keratinocytes, dendritic cells (melanocytes and Langerhans cells), and Merkel cells.

The keratinocytes, or keratin-forming cells, are by far the most common and develop into four identifiable layers of the epidermis (Fig. 1-2). From inside out, they are as follows:

Basal layer	
Spinous layer	Living epidermis
Granular layer	
Keratin layer	Dead end-product

The basal layer lies next to the dermis. This layer can be thought of as the stem cell layer of the epidermis, which is capable of progressive maturation into cell forms higher in the epidermis. Normally, 3 or 4 weeks are required for the epidermis to replicate itself by the processes of division and differentiation. This cell turnover is greatly accelerated in diseases such as psoriasis, in which the turnover rate may be as short as 2 to 3 days.

The spinous layer, or stratum malpighii, is made up of several layers of epidermal cells, which have a polyhedral shape. The cells of this layer are connected by intercellular bridges, which may be seen in routine sections.

The granular layer is composed of flatter cells containing protein granules called *keratohyalin granules*. In lichen planus, the granular cell layer is focally increased.

The outermost layer of the epidermis is the *keratin (cornified) layer*. It is made up of stratified layers of dead keratinized cells that are constantly shedding (Fig. 1-3). The protein in these cells is called *keratin* and is capable of absorbing vast amounts of water. This is readily seen during bathing, when the skin of the palms and the soles becomes white, swollen, and wrinkled. The keratin layer provides a major barrier of protection for the body. Mucous membranes, such as the oral and vaginal mucosa, do not have granular or keratin layers.

Immediately beneath the basal layer is the interface between the epidermis and the dermis, known as the basement membrane zone or dermal–epidermal junction. It is difficult to visualize in routine hematoxylin and eosin stained sections but can clearly be seen as a thin band with periodic acid-Schiff (PAS) stains, because of the presence of mucopolysaccharides. Ultrastructurally, the basal cells are attached to the basement membrane by hemidesmosomes. Beneath the basal cells is an electron-clear layer known as the lamina lucida. Below this is a more electron-dense layer known as the lamina densa, which consists predominantly of type IV collagen. Anchoring filaments extend through the basement membrane zone to connect the surface membranes of the basal cells to the lamina densa. There are anchoring fibrils that attach the lamina densa to the papillary dermis.

Several blistering diseases occur because of defects in the basement membrane zone. Bullous pemphigoid antigens are present within the hemidesmosomes of the basement membrane zone. Circulating IgG antibodies bind to these antigens, resulting in the subepidermal blistering disease bullous pemphigoid. Epidermolysis bullosa represents a heterogeneous group of noninflammatory blistering disorders that can be divided into three subtypes based on the location of the blister. In epidermolysis bullosa simplex, the blister usually occurs through the basal cell layer. In the junctional form, it occurs between the basal cells and the lamina lucida,

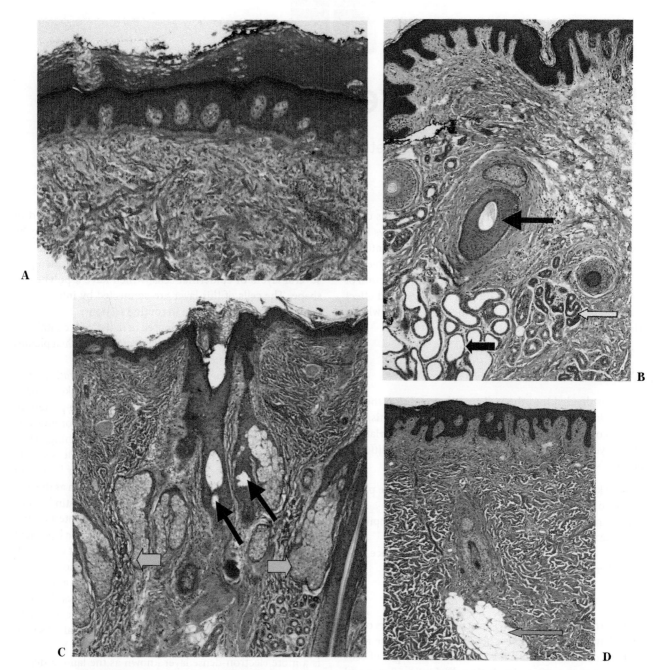

FIGURE 1-1: Histology of the skin. Photomicrographs from four different areas of the body: palm **(A)**, axilla **(B)**, face **(C)**, and back **(D)**. Note the variations in the histologic features: thickened keratin layer from the palm **(A)**, **(B)** multiple glandular elements from the axilla (hair follicle, *thin black arrow*; apocrine gland, *thick black arrow*; eccrine gland, *yellow arrow*), **(C)** numerous pilosebaceous units from the face (hair follicles, *thin arrows*; sebaceous glands, *thick arrows*), and **(D)** thick dermis from the trunk (subcutaneous fat, *arrow*). (Courtesy of Dr. K. Watson.)

probably because of a defect in the hemidesmosomes. In the dermolytic form, the blister occurs beneath the lamina densa in the area of the anchoring fibrils.

The *melanin-forming cells*, or *melanocytes*, are sandwiched between the more numerous keratin-forming cells in the basal layer. In routine hematoxylin and eosin stained sections, melanocytes have small, dark nuclei and clear cytoplasm, which is the result of shrinkage artifact. Approximately 10% of the cells in the basal layer are melanocytes. However, this varies according to the body site and ethnic background of the individual. These melanocytes are dopa-positive because they stain darkly after contact with a solution of levorotatory 3,4-dihydroxyphenylalanine, or *dopa*. This laboratory reaction closely simulates physiologic melanin formation, in which the amino acid tyrosine is oxidized by the enzyme tyrosinase to form dopa. Dopa is then further changed, through a series of complex metabolic processes, to melanin. In dermatopathology practices, melanocytes are most commonly recognized

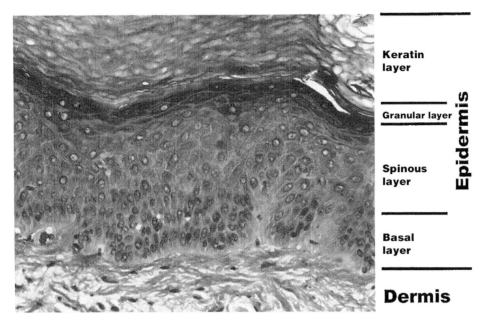

Keratin layer

Granular layer

Spinous layer

Basal layer

Epidermis

Dermis

FIGURE 1-2: Histology of the epidermis. A photomicrograph from the palm. (Courtesy of Dr. K. Watson.)

by showing positive cytoplasmic immunoreactivity for S-100 protein, HMB-45, and Melan-A (MART-1), which may be useful in the diagnosis of melanocytic tumors such as malignant melanoma. SOX-10 and MiTF are two other immunohistochemical markers, which stain the nucleus of melanocytes. Melanocytes may also be recognized using silver stains because melanin is both argyrophilic and argentaffin positive. For example, the Fontana–Masson histochemical stain results in black cytoplasmic granules within melanocytes because of the ability

of melanin to reduce ammoniated silver nitrate. Melanin may also be bleached, which is useful in identifying the neoplastic melanocytes that are obscured in heavily pigmented tumors such as some subtypes of blue nevi.

Melanin pigmentation of the skin, whether increased or decreased, is influenced by many local and systemic factors (see Chapter 30). Melanocyte-stimulating hormone from the pituitary is the most potent melanizing agent. Melanin is transferred from melanocytes to basal keratinocytes. Skin

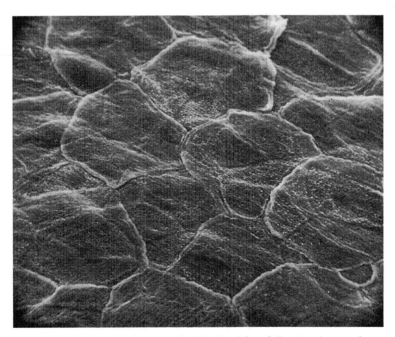

FIGURE 1-3: Keratin-layer cells. Underside of the top layer of epidermal keratin-layer cells on Scotch tape stripping is seen with Cambridge Mark II Stereoscan at 1,000×. (Courtesy of Drs. J. Arnold, W. Barnes, and G. Sauer.)

color is largely related to the amount of melanin present in basal cells. Exposure to ultraviolet light results in increased melanocyte concentration and function.

Langerhans cells are found scattered evenly throughout the epidermis. They are bone marrow–derived mononuclear cells. They are involved in cell-mediated hypersensitivity, antigen processing and recognition, stimulation of immune-competent cells, and graft rejection. Sunlight suppresses their immune function. Their number is decreased in certain skin diseases, such as psoriasis. Staining with membrane adenosine triphosphatase and monoclonal antibodies such as S-100 protein and CD-1 a can be done for identification. Electron microscopy reveals that these cells contain characteristic racquet-shaped Birbeck granules. These cells proliferate in the disease Langerhans cell histiocytosis (formerly known as histiocytosis X), which may be isolated to the skin or may be part of a larger systemic process.

Merkel cells are located within the basal layer but may also be found within hair follicles and sweat ducts. They are assumed to function as touch receptors and are associated with fine unmyelinated nerve fibers. They are inconspicuous in routine sections. They may be recognized using immunostains for the neuroendocrine markers neuron-specific enolase (NSE), chromogranin, and synaptophysin. Ultrastructurally, they contain dense core neurosecretory granules. They give rise to primary neuroendocrine carcinoma of the skin (Merkel cell carcinoma).

Dermis

The dermis consists of connective tissue, cellular elements, and ground substance. It has a rich vascular and nerve supply and contains pilosebaceous, apocrine, and eccrine structures. Anatomically, it is divided into two compartments. The first contains thin collagen fibers, delicate elastic fibers, numerous capillaries, and abundant ground substance, which form a thin layer beneath the epidermis (papillary dermis) and surrounding adnexal structures (periadnexal dermis). Together, these are regarded as a single unit called the *adventitial dermis*. This is an important unit because it is altered together with the adjacent epithelium in many inflammatory diseases. The second compartment, known as the *reticular* or *deep dermis*, is composed of thick collagen bundles with intertwined elastic fibers. The reticular dermis is thick and comprises the bulk of the dermis. It contains less ground substance, vascular spaces, and cellular elements than the thin adventitial dermis.

The *connective tissue* component of the dermis consists of collagen fibers, including reticulin fibers and elastic fibers. These fibers contribute to the support and elasticity of the skin.

Two different types of collagen are present within the dermis. Type I collagen is predominantly found within the thick fibers of the reticular dermis. Type III collagen, also known as *reticulin*, is largely found within the thin fibers of the papillary and periadnexal dermis. These reticulin fibers are not visible in routine hematoxylin and eosin stained sections, but can be identified with silver stains. They are abundant in certain pathologic conditions such as granulomas, syphilis, sarcoidosis, and some mesenchymal tumors. The proteins present in collagen fibers are responsible for nearly one-fourth of a person's overall protein mass. If tannic acid or the salts of heavy metals, such as dichromates, are combined with collagen, the result is leather.

Elastic fibers are thinner than most collagen fibers and are entwined among them. They are composed of the protein elastin. Elastic fibers do not readily take up acidic or basic stains, such as hematoxylin and eosin, but they can be identified with the Verhoeff–van Gieson stain.

Cellular elements of the dermis include fibroblasts, endothelial cells, mast cells, and a variety of miscellaneous cells, including smooth muscle, nerve, and hematopoietic cells. The hematopoietic cells include lymphocytes, histiocytes (macrophages), eosinophils, neutrophils, and plasma cells. These hematopoietic cells are increased in numerous inflammatory diseases of the skin.

Fibroblasts form collagen and produce ground substance. They are involved in immunologic and reparative processes. Fibroblasts are increased in numerous types of skin disorders.

Mast cells are derived from bone marrow stem cells. They are present in normal skin in small numbers and are usually concentrated around blood vessels, particularly postcapillary venules. They have intracytoplasmic basophilic metachromatic granules containing heparin and histamine. The granules do not stain with routine hematoxylin and eosin, but may be seen with colloidal iron, toluidine blue, and Alcian blue stains. Mast cells are increased in many different inflammatory dermatoses, but play a particularly important role in urticarial eruptions. Urticaria occurs when mast cells and basophils are degranulated, resulting in vascular permeability and tissue edema. Mast cell degranulation also plays a role in activating other inflammatory cells to the area of tissue injury.

Neoplastic proliferations of mast cells may form papules, plaques, and nodules within the skin, known as cutaneous mastocytosis (*urticaria pigmentosa*). They may also have a telangiectatic appearance, as in telangiectasia macularis eruptiva perstans (TMEP). In addition to metachromatic staining mentioned in the previous paragraph, these proliferations of mast cells show positive immunoreactivity for human mast cell tryptase and CD117, which may be useful in differentiating mast cell proliferations from other cutaneous neoplasms, such as Langerhans cell histiocytosis and leukemia cutis.

Histiocytes (macrophages) are present in only small numbers in the normal skin. However, in pathologic conditions, they migrate to the dermis as tissue monocytes. They play a predominant role in the phagocytosis of particulate matter and bacteria. Under special pathologic conditions, they may form giant cells. They are also involved in the immune system by phagocytizing antigens.

Lymphocytes and plasma cells are found in only small numbers in normal skin, but are significantly increased in pathologic conditions, such as increased plasma cells in syphilis.

The *ground substance* of the dermis is a gel-like amorphous matrix not easily seen in routine sections, but it may be identified with colloidal iron and Alcian blue stains. It is found in greatest concentration within the adventitial dermis, particularly around adnexal structures. There are variable

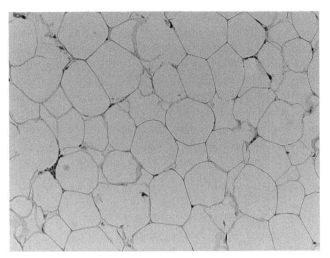

FIGURE 1-4: White adipose tissue. (Courtesy of Dr. K. Watson.)

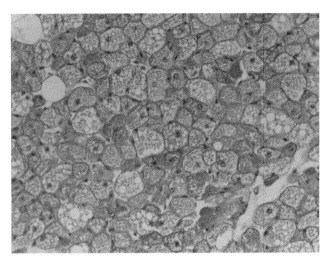

FIGURE 1-5: Brown adipose tissue. (Courtesy of Dr. K. Watson.)

amounts of ground substance in different areas of the body, with increased concentrations within the fingers and toes. The ground substance contains proteins, mucopolysaccharides, soluble collagens, enzymes, immune bodies, and metabolites. It has the capacity to bind water, allowing the movement of nutrients through the dermis, and it provides bulk, contributing to the malleability of the skin.

Subcutaneous Tissue

The subcutaneous tissue constitutes the largest volume of adipose tissue in the body. The adipose tissue is organized into lobules by fibrous septa, which contain most of the blood vessels, nerves, and lymphatics. The thickness of the subcutaneous fat varies from one area of the body to another. It is especially thick in the abdominal region and thin in the eyelids and scrotum. The subcutaneous tissue serves as a receptacle for the formation and storage of fat as well as a site of highly dynamic lipid metabolism for nutrition. It also provides protection from physical trauma and insulation from temperature changes.

Most of the fat in the body consists of white adipose tissue (Fig. 1-4). The white fat cells are derived from mesenchymal cells, as are fibroblasts. They store triglycerides, which can be broken down into fatty acids and used for energy by other tissues such as muscle. White adipose tissue is increased in obesity.

There is a second distinct type of adipose tissue, known as brown fat, which is found predominantly in human newborns and also hibernating animals (Fig. 1-5). Brown fat cells have a different appearance than white fat cells. They are smaller, contain multiple small lipid droplets, and have increased numbers of mitochondria. Recent studies using fluorodeoxyglucose positron emission tomography (PET) suggest that a significant percentage of adult humans have active brown adipose tissue. Brown fat has a different function than white fat. It is involved in energy expenditure that is responsible for generating heat, protecting body temperature in human newborns without shivering. It may also be useful in protecting against obesity. Brown fat may develop from a common precursor to skeletal myocytes.

Lipomas are benign tumors composed of mature fat cells identical to white adipose tissue in the subcutaneous fat. Hibernoma is a benign tumor composed of fat cells resembling brown fat.

VASCULATURE

The skin contains a rich vascular network that provides blood volume far exceeding its nutritional needs. In fact, the vascularization is so extensive that it has been postulated that its main function is to regulate heat and blood pressure of the body, and to provide nutrition to the skin as a secondary function. The vascular plexus arises from thick arteries within the subcutaneous fat. There are two major plexuses, which run parallel to the epidermis, one within the deep dermis near the dermal–subcutaneous junction and one within the superficial (papillary) dermis. There are vertically oriented perforating branches that connect the two plexuses and provide blood to surrounding dermal appendages. Perivascular inflammation surrounding the superficial and deep plexuses occurs in many types of "dermatitis," and this pattern of inflammation may be used as a method of classification of inflammatory disorders of the skin. Inflammatory reactions involving the superficial vascular plexus may result in erythema.

The vascular plexuses consist of a mixture of arterioles, venules, and capillaries. Most of the exchange of water, oxygen, and nutrients with the skin occurs through thin capillaries and venules. The skin also contains an extensive lymphatic network that is independent of the vascular plexus. No blood vessels or lymphatics are present within the epidermis.

A special vascular body, the glomus, deserves mention. The glomus body is most commonly seen on the tips of the fingers and toes and under the nails. Each glomus body consists of a venous and arterial segment, called the *Sucquet–Hoyer canal*. This canal represents a short-circuit device that connects an arteriole with a venule directly, without intervening capillaries. The result is a marked increase in the blood flow through the skin. If this body grows abnormally, it forms an often painful, red, benign glomus tumor, commonly beneath the nail.

NERVE SUPPLY

The skin is a major sensory organ with millions of nerve endings receiving stimulation from the surrounding environment. Sensory and autonomic nerves within the peripheral nervous system permeate the dermis with tiny nerve fibers, which may be myelinated or unmyelinated. These tiny nerve fibers are not visible in routine hematoxylin and eosin stained sections. Only larger myelinated nerve fibers and specialized nerve-end organs are discernible. Special stains are required to visualize the small nerve fibers, such as silver impregnation techniques (Bielschowsky or Bodian stains) or immunoperoxidase stains such as neurofilament protein, which stains axons, and S-100 protein, which stains Schwann cells. The nerve fibers are variably distributed, resulting in regional variations in sensation. They are very prominent on the palms, soles, and fingers, and within mucocutaneous areas.

Numerous tiny unmyelinated sensory nerves with free nerve endings are present within the papillary dermis and surrounding hair follicles. They mediate the sensations of temperature, touch, pain, and itching. Some of the free nerve endings extend into the basal epidermis and contact Merkel cells.

> ### SAUER'S NOTES
>
> *Itching* is the most important presenting symptom of an unhappy patient. It may be defined simply as the desire to scratch. Itching, apparently, is a mildly painful sensation that differs from pain in having a lower frequency of impulse stimuli. The release of proteinases (such as follows itch-powder application) may be responsible for the itch sensation. The pruritus may be of a pricking or burning type and can vary greatly from one person to another. Sulzberger called abnormally sensitive people *itchish*, analogous to *ticklish*. Itching can occur without any clinical signs of skin disease or from circulating allergens or local superficial contactants. The skin of atopic or eczema patients tends to be more itchy. Scratching makes the itching worse. This results in a perpetual itch-scratch cycle.

Sensory nerves in hairless skin, such as the palms and soles, and at the mucocutaneous junction terminate in specialized end organs, known as Meissner corpuscles, Vater–Pacini corpuscles, and mucocutaneous end organs. Meissner corpuscles are most numerous on the fingertips, palms, and soles, where they sense touch and vibration. They are composed of S-100–positive laminated, flattened Schwann cells. Vater–Pacini corpuscles are most numerous within the deep dermis and subcutaneous fat of the feet and hands, and they sense pressure and tension. They are large, measuring up to 1 mm in diameter, and are composed of outer spherical layers of perineurial cells and an inner nerve fiber with accompanying Schwann cell.

Sympathetic autonomic nerve fibers supply blood vessels, arrector pili muscles, apocrine glands, and eccrine glands. Adrenergic fibers carry impulses to the arrector pili muscles, which produce gooseflesh if they are stimulated. This is caused by traction of the muscle on the hair follicles to which it is attached. Cholinergic fibers, if stimulated, increase sweating and may cause a specific type of hives called *cholinergic urticaria* (see Chapter 11). Sebaceous glands do not contain autonomic fibers but are controlled by endocrine stimulation.

APPENDAGES

The appendages of the skin include both the cornified appendages (hairs and nails) and the glandular appendages.

Hair Follicles

Hairs are produced by the hair follicles, which develop from germinative cells of the fetal epidermis. Because no new hair follicles are formed after birth, the different types of body hairs are manifestations of the effect of location as well as external and internal stimuli. Hormones are the most important internal stimuli influencing the various types of hair growth. There are three main types of hairs: (1) *Lanugo hairs:* fine, lightly pigmented hairs covering the body of the fetus, (2) *Vellus hairs* ("peach fuzz"): short, fine hairs that replace lanugo hairs and cover most of the body but are barely noticeable, and (3) *Terminal hairs:* long, coarse hairs present in the adult, which are prominent on the scalp, beard, pubic, and axillary regions. Terminal hairs convert into vellus hairs in male pattern baldness. Vellus hairs develop into terminal hairs in hirsutism. The palms, soles, lips, and some genital areas do not contain hair follicles.

Hair growth is cyclic, with a growing (anagen) phase (Fig. 1-6) and a resting (telogen) phase. The *catagen cycle* is the transition phase between the growing and resting stages and lasts only a few weeks. The duration of hair growth varies in different areas of the body. Approximately 90% of normal scalp hairs are in the growing (anagen) stage, which can last between 3 and 6 years or more, depending on the location. Ten percent of hairs are in the resting (telogen) stage, which lasts approximately 60 to 90 days. However, systemic stresses, such as childbirth, or systemic anesthesia, may cause hairs to enter a resting stage prematurely. This *postpartum* or *postanesthetic effect* is noticed most commonly in the scalp when these resting hairs are depilated during combing or washing, and the thought of approaching baldness causes sudden alarm.

Hair follicles may be thought of as an invagination of the epidermis, with its different layers of cells. The hair follicle can be divided into three areas: (1) *infundibulum*, which extends from the follicular orifice to the entrance of the underlying sebaceous gland, (2) *isthmus*, which extends from the orifice of the sebaceous gland to the insertion of the erector pili muscle, and (3) *inferior segment*, which consists of the follicle below the insertion of the erector pili muscle.

The inferior portion of the follicle includes the hair bulb, which contains matrix cells. These cells perform a similar function to the basal cells of the epidermis. They are responsible

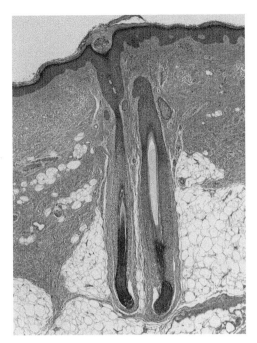

FIGURE 1-6: Anagen hairs with hair bulb and matrix cells. (Courtesy of Dr. K. Watson.)

for the development of the hair shaft. Melanocytes are present in the matrix and determine the color of hair.

There are approximately 100,000 anagen follicles on the normal scalp with tremendous protein-synthesizing capacity. At the rate of scalp hair growth of 0.35 mm/day, more than 100 linear feet of scalp hair is produced daily. The density of hairs in the scalp varies from 175 to 300 hairs/cm^2. Up to 100 hairs may be normally lost daily.

SAUER'S NOTES

1. Shaving of excess hair, as women do on their legs and thighs, does not promote more rapid growth of coarse hair. The shaved stubs appear coarser, but if allowed to grow normally, the hairs appear and feel no different than before.
2. The value of intermittent massage to stimulate scalp hair growth has not been proved.
3. Hair cannot turn gray overnight. The melanin pigmentation, which is distributed throughout the length of the nonvital hair shaft, takes weeks to be shed through the slow process of hair growth.
4. Heredity is the greatest factor predisposing to baldness, and an excess of male hormone may contribute to hair loss. Male castrates do not become bald.
5. Common male pattern baldness cannot be reversed by over-the-counter "hair restorers." Minoxidil solution (Rogaine), which is sold over the counter, is beneficial for a limited percentage of patients, and finasteride (Propecia) pills, available by prescription, are helpful for most patients.

Nail Unit

The nail unit consists of a nail plate and the surrounding soft tissues, which include the nail matrix, proximal and lateral nail folds, nail bed, cuticle, and hyponychium (Fig. 29-1). The nail plate covers the dorsal distal aspect of the fingers and toes, and ranges between 0.3 and 0.75 mm in thickness. It inserts into grooves in the skin that are present proximally and laterally. The plate is produced by the nail matrix, which is located at the proximal end of the plate insertion, ventral to the proximal nail fold. The matrix extends distally to the lunula, which is a crescent-shaped white area under the proximal nail plate, particularly prominent on the thumb and less prominent on the remaining fingers. The nail plate lies on the nail bed. The epithelium of the nail bed produces a small amount of keratin, which tightly adheres to the overlying nail plate. The dermis of the nail bed is richly vascular, resulting in a pink appearance and blanching when compressed. Glomus bodies are also present, which aid in temperature control of the digits. The cuticle represents the cornified layer of the proximal nail fold and serves to seal off and protect the nail matrix. The hyponychium consists of cornified epidermis located at the distal end of the nail bed beneath the distal free edge of the nail plate.

The nail unit is an invagination of the epidermis, similar to the hair follicle. Both have a matrix that produces the protein keratin. The nail plate consists almost entirely of keratin, similar to the hair shaft and cornified layer of the epidermis. Unlike hair growth, which is periodic, nail growth is continuous. Nail growth proceeds at about one-third of the rate of hair growth, or about 0.1 mm/day. It takes about 3 months to restore a removed fingernail and about three times that long for the regrowth of a new toenail. Nail growth can be inhibited during serious illnesses or in old age, increased through nail biting or occupational trauma, and altered because of a variety of diseases and medications.

Glandular Appendages

The three types of glandular appendages of the skin are the sebaceous glands, apocrine glands, and eccrine glands (Fig. 1-7).

The *sebaceous glands* are present everywhere on the skin, except the palms and the soles. In most areas, they are associated with hair follicles. There are sebaceous glands that are not associated with hair follicles, such as the buccal mucosa and vermillion border of the lip, nipple and areola of the breast, labia minora, and eyelids (meibomian glands). The sebaceous glands are holocrine glands, forming their secretions through the disintegration of the entire glandular cell. The secretion from these glands is evacuated through the sebaceous duct to a follicle that may contain either a large terminal hair or a vellus hair. This secretion, known as *sebum*, is not under any neurologic control, but is a continuous outflow of the material of cell breakdown. The sebum covers the skin with a thin lipoidal film that is mildly bacteriostatic and fungistatic and retards water evaporation. The scalp and the face may contain as many as 1,000 sebaceous glands per square centimeter. The activity of the gland increases markedly at the age of puberty,

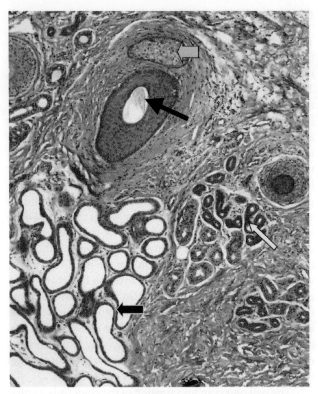

FIGURE 1-7: Histology of the glands of the skin. A photomicrograph from the axilla (hair follicle, *long black arrow*; apocrine glands, *short black arrow*; sebaceous gland, *short blue arrow*; eccrine glands, *yellow arrow*). (Courtesy of Dr. K. Watson.)

and, in certain people, it becomes plugged with sebum, debris, and bacteria to form the blackheads and pimples of acne.

Apocrine glands are found in the axillae, genital region, breast, external ear canal (ceruminous glands), and eyelid (Moll glands). They do not develop until the time of puberty. They consist of a coiled secretory gland located in the deep dermis or subcutaneous fat and a straight duct that usually empties into a hair follicle. The function of the secretions is unknown; however, they may act as pheromones. They are responsible for the production of body odor (the infamous "BO"). Any emotional stresses that cause adrenergic sympathetic discharge produce apocrine secretion. This secretion is sterile when excreted, but undergoes decomposition when contaminated by bacteria from the skin surface, resulting in a strong and characteristic odor. The purpose of the many cosmetic underarm preparations is to remove these bacteria or block the gland's excretion. The apocrine glands are involved in *hidradenitis suppurativa*, an inflammatory process that results from follicular obstruction

and retention of follicular products, which usually occurs in patients with the acne–seborrhea complex.

Eccrine sweat glands are distributed everywhere on the skin surface, with the greatest concentration on the palms, soles, and forehead. They develop as a downgrowth from the primitive epidermis. They are composed of coiled secretory glands, a coiled duct, a straight duct, an intraepidermal coil, and an eccrine pore. The eccrine sweat glands and the vasculature of the skin serve in the maintenance of stable internal body temperature, despite marked environmental temperature changes. They flood the skin surface with water for cooling, and the blood vessels dilate or constrict to dissipate or conserve body heat. Their prime stimulus is heat, and their activity is under the control of the nervous system, usually through the hypothalamus. Both adrenergic and cholinergic fibers innervate the glands. Blockage of the eccrine ducts results in the disease known as *miliaria* (*prickly heat*). If eccrine glands are congenitally absent, as in *anhidrotic ectodermal dysplasia*, a life-threatening hyperpyrexia may develop.

ACKNOWLEDGMENT

We acknowledge the valuable assistance of Dean Shepard from St. Luke's Hospital photographic services.

Suggested Readings

Ackerman BA. *Histologic Diagnosis of Inflammatory Skin Diseases*. Philadelphia: Lea & Febiger; 1978.

Barnhill RL. *Textbook of Dermatopathology*. New York: McGraw-Hill; 1998.

Briggaman RA. Epidermal–dermal junction: structure, composition, function and disease relationships. *Prog Dermatol*. 1990;24(2):1.

Farmer RE, Hood AF. *Pathology of the Skin*. Norwalk, CT: Appleton & Lange; 1990.

Fleischer AB. *The Clinical Management of Itching: Therapeutic Protocols for Pruritis*. London: Parthenon Publishing Group; 1998.

Goldsmith L. *Physiology, Biochemistry, and Molecular Biology of the Skin*. New York: Oxford University Press; 1991.

Hurwitz RM, Hood AF. *Pathology of the Skin: Atlas of Clinical-Pathological Correlation*. Stamford, CT: Appleton & Lange; 1997.

Lever WE, Schaumburg-Lever G. *Histopathology of the Skin*. 7th ed. Philadelphia: JB Lippincott; 1990.

Murphy GF, Elder EE. *Atlas of Tumor Pathology: Non-melanocytic Tumors of the Skin*. Washington, DC: Armed Forces Institute of Pathology; 1991.

Nedergaard J, Bengtsson T, Cannon B. Unexpected evidence for active brown adipose tissue in adult humans. *Am J Physiol Endocrinol Metab*. 2007;293:E444–E452.

Nickolof BJ. *Dermal Immune System*. Boca Raton, FL: CRC Press; 1993.

Rosen T, Martin S. *Atlas of Black Dermatology*. Boston: Little, Brown and Company; 1981.

Seale P, Bjork B, Yang W, et al. PRDM16 controls a brown fat/skeletal muscle switch. *Nature*. 2008;454:947–948.

Laboratory Procedures and Tests

Christopher J. Kligora, MD and Kenneth R. Watson, DO

In addition to the usual laboratory procedures used in the workup of medical patients, certain special tests are of importance in the field of dermatology. These include skin tests, fungus examinations, biopsies, and immunologic diagnosis. For special problems, additional testing methods are suggested in the sections on the various diseases.

SKIN TESTS

There are three types of skin tests:

- Intracutaneous
- Scratch
- Patch

The intracutaneous tests and the scratch tests can have two types of reactions: either an immediate wheal reaction or a delayed reaction. The immediate wheal reaction develops to a maximum in 5 to 20 minutes and is elicited in testing for the cause of urticaria, atopic dermatitis, and inhalant allergies. This is a type-I or anaphylactoid type of immunity. The immediate wheal reaction test is seldom used for determining the cause of skin diseases.

The delayed reaction to intracutaneous skin testing is exemplified best by the tuberculin skin test. Tuberculin is available in two forms—as the purified protein derivative test and as a tuberculin tine test (Mantoux). The purified protein derivative test is performed by using tablets that come in two strengths and by injecting a solution of either one intracutaneously. If there is no reaction after the test with the first strength, then the second strength may be employed.

The tuberculin tine test is a simple and rapid procedure using OTK. Nine prongs, or tines, covered with OTK are pressed into the skin. If at the end of 48 or 72 hours, there is more than 2 mm of induration at the site of any prong insertion, the test is positive. There is now a more accurate blood test that is expensive.

Patch tests are commonly used in dermatology, allergy, and immunology offices, and offer a simple and accurate method of determining whether a patient is allergic to any of the testing agents. There are two different reactions to this type of test: a primary irritant reaction and an allergic reaction.

The primary irritant reaction occurs in most of the population if they are exposed to agents (in appropriate concentrations) that have skin-destroying properties. Examples of these agents include soaps, cleaning fluids, bleaches, "corn" removers, and counterirritants. The allergic reaction indicates that the patient is more sensitive than normal to the agent being tested. This test reaction is idiosyncratic and not necessarily related to concentration or dose. It also shows that the patient has had a previous exposure to that agent or a cross-sensitizing agent. This is a type-IV or delayed type of immunity. It is often very helpful in cases of contact dermatitis.

The technique of the patch test is simple, but the interpretation of the test is not. For example, consider a patient presenting with dermatitis on top of the feet. It is possible that shoe leather or some chemical used in the manufacture of the leather is causing the reaction. The procedure for a patch test is to cut out a half-inch square piece of the material from the inside of the shoe, moisten the material with distilled water, place it on the skin surface, and cover it with an adhesive band or some patch-test dressing. The patch test is left on for 48 hours. When the patch-test dressing is removed, the patient is considered to have a positive patch test if there is any redness, papules, or vesiculation at the site of the testing agent. Delayed reactions to allergens can occur, and, ideally, a final reading should be made after 96 hours (4 days), that is, 2 days after the patch is removed. The other alternative is to use a chemical such as a tanning agent that is used in the processing of the leather. The patch test can be used to make or confirm a diagnosis of poison ivy dermatitis, ragweed dermatitis, or contact dermatitis caused by medications, cosmetics, or industrial chemicals. Fisher (1995) and Adams (1990) compiled lists of chemicals, concentrations, and vehicles to be used for eliciting the allergic type of patch test reaction. Most tests can be performed very simply, however, as in the case of the shoe leather dermatitis. One precaution is that the patch must not be allowed to become wet in the 48-hour period. A patch-test kit, T.R.U.E. Test (Glaxo), includes ready-to-apply, self-adhesive allergen tapes. There are other more extensive patch-test trays available, depending on the allergens.

A method of testing for food allergy is to use the Rowe elimination diet. The procedure is to limit the diet to the following basic foods, which are known to be hypoallergenic: lamb,

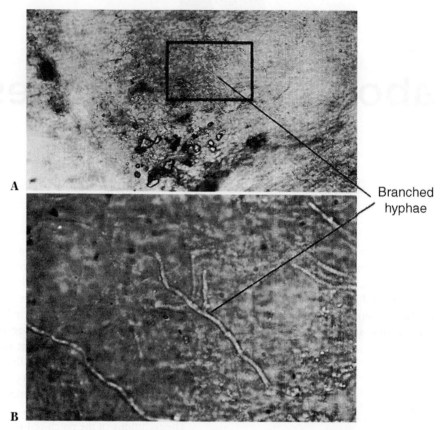

Branched hyphae

FIGURE 2-1: Fungi from a skin scraping as seen with microscope in a KOH preparation. **A:** Low-power lens (100×) view. **B:** High-power lens (450×) view of area outlined above. (Courtesy of Dr. D. Gibson.)

lemon, grapefruit, pears, lettuce, spinach, carrots, sweet potatoes, tapioca, rice and rice bread, corn sugar, maple syrup, sesame oil, gelatin, and salt. The patient is to remain on this basic diet for 5 to 7 days. At the end of that time, one new food can be added every 2 days. The following foods can be added early: beef, white potatoes, green beans, milk (along with butter and American cheese), and white bread with puffed wheat. If there is a flare-up of the dermatitis, which should occur within 2 to 8 hours after ingestion of an offending food, the new food should be discontinued for the present. More new foods are added until the normal diet, minus the allergenic foods, is regained.

Keeping a "diet diary" of all foods, medicines, oral hygiene items, or anything injected or inhaled can sometimes be a retrospective way of identifying an allergen. The skin reaction usually occurs less than 8 hours after ingestion.

FUNGUS EXAMINATIONS

The potassium hydroxide (KOH) preparation is a simple office laboratory procedure for the detection of fungal organisms present in skin and nails. It is performed by scraping the diseased skin and examining the material under the microscope. The skin scrapings are obtained by abrading a scaly diseased

area with a scalpel. If a blister is present, the underside of the blister is examined. The material is deposited on a glass slide and then covered with 20% aqueous KOH solution and a coverslip. The preparation can be gently heated or allowed to stand at room temperature for 15 to 60 minutes. The addition of dimethyl sulfoxide to the KOH preparation eliminates the need to heat the specimen. A diagnostically helpful pale violet stain can be imparted to the fungi if the 20% KOH solution is mixed with an equal amount of Parker Super Quik permanent blue-black ink. Other staining solutions are also available. The slide is then examined microscopically for fungal organisms (Fig. 2-1). A resolution of 10× is usually adequate to see spores and hyphae of dermatophyte fungi.

For culture preparation, a portion of the material from the scraping can be implanted on several different types of agar, including mycobiotic agar, inhibitory mold agar (IMA), BHI (brain hear infusion) with blood, chloramphenicol, gentamicin agar, and Sabouraud's glucose agar. A white or variously colored growth is noted in approximately 1 to 3 weeks (Fig. 2-2).

The species of fungus can be identified by morphology on the culture plate, biochemical characteristics, and microscopic morphology with a lactophenol cotton blue stain of a smear from the fungal colony. A culture media is available that changes color when a pathogen is cultured.

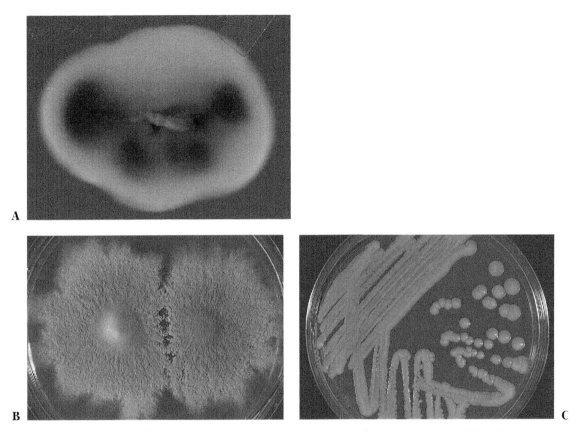

FIGURE 2-2: Fungus cultures: subcultures grown on potato dextrose agar. **A:** *Trichophyton rubrum*. **B:** *Microsporum gypseum*. **C:** *Candida albicans*. (Courtesy of Dr. K. Watson.)

BIOPSIES

The biopsy and microscopic examination of a questionable skin lesion may be invaluable. A definitive diagnosis is nearly always rendered with most pigmented lesions and other cutaneous tumors. In the case of inflammatory lesions, histologic findings may or may not be diagnostic, depending on the disease process, age of the lesion, clinical description of the lesion(s) including extent of involvement, other symptoms and/or medical conditions, and a clinical differential diagnosis. In cases where histologic findings are not diagnostic, at the very least, many pertinent diagnoses on the clinical differential can be excluded. In addition to diagnosis, other useful parameters can be obtained with malignant cutaneous lesions, such as depth of invasion, lymphovascular space invasion, perineural involvement, and adequacy of surgical margins. The quintessential example is malignant melanoma, where most of these factors plus several others may only be assessed histologically and are essential for staging and prognosis.

There are four principal techniques for performing skin biopsies:

1. Surgical excision with suturing
2. Punch biopsy
3. Excision with scissors
4. Shave biopsy

> ### SAUER'S NOTES
>
> 1. The skin biopsy specimen must include adequate tissue for proper interpretation by the pathologist.
> 2. Communication between a pathologist knowledgeable in this disease and the clinician is mandatory for accurate tissue diagnosis.

The decision in favor of one method depends on factors such as location of the biopsy, desired cosmetic result, depth of the diseased tissue, type of lesion to be removed (flat or elevated), and simplicity of technique. For example, vesicles should be completely biopsied in an attempt to keep the roof intact. Scalp biopsy specimens should extend into the subcutis to include the bulbs of terminal follicles. The instruments and materials needed to perform a skin biopsy are discussed in Chapter 6.

Surgical Excision

The technique of performing surgical excision biopsies with suturing of the skin is well known. In general, this type of biopsy is performed if a good cosmetic result is desired and if the entire lesion is to be removed. The disadvantage is that this procedure is the most time consuming of the three techniques, and it is necessary for the patient to return for removal of the sutures. Absorbable sutures can eliminate the need for a return visit. It is important that a sharp scalpel be used to reduce compression artifact and that care is taken not to crush the specimen with the forceps.

Punch Biopsy

Punch biopsies can be done rather rapidly, with or without suturing of the wound. A punch biopsy instrument of appropriate size is needed. Disposable biopsy punches are available. A local anesthetic is usually injected at the site. The operator rotates the instrument until it penetrates to the subcutaneous level. The circle of tissue is then removed. Bleeding can be stopped with pressure or by the use of one or two sutures. An elliptical versus a circular wound results in a neater scar after suturing. The elliptical punch can be produced by stretching the skin perpendicular to the desired suture line before the punch is rotated. Punch biopsies may be inadequate for evaluation of vesiculobullous diseases and must be deep enough to include subcutaneous fat if used for diagnosis of panniculitis or tumors in a subcutaneous location. In most instances, pigmented lesions should not be punched unless they can be completely excised with the punch technique.

Scissors Biopsy

The third way to remove skin tissue for a biopsy specimen is to excise the piece with sharp pointed scissors and stop the bleeding with light electrosurgery, Monsel solution, or aluminum chloride solution. This procedure is useful for certain types of elevated lesions and in areas in which the cosmetic result is not too important. The greatest advantage of this procedure is the speed and the simplicity with which it can be done.

Shave Biopsy

A scalpel or razor blade can be used to slice off a lesion. This can be performed superficially or deeply. Hemostasis can be accomplished by pressure, light electrosurgery, Monsel solution, or aluminum chloride solution. This method is generally not recommended for excision of melanocytic lesions or other potentially malignant tumors where margin assessment is required. However, it can be used for initial evaluation of pigmented tumors if done deep and wide enough. Sometimes a 'scoop shave' or saucerization can be done in an attempt to perform a shave removal of the entire lesion to allow complete evaluation of a pigmented lesion in its entirety without taking the time to perform a complete excision.

Biopsy Handling

The biopsy specimen must be placed in an appropriate fixture, usually 10% formalin. If the specimen tends to curl, it can be stretched out on a piece of paper or cardboard before fixing. Mailing specimens in formalin during winter may result in freezing artifact. This can be avoided by the addition of 95%

ethyl alcohol, 10% by volume. For some procedures, fresh tissue should be taken directly for pathologic processing (fresh tissue, Mohs surgery, direct immunofluorescence), put in sterile saline (for culture of fungi and bacteria, including acid-fast bacteria), viral transport media (for viral culture), Michel's solution (direct immunofluorescence), and occasionally sent frozen on dry ice for special procedures.

CYTODIAGNOSIS

The Tzanck test is useful in identifying bullous diseases such as pemphigus and vesicular virus eruptions (herpes simplex and herpes zoster). The technique and choice of lesions are important. For best results, select an early lesion. In the case of a blister, remove the top with a scalpel or sharp scissors. Blot the excess fluid with a gauze pad, and then gently scrape the floor of the blister with a scalpel blade. Try not to cause bleeding. Make a thin smear of the cells on a clean glass slide. If you are dealing with a solid lesion, squeeze the material between two slides. The slide may be air dried, but it can also be fixed by placing it in 95% ethanol for 15 seconds. Stain the slide with Wright–Giemsa stain (stain for 30 seconds, rinse with water, let dry, and then observe under high-power oil immersion) or hematoxylin and eosin. Pap smear technique can also yield good results.

In addition to skin testing, fungus examination, biopsies, and cytodiagnosis, there are certain tests for specific skin conditions that are discussed in connection with their respective diseases.

ADDITIONAL STUDIES

The deposition of immunoglobulin and complement may be detected by direct immunofluorescence. This is an extremely valuable technique for the diagnosis of lupus erythematosus and autoimmune bullous diseases. It is performed on a frozen section; therefore, the biopsy specimen must be received fresh or in Michel's solution.

Immunohistochemistry is particularly helpful in the accurate diagnosis and classification of neoplasms. It is possible to identify specific antigens in a routinely processed tissue section by attaching a labeled antibody. For example, malignant melanoma may be identified using antibodies directed against S-100 protein as well as other melanoma-specific antigens, such as MART-1, tyrosinase, SOX-10, or MiTF (Fig. 2-3). Different cytokeratin subtypes may be used to help differentiate certain epithelial tumors that are histologically similar. For example, cytokeratin 7 helps to differentiate metastatic small cell carcinoma of the lung from primary Merkel cell carcinoma of the skin, as well as both mammary and extramammary Paget's disease from squamous cell carcinoma in situ (Bowen's disease). Leukocyte common antigen (CD45) labels most lymphomas and leukemias. Multiple other antibodies can be used to distinguish the cell line, diagnosis, and prognosis. CD3, CD4, CD8, CD5, and CD7 are all T-cell markers that can sometimes be used

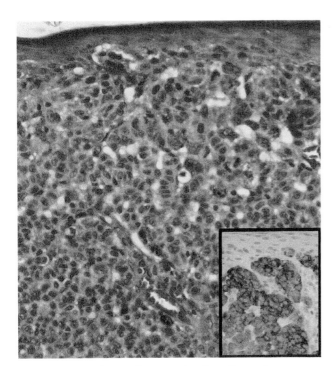

FIGURE 2-3: Photomicrograph of malignant melanoma with positive immunoreactivity for Mart-1 (*inset*). (Courtesy of Dr. K. Watson.)

to distinguish patch-stage mycosis fungoides from benign mimics, such as parapsoriasis and eczema.

DNA technology may be very useful. In situ hybridization allows recognition of specific DNA or RNA sequences using a gene probe in frozen or paraffin tissue sections. For example, a variety of different viruses, including herpes simplex, cytomegalovirus, and a human papillomavirus, can be identified using this technique.

Flow cytometry is another method of identifying specific cell antigens and is generally useful only with lymphomas and leukemias. This test is most commonly performed on lymph nodes, peripheral blood, and bone marrow, but may also be performed on solid organs, such as skin, provided the abnormal cell population is of sufficient quantity. A fresh specimen is needed. Following manipulation of the tissue to tease out the abnormal cells into a liquid media, the individual cells are labeled with antibodies (up to four at once) and passed through a light-scattering source that is able to measure cell size as well as antigen expression. The main advantage that flow cytometry has over tissue immunohistochemistry is the ability to characterize small populations of abnormal cells and to establish monoclonality via the analysis of immunoglobulin light chain expression. Polymerase chain reaction (PCR) may now also be used to establish monoclonality in both fresh and paraffin-embedded tissue. Disadvantages include lengthy time to diagnosis, high cost, and extreme sensitivity to DNA carryover/contamination problems from other specimens. PCR is able to pick up very small populations of clonal cells that may not be truly neoplastic or malignant. PCR is also used to find infectious organisms.

ACKNOWLEDGMENTS

We acknowledge the assistance of Dr. Cindy Essmeyer and members of her staff, Marcella Godinez, M.T., Katrin Boese, M.T., and Tammy Thorne, M.T., in preparation of the section on fungus examination. We also acknowledge the valuable assistance of Dean Shepard, from St. Luke's Hospital photographic services.

Suggested Readings

Ackerman AB. *Histopathologic Diagnosis of Inflammatory Skin Diseases.* Philadelphia: Lea & Febiger; 1978:149.

Adams RM. *Occupational Skin Disease.* Orlando: Grune & Stratton; 1990.

Beare JM, Bingham EA. The influence of the results of laboratory and ancillary investigations in the management of skin disease. *Int J Dermatol.* 1981;20:653–655.

Epstein E, Epstein E Jr. *Skin Surgery.* 6th ed. Philadelphia: WB Saunders; 1987.

Fisher AA. *Contact Dermatitis.* 4th ed. Philadelphia: Lea & Febiger; 1995.

Hurwitz RM, Hood AF. *Pathology of the Skin: Atlas of Clinical-Pathological Correlation.* Stamford, CT: Appleton & Lange; 1998.

Isenberg HD, ed. *Essential Procedures for Clinical Microbiology.* Washington, DC: ASM Press; 1998.

Koneman EW, Roberts GD. *Practical Laboratory Mycology.* 3rd ed. Baltimore: Williams & Wilkins; 1985.

Lever WF, Schaumburg-Lever G. *Histopathology of the Skin.* 7th ed. Philadelphia: JB Lippincott; 1990.

Vassileva S. Immunofluorescence in dermatology. *Int J Dermatol.* 1990;332:153.

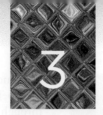

Dermatologic Diagnosis

John C. Hall, MD

This chapter will discuss how to describe primary and secondary skin lesions, common dermatologic conditions associated with different anatomic locations, seasonal skin diseases, military dermatoses, and dermatoses found in patients of color.

PRIMARY AND SECONDARY LESIONS

Most skin diseases have some characteristic primary lesions. It is important to examine the patient closely to find the primary lesion. Commonly, however, secondary lesions that are a direct result of overtreatment (Fig. 3-1), excessive scratching (Fig. 3-2), or infection (Fig. 3-3) have obliterated the primary lesions. Even in these cases, it is usually possible, through careful examination, to find some primary lesions at the edge of the eruption or on other, less irritated areas of the body (Fig. 3-4). Combinations of primary and secondary lesions also occur frequently.

Primary Lesions

- *Macules:* Up to 1 cm and are circumscribed, flat discolorations of the skin (Fig. 3-5A). Examples include freckles, flat nevi, and some drug eruptions.
- *Patches:* Larger than 1 cm and are circumscribed, flat discolorations of the skin. Examples include vitiligo, some drug eruptions, senile freckles, melasma, and measles exanthem.

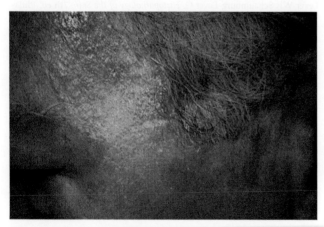

FIGURE 3-1: Vesicular inflammatory contact dermatitis obliterating seborrhea in a man overtreated with tea tree oil.

- *Papules:* Up to 1 cm and are circumscribed, elevated, superficial, solid lesions (Fig. 3-5B). Examples include elevated nevi, some drug eruptions, warts, and lichen planus. A *wheal* (hive) is a type of papule that is edematous and transitory (present <24 hours). Causes of wheals include drug eruptions, food allergies, numerous underlying illnesses, and insect bites.

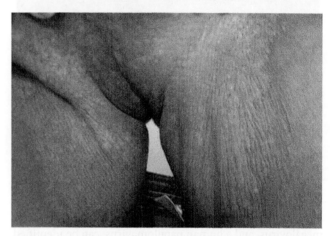

FIGURE 3-2: Dramatic scratching showing erosions and lichenification making the primary lesions of candida impossible to visualize.

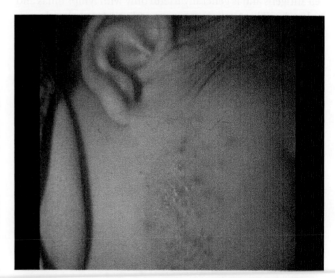

FIGURE 3-3: Secondary infection of the cheek of a child with redness and vesicles hiding the primary papulosquamous seborrheic dermatitis scaling.

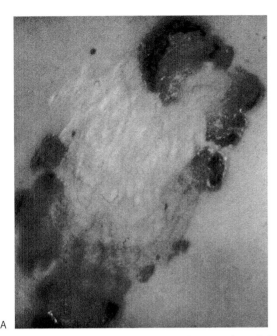
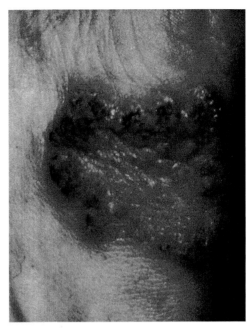

A   B

FIGURE 3-4: Nodular lesions. **A:** Grouped nodular lesions with central scarring (tertiary syphilis). **B:** Grouped warty, nodular lesions with central scarring (tuberculosis verrucosa cutis). (Courtesy of Marion B. Sulzberger, Folia Dermatologica, No. 1, Geigy Pharmaceuticals.)

■ *Plaques:* Larger than 1 cm and are circumscribed, elevated, superficial, solid lesions. Examples include mycosis fungoides and lichen simplex chronicus.

■ *Nodules:* Range in size (up to 1 cm) and are solid lesions with depth. They may be above, level with, or beneath the skin surface (Fig. 3-5C, D). Examples are nodular secondary or tertiary syphilis, basal cell cancers, dermatofibromas, and xanthomas.

■ *Tumors:* Larger than 1 cm and are solid lesions with depth. They may be above, level with, or beneath the skin surface (Fig. 3-5E). Examples include tumor stage of mycosis fungoides and larger basal cell cancers.

■ *Vesicles:* Up to 1 cm in size and are circumscribed elevations of the skin containing serous fluid (Fig. 3-5F). Examples include poison ivy, early chickenpox, herpes zoster, herpes simplex, dyshidrosis, and contact dermatitis.

■ *Bullae:* Larger than 1 cm and are circumscribed elevations containing serous fluid. Examples include pemphigus, bullous pemphigoid, poison ivy, and second-degree burns.

■ *Pustules:* Vary in size and are circumscribed elevations of the skin containing purulent fluid (Fig. 3-5G). Examples include acne, pustular psoriasis, and impetigo.

■ *Petechiae:* Range in size (up to 1 cm) and are circumscribed deposits of blood or blood pigments. Examples are thrombocytopenia, vasculitis, and drug eruptions.

■ *Purpura:* A circumscribed deposit of blood or blood pigment that is larger than 1 cm in the skin. Examples include senile purpura, drug eruptions, bleeding diatheses, chronic topical and systemic corticosteroid use, and vasculitis.

SAUER'S NOTES

1. One of the doctor's tools of the trade is a magnifying lens. *Use it.*

2. A complete examination of the entire body is a necessity when confronting a patient with a diffuse skin eruption or an unusual localized eruption.

3. Touch the skin and skin lesions. You learn a lot by palpating, and patients appreciate that you are not afraid of "catching" the problem. (For the uncommon contagious problem, use precaution.)

4. When in doubt of the diagnosis, verify your clinical impression with a biopsy. The most frequent reason for a successful malpractice suit in dermatology is failure to diagnose.

5. Do not underestimate the importance of adequate lighting.

6. Dermoscopy is a new tool that is mainly used to evaluate pigmented lesions. It combines diascopy and magnification, and is useful in diagnosing melanoma as well as deciding which tumors need a biopsy. Diascopy is a test to observe change in color after compression of a skin condition with a clear plastic or glass slide. If an observer has significant experience in dermoscopy, it is useful when deciding whether a lesion is truly benign or not.

7. There are computerized systems that will soon be available to evaluate multiple variables of pigmented tumors in vivo to decide whether a biopsy is necessary.

8. Serial photography systems have been shown by some authors to be useful when determining which pigmented tumors have changed significantly enough over time to warrant a biopsy.

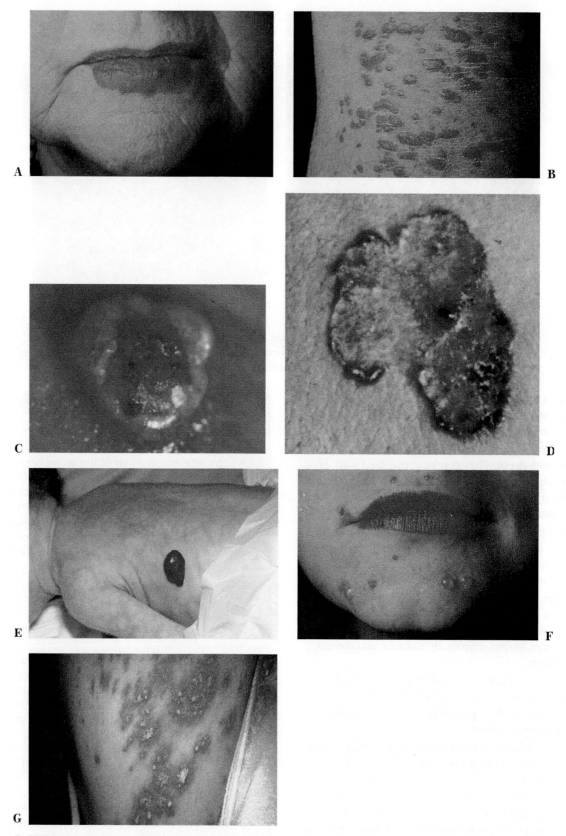

FIGURE 3-5: Primary skin lesions. **A:** Patch on lip (port wine hemangioma). **B:** Papules on knee (lichen planus). **C:** Nodule on lower eyelid (basal cell carcinoma). **D:** Polycyclic nodular lesion (superficial basal cell carcinoma). **E:** Tumor on the left side of an infant (hemangioma). **F:** Vesicles on chin (pemphigus vulgaris). **G:** Pustules, pretibial (pustular psoriasis). (Courtesy of Geigy Pharmaceuticals.)

Secondary Lesions

- *Scales:* Shedding, dead epidermal cells that may be dry or greasy. Examples are seborrhea (greasy) and psoriasis (dry).
- *Crusts:* Variously colored masses of skin exudates of blood, serum, pus, or any combination of these (Fig. 3-6A). Examples include impetigo, infected dermatitis, nummular eczema, or any area of excoriation.
- *Excoriations:* Abrasions of the skin, usually superficial and traumatic. Examples are scratched insect bites, scabies, eczema, and dermatitis herpetiformis.
- *Fissures:* Linear breaks in the skin, sharply defined with abrupt walls. Examples include congenital syphilis, interdigital tinea pedis, and hand eczema.
- *Induration:* Woodiness or hardness as seen in infiltrating tumors such as dermatofibrosarcoma protuberans, cutaneous metastasis, lymphoma, scleroderma, or hypertrophic scars.
- *Ulcers:* Variously sized and shaped excavations in the skin extending into the dermis or often deeper that usually heal with a scar. Examples include stasis ulcers of legs, ischemic leg ulcers, pyoderma gangrenosum, and tertiary syphilis.
- *Scars:* Formations of connective tissue replacing tissue lost through injury or disease. Examples are discoid lupus, lichen planus in the scalp, and third-degree burns.
- *Keloids:* Hypertrophic scars beyond the borders of the original injury (Fig. 3-6B). They are elevated, can be progressive, and usually are the result of some sort of trauma in the skin. Keloids are more common in darker-skinned people. They are common on the upper torso, neck, and with body piercing (especially with piercings of the earlobe). Rarely, keloids can occur spontaneously. Any type of full-thickness skin trauma can heal with a keloidal scar. They are unsightly and can be numb, pruritic, or painful.
- *Lichenification:* A diffuse area of thickening and scaling with a resultant increase in skin lines and markings (Fig. 3-6C). It is often seen in atopic dermatitis or any area chronically rubbed or scratched.

Several combinations of primary and secondary lesions commonly exist on the same patient. Examples are *papulosquamous lesions* of psoriasis, *vesiculopustular lesions* in contact dermatitis, and *crusted excoriations* in scabies.

Special Lesions

Some primary lesions, limited to a few skin diseases, can be called *specialized lesions.*

- *Burrows:* Very thin and short (in scabies) or tortuous and long (in creeping eruption) tunnels in the epidermis.
- *Comedones or blackheads:* Plugs of whitish (whiteheads or closed comedones) or blackish (blackheads or open comedones) sebaceous and keratinous material lodged in the pilosebaceous follicle, usually seen on the face, chest, or back and, rarely, on the upper part of the arms. Examples include acne and Favre–Racouchot on sun-damaged

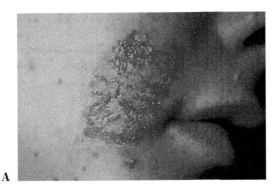

A

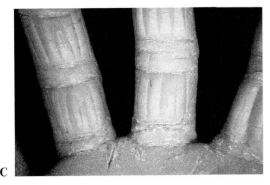

C

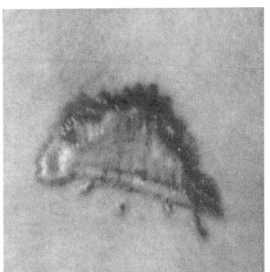

B

FIGURE 3-6: Secondary lesions. **A:** Crust on cheek (impetigo). **B:** Keloid. **C:** Lichenification of flexor fingers in a patient with chronic eczema.

skin in the temporal areas. These are a hallmark of chloracne. Chloracne is caused by exposure to hydrocarbons such as those found in cutting oils and Agent Orange.

- *Cutaneous horn:* A localized spike-shaped area of marked overgrowth of keratin that can stick above the skin half an inch or more. It is quite localized (usually 0.5 to 1 cm in width or less). It most commonly overlies actinic keratoses, but can also overlie seborrheic keratoses, squamous cell carcinomas, warts, porokeratoses, or, less likely, hyperkeratotic basal cell cancers.

- *Flagellate:* Linear whip-like red lesions most often associated with bleomycin therapy but also reported with peplomycin therapy, dermatomyositis, adult-onset Still disease, and Shiitake mushroom dermatitis associated with eating this particular mushroom.

- *Follicular plugs:* Keratin plugs in the hair follicle that are 1 to 3 mm in size and most characteristically seen in lupus erythematosus ("carpet tack sign" seen on the underside of the scale) and lichen planus (more flask-shaped plugs).

- *Mal perforans ulcer:* Seen in diabetics and leprosy patients. There is an associated neuropathy, so the ulcers are painless despite being deep and destructive. They are circular and sharply marginated or "punched out." These ulcers are usually associated with vasculitis; however, ischemic (very painful) and factitial ulcers can also have the same appearance.

- *Milia:* Whitish papules, 1 to 2 mm in diameter, that have no visible opening onto the skin surface. Examples are found in healed burns or superficial trauma sites, healed bullous disease sites, or newborns. They are not uncommon on the face of adults and can become more widespread in newborns.

- *Chancre:* Rounded, usually single, erosions or ulcers often with an exudative surface. These include: anthrax, atypical mycobacterium, blastomycosis (primary cutaneous-type), chancroid, coccidioidomycosis (primary cutaneous-type), cowpox, cutaneous diphtheria, erysipeloid, furuncle, milker's nodule, orf, rat-bite fever (sodoku), sporotrichosis, syphilis (genital but also extragenital), tuberculosis (primary inoculation-type), tularemia, and vaccinia.

- *Striae cutis distensae:* Red, resolving to white, linear areas of atrophy that may be indented. They are seen mainly on the thighs, buttocks, and breasts. They can be seen during rapid weight loss, prolonged use of topical or systemic corticosteroids, bodybuilding (especially with androgen ingestion), Cushing disease, and pregnancy, where it is most pronounced over the abdomen.

- *Telangiectasias:* Dilated superficial blood vessels. Examples include spider hemangiomas, chronic radiodermatitis, basal cell cancer, sebaceous hyperplasia, prolonged chronic sun exposure, necrobiosis lipoidica diabeticorum, and rosacea.

In addition, distinct and often diagnostic changes can occur in the nail plates and the hairs. These are discussed in the chapters relating to these appendages.

DIAGNOSIS BY LOCATION

A physician is often confronted with a patient with skin trouble localized to one part of the body (Figs. 3-7 to 3-10). The following list of diseases with special locations is meant to aid in the diagnosis of such conditions, but this list should not be considered exclusive. Generalizations are the rule, and many rare diseases are omitted. For further information concerning each particular disease, consult the Dictionary-Index located at the end of the book.

- *Scalp:* Seborrheic dermatitis, contact dermatitis, seborrheic keratoses, pilar cysts, psoriasis, folliculitis, pediculosis, and hair loss due to male or female pattern alopecia areata, lichen planopilaris, tinea, chronic discoid lupus erythematosus, telogen effluvium (postpartum alopecia), or trichotillomania.

- *Ears:* Seborrheic dermatitis, psoriasis, atopic eczema, lichen simplex chronicus, actinic keratoses, melanoma, varix, seborrheic keratoses, and squamous cell carcinomas.

- *Face:* Acne, rosacea, impetigo, contact dermatitis, seborrheic dermatitis, folliculitis, herpes simplex, lupus erythematosus, dermatomyositis, nevi, melasma, melanoma (especially lentigo maligna melanoma), basal cell cancer, actinic keratosis, seborrheic keratosis, squamous cell carcinoma, seborrheic keratosis, milia, and sebaceous hyperplasia.

- *Eyelids:* Contact dermatitis due to cosmetics, especially fingernail polish or hair sprays, dermatomyositis, seborrheic dermatitis, atopic eczema, skin tags, syringomas, and basal cell cancer.

- *Posterior neck:* Neurodermatitis (lichen simplex chronicus), seborrheic dermatitis, psoriasis, folliculitis, contact dermatitis, cutis rhomboidalis nuchae, and acne keloidalis nuchae especially in darker-skinned patients.

- *Mouth:* Aphthae, herpes simplex, geographic tongue, syphilis, lichen planus, traumatic fibromas, erythema multiforme, oral hairy leukoplakia, squamous cell cancer, candidiasis, and pemphigus.

- *Axillae:* Contact dermatitis, seborrheic dermatitis, hidradenitis suppurativa, erythrasma, acanthosis nigricans, and Fox–Fordyce disease.

- *Chest and back:* Tinea versicolor, pityriasis rosea, acne, seborrheic dermatitis, psoriasis, secondary syphilis, epidermoid cysts of the back, seborrheic keratoses, senile or cherry angiomas, nevi, and melanomas, especially on the backs of men.

- *Groin and crural areas:* Tinea infection, candida infection, bacterial intertrigo, scabies, pediculosis, granuloma inguinale, warts, skin tags, hidradenitis suppurativa, folliculitis, seborrhea, and inverse psoriasis.

- *Penis:* Contact dermatitis, fixed drug eruption, condyloma acuminata, candida balanitis, chancroid, herpes simplex, secondary syphilis, scabies, balanitis xerotica obliterans, warts, psoriasis, seborrhea, and pearly penile papules.

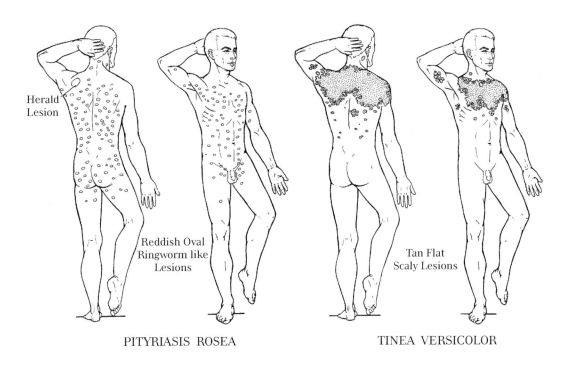

PITYRIASIS ROSEA

TINEA VERSICOLOR

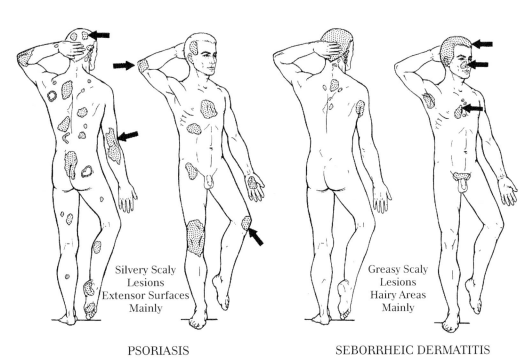

PSORIASIS

SEBORRHEIC DERMATITIS

FIGURE 3-7: Dermatologic silhouettes. Diagnosis by location.

- *Hands:* Contact dermatitis, id reaction to fungal infection of the feet, atopic eczema, psoriasis, verrucae, pustular psoriasis, nummular eczema, erythema multiforme, secondary syphilis (palms), fungal infection, dyshidrotic eczema, warts, and squamous cell carcinoma of the dorsal hands.

- *Cubital fossae and popliteal fossae:* Atopic eczema, contact dermatitis, and folliculitis.

- *Elbows and knees:* Psoriasis, xanthomas, dermatomyositis, granuloma annulare, and atopic eczema.

- *Feet:* Fungal infection, primary or secondary bacterial infection, contact dermatitis from footwear or foot care, atopic eczema, verrucae, psoriasis, erythema multiforme, dyshidrotic eczema, and secondary syphilis (soles of feet).

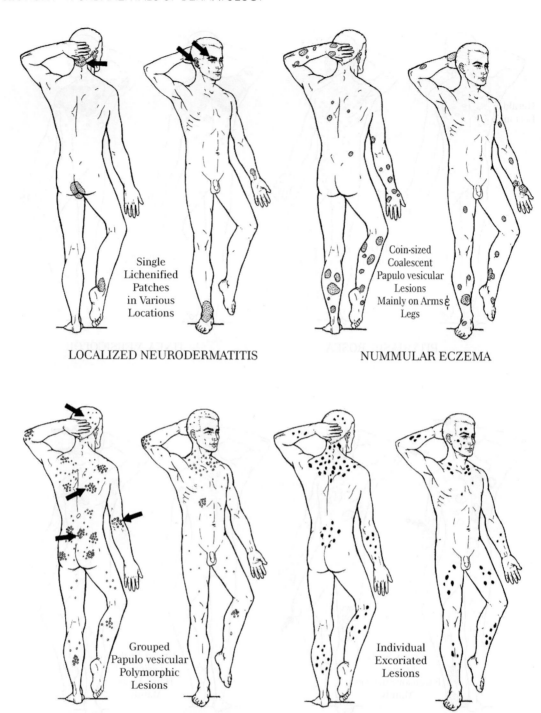

LOCALIZED NEURODERMATITIS

Single
Lichenified
Patches
in Various
Locations

NUMMULAR ECZEMA

Coin-sized
Coalescent
Papulo vesicular
Lesions
Mainly on Arms &
Legs

DERMATITIS HERPETIFORMIS

Grouped
Papulo vesicular
Polymorphic
Lesions

NEUROTIC EXCORIATIONS

Individual
Excoriated
Lesions

FIGURE 3-8: Dermatologic silhouettes. Diagnosis by location.

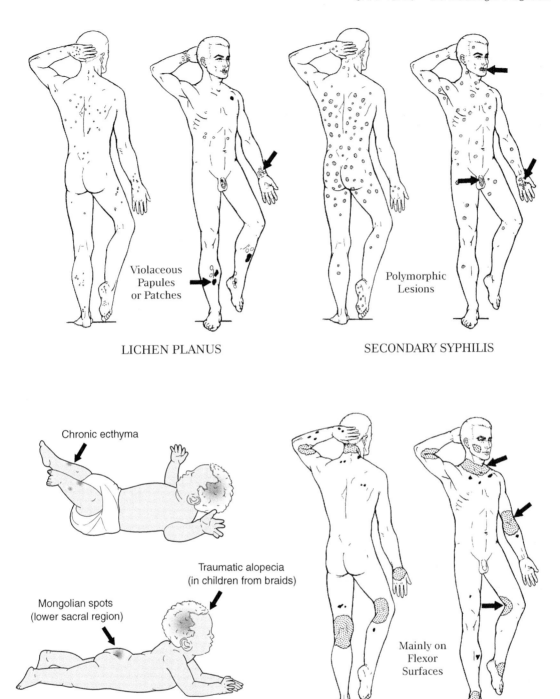

FIGURE 3-9: Dermatologic silhouettes. Diagnosis by location.

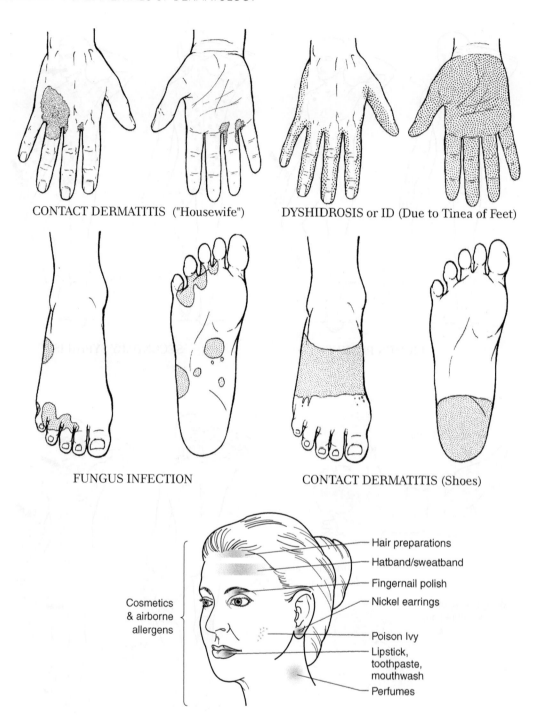

CONTACT DERMATITIS ("Housewife")   DYSHIDROSIS or ID (Due to Tinea of Feet)

FUNGUS INFECTION   CONTACT DERMATITIS (Shoes)

Cosmetics & airborne allergens

Hair preparations
Hatband/sweatband
Fingernail polish
Nickel earrings
Poison Ivy
Lipstick, toothpaste, mouthwash
Perfumes

CONTACT DERMATITIS

FIGURE 3-10: Dermatologic silhouettes. Diagnosis by location.

In diagnosing a rather generalized skin eruption, the following three mimicking conditions must be considered first and ruled in or out by an appropriate history or examination:

1. Drug eruption
2. Contact dermatitis
3. Infectious diseases, such as acquired immunodeficiency syndrome, other viral exanthems, and secondary syphilis

A complete examination of the entire body is a necessity when confronting a patient with a diffuse skin eruption, an unusual localized eruption, and in a patient where malignant melanoma is suspected.

SEASONAL SKIN DISEASES

Certain dermatoses have an increased incidence in various seasons of the year. In a busy doctor's office, a clinician can see "epidemics" of atopic eczema, pityriasis rosea, psoriasis, and winter itch, among others. Knowledge of this seasonal incidence associated with some skin conditions is helpful from a diagnostic standpoint. It is sufficient simply to list these seasonal diseases here, because more specific information concerning them can be found elsewhere in this text. Remember that there are always exceptions to every rule.

Winter

- Atopic eczema
- Irritant contact dermatitis of the hands
- Psoriasis
- Seborrheic dermatitis
- Nummular eczema
- Winter itch and dry skin (xerosis)
- Ichthyosis

Spring

- Pityriasis rosea
- Erythema multiforme
- Acne (flares)
- Viral exanthems

Summer

- Contact dermatitis due to poison ivy
- Tinea of the feet and the groin
- Candida intertrigo
- Miliaria or prickly heat
- Impetigo and other pyodermas
- Polymorphous light eruption
- Insect bites

- Tinea versicolor (noticed after sun tan)
- Darier disease (uncommon)
- Epidermolysis bullosa (uncommon)

Fall

- Winter itch
- Senile pruritus
- Atopic eczema
- Acne (less sun, more stress with school starting)
- Pityriasis rosea
- Contact dermatitis due to ragweed
- Seborrheic dermatitis
- Tinea of the scalp (school children)
- Viral exanthems

MILITARY DERMATOSES

Certain parts of the world continue to be at war, and under its ravages, the lack of good personal hygiene, the lack of adequate food, and the presence of overcrowding, injuries, and pestilence can result in the aggravation of any existing skin disease. In this setting, there is an increased incidence of the following skin diseases:

- Scabies
- Pediculosis
- Syphilis and other sexually transmitted diseases
- Bacterial dermatoses
- Tinea of the feet and the groin
- Pyoderma
- Miliaria
- Leishmaniasis (Middle East)

DERMATOSES OF DARK-SKINNED PATIENTS

The following skin diseases are seen with greater frequency in people of color than in light-skinned patients (Figs. 3-11 and 3-12):

- Keloids
- Dermatosis papulosa nigra (variant of seborrheic keratoses that are dark, small, multiple, facial, and more common in women)
- Pigmentary disturbances from many causes, both hypopigmented and hyperpigmented
- Traumatic marginal alopecia (traction alopecia) (from braids and from heated irons used in hair straightening)
- Seborrheic dermatitis of the scalp, aggravated by grease on the hair
- Ingrown hairs of the beard (pseudofolliculitis barbae)

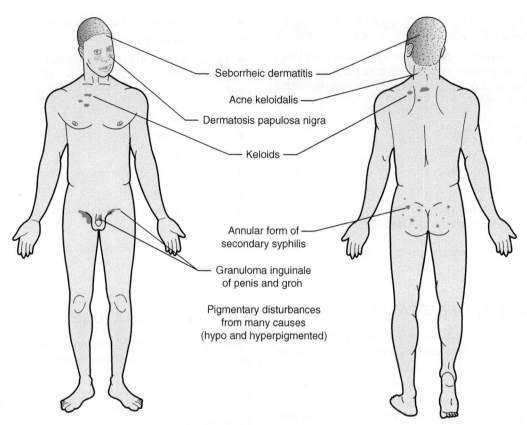

FIGURE 3-11: Dermatologic silhouettes. Conditions more common among dark-skinned patients.

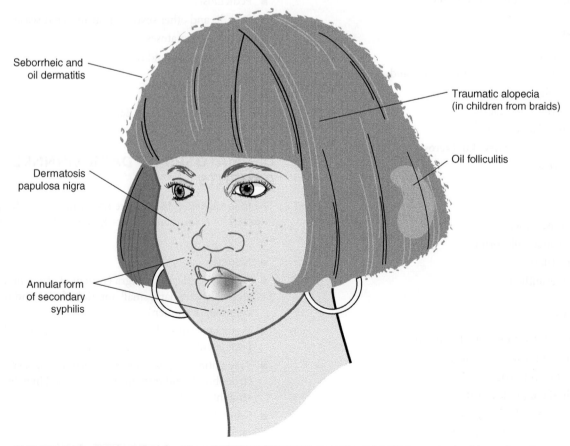

FIGURE 3-12: Dermatologic silhouette. Conditions more common among dark-skinned patients.

- Acne keloidalis nuchae
- Annular form of secondary syphilis
- Granuloma inguinale
- Mongolian spots
- Acral lentiginous melanomas
- Tinea capitis (in children who braid their hair)

On the other hand, certain skin conditions are rarely seen in dark-skinned people:

- Squamous cell or basal cell carcinomas
- Actinic keratoses
- Porokeratosis
- Psoriasis
- Superficial spreading, nodular, and lentigo maligna melanoma
- Scabies

DESCRIPTIVE TERMS OFTEN USED IN DERMATOLOGY

- *Acneiform:* Refers to a resemblance of acne as seen in acne, folliculitis, rosacea, and some drug eruptions such as those due to topical and systemic corticosteroids. It can also be seen with ingestion of iodides or bromides and as part of chloracne due to hydrocarbon exposure.
- *Agminated:* Refers to aggregated in a group such as a clustered group of blue nevi or agminated blue nevi. Another example is a cluster of primary cutaneous follicle center lymphoma, which can appear in a clustered or agminated-type.
- *Annulare or arciform lesions:* Refer to a peripheral circular curving of the lesions seen in diseases such as erythema annulare centrifugum, erythema chronica migrans of Lyme disease, erythema marginatum of scarlet fever, erythema gyratum perstans (which can be associated with underlying malignancy), tinea, impetigo, and psoriasis.
- *Atrophic:* Refers to thinning of the skin as seen in mycosis fungoides with fine superficial "cigarette paper" wrinkling atrophy or deep with a resultant scarring formation as in discoid lupus erythematosus or third-degree burns.
- *Color alterations*
  Hyperpigmented: Increased pigment as seen in postinflammatory hyperpigmentation and residual lesions of lichen planus or dermatitis herpetiformis.
  Hypopigmented: Decreased pigment as seen in pityriasis alba, tinea versicolor after a tan, and postinflammatory hypopigmentation.
  Depigmented: Loss of pigment as in vitiligo or scar.
  Violaceous: Reddish-purple discoloration as seen in vasculitis and the tumors of mycosis fungoides.

Apple-jelly colored: Reddish-brown color seen most often in sarcoidosis, particularly upon pressing the skin with a clear glass slide. This is called diascopy.

Porcelain-white: Stark white color that can be seen in morphea, generalized cutaneous scleroderma, Degos disease, and atrophie blanche or livedoid vasculopathy.

Heliotrope: Refers to violaceous color as seen on upper eyelids in dermatomyositis.

Cayenne pepper: Tiny reddish-brown spots due to hemosiderin staining of the skin, seen most often in the pigmented purpuric dermatoses.

- *Cushingoid:* An appearance seen in patients on high dose, long-term systemic corticosteroids in which the face has a round or moonlike appearance and there is increased central body fat particularly over the back with a "buffalo hump." Acne, striae, rosacea, and hirsutism are also often seen.
- *En cuirasse:* Refers to a shield-like induration usually at the chest wall as seen in scleroderma and infiltrated malignancies, particularly breast cancer.
- *Exophytic:* Protruding from the skin such as in some squamous cell carcinomas, warts, advanced cutaneous lymphoma, and keloids.
- *Filiform:* Refers to tiny filamentous projections that come from a tumor, usually indicative of a filiform wart.
- *Forme fruste:* Refers to an atypical or partial example of a skin disease.
- *Herpetiform:* Means "in a group" and is seen in the blisters of herpes simplex, herpes zoster, varicella, and the autoimmune blistering diseases of dermatitis herpetiformis and impetigo herpetiformis (herpes gestationis).
- *Incognito:* Refers to a hidden skin disease such as in scabies patients who frequently bathe, in dermatitis herpetiformis that is so excoriated that no primary skin lesions can be seen, or in some cases of cutaneous T-cell lymphoma.
- *Keratotic:* Thickening of the horny layer causing dry, heaped up, hard skin such as in keratotic actinic keratosis, squamous cell cancer, keratoderma palmaris et plantaris, chronic palm and sole psoriasis, or eczema (especially lichen simplex chronicus).
- *Linear:* In a line as in poison ivy dermatitis, coup de sabre-type of morphea, lichen striatus, and excoriations.
- *Leonine facies:* A lion-like look to the face with thickening of the normal furrows over the entire face, most often described with cutaneous T-cell lymphoma, leprosy, lichen myxedematosous, or tertiary syphilis.
- *Morbilliform:* Usually used to refer to a measles-like eruption that is symmetric, macular, and consists of 1 cm or smaller, usually red, macules that can become confluent. This is seen most often in morbilliform drug eruptions and viral exanthems, including measles, rubella, and HIV exanthem, among others.

- *Peau d' orange:* A bulging of the skin with an orange-peel look that has a mottled texture and is seen in cutaneous mucinosis such as myxedema, lymphoma of the skin such as T-helper cell lymphoma, other cutaneous malignancies such as breast cancer, and elephantiasis nostra verrucosa such as seen in chronic lymphedema of the lower extremities.

- *Pedunculated:* A narrow stalk-like attachment to the skin as in skin tags.

- *Perifollicular:* Eruptions that seem to be around the hair follicle. This term is often used to describe folliculitis, keratosis pilaris, and follicular eczema.

- *Poikiloderma:* Has three components—fine "cigarette paper" wrinkling atrophy, alternating or lacey hyper- and hypopigmentation, and telangiectasias. This is seen as a result of radiation dermatitis, chronic corticosteroid use topically or systemically, and chronic sun exposure most often seen as poikiloderma of Civatte on the sides of the neck. It is also found in collagen–vascular disease (most commonly lupus erythematosus) as well as in dermatomyositis. It can be a generalized eruption, in which case it is called poikiloderma atrophicans vasculare and is considered by most authorities to be a cutaneous T-cell lymphoma.

- *Psoriasiform:* Resembling psoriasis, as in psoriasis or a psoriasiform plaque of cutaneous T-cell lymphoma.

- *Punched out:* Circular with sharply demarcated edges and full-thickness skin loss and is most often used in relation to an arterial ischemic ulcer, vasculitic ulcer, or mal perforans ulcer.

- *Purpuric:* Purple areas due to bleeding under the skin or purpura. This can be seen in vasculitis, pyoderma gangrenosum, drug eruptions, and brown recluse spider bites.

- *Reticulate:* A lacy distribution of skin lesions as seen in oral lichen planus, the pigmentation of poikiloderma, and the pigmentation seen in erythema ab igne. This can also be referred to as web-like.

- *Scalloped edges:* Circinate or rounded edges as in impetigo and ruptured blisters in bullous diseases.

- *Sclerodermoid:* Indurated skin, often with loss of pigment, and characteristic of scleroderma, scleredema, bleomycin injection sites, pentazocine (Talwin) injection sites, and chronic cutaneous graft-versus-host disease.

- *Telangiectatic:* Covered with telangiectasias as in rosacea, lupus erythematosus.

- *Umbilicated:* A tumor or plaque that has a central indentation or dell. This is often used to describe molluscum contagiosum and can also be seen in sebaceous hyperplasia, basal cell carcinoma, and sometimes in viral blisters such as in herpes simplex or herpes zoster.

- *Varicelliform:* To resemble chickenpox such as in smallpox, chickenpox, herpes zoster, Kaposi's varicelliform eruption, or pityriasis lichenoides et varioliformis of Mucha and Habermann.

- *Varioliformis:* To resemble smallpox as in pityriasis lichenoides et varioliformis acuta or smallpox.

- *Verrucous:* Wart-like in appearance such as in a verrucous keratoacanthoma, squamous cell carcinoma, or wart.

- *Zosteriform:* Refers to the distribution of cutaneous disease in a nerve root distribution. This is seen in herpes zoster, some epidermal and other hamartomatous nevi, and occasionally vitiligo, lichen planus, and others.

Suggested Readings

Archer CB, Robertson SJ. *Black and White Skin Diseases: An Atlas and Text.* Oxford, UK: Blackwell Science; 1995.

Bouchier IAD, Ellis H, Fleming PR. *French's Index of Differential Diagnosis.* 13th ed. London, UK: Butterworth-Heinemann; 1996.

Callen JP. *Color Atlas of Dermatology.* 2nd ed. Philadelphia: W.B. Saunders; 1999.

Du Vivier A. *Atlas of Clinical Dermatology.* 3rd ed. Philadelphia, PA: W.B. Saunders; 2002.

Eliot H, Ghatan Y. *Dermatological Differential Diagnosis and Pearls.* London: Parthenon; 1998.

Fleischer AB Jr, Feldman S, McConnell C, et al. *Emergency Dermatology.* Columbus, OH: McGraw-Hill; 2002.

Goodheart HP. *Goodheart's Photoguide to Common Skin Disorders.* 2nd ed. Philadelphia, PA: Lippincott Williams & Wilkins; 2003.

Habif TP. *Clinical Dermatology.* 4th ed. St. Louis: Mosby; 2004.

Habif TP, Campbell JL Jr, Chapman MS, et al. *Skin Disease: Diagnosis and Treatment.* St. Louis: Mosby; 2001.

Helm KF, Marks JG. *Atlas of Differential Diagnosis in Dermatology.* Philadelphia, PA: W.B. Saunders; 1998.

Hunter J, Savin J, Dahl M. *Clinical Dermatology.* 3rd ed. Oxford, UK: Blackwell Publishing; 2003.

Jackson R. *Morphological Diagnosis of Skin Disease.* Lewiston, NY: Manticore; 1999.

Johnson BL, Moy RL, White GM. *Ethnic Skin: Medical and Surgical.* St. Louis: C.V. Mosby; 1998.

Kerdel FA, Jimenez-Acosta, F. *Dermatology: Just the Facts.* New York: McGraw-Hill; 2003.

Lawrence CM, Cox NH. *Physical Signs in Dermatology.* 2nd ed. St. Louis: Mosby; 2001.

Micali G, Lacarrubba F, eds. *Dermatoscopy in Clinical Practice.* Boca Raton: CRC Press; 2010.

Provost TT, Flynn JA. *Cutaneous Medicine: Cutaneous Manifestations of Systemic Disease.* Hamilton, ON: BC Decker; 2001.

Poyner TF. *Common Skin Diseases.* Oxford, UK: Blackwell Science; 1999.

Ramos-e-Silva M. Ethnic hair and skin: what is the state of science? *Clin Dermatol.* 2002;20:321–324.

Ricketts JR, Rothe MJ, Grant-Kels JM. Cutaneous simulants of infectious disease. *Int J Dermatol.* 2011;50:1043–1057.

Rotstein H. *Principles and Practice of Dermatology.* 3rd ed. Newton, MA: Boston Publishing Co; 1993.

Rycroft RJG, Robertson SJ. *A Color Handbook of Dermatology.* London: Manson; 1999.

Steigleder GK. *Pocket Atlas of Dermatology.* 2nd ed. New York: Thieme; 1993.

Sybert VP. Skin manifestations in individuals of African or Asian descent. *Pediatr Dermatol.* 1996;13:163–164.

Tambosis E, Lim C. A comparison of the contrast stains, Chicago blue, chlorazole black, and Parker ink, for the rapid diagnosis of skin and nail infections. *Int J Dermatol.* 2012;51:935–938.

White GM, Cox NH. *Diseases of the Skin: A Color Atlas and Text.* St. Louis: Mosby; 2000.

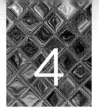

Dermatologic Therapy

John C. Hall, MD

Many hundreds of medications are available for use in treating skin diseases. Most physicians, however, have a few favorite prescriptions that they prescribe day in and day out. These few prescriptions may then be altered slightly to suit an individual patient or disease. Prescription pads printed with commonly used preparations can help save the clinician time and are always legible for the patient. Prescription pads that cannot be photocopied are mandatory. Prescription by computer is becoming the norm.

Treatment of most of the common skin conditions is simpler to understand when the physician is aware of three basic principles as follows:

1. The first principle is to treat the skin lesion by its *type,* more than the cause, influences the kind of local medication used. The old adage "If it is wet, dry it with a wet dressing, and if it is dry, wet it with an ointment" is true in most cases. For example, to treat a patient with an acute oozing, crusting dermatitis of the dorsum of the hand, whether due to poison ivy or soap, the physician should prescribe wet soaks. For a chronic-looking, dry, scaly patch of psoriasis on the elbow, an ointment is indicated because it holds moisture in the skin; an aqueous lotion or a wet dressing is more drying. Bear in mind, however, that the type of skin lesion can change rapidly under treatment. The patient must be followed closely after beginning therapy. An acute oozing dermatitis treated with water soaks can change, in 2 or 3 days, to a dry, scaly lesion that requires an ointment. Conversely, a chronic dry patch may become irritated with greasy ointment and begin to ooze.
2. The second basic principle in treatment is *first do no harm* and never overtreat. It is important for the physician to know which of the chemicals prescribed for local use on the skin are the greatest irritants and sensitizers. It is no exaggeration to say that a commonly seen dermatitis is actually due to patient overtreatment before coming to the office (*overtreatment contact dermatitis*). The patient, many times has gone to the neighborhood drugstore, or to a friend, and used any, and many, of the medications available for the treatment of skin diseases. It is certainly not unusual to hear the patient tell of using an athlete's foot salve for the treatment of the lesions of pityriasis rosea.
3. The third principle is to *instruct the patient adequately regarding the application of the medicine prescribed.* The patient does not have to be told how to swallow a pill, but

does have to be told how to put on a wet dressing. Most patients with skin disorders are ambulatory, so there is no nurse to help them; they are their own nurses. The success or the failure of therapy rests on adequate instruction of the patient or person responsible for the care. Even in

---

SAUER'S NOTES

Skin Diseases Associated with Smoking (Therapy Is Quitting)

1. Smoker's wrinkles—deep facial wrinkles
2. Poor wound healing—especially for flaps and grafts
3. Psoriasis—especially associated with pustular psoriasis
4. Severity of skin cancer—increased risk of basal cancers becoming morpheaform
5. Atopic dermatitis in children whose mothers smoke
6. Arteriosclerotic vascular disease—Buerger disease (Fig. 4-1), ischemic leg ulcers
7. Leukoplakia and squamous cell cancer of the lip and oral mucosa (Fig. 4-2)
8. Condyloma and cervical cancer
9. Increased severity of Raynaud's phenomena and ischemic ulcers
10. Increased neuropathy (especially in diabetics) with mal perforans ulcers (Fig. 4-3)
11. Embolic phenomena—blue toes, livedo reticularis, necrosis with ulcers
12. Decreased effectiveness of antimalarials for cutaneous lupus erythematosus
13. Crohn disease (15% with associated skin disease) incidence and activity
14. Increased nonlymphocytic leukemia systemically including skin
15. Increase in malignant melanoma incidence
16. Possibly less incidence of aphthous ulcers and acne
17. Cutaneous lupus erythematosus
18. Risk of developing contact dermatitis, increase androgenic alopecia, and premature graying of the hair in both men and women
19. Increased necrobiosis lipoidica diabeticorum
20. Increased in urticaria

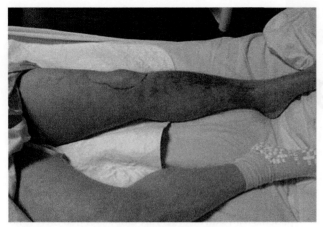

FIGURE 4-1: Erythema, livedo reticular, and early plaques of gangrene in a patient whose only risk factor was a 40-pack year history of smoking. Often referred to as Buerger disease. Patient could not quit smoking and ended up with an above knee amputation.

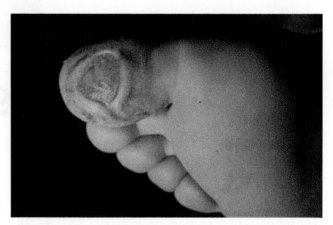

FIGURE 4-3: Punched out ulcer with red base on the plantar surface of the toe. Diabetes is present and smoking will make the associated neuropathy worse and the ability to heal the ulcer more difficult.

hospitals, particularly when wet dressings or aqueous lotions are prescribed, it is wise for the physician to instruct the nurse regarding the procedure.

With these principles of management in mind, let us now turn to the medicine used. It is important to stress that we are endeavoring to present here only the most basic material necessary to treat most skin diseases. For instance, there are many solutions for wet dressings, but Domeboro solution is our preference. Other physicians have preferences different from the drugs listed and their choices are respected, but to list all of them does not serve the purpose of this book.

Two factors have guided us in the selection of medications presented in this formulary. First, the medication must be readily available at most of the drugstores; second, it must be

a very effective medication for one or several skin conditions. The medications listed in this formulary are also listed, in a complete way, in the treatment section for the particular disease. Instructions for more complete use of the medications, however, are as described in this formulary.

FORMULARY

A particular topical medication is prescribed to produce a specific beneficial effect.

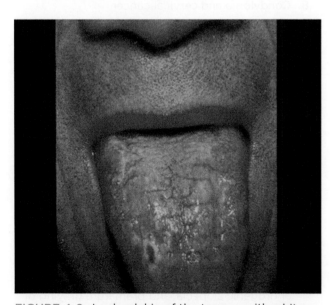

FIGURE 4-2: Leukoplakia of the tongue with white atrophic mucosa and an early erosion. Induration of the tongue was palpable in this smoker who may well get cancer of the tongue if his smoking continues.

SAUER'S NOTES

Local Therapy

1. The type of skin lesion (oozing, infected, or dry), more than the cause, should determine the local medication that is to be prescribed.

2. Do no harm. Begin local therapy for a particular case with mild drugs. The strength of the treatment can be increased if the condition worsens.

3. Do not begin local corticosteroid therapy with the "biggest gun" available, particularly for chronic dermatoses.

4. Carefully instruct the patient or nurse regarding the local application of salves, lotions, wet dressings, and baths. Thin coats of topical medications save money and are as effective as thick coats. Numbers of applications are more important than how thickly the medication is put on. Also, applying medications after hydration such as baths, showers, and hand washing increases penetration and makes topical therapy more effective. Effectiveness can also be increased by occlusion with Saran wrap, or occlusions with cotton socks or cotton dermal gloves.

5. Prescribe the correct amount of medication for the area and the dermatosis to be treated. This knowledge comes with experience.

6. Change the therapy as the response indicates. If a new prescription is indicated and the patient has some of the first prescription left, instruct the patient to alternate using the old and new prescriptions.

7. If a prescription is going to be relatively expensive, explain this fact to the patient.

8. For many diseases, "therapy plus" is indicated. Advise the patient to continue to treat the skin problem for a specified period after the dermatosis has apparently cleared. This may prevent or slow down recurrences.

9. Instruct the patient to telephone you, your nurse, nurse practitioner, medical assistant, or physician assistant if there are any questions or if the medicine appears to irritate the dermatosis.

Effects of Locally Applied Drugs

Anesthetic agents are used in the skin to decrease pain when injections, laser, cryotherapy, electrolysis, excisions, or other procedures are performed. These include lidocaine hydrochloride 3% cream (LidaMantle), 30% to 40% lidocaine compounded in Velvachol or Acid Mantle cream, EMLA cream or disk (2.5% lidocaine and 2.5% prilocaine), and ethyl chloride spray. Anesthetic agents for mucous membranes are used to temporarily ameliorate discomfort from mucous membrane diseases. They include viscous solution of lidocaine (2%) and Hurricaine liquid or gel spray (20% benzocaine); for ophthalmic use, Alcaine solution (0.5% proparacaine) and Pontocaine (0.5% tetracaine) are used.

Antipruritic agents relieve itching in various ways. Commonly used chemicals include menthol (0.25%), phenol (0.5%), camphor (2%), pramoxine hydrochloride (1%), sulfur (2% to 5%), and coal tar solution (liquor carbonis detergens [LCD]) (2% to 10%). These chemicals are added to various bases for the desired effect. Numerous safe and unsafe proprietary preparations for relief from itching are also available. The unsafe preparations are those that contain sensitizing antihistamines, benzocaine, and related—*caine* derivatives. Itch-X gel and spray is over the counter (OTC) and contains 1% pramoxine hydrochloride and 10% benzyl peroxide (Itch-X lotion is OTC, 1% hydrocortisone).

Keratoplastic agents tend to increase the thickness of the horny layer. Salicylic acid (1% to 2%) is an example of a keratoplastic agent that will thicken the horny layer.

Keratolytics remove or soften the horny layer. Commonly used agents of this type include salicylic acid (4% [Salex lotion and cream] to 10%), resorcinol (2% to 4%), urea (20% to 50%), and sulfur (4% to 10%). A strong destructive agent is trichloroacetic acid. Urea in 5% to 10% concentration (Eucerin Plus lotion and Carmol) is moisturizing, whereas in 20% to 50% (Vanamide, Keralac, Carmol) concentration, it is keratolytic. Urea is also available in a nail stick applicator, Kerastick (50%), for onychoschizia and in a Redi-Cloth (Kerol [42%]). α-Hydroxy acids (lactic acid [Lac-Hydrin 5% or 12% cream and lotion or AmLactin and AmLactin XL 12% cream

or lotion]), which are sold over the counter, and glycolic acid (Aqua Glycol is sold OTC in various concentrations and is available as facial cleanser, toner, face cream, shampoo, body cleanser, hand lotion, and body lotion) in 5% to 12% concentrations are moisturizers, whereas in higher concentrations up to 80% are keratolytic and can be used in the office for facial peeling, with caution. Some moisturizers combine ureas and α-hydroxy acids such as U-Kera E (40% urea, 2% glycolic acid) and Eucerin Plus. Kerol Topical Suspension (50% urea with lactic acid and salicylic acid) is keratolytic and can be massaged into callosities for 60 seconds after bath or shower.

Antieczematous agents remove oozing and vesicular excretions by various actions. Soaks for 10 minutes twice a day or clean towels soaked in a solution for 10 minutes twice a day are very effective. The commonest agents include water soaks or compresses (lukewarm to cool), Domeboro solution packets, or dissolvable tablets that are nonprescription, coal tar solution (2% to 5%), hydrocortisone 0.5% to 2% (0.5% and 1% are available without a prescription), and more potent corticosteroid derivatives incorporated in solutions, foams, and creams.

Antiparasitic agents destroy or inhibit living infestations. Examples include permethrin (Elimite or Acticin) cream for scabies, γ-benzene hexachloride (Kwell) cream and lotion for scabies and pediculosis, crotamiton (Eurax) for scabies, and permethrin (Nix) for pediculosis. For scabies and lice, 10% sulfur can be mixed in petrolatum which is effective and very safe, even in infants and pregnant women, but is malodorous and leaves stains.

Antiseptics destroy or inhibit bacteria, fungi, and viruses. Alcohol hand sanitizers are effective on hands and Clorox-containing cleansers are very effective on inanimate fomites such as counters, floors, exam tables, and so on.

Antibacterial topical medications include gentamicin (Garamycin), retapamulin ointment (Altabax), mupirocin (Bactroban), bacitracin (recently found to cause a significant number of cases of contact dermatitis), Polysporin, and neomycin (Neosporin), which causes an appreciable (at least 1%) incidence of allergic contact sensitivity. Soaps, such as Lever 2000 and Cetaphil antibacterial soap, can have extra antibacterial additives.

Antifungal and anticandidal topical agents include miconazole (Micatin, Monistat-Derm), clotrimazole (Lotrimin, Mycelex), ciclopirox (Loprox), econazole (Spectazole), oxiconazole (Oxistat), naftifine (Naftin), ketoconazole (Nizoral), butenafine hydrochloride (Mentax, Lotrimin Ultra), and terbinafine (Lamisil). Sulfur (3% to 10%) is an older but effective antifungal and anticandidal agent. Nystatin is anticandidal but not antifungal.

Antiviral topical agents are acyclovir (Zovirax) ointment or cream and penciclovir (Denavir).

Emollients soften and moisturize the skin surface. Nivea oil, mineral oil, and white petrolatum are good examples. Newer emollients are more cosmetically elegant and effective.

Ointments moisturize the skin. Examples include Vaseline petroleum jelly, Lanolin, Aquaphor, Cetaphil, and Eucerin.

Creams dry the skin but are more cosmetically acceptable than ointments because they do not feel greasy and do not leave oil marks on paper products. Examples are Dermovan and Vanicream. Newer moisturizers attempt to restore the normal skin barrier for protection and to increase penetration of other topicals applied on top of these agents. Three examples are Mimyx, Atopiclair, and CeraVe. CeraVe and Cetaphil RestoraDerm are two examples of increased topical use of ceramides.

SAUER'S NOTES

Locally Applied Generic Products

Advantages: Lower cost—you can prescribe a larger quantity at relatively less expense, and patients appreciate you sharing their concern regarding cost.

Disadvantages: With a proprietary (brand name) product, you are quite sure of the correct potency and bioavailability of the agent, and you know the delivery system and the ingredients in the base.

If you prescribe a proprietary medication when a less expensive generic is available, explain to the patient your reason for doing this.

Types of Topical Dermatologic Medications

Baths

1. Tar bath
   Coal tar solution (USP, LCD) 120.0 mL
   Or Cutar bath oil
   Sig: Add 2 tbsp to a tub of lukewarm water, 6- to 8-in deep.
   Actions: Antipruritic and antieczematous

2. Starch bath
   Limit or Argo starch, small box
   Sig: Add half box of starch to a tub of cool water, 6- to 8-in deep.
   Actions: Soothing; antieczematous and antipruritic
   Indications: Generalized itching and urticaria

3. Aveeno (regular and oilated) colloidal oatmeal bath
   Sig: Add 1 cup to the tub of water.
   Actions: Soothing and cleansing
   Indications: Oilated for generalized itching and dryness of skin, winter, and senile itch. Regular for oozing, draining, wet dermatitis.

4. Oil baths (see section on oils and emulsions) for dry skin.

5. Bleach baths and compresses. For baths, add 1 cup of bleach to full tub of water to soak for several minutes, and add 1 tablespoonful to 1 quart of water to use as compresses for several minutes b.i.d. to treat recurrent recalcitrant *Staphylococcus aureus* folliculitis and secondary infection in atopic dermatitis.

Soaps and Shampoos

1. Dove soaps, Neutrogena soaps, Cetaphil, Basis
   Action: Mild cleansing agents
   Indications: Dry skin or winter itch

2. Dial soap, Lever 2000, Cetaphil antibacterial soap
   Actions: Cleansing and antibacterial
   Indications: Acne, pyodermas

3. Capex shampoo 120.0
   Sig: Shampoo as needed.
   Actions: Anti-inflammatory, antipruritic, and cleansing
   Indications: Dandruff, psoriasis of scalp
   Comment: Contains fluocinolone acetonide, 0.01%

4. Selsun suspension or head and shoulders intensive treatment shampoo 120.0
   Sig: Shampoo hair with two separate applications and rinses. You can leave the first application on the scalp for 5 minutes before rinsing off. Do not use another shampoo as a final cleanser. Contains selenium sulfide.
   Actions: Cleansing and antiseborrheic
   Indications: Dandruff, itching scalp (not toxic if used as directed but poisonous if swallowed, so keep out of reach of small children).

5. Tar shampoos: Tarsum (can be applied overnight or for several hours as a scalp oil and then shampooed out), Polytar, T/Gel (regular and maximum strength), Pentrax, Ionil T, and so on
   Sig: Shampoo as necessary, even daily.
   Actions: Cleansing and antiseborrheic
   Indications: Dandruff, psoriasis, atopic eczema of the scalp

6. Nizoral shampoo 120.0 or Loprox shampoo
   Sig: Shampoo two or three times a week.
   Actions: Anticandidal and antiseborrheic
   Indication: Dandruff, tinea versicolor, and tinea capitis infection
   Comment: Nizoral is available as 1% OTC or as 2% with a prescription.
   Loprox shampoo is similar, with ciclopirox as the active ingredient

7. T-Sal, Salex, and other salicylic acid shampoos
   Indications: Psoriasis and seborrheic dermatitis

Wet Dressings or Soaks

1. Burow's solution, 1:20
   Sig: Add 1 Domeboro tablet or packet to 1 pint of tap water. Cover affected area with sheeting wet with solution and tie on with gauze bandage or string. Do not allow any wet dressing to dry out. It can also be used as a solution for soaks.
   Actions: Acidifying, antieczematous, and antiseptic
   Indications: Oozing, vesicular skin conditions

2. Vinegar solution
   Sig: Add half cup of white vinegar to 1 quart of water for wet dressings or soaks, as described for Burow's solution.
   Indications: Antieczematous, antiyeast, antifungal, antibacterial including antipseudomonas

3. Salt solution
   Sig: Add 1 tbsp of salt to 1 quart of water for wet dressings or soaks, as above.
   Indications: Antieczematous, cleansing

Powders

1. Purified talc (USP), ZeaSORB powder, or ZeaSORB-AF powder 60 (contains miconazole)
   Sig: Dust on locally b.i.d. (supply in a powder can)
   Actions: Absorbent, protective, and cooling
   Indications: Intertrigo, diaper dermatitis
2. Tinactin powder, Micatin powder, ZeaSORB-AF powder, or Desenex powder
   Sig: Dust on feet in the morning
   Actions: Absorbent, antifungal, and antiyeast
   Indications: Prevention and treatment of tinea pedis and tinea cruris as well as candida intertrigo
   Comment: These powders are available OTC.
3. Mycostatin powder 15.0
   Sig: Dust on locally b.i.d.
   Action: Anticandidal
   Indication: Candida intertrigo

Shake Lotions

1. Calamine lotion (USP) 120
   Sig: Apply locally to the affected area t.i.d. with fingers or brush.
   Actions: Antipruritic and antieczematous
   Indications: Widespread, mildly oozing, inflamed dermatoses
2. Nonalcoholic white shake lotion
   a. Zinc oxide 24.0
   b. Talc 24.0
   c. Glycerin 12.0
   d. Distilled water q.s. ad 120.0
3. White shake lotion
   a. Zinc oxide 24.0
   b. Talc 24.0
   c. Glycerin 12.0
   d. Distilled water q.s. ad 120.0
4. Proprietary lotions
   a. Sarna lotion (with menthol and camphor), Sarna for Sensitive Skin contains pramoxine
   b. Cetaphil lotion
   c. Aveeno anti-itch lotion (contains pramoxine)

SAUER'S NOTES

1. Shake lotions 1, 2, and 3 are listed for physicians who desire specially compounded lotions. One or two pharmacists near your office will be glad to compound them and keep them on hand.
2. To these lotions you can add sulfur, resorcinol, menthol, phenol, and so on, as indicated.

Oils and Emulsions

1. Zinc oxide, 40%
   Olive oil q.s. 120.0
   Sig: Apply locally to affected area by hand or brush t.i.d.
   Actions: Soothing, antipruritic, and astringent
   Indications: Acute and subacute eczematous eruptions
2. Bath oils
   Nivea skin oil, α-Keri, Cutar bath oil (contains tar)
   Sig: Add 1 to 2 tbsp to a tub of water. *Caution:* Avoid slipping in tub.
   Actions: Emollient and lubricant
   Indications: Winter itch, dry skin, atopic eczema
3. Hand and body emulsions: A multitude of products are available OTC. Some have petrolatum or phospholipids (Moisturel), some have urea or α-hydroxy acids (Lac-Hydrin lotion 5% OTC, Lac-Hydrin cream and lotion 12% prescription, and AmLactin 12% cream and lotion OTC), Vaseline clinical therapy, Vaseline, petrolatum (Curel), ceramides (CeraVe and EpiCeram Skin Body Emulsion), phospholipids (Moisturel), shea butter (Cetaphil hand cream), lanolin (Eucerin, Nivea, and Aquaphor), and some are lanolin-free.
   Sig: Apply locally as necessary.
   Actions: Emollient and lubricant
   Indications: Dry skin, winter itch, atopic eczema
4. Scalp oil
   Derma-Smoothe/FS oil (fluocinolone acetonide 0.01%) 120.0
   Sig: Moisten scalp hair and apply lotion overnight; wear a plastic cap
   Indications: Scalp psoriasis, lichen simplex chronicus, severe seborrheic dermatitis
5. Baker's P and S Liquid (phenol and sodium chloride)
   Sig: Apply overnight under shower cap as needed for scaling
   Indications: Thick scaling psoriasis

Tinctures and Aqueous Solutions

1. Povidone–iodine (Betadine) solution (also in skin cleanser, shampoo, and ointment) 15
   Sig: Apply with swab t.i.d.
   Actions: Antibacterial, antifungal, and antiviral
   Indication: General antisepsis
2. Gentian violet solution
   Gentian violet, 1%
   Distilled water q.s. 30.0
   Sig: Apply with swab b.i.d.
   Actions: Antifungal and antibacterial
   Indications: Candidiasis, leg ulcers
3. Antifungal solutions
   a. Lotrimin, Mycelex, Loprox, Tinactin, Micatin, Monistat-Derm, and Lamisil spray, among others 30.0
   Sig: Apply locally b.i.d.

b. Fungi-Nail 30.0. Also Kerydin and Jublia
   Sig: Apply locally b.i.d.
   Comment: Contains resorcinol, salicylic acid, para-chlorometaxylenol, and benzocaine in a base with acetic acid and alcohol
c. Penlac nail lacquer (contains ciclopirox)
   Sig: Apply thin coat two times a week; contains ciclopirox
d. Castellani's paint (can be obtained as uncolored): Used for intertrigo

Pastes

1. Zinc oxide paste (USP)
   Sig: Apply locally b.i.d.
   Actions: Protective, absorbent, and astringent
   Indications: Localized crusted or scaly dermatoses

Creams and Ointments

A physician can write prescriptions for creams and ointments in two ways: (1) by prescribing proprietary creams and ointments already compounded by pharmaceutical companies or (2) by formulating one's own prescriptions by adding medications to certain bases, as indicated for the particular patient being treated. For the physician who uses the second method, two different types of bases are used:

SAUER'S NOTES

1. OTC 0.5% or 1.0% Cortaid has proved effective and well tolerated as an emergency nonprescription treatment.
2. Do not use group I topical agents for longer than 2 weeks or more than a 45 g tube per week. A rest period must follow for 2 weeks.
3. Do not overuse the more potent topical steroids because of possible side effects.

SAUER'S NOTES

Compound Preparations

Compound proprietary preparations are frequently prescribed, particularly by family practice physicians and nondermatologic specialists. Physicians should know the ingredients in these compound preparations and should know the side effects. Here are some popular compounds:

Combination Therapies

Mycolog II cream: Contains Nystatin and triamcinolone. *Beware:* It is not beneficial for fungus (tinea) infections; the triamcinolone after long-term use can cause atrophy, striae, and telangiectasia of the skin, especially in intertriginous areas and on the face.

Lotrisone cream: Contains clotrimazole and betamethasone dipropionate. *Beware:* The betamethasone with long-term use can cause atrophy, striae, and dilated vessels, especially in intertriginous areas and

on the face. It also can have significant absorption to cause systemic corticosteroid side effects.

Iodoquinol–hydrocortisone cream (Vytone): Contains iodoquin plus 1% hydrocortisone. *Beware:* The iodoquin causes a moderate yellow stain on skin and clothing.

Cortisporin ointment: Contains 1% hydrocortisone with neomycin, polysporin, and bacitracin. *Beware:* Neomycin allergies can occur infrequently and bacitracin has now also become a significant allergen.

---

1. *Water-washable cream bases:* These bases are pleasant for the patient to use, nongreasy, and almost always indicated when treating intertriginous and hairy areas. Their disadvantage is that they can be too drying. A number of medications, as specifically indicated, can be added to these bases (i.e., menthol, sulfur, tars, hydrocortisone, and triamcinolone).
   a. Unibase
   b. Vanicream
   c. Sarna cream
   d. Cetaphil cream
   e. Unscented cold cream (not water washable)
2. *Ointment bases:* These petroleum jelly–type bases are, and should be, the most useful in dermatology. Although not as pleasant for the patient to use as the cream bases, their greasy quality alleviates dryness, removes scales, and enables the medicaments to better penetrate skin lesions. Disadvantages are that they can flare or cause folliculitis, acne, or rosacea, and they are less cosmetically acceptable because of the greasy feel. Any local medicine can be incorporated into these bases.
   For the physician who wishes to prescribe ready-made, proprietary preparations, these are listed in groups as follows:
   a. White petrolatum (USP)
   b. Zinc oxide ointment (USP), very protective
   c. Aquaphor (contains lanolin)
   d. Eucerin (contains lanolin)
   e. Moisturel (may sting when first applied)
3. *Antifungal ointments and creams:* Lotrimin cream, Lotrimin Ultra cream, Mycelex cream, Spectazole cream, Loprox cream, Tinactin cream, Lamisil cream, Oxistat cream, Naftin cream, Nizoral cream, Mentax cream, and others. *Action:* Antifungal
4. *Antibiotic ointments and creams:* Bactroban ointment or Centany ointment (can get generic mupirocin) and cream, Altabax (retapamulin) ointment, gentamicin ointment and cream, Neosporin ointment, Mycitracin ointment, and Polysporin ointment (antibiotic solutions are discussed in Chapter 15 under acne treatment).
5. *Antiviral ointments for herpes simplex virus infections:*
   a. Acyclovir ointment and penciclovir cream.
   b. Antiviral topicals for genital warts: Topical imiquimod (Aldara, Zyclara) for genital warts use thin coat Monday, Wednesday, and Friday night until dissipated.

c. Polyphenon E (mixture of green tea catechins). Use in a thin coat t.i.d. until clearing, may take up to 4 months.

d. Antiviral topical therapy for plantar warts: 40% salicylic acid plaster, apply overnight and peel away dead skin once a week and stop if there is pain or bleeding.

e. Vinegar soaks have been used with equal parts of water and white vinegar to soak for 5 minutes daily and ointment may be put around the warts to avoid too much drying of noninfected skin.

6. Corticosteroid ointments and creams:

   a. Hydrocortisone preparations (0.5% and 1% hydrocortisone creams and ointments are available OTC and generically)
      - Hytone 1% and 2.5% cream and ointment

   b. Desonide preparations (can be written generically)
      - Tridesilon cream and ointment
      - DesOwen cream and ointment

   c. Triamcinolone preparations (0.5%, 0.1%, 0.025%, 0.01%)
      - Kenalog ointment and cream
      - Aristocort ointment and creams
      - Also available generically

   d. Other fluorinated corticosteroid preparations (see Table 4-1 for a listing of these preparations, which are ranked according to potency).

7. *Corticosteroid antibiotic ointments and creams:* Cortisporin ointment

8. *Corticosteroid antifungal–antiyeast preparations:*

   a. Lotrisone (anticandidal and antifungal), contains betamethasone and clotrimazole

   b. Mycolog II cream and ointment (anticandida), contains triamcinolone and nystatin; generic available

9. *Antipruritic creams and lotions:*

   a. Eurax cream
   b. Sarna lotion
   c. Prax lotion
   d. PrameGel
   e. Doxepin (Zonalon) cream (may cause drowsiness)
   f. Aveeno anti-itch lotion
   g. Eucerin calming cream
   h. Eucerin anti-itch spray

10. *Retinoic acid products:*

    a. Retin-A cream (0.025%, 0.05%, 0.1%) and Retin-A gel (0.01% and 0.025%), Retin-A Micro (0.04% and 0.1%), Retin-A Micro Pump (0.08%, 0.04% and 0.01%), and Renova (0.02%)
       Actions: Antiacne comedones and small pustules (especially the gel) and antiphotoaging
       Indications: Acne of comedonal and small pustular-type; aging wrinkles on face; removal of mild actinic keratoses and prevention of actinic keratoses; and treatment of freckles, molluscum contagiosum, and flat warts

    b. Differin (adapalene gel and cream 0.1% and 0.03%)
       Action: Retinoic acid receptor binder
       Indications: Acne of comedonal and small pustular-type

    c. Avita (tretinoin 0.025%) cream may be less drying
       Action: Antiacne
       Indications: Acne of comedonal and small pustular-type

    d. Tazorac (tazarotene) 30 g 0.1% cream, 100 g 0.05% gel, and 100 g 0.1% gel
       Action: Used for treatment of acne, psoriasis, prevention, and treatment of actinic keratoses, and prevention of skin cancer
       Comment: Expensive and may be irritating

    e. Avage (0.1% tazarotene) cream 30 g
       Action: Approved for acne and may be milder than the same concentration of Tazorac

    f. Refissa (0.05%) is approved for facial wrinkles and hyperpigmentation and it may have a less irritating emollient base.

11. Miscellaneous creams, ointments, and gels:

    a. MetroGel (metronidazole 0.75%) 15.0
       Noritate cream (metronidazole 1%) 30.0
       Indications: Rosacea, perioral dermatitis

    b. Dovonex ointment (also comes as cream and scalp solution) 30.0 or 100.0
       Action: Antipsoriatic
       Comment: Moderately expensive

    c. Aczone (5% avlosulfone [dapsone])
       Action: Antiacne and antirosacea
       Comment: Some authors think a G6PD deficiency test should be done before therapy is initiated

12. Scabicidal and pediculicidal preparations:

    1. Eurax cream and lotion (crotamiton)
       Action: Scabicidal
       Comment: Antipruritic

    2. Kwell (lindane) lotion and cream
       Actions: Scabicidal and pediculicidal

    3. Elimite or Acticin cream
       Action: Scabicidal

    4. Nix Crème rinse
       Indications: Head lice, nits

    5. Ovide (malathion) topical
       Action: Pediculicidal
       Indications: Head lice, nits

    6. Ivermectin oral
       Action: Scabicidal
       Indications: Scabies

13. *Sunscreen creams and lotions:* Paraaminobenzoic acid (PABA) and its esters, such as octyl dimethyl PABA (padimate O), octocrylene, octyl salicylate, methyl anthranilate, avobenzone (Parsol 1789), cinnamates (octyl-methoxycinnamate), oxybenzone (benzophenone-3) are effective ultraviolet light absorbers. Zinc oxide and titanium oxide are light blockers. There are many products on the market. Any sunscreen with a sun protective factor (SPF) of 30 or above offers effective sun-damage protection against short-wavelength ultraviolet light or UVB (290 to 310 nm), if used correctly. There is no equivalent SPF number in the United States for long-wavelength ultraviolet light or UVA, which is also important in photoaging, development of skin precancers and skin cancers, lupus erythematosus, and

TABLE 4-1 • Potency Ranking of Some Commonly Used Topical Corticosteroids

Group I	Group IV	Group VII
Cordran tape	Aristocort ointment 0.1%	Epifoam 1.0%
Diprolene AF cream 0.05%	Cordran ointment 0.05%	Fluocinolone cream 1.0%, 2.5%
Diprolene ointment 0.05%	Cyclocort cream 0.1%	Hydrocortisone cream 1.0%, 2.5%
Diprolene gel 0.05%	Desonide ointment 0.2%	Hydrocortisone lotion 1.0%, 2.5%
OLUX-E foam	Elocon cream 0.1%	
Temovate cream 0.05%	Elocon lotion 0.1%	
Temovate ointment 0.05%	Fluocinolone ointment 0.025%	
Temovate gel 0.05%	Fluocinolone cream 0.2%	
Temovate emollient 0.05%	Halog cream 0.025%	
Temovate solution 0.05%	Halog ointment 0.025%	
Topicort Spray		
Ultravate cream 0.05%	Kenalog cream 0.1%	
Ultravate ointment 0.05%	Kenalog ointment 0.1%	
Vanos (fluocinonide) 0.1% cream	Topicort LP cream	

Group II	Group V
Cyclocort ointment 0.1%	Aristocort cream 0.1%
Diprolene AF cream 0.05%	Betamethasone valerate cream 0.1%
Diprosone ointment 0.05%	Betamethasone valerate lotion 0.1%
Halog cream 0.1%	Cloderm cream 0.1%
Halog ointment 0.1%	Cordran cream 0.05%
Halog solution 0.1%	Cordran lotion 0.5%
Halog-E cream 0.1%	Cordran ointment 0.025%
Lidex cream 0.05%	Cutivate cream 0.1%
Lidex gel 0.05%	Dermatop cream 0.1%
Lidex ointment 0.05%	DesOwen ointment 0.05%
Lidex solution 0.05%	Fluocinolone cream 0.025%
Maxiflor ointment 0.05%	Kenalog cream 0.1%
Psorcon cream 0.05%	Kenalog cream 0.025%
	Kenalog lotion 0.1%
Psorcon ointment 0.05%	Kenalog ointment 0.025%
Topicort cream 0.25%	Locoid cream 0.1%
Topicort gel 0.05%	Locoid ointment 0.1%
Topicort ointment 0.25%	Tridesilon ointment 0.05%

Group III	Group VI
Aristocort cream 0.5%	Aclovate cream 0.05%
Aristocort ointment 0.5%	Aclovate ointment 0.05%
Aristocort A cream 0.5%	Aristocort cream 0.1%
Aristocort A ointment 0.5%	Betamethasone valerate 0.1%
Betamethasone ointment 0.1%	DesOwen cream 0.05%
Cutivate ointment 0.005%	DesOwen ointment 0.05%
Cyclocort lotion 0.1%	DesOwen lotion 0.05%
Diprosone cream 0.05%	Fluocinolone cream 0.01%
Elocon ointment 0.1%	Fluocinolone solution 0.01%
Kenalog cream 0.5%	Kenalog cream 0.025%
Kenalog ointment 0.5%	Kenalog lotion 0.025%
Kenalog ointment 0.5%	Kenalog lotion 0.025%
Maxiflor cream 0.05%	Locoid solution 0.1%
Topicort LP cream 0.5%	Tridesilon cream 0.05%

Note: Group I is the superpotency category. Potency descends with each group, to group VII, which is the least potent (groups II and III are potent corticosteroids; IV and V are midstrength corticosteroids; VI and VII are mild corticosteroids). There is no significant difference between agents within groups II through VII. The compounds are arranged alphabetically within the groups. In group I, Temovate cream or ointment is most potent. (Courtesy of the late Dr. Richard B. Stoughton and Dr. Roger C. Cornell.)

porphyrias and is usually the most important wavelength for photoallergic reactions. Therefore, titanium dioxide, zinc oxide, or avobenzone (Parsol 1789) and probably the two best sunscreens, Antiehelios (Mexoryl SX [expensive]) and Helioplex sufficiently screen out UVA and UVB in a possibly more cosmetically acceptable base.

Sig: Apply to exposed areas before going outside. This should be done at least a half-hour in advance for the best effect. Reapplication is important if exposure to water or significant sweating occurs. After 1 hour, reapplication is advisable. Too thin of an application is a common mistake.

Action: Screening out ultraviolet rays

Indications: Polymorphous light eruption, photoaging, systemic and chronic lupus erythematosus, some cases of dermatomyositis, photoallergy from systemic or topical medications, some types of porphyria, and prevention of skin precancers and skin cancers, especially in light-complexioned people

14. *Antiyeast:* All products listed under *Antifungal* as well as products containing nystatin, which can be used orally, as a cream, as an ointment, with 0.1% triamcinolone (Mycolog II cream and ointment, which can be obtained generically), with various powders (ZeaSORB-AF, which also comes as a drying gel), and with any product which causes skin drying such as Domeboro compresses or ZeaSORB powder.

Aerosols and Foams

Various local medications have been incorporated in aerosol and foam-producing containers. These include corticosteroids (OLUX-E foam, LUXIQ foam), antibiotics (Evoclin foam), antiacne agents (Ovace foam), antirosacea agents (Ovace foam), antifungal agents (Lamisil spray), Retin-A pump, antipruritic medicines (Eucerin spray), and so on. Clobex spray is a class 1 topical corticosteroid.

Kenalog spray (63-g can) and Diprosone aerosol are effective corticosteroid preparations for scalp psoriasis and seborrhea.

Triamcinolone (LUXIQ), clobetasol (OLUX), and clobetasol (OLUXE), which is more of an emollient, are corticosteroid foams and Ovace foam is sodium sulfacetamide foam used for seborrhea, acne, and rosacea. Evoclin is erythromycin foam used to treat acne. Rogaine comes as a foam for hair loss and Verdeso (desonide 0.05%) is a class VI steroid that is now available as a foam.

Corticosteroid Medicated Tape

1. Cordran tape (also comes as a patch)
   Indications: Small areas of psoriasis, neurodermatitis, lichen planus

Medicated Skin Patches

Several are available for transdermal delivery of such agents as nitroglycerin, EMLA patch, and lidocaine patch for topical anesthesia, nicotine antismoking patches, and hormones. More will be developed.

Imiquimod

Imiquimod (Aldara, Zyclara) is used topically for superficial basal cell cancers, actinic keratoses, cutaneous Kaposi sarcoma, molluscum contagiosum, genital warts, and other warts under occlusion. It is being used experimentally for other skin diseases such as Bowen disease, elastosis perforans serpiginosa, cutaneous leishmaniasis, alopecia areata, and lentigo maligna melanoma. Other indications may well become approved with more experience with this topical medication. See section on actinic keratosis therapy in Chapter 30 and wart therapy in Chapter 26.

Local Agents for Office Use

1. Podophyllum in compound tincture benzoin
   Podophyllum resin (USP) 25%

   Compound tincture benzoin q.s. ad 30.0

   Sig: Apply small amount to warts with cotton-tipped applicator every 4 or 5 days until warts are gone. Excess amount may be washed off in 3 to 6 hours of application to prevent irritation.

   Action: Removal of venereal warts

   Comment: Other podophyllum proprietary preparations such as podofilox (Condylox) are marketed.

2. Trichloroacetic acid solution (saturated) or bichloracetic acid
   Sig: Apply with caution with cotton-tipped applicator (have water handy to neutralize within a few seconds).

   Indications: Warts on children, seborrheic keratoses, xanthelasma, sebaceous hyperplasia

3. Modified Unna's boot
   a. Dome-Paste bandage
   b. Gelocast
   c. Compression gelatin bandage with zinc oxide and glycerin then wrap with Coflex flexible wrap
      Indications: Stasis ulcers, localized neurodermatitis (lichen simplex chronicus)

4. Ace bandage, 3- or 4-in wide
   Indications: Stasis dermatitis, leg edema

LOCAL THERAPY RULES OF THUMB

Students and general practitioners state that they are especially confused by doctors' reasons for using one chemical or another for unrelated skin diseases. The answer to this dilemma is not easily given. More often than not, the major reason for our preference is that experience has taught us and those before us that the particular drug works. Some drugs do have definite chemical actions, such as anti-inflammatory, antipruritic, antifungal, or keratolytic actions, and these have been listed in the formulary. But there is no definite scientific explanation for the beneficial effect of some of the other drugs, such as tar or sulfur in cases of psoriasis.

In an attempt to solve this apparent confusion, here are some generalizations summarizing our experience.

Tars (coal tar solution [LCD], 3% to 10%; crude coal tar, 1% to 5%; anthralin, 0.1% to 1%).
These products have the 3 Ss: sting, stain, and stink.
Consider for use in cases of:
Atopic eczema
Psoriasis
Seborrheic dermatitis
Lichen simplex chronicus
Avoid in intertriginous areas (can cause a folliculitis and irritation)

Sulfur (sulfur, precipitated, 3% to 10%)
Consider for use in cases of:
Tinea of any area of the body
Acne vulgaris and rosacea
Seborrheic dermatitis
Pyodermas (combine with antibiotic salves)
Psoriasis
Insect bites in children

Resorcinol (resorcinol monoacetate, 1% to 5%)
Consider for use in cases of:
Acne vulgaris and rosacea (usually with sulfur)
Seborrheic dermatitis
Psoriasis

Salicylic acid (1% to 5%, higher with caution)
Consider for use in cases of:
Psoriasis
Lichen simplex chronicus, localized thick form
Tinea of feet or palms (when peeling is desired)
Seborrheic dermatitis
Avoid use in intertriginous areas.
Menthol (0.25%); phenol (0.5% to 2%); camphor (1% to 2%)

Consider for use in any pruritic dermatoses. Avoid use over large areas of the body.

Hydrocortisone and related corticosteroids (hydrocortisone powder) (0.5% to 2%) and triamcinolone (0.1%, 0.025%, and 0.01%)

Consider for use in cases of: Contact dermatitis of any area
Seborrheic dermatitis

Intertrigo of axillary, crural, or inframammary regions
Atopic eczema
Lichen simplex chronicus
Avoid use over large areas of the body and for prolonged periods. *Fluorinated corticosteroids, locally*

These chemicals are not readily available as powders for personal compounding, but triamcinolone, fluocinolone, and others are available as generic creams and ointments. Consider for use with or without occlusive dressings, in cases of:

Psoriasis, localized to small area (see Chapter 16)
Lichen simplex chronicus (see Chapter 12)
Lichen planus, especially hypertrophic-type

Also anywhere that hydrocortisone is indicated, but limit duration of therapy.
Avoid use over large areas of the body. Class I topical corticosteroids should be used for no more than 14 consecutive days.

QUANTITY OF CREAM OR OINTMENT TO PRESCRIBE

Several factors influence any general statements about dosage: the severity of the dermatosis, whether it is acute or chronic dermatosis, the base of the product (a petrolatum-based ointment spreads over the skin farther than a cream and is more moisturizing), whether it is dispensed in a tube or jar (patients use less from tubes), and the intelligence of the patient.

- 15 g of a cream used b.i.d. treats a mild hand dermatosis for 10 to 14 days.
- 30 g of a cream used b.i.d. treats an arm for 14 days.
- 60 g of a cream used b.i.d. treats a leg for 14 days.

■ 480 to 960 g or 1 to 2 lb of a cream used b.i.d. treats the entire body for 14 days. This is seldom a practical prescription, but unmedicated white petrolatum or a cream base is economical to use over a large surface area. Other therapeutic agents should be used to make the dermatoses less extensive (i.e., internal corticosteroids).

SAUER'S NOTES

1. There are potential side effects from any systemic therapy. Be aware of these possible reactions by being knowledgeable about every drug you prescribe.
2. The risk/benefit ratio for your patient must always be considered.
3. Be aware of cross-reactions with a patient on multiple medications.

SPECIFIC INTERNAL DRUGS FOR SPECIFIC DISEASES

As in all fields of medicine, certain diseases can be treated best by certain specific systemic drugs. These drugs may not be curative, but they should be considered when beginning to outline a course of management for a particular patient. Many factors influence the decision to use or not use such a specific drug. Here follows a list of skin diseases and some systemic medicines considered specific (or as specific as possible) for the disease. For proper dosage and contraindications, check the appropriate sections in this book or in other contemporary books on therapy.

■ *Acne vulgaris or rosacea in the scarring or severe stage:* antibiotics, Nicomide, and in women, spironolactone and birth control pills. For severe cases of cystic acne in men or women without indication of or risk of pregnancy, isotretinoin (Accutane) is indicated.

■ *Acquired immunodeficiency syndrome (AIDS):* Many systemic drugs are used, directed as specifically as possible against opportunistic organisms, tumors, and the human immunodeficiency virus (HIV). Highly active antiretroviral therapy (HAART) is the most effective therapeutic regimen for AIDS. Because of its expense, only 10% of HIV-infected patients worldwide are treated with HAART. This is a critical problem on the African continent.

■ *Alopecia areata:* corticosteroids in any of the four forms—rarely IM or PO corticosteroids.

■ *Atrophie blanche vasculopathy:* pentoxifylline (Trental), anticoagulants such as aspirin, clopidogrel (Plavix), dipyridamole (Persantine), and less commonly warfarin (Coumadin).

■ *Bullous pemphigoid:* systemic and group I topical corticosteroids, tetracycline in combination with niacinamide, dapsone, methotrexate, azathioprine, intravenous immunoglobulin, other immunosuppressives.

■ *Creeping eruption:* thiabendazole, topical or oral.

■ *Dapsone therapy:* Dapsone (avlosulfon) is a sulfonamide derivative of medication used more by dermatology therapy than any other specialty. It has anti-inflammatory immunomodulatory affects thought to be from the drugs blockade of myeloperoxidase. Myeloperoxidase converts hydrogen peroxide (H_2O_2) into hypochlorous acid (HOCL). HOCL is a very potent oxidant generated by neutrophils and causes significant tissue damage.

The most dramatic response of dapsone therapy is seen with dermatitis herpetiformis but the other diseases it has been used to treat in the past are cystic acne, linear IgA dermatosis, PLEVA, Hailey–Hailey disease, Sneddon–Wilkinson disease, bullous systemic lupus erythematosus, pustular psoriasis, palmoplantar pustulosis, subacute cutaneous lupus, erythematosus from recluse spider bite, vasculitis, relapsing polychondritis, intestinal bypass syndrome, disseminated granuloma annulare, pyoderma gangrenosum, generalized granuloma annularae, and acropustulosis of infancy. Worldwide the drug is used as a mainstay of therapy for leprosy.

The toxicity of the drug can be limited by giving cimetidine concomitantly to decrease the risk of anemia, which is very frequent in dapsone therapy. Besides anemia, cutaneous drug eruptions (including TEN) is the most significant side effect to monitor on dapsone therapy which can occasionally also cause elevation of liver enzymes.

Dapsone is usually given in a dosage of 100 mg/day and I add 400 mg of cimetidine twice a day to avoid anemia. If the drug is ineffective or a side effect that is not related to allergy occurs, then I substitute 500 mg of sulfapyridine twice a day. If there is an allergic reaction such as a dapsone induced skin reaction then I do not substitute the sulfapyridine.

■ *Darier disease:* Vitamin A, for controlled periods of time, and possibly isotretinoin and acitretin.

■ *Dermatitis herpetiformis:* Dapsone and sulfapyridine.

■ *Dermatomyositis:* Systemic and topical corticosteroids; immunosuppressive agents. Methotrexate, hydroxychloroquine (Plaquenil), and, when other therapies have failed, intravenous IgG.

■ *Granuloma annulare:* Intralesional corticosteroids.

■ *Herpes simplex:* Acyclovir (Zovirax) topical, oral, or intravenous; famciclovir oral (Famvir); valacyclovir oral (Valtrex); foscarnet sodium intravenous (Foscavir). Suppressive therapy for 1 year is advocated by some to reduce disease severity and transmission. Foscarnet can be used intravenously for resistant cases.

■ *Herpes zoster:* Acyclovir oral or intravenous, famciclovir oral, and valacyclovir oral.

- *Kawasaki syndrome:* Intravenous γ-globulin and aspirin.
- *Lichen simplex chronicus:* Intralesional corticosteroids, topical corticosteroids with or without occlusion.
- *Lupus erythematosus:* For systemic lupus erythematosus, use corticosteroids or immunosuppressive agents with care; for discoid form, use topical and intralesional corticosteroids and hydroxychloroquine or related antimalarials (beware of eye damage). Intravenous IgG can be tried when other treatments have failed.
- *Mycosis fungoides* (T helper cell lymphoma or cutaneous T-cell lymphoma [CTCL]): Psoralens and ultraviolet light (PUVA), narrow band UVB, corticosteroids, antimetabolites, retinoids (bexarotene [Targretin]), denileukin diftitox (for CD25-positive tumors), topical nitrogen mustard, topical bischloroethylnitrosourea (BCNU), electron beam radiation, extracorporeal photophoresis, bone marrow transplant (for end-stage disease when all other therapies have failed), and α_{2b}-interferon.
- *Necrobiosis lipoidica diabeticorum:* Topical and intralesional corticosteroids.
- *Pemphigus:* Corticosteroids systemically, cyclosporine, intravenous immunoglobulin, and antimetabolites. Monoclonal antibodies such as Rituximab have had some reported success (Table 4-2).
- *Pruritus from many causes:* Antihistamines (topical and oral) and tranquilizer-like drugs. Doxepin (Zonalon) cream may be beneficial but can cause drowsiness when used over large areas. Selected cases can be treated with oral corticosteroids.
- *Psoriasis, localized:* Intralesional and topical corticosteroids, tar, Dovonex (calcipotriene) or Vectical (Calcitriol), especially in combination with topical corticosteroids. Occasionally, oral antibiotics such as sulfasalazine or tetracycline or oral antiyeast medications such as ketoconazole are used.
- *Psoriasis, severe:* Corticosteroids topically, PUVA, narrow band UVB, methotrexate, cyclosporine (Neoral), and, in men or postmenopausal or sterile women, acitretin (Soriatane). A whole new class of drugs called *biologicals which block lymphokines produced by T-8 lymphocytes* are now available. These include infliximab (Remicade) intravenously, etanercept (Enbrel) subcutaneously, ustekinumab (Stelara) and alefacept intramuscularly. Etanercept, adalimumab, and infliximab are especially helpful in patients with accompanying psoriatic arthritis. These biologicals are all related to TNF-α (tumor necrosis factor α) blockade, except efalizumab, which blocks the CD11a receptor site. Cosentyx(secukinumab) is an IL-17A blocker. Otezla is a small molecule ant-psoriasis and psoriatic arthritis drug that is oral and less immunosuppresive than the biologics.
- *Pyodermas of skin:* Systemic antibiotics are valuable, when indicated.
- *Sarcoidosis:* Topical, intralesional, and systemic corticosteroids; antimalarials; and, when severe and recalcitrant, methotrexate. Early reports with infliximab and related TNF-α blockers have been promising. Pentoxyphylline (Trental) can be tried.
- *Sporotrichosis:* Saturated aqueous solution of potassium iodide orally and ketoconazole orally.
- *Syphilis:* Penicillin or other antibiotics.
- *Tinea of scalp, body, crural area, nails:* Topical imidazoles, ciclopirox or allylamines (oral and topical); or orally griseofulvin and, for selected cases, orally ketoconazole (Nizoral) and itraconazole (Sporanox).
- *Toxic epidermal necrolysis (TEN) or Stevens–Johnson syndrome:* Stop offending drug and life support measures. Systemic corticosteroids early in high doses may be beneficial but this is controversial and later in the disease may be contraindicated. Cyclosporine or intravenous IgG have been advocated by some authors.
- *Tuberculosis of the skin:* Dihydrostreptomycin, isoniazid, p-aminosalicylic acid, and rifampin.
- *Urticaria:* Oral antihistamines (H1 and H2), oral corticosteroids and, when severe, intramuscular and intravenous corticosteroids, sulfasalazine, dapsone, and combinations of these medications. When associated with other signs of anaphylaxis, such as shortness of breath, subcutaneous epinephrine (i.e., EpiPen) can be used by patients in an emergency.

TABLE 4-2 • Use of Intravenous Immunoglobulin in Skin Diseases

Bullous pemphigoid

Dermatomyositis that is refractory to other treatments

Epidermolysis bullosa acquisita

Graft-versus-host disease

Kawasaki disease (mucous membrane, cicatricial pemphigoid)

Pemphigus foliaceus

Pemphigus vulgaris

Toxic epidermal necrolysis (Stevens Johnson)

Necrotizing fasciitis

Toxic epidermal necrolysis

Pyoderma gangrenosum

SAUER'S NOTES

Real-time teledermatology as well as store-and-forward teledermatology are proven advances in providing care to some areas of the United States and the world where dermatologic care by doctors would not otherwise be accessible.

Suggested Readings

Amor KT, Ryan C, Menter A. The use of cyclosporine in dermatology: part I and II. *J Am Acad Dermatol.* 2010;63(6):925–972.

Arndt KA, Bowers KE. *Manual of Dermatologic Therapeutics.* 6th ed. Philadelphia: Lippincott Williams & Wilkins; 2002.

Bronaugh RL, Maibach HI. *Topical Absorption of Dermatological Products.* New York: Marcel Dekker; 2002.

Buchanan P. *Prescribing in Dermatology.* Cambridge: Cambridge University Press; 2006.

Coenraads PJ. Hand eczema. *N Eng J Med.* 2012;367(19):1829–1837.

Drake LA, Dinehart SM, Farmer ER, et al. Guidelines of care for the use of topical glucocorticosteroids. *J Am Acad Dermatol.* 1996;35:615–619.

El-Azhary RA. Azathioprine: current status and future considerations. *Int J Dermatol.* 2003;42:335–341.

Gelfand EW. Intravenous immune globulin in autoimmune and inflammatory diseases. *N Eng J Med.* 2012;367(21):2015–2026.

Haeck IM, Rouwen TJ, Timmer-de Mik L, et al. Topical corticosteroids in atopic dermatitis and the risk of glaucoma and cataracts. *J Am Acad Dermatol.* 2011;64(2):275–281.

Katz HI. *Dermatologist's Guide to Adverse Therapeutic Interactions.* Philadelphia: Lippincott–Raven; 1997.

Kircik LH, Del Rosso JQ. The treatment of inflammatory facial dermatoses with topical corticosteroids: focus on clocortolone pivalate 0.1% Cream. *J Drugs Dermatol.* 2012;11(10):1194–1198.

Lebwohl MG, Heymann WR, Berth-Jones J, et al. *Treatment of Skin Disease: Comprehensive Therapeutic Strategies.* St. Louis: Mosby; 2008.

Lebwohl MG, Heymann WR, Berth-Jones J, et al. *Treatment of Skin Disease.* 3rd ed. Philadelphia: Saunders-Elsevier; 2009.

Levine N. *Dermatology: Diseases and Therapy.* Cambridge: Cambridge University Press; 2007.

Levine N, Levin CC. *Dermatology Therapy: A to Z Essentials.* New York: Springer; 2004.

Loden M, Maibach HI. *Dry Skin and Moisturizers.* London: Taylor and Francis; 2006.

Olsen EA. A double-blind controlled comparison of generic and tradename topical steroids using the vasoconstriction assay. *Arch Dermatol.* 1991;127:197–201.

Ortiz A, Grando SA. Smoking and the skin. *Int J Dermatol.* 2012;51;250–262.

Paghdal KV, Schwartz RA. Topical tar: back to the future. *JAAD.* 2009;61(2):294–302.

Pazyar N, Yaghoobi R, Bagherani N, et al. A review of applications of tea tree oil in dermatology. *Int J Dermatol.* 2013;52:784–790.

Physicians' Desk Reference. Oradell, NJ: Medical Economics; 2005.

Rawlings AV, Leyden JJ, eds. *Skin Moisturization.* 2nd ed. New York: CRC Press; 2009.

Reddy S, Ananthakrishnan S, Garg A. A prospective observational study evaluating hypothalmic-pituitary-adrenal axis alteration and efficacy of intramuscular triamcinolone acetonide for steroid-responsive dermatologic disease. *J Am Acad Dermatology.* 2013;69(2):226–231.

Scheman AJ, Severson DL. *Pocket Guide to Medications Used in Dermatology.* 8th ed. Philadelphia: Lippincott Williams & Wilkins; 2003.

Shelley WB, Shelley ED. *Advanced Dermatologic Therapy II.* Philadelphia: WB Saunders; 2001.

Wakelin SH. *Handbook of Systemic Drug Treatment in Dermatology.* London: Manson Publishing; 2002.

Werth VP. The safe and approprioate use of systemic glucocorticoids in treating dermatologic disease. *J Am Acad Dermatol.* 2013;68(1):177–178.

Wolverton SE. *Comprehensive Dermatologic Drug Therapy.* Philadelphia: WB Saunders; 2007.

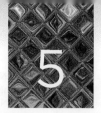

Technologic Applications in Dermatology

Frank C. Koranda, MD, MBA

Technology has expanded the therapeutic options of the doctors. Most of these technologies are office based and are noninvasive or minimally invasive. Some of the most common applications are lasers, intense pulse light (IPL), ultrasound and radiofrequency rejuvenation device, fractional bipolar radiofrequency skin tightening, liposuction, neuromodulators (botulin toxin), lipotransfer, and fat autograft mesenchymal injection (FAMI).

The era of advanced technology in dermatology began 35 to 40 years ago with the introduction of the laser, particularly the carbon dioxide laser. Laser is an acronym for light (L) amplification (A) by the stimulated (S) emissions of radiation (R). The characteristics of laser light are that the light is monochromatic (a single wavelength), collimated (the ray are parallel or non-divergent), and coherent (the rays are in phase) so that they can pass over distances without loss of energy.

CARBON DIOXIDE LASER

When a laser photon of light energy contacts the skin, the light energy is absorbed by water in the tissues and thermal energy is generated. This results in coagulation or vaporization of the tissues with greater energy. The carbon dioxide (CO_2) laser has a wavelength of 1,600 nm in the mid-infra-red spectrum, which is invisible. It is an ablative laser, causing damage to all the tissues because the water content is the laser target. When the CO_2 laser is in focused mode or as a concentrated beam, it can be used as an incisional, cutting instrument with a width of 0.2 mm as compared with the 0.25 mm width of a #15 scalpel blade incision. When the laser cuts, it vaporizes the tissue and there is a smoke plum. In a defocused mode, the CO_2 laser's effect is that of tissue coagulation. In this mode it can seal blood vessels 0.5 mm or less in diameter. The depth of penetration of the CO_2 laser is controlled by the power output measured in watts and by time spent on the target surface. Fluence is the measurement of the energy density applied to the target and is expressed as joules per square centimeter. Because the CO_2 laser is invisible, it is coupled and coaxially aligned with a low-power laser in the visible light spectrum that serves as an aiming device. The helium-neon-aiming laser produces a red light.

The initial CO_2 lasers were of a continuous wave output unless deactivated by the foot control switch. In the early 1990s,

pulsed focused CO_2 lasers were introduced. The goal of pulsing the laser was to decrease the thermal damage to surrounding nontargeted skin. The initial pulsed CO_2 lasers were of 0.1 to 1.0 second in duration. To further reduce thermal energy transfer, ultrapulsed CO_2 lasers were developed to deliver high energy output over a very short duration. The ultrapulsed laser reduces tissue damage by timing the pulse duration to approximate the tissues' thermal relaxation time, that is, the time for a tissue to significantly cool. Another modification of the CO_2 and other lasers is fractional ablation. Instead of causing damage to confluent areas of thermal tissue, fractional lasers delivered the light energy split into thousands of vertical columns of treatment zones leaving as much as 95% of the intervening skin untouched. This is less invasive and healing is faster but more than one treatment may be required.

Listed below are some of the more common conditions the CO_2 laser is used to treat:

- Resurfacing of the face for rejuvenation of the skin and reduction of wrinkles
- Vaporization of actinic cheilitis
- Planning for rhinophyma (Fig. 5-1), angiofibromata of tuberous sclerosis, sebaceous hyperplasia
- Removal of common warts and condylomata acuminatum
- Removal of keloids and hypertrophic scars (Fig. 5-2) which is sometimes followed by intralesional triamcinolone
- Incisional surgery requiring more precision

Currently, there are hosts of other lasers with different wavelength outputs of light energy to correspond to the absorption peaks of the targeted tissue, i.e., tattoos, hair follicles, blood vessels. This is the principle of selective photothermolysis. First, there is a selective absorption of the laser light energy by the targeted tissue; and second, with a brief pulse at high enough power, effective energy is concentrated in the targeted tissue with limited heat dispersal beyond the target. These lasers are designed to prevent collateral damage around the targeted tissue and are classed as non-ablative.

These non-ablative lasers have wavelengths in the visible (400 to 700 nm) to near-infrared (700 to 1,200 nm) spectra. With long wavelengths of laser light, the depth of penetration

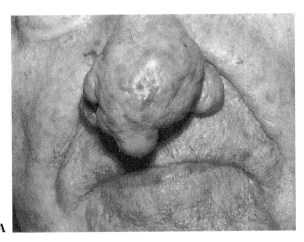
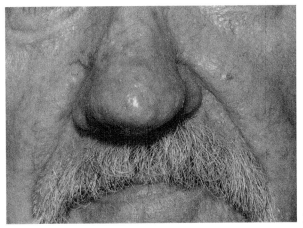

A   **B**

FIGURE 5-1: Rhinophyma before **(A)** and after **(B)** nasal planning with the Coherent CO_2 Ultrapulse laser.

into the skin increases and so does the depth at which the energy is absorbed. The wavelength of laser light selected for treatment is based not only on the absorption spectrum but the depth of the target in the skin. A target may have several peaks of absorption; but for a more deeply located target, a longer wavelength is selected to match one of these peaks, which may not necessarily be the maximum peak. The wavelength must also be different from the absorption peaks of any intervening tissue that could absorb the laser light before it reaches its target.

PULSED DYE LASER

The pulsed dye laser, usually with a 585-nm wavelength and 450-μs or 0.45 ms pulse, has been used extensively for congenital hemangiomas, particularly the port wine stain. (Fig. 5-3) Multiple treatments are required, sometimes more than 20 times. The necessity for retreatment 5 to 8 years after apparently successful treatment is not unusual. Recurrence may be due to blood vessels at a depth beyond the reach of the 585-nm wavelength laser. For deeper penetration, a neodymium:yttrium aluminum garnet (Nd:YAG) laser at 1,064 nm may be directed toward deeper vasculature while sparing

the overlying melanin. This type of laser has also been used for leg vein treatments (Fig. 5-4).

NANOSECOND AND PICOSECOND LASERS

Nanosecond (10^{-9}, one billionth of a second pulse duration) or Q-switched lasers had been the state of the art for tattoo removal (Fig. 5-5). But technology has advanced to the picosecond laser (10^{-12}, one trillionth of a second pulse duration). The advantage of a one trillionth of a second pulse duration is that this concentration of energy has a photomechanical impact more than heat generation effect on the tattoo pigment. The laser breaks the tattoo pigment apart and allows for the body to clear away these smaller particles of pigment. The smaller the particles the more rapidly they are cleared. An analogy is used of breaking rocks apart. The nanosecond laser breaks the rocks into pebbles; the picosecond laser breaks the rocks into grains of sand. The picosecond laser clears away tattoos significantly faster than the nanosecond laser, but multiple treatments are still required. The rapidity of elimination of tattoos also depends on the type of tattoo inks used, the depth to which the inks are placed, and the volume of ink used. There

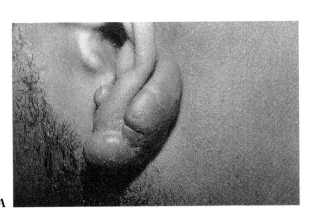
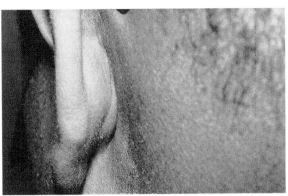

A   **B**

FIGURE 5-2: Keloid of the ear before **(A)** and after **(B)** removal with the Coherent CO_2 Ultrapulse laser.

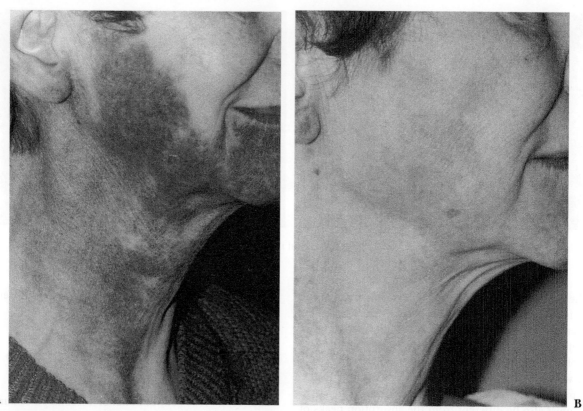

FIGURE 5-3: Congenital port wine stain hemangioma before **(A)** and after **(B)** treatment with candelapulsed tuneable 585-nm dye laser.

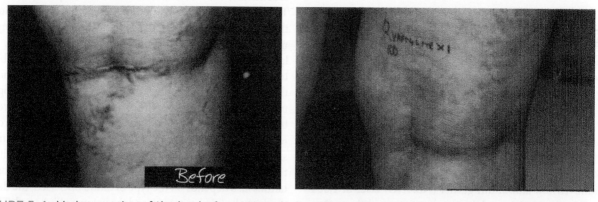

FIGURE 5-4: Varicose veins of the leg before **(A)** and after **(B)** treatment with Lumenis Vasculite laser.

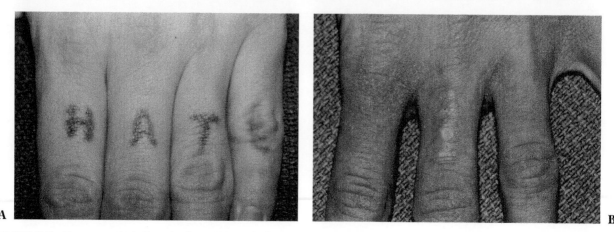

FIGURE 5-5: Homemade tattoo before **(A)** and after **(B)** laser removal.

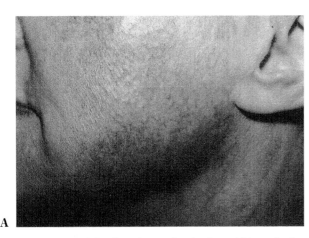 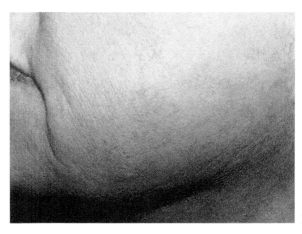

FIGURE 5-6: Facial telangiectasias before **(A)** and after **(B)** treatment with Lumenis Photoderm IPL.

are variations from one tattoo artist to the next and from one tattoo to the next. The skin type of the patient is also a significant factor. The darker the skin, the longer it usually takes in order to avoid hyperpigmentation and hypopigmentation of the overlying skin.

The PicoSure (Cynosure) picosecond dual laser combines two wavelengths, 532 and 755 nm, in one platform, which allows for the treatment of tattoos of all colors with a single machine. In the past, multiple different lasers needed to be used to treat a tattoo with a variety of colors. The company is in the process of adding a 1,064 nm wavelength to the platform for added improvement on darker skin. The PicoSure may also be used to treat acne scars, wrinkles, and nonmalignant pigmentary problems.

HAIR REMOVAL LASERS

Hair removal lasers are usually 694 to 1,064-nm wavelength, so that there is sufficient depth of penetration for absorption by the melanin in the hair follicle. Although the lasers have been touted for the permanent removal of hair, this is an ongoing process to progressively reduce the amount of unwanted hair.

The laser target is melanin so it does not work for very light to white hair.

INTENSED PULSED LIGHT

IPL is not a laser but it functions somewhat like a laser. It is a noncoherent, broad band of wavelength from 500 to 1,200 nm of light generated by a high energy flash lamp. Wavelengths of different bands of light energy are selected for specific targets. For instance a bandwidth of 500 to 670 nm and from 870 to 1,200 nm may be used for vascular lesions. Other bandwidths of light energy may be used for hair removal and for pigment problems. IPL is an all-purpose workhorse and very effective for:

- Facial telangiectasias (Fig. 5-6)
- Vascular component of rosacea
- Poikiloderma of Civatte
- Mottled facial pigmentation (Fig. 5-7)

With the IPL there can also be an improvement in skin tone and a decrease in fine wrinkling (Fig. 5-8). Facial rejuvenation is now a common use for IPL. The photorejuvenation process

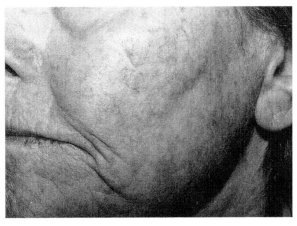 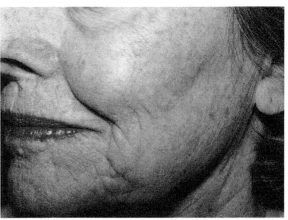

FIGURE 5-7: Actinically damaged facial skin before **(A)** and after **(B)** treatment with Lumenis Photoderm IPL.

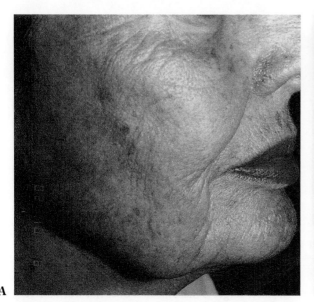
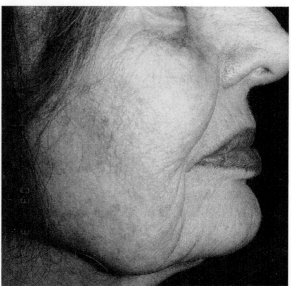

FIGURE 5-8: Photoaged skin of the face before **(A)** and after **(B)** one treatment with Lumenis Photoderm IPL.

is done in a series of four to six IPL treatments usually spaced at 3- to 4-week intervals.

NON-ABLATIVE RADIOFREQUENCY AND ULTRASOUND DEVICES

With these devices either non-ablative radiofrequency energy or ultrasound energy is delivered through the epidermis to the dermis causing no damage to the skin surface. These noninvasive techniques heat the upper to mid-dermis. New collagen formation is stimulated to rejuvenate and tighten the skin. Cooling of the skin and topical anesthetic creams are applied to lessen any discomfort. Discomfort is more noticeable over boney surfaces such as the mandible or the forehead. However there is a lack of predictability of results with both of these types of devices. The degree of improvement is widely variable from no improvement, to little improvement, to noticeable improvement (Fig. 5-9). Rarely is the improvement what is seen in the advertisement photographs.

PROFOUND (SYNERON CANDELA) FRACTIONAL BIPOLAR RADIOFREQUENCY SKIN DEVICE

This new method of skin rejuvenation and tightening produces consistent, predictable results with little downtime and is an office procedure. It has been used not only for tightening of facial and neck skin but for that of the abdomen and arms. The delivery handpiece uses a disposable, one time use cartridge that has an array of five pairs of bipolar microneedles. Each pair of microneedles is coupled to individual radiofrequency generators and to its own temperature sensor for real time temperature control. With bipolar the radiofrequency passes between the tines of the paired microneedles further limiting

collateral damage along with the fractionation. This array of needles is fixed at a length and at an angle so that they can be inserted into the reticular dermis (deep dermis). A bipolar radiofrequency at a set temperature is delivered to the reticular dermis. A common temperature used is 67°C. The fractionation of the treatment makes this a non-ablative device. It is minimally invasive. Precooling of the skin is done before the procedure and then regional blocks and infiltrative local anesthesia are used. Usually the lidocaine is with epinephrine diluted to 1:400,000. Immediate postoperative effects are swelling and some purpura. These resolve in 7 to 10 days. Immediate posttreatment cooling of the skin lessens these effects. It has been demonstrated in several studies that the Profound device stimulates not only significant neocollagenosis but also neoelastogenesis and hyaluronic acid production.

LIPOSUCTION

Liposuction is a technique for recontouring or sculpturing various body areas by fat extraction through various-sized cannulas to which suction is applied. Further modifications include laser assisted. The technique was developed in the late 1970s by Dr. Yves-Gerard Illouz of Paris, France. The earlier methods of performing liposuction were the "dry methods" carried out under general anesthesia. With large volumes of fat removal (greater than 1,500 mL), these procedures were associated with fluid balance problems, necessitating fluid replacement and the need for blood transfusions. In 1986, a dermatologist, Dr. Jeffrey Klein, revolutionized the technique and the safety of liposuction with his work on tumescent liposuction with the infiltration of a large volume of diluted lidocaine with epinephrine in saline solution into the areas to undergo liposuction. With the tumescent technique, blood loss is minimal and it is possible to perform liposuction without general anesthesia. Another dermatologist, Dr. Patrick Lillis,

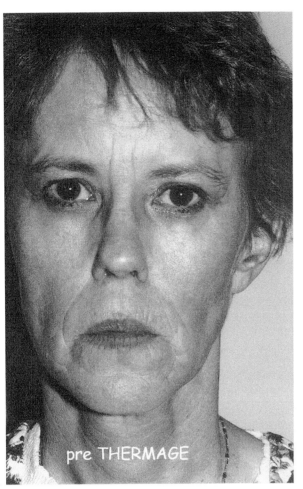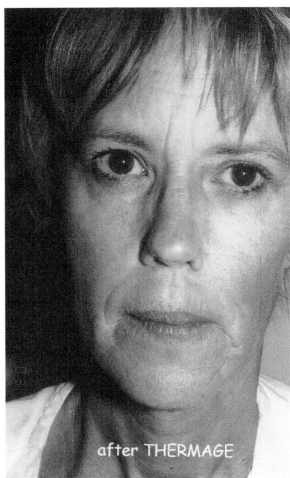

FIGURE 5-9: Facial wrinkling before **(A)** and after **(B)** treatment with Thermage ThermaCool TC.

advanced the tumescent technique by demonstrating the safety of using greater amounts of lidocaine. Although liposuction is most commonly done on the abdomen, thighs, and arms, it is an adjunct in the rejuvenation of the jowls (Fig. 5-10) and the neck (Fig. 5-11).

NEUROMODULATORS—BOTULIN TOXIN TYPE A

Botulin toxin (BT) type A is a neurotoxin from the organism *Clostridium botulinum*, which is the causative agent of botulism. Botulism is associated with food poisoning from improperly sterilized canned goods. BT acts at the presynaptic terminal of motor nerves to block the release of acetylcholine. Death from botulism is caused by paralysis of the diaphragmatic muscles. In 1980, minute doses of BT injected into eye muscles were reported to correct strabismus. Soon BT was used for other neurologic conditions. A husband and wife, Dr. Alastair Caruthers, a dermatologist, and Dr. Jean Caruthers, an ophthalmologist, first used BT for cosmetic purposes in 1988. Dr. Jean Caruthers observed a loss of wrinkles in patients she was treating with BT for blepharospasm.

The most common cosmetic uses of BT are for the upper third of the face to erase horizontal forehead folds, smooth out the vertical folds of the glabella which give a frowning appearance, ablate the "crow's feet" of the lateral orbit, and lift the eyebrows by blocking the depressor muscles (Fig. 5-12). The effect of BT lasts about 4 months and then needs to be reinjected if the individual wishes to maintain the effect. BT has also been used to efface the vertical rhytides of the upper lip, weaken and lessen platysmal neck bands, blunt the marionette line effect of the depressor labii muscles, and get a fuller appearance effect of the lips.

LIPOTRANSFER AND FAT AUTOGRAFT MESENCHYMAL INJECTION

With aging and photodamage, there is a thinning of the epidermis and fracturing and atrophy of dermal tissue. The subcutaneous fat also atrophies. This leads to deepening furrows, particularly in the mesolabial folds and in the marionette lines. But the atrophy is not just skin deep. Muscles atrophy and shorten, and bone is resorbed. The face becomes more narrowed and hollowed compared to the youthful appearance

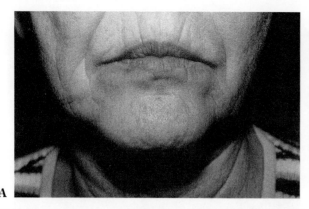
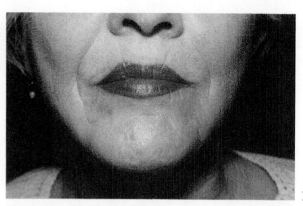

FIGURE 5-10: Jowling of the face and neck fullness before **(A)** and after **(B)** liposuction.

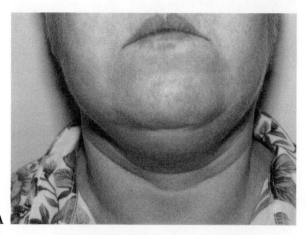
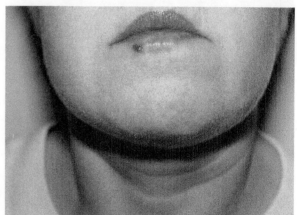

FIGURE 5-11: Neck fullness and lipomatosus before **(A)** and after **(B)** liposuction.

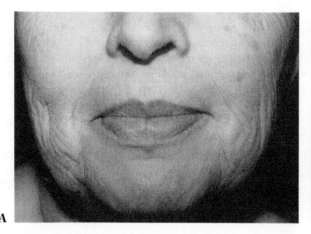
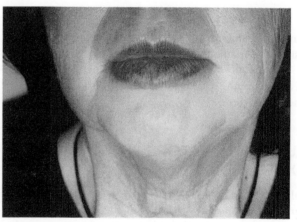

FIGURE 5-12: Periorbital area before **(A)** and after **(B)** BT injection.

of a full, rounded face. Trying to correct this atrophy with a facelift, which pulls up and tightens the skin, does not undress the underlying problem of volume loss. Volume must be replaced and restored for a younger appearing face.

The transfer of autologous fat or fat grafting was first reported in 1893 to fill out scars. Since then, fat grafting or lipotransfer has gone in and out of popularity because of the problems with viability and survival of fat grafts. Fat should be the ideal volume filler since it is readily and widely available on most individuals, it is a living tissue, and it is nonallergenic. Donor sites for fat grafting include the abdomen, the flanks, the thigh, and the lateral knee area. Gentle harvesting of the fat is important and is accomplished with low-pressure aspiration of the fat into a blunt cannula attached to a 10-mL syringe.

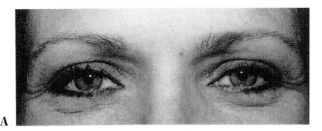 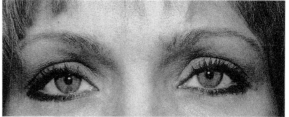

A   B

FIGURE 5-13: Aging face before **(A)** and after **(B)** FAMI.

Once the cannula is introduced into the area of fat harvest, the plunger on the syringe is slowly pulled back creating a low-pressure vacuum. Centrifugation of the fat separates out three layers: a supranatant layer of oily fluid, a middle layer of fat, and an infranatant layer of blood and fluid. The supranatant and infranatant layers are removed and the fat is transferred to 1-mL syringes to which are attached blunt tipped cannulas for the fat injection. The blunt tips reduce the risk of intravascular injection.

Dr. Roger Amar, a French plastic surgeon, has refined the process of lipotransfer with his emphasis on injecting the fat into facial muscles. Muscle tissue is an ideal recipient bed since it is well vascularized to insure viability of the fat graft. Dr. Amar has developed a set of cannulas with different configurations to best accommodate introduction into particular facial muscles. He has coined the term, fat autograft muscle injection for his method (Fig. 5-13).

Various surgeons have observed what appears to be a regeneration of muscles and bone in areas of fat grafting. Adipose tissue has a higher concentration of stem cells or mesenchymal cells than other body tissue. The transfer of stem cells along with the fat cells may explain this phenomenon. Since these stem cells come from the individual, the ethical problem associated with embryonic stem cells does not arise.

SOFT TISSUE FILLERS

A youthful face is a fuller and rounded face as opposed to the narrow and more hollowed face, which develops with sun exposure from both natural sunlight and tanning beds and with aging. Many patients seek this youthful look but also hope to achieve it with minimal downtime and without surgery. This can be accomplished with the injection and accurate placement of the appropriate soft tissue fillers. Over the last 20 years soft tissue fillers have been used increasingly to restore a youthful volume to the face, to lift sagging tissue, and to fill up rhytides and folds. The hyaluronic-based fillers are one of the types most commonly use. Variations among different hyaluronic fillers depend on the viscosity, affinity for water based on concentration of hyaluronic acid, stiffness or 'G' factor, and the various agents used to cross-link these agents of repeating polymer chains of polysaccharides. These characteristics will determine for which application one agent is most appropriate. For the lips where no unevenness or visibility is wanted, an agent with decreased stiffness or low

'G' that is easily spreadable over the area is desired. The filler, Belotero, was designed for this. For the mid-face where lift is needed and for deeper placement, an agent such as Juvaderm Voluma, with increased viscosity and stiffness, would be more appropriate. The hyaluronic fillers join with the natural hyaluronic acid and bind to water and probably stimulate neocollagenosis to produce an increased volume effect. The duration of effect depends on the product and may last from 4 to 24 months. Some of the various lines of hyaluronic fillers are Restylane, Juvaderm, and Belotero. The most frequent side effects with any of the fillers are bruising, mild edema, development of nodules if the volume of the filler is too much or too superficially placed for the type of filler used. Immediate application of cold packs after injection significantly decreases any bruising and swelling. Skin necrosis is a rare complication and immediate treatment with hyaluronidase is indicated if the filler is hyaluronic acid.

Another class of soft tissue augmentation is the stimulating fillers such as Radiesse, which contains calcium hydroxyapatite microspheres. This was initially and still is used for vocal cord incompetence. This filler is indicated for deeper placement requirements. It is not for superficial use such as in the lips, tear trough, or glabella. The calcium hydroxyapatite microspheres are suspended in an aqueous carboxymethylcellulose carrier gel. This gel is absorbed and the hydroxyapatite microspheres trigger a fibroblastic response stimulating neocollagenosis. This volume effect may last 12 to 15 months. Figure 5-14 is of a patient before and after injection with Radiesse. A minimum of two syringes of Radiesse was recommended to be injected, but this was her first time and she was apprehensive. She is very pleased with the results but with more filler, there would have been greater improvement.

Potential side effects are the same with all the fillers including fat. The most serious complication is vascular occlusion. Although rare, it has caused vision loss, stroke, and skin necrosis. Care must be taken to avoid intravascular injection. Knowledge of the facial anatomy is the key.

TEMPERED OPTIMISM

We physicians have the opportunity and the ability to improve the human condition. Technologic advances continue to enhance this capability. But medical treatments have potential risks as well as benefits. With any treatment or procedure, there will always be some patients who have unanticipated

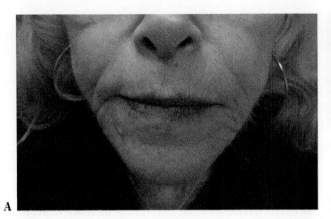
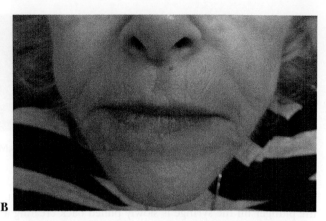

FIGURE 5-14: Hollowed facial appearance before **(A)** and 3 months after **(B)** injection of one syringe of Radiesse.

and untoward sequelae and difficulties despite the best of evaluation, precautions, equipment, material, and technique used. Biologic systems have an inherent unpredictability.

SAUER'S NOTES

New technologies in all fields of medicine are driven not only for the betterment of man but also for financial gain. The medical-industrial complex is a multitrillion-dollar business. In promoting these technologies, photos of the best results and data highlighting the positive results are featured. There is a saying in the military to bear in mind: "Never believe what you hear and only half of what you see."

Suggested Readings

Carniol PJ, Monheit GD. *Aesthetic Rejuvenation Challenges and Solutions: A World Perspective.* London: Informa UK LTD; 2010.

Sykes JM, Trevidic P, Suárez GA, et al. Newer understanding of specific anatomic targets in the aging face as applied to injectables: facial muscles—identifying optimal targets for neuromodulators. *Plast Reconstr Surg.* 2015;136(suppl 5):56S–61S.

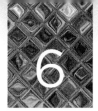

6

Fundamentals of Cutaneous Surgery

Frank C. Koranda, MD, MBA

Our skin, "the gift wrap of life," is the barrier between us and a hostile environment. Skin is the largest organ of the body. Sooner or later, most physicians will have to deal with a tear, cut, or incision into this barrier that will need to be repaired.

INSTRUMENT SELECTION

Quality instruments may be expensive but are usually worth the price and will last with proper care. For most cutaneous surgeries, smaller needle holders such as the Webster function well. The size of the Webster makes it ideal for using a palming technique for holding and manipulation (Fig. 6-1A). The palming technique can be more efficient than using the finger holds or ring holds. Efficiency in surgery is economy of motion. Smooth jaws on the needle holder are less traumatic on precision needles and less apt to cut 5-0 or 6-0 sutures than serrated jaws. For very delicate surgery and for finer sutures such as 7-0, the Castroviejo needle holder may be preferred (Fig. 6-1B). The amount of motion necessary to lock and unlock the Castroviejo is less than that required for a standard needle holder.

Skin should be handled delicately. Gentle handling of skin may require the use of skin hooks such as the single-hook Frazier and the fine double-hook Tyrell. If using pickups to handle a tissue, use Adson forceps with fine teeth or Micro-Adson forceps. Another finer type of forceps is the Bishop-Harmon with teeth (Fig. 6-1C).

For tissue cutting and dissection on the face, Littler scissors are well designed for most situations (Fig. 6-1E). For finer scissors, a Stevens is a good choice (Fig. 6-1E). If larger scissors are needed for undermining and dissection, the Metzenbaum, Malis, or Ragnell scissors may be used (Fig. 6-1D). For precise cutting of sutures and for suture removal, use a straight or curved iris. Another option is the Gradle scissors (Fig. 6-1F).

The No. 3 scalpel handle is used with the Nos. 10, 11, and 15 blades. For a finer incision use a No. 15C blade instead of a No. 15. This blade was originally designed for periodontal surgery. For an even more precise incision, use a Beaver scalpel handle with a No. 6900 or 6400 Beaver blade. This is ideal for the thin, lax eyelid skin.

Standardization of instrument sets will help to prevent the mixing of instruments into the wrong packs. An all-purpose basic cutaneous surgery set may consist of the following instruments:

- Webster needle holder with smooth jaws
- Fine Adson forceps with teeth
- Bishop Harmon forceps with teeth
- Littler scissors for cutting tissue and dissection
- Straight and curved iris scissors for cutting sutures
- Utility scissors for dressings
- Knife Handle No. 3 with etched ruler on handle
- Mosquito, fine curved hemostats (two)
- Towel clip, 3.5 in

SUTURE SELECTION

The two groups of sutures are absorbable and nonabsorbable. The common absorbable sutures are:

- Plain gut
- Chromic gut
- Polyglactin 910 (Vicryl)
- Polyglycolic acid (Dexon)
- Polydioxanone (PDS)
- Polyglyconate (Maxon)
- Poliglecaprone (Monocryl)

Gut sutures are made from the submucosal layer of the small intestine of sheep and the serosal layer of cattle. It undergoes degradation by phagocytosis and creates a variable foreign body response. Plain gut gradually loses its tensile strength over 2 weeks. Chromic gut suture is coated with chromic salts to delay degradation. It has a slightly prolonged tensile strength over plain gut.

Fast-absorbing plain gut is a modification of plain gut that is designed to break down in 4 to 7 days and is used as a skin suture. It comes in 6-0 and 5-0 sizes. The 6-0 fast-absorbing plain gut usually breaks down in 6 to 7 days, but the 5-0 often

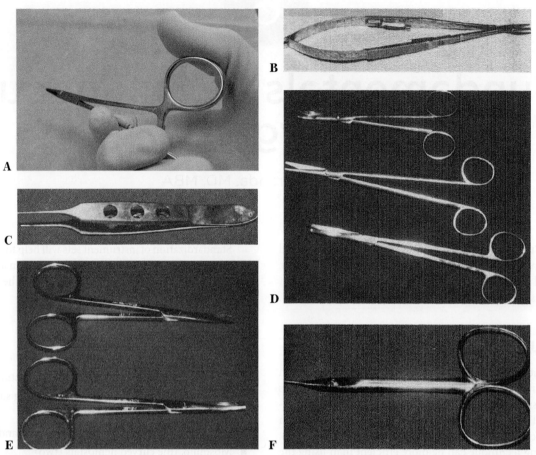

FIGURE 6-1: Surgical instruments. **A:** Webster needle holder, held with palming technique **(B)** Castroviejo needle holder. **C:** Bishop-Harmon ophthalmic forceps. **D:** Top to bottom: Metzenbaum, Malis, and Ragnell scissors. **E:** Top to bottom: Stevens scissors and Littler scissors. **F:** Gradle scissors.

persists for 10 to 15 days. The fast-absorbing sutures are usually easily removed by wiping them over with a Q-tip covered with an antibiotic ointment. At times the fast-absorbing may be more inflammatory than a nylon or silk suture particularly on the eyelids.

Synthetic absorbable sutures undergo degradation by hydrolysis. Vicryl and Dexon sutures are similar, but Vicryl has a better tensile strength profile, maintaining 75% at 2 weeks and 50% at 3 weeks. It is not uncommon for a stitch granuloma to develop with this suture usually where the material is concentrated, at a knot. Rarely an allergic contact dermatitis occurs. Alternatives to these sutures where maintenance of tensile strength over a longer period is required are PDS and Maxon. PDS retains 64% of tensile strength for 6 weeks. Hydrolysis occurs between 180 and 210 days. For subcutaneous facial closure, Monocryl is a good choice, since there is rarely a significant inflammatory response. It is a monofilament as is PDS and usually requires five to six throws on the knot to prevent slippage. Monocryl maintain 50% to 60% of its tensile strength at 1 week and 20% to 30% at 2 weeks.

The major nonabsorbable sutures are silk, nylon, and polypropylene. Silk suture is frequently used on the eyelids and lips, since it is soft and not irritatingly sharp.

Monofilament nylon suture such as Ethilon is a general purpose skin suture. Polypropylene or Prolene is a monofilament suture with an increased memory and high tensile strength. It requires six throws to a knot.

For subcutaneous sutures on the face, usually a 4-0 or 5-0 size suture is used. For skin sutures on the face, usually a 5-0 or 6-0 size suture is used. For more delicate work, 7-0 size may be indicated.

For skin and fascia, use a reverse cutting needle. With the reverse cutting needle, the cutting edge is on the outside of the curve. For facial surgery or for other fine cutaneous surgery, precision point needles are best. There is reduced tissue drag and trauma with these supersmooth, highly honed needles with electropolished tips. In the Ethicon product line, these needles have the code prefix P or PS, (for plastic or plastic surgery). The silhouette of the needle in actual size is shown on the individual suture packet. The P3 needle has good utility for the face. For general cutaneous surgery, an FS (for skin) reverse cutting needle may be used, but there is considerable drag and tissue resistance compared with the P needles with electropolished needle points. The needle should be grasped 1/3 to 1/2 the distance from where the suture is swaged to the needle. The tip of the needleholder should grasp the needle.

When pulling the needle out through the tissue, grasp the needle as far away from the tip as possible to avoid dulling the tip.

TYPES OF STITCHES

Buried Subcutaneous Stitch

The buried subcutaneous stitch is used to close the dead space to prevent hematoma and a nidus for infection (Fig. 6-2). It also reduces the tension on the skin. Burying the knot deep in the tissue decreases the amount of tissue reaction in the more superficial part of the wound so that the major inflammatory response is away from the surface of the incision and less apt to disrupt it.

To bury the knot, the needle first enters through the deep portion of the wound and exits more superficially on the same side. It then enters superficially on the other side of the wound and exits through the deeper tissue on that side of the wound. This is usually an absorbable suture.

Many texts recommend that interrupted subcutaneous sutures be used in case a suture breaks. However, multiple buried sutures, each with a knot, will place a greater mass of foreign body in the tissue and produce a greater inflammatory response. Running a subcutaneous suture poses no difficulty even if the suture breaks, since the friction on the suture and the edema of the tissue secure it.

Simple Skin Stitch

With the simple skin stitch, the suture is passed through the epidermis and dermis from one side to the other (Fig. 6-3). The exit and entry points are usually 2 to 3 mm from the incision edge. A greater "bite" of tissue should be taken more deeply than superficially to help evert the wound edges.

The simple skin stitch functions to approximate and evert the wound edges and to adjust the height of the wound edges so that they are even. If one side of a wound is lower than the other side, a slightly deeper bite should be taken on the lower side for the initial wound height adjustment. The knot is then placed on the lower side of the wound to further finely adjust the height of the wound edges.

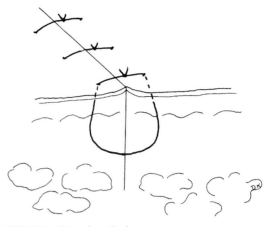

FIGURE 6-3: Simple stitch.

Vertical Mattress Stitch

The vertical mattress stitch tents up the skin edges (Fig. 6-4). This eversion of the edges compensates for contracture that later occurs in the wound which may produce a linear depression. If the wound is not everted sufficiently with simple interrupted stitches or with a simple running stitch, vertical mattress stitches can be placed in the areas not everted.

Horizontal Mattress Stitch

The horizontal mattress stitch is used for the closure of a wound under tension. It can cause strangulation of the skin (Fig. 6-5). Therefore, it may be used with a bolster such as a small piece of a red Robinson catheter through which the exposed suture passes to reduce the pressure on the skin. In general it is not a preferred stitch for facial surgery.

Corner Stitch (Tip Stitch)

The corner stitch is used for v-shaped corners, to prevent necrosis of the skin tip. It is inserted vertically down through the main segment of skin and out through the dermis. It then enters horizontally through the dermis in the tip of the flap and out, and then back up through the main segment of skin (Fig. 6-6). The suture should enter and leave the flap tip in

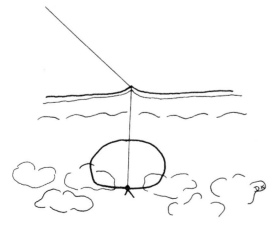

FIGURE 6-2: Buried subcutaneous stitch.

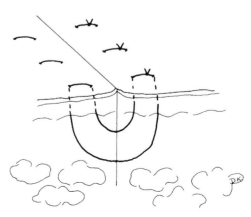

FIGURE 6-4: Vertical mattress stitch.

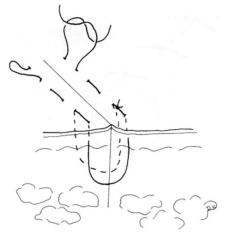

FIGURE 6-5: Horizontal mattress stitch.

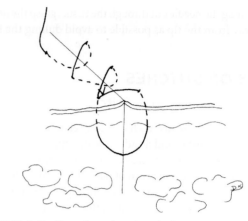

FIGURE 6-7: Running simple stitch.

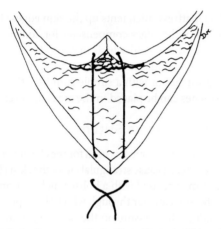
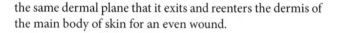

FIGURE 6-6: Corner stitch (tip stitch, half-buried mattress stitch).

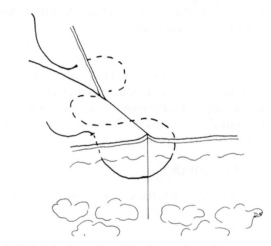

FIGURE 6-8: Running intradermal stitch.

the same dermal plane that it exits and reenters the dermis of the main body of skin for an even wound.

Running Simple Stitch

The running simple stitch is a continuously repeated over and- over stitch that is a rapid method of closure (Fig. 6-7). This stitch can evenly distribute tension along the wound. By adjusting the depth of bite of tissue with each placement of the suture, the height of the wound edges may be adjusted. A running stitch applies less pressure on the skin than numerous individually knotted stitches. This stitch is easier and less traumatic to remove than multiple interrupted stitches.

Running Intradermal Stitch

The running intradermal stitch is placed in the dermis and may be left in place for an extended period without causing cross-hatching of the skin (Fig. 6-8). The suture used may be a permanent type such as Prolene because of its memory and strength or an absorbable type such as PDS or Monocryl depending on the stress on the wound. The suture enters the skin at a point 4 to 5 mm beyond the edge of the incision.

From this point it is brought into the wound and then into the dermis on one side and crosses to the other side. The stitch is continued in a running S pattern staying in the same plane of the dermis from one side to the other. In a long running intradermal stitch that is to be removed, it is wise to have it periodically come through the surface of the skin and then back in through the skin. This allows for removal of the suture in short segments facilitating later removal since the friction on the suture and the healing process tend to secure the suture. With PDS or Monocryl, the need for removal can be avoided.

Although the running intradermal stitch nicely coapts the wound edges, further approximation may be accomplished with a tissue adhesive to the surface of the skin edges.

SUTURE TYING

Sutures should be tied so that they lie down as square knots. The sutures should be tied to coapt the wound edges but not to strangulate. Most err by tying too tightly. One way of avoiding too tightly tied knots is to not snug down the second throw of the suture. Leaving this throw slightly loose also compensates for the tissue edema that develops in wounds. Tying too tightly is a major cause of suture track marks on the skin. Leaving sutures in too long is another factor. Granulomas or microcysts may also form along the suture tract if the suture is left in too long.

HEMOSTASIS

Hemostasis is essential to a good wound healing. A rule of thumb on controlling bleeders is that named vessels should be clamped and ligated, and unnamed vessels may be electro-coagulated. In tying off vessels, use the smallest suture that is practical, usually a 4-0 or 5-0 on the face. The suture should be cut on the knot to leave the least amount of material in the wound that might cause a foreign body reaction.

A biterminal device is usually used for electrocoagulation. The current enters the patient through an active or coagulating electrode. When tissue contact is made, heat is generated and coagulation occurs. The current passes through the patient and out via the dispersing electrode, the grounding pad. The patient usually becomes part of the current circuit.

The grounding pad should be placed as close as possible to the surgical site. If possible, the heart should not be between the active electrode and the grounding pad because it then becomes part of the current pathway. The area of co-agulation should be kept dry with sponging or with suction; bleeding into the area disperses the current and diminishes the coagulation effect.

Biterminal coagulation is not bipolar coagulation. Bipolar coagulation is the system in which a single electrode contains both terminals. With bipolar coagulation forceps, the current passes between the tines of the forceps, coagu-lating the tissue between the tines. Bipolar coagulation is more precise, produces less tissue damage, and does not involve current transmission through the patient. Although jeweler-sized bipolar forceps are sometimes recommended to lessen damage to the tissue, the reverse is usually the case. A bipolar forceps with tines with a larger surface are more efficient in coagulating the tissue between the tines and less apt to cause damage than having to overcoagulate to achieve hemostais with a jeweler forceps.

True electrocautery is essentially a red-hot branding iron that seals blood vessels by the direct application of heat. An electrocautery system uses either low-frequency alternating current or direct current. The current remains in the electrode tip and does not pass into the patient. There are a variety of disposable battery-powered cautery pens.

In the preoperative evaluation, it is important to ask whether the patient has any implanted electrical devices such as a pacemaker, vagus nerve stimulator, or other neurostimulator. The majority of newer pacemakers are defibrillating. With the defibrillating pacemakers, electrocoagulation should not be used until proper protective measures have been undertaken. The manufacturers have toll-free numbers to call for instruc-tions. In the event that there is a question, the cautery pens should be safe because they seal the blood vessels by direct heat and not by electricity.

PATIENT INFORMATION ON POTENTIAL COMPLICATIONS OR SIDE EFFECTS OF SKIN SURGERY

1. *Scar formation:* Scars form whenever there is injury to the skin. Some scars are more noticeable than others. Some individuals are more prone to thickened or keloid scars. Scars in areas of high sebaceous gland concentration and activity such as the nose and forehead are more likely to become widened and depressed even with the most precise closure. Postoperative treatment of the scar may be necessary.

2. *Pain:* Postoperative pain will depend on the extent of surgery and also on the particular individual. Pain med-ications are prescribed and may be taken after surgery if needed. With narcotic pain medications, do not drive, operate machinery, or make important decisions. Alcohol can amplify the effects of pain medications. It is best to eat something solid before pain medications, since they may irritate the stomach and cause nausea.

3. *Bleeding:* Bleeding after surgery can usually be controlled with firm pressure applied continuously to the wound for 20 to 30 minutes by the clock and followed with ice compresses. Some oozing is to be expected. In the case of severe or persistent bleeding, please call the doctor.

4. *Swelling:* Various degrees of swelling will occur. Cold compresses on for 20 minutes and off for 10 minutes for the first 24 to 48 hours will lessen swelling. Elevation of the head at 15 to 20 degrees when lying down or sleeping will help to reduce edema. A reclining chair usually provides a good angle of head elevation.

5. *Bruising:* Bruising around the surgery site will resolve. With surgery of the anterior scalp, forehead, or around the eyes, a black eye may develop within 12 to 72 hours after surgery. Sometimes the eye will swell shut.

6. *Hematoma:* This is a lump that forms under the skin from bleeding after the surgery. It represents a collection of blood.

7. *Infection:* With any injury to the skin or surgery, infection is possible. Therefore, an antibiotic ointment, and some-times antibiotic tablets, may be prescribed at the time of surgery. Wound infections usually occur 4 days after surgery. If you suspect an infection, please call the doctor.

8. *Numbness:* It is common to have numbness in the area of surgery because there are always sensory nerves running through the skin. Usually this numbness will go away in 6 to 12 months. But in some instances, it may be permanent.

9. *Paralysis of nerve:* If a cancer extends into the area of a nerve that controls the movement of muscles, temporary or permanent paralysis may occur. The greatest areas of risk on the face are the temple area where the nerve to the eyebrow and eyelid runs and the lower cheek where the nerve to the lower lip runs.

10. *Wound dehiscence:* In straightforward terms, this means the wound separates or pulls apart. This can happen anywhere, but it is most prone to occur when the wound overlies an area of muscle mass such as on the back or the extremities. If a body movement seems to tug on the wound, stop the movement and relax.

11. *Wound healing:* Not all skin wounds heal ideally. At times a skin repair, graft, or flap may fail to heal well or the wound may seem to lift up or protrude. This may affect part of the wound or the whole wound. Most often, the wound will still heal adequately with treatment. Sometimes additional surgery is required.

PATIENT INSTRUCTIONS FOR SURGERY

1. If you are taking prescribed medications, continue to take them unless instructed otherwise.
2. If you are taking Plavix (clopidogrel) or Coumadin (warfarin), or the newer classes of anticoagulants because of a heart attack, atrial fibrillation, blood clot, heart stent, stroke, or transient ischemic attack, you will usually be able to continue on the medication, although you will probably bleed more and may have a greater chance of postoperative bleeding. If you are taking Coumadin, you may require a blood test international normalized ratio (INR) within a week of surgery. Usually we will not operate if the INR is greater than 2.9.
3. If you are routinely taking aspirin or ibuprofen products such as Motrin, Aleve, or Advil for headaches, pain, or preventive measures, please stop 10 days before surgery. Not necessary for punch, small ellipse or shave biopsy. These products may cause more bleeding during and after surgery. Aspirin and ibuprofen may be present in various products. For instance, aspirin is found in Pepto-Bismol and Alka-Seltzer. Aspirin may be listed as salicylate or salicylic acid. If you have arthritis, celecoxib (Celebrex), an anti-inflammatory drug that does not have an effect on bleeding, can be prescribed. It is used with caution in patients who have cardiovascular disease or risk factors for cardiovascular disease.
4. If you have a pacemaker, it is important that you inform the doctor and specify its type and whether it is a defibrillating pacemaker so that proper precautions can be taken. Please also mention if you have a neurostimulator implant such as a vagus nerve stimulator.
5. If you have any joint replacement implants, you may need antibiotics prior to surgery. If you have had carditis, mitral valve prolapse, or heart valve replacement, you will be prescribed preoperative antibiotics.
6. Two weeks before surgery, stop taking vitamin E and supplements such as garlic, ginger, ginkgo biloba, ginseng, and ephedra. In general, it is best to stop all supplements 2 weeks prior to surgery.
7. Stop smoking for 2 weeks before and for 2 weeks after surgery. It is well documented that smoking causes poor wound healing.
8. Wash your hair the night before or morning of surgery.
9. Shower and wash your face the morning of surgery.
10. Someone should come with you or be available to drive you home.
11. Please arrive at the designated time.
12. If you decide to cancel surgery, please let your surgeon know in enough time so that another patient can be scheduled. However, doctors do understand that illness may occur unexpectedly.
13. If you are apprehensive and require an anti-anxiety medication, it may be prescribed. However, you must sign your operative consent ahead of time or before taking the medication.

PATIENT SAFETY

Whether doing surgery in a hospital, in an ambulatory surgery center, or in the office, a protocol for preventing wrong site, wrong procedure, and wrong person surgery should be instituted. This protocol is referred to as "time out." Time out includes all persons involved in the surgery, which can vary depending on the location (i.e., the hospital vs. the office). In the hospital, it would involve the surgeon, the anesthesiologist, the circulating nurse, and the surgical ("scrub nurse") technician or nurse. In office surgery, it will usually only involve the surgeon and the nurse or medical assistant. Time out is a verification procedure.

The site of surgery should be marked. If multiple surgeons are doing procedures in the same facility, the surgeon's initials will also be placed with a skin marker. The person performing the surgery should mark the site. Marking should occur with the patient involved, awake, and aware, if possible, for cross-verification.

Patient's identity should be verified with two identifiers such as name and birth date. In the operating area, the nurse will again verify the patient's identity, procedure to be done, surgical site, patient's position (if appropriate), and any other pertinent information such as the presence of a pacemaker or other implants. This is done in the presence of the entire surgical team who are to acknowledge that the information is correct. This is similar to a pilot's preflight checklist.

SKIN PREPARATION FOR SURGERY

It is best to shave as little hair as possible; do not shave the eyebrows because they grow very slowly. Prep the skin with Betadine or Hibiclens; do not use Hibiclens around the eye. Use Betadine or Shur-Clens (poloxaner 188) around the eye. Prepare a large enough surgical field so that one may see not only the immediate surgical site but also the relationship to the surrounding anatomic landmarks to be sure that the closure of the wound is not distorting some other structure such as the nose, lip, or eyelid.

Incision lines are marked out before any distortion by infiltrative anesthesia. Round toothpicks dipped in methylene blue or Bonney's blue make a more exact line than most skin marking pens.

ANESTHESIA

Most cutaneous surgery requires only infiltrative or regional block anesthesia. The standard agent, 1% lidocaine, is a safe, rapidly acting, short-duration anesthetic to which allergic reactions are exceedingly rare. By the addition of epinephrine, systemic absorption of lidocaine is lessened, duration of action is significantly prolonged, and a local hemostatic effect is achieved. Optimal vasoconstriction usually occurs in 15 minutes. The available commercial preparations may combine lidocaine with 1:100,000 epinephrine. Patients may react to epinephrine with apprehension, body tremors, diaphoresis, palpitations, tachycardia, and increased blood pressure. These side effects can be decreased or eliminated by diluting the epinephrine to 1:400,000 without significantly changing its efficacy.

The maximum recommended dosage of lidocaine is 500 mg, the equivalent of 50 mL of a 1% lidocaine solution. The earliest sign of toxicity is on the central nervous system (CNS) with mild sedation, which may proceed to seizure activity. Cardiac toxicity usually occurs at twice the level.

Warming the anesthetic agent to room temperature and buffering the lidocaine decreases the discomfort of the injection. Lidocaine is buffered by diluting it 10% with 8.4% sodium bicarbonate.

At the end of the procedure, a longer acting anesthetic 0.25% bupivacaine diluted to 1:400,000 can be injected for a more prolonged anesthesia of 5 to 8 hours. Even after sensation returns, there may be an analgesia that will persist for some time. Toxic limit for bupivacaine is 3 mg/kg. Bupivacaine can cause cardiac toxicity at the same levels needed to cause CNS toxicity. Bupivacaine can bind tightly to myocardial tissue and may trigger dysrhythmias. This is more of a problem in a highly vascular area such as the tonsillar bed. However, intravascular injection should be avoided.

Ropivacaine is another long-acting anesthetic with less potential for cardiac toxicity than bupivacaine. Ropivacaine has a toxic limit of 3 mg/kg. Epinephrine does not decrease its systemic absorption as with lidocaine and bupivacaine. Occasionally a patient may be sensitive to the methyl paraben preservative in lidocaine. Ropivacaine has no preservatives.

PLACEMENT OF INCISIONS

Incisions should be planned so that they are as parallel to or within wrinkle, smile, and expression lines as can be. When there is a lack of definite wrinkles, place the incisions in the direction of relaxed skin tension lines. These lines run at right angles to the contractions of the underlying muscle.

Incision scars may also be camouflaged by placing them at the boundaries of aesthetic and anatomic areas, such as the vermilion junction, the paranasal fold (the junction of the nose and the cheek), the submandibular area, the submental area, the preauricular sulcus, and along the eyebrow or within the hairline.

SKIN INCISIONS

Incisions should be made vertical to the skin surface. Obliquely angled incisions do not coapt as well. An exception to this rule is in the area adjacent to the eyebrows or in the hair. Incisions

placed here should be at an angle that parallels the angle of the hair shaft as it emerges from the skin to avoid transection of the hair follicle.

Even small wounds benefit from undermining equal to the width of the wound to reduce tension. Undermining may be done with a scissor or a scalpel. On the face, the level of undermining is usually just under the dermal plexus. On the scalp, the most effective mobilization of the skin is by undermining between the aponeurosis of Galen and the periosteum, which is a relatively blood-free plane. However, this is below the sensory nerves.

EXCISIONS

The standard excision is fusiform in shape. If the length-to-width ratio is less than 4:1, or if one side is longer than the other, redundant tissue will develop at the corners or ends of the closure. With asymmetric wounds when approximating the tissue, insert the needle at wider intervals on the longer side of the wound than the shorter, approximately a 1:2 ratio. This will eliminate or decrease the amount of redundant tissue. These so-called dog-ears or standing cones of tissue, if small, level out and flatten as the wound undergoes contracture. If large, they should be removed by tenting up the corner of the wound with a skin hook to define the extent of the dog-ear. The dog-ear is incised along its base on one side or the other. The final wound curves toward the side on which the incision is placed. After making the incision along one side of the base of the dog-ear, the flap of tissue that is created is pulled across the incision. Where the base of the redundant tissue crosses the incision, it is transected. The dog-ear is eliminated and closure of the wound is completed (Fig. 6-9).

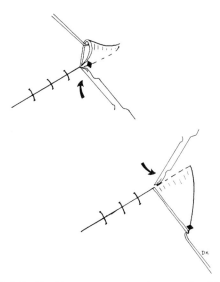

FIGURE 6-9: Tenting up corner of wound with skin hook to define extent of dog-ear.

WOUND DRESSINGS

In the first hours after the incision, a coagulum forms over the wound. Between 12 and 72 hours, there are two spurts of mitotic activity, and epidermal cells begin migrating across the wound. However, if a dried crust forms, it is a barrier to the epidermal migration. Rather than being able to migrate straight and level across the gap between the wound edges, the epidermal cells must find a plane of migration beneath the dried crusts. This leads to a shallow, linear depression in the healed incision.

To prevent wound crusting and the resultant linear trough in the healed wound, an occlusive dressing such as Bio-Occlusive or Tegaderm may be used.

Coating the wounds with an ointment is necessary to prevent drying of the area. Many skin surgeons now prefer Vaseline as the ointment of choice. If an antibiotic ointment is applied, a lesser potent over-the-counter one than a prescription one such as mupirocin, is usually adequate. In New Zealand, overuse of mupirocin has caused an increase in resistant bacteria.

Another method is to coat the wound with a liquid bandage which usually contains 2 octyl cyanoacrylate. Cyanoacrylate is the active ingredient in "crazy glue." Depending on the brand used, it may take 3- to 5-weeks for it to peel off. No ointment is to be applied, since this will hasten its dissolution. If applying a dressing over it, be sure it has dried. Drying completely may take several minutes.

SUTURE REMOVAL

There are no hard-and-fast rules for suture removal. If there is doubt about whether the sutures should be removed, cut every other or third stitch and observe for another day or so. Some guidelines for the timing of suture removal are:

- Face: 7 to 10 days
- Neck: 10 to 12 days
- Back: 14 days
- Abdomen: 7 to 10 days
- Extremities: 10 to 18 days

Wound infections are most apt to develop 4 to 5 days after surgery.

To avoid disrupting the wound, the sutures should be cut with a fine scissor such as a Gradle, iris or with a No. 11 scalpel blade. Pull the suture toward the incision to remove. Pulling the suture away from the incision places traction on the incision line.

WOUND DYNAMICS

Wound Healing

Wound healing is divided into four phases:

- Inflammatory
- Fibroblastic
- Proliferative
- Remodeling

These phases overlap and blend into each other. During the early inflammatory phase, there is vasoconstriction with platelet aggregation. After 5 to 10 minutes of vasoconstriction, there is active venule dilatation and increased vascular permeability, lasting about 72 hours. Within a few hours of these vascular responses, a cellular response occurs. Polymorphonuclear leukocytes migrate into the area. There is a diapedesis of monocytes that transform into tissue macrophages. The macrophage is the dominant cell for the first 3 to 4 days. It initiates the fibroblastic phase.

While the inflammatory phase is still proceeding, the proliferative phase commences. Epidermal cells undergo changes and begin migrating into the wound. By the third day, migration of epidermal cells across an apposed incision is complete. Fibroblasts within the dermis begin to proliferate at 25 to 36 hours after the initial injury. By the fourth day, the fibroblastic phase is heralded by the synthesis of collagen and proteoglycans by the proliferating fibroblasts. Collagen fibers are laid down in a random pattern without orientation.

Overlapping with and toward the latter part of the fibroblastic phase, the remodeling phase begins. This is a phase of differentiation, resorption, and maturation. Fibroblasts disappear from the wound, and collagen fibers are modeled into organized bundles and patterns. This phase may go on for a year or longer.

Wound Contraction

In an open wound healing by second intention, there is an active drawing of the full thickness of the surrounding skin toward the center of the wound. Wound contraction begins during the proliferative phase of wound healing. There is a differentiation of fibroblasts to myofibroblasts, which are responsible for this activity. Wound contraction usually proceeds until the wound is closed or until surrounding forces on the skin are greater than the contractile forces of the myofibroblasts.

Wound Contracture

All wound scars undergo contracture with a resultant shortening along their axes. This process of contracture is due to collagen cross-linking, which occurs during the remodeling phase. Contracture is distinct and different from wound contraction. Intralesional steroids counter the collagen cross-linking.

Wound Strength

By 2 weeks, the wound has gained 7% of its final strength; by 3 weeks, 20%; by 4 weeks, 50%. At full maturation, the healed wound regains about 80% of the strength of the original intact skin.

DOCUMENTATION AND ASSESSMENT

Although success or failure in cutaneous surgery may be readily apparent, it is important to document results with objective photography. After surgery, patients tend to scrutinize their faces and will see asymmetries and blemishes that were always there but did not receive any notice. But the patients may now attribute these imperfections to the surgery.

With consistent, standardized photographs, one may judge progress and analyze techniques and methods. Preoperative and postoperative photographs are essential, as are intraoperative photographs. Photographs are a method of self-assessment and serve as a stimulus and direction for improvement.

SAUER'S NOTES

1. One of the more common complaints after skin surgery is a numbness or altered sensation in the area. This is not a complication but an anticipated result of cutting through the skin. It is best to warn patients of this possibility before surgery and that this alteration in sensation may last for 6 to 12 months and sometimes may be permanent.

2. In areas of high sebaceous gland activity such as the T-area of the face and in patients with acne and rosacea, incisions tend to spread and widen no matter how meticulous and precise the surgery. This is a phenomenon of wound healing. "What the patient is told before surgery is informed consent; what is told after surgery may be taken as an excuse."

3. Beware of the temporal branch of the facial nerve. As it exits the parotid gland at the superior border, it runs a superficial course over the zygomatic arch and into the temporal area. Transection of this branch causes paralysis of the frontalis muscle on that side and drooping of the eyebrow. With any excision in the temporal area, this is a possibility. Forewarn the patient. A drooping eyebrow can be corrected with a browpexy.

4. Beware of the spinal accessory nerve in the posterior triangle of the neck. The spinal accessory nerve pierces through the posterior border of the sternocleidomastoid muscle a little above its midpoint and enters the posterior triangle. The spinal accessory nerve then travels superficially, just below the subcutaneous fat in the investing fascia covering the posterior triangle. There is also a chain of lymph nodes intimately associated with the spinal accessory nerve along its course in the posterior triangle. Paralysis of this nerve causes an inability to raise the arm above the horizontal position. This nerve has been transected by those aware of its superficial location as well as by those unaware. "Good judgment is based on experience, which is based on bad judgment."

5. No matter how careful and diligent the surgeon, the response of biologic systems is not always predictable; and the outcome not always anticipated or desired. "If one wants to be a surgeon, be prepared to cry and to pray."

SKIN CANCER

Skin cancer is the most common type of malignancy in the United States. The major causes of skin cancers are ultraviolet light exposure (both natural sunlight and tanning beds), ionizing radiation, and chemicals such as arsenic. The yearly incidence of skin cancer is 4 to 5 million in Americans. Basal cell carcinoma is the most common type and accounts for 75% to 80% of skin cancers. Squamous cell carcinoma is the next most common form and accounts for 15% to 20%. However, squamous cell carcinoma is more common in immunosuppressed patients, black patients, patients with cancer on the lips and hands, and in patients treated with psoralens and UVA light (long wavelength ultra violet light, 320-400 nm). The third most common type of cancer and usually most likely to be deadly is melanoma. The incidence of melanoma is doubling every 15 years. For a person born in 1930, the risk of melanoma is 1 out of 1,500; if born in 1980, the risk is 1 out of 126; if born in 2007, the risk is 1 out of 63. Risk factors for melanoma, in addition to fair skin and family history, include increased ultraviolet light exposure during the preteen and teen years. If during this time, there is an episode of blistering or painful sunburn, the risks increases. One cannot get a tan without damaging the skin. A major new risk factor over the last thirty years is the increased use of tanning beds. Tanning beds not only promote melanoma but they accelerate the aging process of the skin. If a tanning bed is used 1 to 3 times a year, the risk of melanoma increases by 2-fold; if used 4 to 9 times a year, the risk increases by 4-fold; if used 10 times or more a year, the risk increased 7-fold. A woman who has used a tanning bed once has twice the risk of melanoma than one who has never been in a tanning bed.

SAUER'S NOTES

There is never a good reason to use a tanning bed. It does not protect against burning and tanned skin does not look good when the news of metastatic melanoma is announced to a patient.

Mohs Surgery for the Target Removal of Skin Cancer

Mohs surgery is a precise surgical method combined with histologic mapping for a targeted removal of skin cancer. This procedure was developed by Dr. Frederic Mohs of the University of Wisconsin, Madison.

Mohs surgery provides the greatest assurance of cancer removal along with the most conservative margins of resection. It has the highest cure rates for skin cancer: 97% to 99% for primary skin cancers and 95% to 96% for recurrent skin cancers.

While a medical student at Wisconsin in the 1930s, Frederic Mohs was a Brittingham research assistant in the zoology department. He was studying the inflammatory response of normal tissue and cancerous tissue in rats that were injected with different irritants. He observed that the injection of 20% zinc chloride produced necrosis in the tissue, but that on microscopic examination, histologic detail was preserved. He stated his "eureka" observation: "The chemical had produced fixation in situ."

Over the years, this observation led to his development of a method of skin cancer removal guided by microscopic control. The key to the microscopic control was the preparation of the tissue with compressed horizontal section. This provided complete assessment of all of the deep and perimeter margins. Color coding was applied to the tissue for more precise orientation and a map was made of the location of each specimen. If cancer was identified in any specimen, the exact location would be known and additional resection from that area performed. He published his first article on this method in 1941, entitled "Chemosurgery: a microscopically controlled method of cancer excision." However, chemosurgery with the application of a zinc chloride paste to the skin cancer and subsequent cancer removal and microscopic checking would usually be a several-day ongoing procedure.

In 1974, Dr. Theodore Tromovitch and Dr. Samuel Stegman reported on a significant number of skin cancer patients having microscopically controlled excision routinely using a fresh tissue technique without the zinc chloride fixation. This was accomplished by horizontally compressing the tissue and immediately cutting the specimen into ultrathin sections on a cryostat and staining and mounting the specimens for microscopic analysis. Their study ushered in the present era of Mohs surgery not requiring an in vivo tissue fixation and making it possible to remove most skin cancers during 1 day of surgery.

Mohs surgery is most commonly used for basal and squamous cell carcinomas, but it has found application in the removal of other types of skin cancers and some oropharyngeal cancers.

Prior to the surgery, a definitive diagnosis is established by biopsy. Most procedures may be accomplished under local anesthesia. Photo documentation is commonly done.

Mohs Surgery Method

The mass of clinically evident cancer is removed either by scalpel or curette or both (Figs. 6-10 and 6-11). An advantage of curettage is that cancerous tissue is usually less resistant to the action of the curette than normal tissue. The mechanical

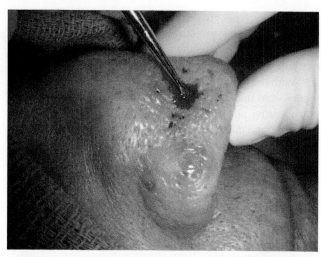

FIGURE 6-11: Curettage of basal cell carcinoma on right tip of the nose.

resistance of normal tissue helps to define the extent of the cancer. After the apparent cancer mass has been removed, the first stage of Mohs surgery is performed.

With the scalpel, a thin underlying layer of tissue is excised from the bed of the cancer along with a 2 to 3 mm perimeter margin (Fig. 6-12). The edges of the excision are beveled at 45 degrees in order to facilitate the histologic processing. Prior to the excision, small hash or reference marks are placed at various points along the perimeter of the excision and into the excision specimen for more precise histologic orientation. A saucerized-type excision is then performed (Fig. 6-13).

The excised specimen is subdivided into smaller pieces as necessary for tissue processing. An excised Mohs surgery layer may consist of one piece or multiple pieces, depending on the size of the cancer. The specimen is laid on grid paper with the patient's name and the specimen's orientation marked (Fig. 6-14). A map of the specimen's shape, subdivisions, reference marks, color coding, and position on the face or other area is drawn (Fig. 6-15).

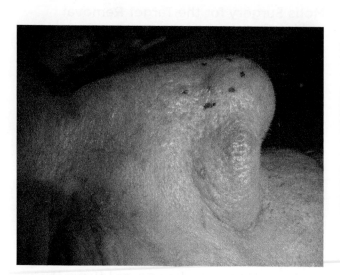

FIGURE 6-10: Basal cell carcinoma, outlined on right tip of the nose.

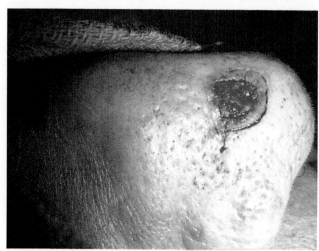

FIGURE 6-12: Area of cancer: right tip of the nose, incised for removal of tissue layer for processing with Mohs technique.

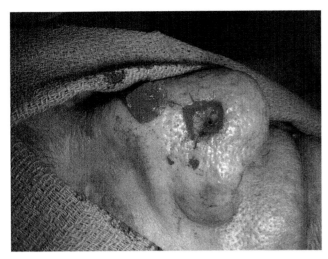

FIGURE 6-13: Tissue layer removed and lying directly above excision site on right tip of the nose.

A temporary dressing is applied to the patient, and the patient is escorted to the waiting area while the specimen is processed in the laboratory. The specimen is transferred to the laboratory where color coding is applied to the edges for further orientation and correlation with the map (Fig. 6-16). Each specimen piece is then inverted and compressed so that the edges are in the same plane as the deep margin. The specimen piece is placed on a cryostat chuck for cutting horizontal microscopic sections and the chuck is fixed in the cryostat (Figs. 6-17 and 6-18). The microscopic sections are usually cut at 4 to 14 μm in thickness depending on the characteristics of the tissue.

The horizontally cut microscopic slides of the excised layers from the perimeter and base of the cancer are the sine qua non of this procedure. To accomplish this requires well-trained technicians.

The processing of the specimens for Mohs surgery requires finely practiced skill to ensure that the specimen's deep and

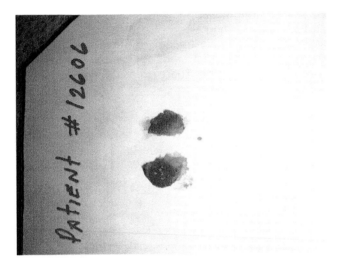

FIGURE 6-14: The specimen of tissue layer that has been subdivided is laid on grid paper with the patient's number for identification and for orientation of specimen as to superior and inferior, left and right.

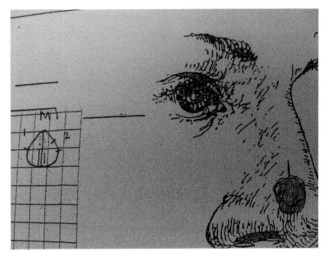

FIGURE 6-16: Map of specimen to the left and diagram of the nose with the area of cancer marked to the right.

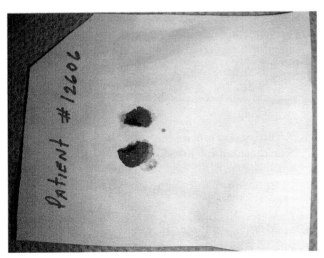

FIGURE 6-15: The specimen on grid paper with color coding applied to the subdivided edges.

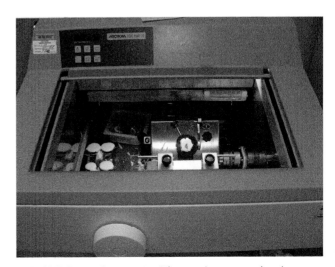

FIGURE 6-17: Cryostat with specimen on chuck.

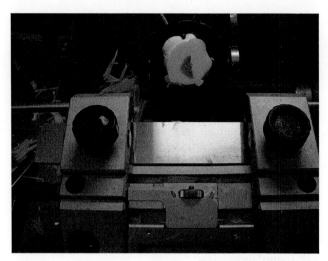

FIGURE 6-18: Close-up of specimen on chuck in cryostat. The microtome blade is below the chuck.

perimeter margins are in the same plane. This skill is time and energy demanding.

Various devices have been designed to facilitate this processing. The innovative CryoHist invented by late Dr. David Rada is a sophisticated apparatus that uses vacuum compression with freezing of the specimen to achieve consistent horizontal cuts (Fig. 6-19).

The microscopic sections are mounted on glass slides and stained, usually with hematoxylin and eosin. After placing cover slips on the labeled slides, they are ready to be examined under the microscope (Fig. 6-20).

The Mohs surgeon serves two roles—first as the surgeon excising the cancer and second as the dermatopathologist microscopically examining the slides of the excised cancer. Because of the need for extensive training in dermatopathology, most Mohs surgeons are dermatologists.

The Mohs surgeon examines the specimen under the microscope and correlates the findings with the map of the

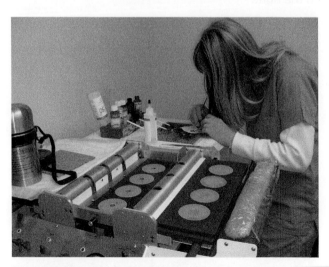

FIGURE 6-19: Rada CryoHist in foreground with a technician preparing the specimen in the background.

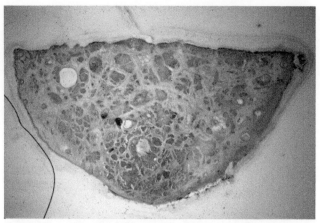

FIGURE 6-20: Microscopic slide of compressed, horizontal section. Along the curved edge of the border is the epidermis. The straight-edged portion of the specimen is where it has been subdivided. There is blue color coding along part of the straight edge, indicating the superior half of the specimen, and red color coding along the other part, indicating the inferior half of the specimen. The area between the curved edge and straight edge is the deep margin of the excision. There is basal cell carcinoma in the central area with close proximity to the middle part of the skin edge. Thus, another layer of excision is required from this area.

excised specimen. If no cancer remains, the patient is ready for either immediate or delayed reconstruction. If residual cancer is identified, the location of the cancer seen on the slide is correlated with the map and the position of the cancer is plotted. A further layer of Mohs surgery is performed in the targeted area of remaining cancer. The process of microscopic processing of horizontal compressed specimens and microscopic examination is repeated. The layered resection of tissue is repeated as is needed in each patient until the perimeter and deep margins are totally clear of cancer cells (Fig. 6-21).

Indications for Mohs Surgery

Various methods are used to treat skin cancers: (1) cryosurgery, (2) curettage and electrodesiccation (scraping and burning), (3) topical creams, (4) radiation therapy, (5) excision, and (6) Mohs surgery.

Mohs surgery can be used for most skin cancers, but there are situations when it should be the major consideration for the method of removal.

1. Recurrent skin cancers (Figs. 6-22 to 6-28)
2. Skin cancers greater than 2 cm in clinical measurement (Figs. 6-29 to 6-32)
3. Morpheaform and sclerosing basal cell carcinomas (Figs. 6-33 to 6-35)
4. Cancers with ill-defined borders (Figs. 6-36 and 6-37)
5. Skin cancers in areas with high recurrence rates: ears, nose, eyelids, and scalp (Figs. 6-38 and 6-39)
6. Cancers induced by radiation therapy
7. Cancers induced by immunosuppression

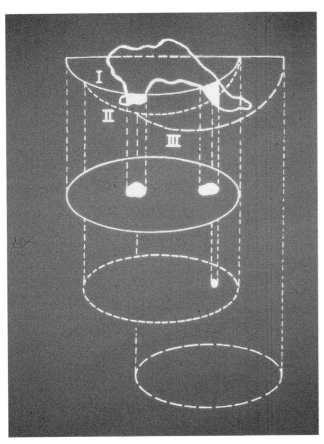

FIGURE 6-21: Diagram of the concept of Mohs surgery with a layer excision of the residual cancer guided by microscopic control.

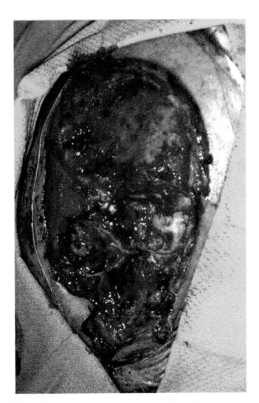

FIGURE 6-23: Resultant wound after Mohs surgery with parotidectomy with facial nerve dissection and mastoidectomy. The facial nerve with its upper and lower divisions is seen in the center area of the wound.

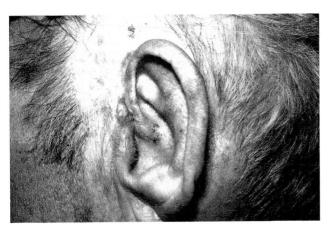

FIGURE 6-22: Recurrent basal cell carcinoma of the left ear. This cancer had been removed on three previous occasions by other doctors.

8. Histologically aggressive cancers: poorly differentiated squamous cell carcinoma, cancer with perineural invasion, metatypical basal cell carcinoma, infiltrating basal cell carcinoma

9. Cancers in critical areas: perioral, genital, hands, feet (Figs. 6-40 to 6-43)

10. Cancers where maximum tissue preservation is required

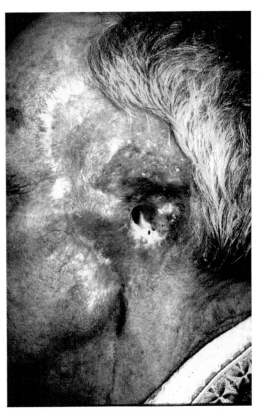

FIGURE 6-24: Area of left ear after full thickness skin graft.

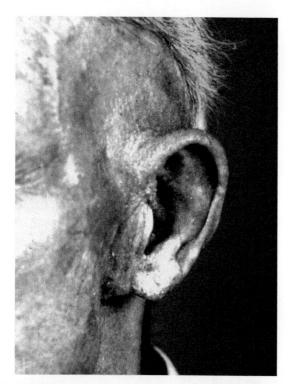

FIGURE 6-25: Prosthetic ear in place.

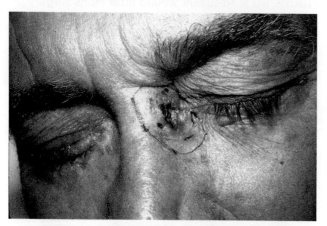

FIGURE 6-26: Recurrent basal cell carcinoma in medial canthus of the left eye.

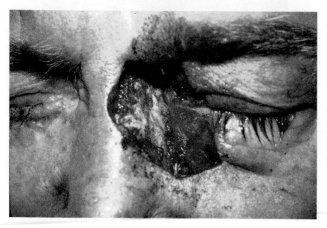

FIGURE 6-27: Wound of medial canthus of the left eye after Mohs surgery.

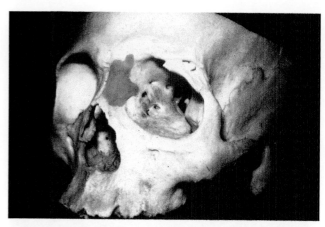

FIGURE 6-28: Skull with red putty, representing the extent of the cancer in Figure 6-26. Cancer of the medial canthus tends to extend along the medial wall of the orbit toward the lamina papyracea. At the lamina papyracea, the cancer may penetrate into the ethmoid sinus.

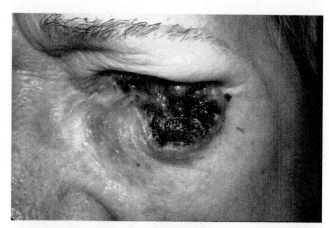

FIGURE 6-29: Primary basal cell carcinoma, greater than 2 cm in size, of the left eyelid and extending onto the bulbar conjunctiva.

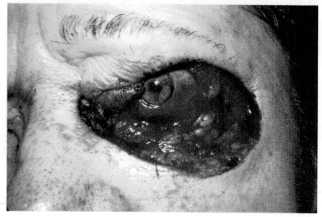

FIGURE 6-30: Extent of basal cell carcinoma of the left eyelid and bulbar conjunctiva after Mohs surgery.

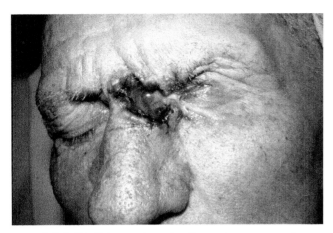

FIGURE 6-31: Primary basal cell carcinoma, greater than 2 cm in size, of the medial canthus infiltrating into the eye and the orbit.

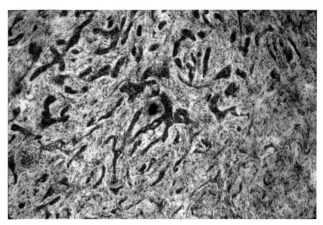

FIGURE 6-34: Histology slide of morpheaform type of basal cell carcinoma displaying an infiltrating, sclerotic pattern with Indian filing of the cancer cells.

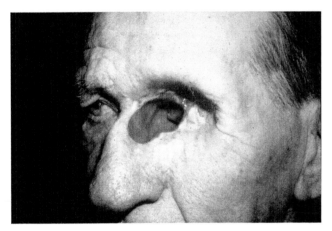

FIGURE 6-32: Extent of cancer in Figure 6-31 after Mohs surgery with orbital exenteration of the eye and ethmoidectomy.

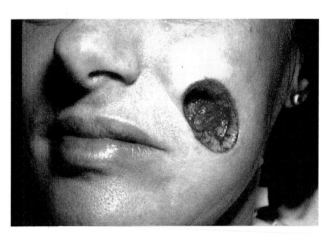

FIGURE 6-35: Extent of morpheaform basal cell carcinoma in Figure 6-33 after Mohs surgery.

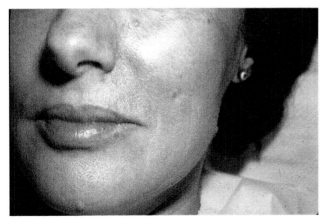

FIGURE 6-33: Morpheaform basal cell carcinoma of the cheek.

Advantages of Mohs Surgery

1. The horizontal compressed frozen sections allow for microscopic examination of the entire perimeter and of all the deep margins.
2. The mapping with microscopic control allows for accurate targeting of residual cancer.
3. There is maximum assurance of cancer removal with minimal sacrifice of normal tissue.

A Personal Note on Frederic E. Mohs, M.D.

Dr. Mohs spent his entire career at the University of Wisconsin in Madison from undergraduate school until his death on July 1, 2002 (Fig. 6-44). He treated his first patient with chemosurgery on June 23, 1936 at the University of Wisconsin Hospital. Today Dr. Mohs' name and his procedure are synonymous. Mohs surgery is practiced throughout the world.

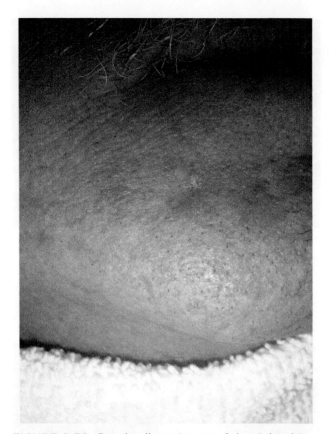

FIGURE 6-36: Basal cell carcinoma of the right chin with ill-defined clinical borders.

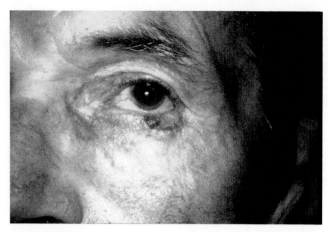

FIGURE 6-38: Primary basal cell carcinoma of the left lateral lower eyelid.

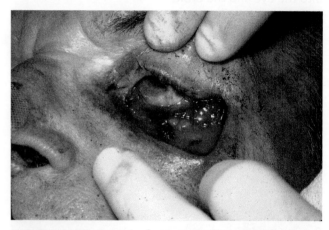

FIGURE 6-39: Extent of cancer in Figure 6-38 after Mohs surgery.

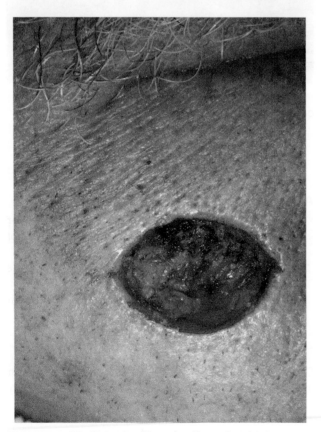

FIGURE 6-37: Extent of basal cell carcinoma in Figure 6-36 after Mohs surgery.

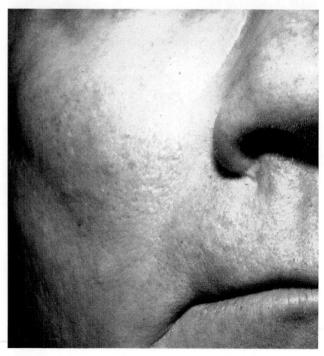

FIGURE 6-40: Basal cell carcinoma of the upper lip at the junction of the ala nasi and nasal sill.

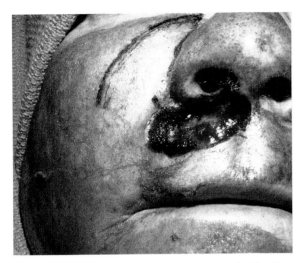

FIGURE 6-41: Extent of cancer in Figure 6-40 after Mohs surgery.

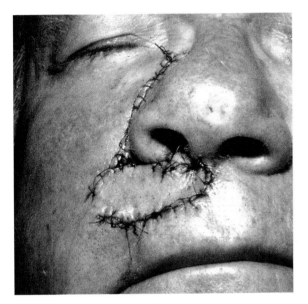

FIGURE 6-42: Reconstruction of the wound in Figure 6-41 with a nasolabial transposition flap.

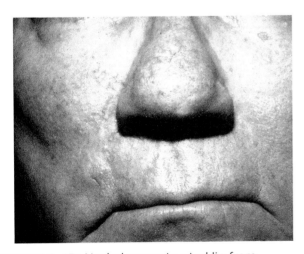

FIGURE 6-43: Healed reconstructed lip from Figure 6-42.

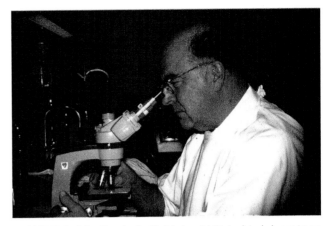

FIGURE 6-44: Frederic E. Mohs, M.D. in his laboratory at the University of Wisconsin.

Dr. Mohs was a very quiet man, but he was focused on his life's mission, which was to continue to improve and perfect his technique, to apply it wherever appropriate, and to teach it to all who were interested (Fig. 6-44).

SAUER'S NOTES

1. Mohs surgery is a method of cancer removal that allows the Mohs surgery specialist to microscopically identify cancer, map out its location, and accurately target the areas that must be removed.

2. When the standard types of frozen sections to check margins are performed by pathologists, the sections are cut vertically. For Mohs surgery, the specimens are compressed so that the perimeter margin and deep margin are in the same plane. The specimen is inverted, placed on the cryostat chuck, and frozen. Horizontal cuts through the undersurface of the specimen for microscopic slides are performed.

3. The horizontal compressed frozen sections with the Mohs technique allow for the microscopic examination of all of the perimeter and of all of the deep margins of the cancer.

Suggested Readings

Gross KG, Steinman HK, Rapini RP. *Mohs Surgery: Fundamentals and Techniques*. St. Louis: Mosby; 1999.

McGregor IA, McGregor AD. *Fundamental Techniques of Plastic Surgery*. Edinburgh: Churchill Livingstone; 1999.

Mohs, FE. Chemosurgery: a microscopically controlled method of cancer excision. *Arch Surg*. 1941;42:279–295.

Mohs FE. *Chemosurgery: Microscopically Controlled Surgery for Skin Cancer*. Springfield: CC Thomas; 1978.

Tromovitch TA, Stegman SJ. Microscopically controlled excision of skin tumors: chemosurgery (Mohs): fresh tissue technique. *Arch Dermatol*. 1974;110:231–232.

Weerda H. *Reconstructive Facial Plastic Surgery*. Stuttgart: Thieme; 2001.

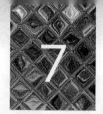

7

Cosmetics for the Physician

Zoe D. Draelos, MD and Marianne N. O'Donoghue, MD

Doctors must be expert in the diagnosis of skin disease and the maintenance of skin, hair, and nail health. This includes understanding the preferred methods of cleansing and moisturizing, safe hair care products, non-damaging nail products, and science-based skin care practices. It is important to examine how cosmetics function and which products might cause adverse reactions.

The U.S. Food and Drug Administration (FDA) defines cosmetics as "(1) articles intended to be rubbed, poured, sprinkled, or sprayed on, introduced into, or otherwise applied to the human body or any part thereof for cleansing, beautifying, promoting attractiveness, or altering the appearance, and (2) articles intended for use as a component of any such article: except that such term shall not include soap." Cosmetics are not presently regulated in the same manner as drugs, however, there is a current trend to consider regulating the introduction of new cosmetic ingredients more carefully. At present, the cosmetics industry voluntarily regulates itself being careful to only make appearance and not functional claims. The Cosmetic Ingredient Review, an independent panel of expert scientists and doctors, studies the safety of cosmetic ingredients and was established to examine all published and voluntarily submitted industry data, and summarize their findings in a safety monograph for each individual ingredient or class of cosmetic ingredients.

In the United States, the labeling of cosmetic products is tightly regulated. It is specified that the manufacturer should label all ingredients in descending order of concentration for all ingredients greater than 1% of the product. Ingredients that comprise less than 1% of the product may be listed in any order, but are usually composed of the colorants, preservatives, and fragrances. The ingredient disclosure can be present on any of the packaging. Cosmetic products intended for sale need a statement of identity, net quantity of content, name and place of the manufacturer or distributor, declaration of ingredient statement, any necessary warning statements, and directions for use.

This means that the physician can trace the origin of any product to which a patient has an adverse reaction. The research and development departments of most cosmetic companies are helpful and knowledgeable, willing to provide patch-testing materials and other advice should adverse events occur. Many cosmetic companies voluntarily report these issues to the FDA to assist in the development of safer cosmetic products.

CLASSIFICATION OF COSMETICS

Cosmetics can be classified into toiletries, skin care products, fragrance products, and colored cosmetics. Each of these products provides a different hygiene or appearance need.

Toiletries

Toiletries include soaps cleansers, shampoos, hair rinses and conditioners, hair dressings, sprays and setting lotions, hair-color preparations, waving preparations, straightening (relaxing) agents, deodorants, antiperspirants, and sun-protective agents. Each of these product categories will be addressed.

Cleansers

The purpose of cleansing is to remove sebum, induce cutaneous desquamation, rinse off airborne pollutant particulates, reduce cutaneous pathogenic organisms, and disrupt any existing cosmetic films. The classic cleanser is soap, which has contributed more to public hygiene and reduced morbidity and mortality than any other substance invented.

Soap consists of a substance made up of fatty acid and an alkaline content resulting in a fatty acid salt with detergent properties. Modern refinements have attempted to adjust the alkaline pH, resulting in less skin irritation, and incorporate substances to reduce calcium fatty acids that create soap scum when used with hard water. There are three types of soap formulations:

1. True soaps composed of long-chain fatty acid alkali salts with a pH between 9 and 10.
2. Combars composed of alkaline soaps to which surface-active agents have been added also with a pH of 9 to 10.
3. Syndet (synthetic detergent) bars composed of synthetic detergents and fillers which contain less than 10% soap and have an adjusted pH of 5.5 to 7.0.

True soaps are rarely used today due to their irritation. Combars are very popular, as most deodorant soaps utilize this formulation. For dermatologic purposes, where patients have sensitive dermatitis skin, syndet bars dominate. Syndets combine excellent cleansing while minimizing damage to the intercellular lipids. Commonly used bar syndet cleansers are sodium cocoate, sodium tallowate, sodium palm kernelate, sodium stearate, sodium palmitate, triethanolamine stearate, sodium cocoyl isethionate, sodium isethionate, sodium dodecyl benzene sulfonate and sodium cocoglyceryl ether sulfonate. Common liquid syndets include sodium laureth sulfate, cocoamido propyl betaine, lauramide DEA, sodium cocoyl isethionate, and disodium laureth sulfosuccinate.

The goal of a cleanser is to remove surface fat soluble and oil soluble dirt without altering the normal acidic pH of the skin, which is between 4.5 and 6.5, while leaving the intercellular lipids intact. No modern cleanser accomplishes this feat creating the diversity of cleansers on the market today. A relatively new cleanser formulation that can more adeptly meet this goal is the body wash or shower gel. These are liquid syndets, usually based on sodium laureth sulfate, that combine cleansing and moisturizing into one step. These products must be used on a puff, which is a woven polyethylene mesh, in order to foam as the conditioning agent prevents foaming. If the body wash is used on a washcloth, excessive product must be used to achieve foaming, defeating the mild cleansing. The puff introduces abundant water and air breaking the body wash emulsion. During the wash phase, there is a low concentration of water and a high concentration of syndet allowing cleansing to occur. However, during the rinse phase, there is a low concentration of body wash and high concentration water. It is during this phase that moisturization occurs as a thin layer of vegetable oil, dimethicone, or a quaternary ammonium compound is left behind on the skin providing protection for the intercellular lipids. For this reason, body washes have great utility for cleansing dermatitic skin.

Shampoos

Shampoos are very similar in formulation to liquid cleansers, except they contain a sequestering agent to prevent precipitated calcium salts, commonly known as soap scum, from depositing on the hair. Shampoos contain the same syndet detergents discussed previously, but they usually combine several surfactants to create the various balances required between cleansing and conditioning. Shampoos contain a principal surfactant for detergent and foaming power, secondary surfactants to condition the hair, and various additives to address specific scalp and hair needs, as well as providing marketing cache. Most shampoos sold today are pH-balanced as the hair shaft cuticle tends to loosen and swell when exposed to alkali detergents.

The largest category of shampoos sold today is conditioning shampoos. These products are formulated much like the body washes discussed previously, where cleansing occurs during the application phase and conditioning occurring during the rinse phase. These shampoos are popular with people who wash their hair frequently or have chemically treated hair as perfectly clean hair is rough, harsh, unable to hold a curl, full

of static electricity, and dull. Sebum is the perfect conditioner, but supports the growth of bacteria and fungus, resulting in dermatologic disease. The goal of shampooing the hair is to remove all of the sebum and then replace the cosmetic value of sebum by coating the hair with the appropriate amount of conditioner to obtain the desired appearance. Oily hair shampoos contain low conditioner concentrations while those for dry hair contain higher amounts of conditioning agents providing for the tremendous variety of shampoos on the market at present.

Medicated shampoos play an important role in dermatology for scalp disease and may contain monographed over-the-counter (OTC) drug ingredients, such as tar, salicylic acid, zinc pyrithione, sulfur, and prescription drug ingredients, such as ketoconazole, clobetasol, and fluocinonide. OTC drug shampoos can only contain one active ingredient and are many times alternated to take advantage of different ingredient benefits. For example, tar is an anti-inflammatory, salicylic acid is an exfoliant, zinc pyrithione and sulfur are anti-fungals. Rotating these shampoos is helpful in exfoliating the scalp while reducing fungal colonization and inflammation.

Conditioners

Conditioners are used following shampooing and rinsed in the shower or applied to towel dried hair and left in. As the application practice suggests, the rinsed conditioners are known as "instant conditioners" while the nonrinsed conditioners are known as "leave in conditioners." Their formulation is very similar, but they are useful as the application method provides for minimal or maximal coating of the hair shaft depending on the intactness of the cuticle or the styling desires of the individual.

The major conditioners for hair possessing a damaged cuticle are cationic surfactants, such as quaternary ammonium compounds, more commonly known in the industry simply as "quats". Quaternary ammonium compounds, especially stearalkonium ammonium chloride, have been used for many years to improve hair manageability by reducing static electricity through charge neutralization. Another category of conditioners is based on polymers, such as polyvinylpyrrolidone (PVP) or vinyl acetate function as film formers to coat the hair shaft smoothing the cuticle and producing increased shine. These polymers are also used to hold the hair in a desired position and are found in styling gels and hairsprays. Conditioners may also contain sunscreens to prevent UV radiation from damaging hair color, but the FDA has determined that no hair care products can make sun protection claims or list an SPF. It is possible for the polymer-based hair care products to resist removal resulting in a product build-up. Using a special anionic shampoo can prevent the hair from developing the limp appearance of over conditioned hair.

The most medically relevant conditioning agents for hair possessing a damaged cuticle are the protein-based conditioners, containing hydrolyzed protein from various sources that can penetrate into the hair shaft during application restoring hair strength by 5% to 7%, depending on the formulation and the degree of cuticular loss. The protein fragments can temporarily reside in the hair shaft cortex and are used to restore hair appearance when the hair has just been permanently dyed or waved.

Finally, styling aids consist of lotions, gels, mousses, or hair spray. These represent products that are applied to towel dried hair and left in place, many times being reapplied to restore or maintain the desired hair style. Most of styling aids contain water, copolymers, polyvinylpyrrolidone, quaternary salts, and fragrance. The polymers impart waterproof qualities to the hair so water contact from perspiration or mild rain does not alter the hair style.

Permanent Waves and Hair Straighteners

The three patterns of hair growth are straight, wavy, and kinky. To change the hair growth pattern of virgin hair permanently, a chemical reaction involving the breaking and subsequent rearrangement of hair disulfide bonds with heat, high pH, or thioglycolates must occur. For hair straightening, the bonds are broken with sodium hydroxide, guanidine hydroxide, lithium hydroxide, heat, or thioglycolates. The hair is chemically treated until the disulfide bonds are broken and then combed straight. The disulfide bonds are reformed with the hair in its new conformation requiring neutralization with hydrogen peroxide, sodium perborate, or potassium bromate. Some of the disulfide bonds cannot be reformed resulting in weakening of the hair shaft manifesting as brittle, easy fractured hair shaft.

The most common form of permanent hair curling or waving is the acid permanent wave based on glycerol monothioglycolate. This permanent wave can be used on fine or color-treated hair with less hair shaft weakening; however, allergic contact dermatitis to glycerol thioglycolate can occur. It is best to administer this permanent wave in a professional salon. Most home permanent waves are based on ammonium thioglycolate, which is less allergenic, but does not produce as tight a curl.

Kinky hair requires the strongest disulfide bond breaking agents as straightening the hair shafts requires more disulfide bond breakage than curling straight hair. The chemicals for hair straightening procedures include lye or non-lye agents, such as sodium, lithium, or calcium hydroxide. These products are best applied in a professional salon as the chemical must be applied to the hair, avoiding the scalp, and removed promptly to prevent burning the skin and over-weakening the hair shafts. Frequent use of hair straightening agents can weaken the hair shaft so it fractures at the point of maximum trauma where it exits the scalp. This can lead to the assumption that the hair is falling out when actually it is breaking off. Discontinuing the straightening or extending the interval between procedures or using a milder straightening chemical may be helpful in preventing further hair loss.

Hair Coloring

The popularity of hair coloring continues to grow with males and females of all ages finding alteration of their natural hair color appealing. The five major types of hair coloring are temporary, gradual, natural, semipermanent, and permanent.

Temporary colors are textile dyes deposited on top of the cuticle temporarily, but can be rubbed off or easily removed with water contact, including perspiration or rain. They allow the user to change hair color until the next water contact from shampooing. Temporary hair dyes are most popular in vivid party colors for creating red, blue, green, etc. hair. They are also used to optically whiten gray/yellow hair by adding a blue/purple dye to create the color of silver. Temporary hair dyes are safe and do not cause allergic contact dermatitis.

Gradual colors contain metallic salts. Gray hair can be gradually dyed brown or black by the combination of lead acetate and sulfur. The chemical reaction results in the formation of salts that precipitate on the outside of the hair shaft allowing a gradual change in color. Unfortunately, the hair looks lusterless and may possess a sulfur odor. The metal precipitate also precludes any other chemical hair processing, such as permanent waving or coloring. Gradual hair dyes are most popular among men who want a gradual color change so as not to call attention to their use of hair dyes.

Semipermanent dyes last from 4 to 8 shampooings and can only dye the hair darker, not lighter. The active ingredients are low molecular weight dyes specifically synthesized for hair coloring. Because the molecules are small, they can penetrate the cuticle and enter the superficial cortex, but the color molecules can also easily diffuse out of the hair shaft. This is why semipermanent dyes wash out with each shampoo or hair/water contact episode. Semipermanent dyes have a low incidence of allergic contact dermatitis, but some of the longer lasting "demipermanent" dyes may have added p-phenylenediame (PPD) and could cause allergic contact dermatitis. Patients should be cautioned to always perform an allergenicity test following the instructions required by law on all hair-coloring products. In addition, it is worthwhile to read the ingredient disclosure for the presence of PPD. Semipermanent dyes are not damaging to the hair shaft and can be used to cover gray if less than 10% of the hairs are gray.

A variant of synthetic semipermanent dyes are the natural or vegetable dyes based on henna from *Lawsonia inermis* plant. Henna dyes are making a comeback, but can only dye the hair red. More commonly, henna is used to decorate the skin for special occasions in Middle Eastern culture. Henna is capable of producing allergic contact dermatitis. Some henna products that are available in a wide color range combine henna with the synthetic semipermanent dyes mentioned previously.

The most popular hair-coloring products for men and women are the *permanent hair dyes*. In permanent hair coloring, an oxidation reduction reaction occurs in the hair cortex with colorless dyestuffs becoming oxidized by hydrogen peroxide. The reaction is p-phenylenediamine + H_2O_2 = amines; amines + couplers = indo dyes. The resulting indo dye molecules are large and cannot diffuse out of the hair cortex making the color permanent. However, permanent hair coloring must be repeated every 4 to 6 weeks as new growth, known as "roots," becomes visible at the scalp. Permanent hair coloring damages the hair structure by weakening hair shaft strength and damaging the cuticle due to ammonia and hydrogen peroxide exposure, both of which swell the cuticular scale. More damage is induced by lightning or bleaching the hair color. Bleaching is a two-step procedure where the natural color, produced by eumelanin, removed with hydrogen peroxide with subsequent re-dyeing to a lighter color. While these are two separate steps, they occur instantaneously when using a permanent dye lighter than the virgin hair color. It is the removal of the natural hair color that produces dramatic structural weakening of the hair shaft.

Permanent hair coloring can be used to dye the hair lighter or darker than the virgin color. This versatility provides for many creative and artistic methods of hair dyeing. One such variant of hair lightning, known as *frosting or highlighting*, consists of taking locks of hair and selectively bleaching them, using 30 or 40 volumes of hydrogen peroxide followed by wrapping the lock in aluminum foil. This allows the hair to be multicolored simulating artificially the highlights induced by color variation in natural hair. Table 7-1 summarizes these hair-coloring techniques.

Skin Care Products

Skin care products include cleansers, moisturizers, cosmetics, and fragrances. This discussion will briefly review each product category.

Moisturizers

Moisturizers are important cosmetics for the doctors to understand as they can improve stratum corneum barrier function and assist in the resolution of dermatitic disease. Moisturizers contain ingredients that physically trap or attract water to the skin while emollients are substances that temporarily make the skin feel smooth and soft. Most moisturizing substances also have some limited emollient characteristics. There are six important categories of moisturizing ingredients: hydrocarbons, waxes, natural lipid polyesters, lightweight esters and ethers, silicone, and ceramides.

Hydrocarbons are some of the oldest and most effective occlusive moisturizers including mineral oil and petrolatum. Because these products contain no water to support bacterial or fungal growth, they can be formulated preservative-free. It has been shown by tagging C^+ atoms that petrolatum actually penetrates into the intercellular spaces of the stratum corneum aiding in barrier repair, however petrolatum is heavy and not aesthetically pleasing, thus creating opportunities for many different moisturizer formulations. In the temperate zones in the winter, however, petrolatum is ideal for hands, feet, and other dry body areas. Cosmetic grade petrolatum is noncomedogenic, but not widely used in facial moisturizers due to its greasiness.

Waxes, such as beeswax, synthetic beeswax, cholesterol, and lanolin, may be combined with petrolatum in therapeutic moisturizers designed for very dry dermatitic skin. These substances usually cause no adverse reaction themselves, but esters of lanolin can occasionally be comedogenic and a source of allergic contact dermatitis.

Natural lipid polyesters retard water loss by integrating with the proteins of the stratum corneum. Short-chain acids such as coconut oil, capric or caprylic triglycerides, esters of lanolin, and synthesized unsaturated fatty acid esters such as sorbitol oleate or lanolin linoleate can be comedogenic because of their interaction with the stratum corneum. Long-chain polyesters are less likely to be comedogenic because of their molecular size, which inhibits skin penetration.

Lightweight esters and ethers, such as isopropyl myristate, also can be comedogenic. They are acceptable if they comprise less than 2% of the formulation. Some of these products act as preservatives at lower concentrations.

Silicone is the emollient with the widest use, especially in products that claim to be oil-free. Silicone is not a vegetable or mineral oil, supporting the oil-free claim, even though it is a clear oily liquid. This inert product is noncomedogenic and is added to reduce the greasiness of petrolatum by improving skin smoothness and softness. Silicone oils, such as dimethicone, amodimethicone, and cyclomethicone, are lubricating, protective, and water repellant. There is no topical absorption of silicone, so safety concerns are minimal and no reports of allergic or irritant contact dermatitis are found.

Synthetic ceramides, mimicking the natural ceramides found in the intercellular lipids, are added to many therapeutic moisturizers to aid in barrier repair. The first step in barrier repair following injury is a burst of ceramide synthesis leading to the concept that providing extra ceramides externally might decrease barrier repair time. Indeed synthetic ceramides can diffuse into the intercellular lipids, but whether or not they are physiologically active is controversial. The extracellular matrix contains ceramides, free sterols (cholesterol), and free fatty acids. Ceramides comprise 40% to 50% of the matrix and are composed of a fatty acid and sphingoid base.

Humectants

Humectants, such as glycerin, sodium pyroglutamic acid, sorbitol, urea, lactic acid, and propylene glycol, absorb water and can moisturize the skin by drawing water from the viable epidermis and dermis to the upper layers of the epidermis. If the skin barrier is damaged, this water will evaporate into the atmosphere further drying the skin. If the humectant is combined with an occlusive agent, such as petrolatum, the water will be trapped and hydrate the skin. This is the mechanism by which most moisturizers function. Good therapeutic moisturizers will contain humectants and occlusive ingredients.

Cleansers and Surfactants

Surfactants are surface-active ingredients that mix the oil and water phases in an emulsion and remove unwanted materials from the skin surface. Surfactants can damage the skin barrier, which is why emulsifiers are the single most common cause of irritant contact dermatitis in leave-on skin care products. The four major types of surfactants are anionic, nonionic, cationic, and amphoteric.

Anionic surfactants are the principal ingredients in shampoos and synthetic detergent liquid soap. Sodium lauryl sulfate is the most commonly used surfactant in liquid cleansers. Other anionic surfactants include alpha olefin sulfonates, Na/K stearate, triethanolamine (TEA)-lauryl sulfate, and sulfosuccinates.

TABLE 7-1 • Coloring Products and Their Key Characteristics

Type of Coloring Product	Recognition	Skill Involved	Type of Dye	Color Change Range	Site of Action	Lasting Quality	Overall Performance	Degree of Abuse of Hair Structure	Potential for Dermatologic Complaints
Temporary color rinses	Multiple-use package	Minimal; apply and dry	High molecular weight acid dyes as used in textiles, and certified food colors in a hydro-alcoholic suspension	Covers gray	Surface of shaft	Poor; removed by shampooing	Poor	Negligible	Negligible
Semi-permanent	Single- or multiple-use package; more viscous than no. 1 to prevent dripping off of hair	Moderate; apply to freshly shampooed hair and leave in place for 15–40 min; skin patch test required	Low molecular weight dyes: nitrophenylene-diamines, nitroaminophenols, aminoanthroquinones in shampoo vehicle or a solvent system	Covers gray; one to three shades on dark side of normal hair color	Penetrates to cortex	Gradually lost through three to five shampoos	Fair	Negligible	Negligible
Permanent Oxidation Type									
Single process	Two-unit system for mixing just before use	Moderate; skin patch test required	Several classes of dyes including PPD intermediates in an alkaline peroxide "shampoo"	Covers gray; two or three shades on each side of normal	Cortex	Permanent; new growth touch-up every 4–8 wk	Excellent	Moderate	Modest
Double process	Same as above	Professional attention necessary	As above, but hair must be previously decolorized (stripped)	Unlimited	Cortex	As above	Excellent	Significant	Moderate; hair breakage; local and systemic peroxide reactions
Progressive	Multiple-use package	None	Metallic salts particularly lead, in solution, cream, or pomade form	Discolors hair only	Surface and some beneath cuticle	As long as product is used regularly	Poor	Minimal	Negligible; a public health problem; incompatible with other chemical hair services
Vegetable	For all practical purposes, this does not exist and is not available.								
Henna	Although true henna is a vegetable dye, its color properties and lasting abilities make it unacceptable. Products are being marketed currently with this name but are actually henna coloring in the second and third categories above.								

Note: The late Dr. Earl Brauer compiled this chart for previous editions of this book.
Abbreviation: p-Phenylenediamine.

The *nonionic surfactants* are gentler than the anionics. They allow for the removal of minerals from hard water and increase the viscosity and solubility of shampoos. They are popular emulsifiers. This category includes sorbitan fatty acids, polysorbates, polyethylene glycol lipids, and lauramine oxide.

The *cationic surfactants* function largely as conditioners for hair, thickeners for shampoo, and hair grooming aids. These include stearalkonium chloride, quaternary ammonium salts, quaternary fatty acids, and amino acids.

The *amphoteric surfactants* contain a balance of positive and negative charges. These are not as aggressive cleansers as the anionic surfactants. Examples of these surfactants are *N*-alkyl-amino acids, betaines, and alkyl imidazoline compounds. Cocamidopropyl betaine, the main surfactant in baby shampoo, is an infrequent cause of allergic contact dermatitis.

Preservatives

Preservatives are second only to fragrance in causing allergic contact dermatitis. They are absolutely necessary, however, to keep skin care products free from contamination. The more water in a formulation, the more preservatives required. Preservatives are classified into three categories: antimicrobials, ultraviolet light absorbers, and antioxidants. Preservative allergenicity is important and can be influenced by the following variables:

- Inherent sensitizing potential
- Concentration in the final product
- Wash-off or leave-on product
- Duration of the skin contact
- State of the epidermal surface when applied
- Body region

Of all these variables, the first two are the most important. Preservatives are mixed and matched depending on whether there is a concern of gram-positive or gram-negative organisms, *Candida* sp, *Pityrosporum ovale*, or fungus. The following is a review of four of the most commonly used groups of preservatives, their efficacies, and their disadvantages.

Formaldehyde and Formaldehyde Releasers: Free formaldehyde is present, especially in shampoos, because of its efficacy against *Pseudomonas aeruginosa*. Because shampoos only remain in contact with the skin for a brief period, allergic contact dermatitis is rare. However, hairdressers, who have prolonged contact with shampoo, are more likely to experience irritant or allergic contact dermatitis. In addition, formaldehyde-allergic patients must avoid permanent press or wrinkle-resistant garments and should wash all new clothing items before wearing as formaldehyde is a common fabric finishing ingredient.

Some preservatives release formaldehyde while in formation. Of the formaldehyde releasing preservatives, *quaternium 15* is number one and *imidazolidinyl urea* is number two in causing allergic contact dermatitis. Other formaldehyde releasers include *BNPD (Bronopol), diazolidinyl urea (Germall II),* and *DMDM hydantoin (Glydant)*. All of these preservatives are very effective against Pseudomonas, which is why they are still in use today despite their issues.

Parabens: Parabens are the least allergenic and most widely used of all preservatives due to their effectiveness against fungi and gram-positive bacteria. They are relatively water insoluble, so are not effective against Pseudomonas sp. Combining two parabens, such as ethyl and methyl paraben, in the same formulation enhances preservative efficacy, but all parabens cross-react. As with the formaldehyde releasers, parabens are more likely to react with dermatitic skin, but sensitization is uncommon with these preservatives. Recently there has been a trend to produce paraben-free skin care products, yet parabens remain one of the most effective and safe skin care preservatives.

Antioxidants: Antioxidants are also incorporated into skin care products to prevent the oils from rancidity. Frequently used antioxidant preservatives include butylated hydroxyanisole (BHA), butylated hydroxytoluene (BHT), triclosan, and sorbic acid. BHA and BHT are present in lipstick and sunscreens, but their widest use is in foods. Triclosan is a disinfectant and preservative in deodorants, shampoo, and soap. Sorbic acid is used often in creams and lotions. It is fungistatic but has poor bacterial inhibition.

Kathon CG (Methylchloroisothiazoline and Methylisothiazolinone): This organic preservative was considered the most complete and safest preservative until the 1990s. It is an odorless and colorless biocide that exhibits microbicidal activity against a wide spectrum of fungi and gram-positive and gram-negative bacteria. Many paraben-free formulations switched to the Kathons, but numerous reports of allergic contact dermatitis have emerged. More than 80 publications in the 1990s reported allergic contact dermatitis to cleansing cream, hair tonics, hair balsam, wash softeners, cosmetics, and moist toilet paper containing Kathons. According to the North American Contact Dermatitis Group, the incidence of allergy to Kathons is 1.9%. To minimize the occurrence of allergic contact dermatitis, the concentration of Kathon should be below 15 ppm in rinse-off products and less than 7.5 ppm in leave-on products. For this reason, Kathons are now recommended for use only in shampoos and instant conditioners that have only brief skin contact.

Fragrance and Fragrance Products

Fragrance is the most common allergen in skin care products. In one study, it accounted for 149 of 536 reactions. Together, fragrance and preservatives accounted for half of all the reactions to cosmetics. Fragrance products include perfume, cologne, toilet water, bathwater additives, bath powder, and aftershave lotions. The most common reaction to fragrance is allergic contact dermatitis, followed by photodermatitis, contact urticaria, irritation, and depigmentation.

The common fragrance allergens are:

- Cinnamic alcohol
- Cinnamic aldehyde
- Hydroxycitronellal
- Isoeugenol
- Oak moss absolute

The most common photoallergen is musk ambrette, but this substance is no longer used as a fragrance. Oil of bergamot is also a photoallergen, but it too is an ingredient of antiquity. Most fragrances currently on the market do contain these natural ingredients, instead relying on synthetic fragrances that do not possess allergenicity issues.

Color Cosmetics

Color cosmetics include foundation, eye makeup (shadow, liner, mascara), lipstick, rouge, blush, and nail enamel. The use of color cosmetics is likened to an artist painting a picture on a canvas.

Foundation is used to give a simple flawless complexion on which other color cosmetics can be applied. Facial foundation is useful for covering issues arising after surgery or to cover facial defects, such as telangiectasias or lentigines. A thicker foundation, known as a concealer, has higher amounts of titanium dioxide and can be dabbed on facial defects for greater camouflaging ability. The concealer can be applied directly to a pigmentation defect, allowed to dry, and then blended over the entire face with a facial foundation. The types of foundation vary in the amount of coverage and moisturizing ingredient content. Foundation can be transparent, imparting only color, translucent, offering more cover, or opaque, offering total coverage.

Foundation formulations can be oil-based, water-based, oil-free, and water-free or anhydrous.

Water-based foundations are oil-in-water emulsions. The pigment is emulsified in a small amount of oil. The primary emulsifier is a soap, for example, TEA or a nonionic surfactant. These are best for normal skin.

Oil-free foundations contain no animal, vegetable, or mineral oils. They contain dimethicone or cyclomethicone as an emollient. These are for people with oily skin and are noncomedogenic, nonacnegenic, and hypoallergenic.

Water-free or anhydrous foundations are waterproof. They contain vegetable oil, mineral oil, lanolin alcohol, and synthetics to form the oil phase. Waxes may be added to make it a cream. High concentrations of pigments may be added to these preparations providing excellent camouflaging abilities. Under these foundations, green or mauve tints can be added to improve red or yellow discoloration. This is important for acne rosacea, laser therapy, and post-cosmetic surgery.

Powders

Powders are applied over facial foundations to improve wear characteristics. The covering ability of face powder ingredients in the order of increasing opacity is: titanium dioxide, kaolin, magnesium carbonate, magnesium stearate, zinc stearate, prepared chalk, zinc oxide, rice starch, precipitated chalk, and talc.

Comedogenicity and Cosmetics

Comedogenicity, especially in facial foundations, is a concern for the doctor and the patient. While cosmetics rarely cause comedone formation, there is a great deal of advertising attention directed to the noncomedogenic claim. The ingredients that are more likely to be comedogenic are cosmetics and they are listed below:

- Isopropyl myristate
- Isopropyl ester
- Oleic acid
- Stearic acid
- Petrolatum (not cosmetic grade)
- Lanolin (especially acetylated lanolin alcohols and lanolin fatty acids)

Not all products containing these ingredients may be comedogenic in all persons, thus testing may be necessary. Much of the comedogenicity reported more than two decades ago was due to the use of contaminated raw materials. All large cosmetic manufacturers now use cosmetic grade mineral oil and petrolatum, which has decreased the reports of comedogenic cosmetics.

Cheek and Lip Cosmetics

Blush adds color and the look of rosy cheeks to the patient's appearance. Similarly, *lipsticks* can also add color and impart an appearance of wellness. Lipsticks are made of waxes that are usually nonallergenic and noncomedogenic, but frequently contain castor oil, a known cause of lip allergic contact dermatitis. Lipstick can also be used to camouflage lip issues associated with aging or disease. For women who have vertical lines above and below the vermilion border, the use of a lip liner can be helpful. This stops the waxy lipstick from "bleeding" into the vertical furrows when the patient eats or drinks. Lip liner is also recommended for women with asymmetry of their lips owing to removal of a tumor, other lip surgery, or lips that are too thin. The desired outline of the lips can be drawn with the pencil or liner and then the color can be filled in.

Eye Cosmetics

Eye makeup—shadow, liner, mascara—can be used to enlarge, brighten, or accentuate the eyes. Because of the need to prevent infection, most eye makeup contains preservatives. These preservatives are listed on the package and patients can check to see if they have had an adverse reaction to them. Generally, the preservatives are ethlenediamine tera acetate (EDTA), British antilewisite (BAL), thimerosal, parabens, quaternium 15, or phenylmercuric acetate/nitrate. Usually, each cosmetic company formulates its products with its specific preservatives. Therefore, a patient who cannot use one company's eye product may be able to use another company's product. Most American eye cosmetics are formulated without fragrance and with the simplest hypoallergenic formula.

Eye shadow can function to conceal flaws or enlarge the eye. Usually, if the patient has an allergic reaction to cream eye shadow, a powder eye shadow is a good substitute.

Eyeliner may help to change the shape of the eye as well as accentuate it. These products usually are waxes and therefore have no adverse reaction. Pencil eyeliner is preferred to liquid eyeliner for a more natural appearance.

Mascara can be water-based or waterproof. The water-based products are healthier for the eyelashes because they can be removed easily with soap and water. Products with lengtheners, however, may add lacquer and may require special solvents to remove the old mascara. Waterproof mascara may have a lower concentration of preservatives and may therefore be less allergenic for some patients. It is necessary to use an eye makeup remover to take mascara off. The use of the special remover may be more traumatic to the eyelashes. Because of this, patients with fragile lashes (e.g., patients with alopecia areata) should wear water-washable mascara. *Eyelash curlers* can be used to give the illusion of longer lashes and conceal blepharochalasis. The patient who is allergic to nickel or rubber should not use this instrument. If the eyelash curler is to be used, it must be used before the mascara is applied.

Nail Polish

Nail enamels, including base coats and top coats, have similar composition. The ingredients in the formulation are:

- *Film former*: nitrocellulose
- *Resin*: toluene sulfonamide/formaldehyde resin, alkyl resins, acrylates, vinyls, polyesters
- *Plasticizers*: camphor, dibutyl phthalate, dioctyl phthalate, tricresyl phosphate
- *Solvents*: alcohol, toluene, ethyl acetate, butyl acetate
- *Colorants*
- *Pearl*: guanine, bismuth oxychloride

The major ingredient that causes allergic contact dermatitis in nail polish is toluene sulfonamide. Butyl and ethyl methacrylate, which are in the glue used for sculptured nails, press-on nails, and nail mending, can also cause allergic contact dermatitis. Cuticle remover (sodium or potassium hydroxide) is left on the cuticle to dissolve dead skin. If left on too long, this product becomes an irritant. The entire nail can be separated from the nail bed by too vigorous use of cuticle remover.

COSMECEUTICALS

Cosmeceuticals is a term well known to doctors and consumers, but this term has no regulatory meaning. Cosmeceuticals are simply cosmetics, however, cosmeceutical implies a product that does more than fragrance and color the skin. For this reason, most cosmeceutical formulations contain a hero ingredient designed to somehow improve the appearance of the skin. Cosmeceutical hero ingredients may include retinoids, antioxidants (vitamins), α-hydroxy acids, and β-hydroxy acids.

Retinoids

In 1984, L.H. Kligman demonstrated that connective tissue could be repaired in the rhino mouse with tretinoin. Subsequently, this was established in humans with a multicenter, double-blind study over a 48-week period. The gold standard for the reversal of photoaging remains topical tretinoin, but because of its irritant potential, many other products have been studied.

Since 1984, many preparations of tretinoin have been formulated. The first products with concentrations of 0.1% were very irritating, leading to subsequent topical formulations of 0.025% and 0.01% tretinoin in creams and gels. These products have been demonstrated in biopsies, photographs, and clinical observations to improve skin appearance. A 4-week treatment with tretinoin in a solution of 50% ethanol and 50% propylene glycol 400 was studied by D.E. Kligman and Z.D. Draelos for rapid retinization of photoaged facial skin. Almost all subjects improved on all measures of clinical grading (fine lines, mottled pigmentation, and surface texture/roughness) by 4 weeks.

Adapalene 0.1% cream and gel is less irritating than tretinoin, but has not been approved for a photoaging indication. Tazarotene cream 0.1% has been studied for photoaging and compared with tretinoin emollient cream 0.05% for efficacy. The results were similar, but the tazarotene cream demonstrated quicker efficacy at weeks 12 and 20 with more aggressive irritation.

Antioxidants

Antioxidants are products that quench free oxygen radicals. These free radicals are formed when oxygen is exposed to sunlight, pollution from combustion, and normal metabolism. Free radicals have a role in skin carcinogenesis, inflammation, and aging. It is the loss of an electron from an oxygen molecule that creates the unstable highly reactive oxygen that damages dermal collagen resulting in the release of matrix metalloproteases, such as collagenase and elastase, and DNA, resulting in the formation of skin cancer. The missing electron can be supplied from an antioxidant that donates the electron, itself becoming oxidized. Naturally occurring antioxidants include vitamins A, B_3 (niacinamide), B_5 (panthenol), C, and E. Other naturally occurring antioxidants include α-lipoic acid, β-carotene, catalase, glutathione, superoxide dismutase, ubiquinone (coenzyme Q_{10}), and plant antioxidants such as green tea polyphenols, silymarin, soy isoflavones, and furfuryladenine. These ingredients have been incorporated into many cosmeceuticals given below:

Niacinamide in aging human skin cells in vitro increases synthesis of collagen, involucrin, filaggrin, and keratin. It increases the biosynthesis of ceramides and other stratum corneum lipids, therefore leading to an improved epidermal barrier and a decrease of transepidermal water loss.

Dexapanthenol is a stable alcohol form of pantothenic acid converted in the skin. It acts as a humectant. It is also used in healing ointments.

Vitamin C promotes collagen synthesis, has antioxidant properties, and has photoprotection from both UVA and UVB. It is anti-inflammatory, lightens hyperpigmentation, and reduces post-laser resurfacing erythema.

Vitamin E is the major antioxidant in scavenging lipid peroxyl radicals. It plays a major role in photoprotection and acts as a humectant. The combination of vitamins C and E is synergized to have a more efficient role in photoprotection and rejuvenation.

Idebenone is a synthetic form of ubiquinone and has been demonstrated to be very effective as an antioxidant.

Rosemary is a substance that is better known as a spice but is a potent antioxidant due to its phenolic deterpines. It has been shown to suppress tumorigenesis in the two-stage cancer model in mice. It also exhibits photoprotection in mice.

Oatmeal is a substance that has always been soothing and anti-inflammatory. It can repair skin and hair damage from ultraviolet radiation, smoke, bacteria, and free radicals.

Olive oil contains polyphenolic compounds that protect against inflammation. It is found in soaps, lip balms, shampoos, and moisturizers. Extra-virgin olive has protected mice after ultraviolet exposure.

Grape seed extract is an antioxidant because of its oligomeric proanthocyanides. These compounds are found in the flavonoid family, which is most famous for green and black tea. This extract helps vascular endothelial growth factor expressed in keratinocytes, which fosters wound healing. It also scavenges free radicals for vitamins C and E.

Tea tree oil is a compound that has been widely used in hair and skin products because of its activity against *Propionibacterium acnes* and trichophytic dermatophytosis. It is very popular in beauty salon products. It has the highest rate of contact dermatitis of the cosmeceuticals. Many reports have come from Great Britain. Its efficacy in antidandruff shampoos needs to be proved.

Coffeeberry extract has been included with green tea since they both contain polyphenols. Green tea is anti-inflammatory and a photoprotector. Coffeeberry is supposed to have more antioxidants than the tea.

α-Hydroxy Acids

Doctors have used lactic acid for many years as a humectant to digest the protein bonds on accumulated keratin opening up water binding sites to allow hydration. The research by Van Scott ushered the rest of the α-hydroxy acids into widespread use. These natural fruit acids exert their influence by diminishing corneocyte cohesion. The most commonly used ingredients are

- *Glycolic acid*: sugarcane
- *Lactic acid*: sour milk
- *Malic acid*: apples
- *Citric acid*: citrus fruits
- *Tartaric acid*: grapes

The α-hydroxy acids have been incorporated into cosmetic formulations for shampoos, soaps, face creams, and body creams. The α-hydroxy acid must be present as an acid to have any effect, meaning that the formulation must be acidic and may cause skin stinging and burning upon application. Many α-hydroxy acid formulations use buffering agents to increase the pH, but this decreases the concentration of the active acid, reducing efficacy. The poor skin tolerability of glycolic acid has largely removed this ingredient from the marketplace at present for facial use although glycolic acid peels remain popular. Other α-hydroxy acids, such as lactic acid, are widely used in moisturizers to exfoliate the body and minimize skin scale.

β-Hydroxy Acids

In the search for a less irritating and stinging compound for creams and peels, the β-hydroxy acid salicylic acid has become popular. Doctors have used this keratolytic agent for years as a monographed OTC acne treatment at concentrations of 2% to 3% and as a keratolytic therapy for warts at concentrations of 10% to 15% in creams and 40% in pastes. Salicylic acid appears to have an anti-inflammatory component and may have less sting and irritancy than glycolic acid. β-Hydroxy acid face peels have also become popular for patients who cannot tolerate glycolic or trichloroacetic acid peels at concentrations between 10% and 40%.

Protein-Based Cosmeceuticals

Protein-based cosmeceuticals have been adapted from wound healing and skin repair studies to skin care products. These proteins purport to increase fibroblast activity, increase protein and collagen syntheses, and produce antioxidant enzymes. These proteins include peptides, copper peptides, and human growth factors.

Peptides

It was discovered in vitro in 1993 that a subfragment of type I collagen could stimulate type I, type III, and fibronectin. Ex vivo studies in full thickness human skin biopsies demonstrated stimulation of collagen I with a pentapeptide consisting of five amino acids that when combined with palmitic acid could penetrate the skin (palmitoyl pentapeptide-3 Pal-KTTKS). In vitro studies demonstrate stimulation of collagen IV and glucosaminoglycans, including hyaluronic acid. The advantages of pentapeptides are that they stimulate matrix formation and are not irritating. Subsequent to this development many different peptides have entered the cosmetic market. Most peptides are used in small quantity in formulation as they are expensive to synthesize and thought to work at a receptor level. More study is required to confirm their utility, especially since they are usually formulated in a moisturizing vehicle that also imparts skin benefits.

Copper Peptides

Copper peptides were developed by attaching the metal copper to a synthetic peptide to enhance wound healing. These wound healing products are applied to an open wound, devoid of the stratum corneum, and are used in Mohs surgery, post-laser procedures, and in the therapy of diabetic ulcers. They are purported to promote vascular, collagen, and elastin formation. Copper peptides are used in facial moisturizers and claim to improve fine lines and wrinkles, surface roughness, and increase skin density.

Human Growth Factors

Human growth factors are an emerging area of cosmeceutical ingredient development. Originally, these growth factors were incorporated into facial moisturizers by including spent human fibroblast growth media in the formulation. The spent media contained over 300 different ingredients, which have never been fully characterized. Now, human growth factors, such as epidermal growth factor can be synthesized in a laboratory to avoid contamination of the product. This also avoids the unpleasant odor imparted by using spent media.

Antiperspirants

Antiperspirants are OTC drugs because they must follow a monograph that specifies the ingredients and concentrations that can be used in acceptable formulations. The monograph also sets forth standards for perspiration control. Antiperspirants contain aluminum salts that act by coagulating the sweat duct protein blocking the secretion of sweat. Effective antiperspirants must reduce sweat by at least 20% in half the people tested. Antiperspirant roll-on formulations provide the best sweat reduction followed by sticks and sprays. Antiperspirants are different from deodorants that reduce armpit odor by containing the antibacterial triclosan and fragrance.

Olfactory reference syndrome is preoccupation with the belief that you have a foul body odor and can be a sign of a significant depressive disorder.

Sunscreens

Sunscreens are incorporated into many cosmetic formulations reclassifying them as OTC drugs. The most active antiaging ingredient in many cosmetics is the sunscreen, which can now be used to substantiate claims to this effect. Cosmetics that have an SPF rating on the bottle must specify the active sunscreen ingredients that were used to obtain the SPF. The SPF value for UVB is the ratio of the UVB dose required to produce the minimal erythema reaction through the applied sunscreen product (2 mg/cm^2) compared with the UVB dose required to produce the same degree of minimal erythema reaction without sunscreen. However, most cosmetics with an SPF of 30+ also possess UVA protection qualities. Sunscreens ingredients are also regulated under a monograph and list the approved sunscreens in the following categories: inorganic sunblocks, organic UVB sunblocks, and organic UVA sunblocks. These ingredients are discussed next.

Inorganic Sunscreen Ingredients

Zinc oxide has been used by lifeguards and children for many years on noses, ear tips, upper cheeks, and shoulders. The advantage of this substance is that it is not allergenic. The disadvantage is that it is messy. With ability to manufacture microfine zinc oxide, the elegance of these formulations has improved to produce less skin whitening. The absorption spectrum of microfine zinc oxide extends from 290 to 400 nm making it a broad spectrum photoprotectant.

Titanium dioxide is also a nonallergenic broad spectrum sunblock. It is available in a small particle micronized form to improve cosmesis with a broad absorption spectrum extending from 290 to 350 nm.

Organic UVB Ingredients

p-Aminobenzoic acid (PABA) and PABA esters (Padimate O, Padimate A, glycerol PABA) were the major sunblocks in the United States until the mid-1980s. Their advantages are that they protect against the 290 to 320 nm wavelength, they are easy to work with cosmetically, the esters are nonstaining, and they bind to the horny layer. If a patient applied these 3 days in a row, he or she might still have protection on the fourth day. The disadvantages are the lack of protection for UVA, cross-sensitivity with benzoin and p-phenylenediamine, and that PABA itself may stain clothing. Today, only Padimate O is readily available. This is used primarily in hair products.

Cinnamates (octyl methoxycinnamate and cinoxate) have largely replaced PABA in many products. These are incorporated into face cosmetics yielding an SPF of 6 to 12. The cinnamates are the most commonly used sunblock in facial cosmetics.

Salicylates (homomenthyl, octyl, triethanolamine) only have an SPF of 3.5 but are excellent additions to formulations to increase SPF protection. Rarely, they may cause photodermatitis.

Octocrylene and phenylbenzimidazole sulfonic acid are two other excellent UVB chemical sunscreens. They can even stabilize avobenzone and are helpful in combination with other sunscreens.

Organic UVA Ingredients

Benzophenones were the chief UVA blockers until recently. Oxybenzone and dioxybenzone have a broad absorption spectrum of 300 to 350 nm. These ingredients are incorporated into compounds easily and are less allergenic than the PABA derivatives. There are many reports of photocontact dermatitis from oxybenzone and occasional reports of contact dermatitis and contact urticaria from dioxybenzone. The most common occurrence of the photocontact dermatitis from these products occurs with intense and very warm sun exposure such as is found near the equator. Many patients can use these products in temperate zones but react while on vacation. Physical sunblocks should then be substituted.

Avobenzone has been available since about 1989 in the United States. It has a spectrum of 310 to 400 nm, with a peak at 358 nm. Because of this spectrum, it is the sunblock of choice for all patients with special UVA needs. Of course, it must be combined with a UVB block for total protection. Octocrylene is used to stabilize the inherently unstable avobenzone allowing for the attainment of longer lasting photostable sunscreen. Ecamsule is a newer photoprotectant ingredient that can improve the broad spectrum coverage of UVA/UVB protectant formulations.

Tanning Products

Self-tanning lotions primarily consist of dihydroxyacetone (DHA). The DHA is a sugar that interacts with the skin protein to produce melanoidins that possess a brown color. The products are safe, but involve a glycation reaction. These products used to be orange and streaky but have been perfected to an even-colored tone by the addition of silicone and increased purity DHA. Self-tanning products have been formulated into sprays available at salons to cover the entire body, but the DHA preferentially adheres to skin areas of accumulated protein, such as calluses and seborrheic keratoses. When using these products, patients should exfoliate with a loofah or cleansing granules before the application to enhance color evenness.

HOW TO TEST FOR COSMETIC ALLERGY

The standard patch test for cosmetic ingredients includes: imidazolidinyl urea, wool (lanolin) alcohols, *p*-phenylenediamine, thimerosal, formaldehyde, colophony, quaternium l5, balsam of Peru, and cinnamic aldehyde. Clearly, there are more ingredients of allergenic potential in cosmetics that are not included. It is best if the Doctor learns to formulate products into patch-test samples independent of the standard patch-test tray. The cosmetics that can be tested without dilution are antiperspirants, blushes, eyeliners, eye shadow, foundations, lipstick, moisturizers, perfumes, and sunscreens. The cosmetics that are volatile and need to be allowed to dry on the patch or chamber before 48-hour occlusion are liquid eyeliner, mascara, and nail enamel. The cosmetics that need to be diluted for testing are soaps, shampoos, shaving preparations, hair dyes, and permanent solution. The doctor will need to determine if the products should be open patch tested or if use testing is more appropriate.

Suggested Readings

Adams RM, Maibach HI. A five-year study of cosmetic reactions. *J Am Acad Dermatol.* 1985;13:1062–1069.

Barel AO, ed. *Handbook of Cosmetic Science and Technology.* 3rd ed.

Darr D, Combs S, Dunston S, et al. Topical vitamin C protects porcine skin from ultraviolet radiation-induced damage. *Br J Dermatol.* 1992;127:247–253.

DeLeo V, Clark S, Fowler J, et al. A new ecamsule-containing SPF 40 sunscreen cream for the prevention of polymorphous light eruption (PMLE): a double-blind randomized, controlled study in maximized, outdoor conditions. *Cutis.* 2009;83:95–103.

Draelos ZD. Alpha-hydroxy acids and other topical agents. *Dermatol Ther.* 2000;13:154–158.

Draelos ZD. *Cosmeceuticals.* 3rd ed. Elsevier; 2015.

Draelos ZD. *Cosmetic Dermatology: Products and Procedures.* 2nd ed. Oxford: Wiley Blackwell; 2015.

Draelos ZD. Cosmetics and cosmeceuticals. In: Bolognia JL, Jorizzo JL, Rapini RP, eds. *Dermatology.* 2nd ed. St. Louis: Mosby; 2008:2304.

Elmets CA, Singh D, Tubesing K, et al. Cutaneous photoprotection from ultraviolet injury by green tea polyphenols. *J Am Acad Dermatol.* 2003;44(3):425–432.

Emerit I, Packer L, Auclair C. *Antioxidants in Therapy and Preventative Medicine.* New York: Plenum Press; 1990:594.

Guin JD. Reaction to cocamidopropyl hydroxysultaine, an amphoteric surfactant and conditioner. *Contact Dermatitis.* 2000;42(5):284.

Jackson EM. Tanning without sun: accelerators, promoters, pills, bronzing gels, and self-tanning lotions. *Am J Contact Dermat.* 1994;5(1):38.

Kligman AM, Dogadkina D, Lavker RM. Effects of topical tretinoin on non-sun-exposed protected skin of the elderly. *J Am Acad Dermatol.* 1993;29:25–33.

Kligman DE, Draelos ZD. High-strength tretinoin for rapid retinization of photoaged facial skin. *Dermatol Surg.* 2004;30(6):864–866.

Larsen WG. Perfume dermatitis. *J Am Acad Dermatol.* 1985;12(1):1–9.

Leyden J. Alpha-hydroxy acids. *Dialogue Dermatol.* 1994;34:3.

Maibach HI, Engasser PG. Dermatitis due to cosmetics. In: Fischer AA, ed. *Contact Dermatitis.* Vol 2986. 3rd ed. Philadelphia: Lea & Febiger; 1986:368–393.

O'Donoghue MN. Cosmeceuticals: bleaching agents and the controversy of hydroquinone. *Dermatol Ther.* 2007;20:307–376.

O'Donoghue MN. Hair care products. In: Olsen EA. *Disorders of Hair Growth, Diagnosis and Treatment.* 3rd ed. New York: McGraw-Hill; 2003:481–496.

Olsen EA, Katz HI, Levin N, et al. Tretinoin emollient cream for photodamaged skin: results of 48-week, multicenter, double-blind studies. *J Am Acad Dermatol.* 1997;37:217–226.

Pathak MA. Sunscreens and their use in the preventative treatment of sunlight-induced skin damage. *J Dermatol Surg Oncol.* 1987;13:739–750.

Pinnell SR. Cutaneous photodamage, oxidative stress, and topical antioxidant protection. *J Am Acad Dermatol.* 2003;48(1):1–19.

Shai A, Maibach HI, Baran R. *Handbook of Cosmetic Skin Care.* 2nd ed. London: Informa UK LTD; 2009.

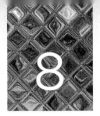

Dermatologic Allergy

Dirk M. Elston, MD and Carly Elston, MD

This chapter will discuss contact dermatitis, occupational dermatoses, atopic eczema, and drug eruptions.

CONTACT DERMATITIS

Contact dermatitis (Figs. 8-1 to 8-4) includes irritant dermatitis and allergic contact dermatitis. Irritant contact dermatitis is more common and occurs after exposure to a highly caustic substance or more commonly as a result of repetitive exposure to low-level irritants. Allergic contact dermatitis requires prior sensitization to an allergen, and then occurs after exposure to very low concentrations of the allergen. Lichenification (accentuation of skin markings, Fig. 8-1) and the histological presence of necrotic keratinocytes suggest irritant dermatitis while microvesiculation (Fig. 8-2) and the histological presence of spongiosis (Fig. 8-3) suggest allergic contact dermatitis. Patch testing will identify allergens to which an individual is allergic, but clinical correlation is required to determine the relevance of each allergen to the presenting dermatitis.

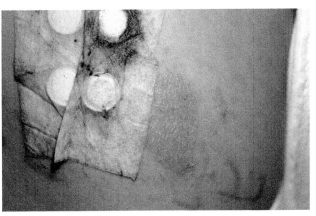

FIGURE 8-2: Positive patch test reaction. Microvesiculation is typical of allergic contact dermatitis.

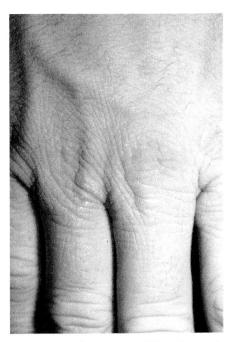

FIGURE 8-1: Lichenification resulting from chronic irritant dermatitis.

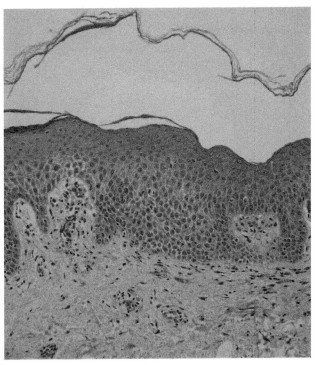

FIGURE 8-3: Spongiosis of the epidermis suggestive of allergic contact dermatitis.

Presentation

Primary Lesions

Irritant dermatitis ranges from mild redness to lichenification, bullae or necrosis depending on the strength of the irritant. Allergic contact dermatitis presents with erythema, edema, vesicles, or bullae. The reaction is usually limited to sites where the contactant touches the skin. However, when the reaction is severe, it can flare beyond these sites of contact. With poison ivy, oak, and sumac, a black stain on skin or clothing can sometimes be seen in a linear pattern where the broken stem or leaf has rubbed against the skin and deposited the oleoresin allergen (Table 8-1).

Secondary Lesions

Crusting is common as a secondary change in lesions of dermatitis. When the local site is severely affected, widespread id eruption may occur. Id reactions may be characterized by dissemination of eczematous patches or vesicles on the palms, soles, and sides of the fingers and toes.

Distribution and Causes

Any agent can affect any area of the body. However, certain agents commonly affect certain skin areas.

- *Face and neck*: cosmetics, soaps, insect sprays, ragweed, perfumes or hair sprays (sides of neck), fingernail polish (eyelids), hat bands (forehead), mouthwashes, toothpaste, lipstick (perioral), nickel metal (under earrings), necklaces and collars (neck), industrial oil (facial chloracne). Eyelid dermatitis can also be caused by topically applied antibiotic ointments (Fig. 8-4).

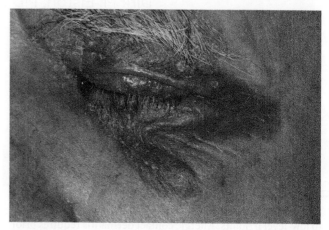

FIGURE 8-4: Allergic contact dermatitis secondary to neomycin.

TABLE 8-1 • Hanifin and Rajka Criteria for Diagnosis of Atopic Dermatitis

Major Criteria	Minor Criteria
Pruritus	Xerosis
Adults: flexural lichenification or linearity	Ichthyosis, palmar hyperlinearity
	Keratosis pilaris
Children: facial or extensor involvement	Type-I skin test reactivity elevated serum IgE
Chronic or chronically relapsing dermatitis	Early age of onset tendency toward skin infections
Atopic history, personal or familial	Nipple eczema cheilitis
	Recurrent conjunctivitis
	Dennie–Morgan fold (accentuated skin line on the lower eyelids)
	Keratoconus
	Anterior subcapsular cataracts
	Orbital darkening
	Facial pallor/facial erythema
	Pityriasis alba
	Anterior neck folds
	Pruritus with perspiration
	Intolerance to wool and lipid solvents
	Perifollicular accentuation (especially in people of color)
	Food intolerance
	Course influenced by environmental/emotional factors
	White dermatographism/delayed blanch

Note: Three major plus four or more minor criteria should be present.

- *Hands and forearms*: soaps, hand lotions, wristbands, computer wrist pads (Fig. 8-5) industrial chemicals, poison ivy, and a multitude of other agents. Irritation from soap often begins under rings as do allergic reactions from nickel (common) (dimethylglyoxime testing can be used to see if nickel is present in a metal object such as jewelry, snaps, and buckles.)

Latex from gloves can cause a contact dermatitis and contact urticarial, and rarely anaphylaxis.

- *Axillae:* Axillary vault: deodorants edges of axillae: detergents, fabric softeners, antistatic agents, and dry cleaning solutions.
- *Trunk:* clothing that is new and not previously cleaned (because it contains a formaldehyde resin), clothing with rubber or metal attached to it (commonly seen on the central abdomen from the metal clasp found in jeans and can lead to an autoeczematous reaction), and transdermal drug patches from the adhesive or the drug.
- *Anogenital region:* douches, dusting powder, diapers in infants or adults, contraceptives, colored toilet paper, topical hemorrhoid preparations, poison ivy, or topicals for treatment of pruritus ani, candida, and fungal infections.
- *Feet:* shoes (Fig. 8-6), foot powders, topical agents for athlete's foot infections.
- *Generalized eruption:* volatile airborne chemicals (paint, spray, ragweed), medicaments locally applied to large areas, bath powders, or clothing (especially if not previously washed).
- *Localized to areas of application or contact:* topical antibiotics (Figs. 8-7 and 8-8), topical antihistamines, reaction to fragrances, preservatives, and rarely even topical corticosteroids.

Course

Irritant dermatitis begins immediately after exposure, while allergic contact dermatitis appears within 2 weeks of the sensitizing exposure, and within 24 to 72 hours of subsequent

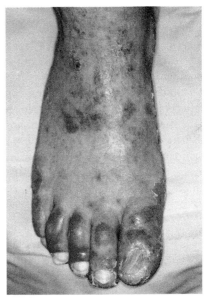

FIGURE 8-6: Allergic contact dermatitis to rubber adhesive used in shoe construction (shoe dermatitis).

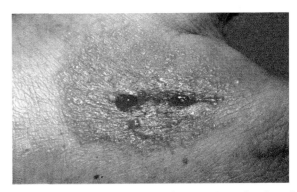

FIGURE 8-7: Allergic contact dermatitis to bacitracin ointment.

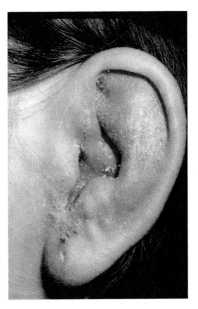

FIGURE 8-8: Allergic contact dermatitis to neomycin in ear drops.

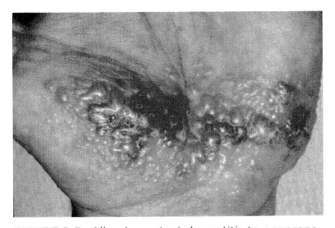

FIGURE 8-5: Allergic contact dermatitis to neoprene rubber in a computer wrist pad.

exposures (usually about 48 hours). The course of an allergic contact dermatitis is roughly 21 days after an isolated exposure. Once established in patients, hypersensitivity reactions are seldom lost. However, years of exposure without a reaction may occur before sensitization takes place.

The blister fluid of a poison ivy reaction contains no allergen, but if the poison ivy oil or other allergen remains on the clothes of the affected person, contact with those clothes of a susceptible person could cause a contact dermatitis. The hair or fur of animals, as well as utensils used in hunting or gardening, can also transfer the allergenic oleoresin of poison ivy, oak, or sumac.

Laboratory Findings

Patch tests (see Chapter 2) are valuable in eliciting the cause of a contact dermatitis. However, careful interpretation is required by the clinician. The patch tests themselves can sensitize a patient. For this reason and typicality of the eruption making a quick diagnosis, patch testing is done to poison ivy, oak, or sumac.

Differential Diagnosis

A contact reaction must be considered and ruled in or out in any case of an eczematous or oozing dermatitis on any body area. Chronic hand dermatitis (Fig. 8-9) may be a manifestation of irritant dermatitis, allergic contact dermatitis, or psoriasis.

Treatment

Treatment for allergic contact dermatitis must be continued for the full 3 week course of the dermatitis. Short courses of corticosteroids, such as a Medrol dose pack, will simply result

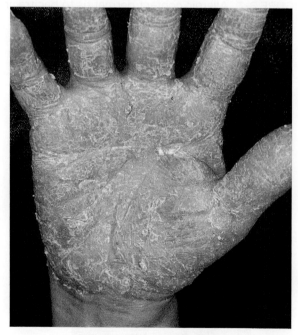

FIGURE 8-9: Chronic hand dermatitis can represent allergic contact dermatitis, irritant dermatitis, or psoriasis.

in a rebound flare of dermatitis once the drug is stopped. Editor's note: I use a 10 day course of prednisone beginning with 50 mg each AM with food and decreasing by 10 mg every 2 days and repeat if necessary.

Treatment of Contact Dermatitis Secondary to Poison Ivy

Case Example: A patient comes to the office with a linear, vesicular dermatitis of the arms and face. He states that he spent the weekend fishing and that the rash broke out the following day. The itching is rather severe but not enough to keep him awake at night. He had "poison ivy" 5 years ago.

First Visit

1. Assure the patient that he cannot pass on the dermatitis to his family or spread it on himself from the blister fluid, but that clothing and tent material used during the trip may be contaminated by the resin. Contaminated fabric should be washed in warm soapy water to remove the allergenic resin.
2. Prescribe Burow's solution to dry an active vesicular dermatitis.
   Sig: Add one packet of powder (Domeboro) to 1 quart of cool water. Wet a wash cloth with the solution and apply to the blistered areas for 20 minutes twice a day. For mild dermatitis, 1% Hydrocortisone cream (1% Hytone [available OTC]), desonide cream, 1% hydrocortisone (HC) Pramosone lotion (contains the antipruritic antihistamine pramoxine) among others. Cheaper OTC pramoxine-containing topicals (Aveeno anti-itch lotions, Sarna for sensitive skin) can also be used.
   Sig: Apply b.i.d. for itching on affected areas.
3. For more severe localized dermatitis, stronger topical corticosteroids (triamcinolone 0.1% cream, fluocinonide 0.05% cream) may be necessary.
4. For more generalized and severe dermatitis, oral prednisone, starting at about 1 mg/kg/day and tapered over 3 weeks or triamcinolone (Kenalog) intramuscular injection 40 to 60 mg IM may be required. Caution the patient about a possible change in insulin requirements in diabetics as well as elevated blood pressure, increased appetite, possible mood alterations, and insomnia.

SAUER'S NOTES

1. In obtaining a history, question the patient carefully about home, over-the-counter (OTC), other physicians', or well-meaning friends' remedies. Contact dermatitis on top of another dermatosis is quite common.
2. Determine the site of the *initial* eruption and think of the agents that touched that area.
3. When prescribing topical therapy, emphasize that all other topical medications should be stopped.

Subsequent Visits

1. Continue the wet packs only as long as there are blisters and oozing.

Barrier creams may decrease dermatitis if applied before exposure; examples include Hydropel and Ivy Block.

A window of up to 2 hours may exist where washing the skin with a surfactant (e.g., Dial soap) and oil-removing compound (e.g., soap or Goop) or a chemical inactivator (e.g., Tecnu) may ameliorate or prevent the contact dermatitis.

Treatment of Chronic Irritant Dermatitis of the Hand Related to Soap

Case Example: A young woman states that she has had a breakout on her hands for 5 weeks. The dermatitis developed about 4 weeks after the birth of her last child. She states that she had a similar eruption after her previous two pregnancies. She has used a lot of local medication of her own, and the rash is getting worse instead of better. The patient and her immediate family never had any asthma, hay fever, or eczema.

Examination of the patient's hands reveals small vesicles on the sides of all of her fingers, with lichenification and erythema with scale, worse under her wedding ring.

First Visit

1. Assure the patient that the hand eczema is not contagious to her family.
2. Inform the patient that soap irritates the skin and is contributing to the dermatitis. Protective gloves can be helpful when extended soap-and-water contact is unavoidable.
3. For body and hand cleanliness, a mild soap, such as Dove or Cetaphil soapless cleanser can be used, followed by a moisturizing cream such as CeraVe.
4. Tell the patient that these prophylactic measures must be adhered to for several weeks after the eruption has apparently cleared, or there will be a recurrence. Injured skin is sensitive and needs to be pampered for an extended time.

OCCUPATIONAL DERMATOSES

Skin disorders represent the second most common group of occupational injuries after repetitive use injury. Irritant dermatitis from chronic low-level exposure is more common than allergic contact dermatitis, but both must be considered and patch testing may be essential.

Management of Industrial Dermatitis

Case Example: A cutting-tool laborer presents with a pruritic, red, vesicular dermatitis of 2 months' duration on his hands, forearms, and face.

1. Obtain a careful, detailed history of his type of work and any recent change, such as use of new chemicals or new cleansing agents or exposure at home with hobbies, painting, and so on. Question him concerning remission of the dermatitis on weekends or while on vacation.
2. Question the patient concerning the first aid care given at the plant.
3. Ask the patient to bring in material safety data sheets for all chemicals contacted.
4. Treatment of the dermatitis with wet compresses and corticosteroids as for other causes of contact dermatitis (see previous discussion). Transferring a patient to a new job in the same work setting where exposure is less intensive may be helpful. Protective clothing such as gloves (being sure not to make the patient too awkward around dangerous machines) or protective barriers (Tetrix, EpiCeram skin barrier emulsion, Pro Q topical) can be beneficial.
5. Most patients are not malingerers, but they do expect and deserve proper care and compensation for their injuries.

ATOPIC ECZEMA

Atopic dermatitis (Fig. 8-10) is a chronic condition that begins in young childhood and can persist into adulthood.

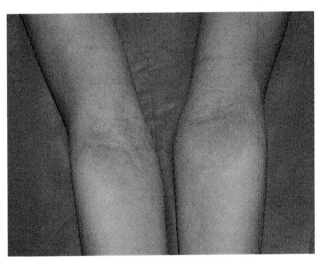

FIGURE 8-10: Atopic dermatitis presents with flexural eczema and lichenification.

Clinical Lesions

- *Infantile form:* blisters, oozing, and crusting, often involving the cheeks and hands.
- *Adolescent and adult forms:* marked dryness, flexural dermatitis, and lichenification.

Course

Atopic dermatitis has been referred to as "the itch that rashes." Patients create the skin manifestations through scratching and rubbing. The infantile form may become milder or even disappears after the age of 3 or 4 years, and approximately 70% of cases clear by puberty. During puberty and the late teenage years, flare-ups or new outbreaks can occur. Thirty percent of patients with atopic dermatitis eventually develop allergic asthma or hay fever.

Causes

The following factors are important:

- *Heredity* is the most important single factor. The family history is usually positive for one or more of the triad of allergic diseases: asthma, hay fever, or atopic eczema.
- *Dryness* of the skin is important. Most often, atopic eczema is worse in the winter owing to the decrease in home or office and outdoor humidity. For this reason, the use of soap and water should be reduced and hot water avoided. Emollients (lanolin-free) can be applied after bathing.
- *Wool* commonly irritates the skin of these patients. Wearing wool or silk clothes may be another reason for an increased incidence of atopic eczema in the winter. Cotton clothes and bed clothing are preferred.
- *Allergy to foods* is a factor that is often overstressed, particularly with the infantile form. Because these patients come from allergic families, allergies of all sorts are common, but the dermatitis is seldom directly related to a food allergy.
- *Emotional stress* aggravates the dermatitis.
- *Concomitant bacterial infection* of the skin, particularly with *Staphylococcus aureus*, is common. Antibiotics only play a role in patients with secondary infection or flares of eczema.
- *Eczema in adults without a history of eczema as a child is not as rare as used to be assumed.*

Differential Diagnosis

- *Allergic contact dermatitis*
- *Psoriasis:* patches localized to extensor surfaces, mainly knees and elbows, with characteristic thick silvery-white scales (see Chapter 16). Nail involvement is not uncommon.
- *Seborrheic dermatitis in infants:* absence of family allergy history; lesions scaly and greasy and often seen in the diaper or intertriginous areas (see Chapter 15).

Treatment of Infantile Form

Case Example: A child, aged 6 months, presents with mild oozing, red, excoriated dermatitis on face, arms, and legs.

First Visit

1. Avoid dietary restrictions, and focus on proper bathing and use of emollients.
2. Avoid exposure of the infant to excessive soaps and to contact with wool. Use mild soap sparingly in soiled areas only. Cool to lukewarm bath water, and short baths followed by liberal applications of emollients such as CeraVe, petrolatum, or Crisco shortening.
3. Corticosteroid ointments are preferred over creams or lotions. Hydrocortisone ointment, 1%, 30.0
   Sig: Apply sparingly once daily to affected areas.
   Comment: 1% Hytone ointment is in a petrolatum base without lanolin. Other proprietary corticosteroid preparations are listed in the Formulary in Chapter 4. In general, low to mid-strength corticosteroids are most appropriate and fluorinated corticosteroids are seldom needed.
4. Diphenhydramine (Benadryl) elixir 90.0 or other sedating antihistamine to help with sleep.
   Sig: Take recommended dose at bedtime.
   Comment: Warn the parent that benadryl may paradoxically stimulate the child.
5. If infection is present, treat with the appropriate systemic antibiotic, such as cephalexin, or dicloxacillin.
6. Pimecrolimus (Elidel) cream and tacrolimus (Protopic) ointment in 0.03% and 0.1% are useful nonsteroidal therapies. They can feel hot on moist skin and aggravate the acute phase of a dermatitis. An initial course of a mid-strength corticosteroid should generally be used initially.

Subsequent Visits: Assess the presence of steroid phobia as well as adherence to "soak and smear" emollient regimens.

Severe or Resistant Cases

1. A pediatric dermatologist may need to prescribe a course of prednisone or cyclosporine. Hospitalization with a change of environment may be necessary for a severe case. Various forms of ultraviolet (UV) light therapy can be helpful, including psoralens and UVA (PUVA), narrow band UVB (TL-01), and broadband UVB, especially in adults. Leukotriene inhibitors such as montelukast may be of benefit in some patients with refractory disease. Early trials with Xolair (omalizumab) and Dapilumab are promising.

NUMMULAR ECZEMA

Nummular eczema (Fig. 8-11) is a common, very pruritic, distinctive, eczematous eruption characterized by coin-shaped (nummular) scaly, vesicular or crusted patches, mainly on the arms and the legs of young and elderly patients.

Presentation

Primary Lesions

Coin-shaped patches of vesicles and papules are usually seen on the extremities and occasionally on the trunk.

Secondary Lesions

Lichenification and bacterial infection do occur.

Course

This is very chronic, particularly in older people. Recurrences are common, especially in fall and winter.

Subjective Complaints

Itching is usually quite severe.

Causes

- History is usually positive for asthma, hay fever, or atopic eczema, particularly in the young adult.
- The low indoor humidity of winter causes dry skin, which intensifies the itching, particularly in elderly patients.

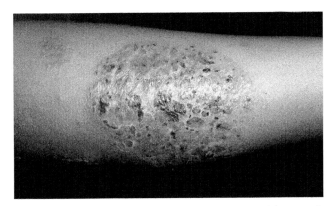

FIGURE 8-11: Nummular eczema presents with round coin-shaped lesions.

Differential Diagnosis

- *Atopic eczema:* mainly in the antecubital and popliteal fossae, not coin-sized lesions (see preceding section).
- *Psoriasis:* not vesicular; see scalp and fingernail lesions (see Chapter 16).
- *Contact dermatitis:* will not see coin-shaped lesions (see beginning of this chapter).
- *Id reaction* from stasis dermatitis of the legs or a localized contact dermatitis: impossible to differentiate this clinically, at times, from nummular eczema, but patient will have a history of previous primary localized dermatitis that suddenly became aggravated and widespread.

Treatment

Case Example: An elderly man presents in the winter with five to eight distinct, coin-shaped, excoriated, vesicular, crusted lesions on the arms and the legs.

First Visit

1. Instruct the patient to avoid excessive use of soaps.
2. Use mild cleansers such as Dove or Cetaphil, and lubricate the skin immediately after every bath or shower with an emollient such as CeraVe, aquaphor, petrolatum or Crisco shortening. Use water as cool as is tolerable to bathe.
3. Corticosteroid ointment 60.0
   Sig: Apply t.i.d. locally.
   Comment: The use of an ointment base is particularly important in the therapy for nummular eczema. Fluorinated corticosteroids are usually needed, at least initially.
   Consider Elidel and Protopic as topical nonsteroid alternatives.

Resistant Cases

1. Add coal tar solution (LCD), 3% to 10%, to the previously mentioned salve.
2. A short course of oral corticosteroid therapy is effective, but relapses are common.
   Rarely, methotrexate or cyclosporine may be required.

DRUG ERUPTIONS

Any drug is capable of causing a skin eruption (Fig. 8-12).

Side effects of topical corticosteroid abuse include: (a) Steroid rosacea. (b) Atrophy, telangiectasias, milia. (c) Purpura, atrophy. (d) Fragility with tearing and cigarette paper wrinkling atrophy.

Patients may not think of over-the-counter medications or herbal remedies of drugs, and it is important to elicit a complete history of ingestants.

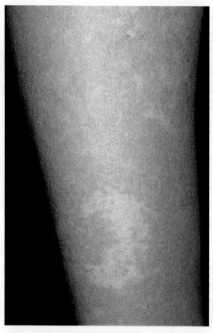

FIGURE 8-12: Morbilliform drug eruptions are commonly related to antibiotics, but drug eruptions can occur with any orally ingested agent.

SAUER'S NOTES

Any patient with a generalized skin eruption should be *carefully* questioned concerning the use of oral or parenteral medicinal drugs. For a minor nonlife-threatening drug eruption, it may not be necessary or advisable to stop a lifesaving drug. The rash may resolve on its own or be controlled with conservative therapy.

Photosensitivity reactions from drugs are covered in Chapter 40. Hepatic drug metabolism pathway involving cytochrome P-450 enzymes defines the most significant and largest group of drug-drug interactions. Adverse drug interactions must always be considered.

Drugs and Associated Dermatoses

Drug eruptions are usually not characteristic for any certain drug or group of drugs, but experience has shown that certain clinical pictures commonly follow the use of certain drugs. Common drugs causing skin eruptions are given in Table 8-2, and common skin eruptions caused by drugs are given in Table 8-3.

Course

The course of drug eruptions depends on many factors, including the type of drug, severity of the cutaneous reaction, systemic involvement, general health of the patient, and efficacy of corrective therapy. Toxic epidermal necrolysis carries a significant risk of mortality. Urticarial reactions may herald the onset of anaphylaxis, and questioning about shortness of breath or trouble swallowing may be important in these patients.

Treatment

1. Eliminate the drug. This is the single most important therapeutic intervention. This simple procedure is often delayed, with resulting serious consequences, because a careful history is not taken. If the eruption is mild and the drug necessary, discontinuation of the drug may not be mandatory.

TABLE 8-2 • Drugs and the Dermatoses They Cause

Drug	Dermatosis/Comments
Accutane	See *isotretinoin*
Acetaminophen (Tylenol)	Infrequent cause of drug eruption; urticaria and erythematous eruptions are noted. Also fixed drug eruption
Adrenocorticotropic hormones (ACTH, prednisone, IM triamcinolone)	Cushing syndrome, hyperpigmentation, acneiform eruptions, rosacea, striae, perioral dermatitis, seborrheic dermatitis–like eruptions, and hirsutism
Allopurinol (Zyloprim)	Erythema, maculopapular rash, and severe bullae (including Stevens–Johnson syndrome and toxic epidermal necrolysis)
Amantadine	Livedo reticularis
Amiodarone	Photosensitivity reaction and blue-gray discoloration of the skin
Amphetamine (Benzedrine)	Coldness of extremities; redness of the neck and shoulders; increased itching in LSC
Ampicillin	See *antibiotics*; flare of morbilliform eruption in over half of patients with infectious mononucleosis
ACE inhibitors	Maculopapular eruption with eosinophilia, pemphigus, a bullous pemphigoid–like eruption, angioedema, rosacea, urticaria, and possibly flare of psoriasis

TABLE 8-2 • Drugs and the Dermatoses They Cause (continued)

Drug	Dermatosis/Comments
Antabuse	Redness of the face and acne
Antibiotics	Various agents have different reactions, but in general: *candida overgrowth* in oral, genital, and anal orifices results in pruritus ani, pruritus vulvae, and generalized pruritus; candida skin lesions may spread out from these foci. Urticaria, morbilliform, and erythema multiforme-like eruptions, particularly from penicillin
	Ampicillin: generalized maculopapular rash, very common in patients with infectious mononucleosis
	Sulfa derivatives: particularly a problem in HIV+ patients. See *streptomycin* and the later section on photosensitivity reactions
Anticoagulants	*Coumadin and heparin*: severe hemorrhagic skin infarction and necrosis
Antineoplastic agents	Skin and mucocutaneous reactions, including alopecia, stomatitis, radiation recall reaction, and erythema
Apresoline (see *hydralazine*)	*Immediate reaction*: pruritus, urticaria, and sweating
Atabrine hydrochloride	*Delayed serum sickness reaction*: urticaria, redness, purpura
Aspirin and salicylates (a multitude of cold, flu, and anti-pain remedies; e.g., Pepto-Bismol)	Urticaria, purpura, bullous lesions
Atabrine	Universal yellow pigmentation; blue macules on the face and mucosa; lichen planus–like eruption
Atropine	Scarlet fever–like rash
Barbiturates	Urticarial, erythematous, bullous, or purpuric eruptions; fixed drug eruptions
Beta-blockers	Alopecia; psoriasis flare
Cetuximab (monoclonal antibody that binds the epidermal growth factor receptor)	Acneiform eruption 3 wk posttherapy in 90% of patients; can consider prophylactic therapy with tetracycline. Used to treat solid tumors. Follicular eruption (80%), painful fissures of fingers and toes (60%), paronychia (30%), telangiectasias, alterations of hair growth and hypopigmentation
Bleomycin	*Antitumor antibiotic*: gangrene, erythema, sclerosis, nail changes, characteristic striate lesions
Captopril	Pemphigus-like eruption; see *ACE inhibitors*
Chloroquine (Aralen)	Follicular eruption ($\frac{1}{3}$ of patients); acneiform eruptions, seborrheic eruptions, nail bed changes
Chemotherapy agents	See *antineoplastic agents;* also see specific drug
Chloral hydrate	Urticarial, papular, erythematous, and purpuric eruptions
Chloroquine (Aralen)	Erythematous or lichenoid eruptions with pruritus and urticaria; ocular retinal damage from long-term use of chloroquine and other antimalarials can be irreversible
Cimetidine	Petechial and purpuric eruptions, especially of the legs; see section on photosensitivity reactions
Chlorpromazine (Thorazine)	Morbilliform rash, increased sun sensitivity, purpura with agranulocytosis, and icterus from hepatitis
	Long-term therapy: slate-gray to violet discoloration of the skin
Cimetidine	Dry, scaly skin
Codeine and morphine	Erythematous, urticarial, or vesicular eruption
Collagen (bovine) injections	Skin edema, erythema, induration, and urticaria at implantation sites
Contraceptive drugs	Chloasma-like eruption, erythema nodosum, hives; some cases of acne are aggravated

(continued)

TABLE 8-2 • Drugs and the Dermatoses They Cause (continued)

Drug	Dermatosis/Comments
Cortisone and derivatives	Allergy (rare); see *ACTH*
Coumadin	See *anticoagulants*
Cyclosporin	Hypertrichosis, sebaceous hyperplasia, acne, folliculitis, epidermal cysts, Kaposi's sarcoma, skin precancers and cancers, gingival hyperplasia, follicular keratosis, palmoplantar paresthesias, and dysesthesias associated with temperature change
Dapsone (avlosulfone)	Red, morbilliform, vesicular eruption with agranulocytosis occurs, occasionally resembling erythema nodosum
Diltiazem	Rare. Photodistributed hyperpigmentation, subacute cutaneous LE, toxic epidermal necrolysis, Stevens–Johnson syndrome, photosensitivity, vasculitis, pruritus, urticaria, and maculopapular dermatitis
Dextran (used in peritoneal dialysis)	Urticarial reactions
Diethylpropion hydrochloride (Tenuate, Tepanil)	Measles-like eruption
Dilantin	See *phenytoin*
Epidermal growth factors	See *cetuximab, erlotinib*
Erlotinib	Follicular eruption (60%), painful fissures in the fingers and toes (40%), paronychia (40%), alterations of hair growth (30%), telangiectasias, and hyperpigmentation
Docetaxel	Cutaneous reactions: up to 70% incidence, beginning usually 2–4 d after treatment with 80% pain or itching; purple-red macules or plaques, often acral, that may peel in 3–4 wk; if worse with repeated doses, this drug may have to be stopped; local hypothermia may be ameliorative; extravasation necrosis, nail loss, supravenous discoloration, subungual abscess, skin sclerosis
	Acral erythrodysesthesia with desquamation: in a few weeks; may worsen each episode and may limit dosage
	Diffuse: (10%) mild scaly erythema with follicular accentuation; does not necessarily recur
	Intertrigo eruption: due to friction from clothing; loose-fitting clothes may help
	Melanotic macules: on trunk or extremities; stomatitis; radiation and sunburn recall
	To ameliorate reactions: 99% DMSO four times a day, oral antioxidants (vitamins E, C, A, and selenium), and oral misoprostol (prostaglandin E, analog)
Estrogenic medications	Edema of the legs with cutaneous redness progressing to exfoliative dermatitis
Feldene	See *piroxicam*
Flagyl	See *metronidazole*
Furosemide	Bullous hemorrhagic eruption
Gold	Eczematous dermatitis of the hands, arms, and legs, or a pityriasis rosea–like eruption; also, seborrheic-like eruption, urticaria, and purpura
Heparin	See *anticoagulants*
Hydralazine (Apresoline)	SLE-like reaction
Hydroxyurea	Dermopathy mimicking cutaneous findings of dermatomyositis; atrophic, erythematous dermatitis over the back of the hands that may be photo-induced; leg ulcers; hyperpigmentation, especially nails (longitudinal bands) and palms

TABLE 8-2 • Drugs and the Dermatoses They Cause (continued)

Drug	Dermatosis/Comments
Ibuprofen (Nuprin, Motrin, Advil)	Bullous eruptions, including erythema multiforme, Stevens–Johnson syndrome, toxic epidermal necrolysis, urticaria, photosensitivity, fixed drug reactions, morbilliform reactions
IVIG (intravenous IgG infusion)	Pompholyx (dyshidrosis)-like eruption 5–7 d after treatment can evolve into a generalized eczematous eruption
Icodextrin (used in peritoneal dialysis)	Psoriasiform dermatosis, acute generalized exanthematous pustulosis
Imipramine	Slate-gray discoloration of the skin
Insulin	Urticaria with serum sickness symptoms; fat atrophy at the injection site
Interferon alpha plus ribavirin for Hepatitis C	Pruritus, xerosis, alopecia, hyperpigmentation, photoallergy, exacerbation of psoriasis and lichen planus, skin necrosis, sarcoidosis, eczematous dermatitis at injection site reaction and possibly erythema gyratum repens
Iodides	See *bromides;* papular, pustular, ulcerative, or granulomatous lesions mainly on acne areas or the legs; administration of chloride hastens recovery
Isoniazid	Erythematous and maculopapular, generalized, purpuric, bullous, and nummular eczema–like; acne aggravation
Isotretinoin	Dry red skin and lips (common); alopecia (rare)
Lasix	See *furosemide*
Lamotrigine	At least 10% with cutaneous drug reactions; may be similar to phenytoin cutaneous drug reactions
Lithium	Acne-like lesions on the body; psoriasis exacerbation
Meclizine hydrochloride (Antivert)	Urticaria
Meprobamate	Small purpuric lesions, erythema multiforme-like eruption
Metronidazole (Flagyl)	Urticaria, pruritus
Minocycline	Skin (muddy skin syndrome), teeth, and scar discoloration
	Rare: hypersensitivity, sickness-like reaction, drug-induced lupus erythematosus, SLE-like syndrome, autoimmune hepatitis, p-ANCA–positive cutaneous polyarteritis nodosa, elastosis perforans serpiginosum, localized cutis laxa, pseudoxanthoma elasticum, anetoderma (primary anetoderma has been associated with antiphospholipid syndrome), bullous pemphigoid
Pentazocine venous	When used as an abused substance it causes deep ulcers along venous access sites with surrounding hyperpigmented woody induration, fibrous myopathy, and puffy hand syndrome
Phenolphthalein (found in 4 Way Cold Tablets, ex-lax, bile salts, and pink icing on cakes)	*Rare syndrome:* hepatitis, exfoliative dermatitis, fever, lymphadenopathy, eosinophilia, lymphocytosis
Morphine	See *codeine;* lichen planus–like eruption; fixed drug eruption, photosensitivity
Nevirapine	Unusually high incidence of potentially life-threatening Stevens–Johnson syndrome; urticaria, erythema multiforme-like eruption, toxic epidermal necrolysis
Penicillin	See *antibiotics*
Procainamide	Lupus-like rash, lichen planus–like rash, pemphigus foliaceus
Psoralens	*Fixed drug eruption:* hyperpigmented or purplish, flat or slightly elevated, discrete, single or multiple patches
	See section on photosensitivity reactions

(continued)

TABLE 8-2 • Drugs and the Dermatoses They Cause (continued)

Drug	Dermatosis/Comments
Phenytoin (Dilantin)	Hypertrophy of gums, erythema multiforme-like eruption; pseudo-lymphoma syndrome, morbilliform reaction
	Fetal hydantoin syndrome: organ defects plus nail hypoplasia
	Note: one of the most common causes of toxic epidermal necrolysis or Stevens–Johnson syndrome along with other antiseizure medications
Propranalol (Inderal)	*Rare*: drug eruption; See *beta-blockers*
Sirolimus	Acneiform eruption that may be recalcitrant to therapy
Psoralens	See section on photosensitivity reactions
Quinidine	Edema, purpura, scarlatiniform eruption; may progress to exfoliative dermatitis
Quinine	Diffuse eruption (any kind)
Rauwolfia alkaloids (reserpine)	Urticaria, photosensitivity reactions, petechial eruptions
Rifampin	Pruritus, urticaria, acne, bullous pemphigoid, mucositis, exfoliative erythroderma, red urine, reddened soft contact lenses
Salicylates	See *aspirin*
Streptomycin	Urticaria; erythematous, morbilliform, and purpuric eruptions
Sulfonamides	Urticaria, scarlatiniform eruption, erythema nodosum, eczematous flare of exudative dermatitis, erythema multiforme-like bullous eruption, fixed eruption; see later section on photosensitivity reactions, morbilliform reaction
	AIDS patients: develop allergic drug eruptions quite often; one of the most common causes of toxic epidermal necrolysis and Stevens–Johnson syndrome
Sulfonylureas	See *sulfonamides* and section on photosensitivity reactions
Suramin	Cutaneous reaction (80%), especially morbilliform, UV light recall (skin eruptions at sites of previous UV exposure), urticaria, "suramin keratoses"
Taxanes (paclitaxel, docetaxel)	Scleroderma-like skin changes, fixed drug, onycholysis, acral erythema, erythema multiforme, pustular eruptions
Tyrosine kinase inhibitors (cetuximab [Erbitux], gefitinib [Iressa], erlotinib [Tarceva], imatinib [Gleevec], panitumumab (Vectibix 90% incidence)	Persistent folliculitis with attributes of both acne and pemphigus in 75% of patients.
Testosterone and related drugs	Acne-like lesions, alopecia in scalp, hirsutism
Tetracycline	Fixed drug eruption, photosensitivity, serum sickness–like reaction Patients <8 y old: teeth staining; see *antibiotics*
Thalidomide	Erythroderma, pustulosis, toxic epidermal necrolysis
Thiazides	See section on photosensitivity reactions
Trimethoprim	Rarely incriminated in drug eruptions
Tumor necrosis factor alpha inhibitors	Psoriasis, vasculitis, lupus-like syndrome, dermatomyositis, and numerous skin infections, most notably Staph. aureus including methicillin resistant Staph. aureus infection
Vitamin A	*Long-term, high-dose therapy*: scaly, rough, itchy skin with coarse, dry, scant hair growth, and systemic changes including liver toxicity
Vitamin D	Skin lesions rare, but headache, nausea, diarrhea, increased urination, and sore gums and joints can be present

TABLE 8-2 • Drugs and the Dermatoses They Cause (continued)

Drug	Dermatosis/Comments
Vitamin B group	Urticaria, pruritic redness, and even anaphylactic reactions can occur after IM or IV administration
	Nicotinic acid: red flush (common—warn patient to eliminate unnecessary alarm), pruritus (common), hives (rare, within 15–30 min of oral ingestion of 50–100 mg)
Warfarin sodium	See *anticoagulants*

Abbreviations: ACTH, adrenocorticotropic hormone; ACE, angiotensin-converting enzyme; DMSO, dimethyl sulfoxide; IM, intramuscular; LSC, lichen simplex chronicus; p-ANCA, perinuclear anti-neutrophil cytoplasmic antibodies; SLE, systemic lupus erythematosus; UV, ultraviolet.

TABLE 8-3 • Dermatoses and the Drugs That Cause Them

Dermatosis	Drug(s)	Comments
Acne-like or pustular lesions	Bromides, iodides, lithium, testosterone, corticosteroids	
Acral erythema	Redness, pain, and swelling of the hands and feet associated with various chemotherapeutic agents including cyclophosphamide, cytosine arabinoside, docetaxel, doxorubicin, fluorouracil, hydroxyurea, mercaptopurine, methotrexate, and mitotane	Most commonly cytarabine, doxorubicin, and fluorouracil Chemotherapy can be continued or briefly interrupted with use of topical corticosteroids
Acute generalized exanthematous pustulosis (AGEP)	Antibiotics especially beta-lactam, (includes penicillin and cephalosporin) can also be caused by viral infections (enterovirus), ultraviolet radiation, and heavy metal exposure (mercury)	It is a severe cutaneous reaction with nonfollicular, pinhead sized pustules, erythema, edema, fever, leukocytosis with neutrophilia. It usually resolves when the causative agent is stopped but it can develop into a toxic epidermal necrolysis-like syndrome.
Actinic keratosis inflammation occurring in patients on systemic chemotherapy	First described with fluorouracil; also doxorubicin, cisplatin, fludarabine, dactinomycin, dacarbazine, and vincristine sulfate	
Alopecia	Amethopterin (methotrexate) and other antineoplastic agents; colchicine, clofibrate, testosterone and other androgens; tricyclic antidepressants; beta-blockers; heparin; progesterone derivatives; coumarin derivatives; isotretinoin	
Angioedema	Aspirin, NSAIDs, ACE inhibitors	
Baboon syndrome	Mercury (most often); also ampicillin, amoxicillin, nickel, erythromycin, heparin, and food additives	Systemic contact dermatitis owing to ingestion, inhalation, or percutaneous absorption; symmetric diffuse acute light red exanthema on the buttocks, anogenital area, major flexural areas of the extremities; peaks at day 2–5 of exposure to the involved drug; resolves within 1 wk

(continued)

TABLE 8-3 • Dermatoses and the Drugs That Cause Them (continued)

Dermatosis	Drug(s)	Comments
DIDMOHS (drug-induced delayed [3–6 wk] multiorgan hypersensitivity syndrome of Sontheimer and Houpt; also called DRESS [drug rash with eosinophilia and systemic symptoms of Bocquet and Roujeau])	Dapsone, carbamazepine, phenobarbital, minocycline, trimethoprim, sulfamethoxazole, procarbazine, allopurinol, terbinafine, thiazide diuretics, diphenylhydantoin	Exanthematous or papulopustular febrile eruption with hepatitis (also possible lung, renal, and thyroid involvement), lymphadenopathy, and eosinophilia
Eczematous eruption	Quinine, antihistamines, gold, mercury, sulfonamides, penicillin, organic arsenic	
Erythema annulare centrifugum	Salicylates, antimalarials, amitriptyline, gold, etizolam	Proximal extremities and trunk with red advancing circinate plaques that may have a dry fine adherent scale in the inner spreading edge. Can be associated with underlying infections, hormonal abnormalities, and underlying malignancies
Erythema multiforme—like eruption	Penicillin and other antibiotics, sulfonamides, phenolphthalein, barbiturates, phenytoin, meprobamate	
Erythema nodosum–like eruption	Sulfonamides, iodides, salicylates, oral contraceptives, dapsone	
Exfoliative dermatitis	Particularly owing to arsenic, penicillin, sulfonamides, allopurinol, barbiturates	In the course of any severe generalized drug eruption
Fixed drug eruption	Phenolphthalein, acetaminophen, barbiturates, organic arsenic, gold, salicylates, sulfonamides, tetracycline, many others	*Fixed drug eruption*: hyperpigmented or purplish; flat or slightly elevated; discrete, single, or multiple patches. Occurs at the same sites on drug challenge
Hyperpigmentation	Contraceptives, atabrine, chloroquine, minocycline, chlorpromazine, amiodarone, bismuth, and gold, silver salts, ACTH, estrogen, adriamycin, AZT, methotrexate	
Hypertrichosis	Oral minoxidil, phenytoin, cyclosporine *Less severe*: oral contraceptives, systemic corticosteroids, psoralens, streptomycin sulfate	
Ichthyosis	Cimetidine, clofazimine, hydroxyurea, cholesterol-lowering agents, nicotinic acid, coenzyme A reductase inhibitors, triparanol	
Keratoses and epitheliomas	Arsenic, mercury, PUVA therapy, immunosuppressive agents	
Lichen planus–like eruption	Atabrine, arsenic, naproxen, gold, others	
Lupus erythematosus	Minocycline, hydralazine, procainamide, isoniazid, chlorpromazine, diltiazem, quinidine	

TABLE 8-3 • Dermatoses and the Drugs That Cause Them (continued)

Dermatosis	Drug(s)	Comments
Linear IgA bullous dermatosis	Vancomycin (most common), furosemide, captopril, lithium, amiodarone, diclofenac, cefamandole, somatostatin, rifampin, topical iodine, phenytoin, trimethoprim, sulfamethoxazole, penicillin G, IL-2, interferon-γ	Often all of mucous membranes and it is very heterogeneous in its cutaneous manifestations. Direct immunofluorescence of perilesional skin shows linear IgA at the basement membrane zone and also occasionally IgG and C3. The diagnosis of drug-induced linear IgA bullous dermatosis is based largely on recent exposure to commonly offending drugs
Lipoatrophies from injections	Corticosteroids (e.g., triamcinolone), insulin, vasopressin, human growth hormone, iron dextran, diphtheria–pertussis–tetanus (DPT) immunization serum, antihistamines, Talwin injection usually due to abuse	
Lipodystrophy	Partial: proteinase inhibitors used to treat AIDS–indinavir or ritonavir plus saquinavir cause decreased subcutaneous fat on the face (cadaveric or cachectic facies) and extremities (pseudomuscular appearance) with increased prominence of the superficial veins, central adiposity with increased abdominal girth (pseudo-obesity), enlargement of breasts, increased dorsal-cervical fat pads (buffalo hump or pseudo-Cushing syndrome)	Increased triglyceride and LDL cholesterol and low HDL cholesterol also occurs
Measles-like eruption	Barbiturates, arsenic, sulfonamides, quinine, many others	
Mucous membrane lesions	*Pigmentation*: bismuth	
	Hypertrophy: phenytoin	
	Erosive lesions: sulfonamides, antineoplastic agents, many other drugs	
Nail changes	*Onycholysis* (distal detachment): tetracycline, apparently owing to a phototoxic reaction	
Neutrophilic eccrine hidradenitis	Bleomycin, chlorambucil, cyclophosphamide, cytarabine, doxorubicin, lomustine, mitoxantrone	
Nicolau syndrome (embolia cutis medicamentosa)	Diclofenac, ibuprofen, iodine, benzathine penicillin, vitamin K, DPT immunizations, antihistamines, interferon-α, corticosteroids	At IM injection site; see Dictionary–Index
Nummular eczema–like eruption	Combination of isoniazid and p-aminosalicylic acid	
Necrosis of the skin	*Localized*: coumarin and heparin derivatives (subcutaneous or intravenous); recombinant interferon-γ	
	Distant: coumarin and heparin derivatives	

(continued)

TABLE 8-3 • Dermatoses and the Drugs That Cause Them (continued)

Dermatosis	Drug(s)	Comments
Ochronosis, exogenous	Topical phenol, quinine injections, topical resorcinol *With prolonged use*: topical hydroquinone, mainly in dark-skinned patients only at the site of application	
Palmoplantar erythrodysesthesia	Chemotherapeutic agents, especially doxorubicin, docetaxel, fluorouracil and cytarabine. Also, epidermal growth factor inhibitors such as sunitinib	Clinically there is tender erythema and swelling of the fingers, toes, palms, and soles. Sometimes there are blisters. Histologically there may be eccrine syringosquamous metaplasia, neutrophilic eccrine hidradenitis or changes similar to graft-vs-host disease
Pemphigoid-like lesions	Furosemide, penicillin, sulfasalazine, ibuprofen	
Pemphigus-like lesions	Rifampin, penicillamine, captopril, pyrazolone derivatives	
Photosensitivity reaction	*Sulfonamides*: sulfonylurea *Hypoglycemics*: tolbutamide (Orinase), chlorpropamide (Diabinese) *Antibiotics*: demethylchlortetracycline (Declomycin), doxycycline (Doryx, Monodox, Vibramycin), griseofulvin (Fulvicin, Grifulvin, Gris-PEG), maxaquin (Lomefloxacin), nalidixic acid (NegGram), tetracycline *Benzofurans*: amiodarone *Chlorothiazide diuretics*: chlorothiazide (Diuril); hydrochlorothiazide; methyclothiazide *Phenothiazines*: chlorpromazine (Thorazine); prochlorperazine (Compazine); promethazine (Phenergan) *Psoralens*: methoxsalen (Oxsoralen); trioxsalen (Trisoralen) *Oxicams*: piroxicam (Feldene)	Several of the newer drugs and some of the older ones cause dermatitis upon exposure to sunlight. These skin reactions can be urticarial, erythematous, vesicular, or plaque-like. The mechanism can be either phototoxic or photoallergic, but this distinction can be difficult to ascertain. This list of *photosensitizing drugs* is rather complete, but also see Chapter 40
Pityriasis rosea-like eruption	Bismuth, gold, barbiturates, antihistamines also see Chapter 40	
Porphyria cutanea tarda exacerbation	Estrogen, iron, ethanol ingestion, hexachlorobenzene, chlorinated phenols, polychlorinated biphenyls; possibly pravastatin	

TABLE 8-3 • Dermatoses and the Drugs That Cause Them (continued)

Dermatosis	Drug(s)	Comments
Pseudolymphoma	Antidepressants, diphenylhydantoin, α-agonists, ACE inhibitors, anticonvulsants, antihistamines, benzodiazepine, beta blockers, calcium channel blockers, lipid-lowering agents, lithium, NSAIDs, phenothiazines, procainamide, estrogen, progesterone	
Pseudoporphyria cutanea tarda (PCT)	NSAIDs (naproxen, nabumetone, oxaprozin, ketoprofen, mefenamic acid, diflunisal), nalidixic acid, tetracycline, chlorothalidone, furosemide, hydrochlorothiazide/triamterene, isotretinoin, etretinate, cyclosporine, 5-fluorouracil, pyridoxine, amiodarone, flutamide, dapsone, aspirin	Skin findings but no biochemical abnormalities. May persist for months after offending drug is stopped, mimics skin findings and skin biopsy of PCT
Psoriasis exacerbation	Lithium, beta-blockers, ACE inhibitors, antimalarials, NSAIDs, terbinafine	
Purpuric eruptions	Barbiturates, salicylates, meprobamate, organic arsenic, sulfonamides, chlorothiazide diuretics, corticosteroids (long-term use)	
Radiation recall	Chemotherapeutic agents, antituberculous medications, Simvastatin, interferon alpha 2b	
Rheumatoid nodulosis, accelerated	Methotrexate	Painful nodules mainly on the hands in long-standing rheumatoid arthritis patients. Dissipates after the drug is stopped.
Scarlet fever–like eruption or "toxic erythema"	Arsenic, barbiturates, codeine, morphine, mercury, quinidine, salicylates, sulfonamides, others	
Seborrheic dermatitis–like eruption	Gold, ACTH	
Stevens–Johnson syndrome	Lamotrigine, valproic acid, penicillin, barbiturates, diphenylhydantoin, sulfonamides, rifampin, NSAIDs, salicylates	
Subacute cutaneous lupus erythematosus	Hydrochlorothiazide, ACE inhibitors, calcium channel blockers, interferons, statins	
Urticaria	Penicillin, salicylates, sera, sulfonamides, barbiturates, opium group, contraceptive drugs, Rauwolfia alkaloids, ACE inhibitors	
Vesicular or bullous eruptions	Sulfonamides, penicillin, mephenytoin	
Whitening of the hair	Chloroquine, hydroxychloroquine	In blonde- or red-haired people

Abbreviations: ACE, angiotensin-converting enzyme; AGEP, acute generalized exanthematous pustulosis; ACTH, adrenocorticotropic hormone; HDL, high-density lipoprotein; IM, intramuscular; LDL, low-density lipoprotein; NSAID, nonsteroidal anti-inflammatory drugs; PUVA, psoralens, and ultraviolet light; AZT, zidovudine.

2. Further therapy depends on the seriousness of the eruption. Morbilliform drug eruptions (measles-like) are the most common type and may resolve with no therapy. An itching drug eruption should be treated with a topical agent such as pramoxine.

3. Toxic epidermal necrolysis is best managed in a burn unit, as fluid and electrolyte balance and monitoring for sepsis are key components of therapy. Intravenous immunoglobulin G has been used in this setting, but data are mixed. Systemic corticosteroids are controversial and best avoided, whereas data on cyclosporine use looks promising. Discontinuation of the offending drug in a timely manner is the most important prognostic factor and can be lifesaving and vision-saving.

SAUER'S NOTES

1. When confronted with any diffuse or puzzling eruption, routinely question the patient regarding *any* medication taken by *any* route.

2. Ask: "Are you taking any vitamins, laxatives, nerve pills, and so forth?" This jogs the patient's memory. Nonsteroidal drugs are used so commonly that you may need to ask specifically about exposure to these drugs.

3. Remember, any ingested chemical agent can cause an eruption, such as toothpaste, mouthwash, breath freshener, and chewing gum.

4. Antiseizure medications, antibiotics, sulfa and sulfa-related drugs, nonsteroidal anti-inflammatory drugs, and allopurinol cause the majority of cutaneous drug eruptions.

All images for this chapter were produced while the author was a full time federal employee. They are in the public domain.

Suggested Readings

Basketter D, Safford B. Skin sensitization quantitative risk assessment: a review of underlying assumptions. *Regul Toxicol Pharmacol*. 2016;74:105–116.

Basketter DA, White IR, McFadden JP, et al. Skin sensitization: implications for integration of clinical data into hazard identification and risk assessment. *Hum Exp Toxicol*. 2015;34(12):1222–1230.

Bhat YJ, Zeerak S, Hassan I. Allergic contact dermatitis to eye drops. *Indian J Dermatol*. 2015;60(6):637.

Brod BA, Treat JR, Rothe MJ, et al. Allergic contact dermatitis: kids are not just little people. *Clin Dermatol*. 2015;33(6):605–612.

Burkhart C, Schloemer J, Zirwas M. Differentiation of latex allergy from irritant contact dermatitis. *Cutis*. 2015;96(6):369, 371, 401.

Dotson GS, Maier A, Siegel PD, et al. Setting occupational exposure limits for chemical allergens-understanding the challenges. *J Occup Environ Hyg*. 2015;12(suppl 1):S82–S98.

Fonacier L. A practical guide to patch testing. *J Allergy Clin Immunol Pract*. 2015;3(5):669–675.

Goldenberg A, Silverberg N, Silverberg JI, et al. Pediatric allergic contact dermatitis: lessons for better care. *J Allergy Clin Immunol Pract*. 2015;3(5):661–667.

Malik M, English J. Irritant hand dermatitis in health care workers. *Occup Med (Lond)*. 2015;65(6):474–476.

Mobolaji-Lawal M, Nedorost S. The role of textiles in dermatitis: an update. *Curr Allergy Asthma Rep*. 2015;15(4):17.

Montgomery R, Stocks SJ, Wilkinson SM. Contact allergy resulting from the use of acrylate nails is increasing in both users and those who are occupationally exposed. *Contact Dermatitis*. 2016;74(2):120–122.

Sipahi H, Charehsaz M, Güngör Z, et al. Risk assessment of allergen metals in cosmetic products. *J Cosmet Sci*. 2015;66(5):313–323.

Stollery N. Allergic reactions. *Practitioner*. 2015;259(1785):34–35.

Wentworth AB, Yiannias JA, Davis MD, et al. Benzalkonium chloride: a known irritant and novel allergen. *Dermatitis*. 2016;27(1):14–20.

Wingfield Digby SS, Thyssen JP. How should we advise patients with allergic contact dermatitis caused by (meth-)acrylates about future dental work? *Contact Dermatitis*. 2016;74(2):116–117.

Wittenberg JB, Canas BJ, Zhou W, et al. Determination of methylisothiazolinone and methylchloroisothiazolinone in cosmetic products by ultra high performance liquid chromatography with tandem mass spectrometry. *J Sep Sci*. 2015;38(17):2983–2988.

Drug Eruptions

Chia-Yu Chu, MD, PhD

The skin is among the parts of the body most commonly affected by adverse drug reactions. Eruptions are observed in 0.1% to 1% of patients treated with most drugs. As such, drug-induced skin eruptions or drug eruptions are relatively common, affecting 2% to 3% of hospitalized patients.

Serious cutaneous drug reactions, as defined by the WHO, occur in approximately 0.1% of these patients, and can lead to disabling sequelae. The incidence of fatalities due to systemic and cutaneous drug reactions among inpatients is estimated at between 0.1% and 0.3%.

Drug eruptions are usually not characteristic for any specific drug or group of drugs, but experience has shown that certain clinical pictures commonly follow the use of certain drugs. A list of drugs that commonly cause skin eruptions is provided in Table 9-1, and a list of skin eruptions that are commonly caused by drugs is provided in Table 9-2.

TABLE 9-1 • Drugs and the Dermatoses They Cause

Drug	Dermatosis/Comments
Accutane	See *isotretinoin*
Acetaminophen (Tylenol)	Infrequent cause of drug eruption; urticaria and erythematous eruptions are noted. Also AGEP and fixed drug eruption.
Adrenocorticotropic hormones (ACTH, prednisone, IM triamcinolone)	Cushing syndrome, hyperpigmentation, acneiform eruptions, rosacea, striae, perioral dermatitis, seborrheic dermatitis–like eruptions, and hirsutism
Afatinib	Follicular eruption (90%), painful fissures in the fingers and toes, paronychia (40%–50%), xerosis, pruritus, alterations of hair growth (trichomegaly, curly hair), telangiectasias, and hyperpigmentation
Allopurinol (Zyloprim)	Erythema, maculopapular rash, DRESS and severe bullae (including Stevens–Johnson syndrome and toxic epidermal necrolysis)
Amantadine	Livedo reticularis
Amiodarone	Photosensitivity reaction and blue-gray discoloration of the skin
Amphetamine (Benzedrine)	Coldness of extremities; redness of the neck and shoulders; increased itching in LSC
Ampicillin	See *antibiotics*; flare of morbilliform eruption in over half of patients with infectious mononucleosis
ACE inhibitors	Maculopapular eruption with eosinophilia, pemphigus, a bullous pemphigoid-like eruption, angioedema, rosacea, urticaria, and possibly flare of psoriasis
Antabuse	Redness of the face and acne
Antibiotics	Various agents have different reactions, but in general: *candida overgrowth* in oral, genital, and anal orifices results in pruritus ani, pruritus vulvae, and generalized pruritus; candida skin lesions may spread out from these foci. Urticaria, morbilliform, and erythema multiforme-like eruptions, particularly from penicillin; DRESS, SJS, and TEN
	Ampicillin: generalized maculopapular rash, very common in patients with infectious mononucleosis
	Sulfa derivatives: particularly a problem in HIV+ patients. See *streptomycin* and the later section on photosensitivity reactions; DRESS, SJS, and TEN

(continued)

TABLE 9-1 • Drugs and the Dermatoses They Cause (*continued*)

Drug	Dermatosis/Comments
Anticoagulants	*Coumadin and heparin*: severe hemorrhagic skin infarction and necrosis
Antineoplastic agents	Skin and mucocutaneous reactions, including alopecia, stomatitis, radiation recall reaction, and acral erythema
Apresoline (see *hydralazine*)	*Immediate reaction*: pruritus, urticaria, and sweating
Atabrine hydrochloride	*Delayed serum sickness reaction*: urticaria, redness, purpura
Aspirin and salicylates (a multitude of cold, flu, and antipain remedies; e.g., Pepto-Bismol)	Angioedema, urticaria, purpura, and bullous lesions
Atabrine	Universal yellow pigmentation; blue macules on the face and mucosa; lichen planus–like eruption
Atropine	Scarlet fever–like rash
Barbiturates	Urticarial, erythematous, bullous, or purpuric eruptions; fixed drug eruptions
β-blockers	Alopecia; psoriasis flare
Bleomycin	*Antitumor antibiotic*: gangrene, erythema, sclerosis, nail changes, characteristic striate lesions
Captopril	Pemphigus-like eruption; see *ACE inhibitors*
Carbamazepine	Maculopapular eruption, DRESS, SJS, and TEN
Cetuximab (monoclonal antibody that binds the epidermal growth factor receptor)	Acneiform eruption or follicular eruption (80%), painful fissures of fingers and toes (60%), paronychia (30%), telangiectasias, alterations of hair growth and hypopigmentation
Chemotherapy agents	See *antineoplastic agents;* also see specific drug
Chloral hydrate	Urticarial, papular, erythematous, and purpuric eruptions
Chloroquine (Aralen)	Erythematous or lichenoid eruptions with pruritus and urticaria; ocular retinal damage from long-term use of chloroquine and other antimalarials can be irreversible
Chlorpromazine (Thorazine)	Maculopapular rash, increased sun sensitivity, purpura with agranulocytosis, and icterus from hepatitis
	Long-term therapy: slate-gray to violet discoloration of the skin
Cimetidine	Dry, scaly skin
Codeine and morphine	Erythematous, urticarial, or vesicular eruption
Collagen (bovine) injections	Skin edema, erythema, induration, and urticaria at implantation sites
Contraceptive drugs	Chloasma-like eruption, erythema nodosum, urticaria; some cases of acne are aggravated
Cortisone and derivatives	Allergy (rare); see *ACTH*
Coumadin	See *anticoagulants*
Cyclosporin	Hypertrichosis, sebaceous hyperplasia, acne, folliculitis, epidermal cysts, Kaposi's sarcoma, skin precancers and cancers, gingival hyperplasia, follicular keratosis, palmoplantar paresthesias, and dysesthesias associated with temperature change
Dapsone (avlosulfone)	Maculopapular eruption, DRESS, SJS, and TEN; occasionally erythema nodosum
Diltiazem	Rare. Photodistributed hyperpigmentation, AGEP, subacute cutaneous LE, SJS, TEN, photosensitivity, vasculitis, pruritus, urticaria, and maculopapular eruption
Dextran (used in peritoneal dialysis)	Urticarial reactions
Diethylpropion hydrochloride (Tenuate, Tepanil)	Measles-like eruption

TABLE 9-1 • Drugs and the Dermatoses They Cause (*continued*)

Drug	Dermatosis/Comments
Dilantin	See *phenytoin*
Docetaxel	Cutaneous reactions: up to 70% incidence, beginning usually 2–4 d after treatment with 80% pain or itching; acral erythema; recall dermatitis; extravasation necrosis, nail loss, supravenous discoloration, subungual abscess, skin sclerosis
	Acral erythrodysesthesia with desquamation: in a few weeks; may worsen each episode and may limit dosage
	Diffuse: (10%) mild scaly erythema with follicular accentuation; does not necessarily recur
	Intertrigo eruption: due to friction from clothing; loose-fitting clothes may help
	Melanotic macules: on trunk or extremities; stomatitis; radiation and sunburn recall
Erlotinib	Follicular eruption (60%), painful fissures in the fingers and toes (40%), paronychia (40%), alterations of hair growth (30%; trichomegaly, curly hair), telangiectasias, and hyperpigmentation
Estrogenic medications	Edema of the legs with cutaneous redness progressing to exfoliative dermatitis
Feldene	See *piroxicam*
Flagyl	See *metronidazole*
Furosemide	Bullous hemorrhagic eruption, drug-induced pemphigoid
Gold	Eczematous dermatitis of the hands, arms, and legs, or a pityriasis rosea-like eruption; also, seborrheic-like eruption, urticaria, and purpura
Heparin	See *anticoagulants*
Hydralazine (Apresoline)	SLE-like reaction
Hydroxyurea	Dermopathy mimicking cutaneous findings of dermatomyositis; atrophic, erythematous dermatitis over the back of the hands that may be photo-induced; leg ulcers; hyperpigmentation, especially nails (longitudinal bands) and palms
Ibuprofen (Nuprin, Motrin, Advil)	Urticaria, photosensitivity, fixed drug reactions, morbilliform reactions, DRESS, SJS, and TEN
IVIG (intravenous IgG infusion)	Pompholyx (dyshidrosis)-like eruption 5–7 d after treatment can evolve into a generalized eczematous eruption
Icodextrin (used in peritoneal dialysis)	Psoriasiform dermatosis, acute generalized exanthematous pustulosis
Imipramine	Slate-gray discoloration of the skin
Insulin	Urticaria with serum sickness symptoms; fat atrophy at the injection site
Iodides	See *bromides;* papular, pustular, ulcerative, or granulomatous lesions mainly on acne areas or the legs; administration of chloride hastens recovery
Isoniazid	Erythematous and maculopapular, generalized, purpuric, bullous, and nummular eczema–like; acne aggravation
Isotretinoin	Dry red skin and lips (common); alopecia (rare)
Lasix	See *furosemide*
Lamotrigine	At least 10% with cutaneous drug reactions; maculopapular eruption, DRESS, SJS, and TEN
Lithium	Acne-like lesions on the body; psoriasis exacerbation
Meclizine hydrochloride (Antivert)	Urticaria

(*continued*)

TABLE 9-1 • Drugs and the Dermatoses They Cause (*continued*)

Drug	Dermatosis/Comments
Meprobamate	Small purpuric lesions, erythema multiforme-like eruption
Metronidazole (Flagyl)	Urticaria, pruritus
Minocycline	Skin (muddy skin syndrome), teeth, and scar discoloration
	Rare: hypersensitivity, DRESS, sickness-like reaction, drug-induced lupus erythematosus, SLE-like syndrome, autoimmune hepatitis, p-ANCA–positive cutaneous polyarteritis nodosa, elastosis perforans serpiginosum, localized cutis laxa, pseudoxanthoma elasticum, anetoderma (primary anetoderma has been associated with antiphospholipid syndrome), bullous pemphigoid
Pentazocine	When used as an abused substance it causes deep ulcers along venous access sites with surrounding hyperpigmented woody induration, fibrous myopathy, and puffy hand syndrome
Phenolphthalein (found in 4-way Cold Tablets, ex-lax, bile salts, and pink icing on cakes)	*Rare syndrome*: hepatitis, exfoliative dermatitis, fever, lymphadenopathy, eosinophilia, lymphocytosis
Morphine	See *codeine;* lichen planus–like eruption; fixed drug eruption, photosensitivity
Nevirapine	Unusually high incidence of potentially life-threatening SJS, TEN; urticaria
Oxcarbazepine	Maculopapular eruption, DRESS, SJS, and TEN
Penicillin	See *antibiotics*
Procainamide	Lupus-like rash, lichen planus–like rash, pemphigus foliaceus
Psoralens	*Fixed drug eruption*: hyperpigmented or purplish, flat or slightly elevated, discrete, single or multiple patches
	See section on photosensitivity reactions
Phenytoin (Dilantin)	Hypertrophy of gums, maculopapular eruption, DRESS, SJS, and TEN
	Fetal hydantoin syndrome: organ defects plus nail hypoplasia
	Note: one of the most common causes of DRESS, SJS, and TEN along with other antiseizure medications
Propranalol (Inderal)	*Rare*: drug eruption; See β-*blockers*
Sirolimus	Acneiform eruption that may be recalcitrant to therapy
Psoralens	See section on photosensitivity reactions
Quinidine	Edema, purpura, scarlatiniform eruption; may progress to exfoliative dermatitis
Quinine	Diffuse eruption (any kind)
Rauwolfia alkaloids (reserpine)	Urticaria, photosensitivity reactions, petechial eruptions
Rifampin	Pruritus, urticaria, acne, bullous pemphigoid, mucositis, exfoliative erythroderma, red urine, reddened soft contact lenses
Salicylates	See *aspirin*
Streptomycin	Urticaria; erythematous, morbilliform, and purpuric eruptions
Sulfonamides	Urticaria, scarlatiniform eruption, erythema nodosum, eczematous flare of exudative dermatitis, maculopapular eruption, DRESS, SJS, TEN, fixed drug eruption; see later section on photosensitivity reactions
	AIDS patients: develop allergic drug eruptions quite often; one of the most common causes of maculopapular eruption, DRESS, SJS, and TEN
Sulfonylureas	See *sulfonamides* and section on photosensitivity reactions
Suramin	Cutaneous reaction (80%), especially morbilliform, UV light recall (skin drug eruptions at sites of previous UV exposure), urticaria, "suramin keratoses"

TABLE 9-1 • Drugs and the Dermatoses They Cause (*continued*)

Drug	Dermatosis/Comments
Taxanes (paclitaxel, docetaxel)	Scleroderma-like skin changes, onycholysis, onychomadesis, acral erythema, erythema multiforme, pustular eruptions
Tyrosine kinase inhibitors (cetuximab [Erbitux], gefitinib [Iressa], erlotinib [Tarceva], afatinib [Giotrif])	Follicular eruption, painful fissures in the fingers and toes, paronychia, alterations of hair growth (trichomegaly, curly hair), telangiectasias, and hyperpigmentation
Testosterone and related drugs	Acne-like lesions, alopecia in scalp, hirsutism
Tetracycline	Fixed drug eruption, photosensitivity, serum sickness–like reaction; patient <8 y old: teeth staining; see *antibiotics*
Thalidomide	Erythroderma, pustulosis, TEN
Thiazides	See section on photosensitivity reactions
Trimethoprim	Rarely incriminated in drug eruptions
Vitamin A	*Long-term, high-dose therapy*: scaly, rough, itchy skin with coarse, dry, scant hair growth, and systemic changes including liver toxicity
Vitamin D	Skin lesions rare, but headache, nausea, diarrhea, increased urination, and sore gums and joints can be present
Vitamin B group	Urticaria, pruritic redness, and even anaphylactic reactions can occur after IM or IV administration
	Nicotinic acid: red flush (common–warn patient to eliminate unnecessary alarm), pruritus (common), hives (rare, within 15–30 min of oral ingestion of 50–100 mg)
Warfarin sodium	See *anticoagulants*

Abbreviations: ACE, angiotensin-converting enzyme; ACTH, adrenocorticotropic hormone; AGEP, acute generalized exanthematous pustulosis; AIDS, acquired immune deficiency syndrome; DRESS, drug reaction with eosinophilia and systemic symptoms; HIV, human immunodeficiency virus; LSC, lichen simplex chronicus; p-ANCA, perinuclear anti-neutrophil cytoplasmic antibodies; SLE, systemic lupus erythematosus; SJS, Stevens–Johnson syndrome; TEN, toxic epidermal necrolysis; UV, ultraviolet.

TABLE 9-2 • Dermatoses and the Drugs That Cause Them

Dermatosis	Drug(s)	Comments
Acne-like or pustular lesions	Bromides, iodides, lithium, testosterone, corticosteroids, EGFR inhibitors	
Acral erythema (see also hand-foot syndrome or palmoplantar erythrodysesthesia)	Various chemotherapeutic agents including cyclophosphamide, capecitabine, cytosine arabinoside, docetaxel, doxorubicin, fluorouracil, hydroxyurea, mercaptopurine, methotrexate, and mitotane	Different from hand-foot skin reaction (HFSR) by symmetric edema and diffuse erythema of the palms and soles which may progress to blistering and necrosis. Chemotherapy can be continued or briefly interrupted with use of topical corticosteroids
Actinic keratosis inflammation occurring in patients on systemic chemotherapy	First described with fluorouracil; also doxorubicin, cisplatin, fludarabine, dactinomycin, dacarbazine, and vincristine sulfate	
Alopecia	Amethopterin (methotrexate) and other antineoplastic agents; colchicine, clofibrate, testosterone and other androgens; tricyclic antidepressants; β-blockers; heparin; progesterone derivatives; coumarin derivatives; isotretinoin	

(*continued*)

TABLE 9-2 • Dermatoses and the Drugs That Cause Them (*continued*)

Dermatosis	Drug(s)	Comments
Angioedema	Aspirin, NSAIDs, ACE inhibitors	
Baboon syndrome; (see also SDRIFE)	Mercury (most often); also ampicillin, amoxicillin, ceftriaxone, penicillin, clindamycin, nickel, erythromycin, heparin, and food additives	Systemic contact dermatitis owing to ingestion, inhalation, or percutaneous absorption; symmetric diffuse acute light red exanthema on the buttocks, anogenital area, major flexural areas of the extremities; peaks at day 2–5 of exposure to the involved allergens; resolves within 1 wk. SDRIFE specifically refers to those cases induced by drugs
Drug reaction with eosinophilia and systemic symptoms (DRESS); also called drug-induced hypersensitivity syndrome (DIHS)	Allopurinol, carbamazepine, phenytoin, lamotrigine, oxcarbazepine, phenobarbital, and the sulfonamides	Exanthematous or papulopustular febrile eruption with hepatitis (also possible lung, renal, thyroid involvement), lymphadenopathy, and eosinophilia
Eczematous eruption	Quinine, antihistamines, gold, mercury, sulfonamides, penicillin, organic arsenic	
Erythema annulare centrifugum	Salicylates, antimalarials, amitriptyline, gold, etizolam	Proximal extremities and trunk with red advancing circinate plaques that may have a dry fine adherent scale in the inner spreading edge. Can be associated with underlying infections, hormonal abnormalities, and underlying malignancies
Erythema multiforme—like eruption	Penicillin and other antibiotics, sulfonamides, phenolphthalein, barbiturates, phenytoin, meprobamate	
Erythema nodosum–like eruption	Sulfonamides, iodides, salicylates, oral contraceptives, dapsone	
Exfoliative dermatitis	Particularly owing to arsenic, penicillin, sulfonamides, allopurinol, barbiturates	In some patients, exfoliative dermatitis may be a manifestation of DRESS
Fixed drug eruption	Phenolphthalein, acetaminophen, barbiturates, organic arsenic, gold, salicylates, sulfonamides, tetracycline, many others	Hyperpigmented or purplish; oval shaped, flat or slightly elevated; discrete, single, or multiple patches. Occurs at the same sites on drug challenge
Hand-foot skin reaction (HFSR)	Multi-kinase inhibitors such as sunitinib, sorafenib or regorafenib	Different from hand-foot syndrome (HFS) by characteristic well demarcated, bean to coin sized, hyperkeratotic, painful plaques with underlying erythema localized to the pressure areas of the hands and feet.
Hand-foot syndrome (HFS) (see also acral erythema or palmoplantar erythrodysesthesia)	Various chemotherapeutic agents including cyclophosphamide, capecitabine, cytosine arabinoside, docetaxel, doxorubicin, fluorouracil, hydroxyurea, mercaptopurine, methotrexate, and mitotane	Different from hand-foot skin reaction (HFSR) by symmetric edema and diffuse erythema of the palms and soles which may progress to blistering and necrosis. Chemotherapy can be continued or briefly interrupted with use of topical corticosteroids.

TABLE 9-2 • Dermatoses and the Drugs That Cause Them (*continued*)

Dermatosis	Drug(s)	Comments
Hyperpigmentation	Contraceptives, atabrine, chloroquine, minocycline, chlorpromazine, amiodarone, bismuth, gold, silver salts, ACTH, estrogen, adriamycin, and methotrexate	
Hypertrichosis	Oral minoxidil, phenytoin, cyclosporine *Less severe*: oral contraceptives, systemic corticosteroids, psoralens, streptomycin sulfate	
Ichthyosis	Cimetidine, clofazimine, hydroxyurea, cholesterol-lowering agents, nicotinic acid, coenzyme A reductase inhibitors, triparanol	
Keratoses and epitheliomas	Arsenic, mercury, PUVA therapy, immunosuppressive agents, vemurafenib, and dabrafenib	
Lichenoid drug eruption (lichen planus–like eruption)	Penicllamine, gold salts, β-blockers, thiazide diuretcis, and antimalarials	
Lupus erythematosus	Minocycline, hydralazine, procainamide, isoniazid, chlorpromazine, diltiazem, quinidine	
Linear IgA bullous dermatosis	Vancomycin (most common), furosemide, captopril, lithium, amiodarone, diclofenac, cefamandole, somatostatin, rifampin, topical iodine, phenytoin, trimethoprim, sulfamethoxazole, penicillin G, IL-2, interferon-γ	
Lipoatrophies from injections	Corticosteroids (e.g., triamcinolone), insulin, vasopressin, human growth hormone, iron dextran, diphtheria-pertussis–tetanus (DPT) immunization serum, antihistamines, Talwin injection usually due to abuse	
Lipodystrophy	Partial: proteinase inhibitors used to treat AIDS–indinavir or ritonavir plus saquinavir cause decreased subcutaneous fat on the face (cadaveric or cachectic facies) and extremities (pseudomuscular appearance) with increased prominence of the superficial veins, central adiposity with increased abdominal girth (pseudo-obesity), enlargement of breasts, increased dorsal-cervical fat pads (buffalo hump or pseudo-Cushing syndrome)	Increased triglyceride and LDL cholesterol and low HDL cholesterol also occurs.
Maculopapular eruption (morbiliform eruption or measles-like eruption)	Antibiotics, nonsteroidal anti-inflammatory drugs (NSAIDs), sulfonamides, and many others	
Mucous membrane lesions	*Pigmentation*: bismuth *Hypertrophy of gums*: phenytoin *Erosive lesions*: sulfonamides, antineoplastic agents, many other drugs	

(continued)

TABLE 9-2 • Dermatoses and the Drugs That Cause Them (*continued*)

Dermatosis	Drug(s)	Comments
Nail changes	*Onycholysis* (distal detachment): tetracycline, apparently owing to a phototoxic reaction	
	Onychomadesis (proximal detachment): Various chemotherapeutic agents including docetaxel, fluorouracil,	
Neutrophilic eccrine hidradenitis	Bleomycin, chlorambucil, cyclophosphamide, cytarabine, doxorubicin, lomustine, mitoxantrone	
Nicolau syndrome (embolia cutis medicamentosa)	Diclofenac, ibuprofen, iodine, benzathine penicillin, vitamin K, DPT immunizations, antihistamines, interferon-α, corticosteroids	At IM injection site; see Dictionary–Index
Nummular eczema–like eruption	Combination of isoniazid and *p*-aminosalicylic acid	
Necrosis of the skin	*Localized*: coumarin and heparin derivatives (subcutaneous or intravenous); recombinant interferon-γ	
	Distant: coumarin and heparin derivatives	
Ochronosis, exogenous	Topical phenol, quinine injections, topical resorcinol	
	With prolonged use: topical hydroquinone, mainly in dark-skinned patients at the site of application only	
Palmoplantar erythrodysesthesia (see also acral erythema or hand-foot syndrome)	Various chemotherapeutic agents including cyclophosphamide, capecitabine, cytosine arabinoside, docetaxel, doxorubicin, fluorouracil, hydroxyurea, mercaptopurine, methotrexate, and mitotane	Different from hand-foot skin reaction (HFSR) by symmetric edema and diffuse erythema of the palms and soles which may progress to blistering and necrosis. Chemotherapy can be continued or briefly interrupted with use of topical corticosteroids.
Pemphigoid-like lesions	Furosemide, penicillin, sulfasalazine, ibuprofen	
Pemphigus-like lesions	Rifampin, penicillamine, captopril, pyrazolone derivatives	
Photosensitivity reaction	*Sulfonamides*: sulfonylurea	A dermatitis upon exposure to sunlight. These skin reactions can be urticarial, erythematous, vesicular, or plaque-like. The mechanism can be either phototoxic or photoallergic, but this distinction can be difficult to ascertain. This list of *photosensitizing drugs* is rather complete, but also see Chapter 40
	Hypoglycemics: tolbutamide (Orinase), chlorpropamide (Diabinese)	
	Antibiotics: demethylchlortetracycline (Declomycin), doxycycline (Doryx, Monodox, Vibramycin), griseofulvin (Fulvicin, Grifulvin, Gris-PEG), maxaquin (Lomefloxacin), nalidixic acid (NegGram), tetracycline	

TABLE 9-2 • Dermatoses and the Drugs That Cause Them (*continued*)

Dermatosis	Drug(s)	Comments
	Benzofurans: amiodarone	
	Chlorothiazide diuretics: chlorothiazide (Diuril); hydrochlorothiazide; methyclothiazide	
	Phenothiazines: chlorpromazine (Thorazine); prochlorperazine (Compazine); promethazine (Phenergan)	
	Psoralens: methoxsalen (Oxsoralen); trioxsalen (Trisoralen)	
	Oxicams: piroxicam (Feldene)	
Pityriasis rosea-like eruption	Bismuth, gold, barbiturates	
Porphyria cutanea tarda (PCT) exacerbation	Estrogen, iron, ethanol ingestion, hexachlorobenzene, chlorinated phenols, polychlorinated biphenyls; possibly pravastatin	
Pseudolymphoma	Antidepressants, diphenylhydantoin, α-agonists, ACE inhibitors, anticonvulsants, antihistamines, benzodiazepine, β-blockers, calcium channel blockers, lipid-lowering agents, lithium, NSAIDs, phenothiazines, procainamide, estrogen, and progesterone	
Pseudoporphyria cutanea tarda	NSAIDs (naproxen, nabumetone, oxaprozin, ketoprofen, mefenamic acid, diflunisal), nalidixic acid, tetracycline, chlorothalidone, furosemide, hydrochlorothiazide/triamterene, isotretinoin, etretinate, cyclosporine, 5-fluorouracil, pyridoxine, amiodarone, flutamide, dapsone, aspirin	Skin findings only without biochemical abnormalities. May persist for months after offending drug is stopped, mimics skin findings and skin biopsy of PCT
Psoriasis exacerbation	Lithium, β-blockers, ACE inhibitors, antimalarials, NSAIDs, terbinafine	
Purpuric eruptions	Barbiturates, salicylates, meprobamate, organic arsenic, sulfonamides, chlorothiazide diuretics, corticosteroids (long-term use)	
Pustulosis, AGEP	Antibiotics (mainly β-lactam); many others	
Radiation recall	Chemotherapeutic agents, antituberculous medications, simvastatin, interferon α-2b	
Rheumatoid nodulosis, accelerated	Methotrexate	Painful nodules mainly on the hands in long-standing rheumatoid arthritis patients. Dissipates after the drug is stopped.
Scarlet fever–like eruption or "toxic erythema"	Arsenic, barbiturates, codeine, morphine, mercury, quinidine, salicylates, sulfonamides, and others	

(continued)

TABLE 9-2 • Dermatoses and the Drugs That Cause Them (*continued*)

Dermatosis	Drug(s)	Comments
SDRIFE	Ampicillin, amoxicillin, ceftriaxone, penicillin, clindamycin, and erythromycin; iodinate contrast media, pseudoephedrine, acetyl salicylic acid, mitomycin C, phenothiazines, valacyclovir, and many other drugs have also been implicated.	Systemic contact dermatitis owing to ingestion, inhalation, or percutaneous absorption of drugs; symmetric diffuse acute light red exanthema on the buttocks, anogenital area, major flexural areas of the extremities; peaks at day 2–5 of exposure to the involved drug; resolves within 1 wk
Seborrheic dermatitis–like eruption	Gold, ACTH	
Stevens–Johnson syndrome (SJS) and toxic epidermal necrolysis (TEN)	Allopurinol, carbamazepine, oxcarbazepine, lamotrigine, phenytoin, penicillin, barbiturates, sulfonamides, rifampin, NSAIDs, salicylates	
Subacute cutaneous lupus erythematosus	Hydrochlorothiazide, ACE inhibitors, calcium channel blockers, interferons, statins	
Urticaria	Penicillin, salicylates, sera, sulfonamides, barbiturates, opium group, contraceptive drugs, Rauwolfia alkaloids, aspirin, NSAIDs, and ACE inhibitors	
Vitiligo or depigmentation	Imatinib, hydroquinone, phenol derivatives	
Whitening of the hair	Chloroquine, hydroxychloroquine	In blonde- or red-haired people

Abbreviations: ACE, angiotensin-converting enzyme; ACTH, adrenocorticotropic hormone; AGEP, acute generalized exanthematous pustulosis; HDL, high-density lipoprotein; IM, intramuscular; LDL, low-density lipoprotein; NSAID, nonsteroidal anti-inflammatory drugs; PUVA, psoralens and ultraviolet light; SDRIFE, Symmetrical drug-related intertriginous and flexural exanthema.

Drug-induced adverse reactions are often classified as type A and type B reactions: The type A classification is intended to refer to predictable side effects that occur as a result of a pharmacologic action of the given drug, whereas type B reactions are regarded as not being predictable.

This chapter will discuss common drug eruptions and also some rare or severe drug eruptions. Most of them are type B reactions and are mainly the result of an allergic reaction. These severe cutaneous adverse reactions (SCARs) include Stevens-Johnson syndrome (SJS), toxic epidermal necrolysis (TEN), drug reaction with eosinophilia and systemic symptoms (DRESS), acute generalized exanthematous pustulosis (AGEP), and generalized bullous fixed drug eruptions (GBFDE). In contrast, some of the drug eruptions related to traditional chemotherapies or targeted anticancer therapies are type A reactions.

It can be stated almost without exception that any drug administered systemically is capable of causing a skin eruption.

SAUER'S NOTES

Any patient with a generalized skin eruption should be *carefully* questioned concerning the use of oral or parenteral medicinal drugs. For a minor non–life-threatening drug eruption, it may not be necessary or advisable to stop the use of a lifesaving drug. The rash may resolve on its own or be controlled with conservative therapy.

SAUER'S NOTES

1. When confronted with any diffuse or puzzling eruption, routinely question the patient regarding *any* medication taken by *any* route.

2. Ask: "Are you taking any vitamins, laxatives, nerve pills, and so forth?" This will jog the patient's memory.

3. Remember, any ingested chemical agent can cause an eruption, even toothpaste, mouthwash, breath freshener, or chewing gum.

4. Antiseizure medications, antibiotics, sulfa and sulfa-related drugs, nonsteroidal anti-inflammatory drugs, and allopurinol cause the majority of cutaneous drug eruptions.

MACULOPAPULAR ERUPTIONS

Clinical Presentation

Drug-induced exanthem or maculopapular eruptions (MPE), often described as "drug rashes" or "drug eruptions" are the most common adverse drug reactions affecting the skin, being responsible for approximately 90% of all drug rashes. The rashes are also referred to as exanthematous or morbilliform (measles-like) eruptions (Fig. 9-1). Such an eruption usually

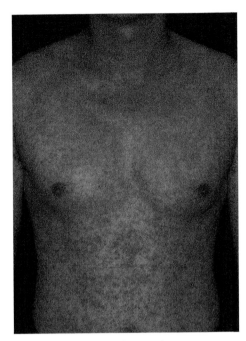

FIGURE 9-1: Drug-induced exanthem or maculopapular eruption consists of erythematous macules or papules, often symmetric.

occurs between 4 and 14 days after a patient begins taking a new medication. However, it can develop sooner, especially in case of rechallenge. The eruption consists of erythematous macules or papules, which are often symmetric. They begin on the trunk and upper extremities, and progressively become confluent. Mucous membranes are usually not involved. Pruritus and low-grade fever are often associated with the eruption, which usually disappears in a few days.

Pathogenesis and Causes

An MPE is usually caused by type-IV hypersensitivity reactions, either type-IVb or IVc. Type-IVb reactions correspond to the Th2-type immune response. Th2 T-cells secrete the cytokines IL-4, IL-13, and IL-5, which promote B-cell production of IgE and IgG4, macrophage deactivation, and mast cell and eosinophil responses, and the high production of the Th2 cytokine IL-5 leads to eosinophilic inflammation. In type-IVc reactions, T-cells can themselves act as effector cells. They emigrate to the skin and can kill keratinocytes. The most commonly prescribed medications, such as antibiotics, nonsteroidal anti-inflammatory drugs (NSAIDs), and sulfonamides, are implicated in most cases.

Management and Prognosis

Treatment is basically supportive, so symptomatic treatments are common practice. The first therapeutic measure is discontinuation of the causative agent, combined with the administration of topical corticosteroid and systemic antipruritic agents. In most instances, the eruption diminishes spontaneously after the drug is withdrawn; however, a few patients may experience a progressive worsening. The

progression of any drug rash should be carefully monitored in the first 48 h to check its course.

URTICARIA/ANGIOEDEMA

Clinical Presentation

Urticaria is characterized by itching, raised, and erythematous wheals, which usually present with a central region of pallor (Fig. 9-2). Individual lesions may enlarge and coalesce with other lesions, and they typically disappear within 24 h. Angioedema is swelling of the deeper dermis and subcutaneous tissues, which may coexist with urticaria in some cases. Angioedema may be disfiguring if it involves the face and lips, or life-threatening if a laryngeal edema or tongue swelling results in airway obstruction. Urticaria or angioedema reactions can be immediate (occurring within hours after exposure) or delayed (occurring days after exposure). These reactions are more common during the first few days of therapy.

Pathogenesis and Causes

Urticaria is mediated by degranulation of the cutaneous mast cell in the superficial dermis, while angioedema results from mast cell activation in the subcutaneous tissues or from non-mast cell-mediated mechanisms. These mechanisms include abnormalities of the complement cascade (i.e., inherited and acquired abnormalities of complement metabolism) and increased activity in vasodilatory kinin pathways. Solitary angioedema without urticaria has been reported to occur in 2 to 10 per 10,000 new users of angiotensin-converting enzyme (ACE) inhibitors and usually affects the mouth or tongue.

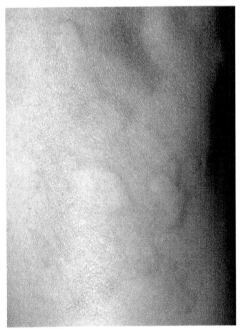

FIGURE 9-2: Urticaria is characterized by itching, raised, and erythematous wheals.

Urticaria and/or angioedema may be manifestations of an IgE-mediated (type-I hypersensitivity) drug reaction. NSAIDs, penicillins, cephalosporins, and sulfonamides are common causes of IgE-mediated drug allergy. IgE-mediated drug reactions may become more severe and progress toward anaphylaxis upon reexposure to the causative agent.

Other drugs, such as the opiate analgesics morphine and codeine, may also cause urticaria due to mast cell degranulation resulting from a non-IgE mediated mechanism. The concomitant use of opiates and vancomycin may increase the frequency of reactions to the latter. The intense flushing of "red man syndrome" seen after rapid vancomycin infusion is also due to direct mast cell activation and may be accompanied by urticaria.

Management and Prognosis

The main course of management involves withdrawal of the causative agent. This can sometimes be combined with use of histamine H1 receptor blockers. Systemic corticosteroids and intramuscular injection of epinephrine (adrenaline) are necessary in an emergency if severe angioedema occurs.

ANAPHYLAXIS

Clinical Presentation

The most severe form of immediate type-I hypersensitivity is anaphylaxis, which is characterized by symptoms affecting multiple organ systems, including pruritus, urticaria, angioedema, laryngeal edema, wheezing, nausea, vomiting, tachycardia, sense of impending doom, and occasional shock.

Drug-related anaphylaxis usually begins a few minutes to a few hours after drug administration.

Pathogenesis and Causes

Anaphylaxis usually results from a type-I hypersensitivity reaction mediated by IgE antibodies through the release of histamine or other mediators of inflammation. Anaphylaxis is much more often related to insect stings. Drugs are the second most common cause of anaphylaxis.

Management and Prognosis

Immediate resuscitation with cardiovascular life support should be provided. Systemic corticosteroids and intramuscular injection of epinephrine (adrenaline) are necessary in the management of anaphylaxis.

HYPERSENSITIVITY VASCULITIS

Clinical Presentation

Vasculitis is defined as inflammation of and damage to the blood vessel wall. Drug-induced vasculitis usually presents as leukocytoclastic vasculitis of cutaneous small vessels (mainly postcapillary venules).

The major clinical findings are numerous palpable purpuras on the lower legs (Fig. 9-3), but such purpuras may also be found on the upper limbs, face, ears, and trunk. Some of the purpuras may be necrotic and form large hemorrhagic blisters or pustules. The constitutive symptoms may include fever, arthralgia, myalgia, and general malaise. Laboratory abnormalities may show low serum complement levels and an elevated erythrocyte sedimentation rate. In most patients, these symptoms and/or findings begin 7 to 10 days after drug exposure. However, the latent period may be as short as 2 to 7 days or longer than 2 weeks with a long-acting drug.

Pathogenesis and Causes

Drugs are the most common cause of hypersensitivity vasculitis, which is usually mediated by a type-III hypersensitivity reaction. The culprit drugs may act as haptens to stimulate an immune response, and then lead to the formation of immune complexes. These immune complexes are deposited in the postcapillary venules and attract neutrophilic leukocytes, which release proteolytic enzymes that can mediate endothelial damage.

The drugs that are most often reported as having caused hypersensitivity vasculitis are hydralazine, minocycline, propylthiouracil, and levamisole.

Management and Prognosis

Discontinuation of the inciting drug should lead to resolution of the signs and diagnosis within a period of days to a few weeks. Bed rest is generally recommended for patients with vasculitis. Patients with more severe reactions may require NSAIDs or corticosteroids.

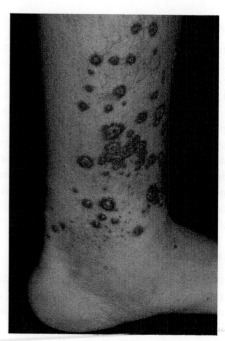

FIGURE 9-3: Palpable purpura on the lower legs.

EXFOLIATIVE DERMATITIS/ ERYTHRODERMA

Clinical Presentation

Erythroderma is defined as chronic scaling erythema involving greater than 90% of the body surface area. Diffuse exfoliation is a characteristic feature of this disease (Fig. 9-4).

Pathogenesis and Causes

Common etiologies of erythroderma include drugs, primary skin disease (atopic dermatitis, psoriasis), and malignancy (especially lymphoreticular malignancy and cutaneous T-cell lymphoma).

Drugs are responsible for approximately 20% of erythroderma cases; common culprit drugs include allopurinol, penicillins, barbiturates, gold salts, arsenic, and mercury. In some patients, exfoliative dermatitis may be a manifestation of DRESS.

Management and Prognosis

Erythroderma is characterized by an increased rate of epidermal turnover, including rapid epidermal cell proliferation and migration, and leads to exfoliation. It represents the most severe manifestation of eczema, psoriasis, and many inflammatory dermatoses. Treatment of erythroderma includes systemic or topical corticosteroids, in combination with systemic antihistamines for pruritus.

ERYTHEMA MULTIFORME

Erythema multiforme (EM), or erythema multiforme majus or major (EMM), is now considered to be a different condition from Stevens-Johnson syndrome (SJS). EM can be diagnosed on the basis of histological features, and is often caused by infections (typically herpes simplex virus or *Mycoplasma pneumoniae*) and has a benign clinical course. However, there are reports of EM in association with the use of medication.

Clinical Presentation

EM is an acute eruption characterized by typical target lesions. Lesions tend to affect the distal extremities, including the palms and soles. Typical target lesions are sharply demarcated papules or plaques made up of three different zones, of which at least two are concentric rings surrounding an erythematous center, with one ring consisting of palpable edema paler than the center (Fig. 9-5). These are distinguished from atypical target lesions that are less well-demarcated and have a less well-defined zonal structure. In atypical target lesions, there are only two zones with an erythematous ring and a central blister (Fig. 9-6).

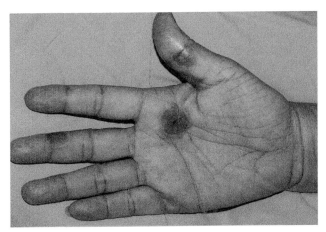

FIGURE 9-5: Typical target lesions have three different zones with two concentric erythematous rings and one paler edematous ring in between.

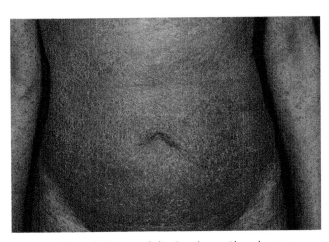

FIGURE 9-4: Diffuse exfoliation in erythroderma.

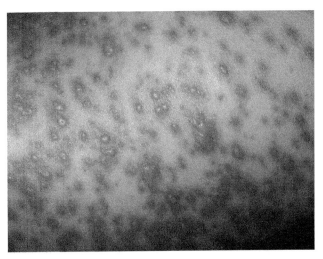

FIGURE 9-6: Atypical target lesions have only two zones with an erythematous ring and a central blister.

STEVENS-JOHNSON SYNDROME AND TOXIC EPIDERMAL NECROLYSIS

Stevens–Johnson syndrome (SJS) and toxic epidermal necrolysis (TEN) are rare, but they constitute the most severe drug-induced skin reactions. The incidence of TEN is estimated to be 0.4 to 1.2 cases/million person-years, and the incidence of SJS 1 to 6 cases/million person-years. Currently, most specialists consider SJS and TEN to be severity variants of the same drug-induced disease.

Clinical Presentation

These disorders are characterized by epidermal necrosis and sloughing of the mucous membranes and skin. The amount of body surface area involved is used to distinguish SJS from TEN; lesions affect less than 10% of the body surface in SJS and greater than 30% of the body surface in TEN. Cases with detachment between 10% and 30% are labeled SJS/TEN overlap. SJS is characterized by a tendency to affect the trunk or generalized dissemination of rather atypical target lesions and maculae (Fig. 9-7).

SJS is characterized by small blisters arising on purple macules. Lesions are widespread and usually predominate on the trunk. Confluence of blisters on limited areas leads to detachment below 10% of the body surface area.

TEN is characterized by the same lesions as SJS but with confluence of blisters leading to positive Nikolsky sign and to detachment of large epidermal sheets on more than 30% of the body surface area (Fig. 9-8).

Patients with SJS or TEN may have high fever. Severe erosions of mucous membranes are almost always found. Systemic manifestations include mild elevation of hepatic enzymes,

intestinal and pulmonary manifestations (with sloughing of epithelia similar to what happens to the skin). Death occurs in 10% of patients with SJS and above 30% of patients with TEN, principally from sepsis.

SAUER'S NOTES

1. Traditionally, the major type of erythema multiforme (EM majus or EM major; EMM) has been equated with SJS, as the changes involving the mucous membranes in EMM cannot be distinguished from the erosions of the mucous membranes seen in SJS and TEN.

2. Nonetheless, EMM and SJS differ in clinical presentation and etiology. While SJS and TEN are almost exclusively induced by drugs, EMM is mainly triggered by infectious agents.

3. EMM is an acute eruption characterized by typical target lesions that consist of sharply demarcated papules or plaques made up of three different zones: at least two concentric rings surrounding an erythematous center, with one ring consisting of palpable edema paler than the center. SJS is characterized by atypical target lesions that have only two zones consisting of an erythematous ring and a central blister.

4. EMM lesions tend to affect the distal extremities, including the palms and soles. SJS lesions are widespread and usually predominate on the trunk.

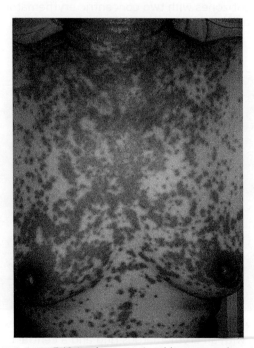

FIGURE 9-7: SJS is characterized by generalized dissemination of atypical target lesions and maculae.

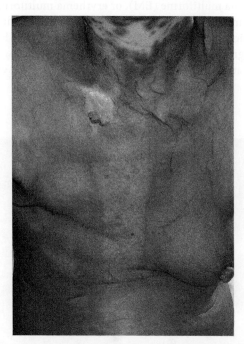

FIGURE 9-8: Toxic epidermal necrolysis is characterized by confluence of blisters leading to detachment of large epidermal sheets on more than 30% of the body surface area.

Pathogenesis and Causes

Drugs are responsible for at least 70% of cases. The risk of developing SJS or TEN is increased in HIV-infected patients.

The immunopathological pattern of early lesions suggests a cell-mediated cytotoxic reaction against epidermal cells. After exposure to the causative agent, antigen-presenting cells present the cognate antigen, causing activation of specific CD4 and CD8 T cells. Once activated, these T-cells, referred to as drug-specific T-cells, proliferate and then migrate into the dermis and epidermis. Drug-specific cytotoxic T-cells expressing the skin homing receptor cutaneous lymphocyte-associated antigen are observed in the development of cutaneous lesions. Cytokines such as interferon (IFN)-γ, tumor necrosis factor (TNF)-α, Fas-ligand, and most importantly, granulysin, could participate in the massive and widespread apoptosis of epidermal cells. Genetic susceptibility could also play an important role in SJS and TEN. For example, a strong association has been reported in Han Chinese between the human leukocyte antigen HLA-B*1502 allele and SJS induced by carbamazepine, and between the HLA B*5801 allele and SJS induced by allopurinol.

Management and Prognosis

Treatment of SJS and TEN is mainly symptomatic, consisting of nursing care, pain control, maintenance of fluid and electrolyte balance, and nutritional support. Early withdrawal of all potentially responsible drugs is mandatory. Short courses of corticosteroids in the early stage of the disease have been advocated, but their effectiveness has never been demonstrated in controlled trials. High-dose intravenous immunoglobulins have been proposed to be a promising treatment modality, but conflicting results have been reported.

SAUER'S NOTES

1. SJS/TEN is a potentially life-threatening disease. As soon as the diagnosis of SJS or TEN has been made, the severity and prognosis of the disease should be rapidly determined to define the appropriate medical setting for management.
2. A prognostic scoring system called SCORTEN based on seven independent, easily measured clinical and laboratory variables has been validated for use on days one and three of hospitalization for SJS/TEN.
3. The seven variables upon which the SCORTEN system is based include (1) age ≥ 40 years, (2) having evolving cancer or hematological malignancies, (3) body surface area detached $\geq 10\%$, (4) tachycardia ≥ 120/minute, (5) serum urea >10 mmol/L, (6) serum glucose >14 mmol/L, and (7) serum bicarbonate <20 mmol/L. Each variable accounts for 1 point.
4. The SCORTEN score calculated within 24 hours of hospital admission is inversely correlated to the survival of patients with TEN: 0 to 1, 94%; 2, 87%; 3, 53%; 4, 25%; ≥ 5, 17%.
5. Patients with a SCORTEN score of 0 or 1 and without rapidly progressing disease may be treated in general wards, while patients with more severe disease and a SCORTEN score ≥ 2 should be transferred to intensive care units or burn units if available.

DRUG REACTION WITH EOSINOPHILIA AND SYSTEMIC SYMPTOMS (DRESS)

Drug reaction with eosinophilia and systemic symptoms (DRESS), or drug-induced hypersensitivity syndrome (DIHS), or drug induced delayed multiorgan hypersensitivity syndrome (DIDMOHS), are severe adverse drug reactions characterized by fever, generalized skin eruption, lymphadenopathies, eosinophilia, and visceral organ involvement. This peculiar syndrome was first reported in the literature in 1937, where it was described as exfoliative dermatitis following administration of sulfanilamide. After the 1950s, an increasing number of patients presenting with similar but variable manifestations received diagnoses defined by the drugs that caused the reaction, including phenytoin hypersensitivity, dapsone hypersensitivity (sulfone syndrome), allopurinol hypersensitivity syndrome, and anticonvulsant hypersensitivity syndrome.

Clinical Presentation

DRESS symptoms typically occur 2 to 6 weeks after the initiation of the offending medication; however, reactions may not develop until 3 months later, especially when the syndrome is induced by allopurinol. A high, spiking fever (usually above 38°C) and rash are usually the first signs, and these are followed by other systemic reactions such as cervical, axillary, and inguinal lymphadenopathies, or general malaise. The rash usually begins as a nonspecific morbilliform eruption (Fig. 9-9), which is indistinguishable from other drug reactions, but can progress to a generalized form or even to erythroderma (Fig. 9-10). Facial edema sparing periorbital regions is a common sign for the diagnosis (Fig. 9-11). The cutaneous eruption later becomes confluent and infiltrated with purpuric changes (Fig. 9-12). As the rash resolves, the end-stage involves large sheet desquamation. Occasionally DRESS patients may present with oral erosions, but the symptoms are usually mild, with lip involvement only, in contrast to the extensive erosions seen in SJS/TEN.

Various hematologic abnormalities have been described in patients with DRESS. Atypical lymphocytes and/or hypereosinophilia are the most prominent and characteristic signs.

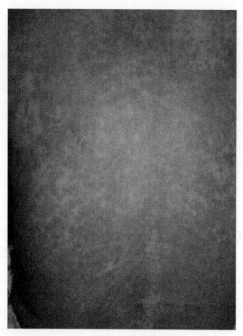

FIGURE 9-9: DRESS rash usually begins as a nonspecific morbilliform eruption.

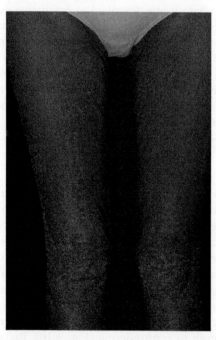

FIGURE 9-10: DRESS may present as erythroderma.

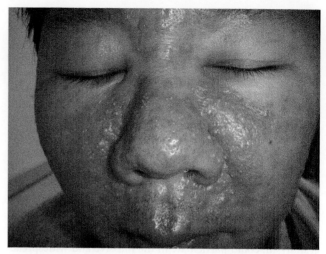

FIGURE 9-11: Facial edema sparing periorbital regions is a characteristic feature of DRESS.

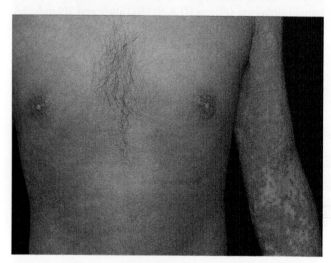

FIGURE 9-12: The cutaneous eruption of DRESS may become confluent and infiltrated with purpuric changes.

Multiple organ involvement is a distinct feature of DRESS. The liver and kidney are the two most frequently involved organs. Anicteric hepatitis presenting as elevated serum alanine aminotransferase is more common in patients with DRESS. Acute liver failure may develop and can contribute to patient mortality. Renal involvement usually presents with increased serum creatinine levels and new-onset proteinuria. Interstitial nephritis, rather than tubular necrosis, is the most common cause of acute renal failure in DRESS patients. The severity of renal dysfunction varies from a mild increase in serum creatinine levels to the development of end-stage renal disease.

The diagnosis of DRESS is complicated, and a detailed scoring system for diagnosis has been proposed by an international expert group (Table 9-3).

Pathogenesis and Causes

The precise pathogenesis of DRESS is complex and not fully understood. It is widely considered to be an immunological reaction to a drug or to its metabolites because of the signs, such as skin eruption, fever, and reappearance of symptoms upon rechallenge with the drug. An increasing amount of evidence from pharmacogenetic studies has shown that the occurrence of this syndrome is determined by the combination of susceptible genetic markers and exposure to specific

TABLE 9-3 • Scoring System of RegiSCAR for Diagnosing DRESS

Assessment/Score	−1	0	1	Comment
Fever ≥38.5°C	No/U	Yes		Acute episodes
Enlarged lymph nodes		No/U	Yes	>1 cm, ≥2 different areas (right side plus left side is not adequate)
Eosinophilia Eosinophils≥700/μL or ≥10% if leukocyte <4,000/μL		No/U	Yes	*Score 2* for extreme eosinophilia Eosinophils ≥1,500/μL or ≥20% if leukocyte <4,000/μL
Atypical lymphocytes		No/U	Yes	
Skin rash				Onset <21 d before hospitalization
Extent >50% body surface area		No/U	Yes	
Rash suggesting DRESS	No	U	Yes	≥2 symptoms: purpuric change, facial edema, infiltration, psoriasiform desquamation
Biopsy suggesting DRESS	No	Yes/U		*Score −1* if results fit any other specific dermatopathologic diagnosis
Organ involvement				Excluding other causes, score max. of 2
Liver: any one criterion		No/U	Yes	ALT>2*UNL, twice on successive dates D-bil.>2*UNL, twice on successive dates AST, T-bil., ALP all>2*UNL, once
Kidney: any one criterion		No/U	Yes	Creatinine>1.5* patient's baseline Proteinuria above 1 g/d
Lung: any one criterion		No/U	Yes	Evidence of interstitial lung (CT, x-ray) Abnormal bronchoalveolar lavage Abnormal blood gases
Muscle/Heart: any one criterion		No/U	Yes	Raised creatine kinase Raised troponin T Abnormalities in the echocardiogram
Pancreas		No/U	Yes	Amylase >2* UNL
Other organs		No/U	Yes	Central nervous system, splenomegaly
Rash resolution ≥15 d	No/U	Yes		
Excluding other causes		No/U	Yes	*Score 1* if ≥3 tests are performed and negative
Hepatitis A, B, C				At least 2 tests are negative and 1 unknown: negative
Mycoplasma/Chlamydia				At least 1 test is negative and 1 unknown: negative
Antinuclear antibody				
Blood culture				Sampling within 3 d after hospitalization
Final score				

Final scores: <2: excluded; 2–3: possible; 4–5: probable; >5: definite
Abbreviations: ALT, alanine transaminase; ALP, alkaline phosphatase; AST, aspartate transaminase; CT, computed tomography; D-bil., direct bilirublin; DRESS, drug reaction with eosinophilia and systemic symptoms; max., maximum; T-bil., total bilirulin; U, unknown; UNL: upper normal limit

drugs. Similar to SJS/TEN, the pathogenesis of DRESS involves drug-specific T-cells, which proliferate and then migrate into the dermis and epidermis. In addition, reactivation of human herpesvirus (HHV)-6 has also been demonstrated to be a specific feature in a certain portion of DRESS patients, and may play some roles in the development of the DRESS symptoms and/ or fluctuations of the disease. Recently, gradual dysfunction of regulatory T-cells has been found to be another feature of DRESS but not SJS/TEN, and this might be associated with increasing risks of developing autoimmune diseases in DRESS patients.

The aromatic antiepileptic agents (carbamazepine, phenytoin, lamotrigine, oxcarbazepine, and phenobarbital), allopurinol, and the sulfonamides are the most frequent causes of DRESS.

Management and Prognosis

The most important treatment for DRESS is an immediate withdrawal of the offending drugs, along with adequate supportive care. Topical corticosteroids or topical antipruritics can be used to relieve cutaneous symptoms, while systemic corticosteroids are the current mainstay of treatment. A recommended starting dose is prednisone 1.0 to 1.5 mg/kg/day. This dosage should be slowly tapered over 6 to 8 weeks to avoid a flare-up of symptoms. Other alternatives include intravenous immunoglobulin, plasmapheresis, or immunosuppressants; however, reports in the literature have shown variable outcomes and inconclusive results.

ACUTE GENERALIZED EXANTHEMATOUS PUSTULOSIS

Acute generalized exanthematous pustulosis (AGEP) is an acute pustular eruption that must be differentiated from pustular psoriasis. Its incidence is estimated to be 1 to 5 cases/million/year.

Clinical Presentation

AGEP is remarkable for its short time to onset (less than 48 hours) after the administration of the suspected drug. It is also characterized by a fever of >38°C, which generally begins the same day as the rash. The clinical presentations include numerous, small, mostly nonfollicular pustules arising on a widespread edematous erythema (Fig. 9-13). The pustules are mainly localized on the skin folds (such as those of the neck, axillae, and groin), trunk, and upper extremities. Leukocytosis with elevated neutrophil count, transient renal failure, and hypocalcemia are frequently seen. The eruption lasts for 1 to 2 weeks and is followed by a superficial desquamation.

Pathogenesis and Causes

AGEP is a T-cell-mediated disease. During the initial stage of AGEP, the vesicles are composed mainly of drug-specific CD4 T-cells and keratinocytes. These cells release increased amounts of CXCL8, a potent neutrophilic cytokine, leading to the chemotaxis of neutrophils into the vesicles, which causes, in turn, the transformation of vesicles into sterile pustules. Analyses of drug-specific CD4 T-cells from patients with AGEP have shown a predominant Th1-type cytokine profile with increased INF-γ and granulocyte/macrophage colony-stimulating factor production. Increased secretion of interferon-γ and granulocyte/macrophage colony-stimulating factor leads to augmented neutrophil survivability, which enhances the formation of sterile pustules. INF-γ and granulocyte/macrophage colony-stimulating factor may induce the release of CXCL8 by keratinocytes, which further leads to neutrophil accumulation.

More than 90% of AGEP cases are drug-induced. Antibiotics (particularly aminopenicillins) and diltiazem are thought to be the main drugs implicated in AGEP. A few cases have been reported to be related to viral infection (enterovirus or parvovirus B19) or hypersensitivity to mercury.

Management and Prognosis

Withdrawal of the causative drug is the main means of managing AGEP, with cases usually resolving spontaneously within 1 to 2 weeks. In some cases, systemic antihistamines and topical corticosteroids may be needed for symptomatic relief.

FIXED DRUG ERUPTIONS

A fixed drug eruption (FDE) is a distinctive reaction characterized acutely by erythematous and edematous plaques with a grayish center or frank bullae, and characterized chronically by a dark postinflammatory pigmentation.

Clinical Presentation

The lesions usually develop less than 2 days after the drug intake. They are characterized by one or a few round, sharply demarcated erythematous and edematous plaques, sometimes with a central blister (Fig. 9-14). The mouth (lips and tongue),

FIGURE 9-13: Numerous, small, and nonfollicular pustules arising on a widespread edematous erythema in AGEP.

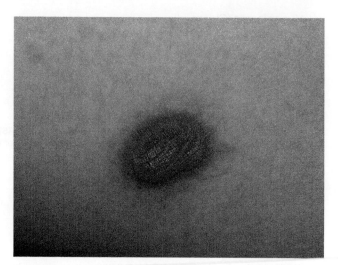

FIGURE 9-14: Fixed drug eruption is characterized by round, sharply demarcated erythematous and edematous plaques, sometimes with a central blister.

genitalia, face, and acral areas are commonly involved sites. The defining features of this eruption include postinflammatory hyperpigmentation and the recurrence of lesions at exactly the same sites with drug reexposure. After several relapses the eruption may involve large areas of the body and become a more severe form of FDE called generalized bullous FDE (GBFDE). Patients with GBFDE can be misdiagnosed as having SJS/TEN (Fig. 9-15), but mucosal involvement is usually absent or mild in GBFDE, and the clinical course is favorable, with rapid resolution in 7 to 14 days after drug discontinuation. A comparison of GBFDE and SJS/TEN is shown in Table 9-4.

Pathogenesis and Causes

The phenomenon of lesions recurring at the previously involved sites has been explained by the discovery of intra-epidermal CD8 T-cells with an effector-memory phenotype being resident in FDE lesions. Sites predisposed to FDE (i.e., the lips, genital areas, or hands) are frequent regions of herpes simplex virus (HSV) reactivation. The occurrence of FDE lesions at previously traumatized sites, such as burn scars and insect bites, have also been well-documented. Intra-epidermal CD8 T-cells with an effector-memory phenotype resident in FDE lesions may mediate protective immunity. Additional recruitment of other inflammatory cells occurs in the late stage of the disease, and then disease activity is downregulated by regulatory T-cells.

The drugs commonly involved in FDE include NSAIDs (acetylsalicylic acid, ibuprofen, naproxen, mefenamic acid), antibacterial agents (trimethoprim-sulfamethoxazole, tetracyclines, penicillins, quinolones, dapsone), barbiturates, acetaminophen (paracetamol), and antimalarials.

Management and Prognosis

The most important treatment for FDE consists of identifying and discontinuing the causative drug. FDE is a self-limited disease, but may cause pigmented lesions in some patients. Topical corticosteroids may be used for symptomatic relief. In patients with GBFDE, adequate supportive care with systemic corticosteroids, similar to the general practice for SJS/TEN patients, may be needed.

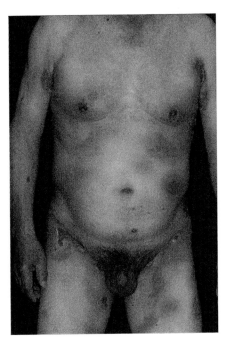

FIGURE 9-15: Patients with GBFDE may mimic SJS/TEN.

TABLE 9-4 • Comparison of Clinical and Pathologic Features Between GBFDE and TEN		
	GBFDE	**TEN**
Clinical Features		
Age	Usually older	All age groups
Previous events	Usually yes	None
Conjunctival involvement	None	Almost all
Constitutional symptoms	Rare	Frequent
Latency of disease onset to drug intake	Short (<3 d)	Long (10–14 d)
Blister lesions	Well demarcated dusky-red patches with blisters/erosions	Symmetrically distributed confluent blisters/erosions
Immuno-Pathologic Features		
Superficial and deep perivascular inflammation	Often	None
Eosinophil infiltration	Often	Usually none
Pigment incontinence	Frequent	Infrequent
Intra-epidermal CD56 cells	Less	More
Intra-epidermal granulysin+ cells	Less	More
Serum granulysin level	Lower	High
Dermal Foxp3+ cells	More	Less

SYMMETRICAL DRUG-RELATED INTERTRIGINOUS AND FLEXURAL EXANTHEMA

SAUER'S NOTES

1. The term "baboon syndrome" is used for describing patients in whom a specific skin eruption resembling the red gluteal area of baboons has occurred after systemic exposure to contact allergens.
2. Baboon syndrome has historically often been equated with a mercury-induced exanthem in patients with previous contact sensitization.
3. Symmetrical drug-related intertriginous and flexural exanthema (SDRIFE) specifically refers to drug-related baboon syndrome with the distinctive clinical pattern.

Clinical Presentation

Symmetrical drug-related intertriginous and flexural exanthema (SDRIFE), or intertriginous drug eruption, is an infrequent type of drug-induced rash. SDRIFE occurs a few hours to a few days after the administration of the offending drug. The rash presents as a sharply demarcated V-shaped erythema in the gluteal/perianal or inguinal/perigenital areas (Fig. 9-16), often with involvement of at least one other flexural or intertriginous fold, in the absence of systemic symptoms.

Five diagnostic criteria have been proposed for SDRIFE as follows:

1. exposure to a systemically administered drug either at the first or repeated dose (excluding contact allergens);
2. sharply demarcated erythema of the gluteal/perianal area and/or V-shaped erythema of the inguinal/perigenital area;
3. involvement of at least one other intertriginous/flexural localization;
4. symmetry of affected areas; and
5. absence of systemic symptoms and signs.

Pathogenesis and Causes

SDRIFE cases represent a distinct subgroup of drug eruptions with very specific involvement sites, and are presumably elicited by an immunological type-IV mechanism similar to that which causes systemic contact dermatitis.

Amoxicillin, ceftriaxone, penicillin, clindamycin, and erythromycin are thought to be implicated in about 50% of cases. Iodinate contrast media, pseudoephedrine, acetyl salicylic acid, mitomycin C, phenothiazines, valacyclovir, and many other drugs have also been implicated.

Management and Prognosis

Treatment includes discontinuing the suspected drug and the use of topical or systemic corticosteroids.

PHOTOSENSITIVE ERUPTIONS

There are two basic types of drug-induced photo eruptions, phototoxic and photoallergic eruptions, which differ in clinical appearance and pathogenesis.

Clinical Presentation

Phototoxic Eruptions

These eruptions typically present as exaggerated sunburn, often a well-demarcated erythema with blisters (Fig. 9-17).

Photoallergic Eruptions

These eruptions are characterized by widespread eczema in the sun-exposed areas, typically the face, upper chest, and dorsal hands (Fig. 9-18).

Pathogenesis and Causes

Phototoxic eruptions are by far the most common drug-induced photo eruptions. They are caused by the absorption of ultraviolet light by the causative drug, which releases energy and

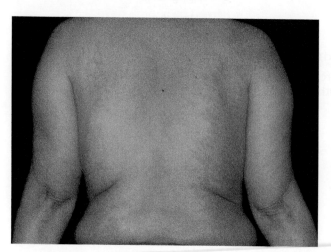

FIGURE 9-16: SDRIFE rash presents as a sharply demarcated, symmetric erythema in the flexor/intertriginous areas.

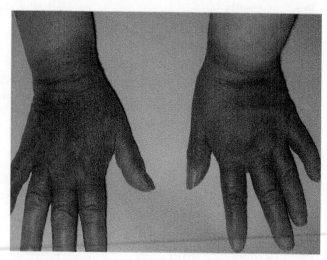

FIGURE 9-17: Phototoxic eruptions typically present as an exaggerated sunburn, often a well-demarcated erythema with blisters.

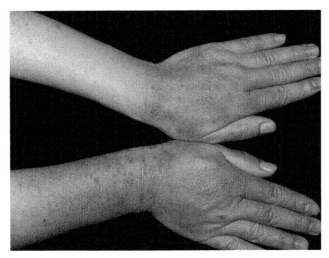

FIGURE 9-18: Photoallergic eruptions are characterized by widespread eczema in the sun-exposed areas. This is a case of photosensitive dermatitis due to diphenhydramine.

damages cells. Ultraviolet A light (UVA) is the wavelength most commonly implicated, although ultraviolet B light (UVB) and visible light can elicit reactions with some drugs. NSAIDs, quinolones, tetracyclines, amiodarone, and the phenothiazines are the most frequent causes of phototoxicity.

Photoallergic eruptions are lymphocyte-mediated reactions caused by exposure to UVA. It is postulated that the absorbed radiation converts the drug into an immunologically active compound that is then presented to lymphocytes by Langerhans cells, causing spongiotic dermatitis (eczema). Most photoallergic reactions are caused by topical agents, including biocides added to soaps (halogenated phenolic compounds) and fragrances such as musk ambrette and 6-methyl coumarin. Systemic photoallergens such as the phenothiazines, chlorpromazine, sulfa products, and NSAIDs can produce photoallergic reactions (i.e., photosensitive dermatitis), although most of their photosensitive reactions are phototoxic.

Management and Prognosis

Treatment includes discontinuing the suspected drug and avoiding sun exposure. Patients with severe skin lesions may need treatment with topical or systemic corticosteroids.

DRUG-INDUCED BLISTERING DISEASES

Autoimmune blistering diseases are a group of disorders in which the body mistakenly attacks healthy tissue, causing blistering lesions that primarily affect the skin and mucous membranes. Certain drugs are known to play a role in the development or aggravation of these disorders. Drug-induced autoimmune blistering diseases may be drug-induced or drug-triggered. The latter term refers to the unmasking of a latent disease by a particular drug.

Clinical Presentation

Drug-Induced Pemphigus

In most cases, drug-induced pemphigus presents as a superficial pemphigus with no mucosal involvement.

Drug-Induced Bullous Pemphigoid (BP)

The clinical manifestations of drug-induced BP include tense vesicles and bullae on an inflammatory base distributed on the arms, legs, and trunk of older patients (Fig. 9-19).

Drug-Induced Linear IgA Bullous Dermatosis (LABD)

LABD could be either idiopathic or drug-induced. Patients with LABD may have various features including erythematous, slightly edematous plaques studded with large, tense bullae on the lateral aspect of the trunk, mimicking BP, or typical "clusters of jewels" consisting of clusters of tense blisters on the erythematous base (Fig. 9-20). Mucosal or conjunctival

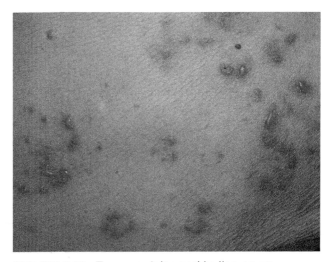

FIGURE 9-19: Tense vesicles and bullae on an inflammatory base distributed on the trunk in a patient of furosemide-induced pemphigoid.

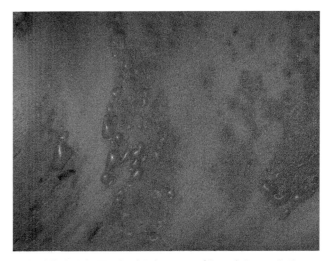

FIGURE 9-20: Typical "clusters of jewels" consisting of clusters of tense blisters on the erythematous base in a patient of LABD.

lesions are not present in drug-induced LABD, but are common in the idiopathic type of LABD.

Pathogenesis and Causes

The drugs most often implicated in drug-induced pemphigus are penicillamine and other thiol (SH) compounds, including captopril or drugs such as piroxicam that are metabolized to thiols. With decreasing use of penicillamine, the incidence of drug-induced pemphigus has been reduced.

Penicillamine and furosemide are the most frequently implicated agents in drug-induced BP, although cases associated with captopril, penicillin and its derivatives, and sulfasalazine also have been reported. Case-control studies have found a significant association between bullous pemphigoid and neuroleptics, loop diuretics, and spironolactone.

LABD is a subepidermal blistering disease characterized by the linear deposition of IgA antibodies at the basement membrane zone. Vancomycin has been identified as the leading culprit in many reports; lithium, cefamandole, captopril, and diclofenac have also been associated with LABD. Spontaneous remission occurs in drug-induced LABD once the offending agent is discontinued.

Management and Prognosis

Treatment includes the discontinuation of the suspected drug and the use of topical or systemic corticosteroids.

> ### SAUER'S NOTES
>
> 1. LABD may present as vesicles and blisters superimposed at the edge of annular lesions, creating a typical "string of beads" sign.
> 2. It may also exhibit a classical "clusters of jewels" appearance consisting of clusters of tense blisters on the erythematous base.

LICHENOID DRUG ERUPTIONS (DRUG-INDUCED LICHEN PLANUS)

Clinical Presentation

Lichenoid drug eruptions are characterized by symmetrically distributed, flat-topped, violaceous, pruritic papules on the trunk and four limbs (Fig. 9-21). The time interval between the initiation of the offending drug and the appearance of the cutaneous lesions varies from months to years.

Pathogenesis and Causes

Persistent activation of CD8 cytotoxic T-lymphocytes against epidermal cells may be the crucial pathologic factor. Plasmacytoid dendritic cells are also thought to be involved in the early phase of lichenoid tissue reactions. They produce large amounts of type-I interferons, such as IFN-α, which mediate the activation of IFN-α secreting cytotoxic T-cells directly or through the maturation of myeloid dendritic cells. Furthermore,

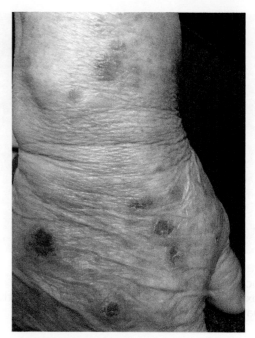

FIGURE 9-21: Lichenoid drug eruptions are characterized by symmetrically distributed, flat-topped, violaceous, pruritic papules.

TNF-α and other inflammatory cytokines/chemokines are also responsible for the amplification of the inflammatory response.

Penicillamine, gold salts, β-blockers, thiazide diuretics, and antimalarials are important common etiologic agents for lichenoid drug eruptions.

Management and Prognosis

Lichenoid drug eruptions generally resolve spontaneously a few weeks to a few months after the discontinuation of the offending drug. Treatment options include topical or systemic corticosteroids.

DRUG-INDUCED LUPUS

Drug-induced lupus includes drug-induced systemic lupus erythematosus (SLE) and drug-induced subacute cutaneous lupus erythematosus (SCLE).

Clinical Presentation

Drug-Induced SLE

Clinical manifestations of drug-induced SLE are mainly systemic, including fever, weight loss, pericarditis, and pleuro-pulmonary inflammation, whereas cutaneous involvement, such as the presence of butterfly malar rash, photoeruptions, and discoid or erythema multiforme-like lesions, is rare. There is no gender predilection. Vasculitis and renal or neurological involvement are rarely associated. The symptoms usually develop >1 year after the medication is administered.

Drug-Induced SCLE

Drug-induced SCLE presents with psoriasiform and annular lesions, usually on the upper trunk and extensor surfaces of the arms, which are indistinguishable from those seen in the idiopathic form of the disease.

Pathogenesis and Causes

Although the pathogenesis of drug-induced lupus is not well understood, genetic predisposition may play a role. Drug-induced lupus is more likely to develop and develops sooner with certain drugs metabolized by acetylation in those patients who are slow acetylators, i.e., those in whom there is a genetically mediated decrease in the hepatic synthesis of *N*-acetyltransferase.

Drugs associated with the highest risk of developing drug-induced SLE are procainamide, hydralazine, minocycline, diltiazem, and penicillamine. Among them, procainamide and hydralazine are metabolized by acetylation. More recent biologic agents such as infliximab and etanercept have also been reported to be definite causes of drug-induced SLE.

Drugs that induce SCLE include thiazide diuretics, calcium channel antagonists, terbinafine, NSAIDs, and griseofulvin. Resolution of the eruption may or may not occur after discontinuation of the drug.

Management and Prognosis

The first step in the treatment is to discontinue the offending medication. Specific manifestations should then be treated until they resolve using the same approaches used in patients with SLE or SCLE. Cutaneous eruptions are treated with topical corticosteroids.

OTHER DRUG ERUPTIONS

Other miscellaneous types of drug eruptions are listed in Table 9.2.

DRUG ERUPTIONS RELATED TO CHEMOTHERAPEUTIC AGENTS

Almost all anticancer chemotherapeutic agents can induce hypersensitivity drug eruptions such as maculopapular eruptions or urticaria. However, conventional chemotherapy may also cause various cutaneous reactions due to its effects on specific cell cycle phases. In this session, some specific drug eruptions related to anticancer chemotherapy will be described.

Clinical Presentation

Acral Erythema

Acral erythema, also known as hand-foot syndrome (HFS) or palmar-plantar erythrodysesthesia, occurs most often in patients with cancer treated with cytosine arabinoside, doxorubicin, capecitabine (an oral 5-fluorouracil derivative), tegafur, liposomal doxorubicin, or docetaxel. Acral erythema is most often characterized by a symmetric edema and erythema of the palms and soles which may progress to blistering and necrosis (Fig. 9-22). Dysesthesia of the involved areas (e.g., paresthesia, tingling, burning, and/or painful sensations) precedes the development of the skin lesions.

Hyperpigmentation

Hyperpigmentation is a common skin toxicity related to anticancer chemotherapy. Pigmentation from chemotherapeutic agents can have a varied appearance, including (1) photodistributed, (2) serpentine supravenous hyperpigmentation (Fig. 9-23), (3) widespread reticulate hyperpigmentation (Fig. 9-24), (4) serpentine streaks in the back and buttocks, and (5) acral pigmentation (Fig. 9-25). The alkylating agents cyclophosphamide, ifosfamide, and thiotepa can also produce

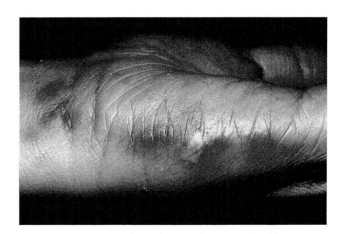

FIGURE 9-22: Acral erythema characterized by a symmetric edema and erythema of the palms and soles may progress to blistering and necrosis.

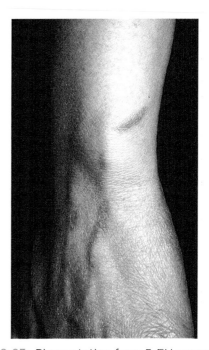

FIGURE 9-23: Pigmentation from 5-FU presents as serpentine supravenous hyperpigmentation.

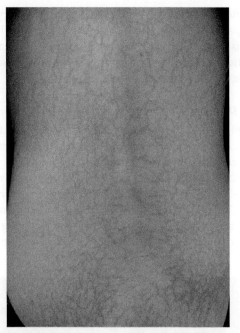

FIGURE 9-24: Widespread reticulate hyperpigmentation due to pemetrexed.

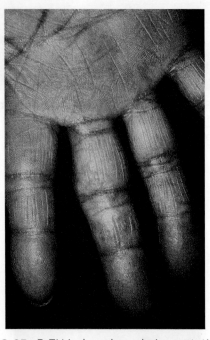

FIGURE 9-25: 5-FU induced acral pigmentation.

hyperpigmentation, while bleomycin can cause flagellate dermatitis and pigmentation. Whip-like erythematous reactions over the trunk or extremities occur in 20% to 30% of patients who are taking bleomycin.

Nail Toxicity

Onycholysis, onychomadesis, Beau lines, onychomelanosis, and subungual hemorrhage are frequently associated with capecitabine, paclitaxel, or docetaxel therapy (Fig. 9-26).

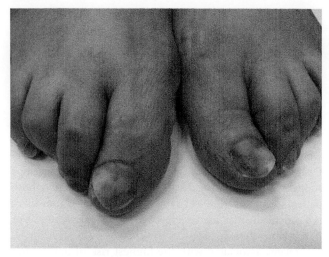

FIGURE 9-26: Nail changes including onycholysis and onychomadesis due to docetaxel.

SAUER'S NOTES

1. Both onycholysis and onychomadesis have been seen in patients receiving taxane therapies.
2. Onycholysis is the detachment of the nail from the nail bed, usually starting at the tip and/or sides.
3. Onychomadesis is the separation of the nail plate from the bed, beginning at the proximal end with subsequent shedding of the nail as the new nail grows.

Radiation Recall Dermatitis Versus Radiation Enhancement

Radiation recall is an acute inflammatory reaction confined to previously irradiated areas that can be triggered when chemotherapy agents are administered after radiotherapy (Fig. 9-27). The most commonly implicated include doxorubicin, docetaxel, paclitaxel, gemcitabine, and capecitabine. If the time interval between the end of radiation and chemotherapy is less than 7 days, such reactions should be considered radiation enhancement or sensitization. Therefore, radiation recall dermatitis should be differentiated by a later occurrence (more than 7 days) after the completion of radiotherapy.

Management and Prognosis

High potency topical corticosteroids are useful for HFS. Cooling of the hands and feet with ice packs both before and during chemotherapy with doxorubicin and taxanes has been found to reduce HFS and nail changes through vasoconstriction.

DRUG ERUPTIONS RELATED TO TARGETED ANTICANCER THERAPIES

Clinical Presentation

Hand-Foot Skin Reaction (HFSR)

The small molecule tyrosine kinase inhibitors sunitinib and sorafenib and others that target angiogenesis are associated with a high incidence of hand-foot skin reaction (HFSR), but the clinical and histologic patterns of HFSR differ from the classic acral erythema caused by conventional cytotoxic agents (Table 9-5). HFSR is characterized by well-demarcated, bean- to coin-sized, hyperkeratotic, painful plaques with underlying erythema localized to the pressure areas of the hands and feet (Fig. 9-28).

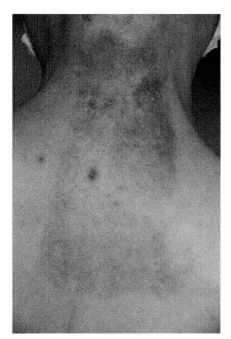

FIGURE 9-27: Radiation recall dermatitis due to docetaxel.

In contrast, acral erythema or HFS is most often characterized by a symmetric edema and diffuse erythema of the palms and soles (Fig. 9-29) which may progress to blistering and necrosis.

Keratotic Lesions

In patients treated with vemurafenib and dabrafenib, 12% and 8% have been reported to develop cutaneous squamous cell carcinoma (SCC) and keratoacanthoma, respectively. Most growths appear 2 to 14 weeks after treatment, and SCC and keratoacanthoma (Fig. 9-30) represent the most common neoplasms. Treatment consists of excision.

Benign keratotic lesions can also be found, and several studies have shown that verrucous keratosis is the most common manifestation.

Photosensitivity

Photosensitivity has been shown to occur in 7% to 12% of patients taking vemurafenib.

Papulopustular Eruptions

Epidermal growth factor receptor (EGFR) inhibitors such as gefitinib, erlotinib, afatinib, and cetuximab generate a unique constellation of skin toxicities, including papulopustular eruptions, hair and nail changes, mucositis, and photosensitivity. The eruption of papules and pustules in a seborrheic distribution is the most common and earliest cutaneous side effect of anti-EGFR agents. Such eruptions consist of folliculocentric pruritic papules evolving into pustules that may coalesce into lakes of pus involving the face (Fig. 9-31), neck, trunk

TABLE 9-5 • Comparison Between Hand-Foot Syndrome (HFS) and Hand-Foot Skin Reaction (HFSR)

	HFS	HFSR
Incidence	1. 6%–89% 2. Doxorubicin plus continuous 5-FU has a highest reported incidence of 89%	1. 4.5%–79% 2. Sorafenib plus bevacizumab has a highest reported incidence of 79%
Clinical presentation	1. Symmetric erythema and edema in palms and soles, accompanied by preceding numbness, itching, or tingling pain (dysesthesia) 2. Can progress to blistering with desquamation, erosion, ulceration, or necrosis	1. Localized, tender lesions over areas subjected to friction or trauma 2. Well demarcated, bean to coin sized, hyperkeratotic, painful plaques with underlying erythema localized to the pressure areas of the hands and feet 3. May appear as well demarcated blisters or ulcers
Histopathology	1. Hyperkeratosis, parakeratosis; epidermal dysmaturation with some dyskeratotic keratinocytes in the epidermis 2. Basal layer vacuolar degeneration or full-thickness necrosis; spongiosis	1. Hyperkeratosis 2. Well-defined band of discohesive dyskeratotic keratinocytes
Causative agents	1. Mainly chemotherapeutic agents 2. Pegylated liposomal doxorubicin, capecitabine, 5-fluorouracil, cytarabine, docetaxel and doxorubicin, other cytotoxic agents	1. Mainly targeted anticancer therapies 2. Multikinase inhibitors (sorafenib, sunitinib, axitinib, pazopanib, regorafenib, bevacizumab, and vemurafenib)

Abbreviations: HFS, hand-foot syndrome; HFSR, hand-foot skin reaction

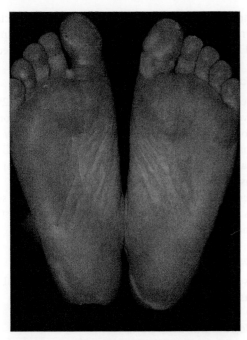

FIGURE 9-28: HFSR is characterized by well demarcated, bean to coin sized, hyperkeratotic, painful plaques with underlying erythema localized to the pressure areas of the hands and feet.

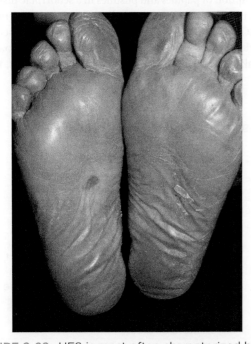

FIGURE 9-29: HFS is most often characterized by a symmetric edema and diffuse erythema of the palms and soles.

(Fig. 9-32), and proximal upper extremities. Rupture of these pustules may lead to crusting and hyperkeratosis.

Pigmentary Changes

Dyspigmentation associated with imatinib use has been described as having a localized, patchy, or diffuse distribution. This is

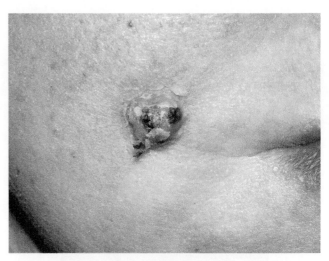

FIGURE 9-30: Keratoacanthoma developed after vemurafenib treatment.

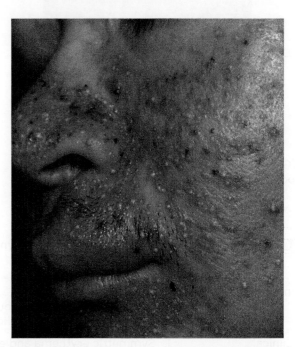

FIGURE 9-31: EGFR inhibitor-induced papulopustular eruptions on the face

consistent with the documented role of c-kit in the physiology of melanocytes, including the regulation of melanogenesis, and the proliferation, migration, and survival of melanocytes.

Hair and Nail Changes

EGFR inhibitors may also induce hair changes such as partial hair loss, curly hair, and trichomegaly; nail changes include paronychia with or without granulation tissue (Fig. 9-33).

Management and Prognosis

High potency topical corticosteroids combined with topical keratolytics, such as urea, are useful for HFSR. Papulopustular eruptions may be managed successfully with topical medications

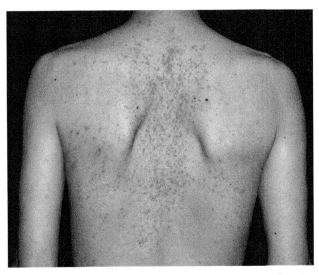

FIGURE 9-32: Papulopustular eruptions on the trunk.

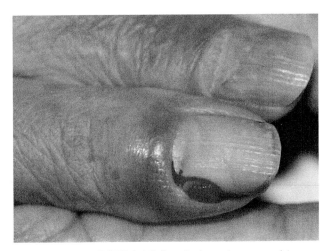

FIGURE 9-33: EGFR inhibitor-induced paronychia with granulation tissue.

alone, including antibiotics, antiseptic creams, and/or low potency topical corticosteroids. Antibacterial soaks (diluted bleach or vinegar in water) are recommended to prevent superinfection of the nail folds. Warm compresses, silver nitrate, topical corticosteroids, and systemic tetracyclines may also be used to reduce periungual inflammation in paronychia.

Suggested Readings

Chen YC, Cho YT, Chang CY, et al. Drug reaction with eosinophilia and systemic symptoms (DRESS): a drug-induced hypersensitivity syndrome with variable clinical features. *Dermatol Sin.* 2013;31:196–204.

Cho YT, Lin JW, Chen YC, et al. Generalized bullous fixed drug eruption is distinct from Stevens-Johnson syndrome/toxic epidermal necrolysis by immunohistopathological features. *J Am Acad Dermatol.* 2014;70:539–548.

Häusermann P, Harr TH, Bircher AJ. Baboon syndrome resulting from systemic drugs: is there strife between SDRIFE and allergic contact dermatitis syndrome? *Contact Dermatitis.* 2004:51:297–310.

Macdonald JB, Macdonald B, Golitz LE, et al. Cutaneous adverse effects of targeted therapies: part I: inhibitors of the cellular membrane. *J Am Acad Dermatol.* 2015;72:203–218.

Macdonald JB, Macdonald B, Golitz LE, et al. Cutaneous adverse effects of targeted therapies: part II: inhibitors of intracellular molecular signaling pathways. *J Am Acad Dermatol.* 2015;72:221–236.

Miller KK, Gorcey L, McLellan BN. Chemotherapy-induced hand-foot syndrome and nail changes: a review of clinical presentation, etiology, pathogenesis, and management. *J Am Acad Dermatol.* 2014;71:787–794.

Mockenhaupt M. Severe drug-induced skin reactions: clinical pattern, diagnostics and therapy. *JDDG.* 2009;7:142–160.

Pichler WJ, Adam J, Daubner B, et al. Drug hypersensitivity reactions: pathomechanism and clinical symptoms. *Med Clin North Am.* 2010;94:645–664.

Reyes-Habito CM, Roh EK. Cutaneous reactions to chemotherapeutic drugs and targeted therapies for cancer: part I. Conventional chemotherapeutic drugs. *J Am Acad Dermatol.* 2014;71:203.e1–203.e12.

Reyes-Habito CM, Roh EK. Cutaneous reactions to chemotherapeutic drugs and targeted therapies for cancer: part II. Targeted therapies. *J Am Acad Dermatol.* 2014;71:217.e1–217.e11.

Roujeau JC, Stern RS. Severe adverse cutaneous reactions to drugs. *N Engl J Med.* 1994;331:1272–1285.

Roujeau JC. Clinical heterogeneity of drug hypersensitivity. *Toxicology.* 2005;209:123–129.

Szatkowski J, Schwartz RA. Acute generalized exanthematous pustulosis (AGEP): a review and update. *J Am Acad Dermatol.* 2015;73:843–848.

Valeyrie-Allanore L, Sassolas B, Roujeau JC. Drug-induced skin, nail and hair disorders. *Drug Safety.* 2007;30:1011–1030.

Ulcer Management: Evaluation and Care

Ingrid Herskovitz, MD, Flor MacQuhae, MD, Olivia Hughes, BS, and Robert S. Kirsner, MD, PhD

A wound can be defined as a disruption in the normal structure and function of the skin and soft tissues. Several etiologies may cause a wound, and wounds can be classified as acute or chronic depending on the duration the wound has been present and the time course of healing. Acute wounds, such as those resulting from traumatic injuries, burns, and surgically created wounds, heal in a timely fashion, following the normal, overlapping stages of wound healing including coagulation, inflammation, proliferation, and remodeling.

WOUND HEALING PHASES

- The coagulation or hemostasis phase involves fibrin, platelets, endothelial cells, and other mediators of the clotting cascade. After injury activated platelets have an increased number of surface receptors, and their subsequent granule release, associated with aggregation, are not only the mainstay for clotting but for wound healing as well. Platelet granules stimulate matrix production and release growth factors such as platelet-derived growth factor (PDGF), transforming growth factor-β (TGF-β), fibroblast growth factor-2 (FGF-2), vascular endothelial growth factor (VEGF), hepatocyte growth factor (HGF), insulin-like growth factor-1 (IGF), and epidermal growth factor (EGF). These growth factors and cytokines such as IL-1α, IL-1β, IL-6, and tumor necrosis factor-α (TNF-α) have downstream effects on fibroblasts, keratinocytes, and endothelial cells throughout the wound healing process and are essential for tissue repair.

- The inflammatory phase (0 to 5 days) starts soon after coagulation. A coordinated cascade of events such as neural input, mast cell degranulation, histamine release, and kinin production causes vasodilatation and increases permeability causing increased blood flow which clinically translates to heat, erythema, swelling, and oftentimes pain with extravasation of proteins and cells from the circulation to the injury site. Specialized cells such as neutrophils and macrophages are recruited to the injury site to remove debris, bacteria,

and damaged tissue, and release pro-inflammatory cytokines that activate keratinocytes and promote wound healing. Macrophages are key cells as they release chemotactic factors, angiogenic factors, and growth factors which recruit other cells (e.g., fibroblasts), induce formation of new blood vessels, and stimulate cellular proliferation and extracellular matrix (ECM) production.

- The proliferative phase (3 to 24 days) leads to granulation tissue formation which is characterized by capillary loops in a matrix of collagen produced in response to PDGF and other growth factors. Fibroblasts migrate into the wound and produce collagen and other components of the ground substance, release cytokines and growth factors such as IL-1 and TNF-α, and fibroblast growth factor-7 (FGF-7) that regulate keratinocyte activity. Cell migration is key and in the important step of migration cells move from the edges into the wound bed along the extracellular matrix through cell adhesion proteins (e.g., integrins) and matrix metalloproteinases (MMPs). The keratinocytes migrate in clusters from the wound edge through "contact guidance" cellular movement, coordinated by mechanical and chemical cues for approximation of wound edges. Keratinocytes from the wound margins and keratinocyte stem cells derived from follicular bulges participate in this process, stimulated by FGF-2, -7, -10, nerve growth factor (NGF), hepatocyte growth factor (HGF), fibrin, plasminogen, and matrix metalloproteinases (MMPs), particularly collagenase, also known as MMP-1. Additionally, keratinocyte proliferation is stimulated by HB-EGF, growth-related oncogene (GRO)-α/CXCL-1 chemokine (C-X-C motif) ligand, IL-6, granulocyte-macrophage colony-stimulating factor (GM-CSF), and nitric oxide. In concert with coverage provided by keratinocytes (reepithelialization), myofibroblasts cause wound contraction. Proteoglycans and glycosaminoglycans (GAG) such as hyaluronic acid, dermatan sulfate, chondroitin sulfate, and heparan sulfate are part of the extracellular matrix and play a role in regulating cellular events, vascular endothelial cells, cytokines, enzymes, and growth factors in the ECM involved in immune function and cellular repair. There is an inter-relation between the immune system and tissue repair as increased heparan sulfate expression has been shown to correlate with the presence of antimicrobial peptides in wounds.

- The remodeling phase (3 weeks to 2 years) is the final step of normal wound healing. Main components for the completion of the wound healing process in this phase are fibroblasts, collagen, MMPs, tissue inhibitors of MMPs, and blood vessels. The process of collagen reorganization takes place primarily mediated by MMPs. Over time type III collagen is replaced by type I collagen. Around 6 months, when the remodeling is most active, the repaired tissue regains 70% to 80% of its pre-injury tensile strength. Fibroblasts phenotypically change into myofibroblasts in response to PDGF, TGF-β, and per-oxisome proliferator-activated receptor (PPAR). This process incurs in wound contraction because of the con-tractile properties of actin filaments within these cells. Reduction in the number of blood vessels and fibroblasts in the wound area result in scar maturation.

Chronic wounds are defined as wounds that do not undergo the normal overlapping stages of wound healing resulting in a lengthy time to function restoration. Chronic wounds may be at different stages of healing because of loss of synchronicity, which in turn causes delay in the healing process. Chronic wounds are not only a physical and psychological burden on patients but also a financial burden on them and on the health care system. Chronic wounds affect populations worldwide, and it is estimated that in the United States alone 6.5 million people are affected. The most common lower extremity ulcers are venous leg ulcers (VLU) related to venous hypertension (with 2% prevalence in developed countries), pressure ulcers (PU) (which ranges from 0.4% to 38% in acute settings and from 0% to 24% in chronic settings) and diabetic foot ulcers (DFU) from vascular disease and neuropathy which occur in 25% of patients with diabetes mellitus, and arterial ulcers (AU) in the absence of diabetes mellitus.

While how fast a wound should heal depends on a variety of factors such as patient age, wound location and cause, chronic wounds are generally present for more than a month and fail to reduce in size without a specific intervention. A good patient history will often reveal important aspects of the patient's health and lifestyle that will enlighten the wound care clinician and direct the diagnosis:

- Ulcer duration and ulcer characteristics (size, depth, site, pain, accompanying edema or lesions, changes of the surrounding skin and exudate, limb temperature, fever)
- History of previous ulceration or trauma, assessment of patient's shoes
- Patient's comorbidities (diabetes mellitus, peripheral vascular disease [PVD], arterial disease, hypertension, vasculitis, malignancy, infectious or inflammatory diseases, neurological conditions, connective tissue dis-eases, varicose veins, deep venous thrombosis, smok-ing, etc.)
- Allergies and medications: antidepressants, antihy-pertensive agents (such as calcium channel blockers, β-blockers, direct vasodilators, antisympathomimetics), hormones, steroids, nonsteroidal anti-inflammatories, glitazones.

After obtaining a thorough history and performing a physical examination, the initial workup should be directed toward these common etiologies (see Table 10-1).

TABLE 10-1 • Initial Management of Chronic Ulcers and Examples

	VLU	DFU	PU	Arterial Ulcer
Location	Distal leg (medially or laterally).	Plantar or lateral foot on pressure points.	Over bony prominences such as sacral, ischial, or calcaneus area.	Distal foot and toes or anterior aspect of leg.
Physical examination	Ulcers are relatively superficial with irregular sloping borders. Base can be exu-dative or dry. Skin changes surround-ing the ulcer include edema, scaling, hyperpigmentation, and thickening of the skin and subcu-taneous tissue.	Varying depth ulcers surrounded by callus. The ulcer is generally not painful. Sensation of the surrounding skin is diminished. There can also be deformity of bones and foot architecture, and the skin around can be scaly due to autonomic neuropa-thy. The ulcer could be infected leading to osteomyelitis.	There are four defined stages for pressure injury that are graded according to the depth of compromised tissues. This lesion can start from the outer layers of skin or from deep structures such as the muscle. They are usually located on the bony prominences or pressure points such as the ischial area, sacral area, and heels.	This is in general the most pain-ful type of ulcer. It has punched out edges and necrosis. Palpations of anterior tibial and dorsalis pedis pulses.

(continued)

TABLE 10-1 • Initial Management of Chronic Ulcers and Examples (continued)

	VLU	DFU	PU	Arterial Ulcer
Main diagnostic steps	Measurement of ankle-brachial index (ABI) and ultrasound guided venous and arterial studies to check integrity of vascular system and the presence of PVD. Hyper-coagulability screen.	Identification of pressure points, if osteomyelitis suspected (deep and recurrent wounds, increasing pain, erythema, edema, temperature, purulent exudates, probing to bone), X-ray of extremity, MRI	Identification of pressure points	Pulse paplaption. Arterial doppler and arterial angiogram. Magnetic resonance angiography (MRA). Ankle-brachial indices (ABI). Toe digital pressures with pulse volume recordings.
Grading system		Wagner grading system **Grade 1:** Superficial diabetic ulcer **Grade 2:** Ulcer extension Involves ligament, tendon, joint capsule or fascia No abscess or osteomyelitis **Grade 3:** Deep ulcer with abscess or osteomyelitis **Grade 4:** Gangrene to portion of forefoot **Grade 5:** Extensive gangrene of foot.	**Stage 1** Intact skin with localized *nonblanchable* erythema. **Stage 2** Partial thickness wound with shallow open ulcer with pink wound bed. **Stage 3** Full thickness tissue loss. Exposed *subcutaneous fat* but bone, tendon, or muscle is not exposed. The presence of *sloughed tissue* may be undermined. **Stage 4** Full thickness tissue loss with exposed *bone, tendon,* or *muscle*. There is often presence of slough and/or *eschar*.	

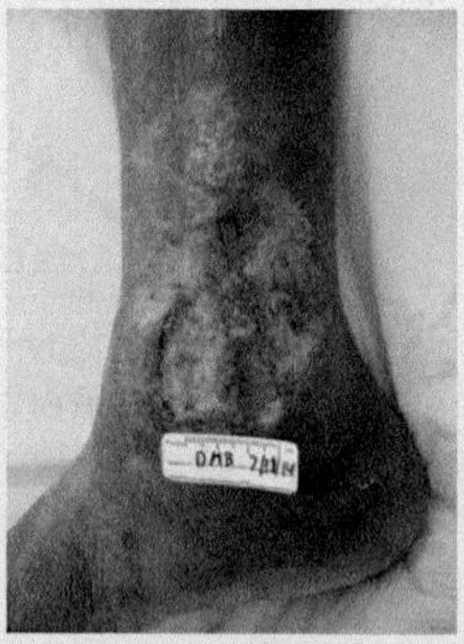

FIGURE 10-1

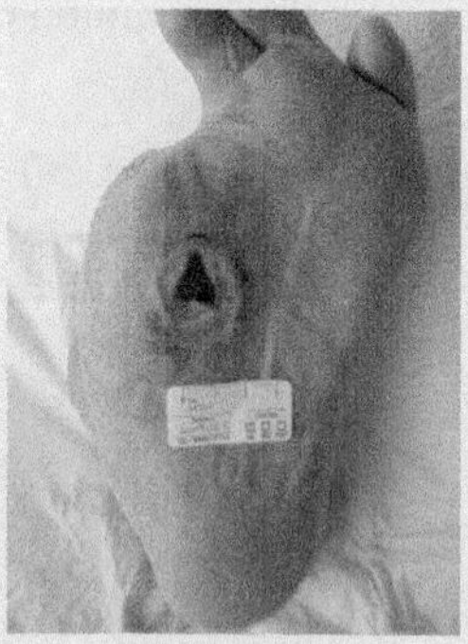

FIGURE 10-2

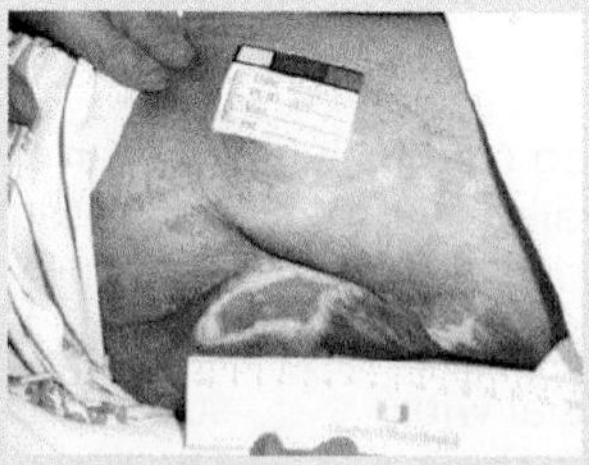

FIGURE 10-3

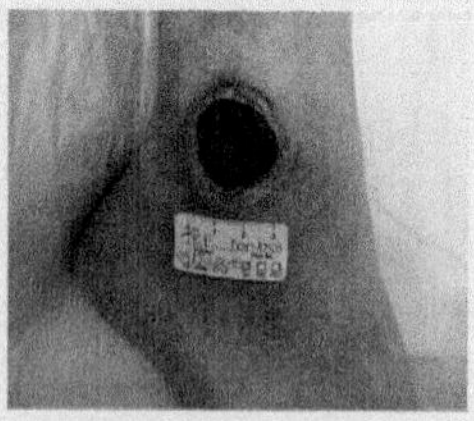

FIGURE 10-4

Abbreviations: DFU, diabetic foot ulcer; MRI, magnetic resonance imaging; PU, pressure ulcer; PVD, peripheral vascular disease; VLU, venous leg ulcer.

PATHOPHYSIOLOGY OF VENOUS LEG ULCERS

VLU are related to chronic venous hypertension which is a product of abnormal retrograde venous blood flow due to incompetent valves and calf muscle pump failure. These lead to increased ambulatory venous pressure which promotes distension of capillary walls and leakage of molecules, such as fibrinogen, into the dermis and subcutaneous tissues. Once fibrinogen leaks out of the capillaries, it polymerizes to form fibrin-creating areas of hardened walls around the capillaries. These cuffs may function like a barrier to the exchange of oxygen and nutrients and may impede the normal transit of growth factors. Other possible causes of delayed healing that occur in patients with venous insufficiency are related to inflammation and leukocyte demargination in the capillaries which act as a physical barrier and release substances such as metalloproteinases, cytokines, free radicals, proteolytic enzymes, and chemotactic factors that negatively affect healing. The disruption of the microcirculation is important in the pathophysiologic process of venous hypertension. The endothelium regulates vascular tone, hemostasis, and coagulation. Processes such as injury, infection, immune diseases, diabetes, genetic predisposition, environmental factors, smoking, and atherosclerosis may damage the vascular wall. The pathologic process begins with increased shear stress on the endothelial cells, causing the release of vasoactive agents and expression of E-selectin, inflammatory molecules, chemokines, and prothrombotic precursors.

The physical examination of a patient's wound with a VLU oftentimes characteristically shows an ulcer of the medial malleolus area that is superficial with irregular borders, with exudate, and with a covering layer of fibrinous material. The skin surrounding the ulcer commonly presents with discoloration, scaling, edema, telangiectasias, induration, and atrophic scars (atrophie blanche) (see Fig. 10-1 in Table 10-1).

Prognostic indicators for ulcer healing are important in identifying potentially slow or non-healing ulcers. These prognostic factors are: a size larger than 5 cm², wound of long duration, and a wound healing rate in the first month of therapy <40%. In the prognosis of VLU, it is expected that after 6 months of treatment, 50% to 70% of patients will be healed.

PATHOPHYSIOLOGY OF DIABETIC FOOT ULCERS

Diabetic neuropathy is the primary underlying condition of DFU and in some patients is associated with peripheral vascular disease.

The neuropathy is a product of nitric oxide production blockade which results in elevated levels of free radicals and reduced vasodilator activity. It is also related to the lower production of neuropeptides such as nerve growth factor, substance P, and calcitonin gene-related peptide. While focus has been on sensory neuropathy, the neuropathy in patients with DFU can be sensory, motor, and/or autonomic. The sensory loss eliminates the protective characteristic of feeling pain, pressure, and heat, facilitating traumatic injury to the affected area. Motor neuropathy together with nonenzymatic glycosylation of periarticular soft tissues leads to limitations in joint mobility, muscle atrophy, ligament stretching, and concomitant foot deformities. The resultant effect is a less biomechanically functioning foot.

Additionally, in DFU physiopathology, there is also a functional ischemia that is likely a consequence of the prolonged inflammatory response in the microcirculation that leads to thickening of the basement membrane impairing the active exchanges between the microcirculation and the interstitium as well as limiting the elastic capacity of capillary walls.

DFU are often painless, usually appear in areas of repetitive trauma on the foot, being therefore more frequent over bony prominences and where the shoe rubs against the foot. The ulcer can be "hidden" under a thick callous or it can be evident with skin slough, a bloody exudate, and/or different depth levels (see Fig. 10-2 in Table 10-1).

There are different systems of classification based on depth, infection, and ischemia that are used, and an example is portrayed in the table below (see Table 10-1).

PATHOPHYSIOLOGY OF PRESSURE ULCERS

PU most often develop with compression of tissues that underlie bony prominences within a short period of time, between 2 and 6 hours. These ulcers can develop from the surface or begin within deeper tissue planes such as the muscle, since the latter is extremely sensitive to pressure-induced ischemia. The main mechanisms of ulcer development are thought to be sustained pressure with perpendicular and tangential forces to the surface, lower skin resistance in the elderly due to changes in composition of the skin, superficial erosions caused by friction, and excessive humidity of the skin related to bodily secretions (sweat, urine).

The physical exam of these ulcers can also show different stages/depths and usually have clear, demarcated, and/or often undermined borders (see Table 10-1). They are located on areas where the patient exerts more pressure in prolonged positions like the heels and the sacral and ischial areas most commonly (see Fig. 10-3 in Table 10-1).

PATHOPHYSIOLOGY OF ARTERIAL ULCERS

AU result from occlusion of the arteries proximal to the developed lesion. Atherosclerosis from lipid deposition on vessel walls is the most common etiology. These compromised vessels are not able to adequately supply the oxygen demand of the tissues leading to ischemia and local necrosis of tissue. This process is further aggravated by hypertension, diabetes mellitus, and smoking. Other causes of arterial compromise are seen but are less frequent and they may be related to collagen tissue disease, malignancies, vasculitis, hemoglobin diseases, etc.

The physical exam of these ulcers often shows a typically small, punched out, necrotic ulcer. Pain, especially when the limb is elevated, and pulses are diminished or absent. Classic ulcers are anterior (which has less arterial redundancy) or distal but may complicate other types of ulcers (see Fig. 10-4 in Table 10-1).

Other relevant causes of extremity wounds are related to vasculitis, malignancy, and pyoderma gangrenosum.

Vasculitis generally occurs in the setting of an inflammatory disease or of a connective tissue disease (such as lupus, polyarteritis nodosa, Churg–Strauss). The lesions in these diseases may present as painful ulcers with nonspecific characteristics such as a wide distribution pattern, punched out or superficial beds, or variation in size. But they are generally associated with systemic symptoms such as fever, malaise, anemia, and immunological markers. In this case, a deep biopsy read by an experienced dermatopathologist is warranted as the diagnosis can be challenging.

Malignancy-associated ulcers can be due to local skin malignancy and as such most commonly occur due to basal cell and squamous cell carcinoma. There can also be wounds that are a consequence of metastatic cancer such as breast cancer and lung cancer. These wounds also tend not to have specific characteristics but tend to come in a large number generally distributed in the trunk. They can be superficial, irregular, coalescent, and bleeding or isolated keratotic inflamed ulcers. Biopsy is warranted to elucidate the origin of the cells in the lesion.

Pyoderma gangrenosum is an inflammatory invasion of neutrophils with painful, rapidly growing ulcers. It is associated with inflammatory bowel disease and other comorbidities including leukemia and collagen vascular diseases.

WOUND CARE OF LOWER LEG ULCERS

Although local wound treatment is important, it is imperative to look at the whole patient, the underlying disease pathophysiology, and the patient-centered concerns before looking at the wound itself.

In order to identify the underlying cause and formulate a complete diagnosis, it is necessary to first perform a comprehensive patient assessment. After the patient assessment comes the wound assessment, which is necessary to outline the wound characteristics which will provide initial information to recognize impediments to the healing process. Furthermore, this is necessary to determine prognosis and create a precise treatment plan.

Based on evidence and practice, several approaches and guidelines have been created and used for wound care purposes. Dressings, cellular and acellular matrices are some examples of wound care treatment options; however, it is vital to individualize patient goals.

Faster and more complete wound healing is one of the major objectives, and this is achieved by providing an optimal wound environment. Wound bed preparation is crucial for wound healing. It includes the use of different methods to evaluate and remove the barriers, so that wound repair can progress normally. The general goal is to achieve a moist and stable wound that has healthy granulation tissue and a well-vascularized wound bed. Both local and systemic factors can delay healing.

Patient Assessment and Patient Concerns

Among the first steps to determine the patient's wound healing capacity is determining the patient's general health status (Table 10-2). Patient assessment is critical for the treatment plan and evaluation of care. It should include:

- Medical history (including past medical history, family history, and social habits)
- Cause of tissue damage
- Medication and allergies
- Comorbidities such as: diabetes mellitus, vascular disease, immunological disease
- Nutrition
- Lifestyle and environment; obesity, tobacco, and alcohol use/abuse
- Mobility, daily activities, occupation
- Inadequate social network, caregiver support
- Psychological assessment for stress and/or depression
- Laboratory assessment

A complete clinical history of the patient is essential. This includes history of present illness, past medical history (PMH), current medications, previous ulcer history, previous and current treatment, etc. Furthermore, laboratory studies should be included in the assessment. These studies include: complete blood count (CBC), comprehensive metabolic panel (CMP), hemoglobin A1c, protein, albumin and pre-albumin levels.

Although the diagnosis in most of the cases can be made by clinical criteria alone, studies suggested that 25% of patients will have ulcers with mixed characteristics; for this reason, noninvasive methods may aid in the diagnosis as well as anatomic and functional evaluation of the venous and arterial system.

Imaging studies are sometimes necessary, especially if osteomyelitis is suspected (x-ray, MRI), to assess blood flow (ankle-brachial index [ABI], venous and arterial ultrasounds). Moreover, a deep tissue biopsy and culture of the lesion might

TABLE 10-2 • Patient Assessment	
Patient Clinical History	**Laboratory Studies**
Past medical history and history of present illness: Previous ulcers, previous treatments, current medications, current diagnosis and treatment, etc.	CBC: RBC, WBC, TLC, Hb, Hct; Glucose, hemoglobin A1c, albumin, pre-albumin, electrolytes, total protein count, hypercoaguability screen.
Imaging	
X-ray, MRI, venous and arterial ultrasounds, other vascular studies if applicable.	Biopsy, culture, special stains.

Abbreviations: CBC, complete blood count; Hb, hemoglobin; Hct, hematocrit; MRI, magnetic resonance imaging; RBC, red blood count; TLC, T-lymphocyte count; WBC, white blood count.

be necessary to assess the presence of an atypical infection and/or other possible atypical etiologies.

In the management of DFUs, the important aspects are: assessment of the diabetic foot; assessment and optimization of vascular supply; local wound care: wound debridement, infection control (detection and treatment), topical antimicrobials, wound dressings; plantar pressure redistribution; and advanced therapies. It is important to evaluate the presence of neuropathic and/or nociceptive pain along with a loss of protective sensation through the Semmes-Weinstein monofilament exam (SWME) (Table 10-3).

Tests and Procedures to Evaluate Low Extremity Ulcers

The ABI (Table 10-4) aids in detecting peripheral vascular disease. It consists in obtainment of the systolic blood pressure from the calf by occluding the pedal arteries with the cuff. The ankle systolic pressure is obtained when the first sound on Doppler ultrasonography is heard after deflation of the cuff.

Then it is compared with the brachial systolic pressure to determine the ABI (a normal ABI value should be >1). If the value is less, this will identify patients with peripheral arterial disease.

Due to normal-false-negative results in the elderly and in diabetic patients, arterial flow should be further assessed with toe-brachial index, transcutaneous oxygen measurement, and pulse volume recordings, among others. Assessment of vascular status is critical as compression therapy is the main treatment for VLUs and beneficial to all well-vascularized limbs. Compression in patients with arterial disease might be contraindicated; it can lead to worsening and, sometimes, to gangrene. Arterial studies can shed a light on whether a more widespread disease is present with involvement of other arteries such as the coronaries. Additionally, vascular studies

are important to assess if the arterial problem in question can be surgically corrected.

The gold standard diagnostic test to determine venous disease is the *color duplex ultrasound*. Not only it is accurate but also noninvasive, reproducible, and provides anatomic and functional data about venous and arterial systems.

Additional tests such as *photo and air plethysmography* allow the clinician to assess whole-limb venous hemodynamics at rest and after exercise. *Invasive venography* is typically used in anticipation of a venous intervention. *Radiography, bone scanning,* and *bone biopsy* are tests that should be always considered if bone infection is suspected, but MRI remains the gold standard for noninvasive tests.

Tissue biopsy should be performed for wounds with an unusual presentation or wounds present for extended period of time without healing. Under microscopic examination, inflammatory, malignant, and infectious etiologies may be detected and tissue should be sent for *tissue culture* as well. In patients with diabetes mellitus, metabolic factors should be assessed including glucose glycated hemoglobin (HbA$_1$c), which is the best indicator of glucose control over a period of time and is associated with a higher potential for suppressing the inflammatory response.

WOUND ASSESSMENT

Wound evaluation includes wound location, evaluating its borders, size, depth, surrounding tissue conditions, onset, and accompanying symptoms (Table 10-5).

There are important questions to ask upon assessing a wound for the first time and on follow-ups:

1. What caused the wound? Obtain with clinical history, physical examination, and support studies if necessary.

TABLE 10-3 • Patient Assessment—Semmes-Weinstein Monofilament Exam (SWME)

SWME test is performed using a single nylon monofilament to check the patient's sensation. The tip of the monofilament is placed perpendicular to the skin, then it is bended over the foot and released (see Figs. 10-5 and 10-6).

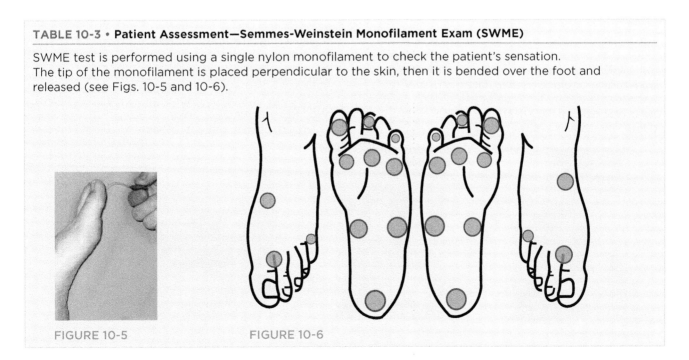

FIGURE 10-5   FIGURE 10-6

TABLE 10-4 • Patient Assessment—Ankle-Brachial Index (ABI)

ABI of the Affected Leg

Screens patients for significant arterial insufficiency.
Identifies patients for whom compression would not be appropriate.

$$\frac{\text{(Higher of 2 Ankle Pressures)}}{\text{(Higher of 2 Brachial Pressures)}} = \text{ABI}$$

>1.3	Abnormally High Range
0.95–1.3	Normal range
0.80–0.95	Compression is considered safe
<0.8	Arterial disease

2. Where is the wound located? Photographs and wound diagram are useful.
3. What does the wound bed and the surrounding skin look like?
4. Does the wound look infected?
5. What is the wound size? For follow-up visits, is the size improving?
6. What are the characteristics and amount of drainage?
7. Are there associated symptoms (pain, pruritus, and edema)? For follow-up visits, is pain improving?

TREATMENT OF LOWER EXTREMITY ULCERS

Treatment of lower extremity ulcers is a difficult task, and not only will it vary based on the type of wound but the success

TABLE 10-5 • Wound Assessment

1. What Caused the Wound?

Venous disease?
Arterial disease?
Pressure ulcer?
Diabetic neuropathic ulcer?
Trauma?
Insect bite?
Animal bite?
Related to obsessive picking in mental illness?

2. Where Is the Wound Located?

To point out the location of the wound(s) (Fig. 10-7).

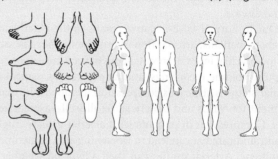

FIGURE 10-7

3. What Does the Wound Bed and Surrounding Skin Look Like?

Pink to red: Viable, living tissue (granulating) (see Fig. 10-8).
Yellow, tan or gray: Slough, fibrinous tissue (see Fig. 10-9).
Dark brown or black: Eschar, necrotic tissue.
Each time describe the type of tissue describe it in percentages (see Fig. 10-10).
(Note: The total is always 100%)

4. Does the Wound Look Infected?

Demonstrated by:
  Pain, swelling, redness, warmth
  Secondary signs
  Delayed or stalled healing
  Increased drainage or exudate
  Increase or change in odor
  Wound bed change in color
  Overall decline in patient's health

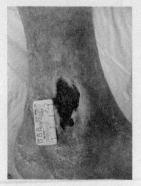

FIGURE 10-8

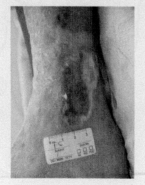

FIGURE 10-9

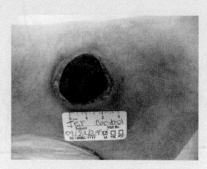

FIGURE 10-10

TABLE 10-5 • Wound Assessment (continued)

5. What Is the Wound Size?

The size will impact the treatment and healing process.
  Correct ways to measure a wound:
    Use a disposable centimeter ruler.
    Measurement consistency is key.
For follow-up visits, is the size improving?
There are two options for traditional wound measurement (Fig. 10-11):

A. Top of the wound is toward the patient's head. The bottom of the wound is toward the patient's feet (see Fig. 10-12).
   Vector 1: Length is measured in cm distal to proximal at the widest distance between the edges.
   Vector 2: Width is measured in cm perpendicular to the previous vector at the widest distance.

B. Regardless of the wound orientation to the patient (see Fig. 10-13).
   Vector 3: Measure the length at the longest distance.
   Vector 4: Measure the width perpendicular to the previous vector.

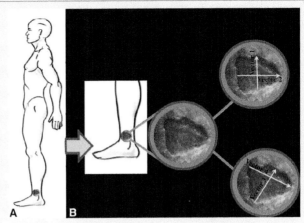

A   B

FIGURE 10-11: Traditional wound measurement. **A:** Top of the wound is toward the patient's head. The bottom of the wound is toward the patient's feet. Vector1: Length is measured in cm distal to proximal at the widest distance between the edges. Vector 2: Width is measured in cm perpendicular to the previous vector at the widest distance. **B:** Regardless of the wound orientation to the patient. Vector 3: Measure the length at the longest distance. Vector 4: Measure the width perpendicular to the previous vector.

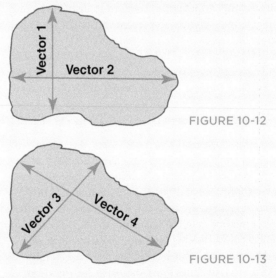

FIGURE 10-12

FIGURE 10-13

Depth should be measured using the deepest part of the wound, perpendicular to the surface of the skin (see Fig. 10-14).
1. Insert cotton-tipped applicator
2. Grasp the applicator with the thumb and forefinger, level with the surface of the skin
3. Measure against a centimeter ruler

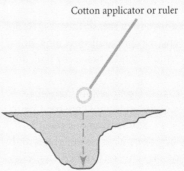

Cotton applicator or ruler

FIGURE 10-14

(continued)

TABLE 10-5 • Wound Assessment (continued)

6. What Are the Characteristics (Type) and Amount of Drainage (Exudate)?	7. Is There Pain Associated with the Wound? (On Follow-up Visits: Is the Pain Improving? Is Associated with Compression Therapy or Other Treatment?): Use Pain Scale.

Type:
  Serous (serum)
  Serosanguinous (serum and blood)
  Sanguineous (bloody)
  Purulent (pus)
Amount:
  Light, moderate, abundant
  Other characteristics: Color, odor
	Wong-Baker FACES (see Fig. 10-15):
	  Pain rating scale
	  Ask the patient to point to the face and number that represents their pain. The pain scale goes from 0 to 10.
	
	FIGURE 10-15

will require a complete patient and wound assessment, having in mind that some patients can present combined etiologies and systemic diseases (Tables 10-6 to 10-8).

Standard wound care (SWC) is a term usually found in the wound care setting. SWC refers to accepted wound care procedures used to treat patients to enhance the healing process.

The standard of care and special care for ulcers include:

- *Edema control:* As health care providers, it is important to educate our patients. There are many goals when treating venous leg ulcers, which include reduction of edema, improvement of pain, ulcer healing, and prevention of recurrence. Bed rest with leg elevation is the simplest method (but least realistic) to help in reversing the effects of venous hypertension. Patients must elevate their legs above the level of the heart for 30 minutes three to four times every day. Also, leg elevation at night decreases swelling and will improve venous circulation. Other methods to decrease edema include lymphedema pumps and compression stockings. In arterial ulcers, leg elevation could worsen the pain and this is a clue for diagnosis.

- *Compression:* In addition to leg elevation, compression therapy is the key and standard of care treatment for vascularized leg ulcers. Studies demonstrate that compression therapy improves ulcer healing rates and by using it after healing prevents recurrence. In the majority of cases, compression therapy is well tolerated without adverse events. But it should be used with caution in patients with medical history of congestive heart failure, because compression of the lower limbs can cause an increase in preload volume worsening their condition. The ideal pressure necessary to overcome venous hypertension is not well defined, but an external pressure of 35 to 40 mm Hg at the ankle is necessary to avoid capillary exudation in patients with venous leg ulcers.

There are two types of compression bandages: inelastic and elastic bandages. Inelastic bandages are rigid. They provide high pressure with muscle contraction (during ambulation), but limited pressure at rest. The example of this type of compression is the "Unna boot," which is a moistened zinc oxide impregnated paste bandage that dries to become inelastic. Unna boots require frequent reapplication as they do not accommodate changes in volume when leg edema is reduced and they have restricted absorptive properties for exudative wounds. Rigid bandage or "Unna boot" can be useful at the early edema reduction phase. On the other hand, elastic bandages accommodate volume changes and provide both resting and working pressures, which is the reason why they are commonly used. Elastic compression bandages not only provide constant pressures (working and resting) but when compared with Unna boots they adapt better to the leg and require less frequent dressing changes.

One of the disadvantages of elastic wraps is that they require training for correct application. They come as single or multilayer bandage systems. A meta-analysis showed that multilayer compression bandages appear to be superior to single-layer bandage systems in patients with venous ulcers. This system includes a wool or cotton layer (for absorption

TABLE 10-6 • Clinical Aspects of the Most Common Types of Ulcers of the Lower Limbs

Wound Type	Pathophysiology	Characteristics	Picture Sample	Therapy
Venous leg ulcer (see Fig. 10-16)	Venous hypertension.	Most common in women than men. Usual location: gaiter area.	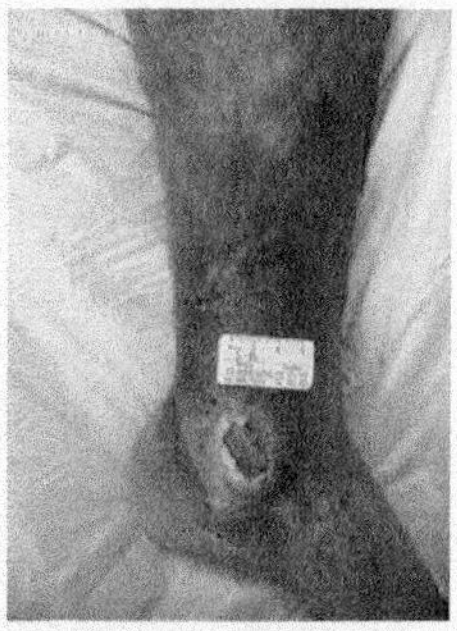 FIGURE 10-16	Leg elevation, compression therapy, aspirin, pentoxifylline, cell and tissue-based therapy. Maintain optimal moisture.
Arterial lower limb ulcer (see Fig. 10-17)	Tissue ischemia. Caused by decreased blood supply, related to arterial disease.	Most common in elderly patients. Usual location: Can be anywhere on the leg, especially the toes and feet, over bony prominences, necrosis present. Abnormal pedal pulses. Typically small, "punched out," well-defined wound borders.	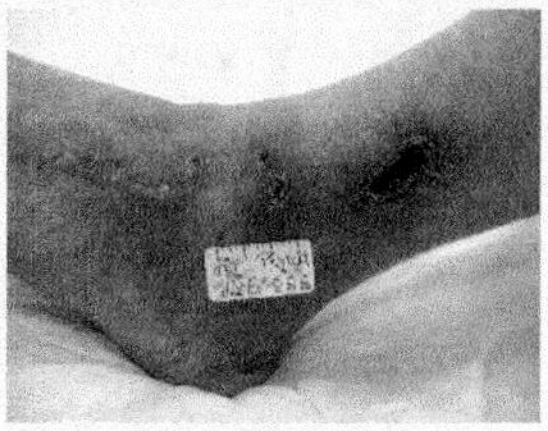 FIGURE 10-17	If perfusion is not adequate, consider vascular consult. If perfusion is adequate, follow protocol based on wound assessment and characteristics. If dry and stable, leave eschar intact.
Neuropathic ulcer (see Fig. 10-18)	Trauma, prolonged pressure.	Most common in patients with diabetes or neurologic disorders. Usual location: Over plantar aspect of foot.	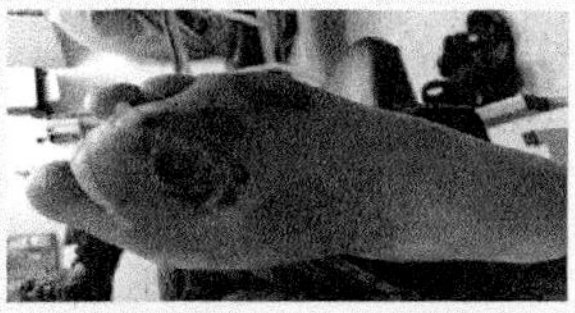 FIGURE 10-18	Off-loading, debridement, topically applied growth factors, tissue-engineered skin.
Pressure ulcer (see Fig. 10-19)	Tissue ischemia and necrosis secondary to prolonged pressure.	Most common in bed-ridden patients. Usual location: Over bony prominence.	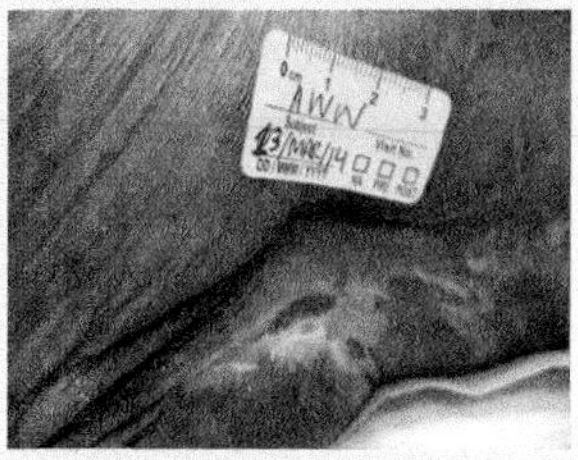 FIGURE 10-19	Goal: Off-loading, proper nutrition, maintain optimal moisture. Surgery consult may be indicated.

TABLE 10-7 • Adjuvant Treatment for Venous Leg Ulcers

Use	Agent
Systemic administration	Pentoxifylline Aspirin
Cellular products	Bilayered living cellular construct (BLCC) (Apligraf, Organogenesis, Canton, MA)
Acellular products	Porcine small intestine submucosa (PSIS) (Oasis, Smith and Nephew, Largo, FL) Poly-N-acetyl glucosamine (pGlcNAc) (Talymed: Marine Polymer Technologies Inc, Danvers, MA) Cadaveric allograft (CA) (AlloDerm; LifeCell Corp., Branchburg, NJ)
Growth factors	GM-CSF
Surgical interventions	Skin grafting
Minimal invasive procedures	Radio frequency endovascular laser ablation

Abbreviation: GM-CSF, granulocyte-macrophage colony-stimulating factor.

TABLE 10-8 • SWC and Special Care for Ulcers: VLUs, DFUs, PUs, etc.

Summary

Debridement (not pyo-derma gangrenous)	Types of debridement: Sharp, pulse, mechanical, chemical, biologic.
Compression	Inelastic compression: Unna boot (with zinc oxide). Elastic compression: Multilayered compression. Compression stockings.
Pain control	Systemic analgesics. Protect ulcer bed with nonadherent pads, topical analgesics, etc. Nonadherent contact dressings.
Edema control	Lymphedema pumps, stockings.
Pressure reduction	Walking boot, total contact cast, off-loading footwear, off-loading devices (special mattress), wheelchair, crutches, etc.

Local Wound Treatment

To clean the wound	Water or saline.
Surrounding wound skin	If dry skin/scaly/irritated: Use skin protectant such as Petrolatum 41%. If irritated: Use skin barrier ointment such as zinc oxide.
Special dressings	If the wound is too dry (hydrate): Hydrogel, Mepilex foam, Mepitil film dressing. Dry to minimal drainage: Hydrofiber dressing, hydroactive gel or patch, hydrogel, honey, foam dressings (gentle). If the wound has minimal drainage (maintain moisture): Hydrocolloids, hydrogel. If the wound is draining moderate or heavy (absorb drainage): Foams, pads, etc. Moderate to heavy drainage: ABD pads, superabsorbent dressings, and alginate wound dressings. If the ulcer margins are macerated (protect skin): Zinc oxide.
Infected wounds	Infection is a clinical diagnosis based on the presence of cardinal signs of inflammation (swelling, pain, redness, warmth, loss of function) and treatment should be initiated without awaiting culture results which are valuable later to assist antibiotic choice if a patient is not improving. Doxycycline, Trimethoprim Sulfamethoxazole, Ciprofloxacin are examples of antibiotic therapy most commonly used in clinic. *Local wound treatment in presence of infection:* Silver sulfadiazine, collagen dressing with silver, alginate wound dressing, foam dressing with silver, silver dressing, iodine gels, mupirocin ointment, collagenase, topical antiseptics, (bacteriostatic wound dressings), odor-absorbent dressings.
Odor control	Charcoal, systemic antibiotic, and local metronidazole unguent are good alternatives.
Undermining/pocket	Fill the space: Packing dressings.
Retainer dressings	Elasticated viscose tubular bandages, tubular elastic dressing retainers.
Dermatitis	Common complication of bandage compression use and exposure to different materials. Can be treated using topical corticosteroids.
Refractory/recalcitrant wounds	Special dressings and advanced therapies (cell and tissue-based therapy).
Advanced therapies	Cellular products (BLCC, DMC), placenta-based products (DHACM, CPM), acellular products (PSIS, pGlcNAc), growth factors (PDGF, GM-CSF). Hyperbaric oxygen therapy: Indications (gas gangrene, chronic non-healing ulcers, diabetic wounds, chronic osteomyelitis, etc).
Other therapies	Growth factors Negative pressure Skin grafting Surgery Others: Pain, malignancy, depression, anxiety.

Abbreviations: BLCC, bilayered cellular construct; CPM, cryopreserved placental membrane; DFU, diabetic foot ulcers; GM-CSF, granulocyte-macrophage colony-stimulating factor; PDGF, platelet-derived growth factor; pGlcNAc, poly-*N*-acetyl glucosamine; PSIS, porcine small intestine submucosa; PU, pressure ulcers; SWC, standard wound care; VLU, venous leg ulcers.

and padding), one or two elastic wraps, and a cohesive wrap. They can be adapted to a wide range of leg sizes and provide sustained pressures of 40 to 45 mm Hg at the ankle, graduating to 17 mm Hg below the knee. After healing, patients using compression therapy should wear graded compression stockings. This is important to prevent ulcer recurrence. Prolonged use and washing of the stockings reduce their compression capability; hence, stockings should be replaced after 3 to 6 months of use.

Patients should receive specific instructions on how to put on compression stockings, which helps with adherence to treatment. Patients who are obese, elderly, arthritic have difficulty in wearing the stockings. Other ways to improve the stocking placement technique are the sock dressing device or other donning devices, which will increase adherence to the treatment.

There are several studies that reveal that nonadherence to compression stockings after healing increase the chances of recurrences. For this reason, as we mentioned before, it is important to educate our patients and emphasize the importance of adherence of compression therapy during and after healing of their wounds.

- *Pain control:* Some patients require compression therapy as standard of care, which sometimes could be painful. If the ulcer in question is painful, protection of the ulcer bed with nonadherent pads, nonadherent contact dressings, and local and systemic analgesics can be beneficial.

- *Pressure reduction:* Most commonly used in patients with DFU, neuropathic ulcers, and PU. Some examples of off-loading devices are: walking boot, total contact cast, off-loading footwear, off-loading devices (special mattress), wheelchair, crutches, etc.

- *Debridement:* This is part of the SWC for chronic wounds and involves the removal of hyperkeratotic skin, senescent cells, necrotic tissue, foreign debris, and bacteria to attain a viable wound bed to promote wound healing. Surgical debridement may promote formation of granulation tissue. There are other types of debridement such as pulse, mechanical, chemical, and biological debridement. Enzyme-debriding agents (chemical debridement) have proteolytic enzyme properties and may accelerate the removal of fibrin. Debridement and removal of calluses in patients with DFU is part of the SWC, but in patients with AU or arterial insufficiency with inadequate blood perfusion, debridement should not be performed. Doppler US of arteries is important in these cases to avoid further complications. Surgical debridement should be avoided in patients in whom pyoderma gangrenosum is suspected as it could incur pathergy and result in increased wound size.

- *Vascular consultation:* In some cases where blood flow studies are abnormal, or when the arterial supply is not sufficient, it is necessary to refer patients to a vascular specialist.

- *Local treatment:* For any type of wound, the first step in local treatment is *wound cleaning* with a non-irritant cleanser or saline solution. After that, identify changes in the skin surrounding the ulcer (*periwound area*): If the skin is dry/scaly/irritated, a skin protectant can be used. If it is *irritated*, a skin barrier topical such as zinc oxide ointment can be used. In presence of contact dermatitis, which is a common complication of bandage compression use and exposure to different materials, the use of a topical corticosteroid may be indicated.

Other local treatment alternatives consist of special wound dressings. The dressing choice will vary accordingly to the aspect of the wound.

- *Make a wound bed inspection:* It is necessary to maintain a proper moist environment. If the wound is too dry, hydrate it using a dressing to increase the moisture, for example, hydrogel. If it is dry or has minimal drainage, hydrofiber dressing, hydroactive gel or patch, hydrogel, honey, foam dressings (gentle) are good options to manage these wounds. If the wound has minimal drainage, maintain moisture using dressings such as hydrocolloids or hydrogel. If the drainage is moderate or heavy, use foams or pads to absorb the drainage. In the presence of moderate to heavy drainage ABD pads, superabsorbent dressings and alginate wound dressings are good options. If the ulcer margins are macerated, protect the skin using zinc oxide or other similar products.

- *If infection is suspected:* Infection is a clinical diagnosis based on the presence of cardinal signs of inflammation (swelling, pain, redness, warmth, loss of function). Treatment should be initiated even before culture results are available. Culture results can be used for later assistance in antibiotic choice in case there is no improvement of the clinical signs. Antibiotics that cover gram positive and gram negatives cocci and bacilli such as Doxycycline, Trimethoprim Sulfamethoxazole, and Ciprofloxacin are examples of antibiotic therapies most commonly used in clinic.

- *Local wound treatment in presence of infection:* Silver sulfadiazine, collagen dressings with silver, alginate wound dressing, foam dressing with silver, silver dressing, iodine gels, mupirocin ointment), collagenase, topical antiseptics (bacteriostatic wound dressings), and odor-absorbent dressings.

- *For odor control:* Charcoal, systemic antibiotic, and local metronidazole unguent are good alternatives.

Some ulcers are deep or have *undermining and pockets* that can be treated by filling the space with packing dressings.

- *Ideal dressing:* While a universal, ideal dressing does not exist, for each patient's wound the best dressing must provide wound protection, comfort to aid in the quality of life for the patient, and remain securely in place during activities. It should be able to manage varying amounts of exudate and should be easy to apply and remove to prevent further damage of the wound or surrounding tissue. Furthermore, it should require a minimal number of changes to diminish disturbance of the healing process and decrease the nursing time and cost.

- *Advanced local therapy:* A tissue-engineered bilayered *cellular construct* (BLCC) (Apligraf, Organogenesis, Canton, MA) is FDA approved for VLU and DFU. It is composed of human-derived fibroblasts and keratinocytes on a bovine type I collagen matrix. BLCC is believed to increase the concentration of growth factors and cytokines.

A monolayer collagen dermal product (CDM) (Dermagraft, Organogenesis, Canton, MA) has been approved for DFU. It is a cryopreserved human fibroblast-derived dermal substitute, composed of fibroblasts, extracellular matrix, and a polyglactin bioabsorbable scaffold. This CDM has been observed to be effective in the treatment of DFUs. Another category of advanced therapies is placenta-based products. Dehydrated human amnion/chorion membrane (dHACM) (Epifix; MiMedx Group Inc., Marietta, GA) and cryopreserved placental membrane (CPM) (Grafix; Osiris Therapeutics, Inc., Columbia, MD) have shown to benefit DFU.

- *Acellular products:* A variety of synthetic and biologic scaffolds are available for treating chronic wounds. One example is a dressing derived from porcine small intestine submucosa (PSIS) (Oasis, Smith and Nephew, Largo, FL). This product has been found to promote angiogenesis and increase host cell migration for growth and wound healing.

  Poly-*N*-acetyl glucosamine (pGlcNAc) is another example. Other examples of acellular products are: Ovine collagen "Endoform," equine type I collagen "Biopad," cadaveric human skin "Alloderm," and hyaluronic acid matrix "Hyalomatrix."

  One growth factor is approved for treating chronic wounds. PDGF (Regranex, Smith and Nephew, Largo Fl) is the only growth factor approved for the treatment of chronic wounds. Other *growth factors* such as GM-CSF are available off-label and can be used as adjuvant therapy to heal wounds.

- *Surgical interventions:* Skin grafting has been used primarily in refractory wounds, such as large or slow-healing venous ulcers. The benefits of graft placement include speeding up of the wound healing process *and* pain reduction.

- *Minimal invasive interventions:* For VLU patients.

- *Radiofrequency endovascular* laser *ablation or ultrasound guided sclerotherapy* can improve venous circulation through varicose venous ablation.

Superficial venous surgery to treat venous leg ulcers when the patient has both superficial and deep venous reflux is controversial. With isolated superficial incompetence, superficial venous surgery may be considered for treatment. The purpose of this procedure is to reduce venous reflux decreasing venous insufficiency. Also, *subfascial endoscopic perforator surgery* is a promising, minimally invasive procedure for certain venous ulcers.

- *Systemic therapy:* The use of Aspirin (300 mg oral daily), in some studies, has shown a positive impact in the rate of healing in venous ulcers.

Pentoxifylline, which is a methylxanthine derivative, is taken 800 mg three times daily and seems to be an effective adjuvant therapy to compression wraps in venous leg ulcer patients. A Cochrane review found that pentoxifylline was superior to placebo in achieving ulcer healing in VLU (RR, 1.70; 95% CI, 1.30 to 2.24). Both were used as adjuvant to compression, where pentoxifylline with compression was superior to placebo with compression (RR, 1.56; 95% CI, 1.14 to 2.13) and as the sole agent (pentoxifylline) without compression (RR, 2.25; 95% CI, 1.49 to 3.39). This may be due to its fibrinolytic properties, its ability to reduce leukocyte adhesion to the vascular endothelium, and its antithrombotic effects. But it can produce severe gastrointestinal side effects such as indigestion, nausea, and diarrhea. I often use only 400 mg twice a day, and it seems to help with less gastrointestinal side effects (JH, editor).

Stanozolol (Sanofi-Winthrop Pharmaceuticals, Morrisville, Pennsylvania) is an androgenic steroid with fibrinolytic properties which does not speed healing, but reduces pain and induration of venous ulcers and lipodermatosclerosis.

- *Other treatment options:* Hyperbaric oxygen therapy has special indications (gas gangrene, chronic non-healing ulcers, diabetic wounds, chronic osteomyelitis, etc). Negative pressure wound therapy is useful in deep acute surgical wound as well as deeper DFUs.

- *Education:* Provide information and educate the patient about the findings, diagnosis, work plan and treatment options.

Gathering and understanding this information is important to provide the best alternatives to patients, and offer better and new treatment options by working as a multidisciplinary team of specialists (dermatologists, vascular surgeons, nurses, physicians, general surgeons, podiatrist, etc). All of these are needed to provide a concise, cost-effective, and comprehensive assessment.

Adherence to compression therapy and maintenance of healing subsequently followed by use of compression stockings are still the key to healing a venous leg ulcer and prevent recurrences, respectively.

Warranting proper management and individualizing an efficacious treatment is important to understand pathophysiologic abnormalities of chronic ulcers. Recognizing standardized approach for wound healing and emergent novel therapeutic approaches for chronic ulcers have offered valuable tools for the management of patients with this condition.

Suggested Readings

Alavi A, Sibbald RG, Mayer D, et al. Diabetic foot ulcers: part I. Pathophysiology and prevention. *J Am Acad Dermatol.* 2014;70(1):1.e1–1.e18; quiz 19–20. doi:10.1016/j.jaad.2013.06.055.

Alavi A, Sibbald RG, Mayer D, et al. Diabetic foot ulcers: part II. Management. *J Am Acad Dermatol.* 2014;70(1):21.e1–21.e24; quiz 45–46. doi:10.1016/j.jaad.2013.07.048.

Ankrom MA, Bennett RG, Sprigle S, et al. Pressure-related deep tissue injury under intact skin and the current pressure ulcer staging systems. *Adv Skin Wound Care.* 2005;18(1):35–42.

Atiyeh BS, Ioannovich J, Al-Amm CA, et al. Management of acute and chronic open wounds: the importance of moist environment in optimal wound healing. *Curr Pharm Biotechnol.* 2002;3(3):179–195.

Blair SD, Wright DD, Backhouse CM, et al. Sustained compression and healing of chronic venous ulcers. *BMJ.* 1988;297(6657):1159–1161.

Burnand K, Clemenson G, Morland M, et al. Venous lipodermatosclerosis: treatment by fibrinolytic enhancement and elastic compression. *Br Med J.* 1980;280(6206):7–11.

De Araujo T, Valencia I, Federman DG, et al. Managing the patient with venous ulcers. *Ann Intern Med.* 2003;138(4):326–334.

Dickey JW Jr. Stasis ulcers: the role of compliance in healing. *South Med J.* 1991;84(5):557–561.

Falanga V. Occlusive wound dressings. Why, when, which? *Arch Dermatol.* 1988;124(6):872–877.

Grey JE, Harding KG, Enoch S. Venous and arterial leg ulcers. *BMJ.* 2006;332(7537):347–350.

Hess CT, Kirsner RS. Orchestrating wound healing: assessing and preparing the wound bed. *Adv Skin Wound Care.* 2003;16(5):246–257; quiz 258–259.

Julien OC, Dye WS, Schneewind J. Surgical management of ulcerative stasis disease of the lower extremities. *AMA Arch Surg.* 1954;68(6):757–768.

Kirsner RS, Mata SM, Falanga V, et al. Split-thickness skin grafting of leg ulcers. The University of Miami Department of Dermatology's experience (1990–1993). *Dermatol Surg.* 1995;21(8):701–703.

Kirsner RS, Vivas AC. Lower-extremity ulcers: diagnosis and management. *Br J Dermatol.* 2015;173(2):379–390. doi:10.1111/bjd.13953.

Kunimoto B, Cooling M, Gulliver W, et al. Best practices for the prevention and treatment of venous leg ulcers. *Ostomy Wound Manag.* 2001;47(2):34–46, 48–50.

Lavery LA, Peters EJ, Armstrong DG. What are the most effective interventions in preventing diabetic foot ulcers? *Int Wound J.* 2008;5(3):425–433. doi:10.1111/j.1742-481X.2007.00378.x.

Lebrun E, Tomic-Canic M, Kirsner RS. The role of surgical debridement in healing of diabetic foot ulcers. *Wound Repair Regen.* 2010;18(5):433–438. doi:10.1111/j.1524-475X.2010.00619.x.

Li J, Chen J, Kirsner R. Pathophysiology of acute wound healing. *Clin Dermatol.* 2007;25(1):9–18.

Margolis DJ, Cohen JH. Management of chronic venous leg ulcers: a literature-guided approach. *Clin Dermatol.* 1994;12(1):19–26.

O'Donnell TF Jr, Passman MA, Marston WA, et al. Management of venous leg ulcers: clinical practice guidelines of the Society for Vascular Surgery and the American Venous Forum. *J Vasc Surg.* 2014;60(suppl 2):3S–59S. doi:10.1016/j.jvs.2014.04.049.

Olivencia JA. Subfascial endoscopic ligation of perforator veins (SEPS) in the treatment of venous ulcers. *Int Surg.* 2000;85(3):266–269.

Partsch H, Mortimer P. Compression for leg wounds. *Br J Dermatol.* 2015;173(2):359–369. doi:10.1111/bjd.13851.

Phillips TJ. Successful methods of treating leg ulcers. The tried and true, plus the novel and new. *Postgrad Med.* 1999;105(5):159–161, 165–166, 173–174 passim.

Samson RH, Showalter DP. Stockings and the prevention of recurrent venous ulcers. *Dermatol Surg.* 1996;22(4):373–376.

Sibbald RG, Orsted H, Schultz GS, et al. Preparing the wound bed 2003: focus on infection and inflammation. *Ostomy Wound Manage.* 2003;49(11):24–51.

Simon DA, McCollum CN. Approaches to venous leg ulcer care within the community: compression, pinch skin grafts and simple venous surgery. *Ostomy Wound Manag.* 1996;42(2):34–38, 40.

Sinclair RD, Ryan TJ. Proteolytic enzymes in wound healing: the role of enzymatic debridement. *Australas J Dermatol.* 1994;35(1):35–41.

Zacur H, Kirsner RS. Debridement: rationale and therapeutic options. *Wounds.* 2002;14(7 suppl F):2E–7E.

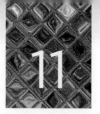

Atopic Dermatitis

Jasna Lipozenčić, MD, PhD and Suzana Ljubojević Hadžavdić, MD, PhD

Atopic dermatitis (AD) is a chronic inflammatory skin disease, characterized by severe pruritus and typical age-specific clinical picture (scaly and oozing plaques on the forehead and face, neck, hands, and flexural area), and is frequently associated with other genetic predisposed atopic diseases such as asthma and/or allergic rhinitis. Urticaria, penicillin allergy, and marked reactions to insect bites are also part of this anaphylactoid or type-I immune disease. The prevalence of AD is rather high, mostly involving children, and affects 2% to 5% of the general population with 10% to 20% or more occurrences in infants and children, and 1% to 3% in adults. There is a wide variation in the prevalence of AD in different populations of the world, and it appears to be increasing.

The course of the disease is characterized by exacerbations and remissions that cannot always be etiologically explained. While majority of the affected individuals have resolution of disease by adolescence, 10% to 30% may then have further episodes in adulthood. A smaller percentage first develops symptoms as adults. Complete remission has been estimated to occur in one-third of patients after 2 years of age and in another one-third after 5 years of age.

The terminology of AD is controversial, with many different names used in different countries, such as neurodermatitis, flexural eczema, Besnier's prurigo, constitutionalis atopica, and atopic eczema. A position statement published by the European Academy of Allergy and Clinical Immunology (EAACI) proposed a new term, "atopic eczema/dermatitis syndrome" (AEDS). The update further suggested that "eczema" could be subclassified as "atopic eczema" and "nonatopic eczema" based on the presence or absence of IgE antibodies.

Despite recent advances in the understanding of the genetics of AD, the pathophysiology remains poorly defined. The pathogenesis of AD is multifactorial. It is widely accepted that a defective skin epidermal barrier results in increased transepidermal water loss (TEWL), as well as increased colonization and penetration by microorganisms and allergens, evoking inflammatory responses. A primary immune dysfunction results in IgE sensitization and a secondary epithelial-barrier disturbance. Mutations in genes encoding filaggrin proteins are believed to be among the genetic contributors to a defective epidermis.

GENETIC ASPECTS

AD is partly caused by a genetic defect in the filaggrin gene *FLG* (leading to barrier dysfunction). It is likely that other genetically determined factors are also involved, such as dysregulation of T helper2 (Th2) cytokine production. Filaggrin plays a key role in epidermal-barrier function, and the barrier dysfunction resulting from mutations of the filaggrin gene may allow increased exposure to allergens, resulting in hyperreactivity to environmental triggers and the induction of IgE autoantibodies.

European Caucasian AD patients, the FLG null mutations R501X and 2282del4 were most frequently associated with the disease. Moreover, it has been shown that in particular AD patients with loss-of-function mutations in the FLG gene suffer from more severe, persistent forms of AD with chronic courses. Interleukin-10 gene (IL10) polymorphisms have been suspected as risk factors for eczema.

Atopic constitution is more frequently transmitted by maternal inheritance. Parental eczema has been shown to confer a higher genetic risk for eczema in subsequent offspring than parental asthma or rhinitis. The odds of developing AD are two- to threefold higher in children with one atopic parent, but increase to three- to fivefold if both parents are atopic.

IMMUNOLOGIC BACKGROUND

AD is frequently associated with immunodeficiency (selective IgA and IgM). Numerous factors are implicated at the onset of the disease. Hyperimmunoglobulinemia E is characteristic of atopic diseases; however, AD is also a consequence of type-IV immune response. The cells infiltrating the skin are predominated by Th2 cell types that produce IL-4, IL-10, and IL-13 and enable differentiation of B lymphocytes and production of IgE and eosinophilia.

There is a Th2 cytokine profile of IL-4, IL-5, and IL-13 in the skin in the acute phase of AD, while Th1/0 with IFN-γ IL-12, and GM-CSF prevail in the chronic phase. There is a significant coordination between AD disease activity and skin eosinophilic cationic protein (ECP) deposition. Moreover, ECP and IL-16 are elevated in the acute AD phase, and IL-10 plays an important immunoregulatory role in atopic as well as nonatopic eczema. In lesional AD skin, there are two types of the high-affinity receptors for IgE-bearing myeloid dendritic cells (DC) (i.e., Langerhans cells (LCs) and inflammatory dendritic epidermal cells [IDECs]), each of which displays a different function in the pathophysiology of AD. Specifically, LCs play a predominant role in the initiation of the allergic immune response and conversion of prime naïve T-cells into Th2 type T-cells with high amounts of IL-4. Furthermore, stimulation of high-affinity receptors for IgE on the surface of LCs by allergens induces the release of chemotactic signals and recruitment of IDECs and T-cells in vitro. Stimulation of high-affinity IgE receptors (FcεRI) on IDECs leads to the release of high amounts of proinflammatory signals, which contribute to the allergic immune response. Keratinocytes play a role in innate immunity by expressing toll-like receptors and by producing antimicrobial peptides in response to invading microbes. AD keratinocytes secrete a unique profile of chemokines and cytokines. Apoptosis of keratinocytes is a crucial event in the formation of eczema (spongiosis in AD). The expression of different immunologic parameters was studied in AD patients since immune dysregulation is a possible key defect in AD. Regulatory T-cells (Tregs) or Th3 cells (CD25+/CD4+) can suppress Th1 as well as Th2 cells. Superantigens of *Staphylococcus aureus* cause defects in Tregs function and promote the skin inflammation. Autoallergens (e.g., Homs 1–5 and DSF 70) are atopy-related autoantigens (ARA) in the setting of AD and other atopic diseases. IgE autoreactivity appears very early (during the first year of life) and is associated with flares in AD. Adhesion molecules may play an important role in the homing of T-cell subsets into allergen-exposed skin of atopic individuals. High expressions of adhesion molecules, especially intracellular adhesion molecules (ICAM)-1 and ICAM-3, E-selectin, and L-selectin, in skin lesions of AD patients revealed that they may play an important role in the pathogenesis of AD. AD is a product of an interaction between various susceptibility genes, host and environmental factors, infectious agents, defects in skin barrier function, and immunologic responses.

SKIN BARRIER DYSFUNCTION

AD is characterized by dry skin and increased TEWL even in nonlesional skin, and fewer ceramides in the cornified envelope of lesional and nonlesional skin are found in AD patients. AD patients develop AD as a result of skin barrier defects that allow for the entry of antigens, resulting in the production of inflammatory cytokines. Changes in the stratum corneum pH in AD skin may impair lipid metabolism in the skin. Such alterations allow the penetration of and increase susceptibility to irritants and allergens, triggering the inflammatory response, cutaneous hyperreactivity, inflammation, and skin damage characteristic of AD. Filaggrin deficiency leads to mild or severe ichthyosis vulgaris. Around 37% of people with AD have clinical evidence of ichthyosis vulgaris. Impaired keratinocyte differentiation and barrier formation allow increased TEWL and the entry of allergens, antigens, and chemicals from the environment to AD.

ENVIRONMENTAL FACTORS

The importance of environmental factors in the development of AD has been increasing. The majority (40% to 65%) of AD patients experience deterioration in the winter, probably due to decreased humidity of the outdoors (due to cold) as well as indoors air due to heating. The aggravation by sun exposure is probably due to a nonspecific intolerance of heat caused by impaired function of sweating in affected skin and induction of itch sweating. Outdoor pollution seems to be one of the major causes of the dramatic increase of atopy in recent years. Chemical compounds and exhaust particles as well as pollens are released into the air and may have indirect effects on the allergic sensitization.

AD is a major contributing factor to occupational irritant or allergic contact dermatitis. Irritants, such as soaps, detergents, and disinfectants, and prolonged exposure to water have an excitatory effect on the impaired barrier layer of atopic skin. Daily washing with soap and water or noxious agent may elicit an irritant contact reaction in atopic individuals. Saliva frequently induces perioral eczema. Contact with wool is a common trigger of irritant contact dermatitis in AD. Other textiles, especially synthetics or dyed fabrics, are sometimes incriminated. Tobacco smoke is also a potent irritator of atopic skin.

Passive smoking also has been linked to IgE responsiveness and increased incidence of asthma as a result of chronic airway inflammation and subsequent enhanced sensitization. Nutritive allergens are primarily important in AD in children. Approximately one-third of children with moderate-to-severe AD have IgE-mediated clinical reactivity to food proteins. The most common allergens in children are egg whites, cow's milk, peanuts, soy, shellfish, and flour. The prevalence of food allergy in AD varies widely from 25% to 60% according to different studies. The timing of solid food introduction or withholding of allergenic foods does not appear to alter the risk of AD. There are also nonspecific irritant reactions predominantly to acid fruit (citrus fruits, tomatoes, etc.) and salty or spicy foods. Aggravation of eczema may also be provoked by food additives. Modification of the maternal or infant diet does not show a protective effect. But, recently published studies of hydrolyzed formula and probiotic supplementation suggest that these could have a beneficial effect in preventing disease development in some high-risk infants who are not exclusively breastfed.

Among airborne allergens, the most important are grass, weeds, tree pollens, animal epidermis, dander allergens (especially cats), house-dust mites, and molds such as *Alternaria spp.* Airborne allergy in AD varies widely according to different studies. While patients with AD are often sensitized to house-dust mites, there is no strong evidence to show that dust mite avoidance strategies prevent AD. The dry skin so characteristic of AD patients favors colonization by *S. aureus*, an organism that is involved in maintaining cutaneous inflammation, as well as being capable of inciting allergic responses in such individuals. This bacterium can be isolated in nostrils and intertriginous regions in 5% to 15% of normal individuals but is found in 64% to 100% of skin lesions in AD patients. It influences the course of the disease via different mechanisms: exotoxins, enzymes, superantigens, and protein A. Bacterial toxins act as superantigens aligned along MHC II and can directly stimulate massive T-cell proliferation.

Malassezia furfur (Pityrosporum ovale) yeast may produce positive skin prick reactions in a higher rate (49%) in patients with AD of the head, scalp, and neck region. It can also be detected in the serum (specific IgE to *P. ovale*) and can provoke positive patch-test reactions. *M. furfur* can induce an eczematous reaction in sensitized AD patients and may be a trigger factor for AD. Patients with AD do not have a major deficiency in defending against viruses. However, some viral skin infections can have a dramatic course. Kaposi's herpetiform (Figs. 11-1 and 11-2) and varicelliform eruptions caused by the spread of herpes and varicella viruses, Epstein–Barr virus, parainfluenza virus, respiratory syncytial virus, and cytomegalovirus infections have been reported to trigger exacerbation of AD. Atopic patients often respond to stress, frustration, embarrassment, or other upsetting events with increased pruritus and scratching. When the higher cortical centers are activated by stress, there is an increased secretion of substance P from the adrenal glands. They serve as brain peptides that are easily released by psychosocial stress, triggering, or exacerbating itching, especially in patients with AD. Histamine is not believed to be the essential mediator of itch in AD. Proteases, kinins, prostaglandins, neuropeptides, acetylcholine, cytokines, and opioids can cause itch or potentiate histamine release into atopic skin. The type of delivery during childbirth (i.e., cesarean or vaginal) does not appear to alter AD risk. No definitive conclusions can be drawn regarding early antibiotic exposure and the risk of AD.

CLINICAL FEATURES

AD is a multifaceted disease. The clinical picture, morphology, and distribution of the skin lesion vary greatly depending on the age of the patient, the ethnic group he or she belongs to (more popular in people of color), the course and duration of the disease, aggravating factors, and possible complications such as superinfection (Fig. 11-3). Its manifestations range from very mild to severe disease.

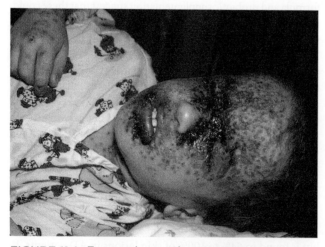

FIGURE 11-1: Eczema herpetiformis (Kaposi's varicelliform eruption) in a 6-year-old boy with a long history of eczema and exposure to herpes simplex on the lip. Excellent response was seen with intravenous acyclovir.

There are three classical stages of disease—infantile, childhood, and adulthood—each of which may show acute, subacute, and/or chronic skin reactions. Acute lesions are characterized by intensely pruritic, erythematous papules and vesicles over erythematous skin, erosions, and serous exudates. Subacute lesions form erythematous, excoriated scaly papules, whereas chronic lesions show red–brown papules and plaques, skin thickening with pronounced skin markings (lichenification) (Figs. 11-4 and 11-5) and nodular papules. All three stages of skin lesions may frequently be present in the same patient.

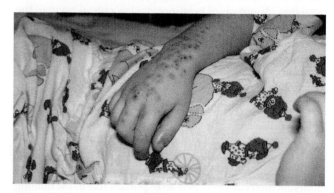

FIGURE 11-2: Same patient, as in Figure 11-1, with vesicular eruption over the arm.

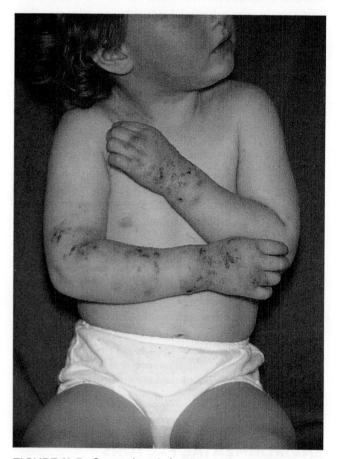

FIGURE 11-3: Secondary infection with crusting, oozing oval lesions over the forearms of a child with childhood eczema.

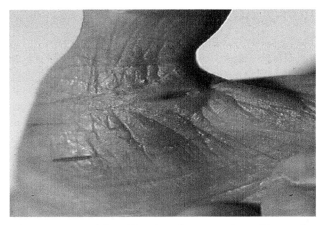

FIGURE 11-4: Lichenification (increased markings of normal skin) over the dorsal surface of the hand in an eczema patient.

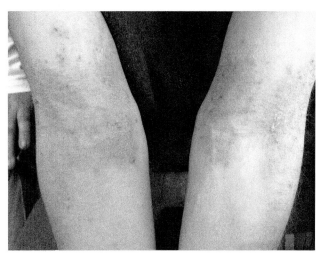

FIGURE 11-6: Antecubital involvement of AD.

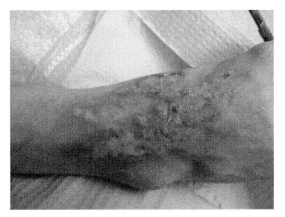

FIGURE 11-5: Well-demarcated lichenified plaque of lichen simplex chronicus over the anterior ankle.

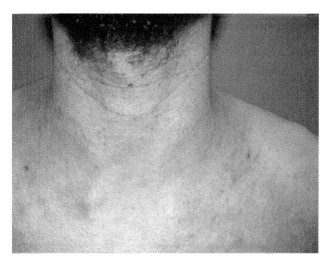

FIGURE 11-7: Lichenification of the neck in the adult AD patient.

In infancy, the characteristic lesions consist of symmetrical, dry, erythematous, scaly plaques with follicular papules on the face, mostly involving the cheeks, forehead, and scalp but not the perioral region. When a child starts to crawl, the lesions extend to the upper trunk, extensor aspect of the upper and lower extremities, and the dorsal aspects of the hands and feet. The diaper region is usually spared due to the moisture retention of diapers. Focal hair loss often results from constant rubbing of the itchy scalp against bedding. Short, thick hairs are a sign of constant rubbing.

The childhood phase, during the second and third years of life, shows a modified clinical picture with characteristic papules and plaques localized primarily in large joint flexures, especially on the neck, elbows, wrists, knees, and ankles. Later in childhood and in adolescence, lesions involving flexural areas persist (Fig. 11-6), including the eyelids, hands, and feet, where pustules are frequently observed. Many children develop a "nummular" (coin-shaped or circular) pattern of AD.

In adults, the disease is characterized by lichenification, chronic course, thickened areas in flexures, on the neck (Fig. 11-7) and eyelids, and chronic facial edema. Localized patches of AD can occur on the nipples, especially in adolescent and young women. The disease has a chronic or chronic-relapsing course, with alternating periods of regression and exacerbation of skin changes with pruritus. In some patients, a seasonal variant of the disease is present, with exacerbations occurring mostly in spring and autumn. Severe pruritus is the main characteristic of AD. It worsens in the evening, during sweating, and by wearing wool clothing.

Keratosis pilaris (Fig. 11-8) is seen most commonly during childhood and presents as small, rough, raised lesions (papules) usually on the upper outer arms, anterior thighs, and sometimes malar areas. **Xerosis** is considered to be the most common dermatosis of atopic individuals. It can persist for life, independent of the activity of atopic symptoms. **Pityriasis alba** is a benign chronic skin disorder that affects some children, usually between the ages of 6 and 12 but may occur up to the age of 20 to 30. Sometimes *Pityriasis alba* can be confused with vitiligo. When an **ichthyosis vulgaris** patient has severe pruritus of flexural involvement, he or she usually has AD. **Dennie–Morgan lines** are symmetrical, prominent folds, extending from the medial aspect of the lower lid. The sign is present in about 70% of atopic children. **Palmoplantar hyperlinearity** is found in people with AD who frequently have a thickening

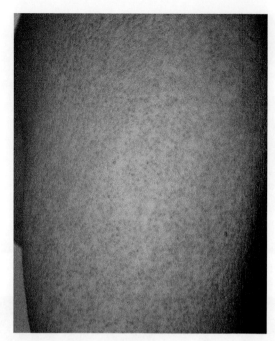

FIGURE 11-8: Keratosis pilaris.

of the skin on the palms and soles with an increase in the number of lines in the skin (hyperlinearity). **Cheilitis** derives from habitual lip-licking (the so-called lip-licker's dermatitis). Cheilitis is noted as a persistent scaliness, usually restricted to the vermilion, but often extending onto the perioral skin. The biggest group of patients with cheilitis has severe AD or at least an atopic diathesis with persistent nodules. **Nipple dermatitis** is noted in 12% to 23% of patients with AD. It is most common in postpubertal girls, often symmetrically, and may occur in breastfeeding women. The very sensitive areolar skin koebnerizes with the slightest rubbing or friction of clothing. Due to chronic rubbing, there is a possible loss of the lateral eyebrow, which is called **Hertoghe's sign.**

DIFFERENTIAL DIAGNOSIS

The diagnosis of AD is usually straightforward but atypical features should prompt the clinician to think about alternatives. In the differential diagnosis, one should think about: chronic inflammatory skin diseases (allergic and irritant contact dermatitis, seborrheic dermatitis, psoriasis), infectious agents (scabies, dermatomycoses) immunologic disorders (dermatitis herpetiformis, pemphigus foliaceus), malignant diseases (cutaneous T-cell lymphoma, histiocytosis X), congenital disorders (Netherton's syndrome, Dubowitz syndrome, erythrokeratodermia variabilis), immunodeficiencies (Wiskott-Aldrich syndrome, DiGeorge syndrome, hyper-IgE syndrome, severe combined immunodeficiency (SCID), ataxia telangiectasia), metabolic diseases (phenylketonuria, tyrosinemia, histidinemia, zinc deficiency, pyridoxine (vitamin B_6) and niacin deficiency, multiple carboxylase deficiency).

HISTOLOGIC FEATURES

The histology is mainly noncontributive to the diagnosis, as there are no definite features allowing us to distinguish between AD and other forms of eczema. The eczematous eruptions all manifest T-cell proinflammatory mediator involvement, but they may be quite different clinically. Acute eczematous lesions are characterized by marked epidermal intercellular edema (spongiosis). Chronic lichenified lesions are characterized by an acantholytic epidermis with elongation of the rete ridges, parakeratosis, and only minimal spongiosis. Those chronic lesions have an increased number of IgE-bearing LCs and IDECs in the epidermis, and macrophages dominate the dermal mononuclear cell infiltrate. These lesions also contain eosinophils.

DIAGNOSIS

AD has a wide spectrum of dermatological manifestations and no definitive diagnostic test. The diagnosis of AD is made clinically and is based on morphology and distribution of the skin lesions, and associated clinical signs. Well-defined diagnostic criteria are important in the diagnosis of AD, and diagnostic criteria developed by Hanifin and Rajka (see Table 8-1) are still widely accepted. Skin biopsies are not essential for the diagnosis, but they can exclude other diagnoses in adults. Elements contributing to the establishment of the diagnosis of AD are compiled from patient history, clinical findings, skin tests, and laboratory investigations.

LABORATORY FINDINGS

Laboratory tests are chosen based on the history data and physical examination. The investigation of exacerbating factors in AD involves a patient history, specific skin and blood tests, and challenge tests, depending on the degree of disease severity and on the suspected factors involved. The atopy patch test (APT) was introduced to assess sensitization to inhalant and nutritive allergens in AEDS patients. APTs are performed with self-made food material applied to the back with large test chambers for 48 to 72 hours. Food APT are not standardized for routine use. So far, APTs have improved the accuracy of skin testing in the diagnosis of allergy to cow's milk, egg, cereals, and peanuts in AD patients.

Cytokine responses to allergens can be detected in cord blood mononuclear cells (CBMC), suggesting allergen priming in utero.

Sensitization to inhalant allergens (e.g., dust, mites, animal dander, and pollen) can be detected by skin prick tests (SPTs) (if the skin is free from eczema) or by measuring specific IgE antibodies.

Contact sensitization to topical medications frequently occurs in AD patients, especially in adults. The possibility of contact allergy needs to be ruled out by patch testing. There is currently no reliable biomarker that can distinguish the disease from other entities. The most commonly associated laboratory feature, an elevated total and/or allergen-specific serum IgE level, is not present in about 20% of the affected individuals.

SCORAD (*Scoring Atopic Dermatitis*) is an international severity criteria of AD. These criteria grade the rash areas, severity of rash elements such as erythema, edema, papule, exudation, crust, lichenification, scratch marks, xerosis cutis, and subjective symptoms such as itch and insomnia.

TREATMENT

Successful management of AD requires a different approach involving skin care, identification and elimination of flare factors, anti-inflammatory treatment as well as education of the patient or patient's parent and family. General measures of prevention and treatment of AD include avoiding those factors that have been identified as potential causes of disease exacerbations. This implies avoidance of skin contact with wool, synthetic materials, and foods that can induce irritation (e.g., citrus fruit or tomatoes). Patients are advised to avoid staying in smoky areas and to reduce exposure to house dust, feather, and animal hair.

Skin care includes appropriate skin hygiene, which is of paramount importance. Understanding the importance of continued emollient usage to maintain optimal skin barrier function even when the skin is clear can prevent flares.

Patients with hypersensitivity to a nutritive allergen are recommended to comply with an appropriate dietary regimen. When prescribing diets for children, it should be borne in mind that inappropriate diet may lead to malnutrition while even a minimal dietary deficit may cause changes in immune response. It should be emphasized that hypersensitivity to food allergens is mostly diagnosed in children, whereas hypersensitivity to inhalant allergens and development of contact allergic dermatitis predominate in older patients.

Early ear-piercing and use of nickel-releasing jewelry has been found to be associated with a significantly elevated risk of nickel-contact allergy in young girls.

Topical Therapy

The skin must be cleansed thoroughly, but gently and carefully to get rid of crusts and mechanically eliminate bacterial contaminants in the case of bacterial superinfection. Skin care preparation should be applied over the skin within 3 minutes (3-minute rule) of bathing; otherwise, bathing will lead to skin drying instead of desirable skin hydration. The application of moisturizers increases hydration of the skin, they lessen symptoms and signs of AD, including pruritus, erythema, fissuring, and lichenification, and their use decreases the amount of prescription anti-inflammatory treatments required for disease control. The quantities of emollients required are usually high (150 to 200 g/week in young children, up to 500 g in adults). The short duration of the bath (only 5 minutes) and the use of bath oils (last 2 minutes of bathing) are aimed at avoiding epidermal dehydration. Bathing is also important because the penetration of corticosteroids into the hydrated

skin is best after bathing. Adding sodium hypochlorite (bleach) with one-half to one cup to the bath-water seems very important because of its bacterial count inhibiting activities. It can be irritating. Soaps with minimum defatting activity and a neutral pH are preferred. The use of oily baths followed by neutral preparations for skin ointment and hydration (creams, ointments, and emulsions) several times a day and continuously is necessary in most AD patients. The higher the degree of the skin dryness, the greater the frequency of preparation usage. Preparations with the addition of urea, omega fatty acids, lipids, zinc, and copper are used for this purpose. The emollient should be applied first when it is a cream, 15 minutes before the anti-inflammatory topical is applied and when it is an ointment, 15 minutes after. Patients with acute, oozing and erosive lesions, and children in particular, sometimes do not tolerate standard topical application, and may first be treated with 'wet wraps' until the oozing stops.

Local corticosteroid preparations remain the most important agents in the management of AD patients for their anti-inflammatory and antipruritic action. Application amount of topical anti-inflammatory therapy should follow the finger-tip unit (FTU) rule (Fig. 11-9). A FTU is the amount of ointment expressed from a tube with a 5-mm diameter nozzle and measured from the distal skin-crease to the tip of the index finger (approximately 0.5 g). This is an adequate amount for application to two adult palm areas, which is approximately 2% of an adult body surface area. The potent corticosteroids should be avoided on the face, the genitalia, and the intertriginous area. With mild disease activity, a small amount of topical corticosteroids two to three times weekly (monthly amounts in the mean range of 15 g in infants, 30 g in children, and up to 60 to 90 g in adolescents and adults) achieves good maintenance.

Wet-wrap therapy (WWT) is one method to quickly reduce AD severity, and is often used in the setting of significant flares and/or recalcitrant disease. The use of wet-wrap dressings with diluted corticosteroids for up to 14 days (usual is up to 3 days) is a safe treatment of severe and/or refractory AD. Usually, anti-inflammatory topical therapy is administered only to

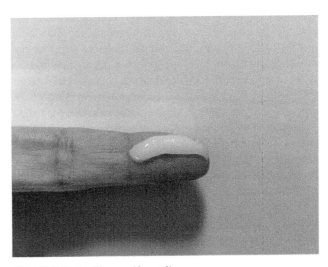

FIGURE 11-9: Finger-tip unit.

the lesional skin and is stopped or tapered down once visible lesions are cleared. This traditional, reactive approach has been challenged recently by the proactive treatment concept, which is defined as a combination of predefined, long-term, low dose, anti-inflammatory treatment applied to previously affected areas of skin in combination with liberal use of emollients on the entire body and a predefined appointment schedule for clinical control examinations. The proactive, usually twice weekly treatment regimen is started after all lesions have successfully been treated by an intensive, usually twice daily treatment approach in addition to ongoing emollient therapy for previously unaffected skin. **Topical calcineurin inhibitors** are steroid-free preparations, which have an immunomodulatory effect. Tacrolimus is approved for moderate-to-severe disease, whereas pimecrolimus is indicated for mild to moderate AD. They are both indicated for the short-term or intermittent long-term treatment of AD in patients older than 2 years of age who are unresponsive to conventional therapy. Their main advantage over corticosteroids is that these agents do not cause skin atrophy and telangiectasia because they do not affect collagen synthesis. They are especially useful for facial and intertriginous lesions. **Topical antipruritics** and antihistamines, including calamine plus diphenhydramine in shake lotions, and more recently in gels, plus promethazine creams, pramoxine, camphor, and menthol, among others, may provide transient itch reduction.

Topical antihistamines have been tried for the treatment of AD but unfortunately have demonstrated little utility and are not recommended.

Capsaicin 0.025% cream acts on substance P release and has an antipruritic effect. There is preliminary evidence that capsaicin is useful in the treatment of AD itch but further trials are needed before an evidence-based recommendation can be given.

Coal tar preparation may have antipruritic and anti-inflammatory effects on the skin, but there are no adequate data to make a recommendation regarding the use of coal tar topical agents for treating AD patients.

Local anesthetics such as benzocaine, lidocaine, polidocanol, as well as a mixture of prilocaine and lidocaine are widely used as short-term effective topical antipruritics. Case series described the efficacy of a combination of polidocanol and 5% urea, but controlled clinical trials investigating the antipruritic effects of local anesthetics in AE are pending.

S. aureus, in particular, is a frequent culprit and colonizer of the skin in AD. Its presence, even without overt infection, appears to trigger multiple inflammatory cascades, via toxins that act as superantigens and exogenous protease inhibitors that further damage the epidermal barrier and potentiate allergen penetration. In cases of localized pyodermal lesions, **local antibiotics**, mostly mupirocin, are applied. The addition of a topical antibiotic to a topical steroid reduces the amount of *S. aureus* isolated from the skin, but topical antimicrobial preparations are not generally recommended in the treatment of AD. The long-term application of topical antibiotics is not recommend due to the risk of increasing resistances and sensitizations.

The yeast *M. furfur* is efficiently eliminated by using a ketoconazole shampoo or with miconazole alone or in combination with hydrocortisone.

Systemic Management

Infectious Agents

Skin infections with *S. aureus* are rather common in AD patients (Fig. 11-3). Oral antibiotics have no benefit on the skin condition in AD as long as skin lesions are not obviously superinfected. A short-term treatment with systemic antibiotics (erythromycin, azithromycin, and cephalosporin) may be beneficial if the skin is obviously superinfected with bacteria. Infection with herpes simplex virus is a severe and life-threatening complication of AD (Figs. 11-1 and 11-2) and requires acyclovir or valacyclovir.

Antihistaminics

Systemic antihistamines are widely used in acute flares against itch. They may be helpful to decrease pruritus and permit sleep during flares, however only a few randomized controlled trials have been conducted and they have, in the majority, shown only a weak or no effect in decreasing pruritus There is insufficient evidence to recommend the general use of antihistamines as a part of treatment of AD. Nonsedating antihistamines are not recommended as a routine treatment for AD in the absence of urticaria or other atopic conditions such as rhinoconjunctivitis and allergic asthma. The first generation of sedative antihistamines (hydroxyzine, clemastine fumarate, dimetinden maleate) may allow a better sleep pattern in acute situations with exacerbations of eczema. Non-sedating antihistamines (loratadine, cetirizine, fexofenadine) demonstrated no or only weak relief of pruritus in AD patients.

Systemic Corticosteroids

The use of systemic corticosteroids is only advised in a short course for acute flare-ups. In children, a short course of oral corticosteroids at a dosage of 0.5 to 1 mg/kg body weight of prednisone or equivalent dose of prednisolone can be used in those whose disorder cannot be controlled by topical therapy, but long-term use should be avoided. Treatment in adults is usually begun with prednisone at dosages of 0.5 to 1 mg/kg/day (usually 40 to 80 mg/day) in a single morning dose or in two divided doses for a period of about 1 week, and then rapidly tapered.

Phototherapy

Phototherapy is a second-line treatment, after failure of first-line treatment (emollients, topical steroids, and topical calcineurin inhibitors). Natural sunlight is frequently beneficial to patients with AD. However, if the sunlight occurs in the setting of high heat and humidity, thereby triggering sweating and pruritus, it may be deleterious to patients. Heliomarinotherapy (sun and sea therapy) is also useful. UVB (short wavelength or ultraviolet B, 290 to 320 nm) or combined UVA (long wave or ultraviolet A, 320 to 400 nm) and UVB exposure is efficacious in AD patients. High daily doses of UVA1 (340 to 400 nm) are even more efficacious, and it is to be preferred in severe cases. Narrow-band UVB is to be preferred to broad-band UVB. Photochemotherapy with oral photosensitizer methoxypsoralen (MOP) followed by UVA exposure (psoralen and ultraviolet A radiation (PUVA) therapy) may be indicated in patients with severe, widespread AD with failure of topical steroid therapy or significant corticosteroid side effects. Topical application of 0.3% 8-MOP ointment (PUVA cream therapy) could be used to treat palmoplantar AD lesions. Close monitoring for skin cancer is indicated. Phototherapy is not indicated in the acute stage of AD (except UVA1, which is also effective in managing AD flares), but is more apt to treat chronic, pruritic, lichenified forms, and should not be prescribed in those patients who experience a worsening of their dermatosis during sun exposure. Topical steroids and emollients should be considered at the beginning of phototherapy to reduce flare-up.

Cyclosporine

Cyclosporine (CSA) is a potent immunosuppressive drug that acts primarily on T-cell receptors by suppressing cytokine transcription. Severe AD patients, refractory to topical corticosteroid therapy, can benefit from treatment with oral cyclosporine (3 to 5 mg/kg/day, standardly 150 to 300 mg/day in adults) for 8 weeks or 3 months. Data on relapse after CSA discontinuation are limited. Patients receiving CSA should be monitored for potential adverse effects that include: infection, nephrotoxicity, hypertension, tremor, hypertrichosis, headache, gingival hyperplasia, and increased risk of skin cancer and lymphoma.

Azathioprine

Azathioprine may be used (off label) in AE patients, if cyclosporine is either not effective or contraindicated. Dosage of the medication ranges from 1 mg/kg/day to 3 mg/kg/day. Patients with deficient activity of the enzyme thiopurine methyltransferase (TPMT) have an increased risk for myelosuppression from azathioprine use, so before starting therapy TPMT deficiency should be excluded. Onset of action with azathioprine is typically slow, with benefits apparent 2 to 3 months after onset of treatment.

Methotrexate

Methotrexate (MTX) may be used (off label) for treatment of AE in adults, if cyclosporine is not effective or not indicated. There are no trial data for its use in children or adolescents. MTX is usually given as a single weekly dose. The dose range for MTX in patients with AD is between 7.5 and 25 mg weekly. Divided dosing, given every 12 hours for 3 doses, is an alternative method for dosing MTX.

Interferon Therapy

INF-γ is known to suppress IgE responses and downregulate Th2 proliferation and function. The treatment with recombinant INF-γ results in clinical improvement and decreases total circulating eosinophil counts (10 to 100 μg/m^2).

Extracorporeal Photopheresis

This treatment consists of the passage of psoralen-treated leukocytes through an extracorporeal UVA light system. It could be used in severe AD patients who are resistant to the therapy.

Allergen Immunotherapy

Available evidence of the effectiveness of immunotherapy with aeroallergens in the treatment of AD is mixed. The best evidence so far is available for allergen specific immunotherapy (ASIT) with house-dust mite allergens.

Other

Mycophenolate mofetil (MMF) is indicated in the management of resistant forms of AD and is behind cyclosporine in AD management. MMF has a better safety profile than cyclosporine or azathioprine, but controlled studies are needed to prove efficacy.

Leukotriene Antagonists

Leukotriene antagonists (montelukast and zafirlukast) are useful for the treatments of asthma and allergic rhinitis. In AD therapy, they are not fully elucidated. Zafirlukast is approved in AD and asthma for adolescents and adults. In chronic AD, montelukast achieved little success. Montelukast administrated 5 mg daily for 4 weeks in a clinical double-blind study of moderate to severe AD in young patients (6 to 16 years) showed a significant decrease in severity, but in another study with severe AD and different doses (5, 10, and 20 mg), there was only partial improvement (relief of pruritus and erythema) in very few patients. AD patients failed to show any benefit from leukotriene receptor antagonist therapy.

Bioengineered Immunomodulators

Most of the new approaches aim at inhibiting components of the allergic inflammatory response, including cytokine modulation (e.g., TNF inhibitors), blockade of inflammatory cell recruitment (chemokine receptor antagonists, cutaneous lymphocyte antigen inhibitors), and inhibition of T-cell activation (alefacept). Bioengineered immunomodulators are in the clinical trial phase for AD treatment. They change the immune profile from Th1 to Th2 or block cytokines. These agents are currently under clinical trials for psoriasis and psoriatic arthritis.

Biologics

In patients with severe AE refractory to topical and systemic treatment, a therapy with biologics (omalizumab, rituximab, alefacept) can be considered. None of the biologics have been approved for the therapy of AE yet.

IgE-blocking antibody omalizumab is a recombinant human monoclonal antibody. Omalizumab specifically binds to the high-affinity FceRI domain of free circulating IgE, and thus prevents binding of free serum IgE to mast cells and other effector cells, has shown some promise in treating patients with AD and elevated IgE. The role of omalizumab in dermatology and for AD is probably best directed toward patients who have high levels of IgE and in whom the IgE is an etiologic factor for their disease.

SAUER'S NOTES

1. Atopic diseases have given medicine a unique chance to study the intricacies of the immune system as this chapter illustrates.
2. An increase in atopic illness, most notably asthma and eczema, continues to be a major health problem of the new century.
3. Do not underestimate the importance of a well-maintained doctor–patient relationship in dealing with patients and their families in this very chronic and often frustrating group of diseases.

SAUER'S NOTES

Food intolerance should not be confused with food allergy. Food intolerance is when the digestive system cannot breakdown food usually manifests as diarrhea, stomach pain, and vomiting. Food allergy can be serious and occur within minutes of ingesting the food resulting in hives, airway swelling, or true anaphylaxis. The foods to be considered are nuts especially peanuts and fish, especially shellfish. Food allergies causing eczema is rare in our experience "editors" but can be a significant factor in a minority of patients.

CONCLUSION

AD develops as a consequence of complex etiology and pathogenesis. The severity and extent of skin lesions and deviation in laboratory parameters, especially immunologic ones, may greatly differ from patient to patient. A consensus will have to be established in the near future on the new criteria defining AD, based on the model set 35 years ago by Hanifin and Rajka. The increasing prevalence of this disease worldwide underlines the role of prevention, recognition, and optimal treatment of the many patients with AD.

Suggested Readings

Akdis CA, Akdis M, Bieber T, et al. Diagnosis and treatment of atopic dermatitis in children and adults: European Academy of Allergology and Clinical Immunology/American Academy of Allergy, Asthma and Immunology/PRACTALL Consensus Report. *Allergy.* 2006;61:969–987.

Brian S Kim. Atopic dermatitis. In: *Medscape.* http://emedicine.medscape.com/article/1049085-overview. Accessed November 29, 2015.

Cookson WO, Moffatt MF. The genetics of atopic dermatitis. *Curr Opin Allergy Clin Immunol.* 2002;2:383–387.

Eichenfield LF, Tom WL, Chamlin SL, et. al. Guidelines of care for the management of atopic dermatitis: section 1. Diagnosis and assessment of atopic dermatitis. *J Am Acad Dermatol.* 2014;70(2):338–351.

Ellis CN, Mancini AJ, Paller AS, et al. Understanding and managing atopic dermatitis in adult patients. *Semin Cutan Med Surg.* 2012;31(3 suppl):S18–S22.

Hanifin J, Rajka G. Diagnostic features of atopic dermatitis. *Acta Derm Venereol (Stockh).* 1980;92(suppl):44–47.

Lipozenčić J, Ljubojević S. Atopic dermatitis. *Rad Med Sci.* 2008;449(32):77–103.

Lipozenčić J, Wolf R. Atopic dermatitis: an update and review of the literature. *Dermatol Clin.* 2007;25:605–612.

Möhrenschlager M, Darsow U, Schnopp C, et al. Atopic eczema: what's new? *J Eur Acad Dermatol Venereol.* 2006;20:503–513.

Novak N, Bieber T, Leung DY. Immune mechanisms leading to atopic dermatitis. *J Allergy Clin Immunol.* 2003;112:S128–S139.

Paštar Z, Lipozenčić J, Ljubojević S. Etiopathogenesis of atopic dermatitis—an overview. *Acta Dermatovenerol Croat.* 2005;13:54–62.

Peng W, Novak N. Pathogenesis of atopic dermatitis. *Clin Exp Allergy.* 2015;45(3):566–574.

Ring J, Alomar A, Bieber T, et al. Guidelines for treatment of atopic eczema (atopic dermatitis), part I. *J Eur Acad Dermatol Venereol.* 2012;26(8):1045–1060.

Ring J, Alomar A, Bieber T, et al. Guidelines for treatment of atopic eczema (atopic dermatitis), part II. *J Eur Acad Dermatol Venereol.* 2012;26(9):1176–1193.

Ring J, Huss-Marp J. Atopic eczema. *Karger Gazette.* 2004;67:7–9.

Rudikoff D, Cohen SR, Scheinfeld N, eds. *Atopic Dermatitis and Eczematous Disorders.* Boca Raton: CRC Press; 2014.

Scheinfeld NS, Tutrone WD, Weinberg JM, et al. Phototherapy of atopic dermatitis. *Clin Dermatol.* 2003;21:241–248.

Schultz Larsen F, Hanifin JM. Epidemiology of atopic dermatitis. *Immunol Allergy Clin North Am.* 2002;22:1–24.

Sidbury R, Davis DM, Cohen DE, et al. Guidelines of care for the management of atopic dermatitis: section 3. Management and treatment with phototherapy and systemic agents. *J Am Acad Dermatol.* 2014;71(2):327–349.

12

Pruritic Dermatoses

John C. Hall, MD

Pruritus, or itching, brings more patients to the physician's office than any other skin disease symptom. Itchy skin is not easily cured or even alleviated. Decreased quality of life due to pruritus can be as significant as pain. Many hundreds of proprietary over-the-counter and prescription drugs are touted as effective anti-itch remedies, but none is 100% effective. Many are partially effective, but it is unfortunate that the most effective locally applied chemicals frequently irritate or sensitize the skin.

Pruritus is a symptom of many of the common skin diseases, such as contact dermatitis, atopic eczema, seborrheic dermatitis, hives, scabies, insect bites, some drug eruptions, and many other dermatoses. Relief of itching is of prime importance in treating these diseases.

In addition to the pruritus that occurs as a symptom of many skin diseases, there are other clinical forms of pruritus that deserve special consideration. These special types include *generalized pruritus* of the winter, senile, and essential varieties, and *localized pruritus* of the lichen simplex–type, which affects the ears, anal area, lower legs in men, back of the neck in women, and genitalia. Localized pruritus of unknown etiology should alert one to the possibility of underlying peripheral nerve or central nervous system pathology.

GENERALIZED PRURITUS

Diffuse itching of the body without perceptible skin disease usually is due to winter dry skin or senile skin.

> ### SAUER'S NOTES
>
> When the presenting complaint is a generalized itching of the skin, always stroke the skin on the forearm with your nail or a tongue depressor. After 5 minutes or so, if there is a wheal reaction at the stroking site, you have a diagnosis of dermographism. This is a common problem that is easily overlooked.

Winter Pruritus

Winter pruritus, or pruritus hiemalis, is a common form of generalized pruritus, although most patients complain of itching confined mainly to their legs. Every autumn, a certain number of elderly patients, and occasionally young ones, walk into the physician's office complaining bitterly of the rather sudden onset of itching of their legs. Men often also itch around the waist. These patients have dry skin caused by the low humidity in their furnace-heated homes, or occasionally from the low humidity resulting from cooling air conditioning. Clinically, the skin shows excoriations and dry, curled, scaling plaques resembling a sun-baked, muddy beach at low tide. The dry skin associated with winter itch is to be differentiated from *ichthyosis*, a congenital, inherited dermatosis of varying severity, which is also worse in the winter. Treatment of winter pruritus consists of the following:

1. Bathing should involve as cool water as possible and as little soap as possible. Soap can be limited to the face, axillae, groin, genitalia, hands, and feet.

2. Bland soap, such as Dove, Oilatum, Cetaphil, or Basis, is used sparingly.

3. Oil, such as Lubath, RoBathol, Nivea, or Alpha Keri, is added to the bath water. (The patient should be warned to avoid slipping in the tub.) The oil can be rubbed on after a shower.

4. Emollient lotions are beneficial, such as Complex 15 (phospholipid), CeraVe (ceramides), Curel (petrolatum), Eucerin, Aquaphor (esterified lanolin, quite greasy), Pen Kera, or Moisturel (not as greasy and noncomedogenic). α-Hydroxy acid preparations include AmLactin 12% cream and lotion (over-the-counter), Lac-Hydrin 5% (over-the-counter), Lac-Hydrin 12% (prescription only), and Eucerin Plus. Urea products (in these higher concentrations may be irritating except on palms or soles) that are beneficial include Kera Lotion (35%), Keracream (40%), Vanamide (40%), Carmol 40 cream and lotion (40%), and Eucerin Plus lotion (also has lactic acid as an α-hydroxy acid). Lubricants should be applied immediately after bathing for the most benefit.

5. A low-potency corticosteroid ointment applied twice daily is effective. Triamcinolone ointment 0.1% is midpotency and very inexpensive. A 1% hydrocortisone can be mixed with any of the mentioned moisturizers or used as a nonspecific ointment.

6. Oral antihistamines are sometimes effective, such as chlorpheniramine (Chlor-Trimeton), 4 mg h.s. or q.i.d, or diphenhydramine (Benadryl), 50 mg h.s. There are newer nonsedating antihistamines such as Claritin 10 mg q.d. (over-the-counter), Clarinex 10 mg q.d., Zyrtec

(may be slightly sedating and also more effective) 10 mg q.d., and Allegra 60 or 180 mg q.d. Some doctors do not think that the nonsedating antihistamines are as effective as the sedating antihistamines. A commonly used sedating antihistamine is hydroxyzine, 10 mg every 8 hours while awake. The dose can be titrated to 25, 50, or rarely 100 mg. The soporific effect, or drowsiness, often becomes less severe with prolonged use.

7. Doxepin (Sinequan) starting at 10 mg/day and working up to 50 mg/day has been used with some success but can be sedating.

8. Neurontin (Gabapentin) 300 mg/day and over weeks to months working up to doses as high as 1,800 mg/day in divided doses has been shown to be successful by some authors.

9. Ultraviolet light in the form of psoralens and ultraviolet light (PUVA) (increases risk of skin malignancy) and narrowband UVB may be beneficial.

10. Mu-opioid receptor antagonists such as naloxone, nalmefene, and naltrexone can be used in difficult cases.

Senile Pruritus

Senile pruritus is a resistant form of generalized pruritus in the elderly patient. It can occur at any time of the year and may or may not be associated with dry skin. There is some evidence that these patients have a disorder of keratinization. This form of itch occurs most commonly on the scalp, shoulders, sacral areas, and legs. Clinically, some patients have no cutaneous signs of the itch, but others may have linear excoriations. *Scabies* should be ruled out, as well as the diseases mentioned under the next form of pruritus to be considered, essential pruritus.

Treatment is usually not very satisfactory. In addition to the agents mentioned previously in connection with winter pruritus, the injection of 40 mg of triamcinolone acetonide suspension (Kenalog-40) intramuscularly every 4 to 6 weeks for two or three injections is quite beneficial. I do not like to repeat this more often than three to four times a year to avoid systemic corticosteroid side effects. Topical antipruritic agents can be used, such as pramoxine hydrochloride (Pramosone with either 1% or 2.5% hydrocortisone is a prescription or Aveeno anti-itch lotion, which is available over-the-counter). Menthol (0.5%), phenol (0.5%), or sulfur (2% to 5%) can be added to any appropriate base (see Chapter 4).

Essential Pruritus

Essential pruritus is the rarest form of the generalized itching diseases. No person of any age is exempt, but it occurs most frequently in the elderly patient. The itching is usually quite diffuse, with occasional "bites" in certain localized areas. All itching is worse at night, and no exception is made for this form of pruritus. Before a diagnosis of essential pruritus is made, the following diseases must be ruled out by appropriate studies:

- Drug reaction
- Diabetes mellitus
- Uremia

- Lymphoma (mycosis fungoides, leukemia, or lymphoma [especially Hodgkin disease]), as a paraneoplastic syndrome from any metastatic underlying malignancy
- Primary sclerosing cholangitis, which has very severe pruritus
- Liver disease (especially hepatitis B or C even without jaundice)
- Bullous pemphigoid before the blisters are present
- AIDS and other immunosuppressed states
- Stress or more severe psychiatric illness such as psychosis or parasitophobia
- Hyperthyroidism
- Post–brain tissue damage such as a stroke, brain cancer, or trauma
- Intestinal parasites
- Intrahepatic cholestasis of pregnancy—early diagnosis in the second half of pregnancy with elevation of total serum bile acids should prompt early treatment with ursodeoxycholic acid
- Telangiectasia macularis eruptiva perstans (may need skin biopsy to find)
- Cutaneous T-cell lymphoma "incognito" (may need skin biopsy to find)
- Drugs, especially opiates such as morphine

Treatment is the same as for senile and winter pruritus. Narrowband UVB is a safe and sometimes effective nonspecific treatment for pruritus. For more recalcitrant severe cases, here is a list of other therapies that can be tried: psychotherapy (including hypnosis), acupuncture, in dialysis patients more intense and magnesium-free dialyses, systemic metronidazole (primary sclerosing cholangitis), ursodeoxycholic acid (primary biliary cirrhosis), sertraline (75 to 100 mg daily), naltrexone (12.5 mg to start and up to 50 mg daily), rifampicin (150 mg t.i.d.), ondansetron (8 mg t.i.d.), gabapentin, nalfurafine, ketotifen, cholestyramine (liver and gallbladder disease), oral activated charcoal, thalidomide, intravenous lidocaine, bupropion, doxepin (10 to 30 mg h.s.), and pimozide.

LOCALIZED PRURITIC DERMATOSES

Lichen Simplex Chronicus

Other common terms for lichen simplex chronicus (LSC) include localized neurodermatitis and lichenified dermatitis. There are pros and cons for all the terms.

LSC (Fig. 12-1) is a common skin condition characterized by the occurrence of single or, less frequently, multiple patches of chronic itching and thickened, scaly, dry skin in one or more classic locations. It is unrelated to atopic eczema according to some experts, but others feel it is an adult form of eczema.

Primary Lesions

This disease begins as a small, localized, well-demarcated, pruritic papule, or patch of dermatitis that might have been

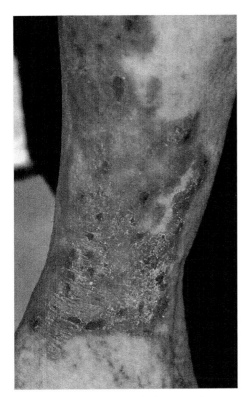

FIGURE 12-1: Localized LSC of the leg. This is a common location. Note the lichenification and excoriations owing to the marked pruritus. (Courtesy of K.U.M.C.; Duke Labs, Inc.)

an insect bite, chigger bite, contact dermatitis, or other minor irritation that may or may not be remembered by the patient. Because of various etiologic factors, a cycle of itching, scratching, more itching, and more scratching supervenes, and a chronic dermatosis develops. Emotional stress is thought to lower the itch threshold and cause exacerbation of the disease. The itching is intense and paroxysmal in nature.

Secondary Lesions

These include excoriations, lichenification, and, in severe cases, marked verrucous thickening of the skin, with pigmentary changes. In severe cases, healing is bound to be followed by some scarring.

Presentation and Characteristics

Distribution*:* This condition is seen most commonly at the hairline of the nape of the neck and on the wrists, the ankles, the ears (see external otitis), anal area (see pruritus ani), and so on (Fig. 12-2).

Course: This disease is chronic and recurrent. Most cases respond quickly to potent topical corticosteroid treatment, but some can last for years and defy all forms of therapy.

Subjective Complaints: The primary symptom is intense itching, often paroxysmal, that is usually worse at night, occurs even during sleep, and may awaken the patient.

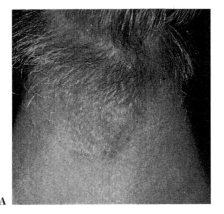

A

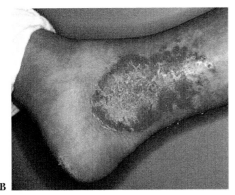

B

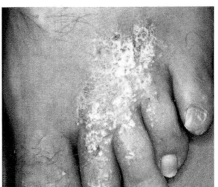

C

FIGURE 12-2: Localized LSC in the occipital area of the scalp **(A)**, of the medial aspect of ankle following lichen planus of the area **(B)**, and on the dorsum of the foot **(C)**. (Courtesy of Duke Labs, Inc.)

Causes: The initial cause (a bite, stasis dermatitis, contact dermatitis, seborrheic dermatitis, tinea cruris, psoriasis) may be very evanescent, but it is generally agreed that the chronicity of the lesion is due to the nervous habit of scratching. It is a rare patient who does not volunteer the information or admit, if questioned, that the itching is worse when he or she is upset, nervous, or tired. Why some people with a minor skin injury respond with the development of a lichenified patch of skin and others do not is possibly due to the personality of the patient or in an atopic patient due to an increased release of antihistamines with an exaggerated triple response of Lewis beginning the chronic itch–scratch cycle.

Age Group: It is very common to see localized neurodermatitis of the posterior neck in menopausal women. Men often prefer the lower leg or ankle. Other clinical types of neurodermatitis are seen at any age.

Family Incidence: This disorder may be unrelated to allergies in the patient or family, thus differing from atopic eczema. Atopic people are more "itchy," however, and, as mentioned, some authors feel the two diseases are a continuum.

Related to Employment: Recurrent exposure and contact to irritating agents at work can lead to LSC.

Differential Diagnosis

- *Psoriasis:* Several patches on the body in classic areas of distribution; family history of disease; classic silvery whitish scales; sharply circumscribed patch; itching may be intense, especially in the scalp and perianal areas, but it is often minimal (see Chapters 15 and 17).
- *Atopic eczema:* Allergic history in patient or family; multiple lesions; classically seen in cubital and popliteal areas and face (see Chapter 8).
- *Contact dermatitis:* Acute onset; contact history positive; usually red, vesicular, and oozing; distribution matches site of exposure to contactant; may be acute contact dermatitis overlying LSC owing to overzealous therapy (see Chapter 8).
- *Lichen planus, hypertrophic form on anterior tibial area:* Lichen planus in mouth and on other body areas; biopsy specimen usually characteristic (see Chapter 17).
- *Seborrheic dermatitis of scalp:* A diffuse, scaly, greasy eruption that does not itch as much and is better in summer (see Chapter 17).

Treatment

Case Example: A 45-year-old woman presents with a severely itching, scaly, red, lichenified patch on the back of the neck at the hairline.

First Visit

1. Explain the condition to the patient, and tell her that the medicine is directed toward stopping the itch. If this can be done, and if she cooperates by keeping her hands off the area, the disease will disappear. Emphasize the effect of scratching by stating that if both arms were broken, the eruption would be gone when the casts were removed. However, this is not a recommended form of therapy. Do not blame the patient for this disease in your zeal to explain the importance of keeping hands off.
2. For severe bouts of intractable itching, prescribe ice-cold Burow's solution packs.
   Sig: Add 1 packet of Domeboro powder to 1 quart of ice-cold water. Apply cloth wet with this solution for 15 minutes PRN.
3. A moderate-potency corticosteroid ointment or emollient cream 15.0.
   Sig: Apply q.i.d., or more often, as itching requires. The moderate-potency fluorinated corticosteroid creams (Synalar, Cordran, Lidex, Diprosone, Cutivate) can be used under an occlusive dressing of plastic wrap on extremity lesions. The dressing can be left on overnight.
   Warning: Long-term occlusive dressing therapy with corticosteroids can cause atrophy of the skin.

Subsequent Visits

1. Add menthol (0.25%) or coal tar solution (3% to 10%) to above ointment or cream for greater antipruritic effect.
2. Intralesional corticosteroid therapy is a very effective and safe treatment. The technique is as follows: use a 1-in long No. 26 needle or 30½ needle and a Luer-Lok-type tuberculin syringe. Inject 3 or 5 mg/mL of triamcinolone parenteral solution (Kenalog-10 or Aristocort intralesional suspension diluted with normal saline or xylocaine with or without epinephrine) intradermally or subcutaneously, directly under the skin lesion. Do not inject all the solution in one area, but spread it around as you advance the needle. Usually 1 mL or less is injected each time. The injection can be repeated every 3 or 4 weeks as necessary to eliminate the patch of dermatitis.
   Warning: A complication of an atrophic depression at the injection site can occur. This usually can be avoided if the concentration of triamcinolone in one area is kept low, and when it occurs, it usually disappears after months.

Resistant Cases

1. An antihistamine or anti-anxiety agent orally.
2. Prednisone 10 mg.
   Sig: 1 tablet q.i.d. for 3 days, then 2 tablets every morning for 7 days.
3. Dome-Paste boot or Coban wrap. Apply in office for cases of neurodermatitis localized to the arms and legs. This is a physical deterrent to scratching. Leave on for 1 week at a time.
4. Psychotherapy is of questionable value and patients may be offended by the suggestion.

External Otitis

External otitis is a descriptive term for a common and persistent dermatitis of the ears owing to several causes. The agent most frequently blamed for this condition is "fungus," but pathogenic fungi are rarely found in the external ear. The true causes of external otitis, in order of frequency, are as follows: seborrheic dermatitis (which is now felt to be related to *Pityrosporum ovale* yeast infection), LSC, contact dermatitis, atopic eczema, psoriasis, *Pseudomonas* bacterial infection (which is usually secondary to other causes), and, lastly, fungal infection, which also can be primary or secondary to other factors. For further information on the specific processes, refer to each of the diseases mentioned.

> ### SAUER'S NOTES
>
> 1. Many cases of acute ear dermatitis are aggravated by an allergy to the therapeutic cream, such as Neosporin, or the ingredients in the base.
> 2. A corticosteroid in a petrolatum base eliminates this problem.
> 3. Use 1% Hytone ointment, DesOwen ointment, or Tridesilon ointment. Author prefers Cloderm cream.

Treatment

Treatment should be directed primarily toward the specific cause, such as care of the scalp for seborrheic cases or avoidance of jewelry for contact cases. When the primary cause has been addressed, however, certain special techniques and medicines must be used in addition to clear up this troublesome area.

Case Example: An elderly woman presents with an oozing, red, crusted, swollen left external ear, with a wet canal but an intact drum. A considerable amount of seborrheic dermatitis of the scalp is confluent with the acutely inflamed ear area. The patient has had itching ear trouble off and on for 10 years, but in the past month, it has become most severe.

First Visit:

1. Always inspect the canal and the drum with an otoscope. If excessive wax and debris are present in the canal, or if the drum is involved in the process, the patient should be treated for these problems or referred to an ear specialist. An effective liquid to dry up the oozing canal is as follows:
   Hydrocortisone powder 1%
   Burow's solution, 1:10 strength q.s. 15.0
   Sig: Place two drops in ear t.i.d.
2. Burow's solution wet packs
   Sig: Add 1 packet of Domeboro powder to 1 quart of cool water. Apply wet cloths to external ear for 15 minutes t.i.d.
3. Corticosteroid ointment 15.0
   Sig: Apply locally to external ear t.i.d., not in canal.

Subsequent Visits

Several days later, after decreased swelling, cessation of oozing, and lessening of itching, institute the following changes in therapy:

1. Decrease the soaks to once a day.
2. Sulfur, ppt. (parts per thousand) 5%
3. Corticosteroid ointment q.s. 15.0
   Sig: Apply locally t.i.d. to ear with the little finger, not down in the canal, or with a cotton tip applicator.

For persistent cases, a short course of oral corticosteroid or antibiotic therapy often removes the "fire" so that local remedies are effective.

Pruritus Ani

Itching of the anal area is a common malady that can vary in severity from mild to marked. The patient with this very annoying symptom is apt to resort to self-treatment and therefore delay the visit to the physician. Usually, the patient has overtreated the sensitive area, and the immediate problem of the physician is to quiet the acute contact dermatitis. The original cause of the pruritus ani is often difficult to ascertain.

Pruritic diseases common in this area are seborrheic dermatitis, psoriasis, lichen sclerosis et atrophicus, candidiasis, tinea, pinworms (especially in children), and hemorrhoids in adults.

Presentation and Characteristics

Primary Lesions: These can range from slight redness confined to a very small area to an extensive contact dermatitis with redness, vesicles, and oozing of the entire buttock.

Secondary Lesions: Excoriations from the intense itching are very common, and after a prolonged time, they progress toward lichenification. A generalized papulovesicular id eruption can develop from an acute flare-up of this entity.

Course: Most cases of pruritus ani respond rapidly and completely to a proper management, especially if the cause can be ascertained and eliminated. Every physician, however, will have a patient who will continue to scratch and defy all therapy.

Causes: The proper management of this socially unacceptable form of pruritus consists in searching for and eliminating the several factors that contribute to the persistence of this symptom complex. These factors can be divided into general and specific etiologic factors.

> ### SAUER'S NOTES
>
> 1. Do not prescribe a fluorinated corticosteroid salve for the anogenital area. It can cause telangiectasia and atrophy of the skin after long-term use.
> 2. One of my favorite medications for pruritus ani or genital pruritus is 1% Hytone ointment applied sparingly locally two or three times a day. The petrolatum base is well tolerated.

3. If the anogenital pruritus is resistant to therapy and especially if the involvement is unilateral, a biopsy should be performed to rule out Bowen's disease or extramammary Paget's disease. Although psychologically disconcerting to the patient, this is a simple area to biopsy with curved iris scissor after local anesthesia has plumped up the skin. It heals rapidly and can be extremely important to be sure a serious malignancy has not been missed.

4. A short burst of systemic corticosteroids may be necessary to break the itch–scratch cycle. An example of this would be 10 days of prednisone beginning with 50 mg each morning and decreasing by 10 mg every 2 days until gone. Thirty 10 mg tablets is the full 10-day course and no refills should be given.

General Factors

- *Diet:* The following irritating foods should be removed from the diet: chocolate, nuts, cheese, and spicy foods. Coffee, because of its stimulating effect on any form of itching, should be limited to 1 cup a day. Rarely, certain other foods are noted by the patient to aggravate the pruritus.

- *Bathing:* Many patients have the misconception that the itching is caused by uncleanliness. Therefore, they resort to excessive bathing and scrubbing of the anal area. This is harmful and irritating, and must be stopped.

- *Toilet care:* Harsh toilet paper contributes greatly to the continuance of this condition. Cotton or a proprietary cleansing cloth (e.g., Tucks) must be used for wiping. Mineral oil or Balneol lotion can be added to the cotton if necessary. Rarely, an allergy to the pastel tint in colored toilet tissues is a factor causing pruritus.

- *Scratching:* As with all the diseases of this group, chronic scratching leads to a vicious cycle. The chief aim of the physician is to give relief from this itching, but a gentle admonishment to the patient to keep hands off is indicated. With the physician's help, the itch–scratch cycle can be broken. The emotional and mental personality of the patient regulates the effectiveness of this suggestion.

Specific Etiologic Factors

- *Oral antibiotics:* Pruritus ani from oral antibiotic therapy is seen frequently. It may or may not be due to an overgrowth of *Candida* organisms. The physician who automatically questions patients about recent drug ingestion will not miss this diagnosis.

- *LSC:* It is always a problem to know which comes first, the itching or the "nervousness." In most instances, the itching comes first, but there is no denying that once pruritus ani has developed, it is aggravated by emotional tension and "nerves." However, only the rare patient has a "deep-seated" psychologic problem.

- *Psoriasis:* In this area, psoriasis is common. Usually, other skin surfaces are also involved.

- *Atopic eczema:* Atopic eczema of this site is rather unusual. A history of atopy in the patient or family is helpful in establishing this cause.

- *Fungal infection:* Contrary to old beliefs, this cause is quite rare. Clinically, a raised, sharp, papulovesicular border is seen that commonly is confluent with tinea of the crural area or buttocks. If a scraping or a culture reveals fungi, then local or systemic antifungal therapy is indicated for cure.

- *Worm infestation:* In children, pinworms can often be implicated. A diagnosis is made by finding eggs on morning anal smears, by applying scotch tape to the anal orifice and viewing the worms under the microscope, or by seeing the small white worms when the child is sleeping. Worms are a rare cause of adult pruritus ani.

- *Hemorrhoids:* In the lay person's mind, this is undoubtedly the most common cause. Actually, it is an unimportant primary factor but may be a contributing factor. Hemorrhoidectomy alone is rarely successful as a cure for pruritus ani.

- *Cancer:* This is a very rare cause of anal itching, but a rectal or proctoscopic examination may be indicated, especially in men who have sex with men.

Treatment

Case Example: A patient states that he has had anal itching for 4 months. It began after a 5-day course of an antibiotic for the "flu." Many local remedies have been used; the latest, a supposed remedy for athlete's foot, aggravated the condition. Examination reveals an oozing, macerated, red area around the anus.

First Visit

1. Initial therapy should include removal of the general factors listed under *Causes* and giving instructions as to diet, bathing, toilet care, and scratching.

2. Burow's solution wet packs
   Sig: Add 1 packet of Domeboro to 1 quart of cool water.
   Apply wet cloths to the area b.i.d. while lying in bed for 20 minutes, or more often if necessary for severe itching. Ice cubes may be added to the solution for more anti-itching effect.

3. Low-potency corticosteroid cream or ointment q.s. 15.0
   Sig: Apply to area b.i.d.

4. Diphenhydramine, 50 mg
   Sig: 1 capsule h.s. (for itching and sedation).
   Comment: Available over-the-counter.

Subsequent Visits

1. As tolerated, add increasing strengths of sulfur, coal tar solution, or menthol (0.25%) or phenol (0.5%) to the above cream, or to Vytone cream with hydrocortisone 1% and iodoquinol (can be given in a cheaper generic formulation).

2. Intralesional corticosteroid injection therapy is very effective. Usually, the minor discomfort of the injection is quite well tolerated because of the patient's desire to be cured. The technique is described in the section on LSC. Use only 3 mg/mL triamcinolone or lower concentration.

Genital Pruritus

Itching of the female vulva or the male scrotum can be treated in much the same way as pruritus ani if the special considerations discussed in this section are borne in mind.

Vulvar Pruritus

Etiologically, vulvar pruritus is caused by *Candida* or *Trichomonas* infection; contact dermatitis from underwear, douche chemicals, contraceptive jellies, and diaphragms; chronic cervicitis; neurodermatitis; menopausal or senile atrophic changes; lichen sclerosus et atrophicus; bacillary vaginosis; or leukoplakia. Pruritus vulvae is frequently seen in patients with diabetes mellitus and during pregnancy.

Treatment can be adapted from that for pruritus ani (see preceding section) with the addition of a daily douche, such as 2 tbsp of vinegar to 1 quart of warm water.

Vulvodynia is a difficult problem to manage. The sensation of burning and pain in the vulvar area is not uncommon and requires careful etiologic evaluation. Most cases can be managed as a contact dermatitis, but there is a strong psychologic element. A minimal dose of haloperidol (Haldol), 1 mg b.i.d., amitriptyline (Elavil), 10 mg h.s., or (doxepin) (Sinequan), 10 mg h.s. is occasionally indicated and effective. Larger doses may be necessary. Scrotodynia is a similar variant in men and pudendal nerve disease should be considered in the differential diagnosis especially in bicycle enthusiasts.

Scrotal Pruritus

Etiologically, scrotal pruritus is due to tinea infection; contact dermatitis from soaps, powders, or clothing; or LSC (Fig. 12-3). Treatment is similar to that given for pruritus ani in the preceding section.

Notalgia Paresthetica

Notalgia paresthetica is a moderately common localized pruritic dermatosis that is usually confined to the middle upper

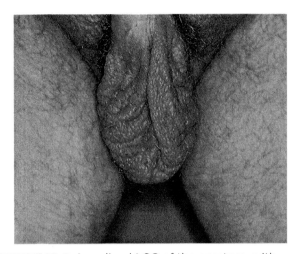

FIGURE 12-3: Localized LSC of the scrotum, with marked lichenification and thickening of the skin. (Courtesy of Duke Labs, Inc.)

back or scapular area off to one side of the spine. A pigmented patch may be formed by the chronic rubbing. Spinal nerve impingement has been suggested as the etiology by some authors. Zonalon cream four times a day may be helpful, but when applied over large areas, it may cause drowsiness. Some evidence exists for a hereditary factor. EMLA (eutectic mixture of lidocaine 2.5% and prilocaine 2.5%) anesthetic cream and capsaicin (Zostrix) cream may be beneficial.

Suggested Readings

Curtis AR, Tegeler C, Burdette J, et al. Holistic approach to treatment of intractable central neuropathic itch. *J Am Acad Dermatol*. 2011;64(5):955–959.

Fleischer A. *The Clinical Management of Itching*. New York, NY: Parthenon Publishing Group; 2000.

Kam PC, Tan KH. Pruritus—itching for a cause and relief? *Anaesthesia*. 1996;51(12):1133–1138.

Stein SL, Cifu AS. Management of atopic dermatitis. *JAMA*. 2016;315(14):1510–1512.

Yosipovitch G, Bernhard JD. Chronic pruritus. *N Eng J Med*. 2013;68(17):1625–1634.

Yosipovitch G, David M. The diagnostic and therapeutic approach to idiopathic generalized pruritus. *Int J Dermatol*. 1999;38:881–887.

Yosipovitch G, Greaves MW, Fleischer A, et al. *Itch: Basic Mechanisms and Therapy*. New York, NY: Marcel Dekker; 2004.

Vascular Dermatoses

John C. Hall, MD

Urticaria, erythema multiforme and its variants, and erythema nodosum are included under the heading of vascular dermatoses because of their vascular reaction patterns. Stasis dermatitis is included because it is a dermatosis owing to venous insufficiency in the legs. Vasculitis is due to inflammation on the arterial side of the vascular tree in small or large vessels. Pigmented purpura is due to microvascular capillary leakage of red blood cells and hence causes hemosiderin staining in a prone patient. It is called a benign hemosiderosis in contrast to the "malignant" type of hemosiderosis seen in hemochromatosis, where internal organs (especially the liver) may be involved. Pyoderma gangrenosum is an ulcerative inflammatory disease, mainly of the lower extremities. Cutaneous necrosis is end-stage vascular compromise with gangrenous disease.

Another group of inflammatory diseases are called autoinflammatory diseases which differ from autoimmune diseases in that no specific antibodies have been discovered in the skin or in the blood. They are characterized by recurrent fever and inflammatory disease of joints, skin, muscles, and eyes. Disease in which a genetic link has been made includes familial Mediterranean fever (FMF). Hyper-IgD syndrome (HIDS), tumor necrosis factor receptor associated autoinflammatory syndrome (TRAPS), cryopyrin-associated periodic syndromes (CAPS), Blau syndrome, pyogenic sterile arthritis, pyoderma gangrenosum, and acne syndrome (PAPA syndrome). No genetic link has been found with some of these syndromes and these include periodic fever, aphthous stomatitis, pharyngitis, and adenitis, (PFAPA syndrome), Majeed syndrome which is characterized by recurrence of multiple osteomyelitis (CRMO), congenital dyserythropoietic anemia, and neutrophilic

dermatosis. For more specific findings, look up each syndrome in the Dictionary–Index. These autoinflammatory syndromes are also considered synonymous with periodic syndromes.

URTICARIA

The commonly (10% to 25% of population at some time in life) seen entity of urticaria (Fig. 13.1), or hives, can be acute or chronic, and due to known or unknown causes. Numerous factors, both immunologic and nonimmunologic, can be involved in its pathogenesis. The urticarial wheal results from liberation of histamine from tissue mast cells and from circulating basophils.

Nonimmunologic factors that can release histamine from these cells include:

- Chemicals
- Various drugs (including morphine and codeine)
- Ingestion of fish (especially shellfish), nuts (especially peanuts), and other foods
- Bacterial toxins
- Physical agents

An example of the type of wheal caused by physical agents is the linear wheal produced by light stroking of the skin, known as *dermographism*. (Consult the Dictionary–Index at the end of the book for the triple response of Lewis reaction.)

Immunologic mechanisms are probably involved more often in acute than in chronic urticaria. The most commonly considered of these mechanisms is the type-I hypersensitivity

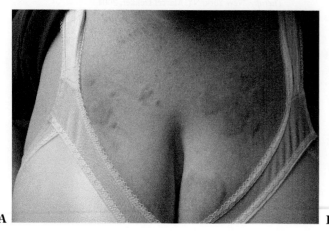

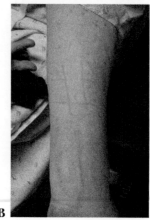

FIGURE 13.1: **A:** Elevated pink plaques on the breasts of a lady with severe stress. They would come and go in a matter of hours. **B:** Linear streaks of dermographism on the forearm and rubbing with the stick end of a Q tip.

state, which is triggered by polyvalent antigen bridging that involves two specific immunoglobulin (Ig) E molecules that are bound to the mast cell or basophil surface (see Chapter 11).

Lesions

Pea-sized red papules to large circinate patterns with red borders and white centers, that can cover an entire side of the trunk or the thigh, may be noted. Vesicles and bullae are seen in severe cases, along with hemorrhagic effusions. A severe form of urticaria is labeled *angioedema*. It can involve an entire body part, such as the lip or the hand. Edema of the glottis and bronchospasm are serious complications and are true medical emergencies.

Presentation and Characteristics

Course

Acute cases may be mild or explosive but usually disappear with or without treatment in a few hours or days. The chronic form has remissions and exacerbations for months or years. One definition of chronic urticaria is one episode at least twice a week for 6 weeks.

Causes

After careful questioning and investigation, many cases of hives, particularly of the chronic-type, are concluded to result from no apparent causative agent. Other cases, mainly the acute ones, have been found to result from the following factors or agents:

- *Drugs or chemicals:* Penicillin and derivatives are probably the most common causes of acute hives, but any other drug, whether ingested, injected, inhaled, or, rarely, applied on the skin, can cause the reaction (see Chapter 8).
- *Foods:* Foods are a common cause of acute hives. The main offenders are seafood, nuts, chocolate, strawberries, cheeses, pork, eggs, wheat, and milk. Chronic hives can be caused by traces of penicillin in milk products (Fig. 13.1A).
- *Insect bites and stings:* Insect bites, stings from mosquitoes, fleas, or spiders, and contact with certain moths, leeches, and jellyfish may cause hives.
- *Physical agents:* Hives can result from heat, cold, radiant energy, vibration, water, and physical injury. *Dermographism* is a term applied to a localized urticarial wheal produced by scratching the skin in certain people (Fig. 13.1B).
- *Inhalants:* Nasal sprays, insect sprays, dust, feathers, pollens, and animal dander are some common offenders.
- *Infections:* A focus of infection is always considered, sooner or later, in chronic cases of hives, and in unusual instances it is causative. The sinuses, teeth, tonsils, gallbladder, and genitourinary tract should be checked.
- *Internal disease:* Urticaria has been seen with liver disease, intestinal parasites, cancer, rheumatic fever, lupus erythematosus, vitiligo, pernicious anemia, rheumatoid arthritis, and others.

- *Nerves:* After all other causes of chronic urticaria have been ruled out, there remain a substantial number of cases that appear to be related to nervous stress, worry, or fatigue. These cases benefit most from the establishment of good rapport between the patient and the physician.
- *Contact urticaria syndrome:* This uncommon response can be incited by local contact on the skin of drugs and chemicals, foods, insects, animal hair or dander, and plants.
- *Cholinergic urticaria:* Clinically, small papular welts are seen that are caused by heat (hot bath), stress, or strenuous exercise.

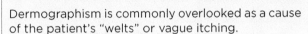

SAUER'S NOTES

Dermographism is commonly overlooked as a cause of the patient's "welts" or vague itching.

Differential Diagnosis

- *Erythema multiforme:* Systemic fever, malaise, and mouth lesions are noted in children and young adults.
- *Dermographism:* A common finding in young adults, especially those who present complaining of welts on their skin or vague itching of the skin with no residual lesions. To make the diagnosis, stroke the skin firmly to see if an urticarial response develops. The course can be chronic, but hydroxyzine, 10 mg b.i.d. or t.i.d., is quite helpful. (Warn the patient about the possibility of drowsiness.) Nonsedating antihistamines can also be tried.
- *Urticarial vasculitis:* Lesions may last more than 24 hours, may be painful, leave a bruise or hyperpigmentation, and be associated with hypocomplementemia and systemic lupus erythematosus. Skin biopsy is confirmatory.

Treatment

Case Example: A patient presents for a case of acute hives due to penicillin injection 1 week previously for a "cold."

1. Colloidal bath
   Sig: Add 1 cup of starch or oatmeal (Aveeno) to 6 to 8 in of lukewarm water in the tub. Bathe for 15 minutes once or twice a day.
2. Sarna lotion, Aveeno Anti-itch lotion, or PrameGel or any pramoxine-containing topical over the counter (OTC).
   Sig: Apply PRN locally for itching.
3. Hydroxyzine (Atarax), 10 mg #30
   Sig: Take 1 tablet t.i.d., a.c. (warn of drowsiness).
4. Diphenhydramine (Benadryl), 50 mg
   Comment: Available OTC
5. Nonsedating antihistamines can also be used

6. Betamethasone sodium phosphate (6 mg/cc Celstone Soluspan), 3 mg/cc
   Sig: Inject 1 to 1.5 cc intramuscularly

For a more severe case of acute hives:

1. Diphenhydramine injection
   Sig: Inject 2 mL (20 mg) subcutaneously.
2. Epinephrine hydrochloride
   Sig: Inject 0.3 to 0.5 mL of 1:1,000 solution subcutaneously.
3. Prednisone tablets, 10 mg #30
   Sig: Take 5 tablets every 2 days and decrease by 1 tablet every 2 days for a 10-day course.

For treatment of a patient with chronic hives of 6 months' duration when cause is undetermined after careful history and examination:

1. Hydroxyzine (Atarax), 10 to 25 mg #60
   Sig: Take 1 tablet t.i.d. depending on drowsiness and effectiveness. Continue for weeks or months.
2. Clemastine (Tavist) 1.34 or 2.68 mg #30
   Sig: Take 1 tablet b.i.d., available OTC.
3. Cyproheptadine (Periactin) 4 mg #60
   Sig: One tablet by mouth t.i.d.
4. Loratadine (Claritin) now OTC 10 mg #30
   Sig: Take 1 tablet once a day.
5. Cetirizine (Zyrtec) 5 or 10 mg #30
   Sig: Take 1 tablet once a day.
6. Fexofenadine (Allegra), 60 or 180 mg #30
   Sig: Take 1 tablet once a day.
7. Cimetidine (Tagamet), 300 mg #60
   Sig: Take 1 tablet t.i.d. (200, 400, or 800 mg).
   Comment: This H_2 blocker is of benefit in some cases and can be added to H1 blockers.
8. Suggest avoidance of seafood, nuts, chocolate, cheese, and other milk products, strawberries, pork, excessively spicy foods, and excess of coffee or tea.
9. Keep a diet diary of everything ingested (including all foods, all medicines, even OTC, candy, menthol cigarettes, chewing gums, chewing tobacco, mouthwash, and breath fresheners) and then see what items were used 12 to 24 hours before the episode of hives occurred.
10. A mild sedative or tranquilizer such as meprobamate, 400 mg t.i.d., or chlordiazepoxide (Librium), 5 mg t.i.d., may help.
11. Doxepin (Sinequan) 10 mg #60
    Sig: 1 tablet t.i.d.
    Comment: This is a tricyclic antidepressant with potent antihistaminic properties. It can cause drowsiness, dry mouth, and other side effects of this classification of drugs.
12. Immunosuppressive drugs such as prednisone are unfortunately necessary in severe cases.
13. Zaditor (ketotifen fumarate) is a mast-cell stabilizer with benefits in severe cases, but I have not used this drug.
14. Sulfasalazine (500 mg increased up to 4,000 mg by increasing by 500 mg each week) has been reported in chronic idiopathic urticaria to be a steroid-sparing or steroid-replacing drug in one report.

ERYTHEMA MULTIFORME

The term *erythema multiforme* introduces a flurry of confusion in the mind of any student of medicine. It is our purpose in this section to attempt to dispel that confusion. Erythema multiforme, as originally described by Hebra, is an uncommon, distinct disease of unknown cause characterized by red iris-shaped or bull's eye–like macules, papules, or bullae confined mainly to the extremities, the face, and the lips (Fig. 13.2). It can be accompanied by mild fever, malaise, and arthralgia. It occurs usually in children and young adults in the spring and the fall, has a duration of 2 to 4 weeks, and is frequently recurrent for several years.

The only relation between Hebra's erythema multiforme and the following diseases or syndromes is the clinical appearance of the eruption.

- *Stevens–Johnson syndrome* is a severe and rarely fatal variant of erythema multiforme. It is characterized by high fever, extensive purpura, bullae, ulcers of the mucous membranes, and, after 2 to 3 days, ulcers of the skin. Eye involvement can result in blindness. It can be related to drugs and its severest form is considered by some to be the same as toxic epidermal necrolysis (see Chapter 21).
- *Erythema multiforme bullosum* is a severe, chronic, bullous disease of adults (see Chapter 18). There is an opinion that this syndrome is completely separate from erythema multiforme. More macular truncal lesions and more epidermal necrosis and less infiltrate may be seen in Stevens–Johnson syndrome (toxic epidermal necrolysis). Sulfonamides, anticonvulsant agents, allopurinol, chlormezanone, and nonsteroidal

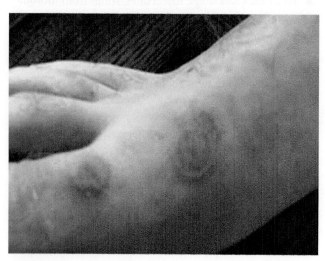

FIGURE 13.2: Oval "bull's eye" or "target" circles on the dorsal foot.

anti-inflammatory drugs commonly cause erythema multiforme bullosum.

- *Erythema multiforme–like drug eruption* is frequently due to phenacetin, quinine, penicillin, mercury, arsenic, phenylbutazone, barbiturates, trimethadione, phenytoin, sulfonamides, and antitoxins (see Chapter 8).

- *Erythema multiforme–like eruption* is caused rather commonly as part of a herpes simplex outbreak and in conjunction with rheumatic fever, pneumonia, meningitis, measles, Coxsackievirus infection, pregnancy, and cancer. It also occurs after deep x-ray therapy and as an allergic reaction to foods.

Differential Diagnosis

- The *erythema perstans* group, or figurate erythemas, includes over a dozen clinical entities with impossible-to-remember names. (See Dictionary–Index under *erythema perstans*.) All have various-sized erythematous patches, papules, or plaques with a definite red border and a less active center, forming circles, half circles, groups of circles, and linear bands. Multiple causes have been ascribed, including tick bites; allergic reactions; fungal, bacterial, viral, and spirochetal infections; and internal cancer. The duration of and the response to therapy vary with each individual case.

- *Erythema chronicum migrans* is the distinctive cutaneous eruption of the multisystem tick-borne spirochetosis Lyme disease. The deer tick, *Ixodes dammini*, is the vector for this spirochete. Early therapy with doxycycline or ampicillin may prevent late manifestations of the disease (see Chapter 25).

- *Reiter's syndrome* is the triad of conjunctivitis, urethritis, and, most important, arthritis, that occurs predominantly in men and lasts about 6 months. The skin manifestations consist of psoriasiform dermatitis, which is called *balanitis circinata* on the penis and *keratoderma blennorrhagica* on the palms and soles.

- *Behçet's syndrome* consists of the triad of genital, oral, and ophthalmic ulcerations seen most commonly in men; it can last for years, with recurrences. Other manifestations include cutaneous pustular vasculitis, synovitis, and meningoencephalitis. It is more prevalent in eastern Mediterranean countries and Japan. Skin hypersensitivity to trauma or pathergy is observed with sterile pustular formation 24 to 48 hours after an intradermal needle prick.

- *Urticaria:* Clinically, urticaria may resemble erythema multiforme, but hives are associated with only mild systemic symptoms. It can occur in any age group; iris lesions are unusual. Usually, it can be attributed to penicillin or other drug therapy, and it responds rapidly but often not completely to antihistamine therapy (see first part of this chapter). It is evanescent and dissipates or moves to a new area in less than 24 hours.

Treatment

Case Example: A 12-year-old boy presents with bull's eye–like lesions on his hands, arms, and feet, erosions of the lips and mucous membranes of the mouth, malaise, and a temperature of 101°F (38.3°C) orally. He had a similar eruption last spring.

1. Order bed rest and increased oral fluid intake.
2. Acetaminophen (Tylenol), 325 mg OTC
   Sig: Take 1 to 2 tablets q.i.d.

   Prednisone, 10 mg #16

   Sig: Take 2 tablets stat and then 2 tablets every morning for 7 days.
3. For severe cases, such as the Stevens–Johnson form, hospitalization is indicated, where intravenous corticosteroid therapy (debatable), intravenous fluid replacement infusions, immunoglobulin, and other supportive measures can be administered.

ERYTHEMA NODOSUM

Erythema nodosum is an uncommon reaction pattern seen mainly on the anterior tibial areas of the legs (Fig. 13.3). It appears as erythematous nodules in successive crops and is preceded by fever, malaise, and arthralgia.

Presentation and Characteristics

Primary Lesions

Bilateral, red, tender, rather well-circumscribed nodules are seen mainly on the pretibial surface of the legs and, rarely, on the arms and the body. Later, the flat, indurated lesions may

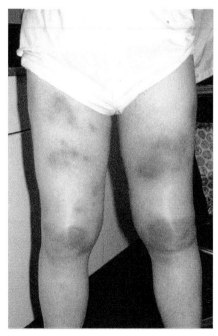

FIGURE 13.3: Erythema nodosum with deep red/brown, indurated, painful areas on the anterior lower extremities.

become raised, confluent, and purpuric. Only a few lesions develop at one time.

Secondary Lesions

The lesions never suppurate or form ulcers but can heal with a bruise.

Course

The lesions last several weeks, but the duration can be affected by therapy directed to the cause, if it is known. Relapses are related to the cause. The lesions can be idiopathic and have a chronic course.

Causes

Careful clinical and laboratory examinations are necessary to determine the cause of this toxic reaction pattern. The following tests should be performed:

- Complete blood cell count
- Erythrocyte sedimentation rate
- Urinalysis
- Strep screen, serum pregnancy test, angiotensin-converting enzyme, tuberculin skin test
- Serologic test for syphilis
- Chest x-ray
- Specific skin tests, as indicated

The causes of erythema nodosum are

- Streptococcal infection (rheumatic fever, pharyngitis, scarlet fever, and arthritis)
- Fungal infection (coccidioidomycosis, trichophyton infection)
- Pregnancy or oral contraceptives
- Sarcoidosis
- Lymphogranuloma venereum
- Syphilis
- Chancroid
- Drugs (contraceptive pills, sulfonamides, iodides, bromides, and echinacea herbal therapy)
- Hepatitis C
- HIV infection
- Celiac disease
- Carcinoid syndrome
- Tuberculosis

It is rare in children, but when it occurs, group A β-hemolytic streptococcal infection (which may be occult) is the most common cause. Oral contraceptives are a common cause in adult women. It is not uncommon to be unable to find a cause.

Age and Gender Incidence

The disorder occurs predominantly in adolescent girls and young women.

Laboratory Findings

Histopathologic examination reveals a nonspecific but characteristically localized inflammatory infiltrate in the subcutaneous tissue, and in and around the veins.

Differential Diagnosis

- *Erythema induratum:* Chronic vasculitis of young women that occurs on the posterior calf area and often suppurates; biopsy shows a tuberculoid-type infiltrate, usually with caseation. A tuberculous causation has been suggested.

- *Necrobiosis lipoidica diabeticorum:* A cutaneous manifestation of diabetes mellitus, characterized by well-defined patches of reddish-yellow atrophic skin, often with overlying telangiectasias primarily on anterior areas of the legs. The lesions can ulcerate; biopsy results are characteristic, but biopsy may not be indicated because of the possibility of poor healing and the characteristic clinical presentation (see Chapter 42).

- *Periarteritis nodosa:* A rare, sometimes fatal, arteritis that most often occurs in men. Twenty-five percent of patients show painful subcutaneous nodules and purpura, mainly of the lower extremities, which often show livedo reticularis. It is a multiorgan system disease; renal failure is often a component. There is also a cutaneous variety. Positive p-ANCA blood test is needed for diagnosis.

- *Superficial thrombophlebitis migrans (Buerger disease):* An early venous change of Buerger disease commonly seen in male patients, with painful nodules of the anterior tibial area. Biopsy is of value. Smoking has been suggested as an important contributing factor.

- *Nodular panniculitis or Weber–Christian disease:* Occurs mainly in obese middle-aged women. Tender, indurated, subcutaneous nodules and plaques are seen, usually on the thighs and the buttocks. Each crop is preceded by fever and malaise. Residual atrophy and hyperpigmentation occur.

- *Leukocytoclastic vasculitis:* Includes a constellation of diseases, such as allergic angiitis, allergic vasculitis, necrotizing vasculitis, and cutaneous systemic vasculitis. Clinically, palpable purpuric lesions are seen, most commonly on the lower parts of the legs. In later stages, the lesions may become nodular, bullous, infarctive, and ulcerative. Various etiologic agents have been implicated, such as infection, drugs, and foreign proteins. Treatment includes bed rest, pentoxifylline (Trental), corticosteroids, and other immunosuppressive drugs (see Chapter 9).

For completeness, the following six rare syndromes with *inflammatory nodules of the legs* are defined in the Dictionary–Index:

1. Subcutaneous fat necrosis with pancreatic disease
2. Migratory panniculitis

3. Allergic granulomatosis
4. Necrobiotic granulomatosis
5. Embolic nodules from several sources
6. Lipoatrophic panniculitis

Treatment

1. Treat the cause, if possible.
2. Rest, local heat, and aspirin are valuable. The eruption is self-limited if the cause can be eliminated.
3. Chronic cases can be disabling enough to warrant a short course of corticosteroid therapy. Some cases have benefited from naproxen (Naprosyn), 250 mg b.i.d. (or other nonsteroidal antiinflammatory drugs), for 2 to 4 weeks.

STASIS (VENOUS) DERMATITIS AND ULCERS

Stasis dermatitis is a common condition owing to impaired venous circulation in the legs of older patients (Fig. 13.4). Almost all cases are associated with varicose veins, and because the tendency to develop varicosities is a familial characteristic, stasis dermatitis is also familial. The medial malleolar area of the ankle is the most common location. Stasis ulcers can develop in the impaired skin. They are commonly accompanied by brownish discoloration, pruritus, excoriations, and dry, fine adherent scales. Late in the disease edema may be accompanied by lymphedematous blebs (elephantiasis verrucosa) and leakage of a serous thick yellow lymph fluid. Numerous conditions are associated with stasis dermatitis (Table 13-3).

Presentation and Characteristics

Primary Lesions

Early cases of stasis dermatitis begin as a red, scaly, pruritic patch that rapidly becomes vesicular and crusted owing to scratching and subsequent secondary infection. Bacterial infection may be responsible for the spread of the patch and the chronicity of the eruption. Edema of the affected ankle area

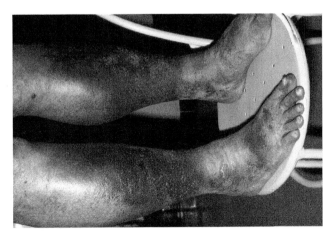

FIGURE 13.4: Severe stasis dermatitis with brawny hyperpigmentation, edema, and dry, adherent scale.

results in a further decrease in circulation and, consequently, more infection. The lesions may be unilateral or bilateral.

Secondary Lesions

Three secondary conditions can arise from untreated stasis dermatitis:

- *Hyperpigmentation:* This is inevitable following the healing of either simple or severe stasis dermatitis of the legs. This reddish-brown increase in pigmentation is slow to disappear, and in many elderly patients it never does so.
- *Stasis ulcers:* These can occur as the result of edema, trauma, deeper bacterial infection, or improper care of the primary dermatitis.
- *Infectious eczematoid dermatitis:* This can develop on the legs, the arms, and even the entire body, either slowly or as an explosive, rapidly spreading distant, symmetric, autoeczematous, or "id" eruption (see Chapter 21).

SAUER'S NOTES

Leg Ulcer Mantras

1. Look for underlying disease.
2. Look for an underlying malignant tumor, that is, basal cell cancer, squamous cell cancer, and melanoma.
3. Look for clotting disorders.
4. Look for causes of ischemia, that is, arteriosclerotic vascular disease.
5. Look for an infection (primary or secondary).
6. Look for contact dermatitis.
7. Always consider a skin biopsy as part of the evaluation.

Course

The rapidity of healing of stasis dermatitis depends on the age of the patient and other factors listed under *Causes*. In elderly patients who have untreated varicose veins, stasis dermatitis can persist for years with remissions and exacerbations. If stasis dermatitis develops in a patient in the 40- to 50-year age group, the prognosis is particularly bad for future recurrences and possible ulcers. Once stasis ulcers develop, they can rapidly expand in size and depth. Healing of the ulcer, if possible for a given patient, depends on many factors. Ulcers less than 1 year old, less than 5 cm^2, and ulcers that show significant healing after 3 weeks are more likely to heal by compression and bioocclusive dressings alone. Grafting procedures may be necessary for other venous leg ulcers. Negative pressure devices have shown promise.

Causes

Poor venous circulation owing to the sluggish blood flow in tortuous, dilated varicose veins with incompetence of the venous valves in the distribution of the greater saphenous vein (medial ankle) is the primary cause. If the factors of obesity, congestive heart failure, renal failure, lack of proper rest or care of the legs, pruritus, secondary infection, low protein diet, and old age are added to the circulation problem, the result can be a chronic, disabling disease. Table 13-1 lists tests for nonhealing ulcers.

Differential Diagnosis

- *Contact dermatitis:* Taking a careful history is important especially regarding nylon hose, new socks, contact with ragweed, high-top shoes, and so on, appears where contactant has touched the skin; no venous insufficiency is noted.
- *Lichen simplex chronicus:* Thickened, dry, very pruritic plaque; no venous insufficiency is found (see Chapter 12).
- *Atrophie blanche:* Characterized by small ulcers that heal with irregular white scars; seen mainly over the ankles and legs. Telangiectasis and hyperpigmentation surround the scars. This arterial vasculopathy can respond to pentoxifylline (Trental). Another name for it is segmental hyalinizing vasculopathy. Anticoagulants such as aspirin, Plavix (clopidogrel), Persantine (dipyramidole), and Coumadin may be beneficial. Underlying clotting disorders need to be searched for with a hypercoagulability panel.
- *Arterial or ischemic ulcers:* These are usually more punched out and painful. Intermittent claudication and nighttime pain are relieved by exercise. Arterial duplex ultrasound or arteriography may be necessary to diagnose these ulcers. Revascularization procedures may be indicated, and compression therapies can be counterproductive.

- *Drug eruptions:* These are often worst and first appear on lower legs, and are usually sudden in appearance. Recent use of a new drug is a helpful indication, but the eruption can be from a drug that has been taken for a longer period of time. The clinical manifestations are protean.

Differential diagnosis for stasis ulcers includes:

- Pyodermic ulcers
- Arterial ulcers (such as mal perforans of diabetes)
- Periarteritis nodosa
- Necrobiosis lipoidica ulcers
- Pyoderma gangrenosum
- Malignancies (especially squamous cell carcinoma)
- Ulcers from autoimmune diseases especially lupus erythematosus
- Vasculitis

Blood tests, cultures, and biopsies help to establish the type of ulcer. Never underestimate the value of a complete history and physical examination. Imaging studies such as a venous and/or arterial Doppler study or angiography are often necessary.

Treatment of Stasis Dermatitis

Case Example: A 55-year-old laborer presents with scaly, reddish, slightly edematous, excoriated dermatitis on the medial aspect of the left ankle and leg of 6 weeks' duration.

1. Prescribe rest and elevation of the leg as much as possible by lying in bed. The foot of the bed should be elevated 4 in by placing two bricks under the legs. Attempt to elevate the leg when sitting. Avoid prolonged standing or sitting with the legs bent. Taking time to walk on a long train, car, or plane trip is a good idea. Work restrictions may be necessary.
2. Burow's solution wet packs
   Sig: Add 1 packet of powder to 1 quart of warm water. Apply cloths wet with this solution for 30 minutes b.i.d.
3. An antibiotic and corticosteroid ointment mixture q.s. 30.0
   Sig: Apply to leg t.i.d.

For more severe cases of stasis dermatitis with oozing, cellulitis, and 3+pitting edema, the following treatment should be ordered in addition:

1. Hospitalization or enforced bed rest at home for the purpose of (1) applying the wet packs for longer periods of time and (2) strict rest and elevation of the leg.
2. A course of an oral antibiotic.
3. Prednisone, 10 mg #36
   Sig: Take 2 tablets b.i.d. for 4 days, then 2 tablets in the morning for 10 days.
4. Ace elastic bandage, 4-in wide, No. 8

After the patient is discharged from the hospital and ambulatory, give instructions for the correct application of an ace bandage or a properly measured pressure garment to the leg before arising in the morning. This helps to reduce the edema that could cause a recrudescence of the dermatitis. Pressure dressing should either be knee-high or thigh-high.

TABLE 13-1 • Tests for Hypercoagulability in Nonhealing Leg Ulcers
Activated partial thromboplastin time (aPTT)
Anticardiolipin antibody
Antithrombin III
Complete blood count (CBC)
Cryoglobulins
Factor II (prothrombin)
Factor V (Leiden)
Homocysteine (methylenetetrahydrofolate reductase)
Immunoglobulin electrophoresis
Lupus anticoagulant
Prothrombin time (PTT)
Protein C and protein S
Sickle cell
Thrombin time

Treatment of Stasis Ulcer

As for any chronic difficult medical problem, there are many methods touted for successful management.

Case Example: Consider a 75-year-old obese woman on a low income who has a 4-cm ulcer on her medial right ankle area with surrounding dermatitis, edema, and pigmentation.

1. *Manage the primary problem or problems:* Attempt to remedy the obesity, make sure there is adequate nutrition, and treat systemic or other causes of the ulcer.
2. *Correct the physiologic alterations:* Control the edema with adhesive flexible bandages of adequate width (4-in wide usually) and with correct application from foot up to knee. A Jobst-type support stocking or pump may be indicated in resistant cases.
3. *Treat contributing factors:* Control the dermatitis, itching, and infection.
4. *Promote healing:* Occlusion of the ulcer has been proven to accelerate healing. Unna's boots, adhesive flexible bandage dressings, and polyurethane-type films have been used with success. Enzymatic granules have their proponents as do collagen granules and Granulex. Accuzyme, which contains papain and urea, that is an example of a topical debriding agent.
5. *Skin grafting may be indicated in deep, stubborn ulcers:* Artificial skin substitutes such as Apligraf may be used.
6. *Hyperbaric oxygenation:* This may be helpful for many different types of ulcers where available but is usually used for ischemic ulcers. Claustrophobia and tympanic membrane rupture are two significant side effects.
7. *Topical negative pressure devices:* This is also called vacuum-assisted closure and consists of a fenestrated evacuation tube embedded in a foam dressing and covered with an airtight dressing. Then, a vacuum source attached to the tube applies continuous or intermittent subatmospheric pressure at 100 to 125 mm Hg. The wound needs debridement before beginning this therapy, and the gauze should be changed at least every other day.
8. *Alginate dressings (Kaltostat, Sorbsan, Tegagen, AlgiSite, Aquacel Hydrofiber):* These are derived from brown seaweed and are very absorbent. They are available as ropes or pads. Care must be taken not to overdry the ulcer.
9. *Foams:* Foams (3M Adhesive foam, Lyofoam C, Allevyn hydrocellular dressing, Allevyn cavity dressing) and hydrocolloids (Tegasorb, Mepitil, Mepilix, Mepiliex Ag, Mepilix Foam, DuoDERM CGF, Comfeel Plus) can be used when moderate absorption is desired.
10. *Collagen products:* Collagen products such as Promogran, Oasis wound matrix, and Cymetra are sometimes used for recalcitrant leg ulcers.
11. *Silver ion dressings:* Silver ion dressings (silver sulfadiazine, Aquacel Ag Hydrofiber, Acticoat 7, Actisorb Silver 220, Silverlon wound contact dressing, SilvaSorb, Silvercel), although causing discoloration and some irritation, are helpful in ulcers where infection is suspected.
12. *Regranex:* This is a topical recombinant human platelet growth factor touted by some authors.
13. *"Short-contact" tretinoin solution (0.05%):* This can cause irritation but has been used to attempt to increase granulation tissue.
14. *Hydrogels:* Hydrogels (Restore hydrogel, Carrasyn hydrogel, SAF-gel, Curagel, XCell cellulose dressing) are mainly helpful in hydrating wounds.
15. *Topical options:* The array of topical options for ulcers is confusing, and they are often very expensive. The author frequently uses Johnson & Johnson advanced healing adhesive pads, which are cheap and easy to use (the pad is left on until it falls off in a few days). Be sure the wound is not infected and has been debrided either mechanically or with debriding pad topicals.

Here is the technique we would use for this case example. The diagnosis is stasis or venous ulcer.

1. Advise a multiple vitamin and mineral supplement tablet once a day, including zinc and magnesium.
2. Elevate the leg as much as possible when lying down prone.
3. Erythromycin, 250 mg #100
   Sig: Take 2 to 3 tablets a day until ulcer is healed.
   Comment: Infection is common. Culture to determine appropriate antibiotic to use is more scientific but streptococci, staphylococci, and occasionally psuedomonas are the only bacteria that need to be treated.
4. Prednisone, 10 mg #60
   Sig: Take 1 tablet every morning.
   Actions: Antipruritic, anti-inflammatory
5. Apply an *occlusive dressing* in the office. If there is a lot of drainage and debris, the frequency of dressing changes should be every 3 to 4 days at first, then weekly. Use a footrest stand for the leg. Keep a record of the size of the ulcer.
   a. Apply Bactroban ointment to a Telfa dressing.
   b. Place gauze squares in four layers over the Telfa dressing.
   c. Apply adhesive flexible bandage wrap over the gauze, down to the foot arch, and up to below the knee, more firmly wrapped distally. Do not apply too tightly at first.
   d. Wrap an adhesive flexible bandage, 4-in wide, over the Coban.
   e. Leave the dressing on for 3 to 7 days, and then reapply.
6. Pentoxifylline (Trental) at a dosage of 1,200 to 2,400 mg and divided into three doses per day with food has been shown to be beneficial. Gastrointestinal upset is common.
7. Another variant of occlusive dressing is as follows:
   a. ZeaSORB powder on the ulcer.
   b. Midstrength cortisone cream around the ulcer.
   c. Zinc oxide wrap around the entire leg with a tighter wrap distally.
   d. Flexible adhesive bandage as a second wrap. Change every week, and keep dry.

No management of a venous stasis ulcer is 100% effective, but this routine with modifications is the one we use. If an ulcer is stable or decreasing in size after 4 weeks the current treatment should be continued. If it is enlarging, then alternate therapy, including surgery, should be considered.

An infection of a chronic wound should always be watched for and may be heralded by increasing pain but the Levine technique of culturing which consists of rotating the wound swab over 1 cm area of the wound is superior to the Z-technique which involves rotating the swab between the fingers in a zigzag fashion across the wound without touching its edge.

After the ulcer has healed, which takes many weeks, advise the patient to wear an elastic bandage or support hose constantly during the day, primarily as protection against injury of the damaged and scarred skin, and to decrease recurrent edema.

PURPURIC DERMATOSES

Purpuric lesions are caused by an extravasation of red blood cells into the skin or mucous membranes. The lesions can be distinguished from erythema and telangiectasia by the fact that purpuric lesions do not blanch under pressure applied by the finger or by a clear glass slide (diascopy) (Fig. 13.5).

- *Petechiae* are small, superficial purpuric lesions. These are most often a sign of platelet deficiency or malfunction.
- *Ecchymoses,* or bruises, are more extensive, round or irregularly shaped purpuric lesions often seen in the elderly (senile purpura), patients on chronic topical or systemic corticosteroids, and patients on anticoagulants.
- *Hematomas* are large, deep, fluctuant, tumor-like hemorrhages in the skin.

The purpuras can be divided into the *thrombocytopenic* forms and the *nonthrombocytopenic* forms.

- *Thrombocytopenic purpura* may be idiopathic or secondary to various chronic diseases or to drug sensitivity. The platelet count is below normal, the bleeding time is prolonged, and the clotting time is normal, but the clot does not retract normally. This form of purpura is rare.

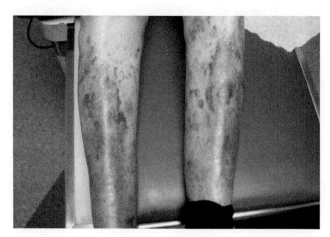

FIGURE 13.5: Dramatic purple/red macular areas of purpura in a patient on long-term systemic corticosteroids.

- *Nonthrombocytopenic purpura* is more commonly seen. *Henoch–Schönlein purpura* is a form of nonthrombocytopenic purpura most commonly seen in children that is characterized by recurrent attacks of purpura accompanied by arthritis, hematuria, IgA glomerulonephritis, and gastrointestinal disorders. Approximately 75% of the time it only involves the skin. If the skin biopsy is done precisely at the correct time, leukocytoclastic vasculitis and IgA can be seen deposited in the vessel wall.

The ecchymoses, or *senile purpura*, seen in elderly patients after minor injury are very common. Ecchymoses are also seen in patients who have been on long-term systemic corticosteroid therapy and also occur after prolonged use of the high potency corticosteroids locally and from corticosteroid nasal inhalers. Anticoagulants make these more common. Another common purpuric eruption is known as *stasis purpura*. These lesions are associated with vascular insufficiency of the legs and occur as the early sign of this change, or they are seen around areas of stasis dermatitis or stasis ulcers. Frequently seen is a petechial drug eruption owing to chlorothiazide diuretics.

PIGMENTED PURPURIC ERUPTIONS

A less common group of cases are those seen in middle-aged adults, classified under the name *pigmented purpuric eruptions*. They are usually asymptomatic, but some cases of pigmented purpuric eruptions are pruritic. The cause is unknown. Most cases have a positive tourniquet test, but other bleeding tests are usually normal. Clinically, these patients have grouped nonblanchable petechial lesions that begin on the legs and extend up to the thighs, and occasionally up to the waist and onto the arms. They turn into a brown cayenne pepper–like nonpalpable discoloration that fades over weeks to months.

Some clinicians are able to separate these pigmented purpuric eruptions into:

- Purpura annularis telangiectodes (Majocchi disease)
- Progressive pigmentary dermatosis (Schamberg disease)
- Pigmented purpuric lichenoid dermatosis (Gougerot and Blum disease)

Majocchi disease commonly begins on the legs but slowly spreads to become generalized. Telangiectatic capillaries become confluent and produce annular or serpiginous lesions. The capillaries break down, causing purpuric lesions. Schamberg disease is a slowly progressive pigmentary condition of the lower part of the legs that fades after a period of months but may recur. The Gougerot and Blum form is accompanied by severe itching and eczematous changes. Otherwise, it resembles Schamberg disease.

Treatment

For these pigmented purpuric eruptions, therapy may not be necessary. Occlusive dressing therapy with a corticosteroid cream can be beneficial, or support garments can be used for prevention. For resistant cases, prednisone, 10 mg, 1 to 2 tablets in the morning for 3 to 6 weeks is indicated.

PYODERMA GANGRENOSUM

Pyoderma gangrenosum is a painful ulcerative disease, usually of the lower extremities.

Lesions

It begins as a pustule, but over days to weeks, it turns into a boggy, bluish-black ulcer with rolled edges. There are sometimes satellite pustules, which then also ulcerate. The edges are erythematous and undermined, and the extent of the ulcer is often more extensive than what is first suspected. It exhibits pathergy, which means it can occur at any site of trauma.

Presentation and Characteristics

It is usually relentless and chronic unless treated aggressively and may occur at sites other than the lower extremities and around ostomy sites. Treatment of the underlying condition can, but does not always, result in resolution of the disease.

Causes

Inflammatory bowel disease (50% of the time it is associated with Crohn's and 50% of the time it is associated with ulcerative colitis) is an underlying association in one-third of cases. Approximately 1.5% to 5% of inflammatory bowel disease patients have pyoderma gangrenosum. In 7% to 10% of pyoderma gangrenosum cases there is an associated underlying malignancy. Leukemia is the commonest and is a bad prognostic sign, with 25% of cases being fatal within 12 months after the diagnosis of pyoderma gangrenosum. In polycythemia vera, if pyoderma gangrenosum develops there is an increased chance of leukemia developing. Waldenström macroglobulinemia, multiple myeloma, myelofibrosis, lymphoma, and metastatic solid tumors can also be underlying diseases.

Sporadic associations with other underlying illnesses include chronic active hepatitis, thyroid disease, hidradenitis suppurativa, cystic acne, sarcoidosis, diabetes mellitus, systemic lupus erythematous, rheumatoid arthritis, AIDS, and Takayasu arteritis.

A few clinical subtypes are more apt to be related to certain underlying conditions.

1. *Ulcerative:* Most common, usually associated with underlying disease, especially inflammatory bowel disease. Very painful, spreads rapidly, and needs aggressive therapy. May be associated with arthritis (especially large joint and monoarticular) and increased IgA (up to 10%).
2. *Pustular:* Grouped pustules on a red base. Toxic patients with acute inflammatory bowel disease. May clear if inflammatory bowel disease is controlled.
3. *Bullous:* Superficial bullae and superficial ulcer with surrounding erythema associated with myeloproliferative disease especially leukemia. Systemic treatment is required.
4. *Vegetative:* It is relatively painless, vegetative, superficial single, slower progression without undermining border

and without underlying illness. Treatment is less aggressive and sometimes can be achieved even with local modalities.

Differential Diagnosis

- *Brown recluse spider bite:* Rapid (within hours) necrosis without ulceration. No underlying illness. Single lesion. More common in the Midwestern part of the United States, that is, Missouri spider.
- *Purpura fulminans:* Toxic patient with widespread areas of necrosis without ulceration. Underlying disseminated intravascular coagulopathy (DIC). Rapid decline and often fatal.
- *Stasis ulcer:* Stasis dermatitis of the lower extremities over the medial malleolus (distribution of greater saphenous vein) with varicosities, edema, and dyspigmentation. Slow in onset and chronic course with little or no pain even though size can be large and depth can be to the tendon of the ankle.
- *Necrotizing fasciitis:* Patient may be very toxic, especially as disease progresses. There are deep gangrenous plaques that may be very painful or anesthetic with rapid spread. It is not infrequently fatal.
- *Vasculitis:* Clinically with palpable purpura and histologically with vasculitis (fibrinoid necrosis of vessel walls and perivascular neutrophils with leukocytoclasis). May not ulcerate or ulcerate much later (weeks to months).

Treatment

Local

1. Avoid aggressive debridement and skin grafting since pathergy may occur.
2. Intralesional corticosteroid (4 to 6 mg/cc triamcinolone) around and under ulcers can help stop spread and start healing.
3. Class I (clobetasol ointment under occlusion) may be beneficial, and topical tacrolimus has been tried.

Systemic

1. High-dose systemic corticosteroids (40 to 60 mg of prednisone daily; taper off over weeks depending on response to therapy).
2. Begin a corticosteroid-sparing agent such as minocycline (100 mg b.i.d.), avlosulfone (100 mg/day), sulfapyridine (500 mg b.i.d.), sulfasalazine (500 mg b.i.d.), azathioprine (50 mg b.i.d.), mycophenolate mofetil, methotrexate, cyclosporine, and tacrolimus.

Biologic agents that have been used with success include most notably etanercept and adalimumab. Omalizumab has been reported as beneficial. Other therapies include IVIG intravenous and subcutaneous and an older treatment of SSKI (supersaturated solution of potassium iodide).

Telangiectasias

Telangiectasias are abnormal, dilated small blood vessels. Telangiectasias are divided into *primary forms*, in which the causes are unknown; and *secondary forms*, which are related to some known disturbance. The primary telangiectasias include the simple and compound hemangiomas of infants, essential telangiectasias, and spider hemangiomas (see Chapter 41). Diseases with numerous telangiectasias include:

- Cirrhosis of the liver
- Osler–Weber–Rendu disease, which also has mucous membrane involvement
- Lupus erythematosus
- Scleroderma
- Dermatomyositis
- Cutaneous polyarteritis
- Metastatic carcinoid syndrome
- Ataxia telangiectasia
- Angiokeratoma corporis diffusum
- Telangiectasia macularis eruptiva perstans
- Rosacea
- Overlying basal cell cancers and sebaceous hyperplasia
- Overlying necrobiosis lipoidica diabeticorum

Unilateral nevoid telangiectasia syndrome can be congenital or acquired. The acquired form appears when increased estrogen levels occur in women during puberty or pregnancy or in cirrhosis. C3, C4, and trigeminal dermatomes are most commonly involved.

Hereditary benign telangiectasia is an uncommon autosomal dominant disorder with generalized telangiectasias at an early age, especially on sun-exposed areas. There is no mucosal involvement.

Secondary telangiectasia is very commonly seen on the fair-skinned person as a result of aging, chronic topical and systemic corticosteroid use, and chronic sun exposure. X-ray therapy and burns can also cause telangiectasias.

Treatment for secondary telangiectasias can be accomplished quite adequately with very light electrosurgery to the vessels, which is usually tolerated without anesthesia, or for many extensive lesions, use of laser therapy or intense pulsed light therapy is helpful. Injectable sclerosing agents are available for therapy on the lower legs, as are endovascular laser and vessel ligation.

VASCULITIS

Inflammation of the blood vessels (vasculitis) (Fig. 13.6) commonly affects the skin and has numerous underlying causes. It can only be cutaneous (Gougerot and Ruiter type), but often involves other organs, most commonly the joints, kidney, and gastrointestinal tract and rarely the nervous system, eye (temporal arteritis), heart, and respiratory tract. Diagnosis is confirmed by biopsy and then appropriate tests need to be done to look for underlying causes (Table 13-2). Vasculitis classification (Table 13-3) is complex, but it can be helpful in trying to find an underlying cause (Table 13-4). Laboratory evaluation is important (Table 13-5).

Presentation and Characteristics

Primary Lesions

Palpable purpura is the classic clinical appearance. Varying shades of bluish-red discoloration may be firmly indurated or difficult to feel. Lesions can be large (many centimeters) or quite small (several millimeters) with a petechial look. The dependent areas are the location where they are most commonly seen—legs on ambulatory patients and the buttocks and back in bedridden patients.

Secondary Lesions

As the vascular damage progresses, blisters, nodules, ulcers, necrosis, and gangrene may occur. Livedo reticularis (see Dictionary–Index) is a bluish-red, netlike appearing condition that can be associated with vasculitis.

Course

The disease may be very chronic and long lasting, such as in lupus erythematosus, or acute and self-limited, such as in Henoch–Schönlein purpura (see Chapter 42). Early diagnosis and therapy can prevent renal failure or bowel necrosis.

Causes

See Table 13-2.

Differential Diagnosis

- *Urticaria:* Evanescent, very pruritic.
- *Thrombophlebitis:* There are varicosities and stasis changes and positive Doppler studies in this localized distribution of a vein almost always in the lower extremity below the knee.
- *Erythema nodosum:* May be impossible to tell without a deep skin biopsy, especially in female patients. A deep nodule is present, usually only in a pretibial location.
- *Petechia:* Small, uniform, single-color, nonpalpable lesions associated with decreased platelets.
- *Schamberg disease* (benign pigmented purpura, benign hemosiderosis): Cayenne pepper–colored tiny lesions. No underlying illness. Skin biopsy differentiates. Usually below the knees, but it can rarely be generalized. For several variations, see hemosiderosis in the Dictionary–Index and discussion under petechiae in this chapter.
- *Panniculitis:* Lesions very deep and nodular. May have elevated amylase and lipase when associated with pancreatitis.
- *Cellulitis:* Lesions warm and tender. Elevated white blood cell count with fever. May have proximal, tender, red, linear lymphatic involvement. Lymph nodes may be enlarged.
- *Insect bites:* Very pruritic. History of exposure to insects; acute in onset. Can be excoriated and chronic.

Treatment

Systemic corticosteroids are the mainstay of early therapy. Corticosteroid-sparing drugs including colchicine, dapsone, azathioprine, methotrexate, Cytoxan (drug of choice for Wegener granulomatosis), intravenous γ-globulin, antimalarials, and plasmapheresis have all been used.

LIVEDO VASCULOPATHY (ATROPHIE BLANCHE, SEGMENTAL HYALINIZING VASCULOPATHY)

This disease was at one time thought to be a vasculitis of immune origin and occasionally mimics a true vasculitis. The pathogenesis begins with the deposition of fibrin within

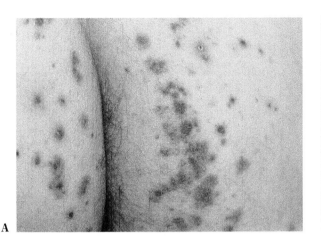
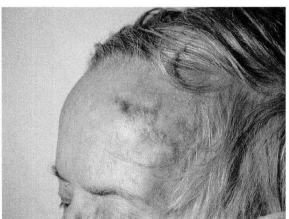
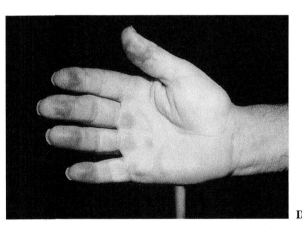

FIGURE 13.6: Forms of vasculitis. **A:** Vasculitis on the buttock of a patient with renal and gastrointestinal vasculitis. Bedridden patient often erupts first on the buttock. **B:** Vasculitis of the lower extremity owing to mixed cryoglobulinemia. Patient was worse in cold weather. **C:** Temporal arteritis. Systemic corticosteroids were used to prevent blindness. **D:** Fingers showing vasculitis in a patient with Wegener's granulomatosis. **E:** Livedo reticularis pattern of vasculitis. This patient has systemic lupus erythematosus. **F:** Vasculitis of the feet. Lower extremities are the location where it is most common in ambulatory patients. **G:** Widespread, drug-induced vasculitis owing to ampicillin. **H:** Vasculitis of the hand in a patient with rheumatoid arthritis.

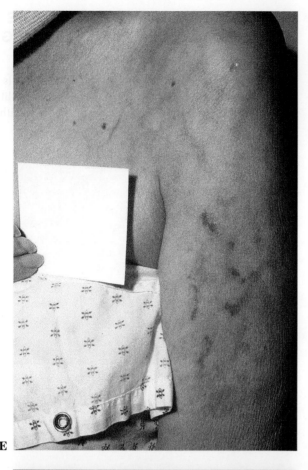

E

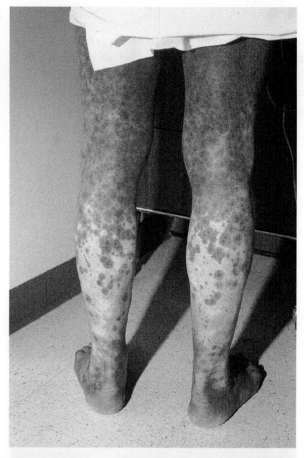

G

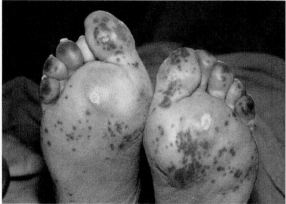

F

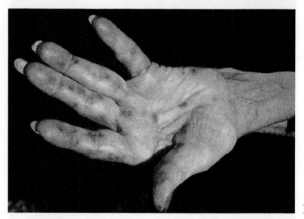

H

FIGURE 13.6: (continued)

the vessel walls without inflammation or immune complex deposition. Later biopsy specimens show a secondary vasculitis. Therefore, biopsy of early disease is essential for correct diagnosis and, subsequently, the correct therapy. Livedo vasculopathy may be seen in association with stasis dermatitis or collagen–vascular disease.

Presentation and Characteristics

Primary Lesions

There are recurrent, chronic, painful, stellate-shaped ulcers over lower extremities (especially over the lower medial ankles and

malleoli). They heal slowly with characteristic porcelain-colored, stellate-shaped atrophic scars with surrounding ectatic blood vessels and reddish-brown hyperpigmentation.

Secondary Lesions

Cellulitis with pain, swelling, redness, and warmth of surrounding skin can occur.

Course

The disease is very chronic and without proper therapy can slowly progress to involve larger areas of the lower extremities

TABLE 13-2 • Venous Versus Ischemic Leg Ulcers

	Venous Ulcers	Ischemic Ulcers
Symptoms	Itching	Pain (often severe with tenderness)
	Asymptomatic	
Clinical	Stasis dermatitis	Induration, redness
	Scaling	Pulses diminished or absent
	Hyperpigmentation	Intermittent claudication
	Edema, varicosities	Decrease pain upon exercise
Ulcer appearance	Ragged edge	Sharp edge, "punched out"
	Exudative base	Dry crusted or clean base
Ulcer location	Medial malleolus (distribution of greater saphenous vein)	Pretibial
Radiographic	Abnormal venous Doppler	Abnormal arterial Doppler and arterial angiogram
Mainstay of therapy	Pressure dressing	Arterial surgical repair
History	Thrombophlebitis, obesity, diabetes, vein or lymphatic obstruction or disruption from blood clots, infection, or surgery	Arteriosclerotic vascular disease including heart, cerebrovascular, and peripheral arterial vascular disease

TABLE 13-3 • Types of Vasculitis

1. Leukocytoclastic vasculitis (hypersensitivity angiitis or allergic vasculitis)
   A. Idiopathic
   B. Drug induced
   C. Hypocomplementemic vasculitis (often urticarial)
   D. Essential mixed cryoglobulinemia
   E. Hyperglobulinemic purpuras (Waldenström macroglobulinemia)
2. Rheumatic vasculitis
   A. Systemic lupus erythematosus
   B. Rheumatoid vasculitis
   C. Dermatomyositis
3. Granulomatous vasculitis
   A. Eosinophilic granulomatosis with polyangiitis (Churg–Strauss)
   B. Granulomatosis with polyangiitis (Wegener's Granulomatosis)
   C. Lymphomatoid granulomatosis
4. Polyarteritis nodosa
   A. Classic type
   B. Cutaneous type
5. Giant cell arteritis
   A. Temporal arteritis
   B. Takayasu disease

TABLE 13-4 • Conditions Associated with Stasis Ulcers

Previous surgery (including joint replacements, vessel harvesting, and fracture)

Diabetes mellitus

Venous insufficiency and thrombophlebitis

Anemia

Prolonged standing or sitting with legs bent

Obesity

Poor nutrition (lack of sufficient vitamins A, C, E, selenium, zinc, copper, thiamine, pantothenic acid, and manganese)

Neuropathy

Immunosuppression

Cause

A disorder of coagulation with elevated fibrinopeptide, decreased plasminogen activator, and abnormal platelet functions are all considered possibilities.

Differential Diagnosis

- *Stasis dermatitis:* Stellate scar less common; does have dramatic hyperpigmentation following eczematous dermatitis, often with edema and varicosities. Vasculitis more widespread and can be multisystem. Different biopsy with true vasculitic inflammatory changes seen early in course. Atrophie blanche scars less common.

but is rare above the knee. Although treatment can halt the disease ulcers and pain, the scars and dilated vessels as well as the hyperpigmentation remain.

TABLE 13-5 • Basic Laboratory Evaluation of Vasculitis

Urine analysis (most crucial test because early asymptomatic renal disease can be detected and progression to renal failure prevented)

Stool screen for occult blood (stool Guaiac)

Complete blood count with platelets and coagulation screen

Hypercoagulability studies may be indicated such as anticardiolipin and antiphospholipid antibodies, complement levels, homocysteine, factor V Leiden, that is, hypercoagulability screen and hematology consult

Antinuclear antibody, rheumatoid factor, liver enzymes, hepatitis screen, cryoglobulins, cryofibrinogen, and immunoglobulins

Antineutrophil cytoplasmic antibody (ANCA) that is positive in Granulomatosis with polyangiitis (c-ANCA)

Polyarteritis nodosa (p-ANCA)

Microscopic polyangiitis (p-ANCA)

Eosinophilic granulomatosis with polyangiitis (p-ANCA)

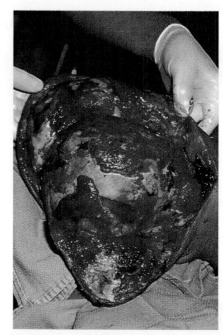

FIGURE 13.7: Necrotizing fasciitis of the scalp showing extensive necrosis that eventually went even beyond the margins shown here. Group A beta streptococci was cultured. The patient walked out of the hospital with full recovery.

Treatment

First Visit

1. Aspirin, 81 mg/day with food
2. Dipyridamole (Persantin)
3. Pentoxifylline (Trental), 400 mg b.i.d. with food
4. Any combination of the first three

Second Visit

1. Warfarin is probably the best choice of more aggressive anticoagulation therapy.
2. Can combine warfarin with 1, 2, or 3 from the previous list.
3. Heparin can be given subcutaneously, but it is expensive and has greater risk of bleeding.
4. More experimental therapies include tissue plasminogen activator and fluindione.
5. Topical dapsone therapy has been tried by some authors with success.

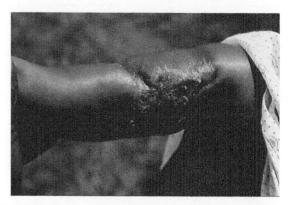

FIGURE 13.8: *Mycobacterium ulcerans* in an African child at the time of debridement. (Courtesy of Dennis Palmer, MD.)

ACUTE CUTANEOUS NECROSIS

This group of diseases (Figs. 13.7 to 13.17) can be defined by sudden onset, painful areas of full-thickness skin loss and gangrene. They have a variety of causes but a similar looking end-stage of black, necrotic, gangrenous tissue.

Presentation and Characteristics

Primary Lesions

These are most commonly seen in the lower extremities. The center is dusky gray or black with induration and often severe pain. An advancing edge of erythema indicates areas of eventual spread of the tissue destruction. Debridement of tissue is often very extensive, and sometimes amputation is required.

Secondary Lesions

Ulcerations with or without secondary infections may occur, and significant scar formation is the rule.

Course

Systemic disease is not uncommon and a lethal outcome may result. Early, aggressive therapy can ameliorate mortality and morbidity in some cases.

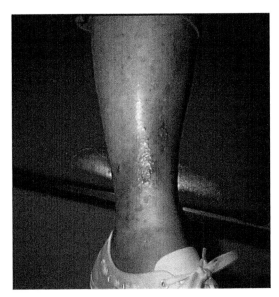

FIGURE 13.9: Necrotic ulcer on the leg in a patient with antiphospholipid syndrome.

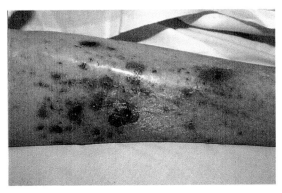

FIGURE 13.10: Emboli with necrosis on the leg of an elderly male after arteriogram of the iliac artery.

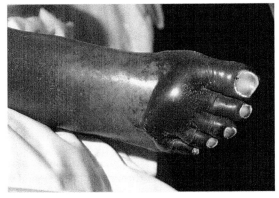

FIGURE 13.11: Coumadin necrosis on day 3 of Coumadin therapy resulting in partial amputation of the foot.

Causes

The causes include Coumadin necrosis, calciphylaxis, spider bite (most commonly the brown recluse in the United States), hypercoagulability states, necrotizing fasciitis, pyoderma gangrenosum, vasculitis, *Mycobacterium ulcerans* (tropical areas), purpura fulminans, embolic phenomena, arteriosclerotic

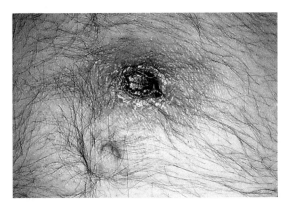

FIGURE 13.12: Echthyma gangrenosum on the umbilicus of a patient with pseudomonas sepsis.

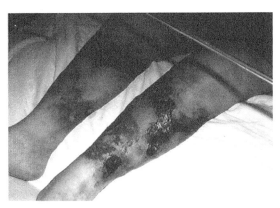

FIGURE 13.13: Calciphylaxis in an elderly woman who refused further hemodialysis due to the severity of her pain and died of renal failure.

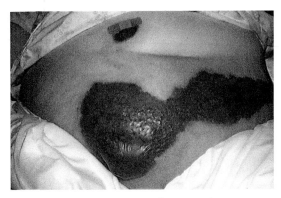

FIGURE 13.14: Heparin necrosis at a subcutaneous heparin injection site on the abdomen of a pregnant woman. Heparin is given as prophylaxis to prevent thrombophlebitis.

occlusive disease (Buerger disease is an example), ecthyma gangrenosum (usually due to pseudomonas sepsis), and *Vibrio vulnificus* infection.

Differential Diagnosis

■ *Coumadin necrosis (Fig. 13-11):* Over 90% of cases occur between days 3 and 5 after Coumadin therapy has been started. It can occur with any Coumadin

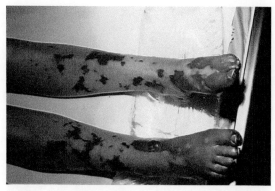

FIGURE 13.15: Purpura fulminans (symmetrical peripheral gangrene) in a woman with DIC due to sepsis. Partial amputation of both feet was required.

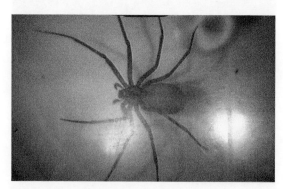

FIGURE 13.16: *Loxosceles reclusus* (brown recluse) spider with characteristic violin on the dorsal surface.

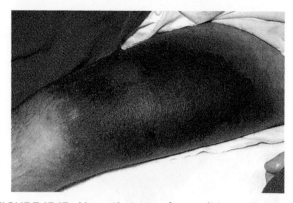

FIGURE 13.17: Necrotic type of vasculitis on the anterior thigh in an HIV patient.

derivative. It most often occurs on areas with large amounts of subcutaneous fat. Only one or two areas are usually involved. Biopsy with fibrin thrombi and minimal inflammation is useful.

- *Heparin necrosis (Fig. 13-14):* Usually occurs within weeks of beginning heparin. Occurs most often at subcutaneous injection sites but can be widespread at sites distant to both IV and subcutaneous heparin. Seen with any type of heparin as part of heparin-induced

thrombocytopenia (HIT) syndrome with antiplatelet antibodies present.

- *Calciphylaxis (Fig. 13-13):* Seen in end-stage renal patients, usually on the lower extremities. Exquisite pain with large areas involved and there is at least 50% mortality.
- *Spider bites:* Occurs in ambulatory patients without underlying disease. Mainly affects lower extremities, and spider (especially brown recluse in the United States [Fig. 13-16]) is usually not seen. Patient is ambulatory and usually not toxic.
- *Hypercoagulability states:* Often asymmetric with small, multiple distal sites, and livedo reticularis.
- *Necrotizing fasciitis (Fig. 13-7):* Patient is very toxic with a marked increase in creatine phosphokinase (CPK). May have a history of trauma. The disease may be very painful early and anesthetic late. Affects a single, very large area with rapid spread over hours. Common in groin or genital area (Fournier gangrene).
- *Pyoderma gangrenosum:* Primarily an ulcerative disease. It is a marker of underlying disease. See earlier in the chapter.
- *Vasculitis:* Often not gangrenous. Palpable purpura also present. See earlier in the chapter.
- *M. ulcerans (Fig. 13.8):* Endemic in tropical Africa. Not painful, and patient is not toxic. It is not usually life threatening.
- *Purpura fulminans (Fig. 13.15):* Patient is toxic and usually septic. There is symmetrical peripheral gangrene with rapid downhill course and DIC.
- *Emboli:* There are multiple, small distal lesions with livedo reticularis and a history of cardiac or orthopedic procedure. Watch for related renal embolic phenomena with renal failure (blood in urine and increased creatinine).
- *Arteriosclerotic vascular occlusion:* Necrosis follows distribution of artery. Angiographic studies may be diagnostic. History of arteriosclerosis.
- *Ecthyma gangrenosum (Fig. 13.12):* Septic patient with blood culture positive for *Pseudomonas aeruginosa* in most cases. May have single or multiple sites of involvement. Likes anogenital site.
- *Vibrio vulnificus infection:* Very toxic patient with a history of raw ingestion by eating raw shellfish, by swallowing infected water, or through an open wound while swimming in coastal waters.

Treatment

Following these patients with surgical as well as medical consultation is warranted.

1. *Coumadin necrosis:* Can continue Coumadin but would not restart. May need to debride later.
2. *Heparin necrosis:* Stop heparin immediately and permanently. May need to debride later.

TABLE 13-6 • Underlying Conditions Associated with Cutaneous Necrosis

Diseases	Underlying Condition
Coumadin necrosis	Obesity, female, decreased amount or function of protein C or S in all cases
Heparin necrosis	Heparin-induced thrombocytopenia, heparin-induced antiplatelet antibodies
Calciphylaxis	End-stage renal disease (almost all cases)
Spider bites	Outpatient setting, patient not ill
Hypercoagulability states	See Table 13-2, clotting disorders, polycythemia, cryoglobulinemia, Waldenström macroglobulinemia, hyperimmunoglobulinemia
Necrotizing fasciitis	Cellulitis (most often Group A streptococci) in all cases, postop, rarely during pregnancy, diabetes (40% to 50%), underlying cancer +/− chemotherapy, varicella (especially in children), renal dialysis, use of NSAIDs, AIDS, traumatic wound
Pyoderma gangrenosum	See earlier in this chapter
Vasculitis	See earlier in this chapter
Mycobacterium ulcerans	Endemic tropical African infection
Purpura fulminans	DIC in almost all cases usually caused by sepsis, may have abnormalities of protein C or S
Embolic phenomena	Associated with orthopedic, arterial, or cardiac procedures
Arteriosclerotic occlusive disease	Arteriosclerotic disease elsewhere (heart, kidney, brain, peripheral arteries), smoking, obesity, diabetes, hyperlipidemia, family history, sedentary lifestyle, and hypertension
Echthyma gangrenosum	*Pseudomonas aeruginosa* sepsis in almost all cases, HIV, chemotherapy, neutropenia, predisposing antibiotic, underlying cancer, IV drug abuse, agammaglobulinemia
Vibrio vulnificus infection	Always swimming in contaminated water (via aspiration, swallowing, or a wound) or eating contaminated raw shellfish (especially oysters), often on systemic corticosteroid treatment, and alcoholic liver disease

3. *Calciphylaxis:* Take sodium thiosulfate (12.5 to 50 g three times a week) IV. If hyperparathyroid consider parathyroidectomy. Hyperbaric oxygen, increased low calcium dialysis, bisphosphonates, and cinacalcet have all been tried.

4. *Spider bites:* Prednisone (50 mg each arm for 2 days and decrease by 10 mg every 2 days for a 10-day course) or dapsone (100 mg each day for 3 to 5 days) can be tried. Debride late, if at all. Ace wrap, ice compresses, and elevation are the old standby.

5. *Hypercoagulable state:* See if your hematologist is in the office and perform a hypercoagulability screen.

6. *Necrotizing fasciitis:* Emergency, aggressive debridement, and emergency IV antibiotics of vancomycin and/or clindamycin (while awaiting cultures) are undertaken. Hyperbaric oxygenation, if available, has been used.

7. *Pyoderma gangrenosum:* See earlier in the chapter. Take systemic corticosteroids early and begin steroid-sparing drug for long-term use.

8. *Vasculitis:* See earlier in the chapter. Take systemic corticosteroids early to save skin and renal function.

9. *M. ulcerans:* Debridement and possible anti-mycobacterium therapy (may be unavailable in jungle) can be undertaken.

10. *Purpura fulminans:* Treat DIC and sepsis or other underlying condition. Debride as needed.

11. *Embolic phenomena:* Anticoagulation may be helpful. Renal compromise may be unavoidable.

12. *Arteriosclerotic occlusive disease:* Consider arterial repair and then consider anticoagulation.

13. *Ecthyma gangrenosum:* Treat sepsis early and debride later if necessary.

14. *Vibrio vulnificus:* Emergency debridement and emergency IV antibiotics, especially tetracyclines and penicillins (cephalosporins and chloramphenicol have also been used).

HAND ECZEMA

Dermatitis of the hands is very common and affects up to 4% to 5% of the population and deserves a brief discussion as it overlaps numerous chapters. It can be very mild or severe enough to interfere with normal use of the hands including usage at a job with significant disability. The numerous etiologies are enumerated in Table 13-7.

TABLE 13-7 • Causes of Hand Eczema

i. Chronic hand eczema of unknown ideology
ii. Work-related hand eczema
   a. Allergic
   b. Toxic
   c. Stress-related
iii. Dermatitis-related to nonoccupation causes
   a. Allergic
   b. Irritant
iv. Fungal disease
   a. Dry moccasin type
   b. Vesicular type
   c. ID reaction from inflammatory disease elsewhere on the skin, especially inflammatory tinea pedis
v. Stress-related
   a. Dyshidrotic Eczematous dermatitis
   b. Excessive compulsive disorder—most notably frequent hand washing
vi. Skin diseases with manifestations on the hands
   a. Psoriasis
   b. Lichen planus
   c. Pityriasis rubra pilaris
   d. Epidermolysis bullosa (especially Weber-Cockayne variant)
   e. Atopic dermatitis
   f. Exfoliative erythroderma
   g. Drug eruption

Presentation and Characteristics

Primary Lesions

Dry fissured dermatitis is most common in eczema. Dry fine adherent scale in the lines of the skin is most common with dry type tinea pedis and frequently involves one hand rather than two. Dyshidrotic eczema tends to be basically vesicular with tiny vesicles along the palms and sides of fingers. Psoriasis may present simply as a dry fissured dermatitis or the more classic silvery white psoriasiform scale on flexor fingers, palms. Psoriasis is also common on the backs of hands and especially the knuckles. Contact dermatitis is either irritant or allergic, and mimics irritant and allergic skin reactions elsewhere. Blistering particularly on the backs of hands can occur with either allergic or irritant contact dermatitis and more fissured dermatitis tends to be on flexor fingers and palms. No matter what disease is involved, fissuring of the fingertips tends to be common and these fissures can be painful. Secondary infection in any hand eczema is not rare and cultures for strep and staph, and appropriate antibiotics usually of the oral variety are adequate for a minimum 6 to 10 day course.

Secondary Lesions

Any involvement of the hands frequently can also involve the feet during the course of the hand dermatitis and may be simultaneous with the hand disease. Secondary lesions demonstrate increased redness, tenderness, deep fissures, and infection.

Infections should be treated appropriately with antibiotics for strep or staph, usually oral and for a minimum of 10 days is adequate. Always consider a possible cause, either allergic or irritant, maybe from topicals the patient has already used. The patient could have bought it OTC or been prescribed by another physician and that should always be considered in the differential diagnosis.

Course

The disease is often extraordinarily chronic and recalcitrant to therapy. Careful instruction on exactly how to take care of the skin of the hands is often necessary. Causes: see Table 13-7.

Fungal culture will help rule a fungal infection in or out. Significant disease of other etiologies elsewhere may help with the diagnosis, such as psoriasis or lichen planus. Detailed history of exposure to chemicals, solvents, and irritants should be obtained in both the work and the home environment. Other than a fungus, which is treated appropriately with oral and/or topical fungal medications there are general rules of therapy for hand eczema or chronic hand dermatitis. Avoidance of hot water may be helpful and the use of topical corticosteroids or calcineurin inhibitor when a flare and even a systemic steroids when a severe flare may be indicated. Emollients containing Ceramide, α-hydroxy acids, β-hydroxy acids (salicylic acid), occasionally tar preparations, and various other topicals especially in an ointment base. It is important to apply the therapies often especially after bath, shower, or washing the hands.

It is important to let the patient know your expectations of the disease that it may not be curable and may be chronic and recurrent. Patch testing may be helpful in finding an allergen either at work or at home. When lichenified skin is fissured, Cordran tape overnight can be helpful. When the skin is very dry, soak for 3 to 5 minutes with a 1 or 2 capfuls of Cutar and water or oilated Aveeno and then application of an ointment or emollient. Sometimes applications of medication especially steroids under occlusion wearing white gloves overnight is beneficial or wet wraps for 5 to 10 minutes over hands and fingers over a steroid ointment can also be very beneficial.

Suggested Readings

Cherry G. *The Oxford European Wound Healing Course Handbook*. Oxford: Oxford University Press; 2002.

El-Kehdy J, Haneke E, Karam PG. Pyoderma gangernosum: a misdiagnosis. *J Drugs Dermatol*. 2013;12(2):228–230.

Ghersetich I, Panconesi E. The purpuras. *Int J Dermatol*. 1994;33:1.

Greaves MW, Kaplan AP. *Urticaria and Angiodema*. New York: Marcel Dekker; 2004.

Hairston BR, Davis MD, Pittelkow MR, et al. Livedoid vasculopathy: further evidence for procoagulant pathogenesis. *Arch Dermatol*. 2006;142:1413–1418.

Henz BM, Zuberbier T, Grabbe J, et al. *Urticaria: Clinical, Diagnostic, and Therapeutic Aspects*. New York: Springer-Verlag; 1998.

Kaplan AP, Greaves MW. Angioedema. *J Am Acad Dermatol*. 2005;53(3):373–388.

Li J, Chen X, Zhao S, et al. Demographic and clinical characteristics and risk factors for infantile hemangioma. *Arch Dermatol*. 2011;147(9):1049–1056.

Nazarian RM, Van Cott EM, Zembowicz A, et al. Warfarin-induced skin necrosis. *J Am Acad Dermatol*. 2009;61(2):325–332.

Ng AT, Peng DH. Calciphylaxis. *Dermatol Ther*. 2011;24:256–262.

Nussinovitch M, Prais D, Finkelstein Y, et al. Cutaneous manifestations of Henoch–Schönlein purpura in young children. *Pediatr Dermatol*. 1998;15:426–428.

Ollert MW, Thomas P, Korting HC, et al. Erythema induratum of Bazin: evidence of T-lymphocyte hyperresponsiveness to purified protein derivative of tuberculin: report of two cases and treatment. *Arch Dermatol*. 1993;129:469–473.

Reichrath J, Bens G, Bonowitz A, et al. Treatment recommendations for pyoderma gangrenosum: an evidence-based review of the literature based on more than 350 patients. *J Am Acad Dermatol*. 2005;53(2):273–283.

Sokumbi O, Wetter DA. Clinical features, dianosis, and treatment of erythema multiforme: a review for the practicing dermatologist. *Int J Dermatol*. 2012;51:889–902.

Stein SL, Miller LC, Konnikov N. Wegener's granulomatosis: case report and literature review. *Pediatr Dermatol*. 1998;15:352–356.

Strazzula L, Nigwekar SU, Steele D, et al. Intralesional sodium thiosulfate for the treatment of calciphylaxis. *JAMA Dermatol*. 2013;149(8):946–949.

Thornsberry LA, LoSicco KI, English JC. The skin and hypercoagulable states. *J Am Acad Dermatol*. 2013;69(3):450–462.

Valencia IC, Falabella A, Kirsner RS, et al. Chronic venous insufficiency and venous leg ulceration. *J Am Acad Dermatol*. 2001;44:401–421.

Wysong A, Venkatesan P. An approach to the patient with retiform purpura. *Dermatol Ther*. 2011;24:151–172.

Zimmet SE. Venous leg ulcers: modern evaluation and management. *Dermatol Surg*. 1999;25(3):236–241.

14

Vasculitis

Kristen Fernandez, MD and Kari L. Martin, MD

Vasculitis is an all-encompassing term meaning inflammation of the blood vessels. This can lead to infarct and thrombosis resulting in tissue ischemia, or may lead to weakening of the vessel walls, rupture and hemorrhage. The clinical manifestations, pathophysiology, diagnosis and management of these diseases contain a significant amount of overlap, but there are also key characteristic differences to be aware of.

CLASSIFICATION

There are a variety of ways to classify vasculitis. Perhaps the easiest way is by the size of vessels affected during the disease process. In general, these are broken down into small, medium, and large sized vessels as well as a mixed category, which usually involves small and medium sized vessels. This chapter will cover primary vasculitis disorders. Vasculitis may also be induced by infections, connective tissue disease, medications or other substances and is then termed secondary vasculitis (Table 14-1).

TABLE 14-1 • Classification of Vasculitis

Small Vessel Vasculitis

ANCA-associated

  Microscopic polyangiitis

  Granulomatous with polyangiitis (Wegener's)

  Eosinophilic granulomatosis with polyangiitis (Churg-Strauss)

Immune complex associated

  Anti-glomerular basement membrane disease

  Cryoglobulinemic vasculitis

  IgA vasculitis (Henoch-Schönlein purpura)

  Hypocomplementemic urticarial vasculitis (anti-C1q vasculitis)

  Cutaneous leukocytoclastic vasculitis

Medium Vessel Vasculitis

Polyarteritis nodosa

Kawasaki disease

Large Vessel Vasculitis

Takayasu arteritis

Giant cell arteritis (Temporal arteritis)

PATHOPHYSIOLOGY AND CLINICAL PRESENTATION

Small Vessel Vasculitis

ANCA-Associated Vasculitis

Anti-neutrophil cytoplasmic antibodies (ANCA) are a heterogeneous group of antibodies which may be seen under immunofluorescence in one of three patterns: cytoplasmic (cANCA), perinuclear (pANCA), or in an atypical pattern (aANCA). It is still unclear what causes the formation of these antibodies, but it is hypothesized that a genetic predisposition along with the right environmental trigger may lead to the development of ANCA antibodies. These antibodies activate neutrophils and macrophages, which then may also promote downstream activation of T or B lymphocytes or eosinophils, a major player especially in eosinophilic granulomatosis with polyangiitis (EGPA).

Microscopic Polyangiitis: Microscopic polyangiitis (MPA) is classically caused by non-granulomatous inflammation of the kidneys and lungs. Many patients also have fever, maylagias, arthralgias, and weight loss. Mono- and polyneuropathies may also be seen when neural involvement occurs. Cutaneous manifestations include purpura, digital gangrene, and ulcers.

Granulomatosis with Polyangiitis (Wegener's): Granulomatosis with polyangiitis (GPA) is characterized by inflammation of the upper and lower respiratory tract as well as small and sometimes medium vessels of the skin and kidneys. Patients may present with nasal symptoms varying from epistaxis to complete cartilaginous destruction and saddle nose deformity. The oral mucosa may be involved with gingival hyperplasia, ulcers of the tongue, palate, gums or buccal mucosa, or cobblestone lesions on the palate. Patients may have fever, arthralgias and malaise, but these are often absent in early, localized disease. Pulmonary involvement is common and may be asymptomatic and only noted on imaging, or may present as cough or hemoptysis. Glomerulonephritis and ocular inflammation may also be seen. The cutaneous lesions in GPA may be common vasculitis morphologies such as skin ulcers, bullae, and nodules or nail infarcts, or rare morphologies like verrucous papules.

Eosinophilic Granulomatosis with Polyangiitis (Churg-Strauss): Characteristically, eosinophilic granulomatosis with polyangiitis (EGPA) consists of adult-onset asthma, eosinophilia and allergic rhinitis in the prodromal phase. The second phase is the eosinophilic phase which involves peripheral eosinophilia and eosinophilic infiltration of various organs. Finally, the last phase is that of vasculitis. Eosinophilic granulomatous inflammation and sometimes necrosis of the airways and other organs ensues. These same eosinophilic granulomas and necrosis affect the small and medium sized vessels of the skin and may be seen as nodules, urticaria or ulcers in 30% to 60% of patients. The vasculitis in EGPA may also involve nerves, heart, lungs, gastrointestinal tract, and kidneys. Neurologic involvement is typically seen as multiple mononeuropathies or symmetric polyneuropathy. Arthralgias and myalgias are also common. Cardiac involvement may be severe and is the cause of death in 50% of patients.

Immune Complex

Anti-glomulerular Basement Membrane disease (Goodpasture Syndrome): Anti-glomerular basement membrane antibodies against type IV collagen are pathogenic in patients with this syndrome. Patients classically present with glomerulonephritis and pulmonary hemorrhage, but not typically cutaneous disease.

Cryoglobulinemic Vasculitis: Cryoglobulins are immune complexes that precipitate at temperatures less than 37°C and dissolve again when warmed above 37°C. They may lead to inflammation of the small vessels of the skin, joints, kidneys and nerves termed cryoglobulinemic vasculitis (CryoVas). Type I cryoglobulins are single monoclonal immunoglobulins related to an underlying B-cell lymphoproliferative disorder. Types II and III cryoglobulins are termed mixed cryoglobulins, and are polyclonal immunoglobulin G (IgG) with or without monoclonal immunoglobulin M (IgM). These types of mixed CryoVas are most commonly caused by hepatitis C virus (HCV) infection.

The clinical presentation of CryoVas varies from mild symptoms such as fatigue and purpura to fulminant widespread vasculitis. Some patients may note worsening or onset of symptoms after exposure to cold, but many do not. Cutaneous symptoms are seen in approximately 85% of patients with HCV negative CryoVas and 75% of those with HCV. This may present as purpura, necrosis, ulceration, or livedo. These signs classically begin on the lower limbs and then extend to the abdomen, trunk, or upper limbs. Arthralgias, polyneuropathy, cognitive impairments, glomerulonephritis, and sicca syndrome may all occur as well.

IgA Vasculitis (Henoch-Schönlein Purpura): IgA vasculitis, also known as Henoch-Schönlein purpura (HSP) is often a widespread vasculitis involving the skin, gastrointestinal tract, kidneys, and joints. The lungs and nervous system may also be rarely involved. It is most commonly seen in children ages 3 to 10 years of age, but may also be seen in adults. Patients may have a preceding upper respiratory infection followed by a prodrome of headache, anorexia, and fever. Patients then develop abdominal pain, vomiting, arthralgias, subcutaneous or scrotal edema, hematuria and bloody stools. The hallmark cutaneous findings are palpable purpura usually beginning on the ankles or lower legs which may progress to the thighs, buttocks, abdomen or rarely diffusely (Fig. 14-1).

Adult patients with HSP may differ in their clinical presentation from children. Adults are less likely to have a preceding upper respiratory infection and more likely to have renal involvement at presentation. Adults are also more likely to have resulting chronic renal insufficiency.

Hypocomplementemic Urticarial Vasculitis (Anti-C1q Vasculitis): The more common entity of urticarial vasculitis is a fixed urticarial eruption which corresponds usually to a leukocytoclastic, self-limited vasculitis with normal complement levels and is usually kept just to the skin. Alternatively, hypocomplementemic urticarial vasculitis (HCUV) is a systemic process resulting in arthritis, angioedema, eye symptoms, asthma, and obstructive pulmonary disease and is seen virtually only in women. Some patients may also have glomerulonephritis, Jaccoud's arthropathy (hand deformities including swan neck deformity, Z deformity of the thumb, and ulnar deviation of the fifth digit) and valvular heart disease. Anti-C1q antibodies are thought to be pathogenic. These antibodies are also common in patients with systemic lupus erythematosus (SLE), and many patients with HCUV will over time meet diagnostic criteria for SLE as well. Occasionally gammopathies, Sjögren syndrome, serum sickness or viral infection (classically hepatitis C) may also underlie urticarial vasculitis or HCUV.

Cutaneous Leukocytoclastic Vasculitis: The hallmark finding in cutaneous leukocytoclastic vasculitis (LCV) is palpable purpura. It may vary in size from pinpoint to over a centimeter and may also become vesicular, bullous or pustular (Figs. 14-2 and 14-3). Ankles and lower legs are common sites, but LCV

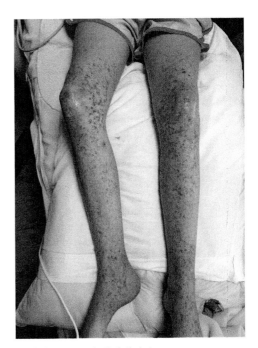

FIGURE 14-1: Henoch Schönlein purpura.

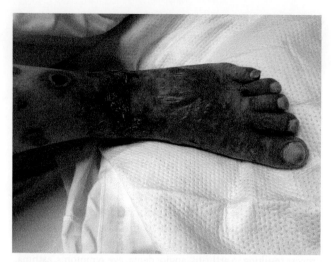

FIGURE 14-2: Bullous leukocytoclastic vasculitis.

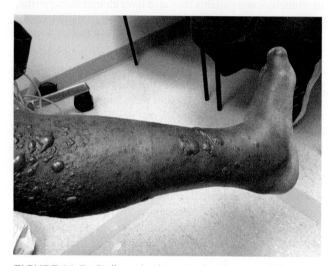

FIGURE 14-3: Bullous leukocytoclastic vasculitis.

may occur anywhere. Other than fever and mild arthralgias, systemic symptoms are rare.

It is most often preceded by a new medication or infectious process. This is thought to produce immune complexes which deposit in blood vessels. Complement is then activated and a variety of inflammatory cytokines are released. Most cases of LCV are self-limited, but few can be recurrent, in which case, a chronic underlying cause should be sought.

Medium-Vessel Vasculitis

Polyarteritis Nodosa

Non-granulomatous inflammation of medium-sized vessels constitutes polyarteritis nodosa (PAN). It is often an idiopathic disease, but may be associated with hepatitis B virus (HBV) infection in some patients. In these cases, it is likely that the vessel inflammation is secondary to HBV induced immune complexes that are trapped in vessel walls. PAN may also be associated with hairy cell leukemia, cryoglobulinemia, myelodysplastic syndrome, rheumatoid arthritis, Sjögren syndrome, and other hematologic malignancies.

The clinical presentation with PAN varies greatly. Many systems may be involved: skin, kidney, joints, gastrointestinal tracts, and nerves. Given that medium sized vessels are involved, the clinical presentation of varying systems differs from small vessel vasculitides. For example, in PAN, renal involvement presents as renal infarcts, renal artery stenosis or microaneurysms and the glomerulus is typically spared. Skin disease may present as purpura, livedo reticularis, skin infarctions, nodules, or peripheral gangrene.

Kawasaki Disease

The diagnosis of Kawasaki disease is done when a child has fever for 4 days along with at least four of the following clinical findings: skin eruption, stomatitis, chelitis, edema of the hands and feet, conjunctival injection and cervical lymphadenitis. The skin manifestations can vary immensely and may be a desquamating perianal eruption, erythema multiforme-like lesions, macular, urticarial, papular or pustular. Systemic complications may include intestinal pseudo-obstruction, facial nerve palsies, digital gangrene and coronary artery aneurysms. It has been hypothesized that Kawasaki disease is due to an infectious trigger in genetically susceptible people, but the details remain to be identified.

Large Vessel Vasculitis

Takayasu Arteritis

A vasculitis of the great vessels of the aortic arch, Takayasu arteritis is most common in young women. Cutaneous lesions are rare, but may include hair thinning, skin atrophy, an associated necrotizing small vessel vasculitis, erythematous nodules or pyoderma gangrenosum-like ulcerations.

Giant Cell Arteritis

Giant cell arteritis most commonly affects the temporal vessel of adults over the age of 50 years. It leads to unilateral headache and tenderness of the scalp overlying the affected vessel. Fever, anemia, polymyalgia rheumatica, and even blindness may occur. Cutaneous manifestations are rare but may include ulceration of the skin overlying the affected vessel(s).

DIAGNOSTIC APPROACH

Eliciting the specific type of vasculitis often requires a complete diagnostic workup, including history and physical, laboratory evaluation, and biopsy, as the degree and location of inflammation often differ between the different types of vasculitis, as well as between individual patients. A through workup will help detect signs of inflammation, the type and extent of organs involved, and potential secondary causes of vasculitis.

History

Cutaneous vasculitis may affect the skin only, or it may be associated with collagen vascular disorders, infections (including hepatitis), paraprotenimia or malignancy, or medications. History is critical in determining if a patient has a history of new medication exposure (prescription or over-the-counter) or an established diagnosis of one of the above disorders.

Additionally, a complete review of systems should be obtained, specifically noting the presence or absence of fevers/chills, arthralgias/myalgias, abdominal pain or change in bowel movements, such as diarrhea, melena, or hematochezia, hematuria, cough, sinusitis or hemoptysis. It is also useful to ask about recent travel and illicit drug use.

Physical Examination

Physical examination can be very helpful in distinguishing between small and medium vessel vasculitis, both of which can demonstrate cutaneous involvement. Palpable purpura is the classic cutaneous physical exam finding of small-vessel vasculitis. Palpable purpura most often is present as firm, purpuric 1 to 3 mm papules distributed in dependent areas, such as the lower legs, in areas of pressure, such as under tight clothing or a waistband, and can demonstrate koebnerization. The papules can sometimes coalesce to form plaques, at which point ulceration or bullae can be seen.

More rarely, urticaria can be seen in small-vessel vasculitis, but the features are different than in traditional urticaria (Fig. 14-4), as the urticarial wheals often last for greater than 24 hours and demonstrate more of a burning sensation than pruritus.

In medium-vessel vasculitis, one can see purpura in a retiform distribution. Livedo racemosa or reticularis can also be seen in medium-vessel vasculitis, indicative of slow flow of the underlying vessels (Fig. 14-5). As mentioned above, ulceration and bullae can be seen at times in the palpable purpura of small-vessel vasculitis; however this is much more commonly seen in small-vessel vasculitis.

Laboratory Evaluation

Laboratory evaluation is helpful in cutaneous vasculitis to (1) determine presence or extent of systemic involvement and (2)

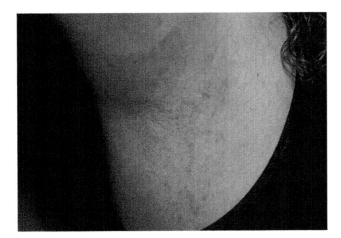

FIGURE 14-4: H&E 20×. Fibrin deposition in small vessels with neutrophilic infiltrate and leukocytoclasia.

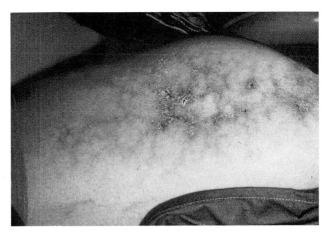

FIGURE 14-5: Urticarial vasculitis on the anterior neck mimicking hives but more persistent with more burning rather than itching. Biopsy showed LCV.

evaluate for an underlying disease as the cause of vasculitis. Baseline tests should include:

- complete blood count with differential
- basic metabolic panel (to monitor for renal involvement)
- urinalysis (also to monitor for renal involvement)
- erythrocyte sedimentation rate

In patients without an identifiable cause of vasculitis, further workup might include:

- hepatitis B and C serologies
- ANA panel
- ANCA panel
- serum protein electrophoresis (to rule out underlying paraproteinemia)
- cryoglobulins

Biopsy

Skin biopsy remains the gold standard in establishing the diagnosis of cutaneous vasculitis. Ideally, the biopsy will extend to subcutis and be sampled from the earliest purpuric papule. A high-yield biopsy specimen should guide classification of vasculitis based on both the size of vessels affected and the dominant inflammatory cell (neutrophilic, lymphocytic, or eosinophilic).

Classically in leukocytoclastic vasculitis (LCV), pathology would demonstrate disruption of small vessels by inflammatory cells, deposition of fibrin within the lumen, and/or vessel wall with karyorrhectic nuclear debris (Fig. 14-6). Most of the inflammation in LCV should be driven by neutrophils. In contrast, medium-vessel vasculitis can be identified solely by infiltration of the vessel wall by inflammatory cells. Extravasation of red blood cells and necrosis are supportive, but not diagnostic of vasculitis. Ideally, direct immunofluorescence would also be performed, as IgA driven disease can indicate a higher probability of systemic involvement.

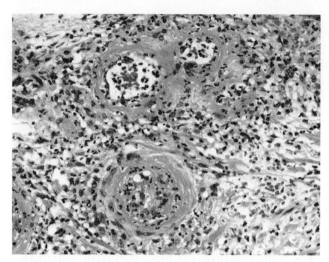

FIGURE 14-6: Livedo reticularis over the anterior thigh with early erosive necrotic areas appearing in a net-like vascular pattern.

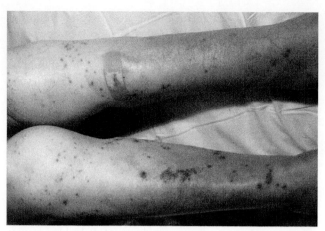

FIGURE 14-7: Clinically mild cutaneous vasculitis with palpable purpura and petechiae, however, underlying renal disease was severe, indicating the importance of evaluating for underlying systemic disease whenever vasculitis is suspected. The bandage covers the biopsy site where LCV was the histologic diagnosis.

TREATMENT

Given that the prognosis of cutaneous vasculitis can range from benign and self-limited, as is often the case in leukocytoclastic vasculitis, to severe or recurrent disease, it is not surprising that treatment of vasculitis ranges from observation only to systemic immunosuppressive therapy.

For leukocytoclastic vasculitis and other small-vessel vasculitities, eliminating the underlying cause (i.e., medication or treating an infection) should resolve the skin disease within 2 to 3 weeks. Since dependent areas, such as the lower legs, are often worst affected, compression devices can be helpful. For ulcerations/bullae, one should consider local wound care with emollients and occlusive dressings. A course of oral corticosteroids should be considered for ulcerative/bullous LCV to decrease progression of disease. For more severe cases of LCV, dapsone and colchicine have for many years demonstrated moderate effectiveness.

Patients with severe systemic involvement in LCV (Fig. 14-7) or those with more severe types of vasculitis will likely require high doses of corticosteroids (1 to 2 mg/kg/d). Further addition of immunosuppressive therapy should be considered; treatment options include cyclophosphamide, azathioprine, methotrexate, and mycophenolate mofetil. Most recently, rituximab has been used with good success and has proven more effective than cyclophosphamide specifically for ANCA-associated vasculitis.

Suggested Readings

Cacoub P, Comarmond C, Domont F, et al. Cryoglobulinemia vasculitis. *Am J Med.* 2015;128(9):950–955.

Callen JP. Colchicine is effective in controlling chronic cutaneous leukocytoclastic vasculitis. *J Am Acad Dermatol.* 1985;13(2 pt 1):193–200.

Carlson JA. The histological assessment of cutaneous vasculitis. *Histopathology.* 2010;56(1):3–23.

Ghetie D, Mehraban N, Sibley C. Cold hard facts of cryoglobulinemia. *Rheum Dis Clin North Am.* 2015;41(1):93–108.

Gioffredi A, Maritati F, Oliva E, et al. Eosinophilic granulomatosis with polyangiitis: an overview. *Front Immunol.* 2014;5:549.

Gonzalez-Gay MA, Garcia-Porrua C, Salvarani C, et al. Cutaneous vasculitis: a diagnostic approach. *Clin Exp Rheumatol.* 2003;21(6 suppl 32):S85–S88.

Sharma A, Dogra S, Sharma K. Granulomatous vasculitis. *Dermatol Clin.* 2015;33(3):475–487.

Stone JH, Merkel PA, Spiera R, et al. Rituximab versus cyclophosphamide for ANCA-associated vasculitis. *N Engl J Med.* 2010;363(3):221–232.

Seborrheic Dermatitis, Acne, and Rosacea

John C. Hall, MD

Seborrhea dermatitis, acne, and rosacea all tend to occur in patients with oily skin. They occur in areas where the oil glands are the largest and most plentiful such as the scalp, face, central chest, and upper back. Response to therapy is better with substances that remove oil and are worsened by substances that are oily. Many therapies are beneficial for all three diseases.

SEBORRHEIC DERMATITIS

Seborrheic dermatitis, in our opinion, is a synonym for *dandruff*. The former is the more severe manifestation of this dermatosis. Seborrheic dermatitis is exceedingly common on the scalp, but less common on the other areas of predilection: ears, face, sternal area, axillae, intergluteal area, and pubic area (Figs. 15-1 and 15-2). It occurs as part of the acne seborrhea complex. Dandruff is spoken of as oily or dry, but it is all basically oily. If dandruff scales are pressed between two pieces of tissue paper, an oily residue is expressed, leaving a mark on the tissue.

Certain misconceptions that have arisen concerning this common dermatosis needs to be corrected. Seborrheic dermatitis cannot be cured, but remissions for varying amounts of time do occur naturally or as the result of treatment. Seborrheic dermatitis does not cause permanent hair loss or baldness unless it becomes grossly infected. Seborrheic dermatitis is not contagious. The cause is unknown, but an important etiologic factor is the yeast *Pityrosporum ovale*.

Seborrheic dermatitis in AIDS patients can be widespread and recalcitrant to therapy. It can be severe and is common in patients with Parkinson disease.

Presentation and Characteristics

Primary Lesions

Redness and scaling appear in varying degrees. The scale is of the greasy type (see Fig. 13-1).

Secondary Lesions

Rarely seen are excoriations from severe itching and secondary bacterial infection. Lichen simplex chronicus can follow a chronic itching and scratching habit.

Course

Exacerbations and remissions are common, depending on the season, treatment, and age and general health of the patient. A true cure is impossible.

Seasonal Incidence

This condition is worse in colder weather, presumably due to lack of summer sunlight.

Age Incidence

Seborrhea occurs in infants (called *cradle cap*), but usually disappears by the age of 6 months (Fig. 15-3). It may recur again at puberty.

Differential Diagnosis

Scalp Lesions

- *Psoriasis:* Sharply defined, silvery-white, dry, scaly patches; typical psoriasis lesions on the elbows, knees, nails, or elsewhere (see Chapter 16).
- *Lichen simplex chronicus:* Usually a single patch on the posterior scalp area or around the ears; intense itching; excoriation; thickening of the skin (see Chapter 12).
- *Tinea capitis:* Usually occurs in a child; broken-off hairs, with or without pustular reaction; some types of fluoresce under Wood light; positive culture and potassium hydroxide mount (see Chapter 28).
- *Atopic eczema:* Usually occurs in infants (where it spares the diaper area) or children; diffuse dry scaliness; eczema also on face, arms, and legs; atopic personal and family history (see Chapter 12).

Face Lesions

- *Systemic lupus erythematosus:* Faint, reddish, slightly scaly, "butterfly" eruption, aggravated by sunlight, with fever, malaise, arthritis, Raynaud and positive antinuclear antibody test (see Chapter 41).
- *Chronic discoid lupus erythematosus:* Sharply defined, red, scaly, atrophic areas with large follicular openings with keratotic plugs, resistant to local therapy, often leaves scars (see Chapter 41).

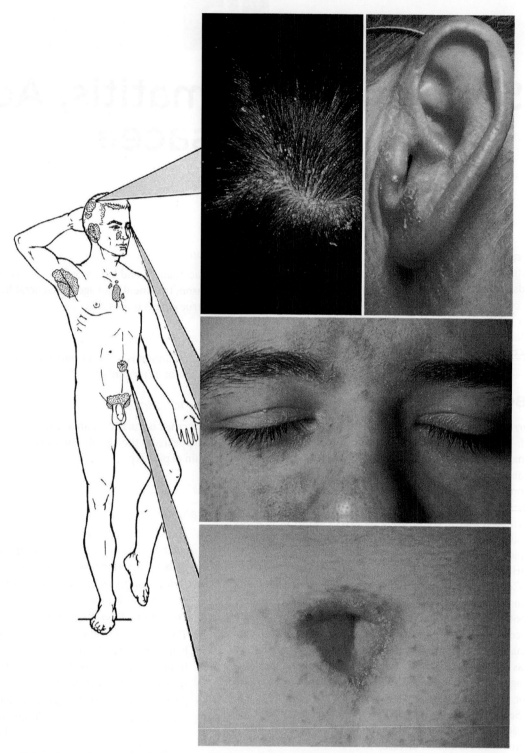

FIGURE 15-1: Seborrheic dermatitis. (Courtesy of Owen Laboratories, Inc.)

Body Lesions

- *Tinea corporis* (see Chapter 28)
- *Psoriasis* (see Chapter 16)
- *Pityriasis rosea* (see Chapter 17)
- *Tinea versicolor* (see Chapter 17)

Treatment

Case Example: A young man presents with recurrent red, scaly lesions at the border of the scalp and forehead and diffuse, mild, and whitish scaling throughout the scalp.

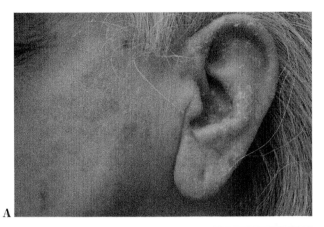

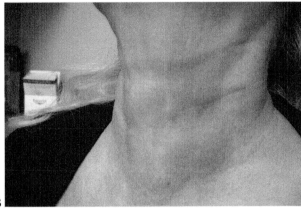

FIGURE 15-2: **A:** Seborrhea with a well-demarcated salmon-pink preauricular plaque and redness with fine adherent greasy scale over ear. **B:** Seborrhea over the anterior neck with papulosquamous dermatitis accentuated in the fold of the skin. This intertriginous-type location is characteristic.

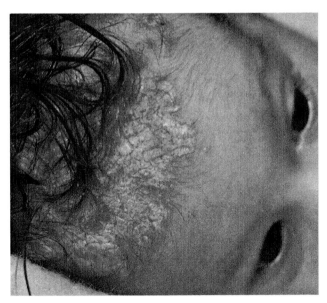

FIGURE 15-3: Seborrheic dermatitis of infancy. This is one of the causes of "cradle cap." (Courtesy of Smith Kline & French Laboratories.)

1. Management of cases of dandruff must include explaining the disease and stating that it is not contagious, that there is no true cure, that it does not cause baldness, and that there are seasonal variations. Therapy can be very effective, but only for keeping the dandruff under control.

2. With this information in mind, tell the patient that shampooing offers the best management. There are several shampoos available, and the patient may have to experiment to find the most suitable one. The following types can be suggested:

   Selenium sulfide 2.5% suspension (Selsun; Head and Shoulders Intensive Treatment, which is available over the counter; Selseb prescription shampoo, which also contains urea and zinc pyrithione) 120.0.

   Sig: Shampoo as frequently as necessary to alleviate itching and scaling. Use no other soap. Refill prescription p.r.n.

   Additional shampoos:

   Sig: Shampoo as frequently as necessary to keep scaling and itching to a minimum.

   - Tar shampoos, such as Ionil T, Tarsum, Reme-T, Pentrax, X Seb T, T-Gel, and T-Sal (a salicylic acid shampoo).
   - Zinc pyrithione shampoos, such as Zincon, Head & Shoulders, and DHS Zinc.
   - Ketoconazole (Nizoral) shampoo (over the counter) and as a higher percentage it is available as a prescription, Loprox shampoo, Capex shampoo (contains fluocinolone, by prescription) or Clobex shampoo (contains clobetasol and should be used Monday, Wednesday, and Friday by prescription).

3. Triamcinolone (Kenalog) spray, 63 mL.

   Sig: Apply sparingly to scalp at night. Squirt the spray through a plastic tube that is supplied.

   Comment: A spray is less messy on the scalp than a corticosteroid solution, but solutions are available.

4. A low-potency corticosteroid cream 15.0.

   Sig: Apply b.i.d. locally to body lesions. A good combination is 1% HC and 2% sulfur in Vanicream. Generic Vytone cream is another safe therapy.

5. Ketoconazole 2% cream 15.0 (available over the counter).

   Sig: Apply b.i.d. on scalp or body lesions.

   Comment: This is a corticosteroid-sparing agent.

   Ciclopirox (Loprox shampoo) and sodium sulfacetamide (Ovace) wash, used as a shampoo, may also be used.

6. 5% LCD (liquor carbonis detergens), 3% salicylic acid in betamethasone solution is another example to apply twice a day to the scalp.

7. Fluocinolone 0.01% solution is popular because it is mixed in propylene glycol, which kills yeast.

8. Pimecrolimus (Elidel) cream and tacrolimus ointment 0.1% and 0.3% (Protopic) can be used in a thin coat b.i.d. without topical corticosteroid side effects.

9. Foam preparations such as sodium sulfacetamide foam (Ovace), betamethasone valerate (Luxiq) foam, or clobetasol (Olux) foam may be beneficial b.i.d. and after shampooing. Avoid overuse of triamcinolone and especially clobetasol.

SAUER'S NOTES

1. Do not prescribe a fluorinated corticosteroid cream for long-term use on the face or in intertriginous areas.
2. Reiterate that there is no cure for seborrheic dermatitis; long-term management is necessary.
3. Reassure the patient that seborrheic dermatitis does not cause permanent hair loss.

ACNE

Acne vulgaris is a common skin condition of adolescents and young adults. It is characterized by any combination of comedones (blackheads and whiteheads), pustules, cysts, and scarring of varying severity (Figs. 15-4 to 15-6).

Severe cystic acne is called *acne conglobata*. When accompanied by systemic symptoms such as arthralgia, leukocytosis, and fever, the term *acne fulminans* is used. *Hidradenitis suppurativa*, also termed *acne inversa*, is a debilitating disease of deep undermining cysts and fistulas in the axillary, inguinal, and perirectal areas. Treatment is difficult and includes surgery, antibiotics, and isotretinoin (Accutane). Pyoderma gangrenosum can be confused with and associated with acne conglobata, acne fulminans, and hidradenitis suppurativa.

Dissecting cellulitis of the scalp (perifolliculitis capitis abscedens et suffodiens) is an inflammatory disease of the scalp with undermining cysts and fistulas of the scalp resulting in scarring alopecia. Treatment is difficult but antibiotics, surgery, laser, x-ray, isotretinoin, azathioprine, dapsone, colchicine, methotrexate, and systemic and intralesional corticosteroids may be helpful.

Acne conglobata, hidradenitis suppurativa, and dissecting cellulitis of the scalp have been referred to as the *follicular occlusion triad*. Pilonidal sinus is added by some authors to make this a tetrad.

Presentation and Characteristics

Primary Lesions

Comedones, papules, pustules, and, in severe cases, cysts occur.

Secondary Lesions

Pits and scars are evident in severe cases. Excoriations of the papules are seen in some adolescents, but most often they appear as part of the acne of women in their 20s and 30s. When severe, it is called *acne excoriae des jeunes filles*. This disease may have few or no primary acne lesions. It is difficult to treat, but some authors recommend selective serotonin reuptake inhibitors as antiobsessive-compulsive therapy.

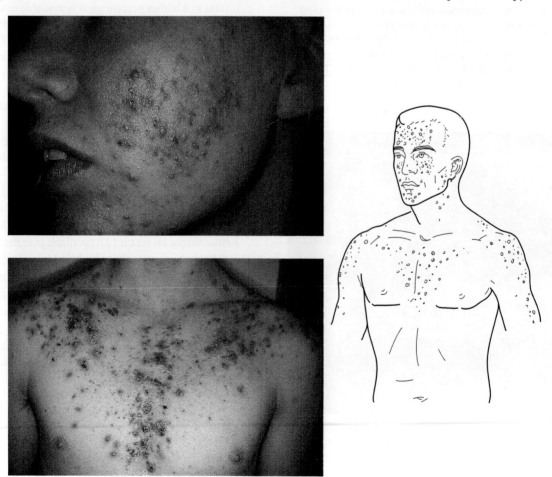

FIGURE 15-4: Acne of the face and chest.

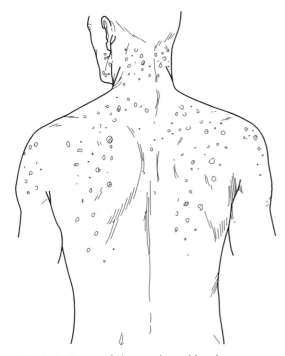

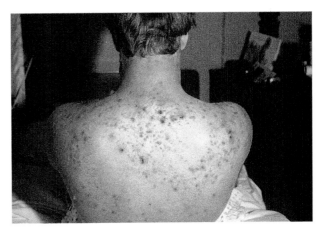

FIGURE 15-5: Acne of the neck and back.

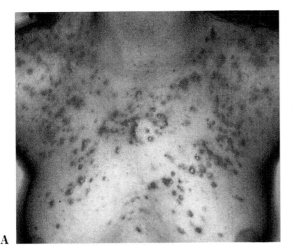

A

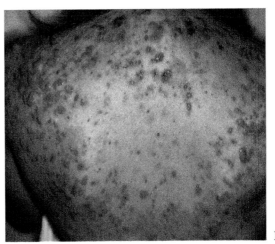

B

FIGURE 15-6: Severe acne vulgaris of the chest **A:** and back **B:** of a 15-year-old girl. (Courtesy of Hoechst-Roussel Pharmaceuticals, Inc.)

Distribution

Acne occurs on the face and neck and, less commonly, on the back, chest, and arms. More rare locations are the scalp, buttocks, and upper legs.

Course

The condition begins at ages 8 to 12 years, or later, and lasts, with new outbreaks, for months or years. It subsides in most cases by the early 20s, but occasional flare-ups may occur for years. Cases tend to start earlier and be more prolonged in women. This variation between sexes is most likely hormonally related. The residual scarring varies with severity of the case, individual susceptibility, and response to treatment.

Subjective Complaint

Tenderness of the large pustules and itching may be reported (rarely). Emotional upset is common as a result of the unattractive appearance.

Causes

The following factors are important:

- Heredity
- Hormonal balance
- Increased heat and sweat such as with increased exercise
- A hot, humid environment due to climate, workplace, or place of exercise
- Diet (high glycemic diets may play a role)

- Use of oily cosmetics
- Sometimes exposure to oils at the workplace

In a case of severe adult acne, one should rule out an endocrine disorder. Hirsutism or abnormal menstrual periods in women are clues. Androgen abuse in male athletes can be causative.

Season

Most cases are better during the summer due to ultraviolet light exposure.

Contagiousness

Acne is not contagious.

Differential Diagnosis

- *Drug eruption:* Note history of ingestion of lithium, corticosteroids, iodides, bromides, trimethadione, and antiestrogens used to treat estrogen receptor-positive breast cancer, testosterone (including anabolic steroids used by athletes and body builders), lithium and corticosteroids administered topically, orally, and intramuscularly (see Chapter 9).
- *Contact dermatitis from industrial oils* (see Chapter 9).
- *Perioral dermatitis* (Fig. 15-7): Red papules, small pustules, and some scaling on chin, upper lip, and nasolabial fold found almost exclusively in women. There is a perioral halo of clear skin. The cause is unknown. Corticosteroid creams locally, initially improve but eventually aggravate the eruption and usually should not be prescribed. Tetracycline, orally, as for acne, is the therapy of choice. Metronidazole gel (MetroGel) is an alternative local therapy for children under 12 years of age. Also, topical erythromycin and topical clindamycin formulations may be helpful. Some authors think this should be called *periorificial dermatitis* because it can occur around the eyes, the nares, and in the diaper area often associated with topical corticosteroid abuse. With time the eruption can become granulomatous.

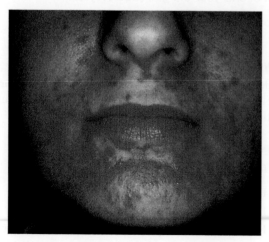

FIGURE 15-7: Perioral dermatitis. (Courtesy of Hoechst-Roussel Pharmaceuticals, Inc.)

- *Adenoma sebaceum:* Rare; associated with epilepsy and mental deficiency. There are 2- to 4-mm papules over central face without comedones, pustules, or cysts.

Treatment

Case Example: An 11-year-old patient presents with a moderate amount of facial blackheads and pustules.

First Visit

1. Give instructions regarding skin care (see Patient Education Sheet, "What You Should Know About Acne"). Stress to the patient and the parent that not one factor but several (heredity, hormones, diet, stress, season of the year, and greasy cosmetics) influence acne breakouts. Some of these factors cannot be altered.

2. *Bar soap:* The affected areas should be washed twice a day with a washcloth and a noncreamy soap, such as Dial, Neutrogena for acne-prone skin, or Purpose.

3. Sulfur, ppt., 6%
   Resorcinol, 4%
   Colored alcoholic shake lotion (see Formulary in Chapter 4) q.s. 60.0.
   Sig: Apply locally at bedtime with fingers.
   Comment: Proprietary products similar to the above lotion include Sulfacet-R, Novacet lotion, Klaron lotion, Ovace cream, gel and cleanser, Plexion cream and cleanser, and Seba-Nil liquid and cleanser.

4. Benzoyl peroxide preparations
   Benzoyl peroxide gel (5% or 10%) as in Benzagel, Desquam-X, Benzac-W, Panoxyl, Persa-Gel, Brevoxyl, Zoderm (also contains urea to decrease dryness), Benziq (with glycerin to decrease drying, comes as a wash and gel [5.25%] or LS Gel [2.75%]), and others. Some of these are also available as emollient gels.
   Sig: Apply locally once a day.
   Comment: Some dryness of skin is to be expected. Fabric can be bleached by the benzoyl peroxide.

5. Tretinoin (Retin A) gel (0.01% or 0.025%) or cream (0.025%, 0.05%, or 0.1%) is available generically, tretinoin (Retin A Micro 0.04% and 0.1%), tretinoin (Avita). Retin A micro is also available in a pump formula of 0.1% and 0.04%.
   Sig: Apply locally once a day at night. Patient toleration varies considerably. These products may take several weeks to become less irritating and may make the acne flare within these few weeks before improvement begins. Some authors recommend to use only for a night to avoid sun sensitivity.
   Comment: Especially valuable for comedonal acne.

6. Local antibiotic solutions, pledgets, and gels.
   Clindamycin 1% (also as a gel called Clindagel) or erythromycin 2% lotion q.s. 30.0.
   Sig: Apply locally once or twice a day.

7. Adapalene (Differin) cream 0.1% q.s. 15 g (Differin Gel [0.3%] can be used if irritation is a problem). Differin lotion 0.1%. The Differin lotion comes in a pump dispenser.

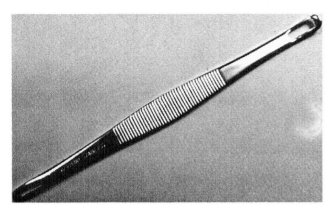

FIGURE 15-8: Comedone extractor. The most frequently used instrument in my office. Firm but gentle pressure with the smaller end over a comedone forces the comedone out of the sebaceous gland opening. Gentle opening of the pimple with an 11 Bard Parker blade before using the comedone extractor may be helpful.

Sig: Thin coat each night.

Comment: May be less irritating and more effective than Retin A.

8. Remove the blackheads with a comedone extractor (Fig. 15-8) in the office.

9. Sulfur preparations with low incidence of odor or drying such as Klaron, Novacet, Ovace (cream, gel, foam, or cleanser), Plexion TS (also comes as a cleanser), thin coat b.i.d.

10. Benzoyl peroxide plus antibiotic; lasts longer if kept refrigerated. The benzoyl peroxide helps prevent antibiotic resistance and is synergistic with the antibiotic. Can bleach fabric. Benzamycin (benzoyl peroxide plus erythromycin), Benzaclin (benzoyl peroxide plus clindamycin), thin coat b.i.d.; and Duac (benzoyl peroxide plus clindamycin), thin coat b.i.d. It does not need to be refrigerated.

11. Akne-mycin ointment and Cleocin T lotion may be good options in patients with dry sensitive skin.

12. Ziana (clindamycin phosphate 1.2% and tretinoin 0.25%) Gel 30 and 60 g tubes. Thin coat q.h.s. This is a combination of antibiotic and retinoid, which may be more convenient than two different applications.

13. (Epiduo) Adapalene-BPO is a single daily application of 0.1% adapalene and 2.5% benzoyl peroxide in a gel base. Irritation potential is similar to adapalene alone.

14. Vanoxide HC has 5% benzoyl peroxide and is in a moisturizing lotion with 0.5% hydrocortisone to decrease irritation.

15. Atralin Gel (0.05% tretinoin) is a low concentration of tretinoin used to decrease irritation.

16. Aczone (dapsone) gel 5% has been used to treat acne but can stain skin and hair yellowish and is expensive.
    Sig: Thin coat twice a day.

17. Acanya Gel (clindamycin phosphate 1.2% and benzoyl peroxide 2.5%).
    Sig: Thin coat once a day.

WHAT YOU SHOULD KNOW ABOUT ACNE[1]

Acne is a disorder in which the oil glands of the skin are overactive and the duct of the oil gland is unable to drain the extra oil. It usually involves the face and frequently the chest and the back, because these areas are the richest in oil glands. When an oil gland opening becomes plugged, a blackhead is formed and irritates the skin in exactly the same way as any other foreign body, such as a sliver of wood. This irritation takes the form of red pimples or deep, painful cysts. This inflammation may destroy tissues and, when healed, may result in permanent scars.

The tendency to develop acne runs in families, especially those in which one or both parents have oily skin. Acne is aggravated by certain foods (especially highly glycemic foods, which contain large amounts of refined sugar), improper care of the skin, lack of adequate sleep, and nervous tension. In girls, acne is usually worse before a menstrual period. Even in boys, acne flares on a cyclic basis. Any or all of these factors can exaggerate the tendency of the oily skin to develop acne. Therefore, the prevention of acne depends on correcting not one but several of these factors.

Because acne is so common, is not contagious, and does not cause loss of time from school or work, many people tend to ignore it or regard it as a necessary part of growing up. We disagree with this.

REASONS FOR TREATING ACNE

There are at least two very important reasons for seeking medical care for acne. The first is to prevent the scarring mentioned. Once scarring has occurred, it is permanent. Then a patient must go through the rest of life being embarrassed and annoyed by the scars, even though active pimples are no longer present. This scarring may vary from tiny little pits, which are frequently mistaken for enlarged pores, to deep, large, disfiguring pockmarks.

The second reason for starting active treatment for acne, even without scarring, is that the condition may become the source of much psychological disturbance to a patient. Even though the acne may appear to others to be mild and inconspicuous, it may seem very noticeable to the patient and lead to embarrassment, worry, and nervousness.

TREATMENT MEASURES TO BE CARRIED OUT BY THE PATIENT

Cleaning Measures

Your face is to be washed twice a day with soap. Do not scrub too roughly. The physician may suggest a particular soap for use. Do not use any face cream, cold cream, cleansing cream, nourishing cream, or any other kind of grease on the face. This includes the avoidance of so-called "pancake-type" makeup, which may contain oil, grease, or wax. Acne is related to excessive oiliness. You may think your face is dry because of the flakes on it, but these are actually flakes of dried oil or the greasy scaling of seborrhea. Later, when the treatment begins to take effect, your skin will actually become dry, even to the point where it is chapped and tender, especially around the mouth and the sides of the chin. When this point is reached, you will be advised as to suitable corrective measures for this temporary dryness. If the skin becomes red and uncomfortable between office visits, the applied remedy may be discontinued for one or two nights.

Girls may use face powder, dry rouge or blush (not cream rouge), and lipstick, but no face creams. Boys with acne should shave as regularly as necessary and should not use oils, greases, pomades, or hair tonics, except those that may be recommended by the physician. Hair should be dressed only with water.

Many cases of acne are associated with oily hair and dandruff and, for these cases, suitable local scalp applications and shampoos will be prescribed by the physician.

Plenty of rest is important. You should have at least 8 hours of sleep each night. Exercise is usually accompanied by increased activity of the oil glands and an acne flare. Wiping the skin off with a cool damp cloth and showering as soon as possible may be helpful. Moderate sun tanning is beneficial for acne, but a sunburn does more harm than good and all sun exposure adds to the cumulative risk of skin cancer. When you get out in the sun, do not use oily or greasy suntan preparations.

Diet

Recent studies have indicated that high glycemic-load carbohydrates may worsen acne. This is controversial, but I think for completeness and for the patient who wants to try diet therapy, it is important to list the diet. It is advisable to avoid or limit the following foods.

Nuts

Especially avoid peanuts, peanut butter, Brazil nuts, and coconuts. Almonds, walnuts, and pecans can be eaten in moderation.

Milk Products

Avoid whole milk (homogenized) and 2% butterfat milk. You can drink up to two glasses of skim milk a day. Avoid sour cream, whipped cream, butter, margarine (allowed in moderation), rich creamy cheeses, ice cream, and sharp cheeses. Cottage and cheddar cheese are permitted. Sherbet can be eaten.

Fatty Meats

Avoid meats such as lamb, pork, hamburgers, and tender steaks. Fish, chicken, and turkey can be eaten unless fried in coconut oil or animal fat. Mazola oil or other corn oils should be used in cooking. French fried potatoes should be avoided.

Spicy Foods

Reduce as much as possible the use of spicy sauces, Worcestershire sauce, chili, catsup, spicy smoked meats, delicatessen products, and pizzas.

Soft Drinks

Avoid soft drinks particularly ones with high sugar content.

Following this diet does not mean that you should starve yourself. Eat plenty of lean meats, fresh and cooked vegetables, fruits (and their juices), and all breads. Drink plenty of water (4 to 6 glasses) daily. One of the most important things to do is to avoid foods that are highly glycemic.

Medical Treatment of Acne

In addition to the prescribed treatment you apply yourself; there are several aspects of the treatment of acne that must be carried out by the physician or the nurse.

One important method of treatment is the proper removal of blackheads. This is often part of the physician's job. Pimples that have pus in them and are ready to open should be opened by the physician or the nurse. This is done with surgical instruments that are designed for the purpose and do not damage tissue or cause scars. Picking of pimples by the patient can cause scarring and should be avoided. When the blackheads are removed and the pustules opened in the physician's office, the skin heals faster and scarring is minimized.

Tetracycline or other antibiotics are frequently prescribed for the acne patient who is developing scars or pits. This antibiotic therapy may be continued by the physician for many months or even years. Occasionally, one develops an upset stomach, diarrhea, or a genital itch from an overgrowth of yeast organisms. Oral fluconazole (Diflucan) has made control of vaginal yeast infection much easier. If these problems develop, stop the medication and call the physician. Oral spirinolactone is considered the oral agent of choice by many in women. Dizziness (orthostatic hypotension), rare cause of abnormal menses, and avoiding during pregnancy are important considerations.

Here are other important comments about oral tetracycline therapy:

1. Tetracycline may make the skin more sensitive to sunlight. Therefore, if you go skiing or to a sunny climate it may be necessary to lower the dosage or stop the tetracycline 4 days before the trip. This sun sensitivity is more common with doxycycline and less common with minocycline.

2. If a woman is on birth control pills and also on tetracycline, there is the remote possibility that the birth control pills may be less effective. Additional birth control measures are indicated at possible times of conception.

3. Do not take tetracycline or a similar antibiotic if you become pregnant because after the fifth month of pregnancy, it can permanently discolor the teeth of the child.

4. The effectiveness of the tetracycline medication is decreased if iron or milk products are ingested at the same time as the tetracycline capsules. The best rule is for you to take tetracycline 30 minutes before meals or 2 hours after a meal.

5. Serious side effects from long-term therapy are almost nonexistent, but if there is any question concerning an illness and the taking of the antibiotic, call your physician. Do not continue taking an antibiotic unless you are under the continued care of your physician. Stop the antibiotic for acne while taking an antibiotic for another condition.

Other internal medications may be prescribed by the physician for acne, such as vitamin A. For very severe cases of cystic scarring acne, isotretinoin can be prescribed, with suitable precautions. Women of childbearing age should be aware of the fact that isotretinoin can cause birth defects if the woman is or becomes pregnant during therapy.

Ultraviolet light treatments are also beneficial for some cases, but the danger of photodamage must be considered. Newer, long-wave ultraviolet light called intense pulsed light (IPL), blue light and red light therapy appears to be safe and beneficial.

Do not take any other medicines internally while under acne therapy without informing your physician.

CONCLUSION

Do not be discouraged! Treatment is effective in at least 95% of all cases. It may be 4 to 6 weeks before noticeable improvement appears. There may be occasional mild flare-ups, but eventually your skin will improve and you and your friends will notice the difference.

It is very important for you and your parents to realize that your physician cannot shorten the length of time it takes for your oil glands to work normally. This maturing process of your skin can take several years, even into the 20s, 30s, or, for a few persons (especially women) longer.

---

[1]This information is from an instruction sheet that I give to my acne patients. I am well aware of differences of opinion regarding the role of diet in acne, but I am presenting my belief.

Treatment for a Case of Scarring Acne

1. Tetracycline, or similar antibiotic, 250 or 500 mg #100
   Sig: Take 1 capsule q.i.d. for 3 days, then 1 capsule b.i.d. This dose can be continued for weeks, months, or years, or the dose can be lowered to 1 capsule a day for maintenance, depending, of course, on the extent of the involvement. Severe cases respond to 3 to 6 capsules a day.

   Tetracycline should be taken 30 minutes before meals or 2 hours after a meal, and not concurrently with iron or calcium for optimal absorption.

   Comment: Minocycline (Solodyn) is also available as time released at once daily dosing (1 mg/kg) at 45-, 90-, and 135-mg tablets. Other effective antibiotics include erythromycin, 250 mg b.i.d. or t.i.d.; minocycline, 100 mg/day; doxycycline (Monodox is doxycycline monohydrate with a decreased chance of esophageal inflammation; Doryx is a preparation that only needs to be given once a day with a decreased gastrointestinal upset and less photosensitivity), 100 mg b.i.d.; and minocycline (Minocin may be better absorbed), 100 mg b.i.d. Other antibiotics include clindamycin 150 or 300 mg b.i.d. and trimethoprim 100 mg b.i.d. Azithromycin (Zithromax) pulse in a 5-day dose pack 500 mg the first day, 250 mg for 4 days (Z-pack) can be used monthly or bimonthly (low dose doxycycline hyclate [20 mg] is subantimicrobial and may eliminate many side effects of larger doses).

2. Other treatments
   a. Vitamin A (water-soluble synthetic A), 50,000 #100
      Sig: Take 1 capsule b.i.d. for 5 months, then not for 2 months to prevent liver toxicity. Avoid if pregnancy is a possibility.
   b. Abrasive cleansers are recommended by some physicians, but the author does not personally recommend them and thinks they can actually make acne worse.
   c. Large papules or early cysts. Intralesional corticosteroid can be injected with care. Dilute triamcinolone suspension (4 mg/mL) with equal part of saline or lidocaine (Xylocaine) with epinephrine, and inject about 0.1 mL into the lesion. Atrophy can result if too large a quantity or too high a concentration is injected.
   d. Incision of fluctuant acne cysts: *never* incise these widely, but if you believe the pus must be drained, do it through a very small incision and possibly an acne stylet. A zero or ear curette can be useful.
   e. Short-term prednisone systemic therapy is effective for severe cystic acne, especially for acne fulminans, an acute, disabling form of acne.
   f. Isotretinoin: For severe, scarring, cystic acne this therapy has proved very beneficial. The usual dosage is 1 mg/kg/day given for 4 to 5 months. There are many minor and major side effects with this therapy

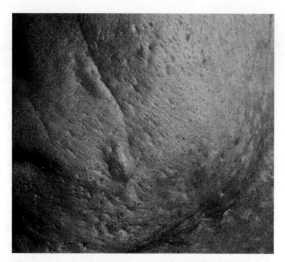

FIGURE 15-9: Acne scars on the cheek.

(notably teratogenic effects in pregnant women), so isotretinoin should only be prescribed by those knowledgeable in its use. Depression may also be a side effect. Some authors have concluded that a lower dose of 20 mg/day can be efficacious with fewer side effects than higher doses for moderate acne. LASIK eye surgery should probably not be done until 6 months after isotretinoin therapy stopped or 6 months before isotretinoin therapy is started. The IPLEDGE program for following patients is mandatory.

3. The residual scarring of severe acne (Fig. 15-9) can be lessened by diamond fraise, or laser resurfacing. There are many other surgical treatments available (see Chapter 5). These procedures are being done by many dermatologists and plastic surgeons.

4. Nicomide, 1 b.i.d. is a vitamin therapy that may be helpful.

5. Spirinolactone 25 or 50 mg b.i.d. may be beneficial in women especially if they flare during the last week of their menstrual cycle.

6. Long-wave ultraviolet light in the form of blue or red light or a combination of the two or IPL therapy. It appears to be safe and can be helpful.

7. Photodynamic therapy with a topical levulinic acid preparation and red light activation.

SAUER'S NOTES

1. For local acne medications, one product can be applied in the morning and a different product at night.

2. To ensure compliance, start with milder agents, increasing the strength as indicated and tolerated.

3. Acne flare-ups occur in cycles—hormonal (females) and seasonal (fall and spring). Keep reminding your patient of these natural flare-ups.

4. "Prom pills." The high school prom (or a wedding or a job interview) is in 1 week. The following will clear much of that inflammatory acne: Prednisone, 10-mg tablets #14
Sig: Take 2 tablets each morning for 7 days.

5. Unfortunately, an appreciable number of men and women continue to have acne into the 20s, 30s, and even later years. Explain this fact to your patients.

ROSACEA

A common pustular eruption with flushing and telangiectasias on the butterfly area of the face may occur in adults especially in the 40- to 60-year-old age group (Fig. 15-10). It is more common in women.

Presentation and Characteristics

Primary Lesions

Diffuse redness, papules, pustules, and, later, dilated venules, m of the nose, cheeks, and forehead, are seen.

Secondary Lesions

Severe, long-standing cases eventuate into the bulbous, greasy, hypertrophic nose characteristic of rhinophyma. More common in men.

Course

The pustules are recurrent and difficult to heal. Rosacea keratitis of the eye may occur. Rosacea is rare in children, but there is a risk of significant eye disease in this population.

Types of Rosacea

1. Erythematotelangiectatic
2. Papulopustular
3. Phymatous
4. Ocular

These are the four common types. More uncommon types include (1) Granulomatous rosacea (2) Rosacea fulminans (pyoderma faciale), and some consider perioral dermatitis a form of rosacea. An unusual form of rosacea called neurogenic rosacea has also been reported in which the patient has neurologic or neuropsychiatric conditions which include tremor, depression, obsessive compulsive disorder (OCD), and complex regional pain syndrome. They may also have collagen vascular diseases, fibromyalgia, and psoriatic arthritis. Marked symptoms of burning, pain, erythema, and flushing sometimes accompanied by facial edema and telangiectasias can also occur. Treatment of both the underlying neurologic conditions as well as the rosacea is warranted.

Causes

Several factors influence the disease:

1. Heredity (oily skin)
2. Excess ingestion of alcoholic beverages, hot drinks, and spicy foods

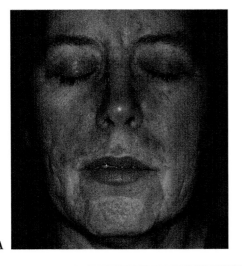
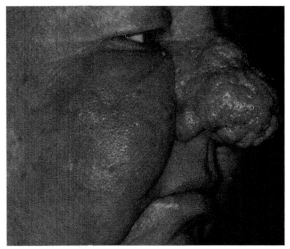
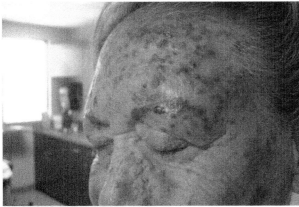
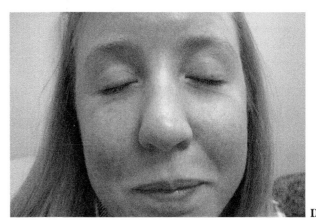

FIGURE 15-10: **A:** Rosacea of a 47-year-old woman. **B:** Rosacea, chronic, with rhinophyma. (Courtesy of Hoechst-Roussel Pharmaceuticals, Inc.) **C:** Severe pustular facial eruption with eyelid involvement. Some experts with call this pyoderma faciale (rosacea fulminans) which is more common in women. **D:** Seborrhea in a young girl mimicking butterfly rash of acute cutaneous lupus erythematous. Note eyelid involvement (marginal blepharitis), and an ANA was negative.

3. *Demodex* mites (may be causative)
4. Increased exercise
5. Increased exposure to hot or cold environment
6. Topical or systemic corticosteroids

Excess sun exposure and emotional stress can aggravate some cases of rosacea.

Differential Diagnosis

■ *Systemic lupus erythematosus:* No papules or pustules; positive antinuclear antibody (ANA) blood test (see Chapter 41).

■ *Boils:* Usually only one large lesion; can be recurrent but may occur sporadically; an early case of rosacea may look like small boils. Bacterial culture shows *Staphylococcus aureus* or group A β-hemolytic strepto-cocci. Responds to anti-*Staphylococcus* antibiotics (see Chapter 24).

■ *Iodide or bromide drug eruption:* Clinically similar, but drug eruption usually is more widespread; history positive for drug (see Chapter 9).

■ *Seborrheic dermatitis:* Pustules uncommon; red and scaly; also in scalp.

■ *Rosacea-like tuberculid of Lewandowsky:* Mimics small papular rosacea clinically and tuberculids histologically, rare; biopsy helpful.

■ *Flushing:* Carcinoid pheochromocytoma, mastocytosis, medullary thyroid carcinoma, climacterium in meno-pausal women and some medications (especially nico-tinic acid).

Treatment

Case Example: A 44-year-old man presents with redness and pustules on the butterfly area of the face.

1. Prescribe avoidance of these foods: chocolate, nuts, cheese, cola drinks, iodized salt, seafood, alcohol, spices, and very hot drinks.
2. Metronidazole gel (MetroGel, Metrocream, Metrolotion, or Noritate cream).
   Sig: Apply thin coat b.i.d. Response to therapy is slow, taking 4 to 6 weeks to benefit.

3. Sulfur, ppt. 6%

   Resorcinol 4%

   Colored alcoholic shake lotion q.s. 60.0

   Sig: Apply to face h.s.

   Similar proprietary lotions are Sulfacet-R lotion Rosac cream (contains a sunscreen), Rosula (contains urea to decrease irritation), sodium sulfacetamide topical preparations, Plexion topical preparations, Novacet lotion, and Avar Green (contains green tint to hide redness).

4. Tetracycline, 250-mg capsules.

   Sig: Take 1 capsule q.i.d. for 3 days, then 1 capsule b.i.d. for weeks, as necessary for benefit. Other antibiotics that can be used, as for acne, include doxycycline, minocycline, and erythromycin.

5. Therapy for *Helicobacter pylori* in the same treatment regimens as for peptic ulcer disease has been tried with some benefit in severe cases.

6. Azeleic acid (Azelex and Finacea) in thin coat b.i.d.

7. Crotamiton (Eurax) lotion in thin coat b.i.d.

8. Subantimicrobial doses of antibiotics (i.e., Oracea [40-mg doxycycline] one each day with food) may be safer (less vaginal yeast infections, less superinfections, less upset stomach, and less photosensitivity) and still be effective.

9. Oral zinc sulfate 100 mg three times a day is safe and has shown benefit according to some authors.

10. Other remedies used include topical tretinoin (may worsen redness), topical tacrolimus, oral sulfate (100 mg b.i.d.), and oral Nicomide (combination of vitamins and minerals).

11. Sun protection may be helpful.

12. Oral β-blockers maybe used to ameliorate the flushing effect when it is severe. β-blockers decrease redness and flushing. An example of this would be carvedilol 6.5 to 6.25 mg 1 to 3 times a day.

13. Mirvaso (bromonidine). This is typically used to help flushing but there may be rebound flushing.

Suggested Readings

Cordain L, Lindeberg S, Hurtado M, et al. Acne vulgaris: a disease of Western Civilization. *Arch Dermatol.* 2002;138:1584–1590.

Drugs for Acne. *Med Lett.* 2016;58(1487):13–15.

Gollnick H, Gunliffe W, Berson D, et al. Management of acne: a report from a global alliance to improve outcomes in acne. *J Am Acad Dermatol.* 2003;49(suppl 1):S1–S37.

Goodman GJ. Treatment of acne scarring. *Int J Dermatol.* 2011;50:1179–1194.

Jemec GBE. Hidradenitis suppurativa. *N Eng J Med.* 2012;366(2):158–164.

Naldi L, Rebora A. Seborrheic dermatitis. *N Eng J Med.* 2009;360(4):387–396.

Acne Scars Classification of Treatment

Leyden JJ. Rosacea update: advances from basic and clinical research. *J Am Acad Dermatol.* 2013;69(6):S1–S57.

Zeichner JA. Evaluating and treating the adult female patient with acne. *J Drugs Dermatol.* 2013;12(12):1418–1427.

Psoriasis

Jeffrey M. Weinberg, MD

PSORIASIS

Psoriasis is a hereditary, papulosquamous skin disorder that affects 1.5% to 2% of the population in Western societies. In the United States, there are 3 to 5 million people with psoriasis, which affects men and women equally.

Psoriasis can have multiple clinical presentations and varies widely among different individuals. It is typically a chronic and recurring disease that is best characterized by well-demarcated erythematous plaques with scaling. The plaques can be localized, which is the most common presentation, and confined to only certain delineated areas of the body. Most commonly plaques are seen on the elbows, knees, and the scalp. The plaques have a characteristic slivery-white scale described as ostraceous (oyster shell appearance), imbricated (shingle-like), crustaceous (like a crustacean shell), dry, and flaky. The scale is the diagnostic feature and not the histologic appearance on biopsy (Fig. 16-1).

There are other variants of psoriasis. In palmoplantar psoriasis, lesions are limited to the soles of the feet and palms of the hands. In contrast, generalized pustular psoriasis and generalized erythrodermic psoriasis (Fig. 16-2) can involve the entire body and be a life-threatening condition, even necessitating hospitalization. It can be seen in association with acute respiratory distress syndrome.

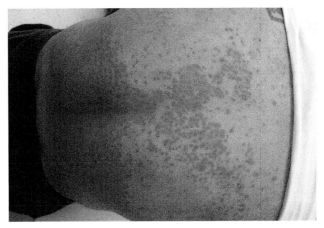

FIGURE 16-2: Exfoliative dermatitis evolving over the back with nonspecific erythema with lack of characteristic scale.

Primary Lesions

Plaque psoriasis: The lesions are well-demarcated, salmon-colored papules and plaques with thick silvery scaling that typically bleeds in a pinpoint distribution when removed (Auspitz sign). Lesions can vary greatly in size and shape in addition to distribution, which may be localized or generalized.

Pustular psoriasis (Fig. 16-3): The lesions are typically yellow pustules that can coalesce and evolve into dark-red crusty lesions.

> **SAUER'S NOTES**
>
> Uncommon manifestations of common diseases are more common than common diseases. This is also true for psoriasis.

Secondary Lesions

Secondary lesions are less common but can include excoriations, lichenification, (thickening) oozing, and secondary infection.

Distribution

Psoriatic patches most commonly occur on the elbows, knees, and scalp, although involvement can occur on any area of the body, including palms, soles, and even nails.

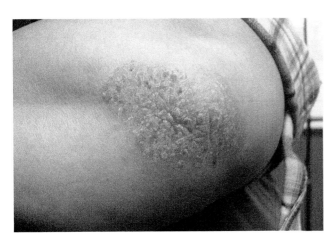

FIGURE 16-1: Silvery-white psoriasiform, well-demarcated plaque with imbricated scale on the elbow. There are pinpoint sites of bleeding (Auspitz sign) seen where the scale has peeled off.

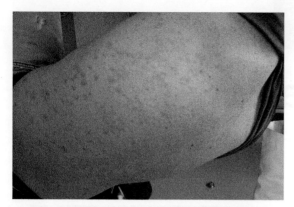

FIGURE 16-3: Drop-shaped round symmetrically distributed psoriasis over the trunk in a patient with streptococcal pharyngitis. This form of psoriasis is seen commonly in older children and young adults and may dissipate or persist.

Course

Psoriasis is typically a chronically recurring disease, although cases of complete resolution do occur. The onset of the disease can occur at any age, but the peaks of onset are in the 20s and 50s.

Causes

While the exact etiology of psoriasis is unknown, there is clearly a hereditary component. When one parent has psoriasis, a child has an 8% chance of having the disease. If both parents have psoriasis, the child's chance of developing psoriasis increases to as high as 41%. Specific human leukocyte antigen (HLA) types have been noted to have a higher frequency of association with psoriasis, specifically HLA-B13, HLA-B17, HLA-Bw57, and most notably HLA-Cw6.

An acute form of psoriasis, guttate psoriasis (Fig. 16-3), characteristically develops in children and younger adults, often follows a streptococcal infection and has characteristic smaller sized, drop-shaped lesions.

Triggering factors include physical trauma, which can elicit the lesions, or any type of excessive rubbing or scratching, which can stimulate the proliferative process. This is referred to as koebnerization or isomorphic response. Aggravating factors include psychologic stress and certain medications such as systemic glucocorticosteroids cessation, oral lithium, antimalarial drugs, systemic interferon, β-blockers, and potentially angiotensin-converting enzyme inhibitors. Alcohol and smoking may also aggravate psoriasis.

Subjective Complaints

Thirty percent of patients present with a complaint of pruritus, especially when psoriasis involves the scalp and anogenital area. Also common are complaints of joint pain, termed psoriatic arthritis, found in 5% to 8% of patients with psoriasis. If minor joint complaints were included some authors would increase this incidence up to 30%. Interestingly, 10% of patients with psoriatic arthritis have no skin manifestations of the disease. Finally, in a rare acute onset of generalized pustular psoriasis called von Zumbusch syndrome, there is associated weakness, chills, and fever.

Season

Exacerbation is typically seen in the winter, most likely due to the lack of sunlight and low humidity. Natural ultraviolet light typically causes psoriatic symptoms to improve.

Age Group

The disease can occur at any age. However, the average onset is typically bimodal, with one peak at approximately 23 years (although in children, mean onset is 8 years) and another at age 55.

Contagiousness

Psoriasis is not contagious.

Relation to Employment

Psoriatic lesions occur more typically in areas of skin injury or repeated skin stress or pressure. This is known as the Koebner phenomenon.

Laboratory Findings

The diagnosis of psoriasis is usually made on clinical grounds, and biopsy is not necessary. If biopsy is performed, histologic findings include the following:

1. Acanthosis: thickening of the skin
2. Increased mitosis of keratinocytes, fibroblasts, and endothelial cells
3. Inflammatory cells in the dermis and epidermis

> **SAUER'S NOTES**
>
> Psoriasis is a clinical diagnosis and not a histologic diagnosis. Many skin diseases are psoriasiform on biopsy.

Differential Diagnosis

1. *Seborrheic dermatitis:* Lesions more yellowish and greasy than those of psoriasis. In the scalp, the scale is usually less thick than in psoriasis. Seborrheic dermatitis and psoriasis can often coexist in some patients (sometimes referred to as sebopsoriasis).
2. *Lichen simplex chronicus:* Usually fewer patches than psoriasis, with less of a thick scale.
3. *Tinea corporis:* Usually a single lesion, with outer scale and central clearing. Potassium hydroxide preparation and fungal culture are positive for fungi.
4. *Psoriasiform drug eruptions:* Check medication history.
5. *Pityriasis rosea:* "Christmas tree" configuration of oval, papulosquamous lesions. Herald patch usually precedes the wider eruption. Superficial fine collarette of scale.
6. *Atopic eczema:* Ask about family history of asthma, allergic rhinitis, and eczema. Involvement typically occurs on flexural surfaces, face, and neck.
7. *Secondary or tertiary syphilis:* These can appear psoriasiform. Inquire regarding history of sexually transmitted diseases and recent symptoms. Check syphilis serology if indicated.

8. *Mycosis fungoides:* Biopsy in chronic cases, especially with involvement of the bathing trunk area.
9. *Nail dystrophy:* Psoriasis is in the differential diagnosis of nail dystrophy. Other entities to consider include onychomycosis, trauma, and lichen planus. The most characteristic nail findings are pitting, onycholysis, oil drop salmon pink spots, and a pink rim at the proximal edge of the onycholysis giving the nail a three colored look (white distally due to onycholysis, pink discoloration more proximal indicating active disease and most proximal the remaining normal nail) (Fig.16-4).
10. Hyperkeratosis of palms and soles (palmar-plantar keratoderma) (Fig 16-5) which can be seen in inherited syndromes, generalized exfoliative dermatitis, pityriasis rubra pilaris, some forms of ichthyosis, eczema, Reiter's syndrome, and occupational dermatoses.

SAUER'S NOTES

Pityriasis rubra pilaris and psoriasis can be impossible to tell apart clinically or histologically.

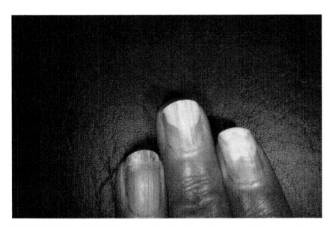

FIGURE 16-4: White onycholysis, salmon-pink proximal rim, and more proximal normal nail forming a tri-colored psoriatic nail. Some mild pitting is also seen.

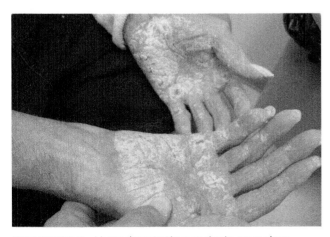

FIGURE 16-5: Hyperkeratotic psoriasis on palms. Silvery-white scale helps to differentiate from other forms of palmar keratoderma.

Treatment

While there is no definitive cure for psoriasis, there are many methods of management that can greatly improve and sometimes almost completely eradicate its skin manifestations, leading to a much improved quality of life. There are many new therapies available or in development for the treatment of the disease.

First Visit of a Patient Presenting With Mild to Moderate Localized Lesions on the Body, Face, or Scalp

For Body Lesions

1. Medium- to high-potency fluorinated corticosteroid cream or ointment
   Sig: Apply b.i.d. to body lesions.
2. Calcipotriene (Dovonex) ointment
   Sig: Apply b.i.d. to body lesions.
3. Calcipotriene and betamethasone dipropionate (Taclonex) ointment or suspension q.d.
4. Tazarotene (Tazorac) gel or cream, 0.05% or 0.1%
   Sig: Apply q.h.s. to body lesions.
5. Intralesional triamcinolone 10 mg/mL
   Sig: Inject subcutaneously to body lesions. This treatment can be very valuable for discrete, recalcitrant lesions.

For Facial (Less Common) and Intertriginous Lesions

1. Low-potency corticosteroid cream or ointment
   Sig: Apply b.i.d. to facial lesions.
2. Pimecrolimus (Elidel) cream 0.1% or tacrolimus (Protopic) ointment 0.03% or 0.01%
   Sig: Apply b.i.d. to facial lesions.

For Scalp Lesions

1. Tar shampoo
   Sig: Shampoo frequently.
2. Topical corticosteroid lotion (Clobex, Diprolene), solution (Cormax, Lidex), or foam (Olux, Luxiq)
   Sig: Apply b.i.d. to scalp.
3. Derma-Smoothe/FS scalp oil
   Sig: Apply overnight to scalp as directed.
4. Calcipotriene (Dovonex scalp solution) 0.0005%
   Sig: Apply b.i.d. to scalp.
5. Tazarotene (Tazorac) gel 0.05% or 0.1%
   Sig: Apply q.h.s. to scalp.
6. Excimer (Xtrac) laser twice weekly for 4 to 10 treatments
7. Bakers P(phenol) and S(sodium chloride) liquid overnight to remove thick scale.

Subsequent Visits of a Patient with Mild to Moderate Localized Psoriasis

1. For body lesions, the potency of the corticosteroid utilized can be increased.

2. Occlusive dressings with corticosteroid can be applied at night and left overnight.
   a. Intralesional corticosteroid therapy can be given whereby individual small lesions are injected with intralesional triamcinolone as discussed previously.
3. Tazarotene (Tazorac) gel or cream, 0.05% or 0.1% as mentioned previously.
4. Ultraviolet therapy: Options include broadband or narrowband ultraviolet B, each three times per week, and oral PUVA (psoralen and ultraviolet A), two to three times per week. PUVA has been associated with an increased risk of squamous cell carcinoma and, with long-term use, melanoma.
5. Excimer (Xtrac) laser twice weekly for 4 to 10 treatments.

First Visit of a Patient With Moderate to Severe Generalized Psoriasis

1. Topical therapies listed for mild to moderate disease are utilized, possibly in combination with other therapies listed below.
2. Broadband or narrowband ultraviolet B, three times per week.
3. PUVA, two to three times per week.
4. Biologic therapies (made by living organisms in a fashion similar to vaccine production).
   a. Etanercept (Enbrel) 50 mg b.i.w. SQ for 3 months, followed by 25 mg b.i.w. This drug can be given as continuous therapy in the long-term and is beneficial for psoriatic arthritis. Injection site reactions have been observed. A purified protein derivative (PPD) skin test or quantiferon gold (QG) blood test should be checked prior to therapy. Exercise caution in patients with multiple sclerosis, congestive heart failure, tuberculosis exposure, and lupus erythematosus. This is immunosuppressive and there is increased risk of infection especially respiratory tract infections. Blocks TNF α.
   b. Infliximab (Remicade) IV 5 mg/kg at weeks 0, 2, and 6, and then every 8 weeks. Infliximab is approved for psoriasis and psoriatic arthritis. As for etanercept, a PPD or QG should be checked prior to therapy. Exercise caution in patients with multiple sclerosis, congestive heart failure, tuberculosis exposure, and lupus erythematosus. Increase in infections as for all TNF inhibitors.
   c. Adalimumab (Humira) 80 mg SQ as a loading dose, followed 1 week later by 40 mg SQ, and then 40 mg SQ every other week. As for other TNF (tumor necrosis factor)-inhibitors, a PPD or QG should be checked prior to therapy. Exercise caution in patients with multiple sclerosis, congestive heart failure, tuberculosis exposure, and lupus erythematosus. Increased infections.
   d. Ustekinumab (Stelara), 45 mg (for patients weighing ≤220 lbs) or 90 mg SQ (for patients weighing >220 lbs) at weeks 0, 4, and then every 12 weeks. A PPD or QG should be checked prior to therapy. Increased infections. Blocks Il-12 and Il-23.
   e. Secukinumab (Cosentyx) 300 mg SQ weekly for 5 weeks, followed by 300 mg SQ monthly. For some patients, a dose of 150 mg may be acceptable. A PPD or QG should be checked prior to therapy. Exacerbation of Crohn's disease was observed in clinical trials. Increased infections. Blocks Il-17a.
   f. Ixekizumab (Taltz) (Blocks Il-27a) see package insert for suggested dosages.
5. Methotrexate: This oral drug can be used weekly. This drug has potential side effects, including liver (higher risk with alcohol ingestion), pulmonary, and bone marrow toxicity. Folic acid decreased risk of these side effects and should be given in all patients. Patients should be monitored closely.
6. Acitretin (Soriatane) therapy 10 to 25 mg q.d. This drug is especially useful in cases of palmoplantar, erythrodermic, and pustular psoriasis (Fig. 16-6). This drug is teratogenic, and a woman cannot become pregnant until 3 years after the drug is discontinued. There are several other potential side effects, including alopecia, bone loss, and hyperlipidemia. Patients should be monitored closely. This drug can be combined with PUVA (Re-PUVA: combination retinoid and PUVA therapy).

Subsequent Visits of a Patient With Moderate to Severe Generalized Psoriasis

1. Continue or rotate therapies as per first visit.
2. Occasionally some of these therapies can be combined. Check the package inserts and published data before combining different systemic therapies.
3. Cyclosporine (Neoral): This oral immunosuppressive therapy is highly effective for short-term, rapid treatment of severe psoriasis. It has many potential toxicities, including hypertension and renal toxicity. Patients should be monitored closely.

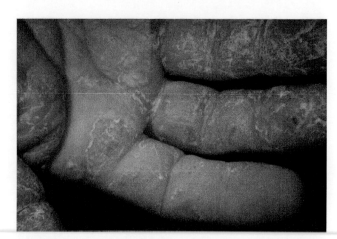

FIGURE 16-6: Desquamating pustules over the palms and flexor figures that are forming painful debilitating erosions.

4. Other biologic therapies: If a patient is nonresponsive to one or more biologic agents, transition to a different agent.

5. Mycophenolate mofetil (CellCept). This oral immunosuppressive drug has been reported to be effective in some patients with psoriasis. There is less organ toxicity with this than with methotrexate or cyclosporine. There is a small increased risk of lymphoma with chronic use of the drug.

6. Apremilast (Otezla) is a new oral small molecule treatment. Gastrointestinal upset is common and the drug is tapered up to 30 mg twice a day over 2 weeks. Not as immunosuppressive. Small risk of depression has been noticed.

7. More small molecules and biologics are being developed such as the small molecule JAK inhibitors (topical and systemic) and the biologic Il-23 blockers.

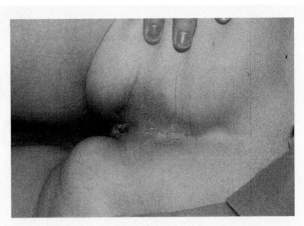

FIGURE 16-7: Inverse psoriasis with loss of scale forming nonspecific erythema in intergluteal cleft. Symmetric (probably not extramammary Paget's or Bowen's disease), without elevated border (probably not tinea), not with fine greasy scale (probably not seborrhea), and no satellite papules or pustules (probably not candida).

Note: Inverse psoriasis (Fig. 16-7) tends to be in intertriginous areas and just as with generalized exfoliative psoriasis the characteristic scale is lost and diagnosis may be difficult. Inverse psoriasis can mimic, or be seen in conjunction with, candidiasis, tinea cruris, seborrhea, and extramammary Paget's disease.

SAUER'S NOTES

Management of Psoriasis

1. Education and support are keys to the treatment of psoriasis. Give written information to the patient regarding the disease and potential treatment options. Carefully counsel patients as to the risks and benefits of their therapies. Encourage the patient to join the National Psoriasis Foundation, which provides comprehensive patient support.

2. Encourage the patient not to pick or scratch their skin or scalp. This can aggravate their psoriasis (Koebner phenomenon).

3. With the use of topical corticosteroids, observe closely for the development of striae and skin atrophy. Avoid high-potency steroids on the face and intertriginous areas.

4. When considering biologic or systemic therapy, patient selection is critical. Take a thorough medical history and review of systems.

5. Remain cognizant of the quality of life and emotional toll of psoriasis. Provide referrals for counseling when appropriate.

6. Psoriasis has been associated with comorbidities that include metabolic syndrome and increased cardiovascular risk. These entities share etiologic features and health outcomes that directly correlate with the severity of psoriatic disease. Therefore these considerations should be part of the evaluation and management of psoriasis patients. Appropriate counseling and/or referral should be made to address potential comorbidities.

Suggested Readings

Boehncke WH, Gladman DD, Chandran V. Cardiovascular comorbidities in psoriasis and psoriatic arthritis: pathogenesis, consequences for patient management, and future research agenda; a report from the GRAPPA 2009 annual meeting. *J Rheumatol*. 2011;38:567–571.

Feely MA, Smith BL, Weinberg JM. Novel psoriasis therapies and patient outcomes, part 1: topical medications. *Cutis*. 2015;95:164–170.

Feely MA, Smith BL, Weinberg JM. Novel psoriasis therapies and patient outcomes, part 2: biologic treatments. *Cutis*. 2015;95:282–290.

Feely MA, Smith BL, Weinberg JM. Novel psoriasis therapies and patient outcomes, part 3: systemic medications. *Cutis*. 2015;96:47–53.

Hugh J, Van Voorhees AS, Nijhawan RI, et al. From the Medical Board of the National Psoriasis Foundation: The risk of cardiovascular disease in individuals with psoriasis and the potential impact of current therapies. *J Am Acad Dermatol*. 2014;70(1):168–177. doi:10.1016/j.jaad.2013.09.020.

Krueger GG, Langley RG, Leonardi C, et al. A human interleukin-12/23 monoclonal antibody for the treatment of psoriasis. *N Engl J Med*. 2007;356:580–592.

Lebwohl M, Bagel J, Gelfand JM, et al. From the Medical Board of the National Psoriasis Foundation: monitoring and vaccinations in patients treated with biologics for psoriasis. *J Am Acad Dermatol*. 2008;58:94–105.

Menter A, Griffiths CE. Current and future management of psoriasis. *Lancet*. 2007;370:272–284.

Naldi L, Griffiths CE. Traditional therapies in the management of moderate to severe chronic plaque psoriasis: an assessment of the benefits and risks. *Br J Dermatol*. 2005;152:597–615.

Weinberg, JM. From the Medical Board of the National Psoriasis Foundation: the risk of cardiovascular disease in individuals with psoriasis and the potential impact of current therapies. *J Am Acad Dermatol*. 2014;70:168–177.

Weinberg, JM, Lebwohl, M, eds. *Advances in Psoriasis: A Multisystemic Guide*. London: Springer; 2014.

Other Papulosquamous Dermatoses

John C. Hall, MD

Papulosquamous eruptions, as indicated by the name, infer elevation and desquamation of the skin. Seborrhea (Chapter 15), the only one of these conditions with a greasy scale, and psoriasis (Chapter 16) are the most common. Most of these conditions are inflammatory, but tinea versicolor is included here due to the similarity of its clinical appearance to the other papulosquamous conditions. Lichen nitidus (see Dictionary–Index) and lichen striatus (see Dictionary–Index) are also considered in the category of papulosquamous skin diseases.

PITYRIASIS ROSEA

Pityriasis rosea is a moderately common papulosquamous eruption, mainly occurring on the trunks of young adults (Figs. 17-1 to 17-3). It is mildly pruritic and occurs most often in the spring and fall.

Presentation and Characteristics

Primary Lesions

Papulosquamous, oval erythematous discrete lesions are seen. A larger "herald patch" resembling a patch of "ringworm" may precede the general rash by 2 to 10 days. A collarette of fine scaling is seen around the edge of the lesions. It begins just inside the pink plaque.

Secondary Lesions

Excoriations are rare. Secondary lesions are the effect of overtreatment or contact dermatitis from topical treatment.

Distribution

The lesions appear mainly on the chest and trunk along Langer lines of cleavage in the skin. Many cases have the oval lesions in a "Christmas tree branches" pattern over the back. In atypical cases, the lesions are seen in the axillae and the groin only. This is sometimes referred to as *inverse pityriasis rosea of Vidal*. Facial lesions are rare in fair-skinned adults but are rather commonly seen in children and people of color.

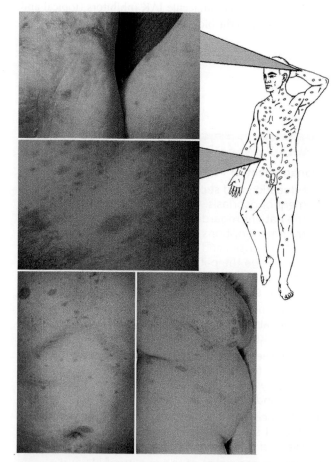

FIGURE 17-1: Pityriasis rosea. (Courtesy of Westwood Pharmaceuticals.)

Course

After the development of the herald patch, new generalized lesions continue to appear for 2 to 3 weeks. The entire rash most commonly disappears within 6 to 8 weeks. Recurrences are rare. There are recurrent and long-lasting variants.

Subjective Complaints

Itching varies from none to severe but is usually mild. Hot showers or baths may exacerbate the itching.

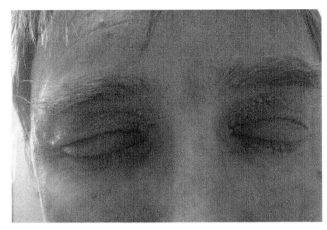

FIGURE 17-2: Severe seborrheic dermatitis of eyelids with swelling redness and greasy nonadherent scale.

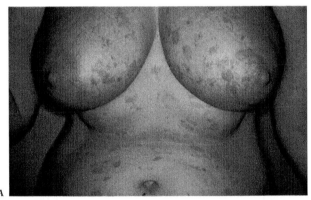

A

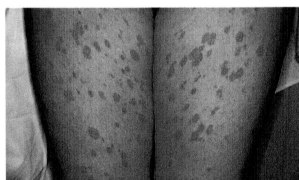

B

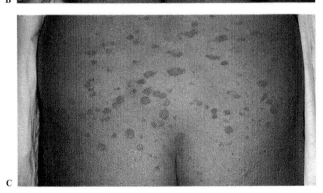

C

FIGURE 17-3: Pityriasis rosea of the chest **(A)**, thighs **(B)**, and buttocks **(C)** of one patient. (Courtesy of Syntex Laboratories, Inc.)

Cause

The cause is unknown. Some authors have incriminated human herpesvirus 6 (HHV-6) and human herpesvirus 7 (HHV-7).

Season

Spring and fall "epidemics" are common.

Age Group

Young adults and older children are most often affected.

Contagiousness

The disease is not contagious.

Differential Diagnosis

- *Tinea versicolor:* Lesions are tannish and irregularly shaped; fungi are seen on scraping and fine, dry, adherent scale becomes apparent when the physician scratches the area with the fingernail.
- *Drug eruption:* No herald patch; positive drug history for gold, bismuth, or sulfa (see Chapter 13).
- *Secondary syphilis:* No itching (99% true); history or presence of genital lesions; positive blood serology; palmar lesions present (see Chapter 29).
- *Psoriasis:* Usually on elbows, knees, and scalp; lesions have a thick, adherent, silvery-white scale.
- *Seborrheic dermatitis:* Greasy, irregular, scaly lesions on the sternum, central face, external auditory canals, scalp, between the buttocks, and on the genitalia (see Chapter 15).
- *Lichen planus:* Lesions are more papular and violaceous; found on the mucous membranes of the mouth and lip; very pruritic and common on flexor wrists.
- *Parapsoriasis:* Rare; chronic form may have fine "cigarette paper" atrophy; can develop into mycosis fungoides (cutaneous T-cell lymphoma [CTCL]).

Treatment

First Visit

1. Reassure the patient that he or she does not have a "blood disease," that the eruption is not contagious, and that it would be rare to get it again.
2. Colloidal bath
   Sig: Add 1 packet of Aveeno oatmeal preparation to the tub containing 6 to 8 in lukewarm water. Bathe for 10 to 15 minutes every day or every other day.
   Comment: Avoid soap and hot water as much as possible to reduce any itching.
3. Use nonalcoholic white shake lotion or Calamine lotion q.s. or any topical with pramoxine (Pramosone lotion, cream, or ointment and, over the counter, Sarna for sensitive skin, among many others)
   Sig: Apply b.i.d. locally to affected areas.
4. If there is itching, prescribe an antihistamine. Cyproheptadine (Periactin), 4 mg #60
   Sig: Take 1 tablet a.c. and h.s.

5. UVB therapy in increasing suberythema doses once or twice a week may be given. The severity is decreased, but itching and disease duration are probably not altered.

Subsequent Visits

1. If the skin becomes too dry from the colloidal bath and the lotion, stop the lotion or alternate it with
   Hydrocortisone cream or ointment, 1% q.s. 60.0
   Sig: Apply b.i.d. locally to dry areas.
2. Continue the ultraviolet treatments.

Severely Pruritic Cases

1. In addition to the above, add
   Prednisone, 5 mg #40
   Sig: Take 1 tablet q.i.d. for 3 days, 1 tablet t.i.d. for 4 days, and then 2 tablets every morning for 1 to 2 weeks, as symptoms of itching demand.
2. Some authors found that acyclovir, 800 mg five times a day for 1 week, early in the course of the disease helps to hasten resolution.

TINEA VERSICOLOR

Tinea versicolor is a moderately common skin eruption with tannish-colored, well-demarcated, circular, scaly patches that cause no discomfort and are usually located on the upper chest and back (Fig. 17-4). It is caused by a lipophilic yeast. Dry scaling can be revealed by stroking the skin with a fingernail (coup d'ongle).

Presentation and Characteristics

Primary Lesions

Papulosquamous or maculosquamous, tan, circular, well-demarcated lesions occur.

Secondary Lesions

Relative depigmentation results because the involved skin does not tan when exposed to sunlight. Skin not exposed to ultraviolet light is slightly hyperpigmented. The hypopigmentation cosmetic defect is obvious in the summer, since the yeast is a monoamine oxidase inhibitor and does not allow tanning, often brings the patient to the office. Hence the name versicolor (varied color).

Distribution

The upper part of the chest and the back, neck, and arms are affected. Rarely are the lesions on the face or generalized.

Course

The eruption can persist for years unnoticed. Correct treatment is readily effective, but the disease usually recurs.

Cause

The causative agent is a lipophilic yeast, *Pityrosporum orbiculare*, which has a hyphal form called *Pityrosporum* or *Malassezia furfur*. These yeasts have also been associated with seborrheic dermatitis and rarely sepsis.

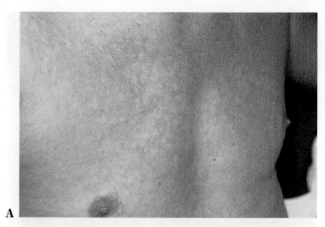
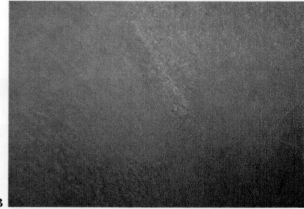

FIGURE 17-4: A: Tinea versicolor on the chest. The dark areas of the skin are the areas infected with the fungus. (Courtesy of K.U. M.C.; Sandoz Pharmaceuticals) **B:** Tinea versicolor on the back with faint pink areas that show fine dry adherent scale on scratching. This is called coup d'ongle or diagnosis with the fingernail.

SAUER'S NOTES

1. It is important to tell the patient that depigmented spots may remain after the tinea versicolor is cured. These can be tanned by gradual exposure to sunlight or ultraviolet light.
2. A topical imidazole cream (clotrimazole, econazole, ketoconazole, miconazole) twice a day topically for 2 weeks, with or without a sulfur soap, can be used. Terbinafine spray (Lamisil) twice a day for 1 week can also be used.
3. Ketoconazole (Nizoral) orally in various short-term regimens and itraconazole (Sporanox) 200 mg orally for 1 week have been used.

Contagiousness

The disease is not contagious and is not related to poor hygiene.

Laboratory Findings

A scraping of the scale placed on a microscopic slide, covered with a 20% solution of potassium hydroxide and a coverslip, shows the hyphae. Under the low-power lens of the microscope, very thin, short, mycelial filaments are seen. Diagnostic grapelike clusters of spores are seen best with the high-power lens. The appearance of spores and hyphae is referred to as "spaghetti and meatballs." The dimorphic organism does not grow on routine culture media.

Differential Diagnosis

- *Pityriasis rosea:* Acute onset; lesions oval with a collarette of fine, adherent, dry scale (see earlier in this chapter).
- *Seborrheic dermatitis:* Greasy scales mainly in hairy areas (see Chapter 15).
- *Mild psoriasis:* Thicker scaly lesions on the trunk and elsewhere (see Chapter 16).
- *Vitiligo:* Because tinea versicolor commonly manifests with hypopigmentation of the skin, many cases are misdiagnosed as vitiligo. This is indeed unfortunate because tinea versicolor is quite easy to treat and has a much better prognosis than vitiligo (see Chapter 40). There is no pigment (depigmentation) in vitiligo and decreased pigment (hypopigmentation) in tinea versicolor. There are no scales in vitiligo.
- *Secondary syphilis:* Lesions are more widely distributed and present on the palms and soles (see Chapter 25).

SAUER'S NOTES

If the pityriasis rosea-like rash does not itch, obtain blood serologic test for syphilis if you have any uncertainty about the diagnosis and especially if palm and sole lesions are present with adenopathy.

Treatment

1. Selenium (Selsun or Head & Shoulders intensive treatment) suspension 120.0
   Sig: Bathe and dry completely. Then apply medicine as a lotion to all the involved areas, usually from the neck down to the pubic area. Let it dry. Bathe again in 24 hours and wash off the medicine. Repeat the procedure again at weekly intervals for four treatments. This can be irritating.

2. Topical imidazole creams such as miconazole (available over the counter), ketoconazole (available over the counter), clotrimazole (available over the counter), econazole (Spectazole), and oxiconazole (Oxistat) twice a day for 2 weeks. Compounding 2% to 5% sulfur may add to the efficacy.

3. If lesions are extensive, 200 mg of ketoconazole orally twice a day for 5 days to cause a remission and on the first day of each month for 6 months beginning April 1 can be used to prevent summer recurrences, which are common in warm, humid climates.
   Comment: Recurrences are rather common and can be easily retreated.

LICHEN PLANUS

Lichen planus is an uncommon, chronic, pruritic disease characterized by violaceous flat-topped papules that are usually seen on the wrists and the legs (Figs. 17-5 to 17-8; see also Fig. 3-1B). The 5 "Ps" are pruritic, polygonal, planar, purple, and papules. If you would like to make it 6, you could add persistent. Mucous membrane lesions on the cheeks or

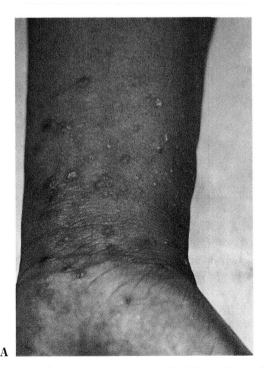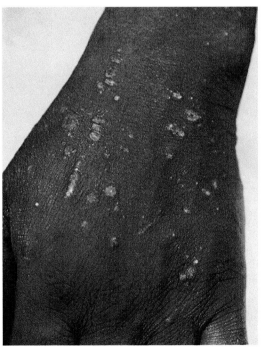

A   **B**

FIGURE 17-5: Lichen planus on the wrist **(A)** and the dorsum of the hand **(B)** in an African-American patient. Note the violaceous color of the papules and the linear Koebner phenomenon on the dorsum of the hand. (Courtesy of E.R. Squibb.)

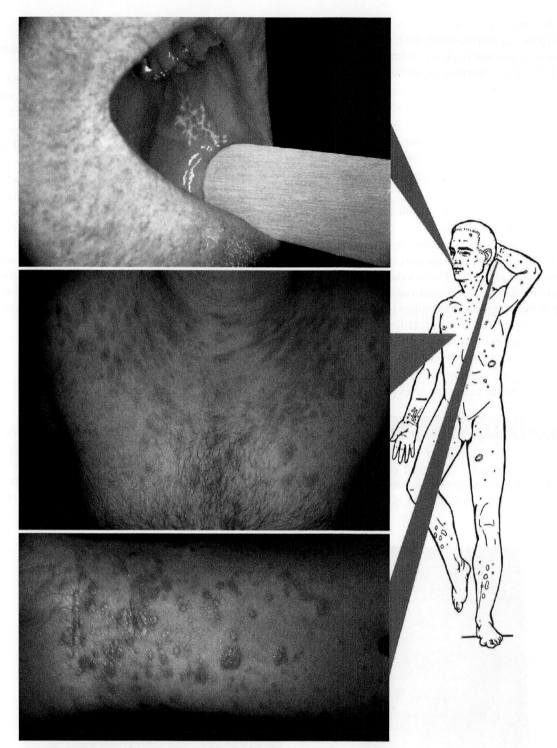

FIGURE 17-6: Lichen planus. (Courtesy of Johnson & Johnson.)

lips are milky white and netlike. Erosions and ulcers on oral mucous membranes are seen in more severe disease, which can make eating and dental hygiene difficult.

Presentation and Characteristics

Primary Lesions

Flat-topped, violaceous papules, and papulosquamous lesions appear. On close examination of a papule, preferably after the lesion has been wet with an alcohol swipe, intersecting small white lines or papules (Wickham striae) can be seen. These confirm the diagnosis. Uncommonly, the lesions may assume a ring-shaped configuration (especially on the penis) or may be hypertrophic (especially pretibial), atrophic, or bullous. On the mucous membranes, the lesions appear as a whitish, lacy network. When mucous membrane involvement is severe, ulcerations may occur and there is an increased occurrence of squamous cell cancer. There is a severe ulcerative form that can occur in the vulvovaginal and rectal area in women and on the soles of the feet in both sexes.

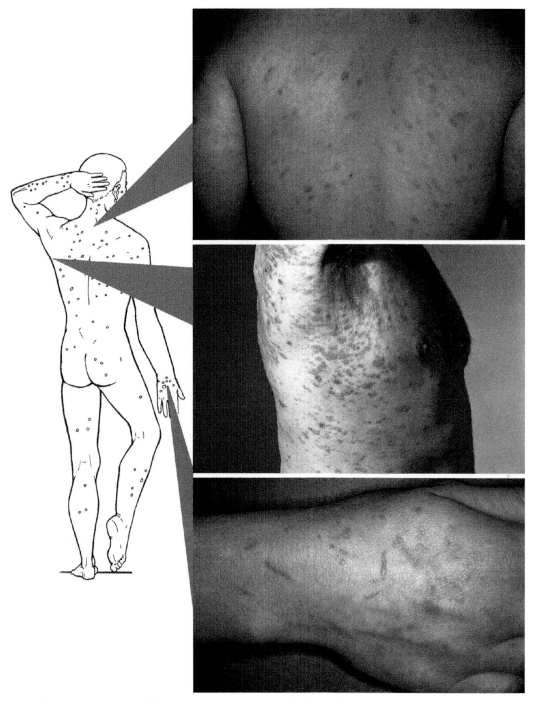

FIGURE 17-7: Lichen planus. Note the Koebner reaction in the lower photograph.

Secondary Lesions

Excoriations and, on the legs, thick, scaly, lichenified patches have been noted. Lesions are often rubbed rather than scratched because scratching is painful.

Distribution

Most commonly, the lesions appear on the flexural aspects of the wrists and the ankles, the penis, and the oral mucous membranes, but they can be anywhere on the body or become generalized.

Course

Outbreak is rather sudden, with the chronic course averaging 9 months in duration. Some cases last several years. There is no effect on the general health except for itching. Recurrences are moderately common (approximately 20%).

Cause

The cause is unknown. The disorder is rather frequently associated with nervous or emotional upsets. It may represent an autoimmune process, and some cases have a distinct pattern

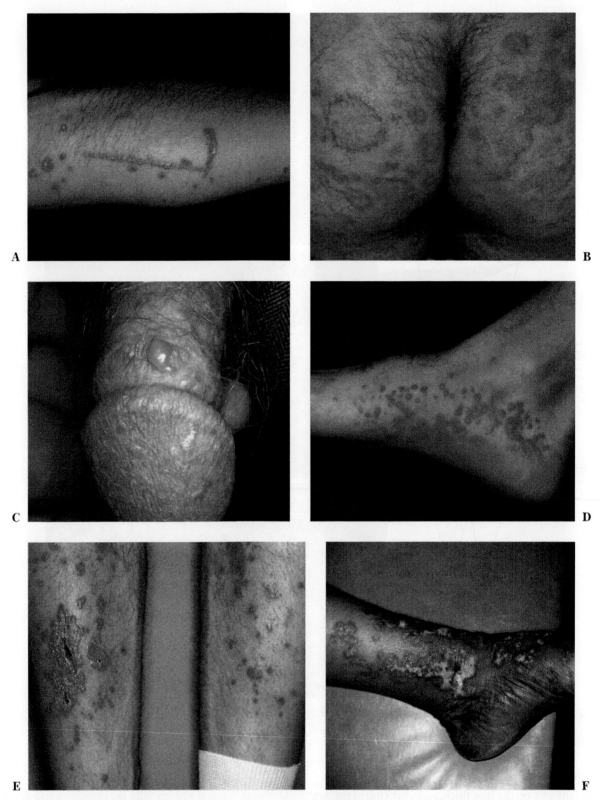

FIGURE 17-8: Lichen planus, unusual variations. **A:** Koebner reaction in scratched areas on the arm. **B:** Atrophic scarring lesions on the buttocks. **C:** Bullous and vesicular lesions on the penis. **D:** Lichen planus on the sole of the foot. **E:** Hypertrophic lesions on the anterior tibial area of the legs. **F:** Hypertrophic lesions on the leg of an African-American woman. (Courtesy of Neutrogena Corp.)

on direct immunofluorescence. Hepatitis C or hepatitis B is present in some cases (possibly up to 20%). This is more common when associated with HIV. There is a rare form flared by the sun (lichen planus actinicus).

Subjective Complaints

Itching varies from mild to severe (severe is more common).

Contagiousness

Lichen planus is not contagious.

Relation to Employment

As in psoriasis, the lichen planus lesions can develop in scratches or skin injuries (Koebner phenomenon).

Laboratory Findings

Microscopic section is quite characteristic.

Differential Diagnosis

- *Secondary syphilis:* No itching; blood serology positive (see Chapter 25).
- *Drug eruption:* History of taking atabrine, arsenic, or gold (see Chapter 13).
- *Psoriasis:* Lesions are more scaly, whitish on the knees and elbows (see Chapter 16).
- *Pityriasis rosea:* Herald patch mainly on the trunk (seen earlier in this chapter).

Lichen planus on the leg may resemble neurodermatitis (usually one patch only; intensely pruritic; no mucous membrane lesions; excoriations; see Chapter 13) or keloids (secondary to injury with no Wickham striae).

Treatment

Case Example: A patient presents with generalized papular eruption and moderate itching.

First Visit

1. Assure the patient that the disease is not contagious, is not a blood disease, and is chronic but not serious. Explain that a hepatitis screen is necessary, since up to 20% of patients may have hepatitis B or hepatitis C.
2. Tell the patient to avoid excess bathing with soap.
3. Suggest a low-potency corticosteroid cream 60.0
   Sig: Apply locally b.i.d.
4. Recommend an over-the-counter antihistamine such as chlorpheniramine, 4 mg #60
   Sig: Take 1 tablet b.i.d. for itching.
   Comment: Warn the patient of drowsiness at the onset of therapy.

Subsequent Visits

1. Occlusive dressing with corticosteroid therapy. This is quite effective for localized cases. I have also found that if occlusive dressings are applied only to the lichen planus on the legs, the rest of the body lesions improve.
2. Meprobamate, 400 mg #100
   Sig: Take 1 tablet t.i.d., *or*
   Chlordiazepoxide (Librium), 5 mg
   Sig: Take 1 tablet t.i.d.
3. It is important in some resistant cases to rule out a focus of infection in teeth, tonsils, gallbladder, genitourinary system, and so on.
4. Corticosteroids orally or by injection are of definite value for temporarily relieving the acute cases that have severe itching or a generalized eruption.
5. Intralesional corticosteroids, especially for localized hypertrophic disease. I use this for oral mucous membrane, vulvovaginal, and rectal disease also.
6. Griseofulvin on rare occasions can decrease disease severity.
7. Treating hepatitis when present can benefit the disease (specifically hepatitis C).
8. Hydroxychloroquine sulfate (Plaquenil) orally can sometimes be helpful. See an ophthalmologist every 6 months to check for retinal toxicity.
9. Topical 0.1% pimecrolimus (Tacrolimus) t.i.d. has shown moderate benefit in one study.
10. Sulfasalazine (500 mg b.i.d.) has been used with success by some authors.
11. High-dose curcuminoids (Turmeric) and ultraviolet B phototherapy have both been used to treat oral lichen planus.

Suggested Readings

Boyd AS, Neldner KH. Lichen planus. *J Am Acad Dermatol.* 1991;25:593–619.

Cribier B, Frances C, Chosidow O. Treatment of lichen planus. *Arch Dermatol.* 1998;134:1521–1530.

Drago F, Broccolo F, Rebora A. Pityriasis rosea: an update with a critical appraisal of its possible herpesviral etiology. *J Am Acad Dermatol.* 2009;61(2):303–318.

Eisen D. The clinical features, malignant potential, and systemic association of oral lichen planus: a study of 723 patients. *J Am Acad Dermatol.* 2002;46:207–214.

Fox BJ, Odom RB. Papulosquamous diseases: a review. *J Am Acad Dermatol.* 1985;12:597–624.

Gonzalez LM, Allen R, Janniger CK, et al. Pityriasis rosea: an important papulosquamous disorder. *Int J Dermatol.* 2005;44:757–764.

Le Cleach L, Chosidow O. Lichen planus. *N Eng J Med.* 2012;366(8):723–732.

Sunenshine PJ, Schwartz RA, Janniger CK. Tinea versicolor. *Int J Dermatol.* 1998;37:648–655.

Granulomatous Dermatoses

John C. Hall, MD

When considered individually, granulomatous diseases are uncommon, but when all of them are considered together, they form a group that is interesting, varied, and ubiquitous.

A *granuloma* is a focal chronic inflammatory response to tissue injury manifested by a histologic picture of accumulation and proliferation of leukocytes, principally of the mononuclear type and its family of derivatives, the mononuclear phagocyte system. The immunologic components in granulomatous inflammation originate from cell-mediated or cell-delayed hypersensitivity mechanisms controlled by thymus-dependent lymphocytes (T-lymphocytes). Five groups of granulomatous inflammations have been promulgated:

- Group 1 is the *epithelioid granulomas*, which include sarcoidosis, tuberculosis in certain forms, tuberculoid leprosy, tertiary syphilis, zirconium granuloma, beryllium granuloma, mercurial granuloma, and lichen nitidus.
- Group 2, *histiocytic granulomas*, includes lepromatous leprosy, histoplasmosis, and leishmaniasis.

- Group 3 is the group of *foreign body granulomas*, including endogenous products (e.g., hair, fat, keratin), minerals (e.g., tattoos, silica, talc), plant and animal products (e.g., cactus, suture, oil, insect parts), and synthetic agents such as synthetic hair and filler substances.
- Group 4 is the *necrobiotic/palisading granulomas*, such as granuloma annulare, necrobiosis lipoidica, rheumatoid nodule, rheumatic fever nodule, cat-scratch disease, and lymphogranuloma venereum.
- Group 5 is the *mixed inflammatory granulomas*, including many deep fungal infections, such as blastomycosis and sporotrichosis, mycobacterial infections, granuloma inguinale, and chronic granulomatous disease.

Most of these diseases are discussed with their appropriate etiologic classifications in the Dictionary–Index. Two of these granulomatous inflammations *sarcoidosis*, group 1, and *granuloma annulare*, group 4, are discussed in this chapter. A classification of granulomas based on etiology is listed in Table 18-1.

TABLE 18-1 • Granulomatous Diseases of the Skin by Etiology	
Infectious	
Deep fungal	Coccidioidomycosis, paracoccidioidomycosis (South American blastomycosis), blastomycosis (North American blastomycosis), histoplasmosis, sporotrichosis, Majocchi granuloma (deep dermatophyte infection)
Bacterial	Tuberculosis, leprosy, atypical mycobacteria, tertiary syphilis, granuloma inguinale, lymphogranuloma venereum, cat-scratch disease
Parasitic	Leishmaniasis
Noninfectious	
Diagnosis	*Etiology*
Necrobiosis lipoidica diabeticorum	Five out of six patients will have or acquire diabetes
Granuloma annulare	Generalized form may be associated with diabetes
Granulomatosis with polyangiitis (formerly Wegener granulomatosis)	Granulomatous vasculitis with renal, lung, and other internal organ involvement
Rheumatoid nodule	Rheumatoid arthritis
Lymphomatoid granulomatosis	Angiocentric lymphoma especially with lung involvement but also renal, skin, and central nervous system involvement

TABLE 18-1 • Granulomatous Diseases of the Skin by Etiology (continued)

Chronic granulomatous disease	Defect of phagocyte NADPH oxidase, which leads to inability to destroy organisms after phagocytosis. Infections with bacteria and fungi occur in skin, lungs, bones, and joints, and sepsis is common
Foreign body granuloma	Many causative agents (see earlier in the chapter)
Granulomatous rosacea	Deep form of rosacea
Granulomatous perioral dermatitis	Deep form of perioral dermatitis
Crohn disease	Inflammatory bowel disease that can rarely involve the skin
Eosinophilic granulomatosis with polyangiitis (formerly Churg–Strauss disease)	Asthma, eosinophilia, and vasculitis in the skin as well as respiratory tract, kidney, gastrointestinal tract, heart, and nerves

SARCOIDOSIS

Sarcoidosis is an uncommon systemic granulomatous disease of unknown cause that affects the skin, lungs, lymph nodes, liver, spleen, parotid glands, and eyes. Less commonly involved organs that indicate more severe disease include the central nervous system, heart, bones, and upper respiratory tract. Any or all of these organs may be involved with sarcoidal granulomas. Lymphadenopathy is the single most common finding. People of color are affected more often than white patients (14:1). Only the skin manifestations of sarcoidosis are discussed here (Fig. 18-1).

Presentation and Characteristics

Primary Lesions

Cutaneous sarcoidosis is a great mimicker of other skin diseases. Superficial lesions consist of reddish papules, apple-jelly colored nodules, and plaques that may be multiple or solitary and of varying size and configuration. Annular forms of skin sarcoidosis are common. These superficial lesions usually involve the face, shoulders, and arms. Infiltration of sarcoidal lesions frequently occurs at scar sites. Subcutaneous nodular forms and telangiectatic, ulcerative, erythrodermic, and ichthyosiform types are rare. Sarcoidosis is often associated with a chronic systemic disease.

Secondary Lesions

Central healing can result in atrophy and scarring.

Course

Most cases of sarcoidosis run a chronic but benign course with remissions and exacerbations. Spontaneous "cure" is not unusual. Erythema nodosum is characteristic of acute benign sarcoidosis (see Chapter 13). Lupus pernio (indurated violaceous lesions on the ears, nose, lips, cheeks, and forehead) and plaques are characteristic of chronic, severe, systemic disease. It is seen most often in women and girls of color.

Causes

The cause of sarcoidosis is unknown.

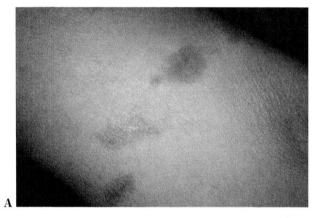

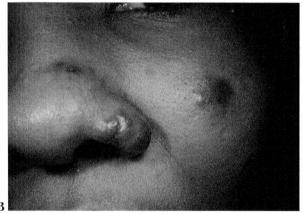

FIGURE 18-1: **A:** Apple jelly red, smooth plaques on the upper leg. Well demarcated and asymptomatic, thus no excoriations or lichenification. **B:** Reddish-brown nodules over the face without ulcerations or excoriations in a person of color.

Laboratory Findings

The histopathologic appearance of sarcoidosis is quite characteristic and consists of epithelioid cells surrounded by Langerhans' giant cells, CD4 lymphocytes, some CD8 lymphocytes, and mature macrophages. No acid-fast bacilli are found, and caseous necrosis is absent. The Kveim test, using sarcoidal lymph node tissue, is positive after several weeks. This is no longer used. Tuberculin-type, candida, and other skin tests are negative (anergic). The total blood serum protein is high and ranges from 7.5 to 10.0 g/dL, mainly because of an increase in the globulin fraction.

Angiotensin-converting enzyme deficiency may be noted.

Differential Diagnosis

- *Other granulomatous diseases:* These can be ruled out by biopsy, culture, and other appropriate studies.
- *Silica granulomas:* Histologically similar; a history of such injury can usually be obtained.

Treatment

For localized skin disease, intralesional corticosteroids (4 to 8 mg/mL triamcinolone) are the treatment of choice at 1- to 2-month intervals. Time appears to cure or cause remission of most cases of sarcoidosis, but corticosteroids and immunosuppressant drugs may be indicated for extensive cases, especially the ones involving the lung, joints, or eye. Hydroxychloroquine and methotrexate may be beneficial. Anecdotal use of allopurinol has been reported. Doxycycline (100 mg b.i.d.) or minocycline (100 mg b.i.d.) has shown benefit in some studies. Other therapies showing some promise are pentoxifylline, isotretinoin, leflunomide, infliximab, and laser.

GRANULOMA ANNULARE

Granuloma annulare is a moderately common skin problem. The usually encountered ring-shaped, red-bordered lesion is often mistaken for ringworm by inexperienced examiners (Fig. 18-2), but there is no scaling. Several clinical variations exist. The two most common are the *localized form* and the *generalized form.* There is also an annular form often seen on the tongue and glans of the penis, a rare linear form, a subcutaneous deep form, a papular variety, and a perforating form mimicking a perforating folliculitis. Some authors have described a subtle patch-type of disease, which is very rare.

Women and girls with granuloma annulare predominate over men and boys in a ratio of 2.5 to 1. No ages are exempt, but the localized form is usually seen in patients in the first three decades of life and the generalized form in patients in the fourth through seventh decades. A granuloma annulare–like eruption has been reported in HIV-positive and chronic Epstein–Barr virus positive patients.

Presentation and Characteristics

Primary Lesions

In both the localized and generalized forms, the lesion is a red, asymptomatic papule with no scaling. The papule may be solitary. Most frequently, the lesion assumes a ring-shaped or arcuate configuration of papules that tend to enlarge centrifugally. Rarely are the rings over 5 cm in diameter. In the localized form of granuloma annulare, the lesions appear mainly over the joints on the hands, arms, feet, and legs. In the much less common generalized form, there may be hundreds of the red

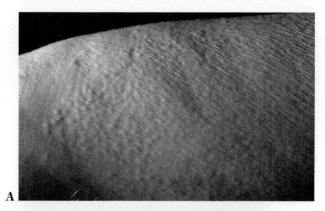

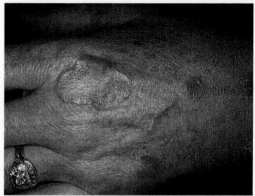

FIGURE 18-2: **A:** Generalized granuloma annulare on the upper proximal to the elbow. Monotonous light pink papules symmetrically cover the trunk and extremities. **B:** Granuloma annulare on the dorsum of the hand. (Courtesy of Hoechst-Roussel Pharmaceuticals Inc.)

or tan papular circinate lesions on the extremities and on the trunk. This is the most common form in HIV-positive patients. Diabetes may be increased in this form.

Secondary Lesions

On healing, the red color turns to brown before the lesions disappear.

Course

Both forms of granuloma annulare can resolve spontaneously after one to several years, but the generalized form is more long lasting. It does not lead to scar formation.

Dyslipidemia may be associated with granuloma annulare particularly in the generalized form.

Causes

The cause is unknown. An immune-complex vasculitis, cell-mediated immunity, and trauma have all been proposed as factors in the disease.

Laboratory Findings

The histopathologic appearance of granuloma annulare is quite characteristic. The middle and upper dermis have focal areas of altered collagenous connective tissue surrounded by an infiltrate of histiocytic cells and lymphocytes. In some cases, these cells infiltrate between the collagen bundles, giving a palisading effect. *Necrobiosis* has been used to describe these changes.

Differential Diagnosis

- *Tinea corporis:* Usually itches and has a scaly red border; the fungus can be demonstrated with a potassium hydroxide scraping or culture (see Chapter 28).
- *Lichen planus, annular form:* Characterized by violaceous flat-topped papules with Wickham striae. Mucous membrane lesions are also often seen.
- *Secondary syphilis:* Can be clinically similar but has a positive serology (see Chapter 25).
- *Other granulomatous diseases:* Can usually be distinguished by biopsy.

There is a subcutaneous form of granuloma annulare that is difficult to distinguish histologically from a rheumatoid nodule or a soft tissue tumor.

Treatment

Localized Form

Some cases respond to the application of a corticosteroid cream for 8 hours overnight with an occlusive dressing such as Saran wrap. Intralesional corticosteroids are effective for cases with only a few lesions. Light liquid nitrogen therapy is sometimes beneficial.

Generalized Form

Numerous remedies have been tried with only anecdotal benefit. Dapsone and hydroxychloroquine have also been used.

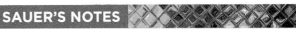

SAUER'S NOTES

1. Biopsy tissue usually needs to be obtained to differentiate between the different granulomatous skin diseases.
2. When trying to distinguish between granulomatous skin diseases, the biopsy must be deep enough to provide an adequate interpretation. A punch or ellipse biopsy, rather than a shave biopsy, needs to be done.
3. Culture for bacteria, acid-fast bacteria, and deep fungi should be done by submitting a portion of the harvested material in sterile saline for culture. If a viral etiology is considered, then a portion of tissue should be collected in viral culture media. This is important since organisms may be sparse in tissue even with appropriate staining and a superficial culture from a swab or skin scraping may be falsely negative.

Suggested Readings

Bagwell C, Rosen T. Cutaneous sarcoid therapy updated. *J Am Acad Dermatol.* 2007;56:69–83.

English JC, Patel PJ, Greer KE. Sarcoidosis. *J Am Acad Dermatol.* 2001;44:725–743.

Haimovic A, Sanchez M, Judson MA, et al. Sarcoidosis: a comprehensive review and update for the dermatologist part I and II. *J Am Acad Dermatol.* 2012;66:699–728.

Hirsh BC, Johnson WC. Concepts of granulomatous inflammation. *Int J Dermatol.* 1984;23:90–100.

Iannuzzi, MC. Sarcoidosis. *N Engl J Med.* 2007;357:2153–2165.

Newman LS, Rose CS, Maier LA. Sarcoidosis. *N Engl J Med.* 1997;336:1224–1234.

Smith MD, Downie JB, DiCostanzo D. Granuloma annulare. *Int J Dermatol.* 1997;36:326–333.

Young RJ, Gilson RT, Yanase D. Cutaneous sarcoidosis. *Int J Dermatol.* 2001;40:249–253.

Urticaria

Saquib R. Ahmed, MD Matthew Dacunha, BS and Anand Rajpara, MD

URTICARIA, ANGIOEDEMA, ANAPHYLAXIS

"Urticaria" comes from the Latin words "Urtica" (nettle) and "Urere" (to burn). Urticaria (Fig. 19-1) is a common skin finding that 15% to 25% of individuals will experience at least once in their lifetime. Urticaria appears as edematous, ill-defined papules that may coalesce into plaques. Generally, lesions are itchy and do not last more than 24 hours at one location. Urticaria can be divided into acute and chronic forms, with the latter being defined as near daily symptoms for more than 6 weeks. Additionally, if a lesion lasts more than 24 hours, urticarial vasculitis is added to the differential diagnosis. Angioedema is a variation of urticaria where the swelling is deeper in the subcutaneous area. Part of anaphylaxis can be obstruction of the airway by angioedema with life-threatening consequences.

Pathogenesis

The mast cell is central to understanding the development and treatment of urticaria. Mast cells are derived from myeloid stem cells and are a type of granulocyte. These granules contain many important preformed enzymes, such as histamine and heparin, and are also capable of synthesis of other cell mediators, such as platelet-activating factor, prostaglandin D2, leukotriene C4, D4, and E4. The release and synthesis of these mediators can vary depending on the stimulus. In urticaria, histamine from mast cells is the major mediator of the condition.

Mast cells contain receptors for IgE and can degranulate by allergen crosslinking due to IgE antibody binding. Activation via IgE requires prior exposure and sensitization to the antigen.

There is also complement-mediated activation of mast cells. In complement-mediated urticaria, immune complexes activate the complement cascade causing the release of anaphylatoxins. Anaphylatoxins can then induce mast cell degranulation.

Some drugs are capable of directly activating mast cells, including: opiates, vancomycin, radiocontrast, and nonsteroidal anti-inflammatory agents (NSAIDS).

The mediators released from mast cells (Table 19-1) can cause vasodilation and increase permeability near the postcapillary venule leading to protein extravasation. Increase in protein extravasation decreases venule oncotic pressure, resulting in tissue edema. Mediators also result in the upregulation of adhesion molecules that allow for inflammatory cells to concentrate in these areas. Increased inflammation results in increased venule permeability and thus increased edema. Localized swelling is the result. Areas of edema that are localized in the superficial portion of the dermis are known as urticaria, whereas edema extending to the deep dermis or subcutaneous layers is known as angioedema (Fig. 19-2). Angioedema most often occurs in soft tissues (eyelids, lips, and genital area), however, urticaria or angioedema may occur simultaneously at one place or in any other location (including the palms and soles, where the patients may feel pain instead of itch). The lesions of urticaria arise through the triple response. The triple response occurs through vasodilation, increase in vascular permeability, and an axon reflex. The axon reflex occurs from sensory nerve fibers releasing substance P. Substance P is a vasodilator and can cause further release of histamine from mast cells.

FIGURE 19-1: Typical wheals of urticaria with elevated edematous erythematous plaques.

TABLE 19-1 • Various Types of Pathogenic Immune Reactions Manifesting on the Skin	
Direct Mediators/ Vasodilators	Indirect Mediators/ Vasodilators
Histamine Prostaglandin D2	Substance P Anaphylatoxins (C3a, C4a, and C5a)
Leukotriene C4 and D4	Histamine-releasing factors
Platelet-activating factor Bradykinin	

infections, antibiotics, or alimentary agents. Complement-mediated serum sickness–like reactions can also result in acute urticaria. Acute urticaria most commonly affects children.

Chronic Urticaria

Wheals can be either small or large. Chronic urticaria is rarely IgE-dependent. It is often due to anti-FcεR autoantibodies (autoimmune) or idiopathic causes. Clinically, patients with chronic urticaria due to anti-FcSymbol StdR autoantibodies are indistinguishable from those that are IgE-dependent. Etiology of chronic urticaria is unknown in 80% of cases and is therefore typically idiopathic. Emotional stress and hot showers, however, are often seen as exacerbating factors. Chronic urticaria predominantly affects adults and is more commonly seen in women than men.

Other Etiologic Types of Urticaria and Angioedema

Physical Urticaria Dermographism

Scratching and abrasions on the skin result in linear urticarial lesions which are pruritic. The lesions arise within minutes and fade in about 30 minutes (Fig. 19-3).

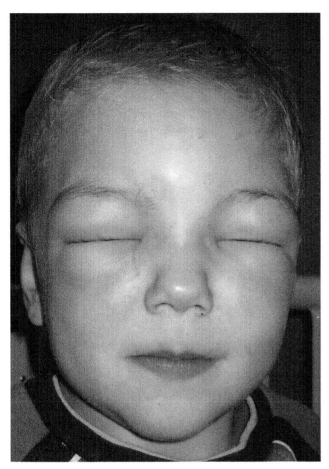

FIGURE 19-2: Swelling of the cheeks and periocular tissue illustrative of angioedema.

Additionally, there are several types of physically induced urticarias including vibratory, pressure, solar, cholinergic, contact, and cold-induced urticaria. It is not fully understood how these physical stimuli lead to mast cell activation and histamine release resulting in urticaria.

Urticaria can be classified into acute (wheals occurring over a period of less than 6 weeks) and chronic (wheals appearing over a period longer than 6 weeks), which can be either intermittent or chronically relapsing with wheals appearing almost every day.

Acute urticaria is most common in children and is often associated with acute viral infection but can also be due to allergies or a drug reaction. Episodes of urticaria lasting greater than 6 weeks are considered chronic and are most likely idiopathic or autoimmune. Triggering factors can be either allergens or infectious diseases of internal organs. Additives in foods can give rise to allergic-type reaction in a subgroup of chronic urticaria patients.

Clinical Types of Urticaria

Acute Urticaria

Wheals tend to be superficial, edematous, and itchy. Acute urticaria is often IgE-dependent and is usually triggered by viral

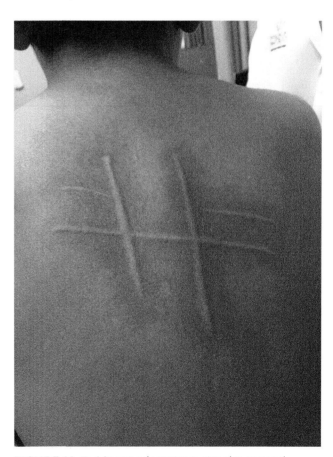

FIGURE 19-3: Linear edematous streaks caused from external scratching of the skin illustrative of dermatographism.

Cold Urticaria/Angioedema

Cold urticaria may be either acquired or inherited, but the acquired form is more common. Acquired cold urticaria may be associated with headache, hypotension, wheezing, syncope, dyspnea, nausea, and diarrhea. In cold urticaria changes in surrounding temperatures and/or contact with cold objects cause an attack of urticaria within minutes. A diagnostic "cold-contact test" can be done via application of ice. Development of a wheal after the ice application would be a positive cold-contact test result. Whealing in cold urticaria typically occurs 2 minutes after exposure upon rewarming. Large hives appear at around 10 minutes. The delay in lesion formation is believed to be due to decreased cutaneous blood flow during the cold exposure. If the entire body is cooled, hypotension and syncope may occur. This puts patients with cold-induced urticaria at risk of drowning.

Cholinergic Urticaria

Cholinergic urticaria has a distinct phenotype presenting with monomorphic, small, punctate papules with a prominent erythematous flare. Lesions may coalesce over time and are stimulated by sweat-inducing stimuli. Such stimuli may include but are not limited to sweat-provoking exercise, hot baths/showers, and outdoor activities. Other known stimuli include drinking alcohol and eating spicy foods. Cholinergic Urticaria is more commonly seen in young adults and rarely in older individuals. In cases of severe exercise–induced cholinergic urticaria, anaphylaxis may develop.

Exercise-Induced Anaphylaxis

Though severe exercise–induced cholinergic urticaria can cause anaphylaxis, exercise-induced anaphylaxis is considered a condition of its own. Exercise-induced anaphylaxis is stimulated by exercise, but not by other means of increasing core temperature such as hot baths. The difference in stimuli can be used to differentiate between exercise-induced anaphylaxis and cholinergic urticaria.

Solar Urticaria

Exposures to UV or visible solar wavelengths induce urticaria with the classic urticarial pruritus and whealing. Different patients do not necessarily react to the same solar wavelengths.

Hereditary Angioedema

Angioedema occurs when the swelling is deeper in the dermis and subcutaneous tissue. Phenotypically, the overlying skin may look distorted. Patients will often complain more about pain than itching. Angioedema can frequently accompany urticaria, but when angioedema occurs by itself the differentia included hereditary angioedema, acquired angioedema, and drug-induced angioedema.

Hereditary angioedema (HAE) occurs in three types. HAE types 1 and 2 refer to inherited C1 esterase inhibitor (C1EI) deficiencies. The C1EI normally prevents a part of the complement cascade from releasing bradykinin. Bradykinin leads to increases in vascular permeability. Screening test for hereditary angioedema will show a low C4. HAE type-I patients are shown to have both low C1EI protein levels and low C1EI functional levels.

Type 2 patients have dysfunctional C1EI in either normal or elevated amounts.

In HAE type 3, individuals have a heterozygous gain-of-function mutation in factor 12 leading to elevated levels of bradykinin. Compared to types 1 and 2, HAE type 3 has a later age of onset and a higher frequency of facial angioedema.

Drug-Induced Angioedema

Many drugs are able to induce angioedema with the most common drugs being NSAIDs and angiotensin-converting enzyme (ACE) inhibitors. ACE inhibitors may be overlooked as a probable cause of angioedema in some patients because angioedema may take over a year to present after the administration of ACE inhibitors.

Acquired Angioedema

Some lymphomas and leukemias may also lead to acquired C1EI deficiencies. Antibodies may form against C1EI or to immune complexes consuming C1q.

Diagnosis

Urticaria is primarily a clinical diagnosis via history and physical examination.

An accurate history is crucial to the diagnosis of urticaria. Patients will report intermittent itchy skin lesions with complete resolution of any individual lesion in a day or two. Since there are many different possible triggers for urticaria, a very detailed history should be taken with a focus on new medications, new foods, recent infections, history of autoimmune disease, and physical factors. Table 19-2 shows common causes of both acute and chronic urticaria.

Physical examination should show several circumscribed, erythematous, and pruritic papules. Wheals and edematous plaques may be either erythematous or skin-colored with a surrounding erythematous halo. Lesions may be localized, regional, or generalized. Angioedema may be present in various locations due to subcutaneous edema.

In some forms of urticaria, there may also be a presentation of fever, such as in cases of viral infection or serum sickness.

TABLE 19-2 • Common Causes of Acute and Chronic Urticaria

Acute	Chronic
Idiopathic ~50%	Idiopathic ~33%
Viral infections ~40%	Autoimmune ~33%
Medications	Physical
Contact dermatitis	Urticarial vasculitis
Transfusion reactions	Infections
Food	

For acute urticaria, a biopsy may show subcutaneous edema, and dilation of vessels. Degranulated mast cells and activated T-helper cells may also be present.

Differential Diagnosis

Arthropod bites, urticarial vasculitis, urticarial bullous pemphigoid, adverse drug reactions, and urticarial contact dermatitis.

Autoantibodies against IgE or the high-affinity IgE receptor have been found that lead to mast cell degranulation; this phenomenon can be shown in the autologous serum test when a wheal develops after injection of a 1/10 dilution of autologous serum (Greaves test). Another subgroup of chronic urticaria when the wheals persist over several days shows leukocytoclastic vasculitis upon histopathologic analysis and is called urticarial vasculitis.

Management

The ideal form of management would be to prevent attacks by eliminating the urticarial trigger (medications, foods, physical factors, etc.). A specific culprit can be difficult to identify, however, and treatment through prevention is not always successful.

Antihistamines are the drugs of choice; sedating antihistamines such as diphenhydramine or hydroxyzine can be given overnight, sometimes also having a beneficial effect on underlying stress reactions with psychosomatic involvement.

During the day, the second generation nonsedating histamine H_1 antagonists may be useful. When urticaria recurs, an allergy workup or workup for an underlying infection may be beneficial. Psychosomatic counseling often is helpful in chronic urticaria. A subgroup of physical urticaria where wheals are induced by mechanical stimuli (pressure), temperature (cold or warm), or radiation (solar urticaria) is difficult to treat.

Contact urticaria is related to a contactant the patient is allergic to, inducing a typical urticarial reaction at the site where the skin touches the allergen.

Urticaria and angioedema may not always be the first signs of anaphylaxis. Patients with acute, severe urticaria can be treated with IV or IM antihistamines as well as steroids. Patients should be observed at least 1 hour after the onset of therapy to make sure that no further symptoms or anaphylaxis develop. Subcutaneous epinephrine such as an EpiPen can be lifesaving.

Suggested Readings

Andrews

Thomas Bieber et al. *Atopic Dermatitis.* 2nd ed.

Bolognia

Fitzpatrick

Jain

make sure the most recent Litt's drug eruption reference manual is listed

Urticaria and Angioedema. 2nd ed. In: Caplan AP, ed.

Dermatologic Parasitology

John C. Hall, MD

Dermatologic parasitology is an extensive subject and includes the dermatoses caused by three main groups of organisms: protozoa, helminthes, and arthropods.

- The *protozoal dermatoses* are exemplified by various forms of trypanosomiases and leishmaniases (see Chapter 50).
- *Helminthic dermatoses* include those due to round-worms (ground itch, creeping eruption, filariasis, and other rare tropical diseases) and those due to flatworms (schistosomiasis, swimmer's itch, and others) (see Chapter 50).
- *Arthropod dermatoses* are divided into those caused by two classes of organisms: the arachnids (spiders, scorpions, ticks, and mites) and the insects (lice, bugs, flies, moths, beetles, bees, and fleas). Lyme disease is caused by a spirochete that is transmitted by a tick and is discussed in Chapter 25. Rickettsial diseases are also tick-borne (see Chapter 24).

In this chapter scabies, pediculosis, and bedbugs are discussed. Scabies are caused by mites, pediculosis is caused by lice, and bedbug is caused by an insect that is usually found in mattresses and furniture. Flea bites, chigger bites, creeping eruption, swimmer's itch, and tropical dermatoses are discussed in Chapter 50.

SCABIES

Scabies (Figs. 20-1 and 20-2) is usually more prevalent in a populace ravaged by war, famine, or disease when personal hygiene becomes relatively unimportant. However, there are unexplained cyclic epidemics of this parasitic infestation. In the 1970s and 1980s, such a cycle plagued Americans. In normal times, scabies is seen in school children, elderly patients in nursing care centers, in poorer populations under crowded conditions, and in sexually active patients with multiple sex partners.

Animal scabies can occur in cats, dogs, foxes, cows, pigs, and other mammals. The disease is sarcoptic mange and is caused by *Sarcoptes scabiei* var. *canis*. Direct contact with an infected animal causes a severe, generalized, polymorphous, pruritic eruption with absence of burrows and a negative wet mount for ova, parasites, or feces. This occurs 24 to 96 hours after exposure, is not associated with human-to-human

transmission, and lasts only 14 to 21 days without further exposure. Treatment is accomplished by topical agents such as permethrin, malathion, or lindane for the pets and anti-pruritic therapy and topical or systemic corticosteroids for the temporary human hosts.

Presentation and Characteristics

Primary Lesions

A burrow caused by the female of the mite *S. scabiei* (see Fig. 20-2) measures approximately 2 mm in length and can be hidden by a secondary eruption. Small vesicles may overlie the burrows. *Scabies incognito* is a form of the disease in which the burrows are not easily identified. It is seen most commonly in patients who are fastidiously clean and bathe at least once a day. *Norwegian*, or *keratotic, scabies* occurs in immunosuppressed patients. Hundreds of organisms create a psoriasiform dermatitis.

Secondary Lesions

Excoriations of the burrows may be the only visible pathologic process. These may be difficult to see, and magnification devices may be helpful. In severe, chronic cases, bacterial infection may be extensive and may take the form of impetigo, cellulitis, or furunculosis.

Residual nodular lesions may persist as an allergic reaction for many weeks or months after the organism is eliminated. They are often recalcitrant to therapy and topical, intralesional, and even systemic corticosteroids may be necessary. Excision may even be necessary. Nodular scabies is not contagious.

Distribution

Most commonly, the excoriations are seen on the lower abdomen and the back, with extension to the pubic, genital, and axillary areas, the legs (ankles especially), the arms (flexor wrists especially), and the webs of the fingers.

> ### SAUER'S NOTES
>
> 1. Scabies should be ruled out in any generalized, excoriated eruption.
> 2. The patient should always be asked if other members of the household itch.

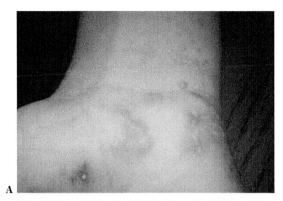

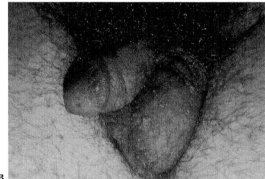

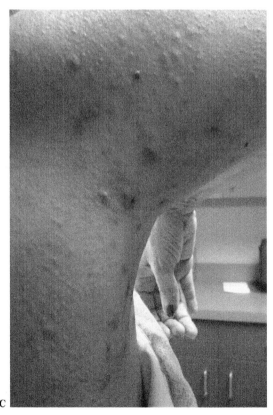

FIGURE 20-1: **A:** Base of palm and flexor wrist with white thread-like burrows with some surrounding erythema. This is a common location to see scabies burrows. **B:** Inflammatory papules on the penis and scrotum quite characteristic of scabies. **C:** Inflammatory papules and nodules on the posterior axillary fold typical of nodular scabies. No organisms are found in this probable immune reaction.

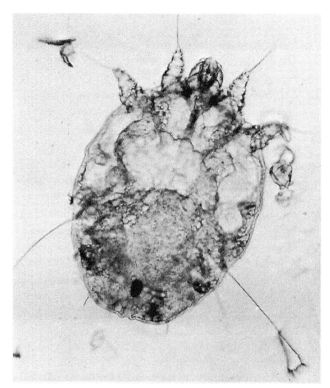

FIGURE 20-2: The female of the mite *Sarcoptes scabiei*. The small, oval, black body near the anal opening is a fecal pellet. Proximal to it is a vague, much larger, oval, pale-edged mass (an egg). (Courtesy of Dr. H. Parlette.)

Subjective Complaints

Itching is intense, particularly at night when the patient is warm and in bed, and the mite is more active. However, many skin diseases itch worse at night, presumably due to a lower-itch threshold when relaxation occurs.

Course

The mite can persist for months and years (7-year itch) in untreated persons.

Contagiousness

Other members of the household or intimate contacts may or may not have the disease, depending on exposure and severity of the infestation.

Laboratory Findings

The female scabies mite, ova, and fecal pellets may be seen in skin scrapings that are done with a No. 15 Bard-Parker blade. The scrapings are done at the site of burrows in the skin or in areas where itching is most severe. The scrapings are then examined under the low-power magnification of the microscope (see Fig. 20-2). Potassium hydroxide (KOH) (20% solution) can be used to clear the tissue. Another method of collection is to scrape the burrow through immersion oil and then transfer the scrapings to the microscopic slides. Skill is necessary to uncover the mite by curetting or scraping.

Differential Diagnosis

- *Pyoderma:* Rule out the concurrent parasitic infestation; positive history of diabetes mellitus; only mild itching (see Chapter 24).
- *Pediculosis pubis:* Lice and eggs on and around hairs; distribution different (see following section).
- *Winter itch:* No burrows; seasonal incidence; elderly patient, usually; worse on legs and back (see Chapter 12).
- *Dermatitis herpetiformis:* Vesicles; urticaria; excoriated papules; eosinophilia; no burrows; characteristic histopathologic appearance; direct immunofluorescence pattern (see Chapter 21).
- *Neurotic excoriations:* Nervous person; patient admits picking at lesions; lesions present in areas where patient can easily reach; no burrows; characteristic stellate hypopigmented scars indicate a prolonged illness.
- *Parasitophobia* (see Chapter 23): Usually the patient brings to the office pieces of skin and debris often carefully stored in a container (match box sign); showing the patient the debris under a microscope helps to convince him or her of the absence of parasites. This is a difficult problem to manage. Pimozide (Orap) or olanzapine (Zyprexa) can be used by a physician experienced in its use. Referral to a psychiatrist is ideal but seldom will the patient consent to this.

SAUER'S NOTES

Scabies

1. I have the patient repeat the medication application in 1 to 7 days, leaving it on again for 12 to 24 hours.
2. Tell the patient that the itching can persist for weeks.
3. Treat all household and sexual contacts (itching or not).

Treatment

Adults and Older Children

1. Inspect or question other members of the family or intimate contacts to rule out the infestation in them. Any household members or intimate contacts must be treated at the same time as the patient to prevent "ping-pong" infestation. This is true even if the itching is not present in contacts.
2. Instruct patient to bathe thoroughly and then apply a scabicide.
3. Permethrin (Elimite, Acticin) 5% cream 60.0 or gamma benzene hexachloride (Lindane, Kwell) 120.0 (not preferred due to toxicity)
   Sig: Apply to the entire body from the neck down. Repeat therapy in 1 week.
4. After 12 to 24 hours, the patient should bathe carefully, and change to clean clothes and bedding.

5. Washing, dry cleaning, or ironing of clothes and bedding are sufficient to destroy the mite. Sterilization is unnecessary.
6. Itching may persist for a few days, even for 2 to 3 weeks or longer, in spite of the destruction of the mite. The itching may be worse for the first several days after treatment. For this apply b.i.d.:
   a. Crotamiton (Eurax) cream q.s. 60.0
      Comment: This cream has scabicidal power and antipruritic action combined.
   b. A topical corticosteroid ointment can be used or, if the pruritus persists, a 10- to 14-day course of systemic corticosteroids may have to be given.
7. If itching persists after 4 weeks, reexamine the patient carefully and repeat the KOH preparation to be sure reinfestation or inadequate treatment has not occurred. Ask if all people who are potential contacts have been treated. It takes a lot of reassurance to convince these itchy patients that they are not still infested with scabies. Repeated unnecessary topical therapy may only increase the itching because these topical agents can act as irritants. Overuse of gamma benzene hexachloride can cause seizures.
8. Oral ivermectin in a single dose is a therapy advocated by some authors. It is helpful in crusted scabies, which also may need keratolytic agents to remove the crusts before using topical therapy.
9. Topical 0.5% Ivermectin has also shown to be quite effective.

Newborns and Infants

1. General instructions are same as for older patients.
2. Lindane lotion used in newborns and infants has caused convulsions.
3. Elimite, Acticin, or Eurax cream 60.0
   Sig: Apply b.i.d. locally to affected areas only
4. Sulfur, ppt. 5%
   Water-washable cream base or Aquaphor q.s. 60.0
   Sig: Apply b.i.d. to affected areas for 3 consecutive days.
   This is a good choice of therapy in pregnant and breastfeeding patients due to its extreme safety. However, it is malodorous and stains clothing.
5. In patients younger than 1 year of age, the bite may occur above the neck. There have been rare reports of disease above the neck in adults. The immunocompromised patient is a candidate for this manifestation.

PEDICULOSIS

Lice infestation affects persons of all ages, but usually those in the lower income strata and military personnel in the field are affected most often because of lack of cleanliness and infrequent changes of clothing. It is also seen as a sexually transmitted disease. Three clinical entities are produced:

- infestation of the hair by the head louse *Pediculus humanus capitis,*
- infestation of the body by *Pediculus humanus corporis,* and

- infestation of the pubic area by the pubic louse *Pthirus pubis* (Fig. 20-3). *P. pubis* infestation can also involve the hairy areas over the abdomen, chest, and eyelids. Because lice bite the skin and live on blood, it is impossible for them to live without human contact. The readily visible oval eggs or nits are attached to hairs or to clothing fibers by the female louse. After the eggs hatch, the newly born lice mature within 30 days. The female louse can live for another 30 days and deposit a few eggs daily.

Presentation and Characteristics

Primary Lesions

The site of the bite is seldom seen because of the secondary changes produced by the resulting intense itching. In the scalp and pubic forms, the nits are found on the hairs, but the lice are found only occasionally. In the body form, the nits and lice can be found after careful searching in the seams of the clothing.

Secondary Lesions

In the scalp form, the skin is red and excoriated, with such severe secondary bacterial infection, in some cases, that the hairs become matted together in a crusty, foul-smelling "cap." Regional lymphadenopathy is common. A morbilliform rash on the body or a generalized papular "id" reaction can be seen in longstanding cases.

In the body form, linear excoriations and secondary infection mask the primary bites. These bites are seen mainly on the shoulders, the belt line, and the buttocks.

In the pubic form, secondary excoriations are again dominant and produce some matting of the hairs. This louse can also infest body, axillary, and eyelash hairs. An unusual eruption on the abdomen, the thighs, and the arms, called *maculae cerulea* because of the bluish-gray, pea-sized macules, can occur in chronic cases of pubic pediculosis.

Differential Diagnosis

Pediculosis Capitis

- *Bacterial infection of the scalp:* Responds rapidly to correct antibacterial therapy (see Chapter 24), culture for bacteria is positive.
- *Seborrheic dermatitis or dandruff:* The scales of dandruff are readily detached from the hair, but oval nits are not so easily removed (see Chapter 15). Nits are easily seen when affected hairs are examined under low power on the microscope.
- *Hair casts (pseudonits):* Resemble nits but usually can be pulled off more easily; no eggs are seen on microscopic examination.

> **SAUER'S NOTES**
>
> All cases of scalp pyoderma must be examined closely for a primary lice infestation.

Pediculosis Corporis

- *Scabies:* May be small burrows; distribution of lesions different; no lice in clothes or nits on hairs (see beginning of this chapter).
- *Senile or winter itch:* History helpful; dry skin, aggravated by bathing; will not find lice in clothes or nits on hairs (see Chapter 12).

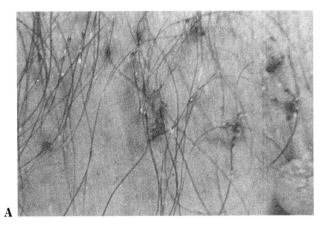

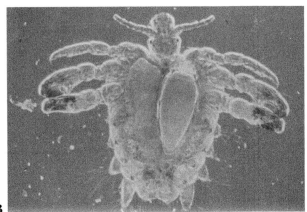

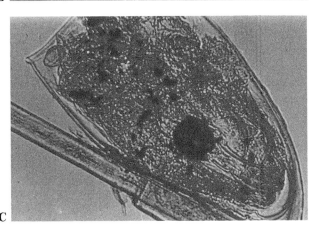

FIGURE 20-3: Pediculosis. **A:** Nits in the pubic areas seen as shiny white nodules on the hair shafts. **B:** Pthirus pubis (pubic louse) seen on a 10× magnification lens of microscope. **C:** Nits of a pubic louse at a 10× magnification. It is flask-shaped and tightly cemented to the hair shaft.

Pediculosis Pubis

- *Scabies:* No nits; burrows in pubic area and elsewhere (see beginning of this chapter).

- *Pyoderma:* Secondary to contact dermatitis from condoms, contraceptive jellies, new underwear, douches—history is important; acute onset, no nits (see Chapter 24).

- *Seborrheic dermatitis:* When in eyebrows and eyelashes, no nits are found. The scaling on the hair is less adherent than the nits in pediculosis (see Chapter 15).

Treatment

Pediculosis Capitis

1. Shampoos or rinses
   a. Permethrin (Nix) cream rinse 60.0
      Sig: Use as a rinse for 10 minutes after shampooing. Only one application is recommended, but I usually recommend repeating in 3 days.
   b. Lindane (Kwell) shampoo 60.0
      Sig: Shampoo and comb hair thoroughly. Leave on the hair for 4 minutes. Repeat medicated shampoo in 3 days. Regular shampoo can be restarted in 24 hours.
   c. Pyrethrins (RID) 60.0
      Sig: Apply to scalp for 10 minutes and rinse off. Apply again in 7 days (nonprescription).
   d. Step Two (formic acid) solution (obtainable without a prescription) can be used to help remove nits from the hairs. Salicylic acid shampoo (T-Sal) may also help remove nits and may be left on overnight at least once.
   e. Permethrin 5% (Elimite) cream 60.0
      Sig: Leave on overnight under shower cap. May be the most effective topical treatment of all for recalcitrant cases.
   f. A single oral dose of ivermectin (Stromectol), 200 (μg/kg, repeated in 10 days may be the most effective oral agent in persistent cases. Some authors are concerned about the safety of this therapy.
   g. Topical malathion (Ovide), available as generic
      Sig: Apply to dry hair for 8 to 12 hours and then shampoo treat 7 to 9 days later if necessary. It is expensive.
   h. Benzoyl alcohol lotion-Ulesfia 5% (Sciele)
      Sig: Apply to dry hair for 10 minutes, then rinse, and repeat 7 days later.
   i. Mayonnaise (not reduced fat) left overnight for three nights is effective and very safe.
   j. Sklice is 0.5% solution of ivermectin in a lotion with fewer than 1% that have irritation of the skin and is successful in about three-fourths of patients. It is applied to the scalp for 10 minutes and then rinsed off.
2. For secondary scalp infection
   a. Trim hair as much as possible and agreeable with the patient.
   b. Shampoo hair daily with a salicylic acid shampoo (T-Sal).
   c. Bactroban or Polysporin ointment 15.0.
      Sig: Apply to scalp b.i.d.

3. Change and clean bedding and headwear after 24 hours of treatment. Storage of headwear for 30 days destroys the lice and nits.
4. Spinosad cream rinse (Natroba) said by some authors to be more effective than permethrin and only requires a single use, however, it is expensive. It is now approved by the FDA for the treatment of head lice in patients greater than 4 years of age.
5. Topical 0.5% Ivermectin has been shown to be quite effective.

Pediculosis Corporis

1. Permethrin 5% (Elimite) cream overnight.
2. Have the clothing laundered or dry-cleaned. If this is impossible, dusting with 10% lindane powder kills the parasites. Care should be taken to prevent reinfestation. Storage of clothing in a plastic bag for 30 days kills both nits and lice.
3. Sulfur 5% to 10% in petrolatum overnight for three nights is effective and very safe. It is malodorous and stains bed clothes.
4. Sklice 0.5% lotion (Ivermectin) a single topical use treatment for head lice in patients greater than 6 months of age. It is expensive and not ovicidal but eggs that are treated die within 48 hours after hatching.

Pediculosis Pubis

Treatment is the same as for the scalp form.

When the disease occurs on the eyelids, sulfacetamide ophthalmic ointment b.i.d. for 5 days is very safe and effective. Petrolatum can also be used in the same fashion.

BEDBUGS

Bedbugs (*Cimex lectularius*) usually present as nighttime papular urticaria. Not every patient has a reaction to the bite. Bedbugs are nocturnal and are attracted to the human host by carbon dioxide, which not all people emit in the same amount, and warmth. Personal cleanliness and good housekeeping are no protection. Bedbugs are visible with the naked eye as tiny reddish-brown insects about the size of a nonengorged tick. The mattress, or more rarely other furniture, is the usual location of the insects. They can also live in cracks in walls.

Presentation and Characteristics

Primary Lesions

Papular urticaria often seen in a row on exposed skin (Fig. 20-4). It often lasts 4 to 6 weeks after the infestation is eliminated.

Secondary Lesions

Honey-colored oozing and crusting may be seen, indicating secondary infection. If continuously scratched, they can last indefinitely and mimic prurigo nodularis. Severe pruritus can result in bruising and bleeding.

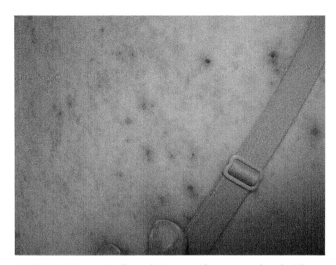

FIGURE 20-4: Bedbug bites on the upper back. They appear as inflammatory clusters of pink papules with a central punctum. This was is a surgery resident who slept in a bed in the hospital for her all night call.

Differential Diagnosis

Urticaria: More evanescent (1 to 2 days or less), scattered, and not in rows. Dermatographism may be present.
Scabies: Has burrows and a positive KOH examination. Finger webs, flexor wrists, and genitalia often affected.

Treatment

1. Symptomatic treatment consists of oral antihistamines, topical antipruritics, topical corticosteroids and, if severe, systemic corticosteroids.
2. The affected mattress, couch, stuffed chair, or other affected furniture is best discarded or fumigation carried out with specific instructions that bedbugs are suspected.
3. Heat treatment is often used by an experienced exterminator since bedbugs have become resistant.

Suggested Readings

Benzyl alcohol lotion for head lice. *Med Lett.* 2009;51(1317):57–59.
Buntin DM, Rosen T, Lesher JL, et al. Sexually transmitted diseases: viruses and ectoparasites. *J Am Acad Dermatol.* 1991;25:527–534.
Centers for Disease Control and Prevention. Scabies in health-care facilities: Iowa. *Arch Dermatol.* 1988;124:837.
Currie BJ, McCarthy JS. Permethrin and ivermectin for scabies. *N Engl J Med.* 2010;362(8):717–725.
Goddard J. *Physician's Guide to Arthropods of Medical Importance.* 2nd ed. Boca Roton, FL: CRC Press LLC; 1996.
Insect repellents. *Med Lett Drugs Ther.* 2016;58(1498):83–84.
Ko CJ, Elston DM. Pediculosis. *J Am Acad Dermatol.* 2004;50:1–12.
Shmidt E, Levitt J. Dermatologic infestations. *Int J Dermatol.* 2012;51:131–141.
Zhu YI, Stiller MJ. Arthropods and skin diseases. *Int J Dermatol.* 2002;41:533–549.

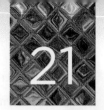

Bullous Dermatoses

John C. Hall, MD

To medical students and practitioners alike, the bullous skin diseases appear most dramatic. One of these diseases, pemphigus, is undoubtedly greatly responsible for the aura that surrounds the exhibition and discussion of an unfortunate patient with a bullous disease. Happy would be the instructor who could behold such student interest when a case of acne or hand dermatitis is being presented.

In almost all cases of bullous diseases, it is necessary to examine a fresh tissue biopsy specimen for deposits of immune reactants, immunoglobulins, and complement components at or near the basement membrane zone. Michel's solution can be used in the place of a fresh tissue specimen. Routine histologic examination of a formalin-fixed biopsy specimen is, of course, also usually indicated.

Four bullous diseases are discussed in this chapter: pemphigus vulgaris, dermatitis herpetiformis, bullous pemphigoid, and erythema multiforme bullosum. However, other bullous skin diseases do occur, and in this introduction they are differentiated from these four.

- *Bullous impetigo:* Bullous impetigo is differentiated from the other bullous diseases by its occurrence in infants and children, rapid development of the individual bullae, presence of impetigo lesions in siblings, bacterial culture positive for *Staphylococcus aureus* and methicillin resistant *Staphylococcus aureus*, and rapid response to antibiotic therapy (see Chapter 24). It can be a recurrent problem in HIV-positive patients in the groin area.

- *Contact dermatitis* caused by poison ivy or similar plants: Bullae and vesicles are seen in a linear configuration. A history of pulling weeds, cleaning out fence-rows, or burning brush is usually obtained, and a past history of poison ivy or related dermatitis is common. It is important to remember that this is a form of delayed hypersensitivity and the time between the exposure causing the eruption and the onset of symptoms can be anywhere from 1 to 2 days to 1 to 2 weeks. This delayed nature of the disease commonly leads to an erroneous diagnosis or a correct diagnosis with inability to establish when the exposure occurred and to therefore eliminate all traces of the plant oil from objects where it may be contacted again and results in another outbreak of the disease. The duration of disease is 10 to 21 days if untreated and is quite uncomfortable (see Chapter 9).

- *Drug eruption:* Elicit drug history (particularly of sulfonamides, nonsteroidal anti-inflammatory drugs [NSAIDs], and antiseizure medications). Fixed drug eruptions are not uncommonly bullous. Fixed drug eruptions are localized, very inflammatory, may blister, leave marked hyperpigmentation, and occur at the same site on drug rechallenge. The eruption usually clears upon discontinuing drugs, but this can be delayed for 2 or more weeks. If the patient is not better within a few days of stopping the drug, this does not mean that the drug is not the cause of the eruption. Bullae appear rapidly (see Chapter 9).

- *Epidermolysis bullosa* (see Chapter 44): This rare, chronic, hereditary skin disease is manifested by the formation of bullae, usually on the hands and the feet, following trauma. The full clinical and immunologic spectra of these diseases are protean in form of inheritance, severity of disease, and tendency to improve with age.

  - The simple form (epidermolysis bullosa simplex) of dominant inheritance can begin in infancy or adulthood with the formation of tense, slightly itchy bullae at sites of pressure that heal quickly without scarring. Forced marches or jogging can initiate this disease in patients who have the heredity factor. Such cases are usually treated erroneously as athlete's foot. The disease is worse in the summer or in climates with high humidity and may be present only at this time. This disease often improves with age.

  - The dystrophic form of recessive inheritance begins in infancy, and as time elapses, the bullae become hemorrhagic, heal slowly, and leave scars that can amputate digits. Death can result from secondary infection and metastatic squamous cell carcinomas. Mucous membrane lesions are more common in the dystrophic form than in the simple form. Treatment is supportive. Gene therapy may be a future modality but has been disappointing so far. Bone marrow transplantation has been tried with some success but further studies are needed. Surgical dressings and skin substitutes (Apligraf) are an important part of care. Various surgical dressings may be helpful. Mepitel, Mepilex, and Mepilex Foam are the dressings I have found especially useful. The blisters should be immediately drained to relieve pain and keep them from enlarging. Secondary infection should be watched for carefully and treated immediately.

- A lethal, nonscarring form is also of recessive inheritance but is usually fatal within a few months (see Chapter 44).

■ *Epidermolysis bullosa acquisita:* An autoimmune response to collagen where skin lesions can appear similar to bullous pemphigoid, cicatricial pemphigoid, and recessive epidermolysis bullosa. Bulla, scarring, and esophageal disease all occur in this acquired illness. Direct immunofluorescence (DIF) is positive in a linear pattern for IgA in the epidermal basement membrane. Dapsone and systemic corticosteroids may be helpful. Trauma can induce blisters that result in scarring.

■ *Familial benign chronic pemphigus* (Hailey–Hailey disease): This is a rare, hereditary bullous eruption that is most common on the neck, groin, and in the axillae (Fig. 21-1). It can be distinguished from pemphigus by its chronicity and benign nature and by its histologic picture. Some consider this disease to be a bullous variety of keratosis follicularis (Darier disease). It is very

painful and can be debilitating. It is caused by a mutation of the *ATP2C1* gene.

■ *Herpes gestationis* (see Chapter 53): This is a vesicular and bullous disease that occurs in relation to pregnancy. It usually develops during the second or the third trimester and commonly disappears after giving birth, only to return with subsequent pregnancies. The histologic features are believed to be significantly distinctive, so this disease can be separated from dermatitis herpetiformis. Immunologic findings of C3 bound to the basement membrane of the epidermis and occasional immunoglobulin (IgG) deposition may be significant. Therapy with systemic corticosteroids is usually indicated.

■ *Porphyria:* The congenital erythropoietic type and the chronic hepatic type (porphyria cutanea tarda) commonly have bullae on the sun-exposed areas of the body (see the Dictionary–Index under *Porphyria*).

■ *Cicatricial pemphigoid:* This disabling but nonfatal bullous eruption of the mucous membranes most commonly involves the eyes. The skin and mucous membranes may be involved, usually in a localized pattern. As the result of scarring, which is characteristic of this disease and separates it from true pemphigus, eyesight is eventually lost. Over 50% of the cases have skin

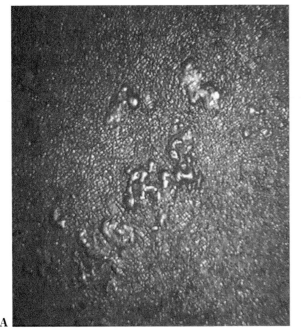

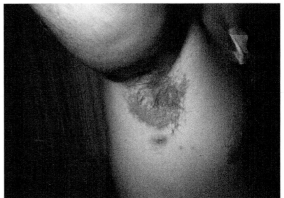

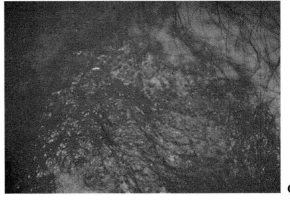

FIGURE 21-1: **A:** Intact confluent vesicles over the back that are usually not seen in Hailey-Hailey disease. **B:** Bright red painful erosions with suggestion of small blistering around the border in the axillae of a patient with Hailey-Hailey. **C:** Painful erosion in the groin, with tiny vesicles along the superior border and lower central area.

lesions. Histologically, the bullae are subepidermal and do not show acantholysis. There is quite a bit of immunologic similarity between this disease and bullous pemphigoid.

- *Linear IgA bullous disease:* Most of the children and adults with this disease differ from classic dermatitis herpetiformis in the morphology and distribution of their lesions, have a poorer response to dapsone, and have linear IgA anti–basement membrane zone antibodies. Classical blisters are seen in a so-called "cluster of jewels" configuration. Also seen are annular grouped papules, vesicles, and bullae. Nontropical sprue is not a part of this illness.

  A drug-induced variant of this disease is seen most often with Vancomycin, but other drugs reported are Phenytoin, Amiodarone, Captopril, and nonsteroidal anti-inflammatory agents. Lesions appear most frequently in children in the perineal and perioral regions. In adults, lesions are seen more often on elbows, knees, and buttock.

- *Incontinentia pigmenti:* The first stage of this rare disease of infants manifests itself with bullous lesions, primarily on the hands and feet (see Chapter 45). This stage may appear in utero and may not be seen clinically.

- *Toxic epidermal necrolysis* (TEN): Most authors consider Stevens–Johnson syndrome a variant of TEN with less skin and more mucous membrane involvement but with the same clinical picture, histology, prognosis, and treatment. This rare disease is characterized by large bullae and a quite generalized Nikolsky sign, in which large sheets of epidermis become detached from the underlying skin with gentle pressure from a finger. The mucous membranes are frequently involved. The patient is toxic. Adults are most commonly affected. Drugs are usually the causative factor, especially in adults. Most commonly implicated are sulfonamides, anticonvulsants, and NSAIDs. There may be a genetic predisposition to this bullous drug reaction. Therapy is supportive, and an appreciable number of cases are fatal. Intravenous immunoglobulins (IVIG) may be lifesaving. Cyclosporine is a preferred mode of therapy by some authors. High-dose systemic corticosteroids are controversial, with opinions ranging from contraindicated to lifesaving if given in very high doses very early in the course of the disease. Some authors would argue that only supportive measures have been shown to be of any benefit. Wound care is essential. Debridement should be avoided. Silver nitrate irrigation and soft gauze dressings (SofSorb gauze, which may be fitted on as a garment) are used in wound care. This is usually done in an intensive care unit because electrolyte and fluid balance is crucial. A central venous line helps greatly in managing these patients. The most crucial factor in survival is stopping any potential offending drug as quickly as possible. Acute graft-versus-host disease can be an identical disease process and should be treated in a similar manner. Mortality for this disease can be significant. A helpful prognostic scoring system is as follows:

Age >40
Underlying malignancy
Heart rate >120
>10% epidermal detachment
BUN >10 mmol/L
Serum glucose >14 mmol/L
Bicarbonate >20 mmol/L

SCORTEN	Mortality
0–1	3.2%
2	12.1%
3	35.3%
4	58.3%
5	>90%

- *Staphylococcal scalded skin syndrome:* Clinically, this disorder is similar to TEN but has been separated from this disease because of the finding that phage group 2 *S. aureus* is the usual cause. In newborns, this formerly was known as Ritter von Ritterschein disease. It also occurs in children and rarely in adults. The prognosis is very favorable. If suspected, antistaphylococcal drugs should be started intravenously immediately. The break in the skin is higher in the epidermis than in drug-induced TEN, and this can be rapidly ascertained with a skin biopsy.

- *Impetigo herpetiformis:* One of the rarest of skin diseases, this disease is characterized by groups of pustules seen mainly in the axillae and the groin, high fever, prostration, severe malaise, and, generally, a fatal outcome. It occurs most commonly in pregnant or postpartum women. It can be distinguished from pemphigus vegetans or dermatitis herpetiformis by the fact that these diseases do not produce such general, acute, toxic manifestations. Laboratory abnormalities include elevated white blood count, elevated sedimentation rate, and low calcium, phosphate, albumin, and vitamin D levels. Bacterial cultures of skin and blood are negative; high-dose (60 to 100 mg q.d.) prednisone and fluid and electrolyte replacement can be lifesaving (see Chapter 53).

In spite of high medical student and general practitioner interest in the bullous skin conditions, the diagnosis and the management of the three main bullous skin diseases, bullous pemphigoid, pemphigus vulgaris, and dermatitis herpetiformis, should be in the realm of the dermatologist. In this chapter, the salient features of these diseases are presented, with therapy briefly outlined.

BULLOUS PEMPHIGOID

Bullous pemphigoid is a chronic bullous eruption most commonly occurring in elderly adults. Bullous pemphigoid can uncommonly occur in children and infants.

Presentation and Characteristics

Primary Lesions

Large tense blisters tend to mushroom out of normal skin and can grow to many centimeters before breaking. The disease can, less commonly, begin with large pruritic erythematous plaques.

Secondary Lesions

When the blisters eventually break down, they leave large superficial erosions that heal without scars. Oral lesions are extremely rare. The urticarial plaques may show excoriations and also heal without scarring.

Course

When untreated, the disease lasts years before resolution.

Causes

Bullous pemphigoid is an idiopathic autoimmune disease that shows antibody deposition at the basement membrane zone of IgG and C3, which recruits neutrophils and eosinophils with destruction of the basement membrane and results in a large subepidermal blister. Serum ELISA test for antigens BP230 and BP180-NC16a. Some drugs such as furosemide, penicillin, sulfasalazine, and ibuprofen can cause a blistering skin disease that mimics bullous pemphigoid but dissipates after the drug is discontinued. There has been one study associating an increased risk of cerebrovascular disease and dementia in patients with bullous pemphigoid.

Laboratory Findings

DIF of IgG and C3 seen at the dermoepidermal junction and indirect immunofluorescence (IF) and circulation IgG may be present. IgG binds to the hemidesmosomal proteins BP antigens 230 (BP230) and 180 (BP180). Subepidermal blisters with invasion of neutrophils and eosinophils are seen. The urticarial plaques are more nonspecific histologically but still have positive DIF. Some studies have suggested an increased incidence of underlying systemic malignancy.

Differential Diagnosis

- *Pemphigus:* See Table 21-1.
- *Dermatitis herpetiformis:* More pruritic; marked response to dapsone; rarely tense blisters; resolves with hyperpigmentation; characteristic DIF
- *Erythema multiforme:* Younger patients with "iris" or "bull's eye" configuration; disease of the palms and soles as well as mucous membrane disease; association with drugs or herpes simplex (in the milder form of the disease) often seen. DIF and IF are negative.

Treatment

This can usually be done as an outpatient.

1. High-dose (50 to 100 mg) prednisone is required for early remission. Other immunosuppressive therapy is begun at the same time and is used on a more chronic basis as the patient is tapered off systemic corticosteroids.
2. Occasionally, tetracycline (500 mg q.i.d.) and niacinamide (500 mg q.i.d.) are helpful alone or as a steroid-sparing regimen.
3. Dapsone (although with a much slower response than in dermatitis herpetiformis) 100 mg/day can occasionally be helpful.

TABLE 21-1 • Differences Between Bullous Pemphigoid and Pemphigus Vulgaris

	Bullous Pemphigoid	Pemphigus Vulgaris
Common age of onset	>70 y; "old man's pemphigus"	40–60 y
Prognosis	Resolves over years	Usually fatal without therapy; lifelong
Clinical characteristics	Large blisters mushroom out of normal skin; can appear urticarial	Fragile blisters break to form confluent erosions; positive Nikolsky sign
Location of blisters	Widespread on skin	Oral lesions common and may be localized to this location
Inheritance	None	Mediterranean; Jewish
Histopathology	Subepidermal blister; neutrophils; eosinophils	Intraepidermal blister
Direct immunofluorescence	Linear IgG, C3 at dermoepidermal junction in bullous and perilesional skin; binding site is proteins of basement membrane zone	IgG around cell surface of keratinocytes; binding site is desmoglein 3
Indirect immunofluorescence	Variable	Present and used to follow disease

4. Azathioprine (50 mg/day or b.i.d.) is a commonly used steroid-sparing agent.
5. Methotrexate (15 mg PO or IM) has been used successfully as a steroid-sparing agent.
6. IVIG has also had success as a single agent or steroid-sparing drug. It is very expensive and must be given intravenously for several days.

PEMPHIGUS VULGARIS

Pemphigus vulgaris is rare. These patients are miserable, odoriferous, and debilitated (Fig. 21-2). Before the advent of corticosteroid therapy, the disease was fatal.

Presentation and Characteristics

Primary Lesions

The early lesions of pemphigus are small vesicles or bullae that appear on apparently normal skin. Redness of the base of the bullae is unusual. Without treatment, the bullae enlarge and spread, and new ones balloon up on different areas of the skin or the mucous membranes. Rarely, mucous membrane lesions may be the main or only manifestation of the disease. Rupturing of the bullae leaves large eroded areas. Nikolsky sign is positive; that is, a top layer of the skin adjacent to a bulla readily separates from the underlying skin after firm but gentle pressure.

Secondary Lesions

Bacterial infection with crusting is marked and accounts, in part, for the characteristic mousy odor. Lesions that heal spontaneously or under therapy do not leave scars.

Course

When untreated, pemphigus vulgaris can be rapidly fatal or assume a slow, lingering course, with debility, painful mouth and body erosions, systemic bacterial infection, and toxemia.

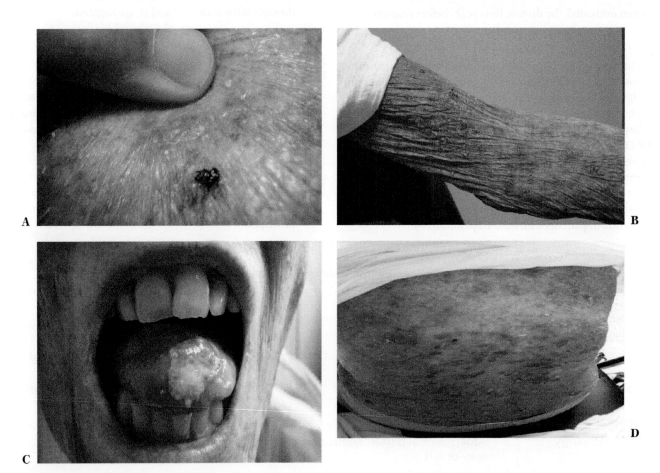

FIGURE 21-2: **A:** Pemphigus on the abdomen with tangential pressure near a ruptured blister peels of the epidermis. This is a positive Nikolsky sign and is also seen in toxic epidermal necrolysis. **B:** Eroded bullae on the flexor forearms in pempigus vulgaris. Note there are no intact blisters since the blister is intraepidermal rather than subepidermal as in bullous pemphigoid. **C:** Pemphigus of the tongue with large eroded area, and white plaque with some epidermis is yet to desquamate. Occasionally pemphigus is only on the mucous membranes. **D:** Paraneplastic pemphigus with all of back covered with erosions. The patients had an underlying lymphoma and the diagnosis was confirmed by direct immunofluorescence. As in this case, mucous membranes of the mouth are involved.

Spontaneous temporary remissions do occur without therapy. The following clinical variations of pemphigus also exist:

- *Pemphigus vegetans:* It is characterized by the development of large granulomatous masses in the intertriginous areas of the axillae and the groin. Secondary bacterial infection, although often present in all cases of pemphigus, is most marked in this form. Pemphigus vegetans is to be differentiated from a granulomatous iododerma or bromoderma (see Chapter 9) and from impetigo herpetiformis (see beginning of this chapter). This type of pemphigus can often be treated more conservatively such as with potent topical corticosteroids.

- *Pemphigus foliaceus* (fogo selvagem): It appears as a scaly, moist, generalized exfoliative dermatitis. The characteristic mousy odor of pemphigus is dominant in this variant, which is also remarkable for its chronicity. The response to corticosteroid therapy is less favorable in the foliaceus form than in the other types (see also Chapter 50 for a Brazilian form). Complementary DNA cloning has shown the autoimmune target to be desmoglein 1. There is some evidence that this may be a disease borne by an insect vector in tropical areas near rivers.

- *Pemphigus erythematosus:* It clinically resembles a mixture of pemphigus vulgaris, seborrheic dermatitis, and lupus erythematosus. The distribution of the red, greasy, crusted, and eroded lesions is on the butterfly area of the face, the sternal area, the scalp, and occasionally in the mouth. The course is more chronic than for pemphigus vulgaris, and remissions are common.

- *Pemphigus herpetiformis:* It appears as grouped vesicles, bullae, or erythematous papules that are very pruritic. DIF of IgG in upper or entire epidermal cell surfaces and circulating IgG autoantibodies are present.

- *Paraneoplastic pemphigus:* It is an often fatal, severe, rare, polymorphous eruption with erosions, bullae, or targetoid lesions and severe mucous membrane disease. DIF shows IgG on all epidermal surfaces and often linear confluent deposits at the dermoepidermal junction; complement may also be on epidermal surfaces. Circulating IgG autoantibodies are present, and 75% of cases have circulating IgG to rat bladder epithelium. Non-Hodgkin lymphoma is the most common underlying malignancy.

- *IgA pemphigus:* It shows flaccid, pruritic vesicles or pustules in an annular pattern with central crusting. It can show neutrophils with IgA DIF, either subcorneal or intraepidermal with less acantholysis. It is more common in females and usually less severe than pemphigus vulgaris with less morbidity and without mucous membrane disease. It responds to dapsone, or if there is sulfa allergy, then methotrexate or retinoids may be helpful. Corticosteroids are usually not helpful, and there may be monoclonal antibodies present.

Some doctors believe that pemphigus foliaceus and pemphigus erythematosus may be distinct diseases from pemphigus vulgaris and pemphigus vegetans.

Causes

The cause of pemphigus vulgaris is unknown, but autoimmunity is a factor. Some cases are associated with underlying malignancy (paraneoplastic pemphigus). Paraneoplastic pemphigus has unique immunofluorescent findings and is usually rapidly fatal. Human herpesvirus 8 has been isolated from the skin lesions of some patients. There is some suggestion that an increased lifetime exposure to penicillin may be associated with increased malignancies. Many drugs have been known to induce pemphigus. These include drugs with a sulfhydryl group such as penicillamine, penicillin, captopril, gold, and piroxicam; drugs that are phenyls such as cefadroxil, aspirin, levodopa, rifampin, and heroin; and nonsulfhydryl nonphenyl drugs such as calcium channel blockers, angiotensin converting enzyme inhibitors, and nonsteroidal anti-inflammatory drugs.

Laboratory Findings

The histopathology of early cases is characteristic and serves to differentiate most cases of pemphigus vulgaris from dermatitis herpetiformis and the other bullous diseases. Acantholysis, or separation of intercellular contact between the keratinocytes, is characteristic. The bulla is intraepidermal. Cytologic smears (Tzanck test) for diagnosis of pemphigus vulgaris reveal numerous rounded acantholytic epidermal cells with large nuclei in a condensed cytoplasm. Antiepithelial autoantibodies against the intercellular substance are found by DIF and IF tests. Fresh tissue biopsy specimens taken from noninvolved skin best show immunoglobulins. IF tests are performed on serum. Complementary DNA cloning shows the autoimmune target to be desmoglein 3.

Differential Diagnosis

See introduction to this chapter as well as the sections on dermatitis herpetiformis and erythema multiforme bullosum.

Treatment

1. If possible, a doctor and internist should be called in to share the responsibility of the care.

2. Hospitalization is necessary for the patient with large areas of bullae and erosions. Mild cases of pemphigus can be managed in the office.

3. Prednisone, 10 mg #100
   Sig: 1 or 2 tablets q.i.d. until healing occurs, then reduce the dose slowly as warranted.
   Comment: Very high doses of prednisone may be needed to produce a remission in severe cases.

4. Local therapy is prescribed to make the patient more comfortable and to decrease the odor by reducing secondary infection. This can be accomplished by the following, which must be varied for individual cases:
   a. Potassium permanganate crystals
      Sig: Place 2 tsp of the crystals in the bathtub with approximately 10-in lukewarm water.
      Comment: To prevent the crystals from burning the skin, they should be dissolved completely in a glass of water before adding to the tub. The solution

should be made fresh daily. The tub stains can be removed by applying acetic acid or "hypo" solution.

   b. Talc

      Sig: Dispense in a powder can. Apply to bedsheets and to erosions twice a day (called a "powder bed").

   c. Polysporin, Bactroban, or other antibiotic ointment q.s.

      Sig: Apply to small infected areas b.i.d.

5. Supportive therapy should be used when necessary. This includes vitamins, iron, blood transfusions, and oral antibiotics. Dapsone and gold therapy can be used with benefit in some cases as a corticosteroid-sparing agent. Methotrexate, azathioprine, cyclosporine, and other immunosuppressive agents are also being used. IVIG may invoke long-term remission in some patients.

6. Nursing care of the highest caliber is a prerequisite for the severe case of pemphigus with generalized erosions and bullae. The nursing personnel should be told that this disease is not contagious or infectious. Surgical dressings such as Mepitel that are not adherent but quite protective may be of great benefit.

7. Mycophenolate mofetil may be an effective and safer immunosuppressive drug according to some authors.

8. Sun avoidance and sunscreen use may be beneficial, especially in pemphigus vulgaris and pemphigus foliaceus.

9. Plasmapheresis has been used with some success.

10. Immunoablative cytoxan has been used in paraneoplastic pemphigus and life-threatening recalcitrant disease.

11. Rituximab, IVIG, and cyclosporine are other immunosuppressive options.

12. Osteoporosis surveillance is indicated because there is an association between pemphigus and osteoporosis independent of systemic corticosteroid use.

DERMATITIS HERPETIFORMIS (DUHRING DISEASE)

Dermatitis herpetiformis is a rare (11.2 per 100,000 in the United States), chronic, markedly pruritic, papular, vesicular,

and bullous skin disease of unknown etiology (Fig. 21-3). It is probably an autoimmune disease and is activated via the alternate complement pathway. The patient describes the itching of a new blister as a burning itch that disappears when the blister top is scratched off. The severe scratching results in the formation of excoriations and papular hives, which may be the only visible pathology of the disease. Individual lesions heal, leaving an area of hyperpigmentation. The typical distribution of the blisters or excoriations is on the scalp, sacral area, buttocks, scapular area, forearms, elbows, and thighs. Large spared areas, especially over the trunk, are sometimes seen. In some cases, the resulting bullae may be indistinguishable from pemphigus or bullous pemphigoid.

The duration of dermatitis herpetiformis varies from months to as long as 40 years, with periods of remission scattered in between. The illness is associated with nontropical sprue. Most patients with dermatitis herpetiformis have nontropical sprue, but it is usually asymptomatic. Some authors have found an association with underlying solid tumors in approximately 10% of patients.

Autoimmune thyroiditis, diabetes mellitus, and T-cell lymphomas are increased. Anemia and osteoporosis can develop from malabsorption.

Laboratory tests should include fixed tissue and fresh tissue biopsy. The DIF shows, in most cases, granular IgA in the dermal papillae of perilesional skin, along with the third component of complement (C3). The finding of endomysial antibodies in the blood is highly specific for the disease. A positive blood test for IgA tissue transglutaminase antibodies (tTGA) is also helpful. An invasive test that can be helpful is gastroduodenoscopy with biopsy, but this is usually not done. Antiendomysial antibodies are present in approximately 60% of patients. A blood cell count usually shows an eosinophilia. This is one disease where a trial of avlosulfon (Dapsone) or sulfapyridine may be not only therapeutic but diagnostic.

Differential Diagnosis

■ *Pemphigus vulgaris:* Large, flaccid bullae; mouth involvement more common; debilitating course; biopsy

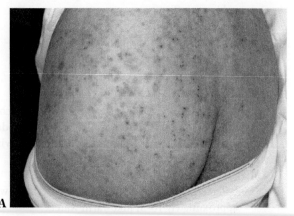
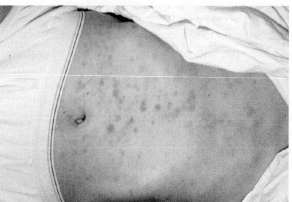

FIGURE 21-3: A: Excoriations over the buttocks with no intact blisters in a patient with dermatitis herpetiformis. The intensity of pruritus can mimic scabies. **B:** Characteristic residual hyperpigmentation over anterior trunk in dermatitis herpetiformis.

specimen characteristic; eosinophilia is uncommon (see *Pemphigus*).

- *Erythema multiforme bullosum:* Bullae usually arise on a red, iris-like base; burning itch is absent; residual pigmentation is minor; course is shorter and palmar–plantar lesions are common (see Chapter 13).

- *Neurotic excoriations:* If this diagnosis is being considered, it is very important to rule out dermatitis herpetiformis. In a case of neurotic excoriations, one usually does not find scalp lesions, blisters, or eosinophilia. Skin lesions are seen only where the patient can reach. If the patient is right handed, then it is often worse on the left side of the body. The skin biopsy is helpful.

- *Scabies:* No vesicles (rarely can occur) or bullae; burrows and lesions are found in other members of the household (see Chapter 20). Potassium hydroxide scraping is diagnostic.

- *Subcorneal pustular dermatosis (Sneddon–Wilkinson disease):* Rare, chronic dermatosis characterized by an annular and serpiginous arrangement of pustules and vesiculopustules on the abdomen, groin, and axillae. Histopathologically, the pustule is found directly beneath the stratum corneum. Dapsone (avlosulfon) or sulfapyridine therapy is effective.

Treatment

A doctor should be consulted to establish the diagnosis and to outline therapy, which consists of local and oral measures to control itching and a course of one of the following quite effective drugs: sulfapyridine (0.5 g q.i.d.) or dapsone (25 mg t.i.d.). Rapid response to these medicines should make the diagnosis suspect. These initial doses should be decreased or increased depending on the patient's response. These drugs can be toxic, and the patient must be under the close surveillance of the physician. The drugs should be avoided in the presence of a G6PD deficiency. Mild to moderate anemia is present in almost all patients on chronic dapsone therapy but is usually well tolerated. Dapsone can cause liver damage and pancytopenia. Cimetidine 800 mg twice a day helps decrease dapsone toxicity. A diet that is gluten free is curative for both the skin and the bowel disease, but it must be maintained for a lifetime and is a very difficult diet to follow. It takes a committed physician and patient to maintain a gluten-free diet. It is estimated that particularly in patients with an onset at age 40 or greater that approximately 10% may go into remission and not need further treatment.

ERYTHEMA MULTIFORME BULLOSUM

Erythema multiforme bullosum (Fig. 21-4) has a clinical picture and course distinct from that of erythema multiforme (Fig. 21-4; see Chapter 11). Many drugs can cause an erythema multiforme bullosum–like picture, but in these cases, the manifestation should be labeled a "drug eruption."

True erythema multiforme bullosum has no known cause. Clinically, one sees large vesicles and bullae usually overlying red, iris-like macules. The lesions most commonly appear on the arms, legs, and face, but can occur elsewhere, including, on occasion, the mouth. Erythema multiforme bullosum can last from days to months.

Slight malaise and fever may precede a new shower of bullae, but for the most part the patient's general health is unaffected. Itching may be mild or severe enough to interfere with sleep.

When the characteristic iris lesions are absent, it is difficult to differentiate this bullous eruption from early pemphigus vulgaris, dermatitis herpetiformis, and bullous pemphigoid. However, the histopathology and immunofluorescence studies are often helpful. DIF and IF studies are negative (Fig. 21-5).

Treatment

These patients should be referred to a doctor or an internist to substantiate the diagnosis and initiate therapy. Corticosteroids orally and by injection are the most effective drugs in use today. For widespread cases requiring hospitalization, the local care is similar to that for pemphigus.

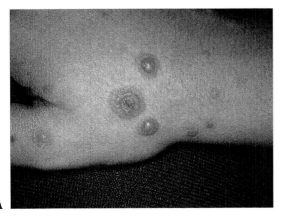
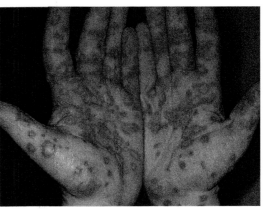

A   **B**

FIGURE 21-4: Erythema multiforme bullosum on the dorsum of the hand **(A)** and on the palms **(B)** 5 days later in the same patient. (Courtesy of Roche Laboratories.)

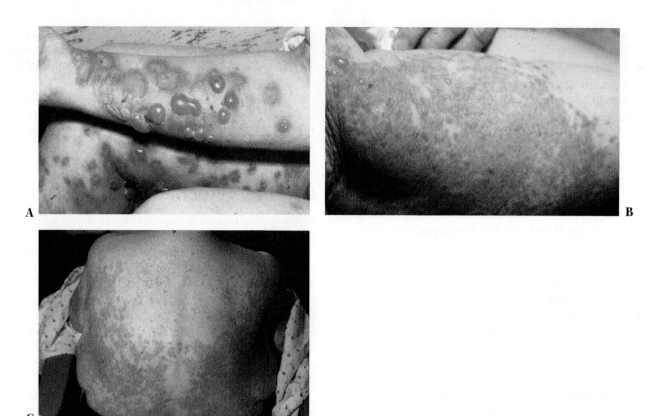

FIGURE 21-5: **A:** Large tense bullae arising on normal skin over the arms and legs. Direct pressure may spread the blister (positive Asboe-Hansen sign). **B:** Large erythematous urticarial plaque distal to elbow on forearm. The clue in might be bullous pemphigoid are the vesicles on the upper right. **C:** Very large areas of symmetrical elevated redness covering the lower back. The condition is very pruritic, as bullous pemphigoid plaques often are, but there are no blisters to help with the diagnosis. Biopsy with DIF is indicated.

SAUER'S NOTES

1. The bullous diseases must be differentiated by biopsy.
2. An intact blister with some edge of normal skin is ideal.
3. Part of the specimen should be sent in formaldehyde and part as fresh tissue or in Michel's solution for DIF.
4. Rapid accurate diagnosis is important because these diseases are not treated the same way and early therapy is important in these sometimes life-threatening and always life-altering diseases.

Suggested Readings

Ahmed AR. Management of autoimmune bullous diseases: pharmacology and therapeutics. *J Am Acad Dermatol.* 2013;69(3):476–477.

Ahmed AR, Kurgis BS, Rogers RS III. Cicatricial pemphigoid. *J Am Acad Dermatol.* 1991;24:987–1001.

Bastuji-Gavin S, Rzany B, Stern RS, et al. Clinical classification of cases of toxic epidermal necrolysis, Stevens–Johnson syndrome, and erythema multiforme. *Arch Dermatol.* 1993;129:92–96.

Bolotin D, Petronic-Rosic V. Dermatitis herpetiformis. *J Am Acad Dermatol.* 2011;64(6):1017–1024.

Cianchini G, Lupi F, Masini C, et al. Therapy with rituximab for autoimmune pemphigus: Results from a single-center observational study on 42 cases with long-term follow up. *J Am Acad Dermatol.* 2012;67(4):617–622.

Diaz LA, Sampaio SA, Rivitti EA, et al. Endemic pemphigus foliaceus (fogo selvagem). *J Am Acad Dermatol.* 1989;20:657–669.

Jordon RE. *Atlas of Bullous Disease.* Philadelphia: WB Saunders; 2000.

Leventhal JS, Sanchez MR. Is it time to re-evaluate the treatment of pemphigus? *J Drugs Dermatol.* 2012;11(10):1200–1206.

Reguiai Z, Tabary T, Maizieres M, et al. Rituximab treatment of severe pemphigus: long-term results including immunologic follow-up. *J Am Acad Dermatol.* 2012;67(4):623–629.

Rogers RS III. Bullous pemphigoid: therapy and management. *J Geriatr Dermatol.* 1995;3:91–98.

Schwartz RA, McDonough PH, Lee BW. Toxic epidermal necrolysis. *J Am Acad Dermatol.* 2013;69:173–184.

Schwartz RA, McDonough PH, Lee BW. Toxic epidermal necrolysis: part II. *J Am Acad Dermatol.* 2013;69(2):187–201.

Stanley JR. Therapy of pemphigus vulgaris. *Arch Dermatol.* 1999;135:76–78.

Zemstov A, Neldner KH. Successful treatment of dermatitis herpetiformis with tetracycline and nicotinamide in a patient unable to tolerate dapsone. *J Am Acad Dermatol.* 1993;28:505–506.

22

Exfoliative Dermatitis

John C. Hall, MD

As the term implies, *exfoliative dermatitis* is a generalized scaling eruption of the skin. The causes are many. This diagnosis should never be made without additional qualifying etiologic terms.

This is a rare skin condition, but many general physicians, residents, and interns occasionally see these cases. Hospitalization serves two purposes; (1) to perform a diagnostic workup, because the cause, in many cases, is difficult to ascertain and (2) to administer intensive therapy under close supervision, especially in cases where the overall condition of the patient is poor. Exfoliative dermatitis can lead to sepsis, high-output congestive heart failure, and dehydration.

Classification of the cases of exfoliative dermatitis is facilitated by dividing them into primary and secondary forms.

PRIMARY EXFOLIATIVE DERMATITIS

These cases develop in apparently healthy persons from no ascertainable cause.

Presentation and Characteristics

Skin Lesions

Clinically, it may be impossible to differentiate this primary form from the one in which the cause is known or suspected. Various degrees of scaling and redness are seen, ranging from fine, generalized, granular scales with mild erythema to scaling in large plaques, with marked erythema (generalized erythroderma) and lichenification. Widespread lymphadenopathy is usually present. The nails become thick and lusterless, and the hair falls out in varying degrees.

Subjective Complaint

Itching, in most cases, is intense. The patient may be toxic and febrile.

Course

The prognosis for early cure of the disease is poor. The mortality rate is high in older patients because of generalized debility and secondary infection.

Causes

Various authors have studied the relationship of lymphomas with cases of exfoliative dermatitis. Some believe the incidence to be low, but others state that 35% to 50% of these exfoliative cases, particularly those in patients older than 40 years, are the result of lymphomas. However, years may pass before the lymphoma becomes obvious.

Laboratory Findings

There are no diagnostic changes, but the patient with a usual case has an elevated white blood cell count with eosinophilia. Biopsy of the skin is not diagnostic in the primary type, but may help to rule out a more specific diagnosis. Biopsy of an enlarged lymph node, in either the primary or the secondary form, reveals lipomelanotic reticulosis (dermatopathic lymphadenopathy), which is benign.

Treatment

Case Example: A 50-year-old man presents with a generalized, pruritic, scaly, erythematous eruption that he has had for 3 months.

First Visit

1. A general medical workup is indicated.
2. A high-protein diet should be prescribed because these patients have an increased basal metabolic rate and catabolize protein.

3. Bathing instructions are variable. Some patients prefer a daily cool bath in a colloid solution for relief of itching (one box of soluble starch or 1 cup of oilated Aveeno to 10 in of bathwater). For most cases, however, generalized bathing dries the skin and intensifies the itching.

4. Provide heating blankets or extra blankets for the bed. These patients lose a lot of heat through their red skin and consequently feel chilly.

5. Locally, an ointment is most desired, but some patients prefer an oily liquid. Formulas for both are as follows:

    a. White petrolatum 240.0

        or a generic corticosteroid ointment, such as triamcinolone 0.025% or 0.1% ointment 240.0

        Sig: Apply locally b.i.d.

        Remember that on large areas of inflamed skin with a defective epidermal barrier, absorption will be dramatic and a systemic corticosteroid effect should be expected.

    b. Zinc oxide 40%

        Olive oil q.s. 240.0

        Sig: Apply locally with hands or a paintbrush b.i.d.

        Comment: Antipruritic chemicals can also be added to this.

6. Oral antihistamine, for example:

    Chlorpheniramine, 8 or 12 mg #100

    Sig: 1 tablet b.i.d. for itching. Warn the patient of possible drowsiness.

    Or for more sedation hydroxyzine 10, 25, or even 50 mg q 8 hours while awake.

Subsequent Visits

1. Systemic corticosteroids: For resistant cases, the corticosteroids have consistently provided more relief than any other single form of therapy. Any of the preparations can be used. For example:

    Prednisone, 10 mg #100

    Sig: 4 tablets every morning for 1 week, and then 2 tablets every morning.

    Comment: Regulate dosage as indicated.

2. Systemic antibiotics may or may not be indicated. Bacterial cultures of the most eroded and inflamed skin should be done even if infection seems unlikely. You might be surprised what you culture.

SECONDARY EXFOLIATIVE DERMATITIS

Most patients with secondary exfoliative dermatitis have had a previous skin disease that became generalized because of overtreatment or for unknown reasons. There always remain a few cases of exfoliative dermatitis in which the cause is unknown but suspected.

Presentation and Characteristics

Skin Lesions

The clinical picture of this secondary form is indistinguishable from the primary form unless some of the original dermatitis is present. As the exfoliation and erythroderma spread, the characteristics of a primary skin disease, such as psoriasis, become harder to ascertain (Fig. 22-1).

Course

The prognosis in the secondary form is better than that in the primary form, particularly if the original cause is definitely known and more specific therapy can be administered.

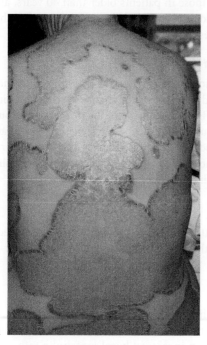

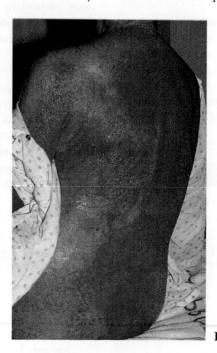

A   B

FIGURE 22-1: Exfoliative dermatitis. **A:** Only at the edge of the large plaques is there a suggestion of psoriasis as the underlying diagnosis. **B:** Exfoliative dermatitis caused by a Dilantin drug eruption.

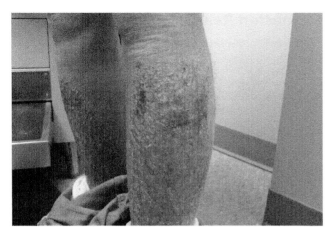

FIGURE 22-2: Generalized exfoliative erythroderma in an adult-onset eczema patient showing erythema, some erosions, and dry medium-sized adherent scale.

Causes

The more common causes of secondary exfoliative dermatitis are as follows:

- Contact dermatitis (see Chapter 12)
- Drug eruption (see Chapter 9)
- Psoriasis (see Chapter 16)
- Atopic eczema (Fig. 22-2) (see Chapter 12)
- Pyoderma or other severe localized inflammation with a secondary id reaction (see Chapter 24)
- Inflammatory fungal disease (i.e., a kerion) with id reaction (see Chapter 28)
- Seborrheic dermatitis, especially in a newborn or an AIDS patient (Fig. 22-3) (see Chapter 15)
- Pityriasis Rubra Pilaris (Fig. 22-4) and Ichthyosis (Fig. 22-5)
- T-cell lymphoma, especially cutaneous T-cell lymphoma (CTCL) (see Chapter 34). A useful rule is that 50% of all patients older than age 50 who have an exfoliative dermatitis have a lymphoma. The Sézary syndrome form of lymphoma is a rare cause of exfoliative dermatitis. It is considered the leukemic form of CTCL. The patient is described as having a "lobster-like" appearance (Fig. 22-6). Sézary syndrome has a very poor prognosis with medium survival of 4 years.
- Internal cancer, leukemia, and other lymphomas.

Treatment

The treatment of these cases consists of a combination of treatment for the primary form of exfoliative dermatitis plus the cautious institution of stronger therapy directed toward the original causative skin condition. This therapy should be reviewed in the section devoted to the specific disease (see the preceding text).

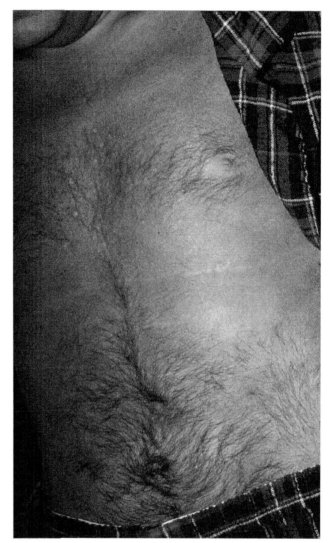

FIGURE 22-3: Generalized redness and scaling in an AIDS patient that represented generalized seborrhea.

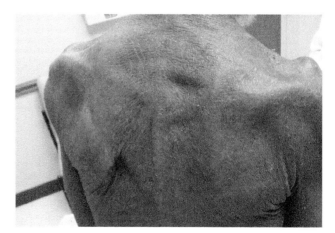

FIGURE 22-4: Exfoliative erythroderma in a patient with pityriasis rubra pillaris.

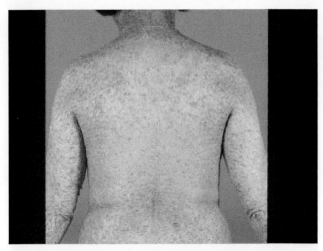

FIGURE 22-5: Generalized exfoliation in a patient with lamellar ichthyosis. Some plate-like scale of primary disease of lamellar ichthyosis can be seen over upper buttocks and extensor arms.

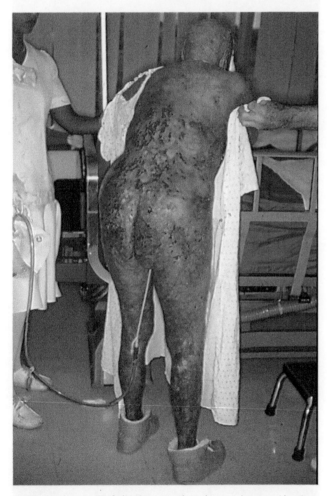

FIGURE 22-6: Exfoliative erythroderma in a patient with CTCL. A search for Sézary cells should be done.

Suggested Readings

Botella-Estrada R, Sanmartin O, Oliver V, et al. Erythroderma. *Arch Dermatol.* 1994;130:1503–1507.

Pal S, Haroon TS. Erythroderma: a clinico-etiologic study of 90 cases. *Int J Dermatol.* 1998;37:104–107.

Rym BM, Mourad M, Bechir Z, et al. Erythroderma in adults: a report of 80 cases. *Int J Dermatol.* 2005;44:731–735.

Sehgal VN, Srivastava G. Erythroderma/generalized exfoliative dermatitis in pediatric practice: an overview. *Int J Dermatol.* 2006;45:831–839.

Wilson DC, Jester JD, King LE Jr. Erythroderma and exfoliative dermatitis [review]. *Clin Dermatol.* 1993;11:67–72.

Psychodermatology

Mio Nakamura, MD and John Koo, MD

Psychodermatology and *psychocutaneous medicine* are unfamiliar terms to many physicians. These terms describe a field of medicine that focuses on the interface between psychiatry and dermatology. In a surprisingly large proportion of dermatologic disorders, the understanding of the psychosocial context is critical for optimal patient management. For example, common skin rashes such as eczema or psoriasis tend to flare up during emotional stress. In some cases, there is no real skin disorder, but the patient targets his or her skin to express an underlying psychopathologic condition. Neurotic excoriations, trichotillomania, and delusions of parasitosis are such examples. Moreover, patients commonly experience a significant negative impact on their psychological stability resulting from the visible disfigurement caused by their skin disorder. Patients with disfiguring skin disorders, such as alopecia areata, vitiligo, and psoriasis, frequently report problems with self-esteem, depression, and social anxiety.

The management of psychodermatologic disorders requires special skills. First, a clinician must evaluate not only the skin manifestation based on the usual dermatologic differential diagnosis but also the underlying psychopathology and the relevant social, familial, and occupational issues. Once a psychodermatologic diagnosis is made, optimal management often requires a dual approach to address both the dermatologic and the psychological aspects. Even in cases where the primary problem is psychopathologic and the skin manifestations are only secondary, supportive dermatologic care is necessary to avoid secondary complications such as infection. More important, it is crucial that the patient does not feel "abandoned." Demonstrating support by treating the dermatologic aspect of the disease may make the patient more accepting of a psychiatric consultation or referral, should there be a need for one. At the same time, it is important for the clinician to try to understand the nature of the underlying psychopathology in order to initiate appropriate psychiatric management. This ranges from providing appropriate psychotropic medication, encouraging the patient to attend stress management courses, and making a formal referral to a psychiatrist (depending on the severity of the underlying psychopathology).

Psychodermatology cases, just like those in any other field of medical practice, can range from mild to severe. While the most difficult and florid cases, such as delusions of parasitosis, are easily recognizable, a large majority of patients have more subtle psychopathologies impacting their skin disease, such as situational stress or mild depression. Therefore, clinicians should be aware of the mind–skin interaction and look for psychological elements in their patients.

CLASSIFICATION

Psychodermatologic disorders can be broadly classified into four categories: psychophysiologic disorders, primary psychiatric disorders, secondary psychiatric disorders, and cutaneous sensory disorders. *Psychophysiologic disorders* are primary skin diseases, such as eczema or psoriasis, which are frequently exacerbated by emotional stress. *Primary psychiatric disorders* refer to psychological issues that manifest as skin findings; there is no primary skin disorder, and all of the manifestations are self-induced. *Secondary psychiatric disorders* are cases in which significant psychological issues develop as a consequence of having a disfiguring skin disorder, including negative impact on self-esteem and body image, depression, humiliation, frustration, and social phobia. Cutaneous sensory disorders are often neurogenic (originating from a nerve with or without neuropathy) or neuropathic (originating from a nerve with structural or functional damage) whereby involvement of the central or peripheral nervous system is suspected, such as cutaneous dysesthesia. In this condition, a patient with no visible rash presents to a clinician with purely sensory skin complaints, such as itching, burning, or stinging.

An extensive medical workup fails to reveal an underlying diagnosis. These patients usually respond better to psychotropic medications than to usual dermatologic therapeutics, such as topical steroids.

It is important to be able to distinguish between these broad categories for several reasons. First, the severity of the underlying psychopathologic condition tends to vary depending on the categories. Psychophysiologic disorders generally involve "milder" psychopathologies, such as situational stress, compared with the primary psychiatric disorders. Second, the approach to patients is frequently different among the categories. For example, in psychophysiologic cases, it is easy to talk to the patient about his or her stress and how it affects the patient's skin disease. On the other hand, in certain cases of primary psychiatric disorder such as delusions of parasitosis or factitial dermatitis in which the patient denies underlying psychiatric disease, patients may not be ready to be confronted with the psychogenic aspect of their condition.

Psychophysiologic Disorders

Psychophysiologic disorders are skin diseases that are often precipitated or exacerbated by emotional stress. Although many dermatologic conditions fall into this category, including eczema, psoriasis, and acne, there are individual differences among patients; there are "stress responders" and "stress nonresponders," depending on whether or not the patient predictably experiences exacerbation of the skin disease with stress.

In "stress responders," the identification of the stressor can be important in treating the primary dermatologic disease. While the issue of stress may not be so important in minor, treatment-responsive dermatologic cases, it may be key in more severe cases. Patients with chronic and recalcitrant dermatoses may be difficult to "turn around" without first addressing stress as an exacerbating factor.

Because patients often feel embarrassed to bring up psychological issues to the physician, it is important for the clinician to ask the patient whether psychological, social, or occupational stress may be contributing to their skin disease. In cases in which psychosocial stress is relatively mild, simple encouragement to find a stress reducer, such as exercise, hobbies, meditation, or other stress management techniques, may suffice. Referral to a therapist or counselor is appropriate if the patient feels it will be beneficial.

If the stress or tension is of significant intensity, it may warrant consideration of medical treatment with an antianxiety agent. There are three general types of agents available to meet these clinical needs. The first type, the benzodiazepines, can be used on an as-needed basis to provide quick relief from anxiety. Generally, an agent with a short half-life, such as alprazolam (Xanax), is recommended. Some of the older agents, such as diazepam (Valium) or chlordiazepoxide (Librium), are more likely to be associated with possible cumulative side effects owing to their longer or unpredictable half-lives. Benzodiazepines should be reserved only for short-term use, as patients may develop tolerance, dependence, and withdrawal after several weeks of continued use.

For cases requiring long-term treatment with an antianxiety agent, there are nonsedating and nonaddicting options, such as buspirone (BuSpar). Owing to its slow onset of action, it cannot be taken on an as-needed basis and may take 4 weeks or more to become effective. A common starting dose is 15 mg daily (7.5 mg twice daily). It can be increased by 5 mg/day every 2 to 3 days to a maximum dose of 60 mg/day. The therapeutic range for most patients is between 15 and 30 mg daily. It is not uncommon for a benzodiazepine to be started in conjunction with buspirone while the therapeutic effect of buspirone is achieved and then tapered off after 2 or 4 weeks.

Antidepressants are the third type of agents used in the treatment of anxiety. Paroxetine (Paxil) is an example of a selective serotonin reuptake inhibitor (SSRI), which is useful in the treatment of not only depression but also chronic anxiety. Common side effects of SSRIs include drowsiness, dizziness, insomnia, weight gain or weight loss, and reduced sexual desire and/or function.

If the intensity and complexity of the anxiety disorder warrant a psychiatric referral, it should be discussed with the patient in a supportive and diplomatic way so as to maximize the chance of the patient accepting the referral as an adjunct to continuing dermatologic therapy.

Primary Psychiatric Disorders

Primary psychiatric disorders are less commonly encountered than psychophysiologic disorders. However, they tend to be more "florid" with a striking presentation.

Delusions of Parasitosis

Delusions of parasitosis belong to a group of disorders called *monosymptomatic hypochondriacal psychosis* (MHP), where seemingly "normal" patients present with a somatic delusional ideation of a hypochondriacal nature. Because of the encapsulated nature of the delusional disorder, these cases are usually quite different from schizophrenia, which involves multiple functional defects, including auditory hallucinations, lack of social skills, flat affect, etc., in addition to delusional ideation.

Delusions of parasitosis is the most common form of MHP encountered by doctors. In this type of MHP, patients firmly believe that their bodies are infested with some type of organism. They frequently present with elaborate ideation involving how these "organisms" mate, reproduce, move in the skin, and, sometimes, come out of the skin or body orifices. Patients often present with the "matchbox" sign, in which bits of excoriated skin, debris, or unrelated insects or insect parts are brought in matchboxes or other containers such as Ziplock bags as proof of infestation (Figs. 23-1 and 23-2). A family member or friend may come in with the patient to confirm the patient's delusion.

Differential Diagnosis: The psychiatric differential diagnosis includes:

- schizophrenia
- psychotic depression

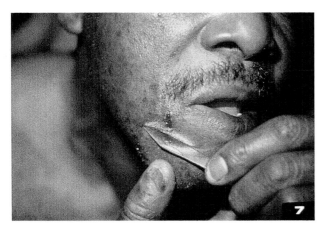

FIGURE 23-1: A man with delusions of parasitosis uses his knife to dig out a "parasite" to demonstrate it to the author (J.K.).

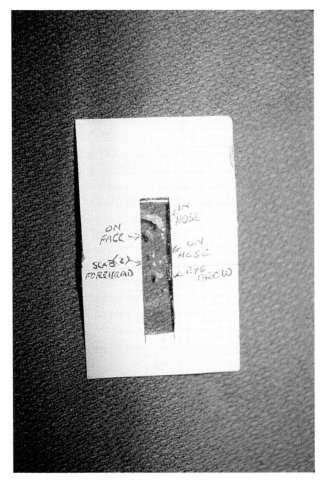

FIGURE 23-2: A carefully constructed specimen board of alleged parasites from a patient with delusions of parasitosis.

■ psychosis with florid mania
■ drug-induced and other forms of psychosis
■ formication without delusions, in which the patient experiences crawling, biting, and stinging sensations without the belief that they are caused by organisms

The other organic forms of psychosis include:

■ vitamin B$_{12}$ deficiency
■ withdrawal from cocaine, amphetamines, or alcohol
■ multiple sclerosis
■ cerebrovascular disease
■ syphilis
■ thyroid dysfunction

If any of the foregoing underlying diagnoses is made, delusions of parasitosis cannot be made. Delusions of parasitosis is a separate psychiatric entity characterized by a very encapsulated ideation where none of the other psychiatric diagnoses with broader underlying manifestations, such as schizophrenia, are involved.

Treatment: Historically, the treatment of choice for delusions of parasitosis is the antipsychotic medication pimozide (Orap). Pimozide has a chemical structure and potency similar to those of haloperidol (Haldol) and has been known to be uniquely effective for this condition by decreasing formication (crawling, stinging, and biting sensations). The dosage used is much lower than that used for schizophrenia. It is generally started at the lowest possible dose of 0.5 or 1 mg and increased by 0.5 or 1 mg/week. By the time the dosage of 3 to 5 mg is reached, most patients experience a significant decrease in formication, as well as the sensations of "organisms" moving in their skin. At the same time, many patients become much less agitated. In younger patients, pimozide can often be continued at the lowest effective dose for several months and then gradually tapered off without necessarily inviting recurrence of symptoms. If the condition recurs, another course of therapy with pimozide can be instituted. In elderly patients, long-term maintenance with a very small dose of pimozide (1 to 2 mg/day) is rarely required.

Just as with many other antipsychotic agents, extrapyramidal signs (EPS) are known side effects of pimozide. The most common of these, namely stiffness and restlessness, can be effectively treated with benztropine (Cogentin) 2 mg up to four times per day as needed. Diphenhydramine (Benadryl) 25 mg can also be used up to four times per day as needed. Although tardive dyskinesia is a possibility with long-term use, the risk appears to be minimal in dermatology patients where a low dose (5 mg/day or less) is generally adequate and often used intermittently. If the patient has a cardiac rhythm disorder, is elderly, or if a dosage higher than 10 mg/day is needed, serial electrocardiograms are required in view of risks of cardiac arrhythmia.

Atypical antipsychotics are also effective in the treatment of delusions of parasitosis. Some of these agents include risperidone (Risperdal), olanzapine (Zyprexa), and quetiapine (Seroquel). The atypical antipsychotics are as effective as conventional antipsychotics for the treatment of psychosis in general. They are better tolerated and have been shown to cause significantly less EPS and tardive dyskinesia in placebo-controlled studies, as well as in clinical practice. Although there have been no randomized controlled trials to evaluate atypical antipsychotics for the treatment of delusions of parasitosis, the safer side-effect profile of atypical antipsychotics may prove useful in the treatment of MHP. It is necessary to mention, however, that atypical antipsychotics can potentially lower the seizure threshold, and thus they should be used with caution in patients with history of seizure disorder.

The greatest disadvantage of atypical antipsychotics in comparison with pimozide is the fact that all atypical antipsychotic agents have psychotic indications, whereas pimozide has no psychiatric indication in the United States. This makes pimozide much more acceptable to patients with delusions of parasitosis who are usually very much averse to any psychotic implications.

Neurotic Excoriations/Factitial Dermatitis

Neurotic excoriations are characterized by self-inflicted excoriations by the fingernails (scratch marks), which may appear as "scooped out" lesions. It is common to see a butterfly distribution on the back in which there is sparing of the interscapular region where the patient is unable to reach. The left side of the back is more involved in a right-handed person, and the opposite is true for a left-handed person. Patients often admit to scratching but cannot control themselves.

Although *neurotic excoriations* and *factitial dermatitis* are sometimes used interchangeably, *factitial dermatitis* should be used more selectively to refer to situations where the patient uses something more elaborate than the fingernails, such as lit cigarette butts, chemicals, or sharp instruments, to damage his or her own skin. Factitial dermatitis tends to be bizarre in shape, depth, and distribution. Patients often do not admit to manipulating the skin but often claim that there is something mysterious causing their disease. In both cases, scarring and infection are common complications.

In cases of neurotic excoriations and factitial dermatitis, the clinician must determine the underlying psychopathology driving such skin manifestations. The most common underlying psychopathologies are major depressive, anxiety, and obsessive–compulsive disorders. In rare cases, patients excoriate their skin in response to a delusional ideation, in which case psychosis is the appropriate diagnosis. Patients with neurotic excoriations are usually suffering from depression or

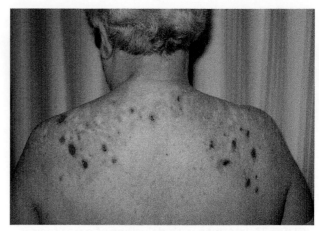

FIGURE 23-3: Multiple neurotic excoriations are present only in the areas easily accessed by the patient's hands on the back of this depressed woman.

anxiety, whereas those with factitial dermatitis tend to hold a delusional ideation (Fig. 23-3).

Treatment: The management of anxiety and delusions/psychosis is as discussed. If the patient has underlying depression driving neurotic excoriations/factitious dermatitis, doxepin (Sinequan) is an effective treatment option. Doxepin is a tricyclic antidepressant with antihistamine effects and is often used by doctors as an antipruritic agent. The antipruritic effect is useful for breaking the itch–scratch cycle, which develops as a result of the patients picking at their nonhealing skin lesions (Fig. 23-4). The sedative/tranquilizing effect of doxepin is also useful because many people with depression who excoriate their skin tend to be agitated ("agitated depression"). The dosage of 100 mg/day or higher is usually required to adequately treat depression. Elderly patients may respond to a lower dose. Of note, the use of doxepin requires all of the usual precautions regarding the use of older tricyclic antidepressants, including the risks of QT prolongation and subsequent cardiac arrhythmias. Similar cardiac considerations have recently been a concern with diphenhidramine (Benadryl) use in the elderly.

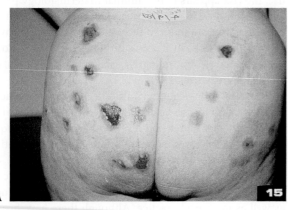
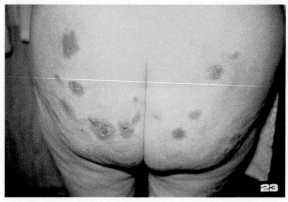

FIGURE 23-4: **A:** Pretreatment photograph of the buttocks of the patient depicted in Figure 23-3. **B:** After 1 week of therapy with doxepin, the patient demonstrates significant improvement in excoriations owing to the antipruritic effect. However, the antidepressant effect of doxepin was not evidenced until later.

Lastly, some cases of factitial dermatitis may in fact be a deliberate manipulation by the patient for secondary gain such as disability benefit or sympathy. If that is the case, the patient has no real psychotic or dermatologic causative factor, and as such, the case is a legal matter involving malingering. This is referred to as Munchausen syndrome, and when another person is involved it is called Munchausen by proxy.

Trichotillomania

Trichotillomania, according to the dermatologic usage of the term, refers to any patient who pulls out his or her own hair. The psychiatric definition of trichotillomania requires the presence of "impulsivity." Trichotillomania is one of the rare psychodermatologic conditions in which a pathologic examination of the skin can be diagnostic. There is a unique change in the hair root called *trichomalacia*, which is seen only in trichotillomania. Therefore, if the patient continues to deny pulling his or her own hair, a scalp biopsy can be helpful in determining the definitive diagnosis.

As with other psychodermatologic cases, the clinician must ascertain the nature of the underlying psychopathology to determine the most appropriate treatment. The most common underlying psychopathology is obsessive–compulsive spectrum behavior, whether or not it formally meets the *DSM-V* criteria for obsessive–compulsive disorder. The other possible underlying psychiatric diagnoses include depression and anxiety, as well as extremely rare cases of delusion. In *trichophobia*, the patient has a delusional belief that there is something in the hair roots that needs to be "dug out" for the hair to grow normally.

Treatment: Treatment is again based on the nature of the underlying psychopathology. Because the most common underlying psychopathology is obsessive–compulsive tendency, medications such as fluoxetine (Prozac), paroxetine (Paxil), fluvoxamine (Luvox), sertraline (Zoloft), and clomipramine (Anafranil) in dosages appropriate for the treatment of obsessive–compulsive disorder can be used. It should be noted that when these medications are used in the treatment of obsessive–compulsive disorder, the dosage tends to be higher than when treating depression. For example, 20 mg/day of fluoxetine or paroxetine is often adequate for the treatment of depression. In contrast, when treating obsessive–compulsive disorder, the required dosage may be 40 to 80 mg/day. In addition, the therapeutic effect when treating obsessive–compulsive disorder takes longer to achieve than when treating depression. The initial response seen in obsessive–compulsive disorder is between 4 to 8 weeks with maximal response by 20 weeks. Once adequate therapeutic response is achieved, therapy should be continued for 6 months to 1 year. Many clinicians have found that a complete remission is unusual. The nonpharmacologic approach includes psychotherapy and behavioral therapy.

Secondary Psychiatric Disorders

Given the visible nature of dermatologic conditions, there is significant psychological and social impact, which affects the quality of life (Fig. 23-5). For example, it is difficult for

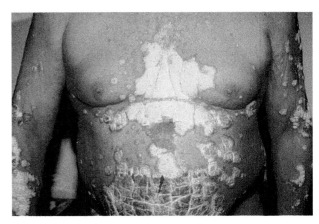

FIGURE 23-5: The disfiguring effects of psoriasis are seen on the arms and torso of this patient with plaque psoriasis. This man experienced severe social, sexual, occupational, as well as psychological impact because of his psoriasis.

patients with skin disorders to get jobs where appearance is important. It is also well documented that patients with visible disfigurement, especially if the condition is perceived to be contagious, are generally treated worse than those with other obvious physical disabilities. It is the clinician's responsibility to explore the patient's psychosocial well-being and determine whether or not intervention is necessary. Although patients may benefit from dermatology support groups or counseling, if any secondary psychopathology is of significant intensity, a referral to a psychiatrist may be warranted.

Cutaneous Sensory Disorders

In cutaneous sensory syndrome, patients present to the clinician with a sensory complaint without any visible skin findings. An extensive workup fails to reveal any underlying medical condition that can be associated with the chief complaint. The sensation can vary from itching, stinging, and biting to other forms of cutaneous discomfort. It is well documented that itching can occur as a manifestation of central nervous system insult, such as multiple sclerosis, brain abscess, brain tumor, or sensory stroke. However, in many cases, it is not possible to demonstrate a focal neurologic deficit. In general, patients with chronic sensory disorders are frustrated because they often do not respond to the usual dermatologic treatment modalities such as topical steroids, emollients, and antihistamines. However, it has been found that these patients frequently do respond to the empiric use of psychotropic medications.

Treatment

If the primary complaint is pruritus, patients often respond to doxepin in doses that are significantly lower than those used for the treatment of depression. Dosages of 10 to 75 mg/day are typically adequate, whether taken at bedtime or in divided doses (Fig. 23-6). The lowest effective dose needed to suppress pruritus should be maintained for several months. In many cases, recurrence of pruritus can be avoided if doxepin is gradually tapered off.

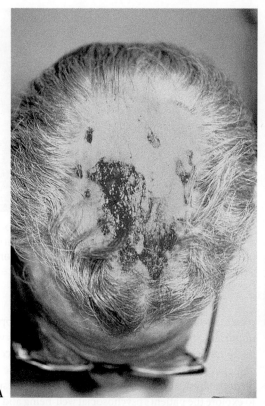 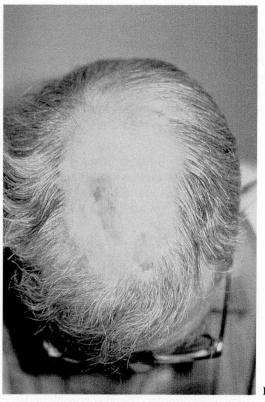

A   B

FIGURE 23-6: **A:** For decades this older man experienced severe, intermittent attacks of scalp pruritus that failed conventional dermatologic therapy and for which no primary skin lesion or systemic organic etiology was ever identified. A mental status examination by the author (J.K.) was entirely negative for any diagnosable psychiatric disorder. **B:** After 2 weeks of empirical treatment with 25 to 50 mg/day of doxepin, the patient experienced complete resolution of pruritus that recurred when doxepin was discontinued. This observation may illustrate a case of central nervous system–mediated pruritus.

If the primary sensory complaint relates to pain or burning, amitriptyline (Elavil), in doses lower than those used to treat depression, is frequently effective. The disadvantage of tricyclic agents is its high side-effect profile, which includes drowsiness, orthostatic hypotension, gastrointestinal symptoms, and cardiac arrhythmia. If the patient cannot tolerate amitriptyline, a newer tricyclic agent such as desipramine (Norpramin) may have lower risks of side effects. If the patient cannot tolerate any tricyclic antidepressants, SSRIs may be effective. However, in contrast to tricyclic agents, the efficacy of SSRIs as analgesics has not been well studied.

In all cases of cutaneous sensory syndrome, it is important to let the patient know prior to initiating therapy that improvement occurs extremely slowly. Fortunately, it is generally possible to find the optimal agent and dosage to resolve the chronic sensory disorder and maintain its effect if the medication is slowly tapered off.

SAUER'S NOTES

If a patient refuses a psychiatric referral, it is the responsibility of the general physician or dermatologist to use pharmacotherapy or psychotherapy to give the patient the best possible care.

Suggested Readings

Bewley A, Taylor RE, Reichenberg JS, et al. *Practical Psychodermatology.* Chichester: Wiley Blackwell; 2014.

Gaston L, Lassone M, Bernier-Buzzanga J, et al. Psoriasis and stress: a prospective study. *J Am Acad Dermatol.* 1987;17(1):82–86.

Ginsburg IH, Prystowsky JH, Kornfeld DS, et al. Role of emotional factors in adults with atopic dermatitis. *Int J Dermatol.* 1993;32:65–66.

Heller MM, Koo JYM. *Contemporary Diagnosis and Management in Psychodermatology.* Longboat Key: Handbooks in Health Care; 2011.

Koo JY, Pham CT. Psychodermatology: practical guidelines on pharmacotherapy. *Arch Dermatol.* 1992;128: 381–388.

Koo JY. Skin disorders. In: Kaplan HI, Saduch BJ, eds. *Comprehensive Textbook of Psychiatry.* 6th ed. Baltimore: Williams & Wilkins; 1995.

Koo JYM. Psychodermatology: a practice manual for clinicians. *Curr Probl Dermatol.* 1995;6:204–232.

Leon A, Levin EC, Koo JY. Psychodermatology: an overview. *Semin Cutan Med Surg* 2013;32(2):64–67.

Nguyen CM, Beroukhim K, Danesh MJ, et al. *Contemporary Diagnosis and Management in Advanced Psychodermatology.* Longboat Key: Handbooks in Health Care; 2015.

Patel V, Koo JY. Delusions of parasitosis; suggested dialogue between dermatologist and patient. *J Dermatol Treat.* 2015;26(5):456–460.

Rapp SR, Feldman SR, Exum ML, et al. Psoriasis causes as much disability as other major medical diseases. *J Am Acad Dermatol.* 1999;41(3):401–407.

Rodriguez-Vallecillo E, Woodbury-Farina MA. Dermatological manifestations of stress in normal and psychiatric populations. *Psychiatr Clin North Am.* 2015;37(4):625–651.

Stein DJ, Mullen L, Islam MN, et al. Compulsive and impulsive symptomatology in trichotillomania. *Psychopathology.* 1995;28:208–213.

Dermatologic Bacteriology

John C. Hall, MD

Bacteria exist on the skin as normal nonpathogenic resident flora or as pathogenic organisms. The pathogenic bacteria cause primary, secondary, and systemic infections. For clinical purposes, it is justifiable to divide the problem of bacterial infection into three classifications (Table 24-1). Some of the diseases listed are of dubious bacterial etiology, but they appear bacterial, may have a bacterial component, can be treated with antibacterial agents, and are, therefore, included in this chapter.

With an alteration in immune capabilities in a person, bacteria and other infectious agents can have erratic behavior. Ordinary nonpathogens can act as pathogens, and pathogenic agents can act more aggressively.

PRIMARY BACTERIAL INFECTIONS (PYODERMAS)

The most common causative agents of the primary skin infections are the coagulase-positive micrococci (staphylococci) and the β-hemolytic streptococci. Superficial or deep bacterial lesions can be produced by these organisms. In managing the pyodermas, certain general principles of treatment must be initiated.

- *Improve bathing habits:* More frequent bathing and the use of bactericidal soap, such as Dial, Cetaphil Antibacterial, or Lever 2000, are indicated. Any pustules or crusts should be removed during bathing to facilitate penetration of the local medications. In rare instances when these infections are recalcitrant to standard therapies, use half to one cup of bleach in a full tub of water to soak daily.
- *General isolation procedures:* Clothing and bedding should be changed frequently and cleaned. The patient should have a separate towel and washcloth.
- *Systemic drugs:* The patient should be questioned regarding ingestion of drugs that can cause lesions that mimic or cause pyodermas, such as iodides, bromides, testosterone, corticosteroids, progesterone, and lithium.
- *Diabetes:* In chronic skin infections, particularly recurrent boils, diabetes should be ruled out by history and laboratory examination.
- *Immunosuppressed patients:* A history of abnormal findings should alert the physician to the increasing number of patients now who are on chemotherapy for cancer, are posttransplant, or have the acquired immunodeficiency syndrome (AIDS).

TABLE 24-1 • Classification of Bacterial Infection
Primary Bacterial Infections
Impetigo
Ecthyma
Folliculitis
Superficial folliculitis
Staphylococcus folliculitis
Chronic noninfectious folliculitis
Folliculitis of the scalp
Superficial—acne necrotica miliaris
Deep scarring—folliculitis decalvans
Folliculitis of the beard
Stye
Furuncle
Carbuncle
Sweat gland inflammations
Erysipelas
Secondary Bacterial Infections
Cutaneous diseases with secondary infection
Infected ulcers
Infectious eczematoid dermatitis
Bacterial intertrigo
Systemic Bacterial Infections
Scarlet fever
Granuloma inguinale
Chancroid
Mycobacterial infections
Tuberculosis of the skin
Leprosy
Gonorrhea
Rickettsial diseases
Actinomycosis

Impetigo

Impetigo is a common superficial bacterial infection seen most often in children. It is the "infantigo" every parent respects.

Primary Lesions

The lesions vary from small vesicles to large bullae that rapidly rupture and discharge a honey-colored serous liquid (Fig. 24-1). New lesions can develop in a matter of hours. The blisters are evanescent and often are not present but leave their oval or scalloped edges.

Secondary Lesions

Crusts form from the discharge and appear to be lightly stuck on the skin surface. When removed, a superficial erosion remains, which may be the only evidence of the disease. In debilitated infants, the bullae may coalesce to form an exfoliative type of infection called *Ritter's disease* or *pemphigus neonatorum*.

Distribution

The lesions occur most commonly on the face but may also be present anywhere else.

Contagiousness

It is not unusual to see brothers or sisters of the patient and, rarely, the parents similarly infected.

Differential Diagnosis

- *Contact dermatitis* caused by poison ivy or oak: Linear blisters and itches severely (see Chapter 8).

- *Tinea of smooth skin:* Fewer lesions; spreads slowly; central clearing; small vesicles in an annular configuration and elevated edge; fungi found on scraping; culture is positive (see Chapter 28).
- *Toxic epidermal necrolysis:* In infants and rarely in adults, massive bullae can develop rapidly, particularly with staphylococcal infection. The severe form of this infection is known as the staphylococcal scalded skin syndrome, which is a type of toxic epidermal necrolysis (see Chapter 21).

SAUER'S NOTES

Body piercing has frequently been associated with localized staphylococcal infection and pseudomonas infection, and rarely bacteremia and endocarditis. Tuberculosis, hepatitis C and B, and even HIV can be transmitted in this way. Noninfectious complications include keloids and allergic dermatitis. This fad should not be recommended, especially in the tongue, lips, navels, nipples, nose, or genitalia.

Treatment

1. Outline the general principles of treatment. Emphasize the removal of the crusts once or twice a day during bathing with an antibacterial soap such as Lever 2000 or chlorhexidine (Hibiclens) skin cleanser.

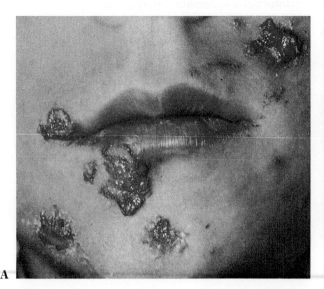
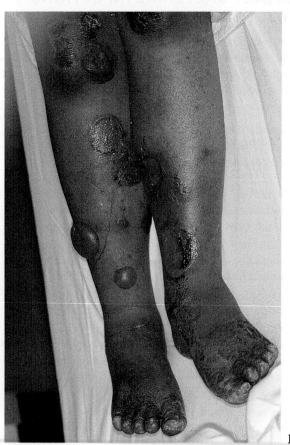

FIGURE 24-1: A: Impetigo of the face. The honey-colored crusts are typical. **B:** Bullous impetigo on the legs of a young child. (Courtesy of Abner Kurtin, Folia Dermatologica, No. 2. Geigy Pharmaceuticals.)

2. Mupirocin (Bactroban) or gentamicin (Garamycin) ointment or Polysporin ointment q.s. 15.0.
   Sig: Apply t.i.d. locally for 10 days. Treat all affected family members or other affected contacts.
3. Oral antibiotics such as a 10-day course of erythromycin, cephalexin, or clindamycin may be necessary.
4. Methicillin-resistant *Staphylococcus aureus* in the community-acquired form (CA-MRSA) now occurs in epidemic proportions. Fortunately, it is often sensitive to sulfamethoxazole with trimethoprim (Septra or Bactrim), clindamycin, or tetracycline derivatives. Abscesses are common and when present, must be treated aggressively by incision and drainage.

The commonest carrier sites for CA-MRSA are, in the following order, external nares, pharynx, inguinal crease, and perineum. To decrease the carrier state, the following measures may be helpful in household contacts or family: change toothpaste, use a mouthwash regularly, change linen daily, mupirocin ointment in nose b.i.d. for 5 days, and clean commonly used surfaces with bleach. It is interesting that eczema, which is frequently infected with staph, is usually methicillin-sensitive *staphylococcus aureus*. A final word on MRSA is that it is now greater than 50% of skin infections in the United States, more pathogenic than other bacterial infections, with significant mortality, more frequently causes abscesses that must be drained to heal, and up to 1/3 of family members will have a carrier state of MRSA, of whom 70% will eventually get a skin infection.

Ecthyma

Ecthyma is another superficial bacterial infection, but is seen less commonly and is deeper than impetigo. It is usually caused by *β*-hemolytic *streptococci* and occurs on the buttocks and the thighs of children (Fig. 24-2).

Primary Lesion

A vesicle or vesiculopustule appears and rapidly changes into the secondary lesion.

SAUER'S NOTES

1. I sometimes add sulfur 5% and hydrocortisone 1% to 2% to the antibiotic cream or ointment for treatment of impetigo and other superficial pyodermas. Many patients with impetigo whom I see have been using a plain antibiotic salve with an oral antibiotic, and the impetigo persists. With this compound salve the impetigo heals.
2. Advise the patient that the local treatment should be continued for 5 days after the lesions apparently have disappeared to prevent recurrences "therapy plus."
3. *Systemic antibiotic therapy:* Some physicians believe that every patient with impetigo should be treated with systemic antibiotic therapy to heal these lesions and also to prevent chronic glomerulonephritis. Erythromycin in appropriate dosages for 10 days would be effective in most cases. Resistance to erythromycin can occur, and then dicloxacillin or cephalexin is effective. Erythromycin-inducible clindamycin resistance is becoming more common. Bacterial sensitivity testing helps to guide appropriate antibiotic therapy. There is a dramatic increase in the United States in community-acquired methicillin-resistant *Staphylococcus aureus* (CA-MRSA), and I am using sulfamethoxazole/trimethoprim as an initial option more often.

Secondary Lesion

This is a piled-up crust, 1 to 3 cm in diameter, overlying a superficial erosion or ulcer. In neglected cases, scarring can occur as a result of extension of the infection into the dermis.

Distribution

Most commonly, the disease is seen on the posterior aspect of the thighs and the buttocks, from where it can spread. Ecthyma commonly follows the scratching of chigger bites.

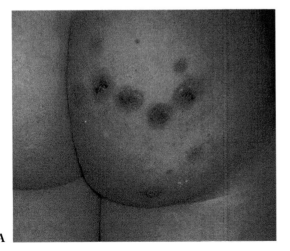 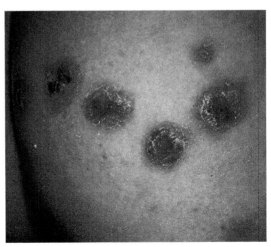

FIGURE 24-2: **A:** Ecthyma on the buttocks of 13-year-old boy. **B:** Close-up of lesions. (Courtesy of Burroughs Wellcome Co.)

Age Group

Children are the most common age group affected.

Contagiousness

Ecthyma is rarely found in other members of the family.

Differential Diagnosis

- *Psoriasis:* Less common in children; whitish, firmly attached scaly lesions, also occur on the scalp, knees, and/or elbows (see Chapter 16).
- *Impetigo:* Much smaller crusted lesions, not as deep (*see* preceding section).

Treatment

1. The general principles of treatment are listed earlier in the chapter. The crusts must be removed daily. Response to therapy is slower than with impetigo, but the treatment is the same for both conditions.
2. *Systemic antibiotics:* If there is a low-grade fever and evidence of bacterial infection in other organs caused by sepsis, one of the antibiotic syrups or tablets can be given orally for 10 days. This is commonly seen in children with extensive ecthyma. It is rarely seen with impetigo.

Folliculitis

Folliculitis is a common pyogenic infection of the hair follicles, usually caused by coagulase-positive *staphylococci* (Fig. 24-3). Seldom does a patient consult the physician for a single outbreak of folliculitis. The physician is consulted because of recurrent and chronic pustular lesions. The patient realizes that the present acute episode clears with the help of nature, but seeks medicine and advice to prevent recurrences. For this reason, the general principles of treatment are listed. The physician must pay particular attention to the drug history and the diabetes investigation. Some physicians believe that a focus of infection in the teeth, tonsils, gallbladder, or genitourinary tract should be ruled out when folliculitis is recurrent.

The folliculitis may invade only the superficial part of the hair follicle, or it may extend down to the hair bulb. Many variously named clinical entities based on the location and the chronicity of the lesions have been carried down through the years. A few of these entities bear presentation here, but most are defined in the Dictionary–Index.

Superficial Folliculitis

The physician is rarely consulted for this minor problem, which is most commonly seen on the arms, scalp, face, and buttocks of children and adults with the acne–seborrhea complex. A history of excessive use of hair oils, bath oils, moisturizers, or suntan oils can often be obtained. The use of these oily agents should be avoided. Culture for *Staphylococcus* or *Streptococcus* may be negative, and in these cases, the same therapeutic regiments that are usually used for acne should

be used. Chronic noninfectious folliculitis is the term I use for this clinical picture.

Folliculitis of the Scalp (Superficial Form)

A superficial form has the appellation *acne necrotica miliaris*. This is an annoying, pruritic, chronic, and recurrent folliculitis of the scalp in adults. The scratching of the crusted lesions occupies the patient's evening hours.

Treatment

1. Follow the general principles of treatment.
2. Selenium sulfide (Selsun, Head & Shoulders Intensive Treatment) suspension shampoo 120.0.
   Sig: Shampoo twice a week as directed on the label.
3. Other shampoos such as T-Sal and sulfur washes, such as Ovace, Plexion, or a generic form of these used as a shampoo, can be tried.
4. Antibiotic and corticosteroid cream mixture q.s. 15.0.
   Sig: Apply to scalp h.s.

SAUER'S NOTES

My routine for *chronic* folliculitis cases includes the following:
1. Sulfur ppt. 5%
   Hydrocortisone 1%
   Bactroban cream q.s. 15.0
   Sig: Apply b.i.d. locally.
2. Long-term low-dose antibiotic therapy can be used, such as erythromycin, 250 mg, q.i.d. for 3 days, then two or three times a day for months.
3. Lichenified papules of excoriated folliculitis respond to superficial liquid nitrogen applications or intralesional corticosteroid injections.

Folliculitis of the Scalp (Deep Form)

The deep form of scalp folliculitis is called *folliculitis decalvans*. This is a chronic, slowly progressive folliculitis with an active border and scarred atrophic center. The end result, after years of progression, is patchy, scarred areas of alopecia, with eventual burning out of the inflammation. It is not a true infection and bacterial cultures are negative. Long-term tetracycline derivatives may be helpful.

Differential Diagnosis

- *Chronic discoid lupus erythematosus:* Redness, hypopigmentation, and hyperpigmentation; enlarged hair follicles with follicular plugs (see Chapter 41).
- *Alopecia cicatrisata* (pseudopelade of Brocq): Rare; no evidence of inflammation. Some authors think this is burned out lichen planus of the scalp.
- *Tinea of the scalp:* It is important to culture the hair for fungi in any chronic infection of the scalp; *Trichophyton tonsurans* group can cause a subtle

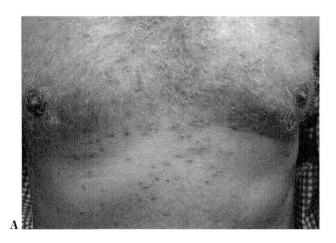
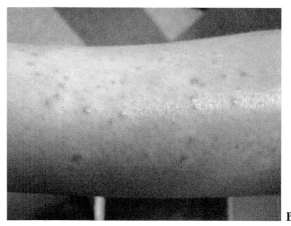
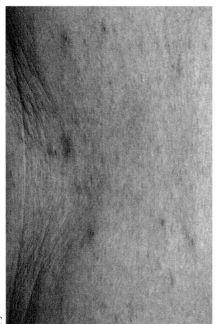
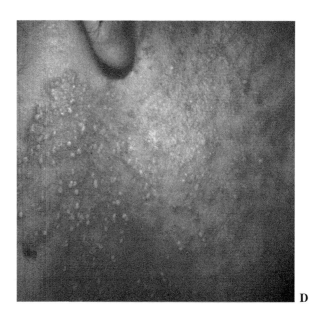
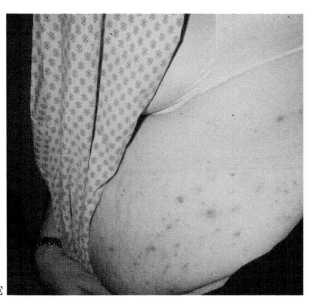

FIGURE 24-3: **A:** Perifollicular papules over chest caused by prolonged use of triamcinolone ointment on chest. The ointment was used for months for eczema. Steroid folliculitis tends to have monotonous papules. **B:** Perifollicular pustules of the pretibial area. Inquiry reveals that new moisturizer or shaving product was being used. Culture is negative for staphylococcus. **C:** MSSA positive folliculitis on chest. Unlike culture negative, there is more inflammation around the pustules. Unlike steroid folliculitis, there is less uniform appearance of individual pustules. **D:** Gram-negative folliculitis on the face and neck in a patient on prolonged oral antibiotics for acne. Pustules culture is gram negative and the pustules are monotonous in appearance. **E:** Hot tub folliculitis due to psuedomas. The patient had been using a hot tub. The papules are more nodular, larger, less uniform in size, and less monotonous. These patients can have malaise and fever.

noninflammatory clinical picture (black dot tinea in children, which is endemic in large urban areas in African American children who braid their hair) (see Chapter 28).

- *Excoriated folliculitis:* Chronic thickened excoriated papules or nodules (can be called *prurigo nodularis*), usually seen on the posterior scalp, posterior neck, anus, and legs. When allowed to heal, whitish scars remain. The inflammation can last for years. Liquid nitrogen applied to the papules is effective, as are intralesional corticosteroids. Occasionally, these patients can be treated with a drug such as a selective serotonin reuptake inhibitor to decrease obsessive–compulsive behavior. Common in dialysis patients and can be seen in hepatitis C and AIDS.

- *Lichen planopilaris:* Scarring lichen planus in the scalp, which is usually characteristic on biopsy. It may have follicular plugging and is characterized by perifollicular cuffing of fine adherent scale and a purplish pink color. Topical or intralesional corticosteroids and antimalarials are often used with success.

Treatment

Results of treatment may be disappointing. Long-term antibiotics, especially tetracycline derivatives, may be helpful; occasionally intralesional corticosteroids may be palliative.

Folliculitis of the Beard

This is the familiar "barber's itch," which was resistant to therapy in the days before antibiotics. This bacterial infection of the hair follicles is spread rather rapidly by shaving.

Differential Diagnosis

- *Contact dermatitis* caused by shaving lotions: History of new lotion applied; general redness of the area with some vesicles (see Chapter 8).

- *Tinea of the beard:* Very slowly spreading infection; hairs broken off; usually a deeper, nodular type of inflammation (Majocchi's granuloma); culture of hair produces fungi (see Chapter 28).

- *Ingrown beard hairs* (pseudofolliculitis barbae): Hair circling back into the skin with resultant chronic inflammation; a hereditary trait, especially in African Americans. Close shaving aggravates the condition. Local antibiotics rarely help, but locally applied depilatories may help. Other local therapy to consider is Retin-A gel and Benzashave (shaving cream with benzoyl peroxide). Permanent hair removal by electrolysis or laser can be helpful. Vaniqa applied twice a day after hair removal can be used to reduce the rate of regrowth of hair. Growing a beard or mustache eliminates the problem. Hairs may also become ingrown in axillae, pubic area, or legs, especially when closely shaved in places with curly hair.

Treatment

1. Follow the general principles of treatment, stressing the use of Dial or other antibacterial soap for washing of the face.

2. Shaving instructions:
   a. Change the razor blade daily or sterilize the head of the electric razor by placing it in 70% alcohol for 1 hour.
   b. Apply the following salve very lightly to the face before shaving and again after shaving. *Do not shave closely.*

3. Antibiotic and hydrocortisone cream mixture q.s. 15.0.
   Sig: Apply to the face before shaving, after shaving, and at bedtime.
   Comment: For stubborn cases, add sulfur 5% to the cream.

4. Oral therapy with erythromycin, 250 mg (can also use cephalexin on clindamycin).
   Sig: one capsule q.i.d. for 7 days, then one capsule b.i.d. for 7 days.

Sty (Hordeolum)

A *sty* is a deep folliculitis of the stiff eyelid hairs. A single lesion is treated with hot packs of 1% boric acid solution and an ophthalmic antibiotic ointment. Recurrent lesions may be linked with the blepharitis of seborrheic dermatitis (dandruff) or rosacea. For this type, vytone or cleansing the eyelashes with Johnson's baby shampoo is indicated. If it is a chronic problem, tetracycline antibiotics short-term or long-term can be used.

Furuncle

A furuncle, or boil (Fig. 24-4), is a more extensive infection of the hair follicle, usually caused by *Staphylococcus*. A boil can occur in any person at any age, but certain predisposing factors account for most outbreaks. An important factor is the acne–seborrhea complex (oily skin and a history of acne and dandruff). Other factors include poor hygiene, diabetes, local skin trauma from friction of clothing, and maceration in obese persons. One boil usually does not bring the patient to the physician, but recurrent boils do.

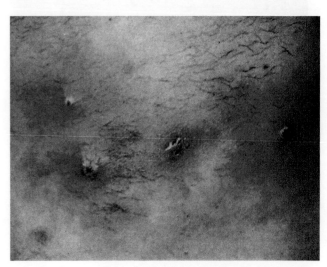

FIGURE 24-4: Multiple furuncles (boils) on the chest. (Courtesy of Abner Kurtin, Folia Dermatologica, No. 2. Geigy Pharmaceuticals.)

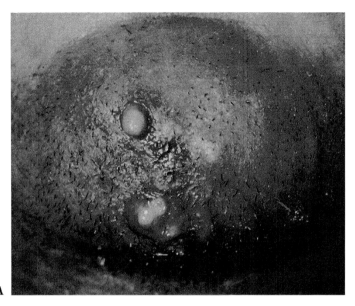
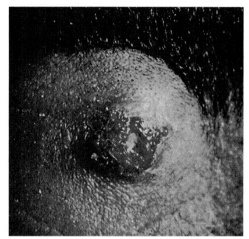

A   B

FIGURE 24-5: **A:** Carbuncle on the chin. Notice the multiple openings. (Courtesy of Abner Kurtin, Folia Dermatologica, No. 2. Geigy Pharmaceuticals.) **B:** Carbuncle on the back of the neck. (Courtesy of J. Lamar Callaway, Folia Dermatologica, No. 4. Geigy Pharmaceuticals.)

Differential Diagnosis
Single Lesion

- *Primary chancre-type diseases:* See list in Dictionary–Index.

Multiple Lesions

- *Drug eruption from iodides or bromides:* See Chapter 8.
- *Hidradenitis suppurativa:* See later in this chapter.

Treatment
Case Example: A young man has had recurrent boils for 6 months. He does not have diabetes, is not obese, is taking no drugs, and bathes daily. He now has a large boil on his buttocks.

1. Burow's solution hot packs.
   Sig: 1 packet of Domeboro powder to 1 quart of hot water. Apply hot wet packs for 30 minutes twice a day.
2. Incision and drainage: This should be done only on "ripe" lesions where a necrotic white area appears at the top of the nodule. Drains are not necessary unless the lesion has extended deep enough to form a fluctuant abscess. If near the rectum, consider a perirectal abscess as the diagnosis. This has a communicating tract with the rectum, which must be treated surgically. Referral to a general surgeon or proctologist is indicated.
3. Oral antistaphylococcal penicillin, such as dicloxacillin or cephalexin, should be prescribed for 5 to 10 days. (Bacteriologic culture and sensitivity studies are helpful in determining which antibiotic to use.) I often now use sulfamethoxazole/trimethoprim empirically to cover MRSA before culture results are known.
4. For recurrent form:
   a. Follow general principles of treatment by use of an antibacterial soap.
   b. Rule out focus of infection in teeth, tonsils, genitourinary tract, and so on.
   c. Begin oral therapy with erythromycin, 250 mg, which is very effective in breaking the cycle of recurrent cases. *Sig:* four capsules a day for 10 days.

Cultures should be done to determine sensitivity and antibiotic choices altered as indicated.

Carbuncle

A carbuncle is an extensive infection of several adjoining hair follicles that drains with multiple openings onto the skin surface (Fig. 24-5). Fatal cases were not unusual in the pre-antibiotic days. A common location for a carbuncle is the posterior neck region. Large, ugly, criss-cross scars in this area in an older patient demonstrate the outdated treatment for this disease, namely multiple bold incisions. Because a carbuncle is, in reality, a multiple furuncle, the same etiologic factors apply. Recurrences are uncommon.

Treatment: Treatment is the same as for a boil (see preceding section) but with greater emphasis on systemic antibiotic therapy.

Sweat Gland Inflammations

Although not true infections, inflammations of the sweat gland are included here because of similar clinical appearance (Fig. 24-6) and similar treatment. Primary eccrine sweat gland or duct infections are very rare. However, prickly heat, a sweat retention disease, frequently develops a secondary bacterial infection. Primary apocrine gland inflammation is rather common. Two types of inflammation exist:

- *Apocrinitis* denotes inflammation of a single apocrine gland, usually in the axilla, and is commonly associated with a change in deodorant. It responds to the therapy

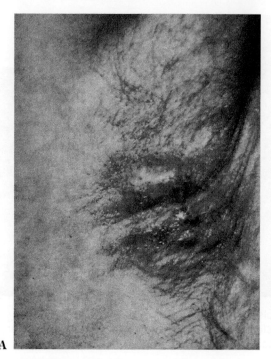
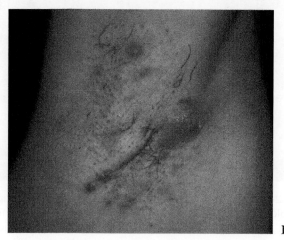

A **B**

FIGURE 24-6: **A:** Sweat gland inflammation of the axilla (hidradenitis suppurativa). (Courtesy of Abner Kurtin, Folia Dermatologica, No. 2. Geigy Pharmaceuticals.) **B:** Hidradenitis suppurativa of the axilla of 6 years' duration. (Courtesy of Burroughs Wellcome Co.)

listed for furuncles. In addition, a lotion containing antibiotic aids in keeping the area dry, such as an erythromycin solution (A/T/S, Erymax, EryDerm, Erycette, T-Stat, Staticin).

■ The second form of apocrine gland inflammation is *hidradenitis suppurativa*. This chronic, recurring inflammation is characterized by the development of multiple nodules, abscesses, draining sinuses, and eventual hypertrophic bands of scars. The most common location is in the axillae, but it can also occur in the groin, perianal, submammary, buttocks, and suprapubic regions. It does not occur before puberty. Etiologically, there appears to be a hereditary tendency in these patients toward occlusion of the follicular orifice and subsequent retention of the secretory products. Two other diseases are related to hidradenitis suppurativa and may be present in the same patient: (1) a severe form of acne called *acne conglobata* and (2) *dissecting cellulitis of the scalp* (see Chapter 13).

Treatment

The management of these cases is difficult. In addition to the general principles mentioned previously, hot packs are used locally, and an oral antibiotic, especially tetracycline, should be given for several weeks.

Plastic surgery or a marsupialization operation is indicated in severe cases. When draining canals or sinuses are present, the marsupialization operation is curative and can be done in the office. After the bridge over the canal has been trimmed away, bleeding is controlled by electrosurgery. These areas can be treated with intralesional corticosteroid injections. Laser therapy has its advocates. Isotretinoin (Accutane) can be tried for 5 to

10 months (see Chapter 15). Biologics including adalimumab and infliximab have been tried. Do not give if there is a chance of pregnancy. Tumor necrosis factor blockers have been used in some patients with success for hidradenitis suppurativa.

Erysipelas

Erysipelas is an uncommon β-hemolytic streptococcal infection of the subcutaneous tissue that produces a characteristic type of cellulitis (Fig. 24-7), with fever and malaise. Recurrences are frequent.

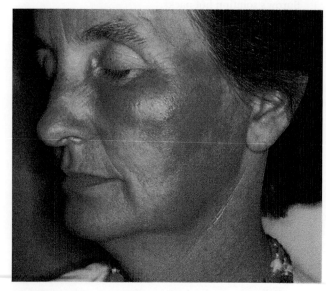

FIGURE 24-7: Erysipelas of the cheek. (Courtesy of Burroughs Wellcome Co.)

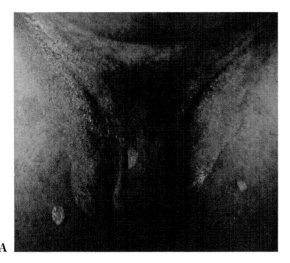 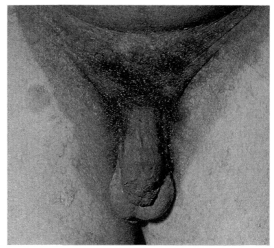

A **B**

FIGURE 24-8: Erythrasma of the crural area with fluorescence under Wood's light **(A)** and in natural light **(B).** (Courtesy of Burroughs Wellcome Co.)

Primary Lesion

A red, warm, raised, brawny, sharply bordered plaque enlarges peripherally. Vesicles and bullae may form on the surface of the plaque. Multiple lesions of erysipelas are rare.

Distribution

Most commonly lesions occur on the face and around the ears (following ear piercing), but no area is exempt. Some authors now think the legs are the most common site.

Course

When treated with systemic antibiotics, response is rapid. Recurrences are common in the same location and may lead to lymphedema of that area, which eventually can become irreversible. The lips, cheeks, and legs are particularly prone to this chronic change, which is called *elephantiasis nostras* or when the area develops a more warty appearance, elephantiasis nostra verrucosa.

Subjective Complaints

Fever and general malaise can precede the development of the skin lesion and persist until therapy is instituted. Elderly patients may present with altered sensorium and somnolence. Pain at the site of the infection can be severe.

Differential Diagnosis

- *Cellulitis:* Lacks a sharp border; recurrences are less common
- *Contact dermatitis:* Sharp border absent; fever and malaise absent; eruption predominantly vesicular and very pruritic rather than painful (see Chapter 8)

Treatment

1. Institute bed rest and direct therapy toward reducing the fever. If the patient is hospitalized, semi-isolation procedures should be initiated. Blood cultures should be considered to rule out sepsis.
2. Give an appropriate systemic antibiotic, such as erythromycin or a penicillin derivative, for 10 days.
3. Apply local, cool, wet dressing, as necessary for comfort.

Erythrasma

Erythrasma is an uncommon bacterial infection of the skin that clinically resembles regular tinea or tinea versicolor (Fig. 24-8). It affects the crural area, axillae, and webs of the toes with flat, hyperpigmented, fine, scaly patches without central clearing or an elevated edge as in tinea cruris. If the patient has not been using an antibacterial soap, these patches fluoresce a striking reddish orange coral color under Wood's light. The causative agent is a diphtheroid organism called *Corynebacterium minutissimum*.

The most effective treatment is erythromycin, 250 mg, q.i.d. for 5 to 7 days. Locally the erythromycin lotions are quite effective (e.g., Staticin, T-Stat, EryDerm, and A/T/S lotion [can be obtained generically]). They are applied twice daily for 10 days.

SECONDARY BACTERIAL INFECTIONS

Secondary infection develops as a complicating factor on a preexisting skin disease. The invasion of an injured skin surface with pathogenic *streptococci* or *staphylococci* is enhanced in skin conditions that are open, deep, oozing, and of long duration.

Cutaneous Diseases with Secondary Infection

Failure in the treatment of many common skin diseases can be attributed to the physician not recognizing the presence of the secondary bacterial infection.

Infected Ulcers

Infected ulcers are deep skin infections owing to an injury or disease that invades the subcutaneous tissue and, upon healing, leaves scars. Ulcers can be divided into primary and secondary ulcers, but most become secondarily infected with bacteria.

Primary Infected Ulcers

Primary ulcers from infection result from the following causes: gangrene owing to pathogenic *streptococci*, *staphylococci*, and *Clostridium* species; syphilis; chancroid; tuberculosis; diphtheria; fungi; leprosy; anthrax; cancer; and lymphomas.

Secondary Infected Ulcers

Secondary ulcers can be related to the following diseases: vascular disorders (arteriosclerosis, thromboangiitis obliterans, Raynaud's phenomenon, phlebitis, and thrombosis); neurologic disorders (spinal cord injury with bedsores or decubiti, central nervous system syphilis, spina bifida, poliomyelitis, and syringomyelia); diabetes; trauma; ulcerative colitis; Crohn's disease; immunosuppression; allergic local anaphylaxis; and other conditions. Finally, there is a group of secondary ulcers called *phagedenic ulcers*, variously described under many different names. These arise in diseased skin or on the apparently normal skin of debilitated persons. These ulcers undermine the skin in large areas, are notoriously chronic, and are resistant to therapy.

SAUER'S NOTES

1. Any type of skin lesion, such as hand dermatitis, poison weed dermatitis, atopic eczema, chigger bites, fungus infection, traumatic abrasion, and so on, can become secondarily infected.
2. The treatment is usually simple: An antibacterial agent is added to the local treatment one would ordinarily use for the dermatosis in question. For extensive secondary bacterial infection, the appropriate systemic antibiotic is indicated, based on bacterial culture and sensitivity studies.

Treatment

1. For primary ulcers, specific therapy is indicated, if available. The response to therapy is usually quite rapid.
2. For secondary ulcers, appropriate therapy should be directed toward the primary disease. The response to therapy is usually quite slow. This is especially true for the decubitus ulcer of the immobile, incontinent person. These must be kept clean and the patient must be kept off the pressure site where the ulcer has developed as much as possible. Early in these ulcers, I use Johnson & Johnson self-healing pads for protection. It is cheap and can be left on and replaced indefinitely.
3. The basic rules of local therapy for ulcers can be illustrated best by outlining the management of a patient with a

stasis leg ulcer (see Stasis [Venous] Dermatitis and Ulcers section in Chapter 13).
   a. Rest of the affected area: If rest in bed is not feasible, then an Ace elastic bandage, 4 in wide, should be worn. This bandage is applied over the local medication and before getting out of bed in the morning. A more permanent support is a modification of an Unna boot (Dome-Paste bandage, Gelocast, or an easy-to-apply and effective adhesive flexible bandage). This boot can be applied for 1 week or more at a time if secondary infection is under control.
   b. Elevation of the affected extremity: This should be carried out in bed and can be accomplished by placing two bricks, flat surface down, under both feet of the bed. (Arteriosclerotic leg ulcers should not be elevated.)
   c. Burow's solution wet packs
      Sig: one packet of Domeboro powder to 1 quart of warm water. Apply wet dressings of gauze or sheeting for 30 minutes t.i.d.
   d. If debridement is necessary, this can be accomplished by enzymes, such as Debrisan, Santyl (collagenase) ointment, Acuzyme, Panafil, or Elase ointment, applied twice a day and covered with gauze. Surgical debridement is often beneficial.
   e. Gentian violet 1%
      Distilled water q.s. 15.0
      Sig: Apply to ulcer b.i.d. with applicator.
      Comment: A liquid is usually better tolerated on ulcers than a salve. If the gentian violet solution becomes too drying, the following salve can be used alternately for short periods.
   f. Bactroban or other antibiotic ointment q.s. 15.0
      Sig: Apply to ulcer and surrounding skin b.i.d.
   g. Long-term erythromycin or cephalexin therapy: 250 mg, one capsule q.i.d. for 14 or more days, then one capsule b.i.d. for weeks, is helpful for chronic pyogenic ulcers. Other systemic antibiotics may be used.
   h. Low-dose oral corticosteroid therapy: prednisone, 10 mg
      Sig: one or two tablets every morning for 3 to 4 weeks, then one tablet every other morning for months. When this is added to the above routine, many indolent ulcers heal.
      Comment: The best treatment for one ulcer does not necessarily work for another ulcer. Many other local medications are available and valuable.
4. Surgical management, such as excision and grafting, may be indicated.
5. Various surgical dressings may be beneficial, such as OpSite, Duoderm, Tegaderm, or Polymem; Johnson & Johnson makes an inexpensive surgical wound dressing.
6. Silver-impregnated topicals and negative pressure therapy are newer therapies.
7. Hyperbaric oxygenation may also be beneficial.

Infectious Eczematoid Dermatitis

The term *infectious eczematoid dermatitis* or *auto eczematous dermatitis* is more often used incorrectly than correctly. Infectious

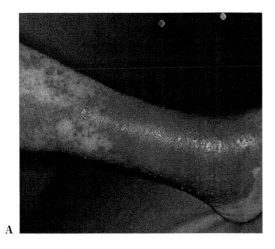
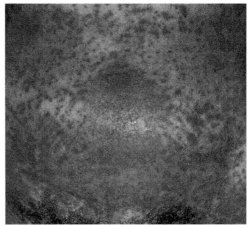
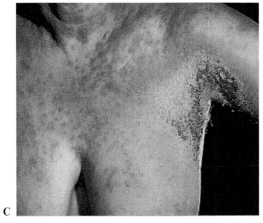

FIGURE 24-9: Bacterial infections of skin. **A:** Infectious eczematoid dermatitis **(B)** from stasis dermatitis of the legs with a spread to the body. **C:** Infectious eczematoid dermatitis in the axilla. (Courtesy of Burroughs Wellcome Co.)

eczematoid dermatitis is an uncommon disease characterized by the development of an acute eruption around an infected exudative primary site, such as a draining ear, mastitis, a boil, or a seeping ulcer (Fig. 24-9). Widespread eczematous lesions can develop at a distant site from the primary infection, presumably owing to an immune phenomenon, and *autoeczematous dermatitis*, or so-called *id reaction*.

> ### SAUER'S NOTES
>
> The primary factor in the management of an ulcer is to not let it happen. This is especially appropriate for decubitus ulcers. Frequent turning of the bedridden patient, air pressure mattresses, and devices to prevent rollover onto the back are helpful.

Primary Lesions

Vesicles and pustules in circumscribed plaques spread peripherally from an infected central source. Central healing usually does not occur, as in ringworm infection.

Secondary Lesions

Crusting, oozing, and scaling predominate in widespread cases.

Distribution

Mild cases may be confined to a small area around the exudative primary infection, but widespread cases can cover the entire body, obscuring the initial cause.

Course

The course depends on the extent of the eruption. Chronic cases respond poorly to therapy. Recurrences are common even after the primary source is healed.

Subjective Complaints

Itching is usually present.

Cause

Coagulase-positive staphylococci are frequently isolated.

Differential Diagnosis

- *Contact dermatitis with secondary infection:* No history or finding of primary exudative infection; history of contact with poison ivy, new clothes, cosmetics, or dishwater; responds faster to therapy (see Chapter 8)

- *Nummular eczema:* No primary infected source; coin-shaped lesions on extremities; clinical differentiation of some cases is difficult (see Chapter 8)
- *Seborrheic dermatitis:* No primary infected source; seborrhea–acne complex, with greasy, scaly eruption in hairy areas (see Chapter 15)
- *Eczematous psoriasis:* A recently described skin ailment with the appearance of diffuse severe nummular eczema, but with a response to therapy mimicking that of psoriasis

Treatment

Case Example: An 8-year-old boy presents with draining otitis media and pustular, crusted dermatitis on the side of the face, neck, and scalp.

1. Treat the primary source—the ear infection, in this case.
2. Apply Burow's solution wet packs
   Sig: one packet of Domeboro powder to 1 quart of warm water. Apply wet sheeting or gauze to the area for 20 minutes t.i.d.
3. Apply antibiotic and corticosteroid cream, such as Bactroban ointment 15.0

   Triamcinolone 0.1% cream 15.0

   Sig: Apply t.i.d. locally, after the wet packs are removed. A patient with a widespread case might require hospitalization, daily mild soap baths, oral antibiotics, or corticosteroid systemic therapy.

Bacterial Intertrigo

The presence of friction, heat, and moisture in areas where two opposing skin surfaces contact each other leads to a secondary bacterial, fungus, or yeast infection.

Primary Lesion

Redness from friction and heat of opposing forces and maceration from an inability of the sweat to evaporate freely leads to an eroded patch of dermatitis.

Secondary Lesion

The bacterial infection may become severe enough to result in fissures and cellulitis.

Distribution

The inframammary region, axillae, umbilicus, pubic, crural, genital, and perianal areas as well as the areas between the toes may be involved.

Course

In certain persons, intertrigo tends to recur each summer.

Causes

The factors of obesity, diabetes, and prolonged contact with urine, feces, and menstrual discharges predispose to the development of intertrigo. AIDS may present with recurrent bullous groin impetigo.

Differential Diagnosis

- *Candidal intertrigo:* Scaling at the border of the erosion with an overhanging fringe of epidermis; presence of surrounding small satellite lesions; scraping and culture reveals *Candida albicans* (see Chapter 28)
- *Tinea:* Scaly or papulovesicular elevated border; scraping and culture are positive for fungi (see Chapter 28)
- *Seborrheic dermatitis:* Greasy red scaly areas, also seen on the scalp. Bacterial intertrigo may coexist with seborrheic dermatitis (see Chapter 15)

Treatment

Case Example: A 6-month-old infant presents with red, pustular dermatitis in the diaper area, axillae, and folds of the neck.

1. Bathe the child once a day in lukewarm water with antibacterial soap. Dry affected areas thoroughly.
2. Double rinse diapers to remove all soap or use disposable diapers.
3. Change diapers as frequently as possible and apply a powder each time, such as Talc, unscented (Zeasorb) 45.0.
4. Hydrocortisone 1%.
   Bactroban ointment q.s. 15.0

   Sig: Apply to affected areas t.i.d. Continue local therapy for at least 1 week after dermatitis is apparently clear—"therapy plus." Allow only two refills of this salve to avoid atrophy of the skin.

SYSTEMIC BACTERIAL INFECTIONS

Scarlet Fever

Scarlet fever is a less common streptococcal infection characterized by a positive streptococcal culture, sore throat, high fever, and a scarlet rash. Less commonly, the skin can be the source of the streptococcal infection. Decreased incidence in recent decades is probably related to different "phase"-type *streptococci.* The skin rash is caused by the production of an exotoxin. Pastia's sign is pink, red, or hemorrhagic transverse lines at the elbow, wrist, or inguinal areas 2 to 3 days after the fever. Pastia's sign occurs before the skin eruption begins and persists after the eruption is gone. The eruption develops after a day of rapidly rising fever, headache, sore throat, and various other symptoms. The rash begins first on the neck and the chest, and rapidly spreads over the entire body, except for the area around the mouth. Close examination of the pale scarlet eruption reveals it to be made up of diffuse pinhead-sized, or larger, macules. In untreated cases, the rash reaches its peak on the fourth day, and scaling commences around the seventh day and continues for 1 or 2 weeks. "Strawberry tongue" is seen at the height of the eruption. Erythema nodosum can also occur.

The presence of petechiae on the body is a grave prognostic sign. Complications are numerous and common in untreated cases. Glomerulonephritis and rheumatic fever with consequent rheumatic heart disease may develop.

Differential Diagnosis

- *Measles:* Early rash on face and forehead, larger macular rash, running eyes, photophobia, cough (see Chapter 26)
- *Drug eruption:* Lack of high fever and other constitutional signs; atropine and quinine can cause an eruption that is clinically similar to scarlet fever (see Chapter 8)

Treatment

Penicillin or a similar systemic antibiotic is the therapy of choice. Complications should be watched for and should be treated early.

Granuloma Inguinale

Before the use of antibiotics, particularly streptomycin and tetracycline, this disease was one of the most chronic and resistant afflictions of humans. Formerly, it was a rather common disease. Granuloma inguinale should be considered a venereal disease, although other factors may have to be present to initiate infection.

Primary Lesion

An irregularly shaped, bright red, velvety appearing, flat ulcer with a rolled border is seen (Fig. 24-10).

Secondary Lesions

Scarring may lead to complications similar to those seen with lymphogranuloma venereum. Squamous cell carcinoma can develop in old, chronic lesions.

Distribution

Genital lesions are most common on the penis, scrotum, labia, cervix, or inguinal region.

Course

Without therapy, the granuloma grows slowly and persists for years, causing marked scarring and mutilation. Under modern therapy, healing is rapid, but recurrences are not unusual.

SAUER'S NOTES

Syphilis must be considered in any patient with a penile lesion. It can be ruled out by darkfield examination (there is rarely anyone qualified to accurately do this test and hence its usefulness has been greatly reduced) or blood serology tests. The serology should be repeated in 6 weeks if clinical suspicion is high because the initial serology in primary syphilis may be negative.

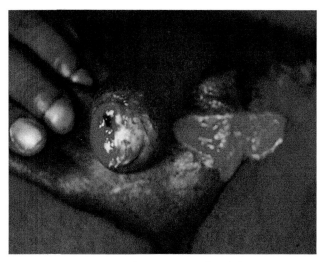

FIGURE 24-10: Granuloma inguinale of the penis and crural area. (Courtesy of Derm-Arts Laboratories.)

Cause

Granuloma inguinale is caused by *Calymmatobacterium granulomatis*, which can be cultured on special media.

Laboratory Findings

Scrapings of the lesion reveal Donovan bodies, which are dark-staining, intracytoplasmic, cigar-shaped bacilli found in large macrophages. The material for the smear can be obtained best by snipping off a piece of the lesion with small scissors and rubbing the tissue on several slides. Wright or Giemsa stains can be used.

Differential Diagnosis

- *Granuloma pyogenicum:* Small lesion; history of injury, usually; short duration; rarely on genitalia; bright red and bleeds easily; no Donovan bodies
- *Primary syphilis:* Short duration; inguinal adenopathy; serology may be positive; spirochetes (see Chapter 29)
- *Chancroid:* Short duration; lesion is small, not red and velvety; no Donovan bodies (see next section)
- *Squamous cell carcinoma:* More indurated lesion with nodule; may coexist with granuloma inguinale; biopsy specific

Treatment

Tetracycline, 500 mg q.i.d., is continued until all the lesions are healed.

Chancroid

Chancroid is a venereal disease with a very short incubation period of 1 to 5 days. It is caused by *Haemophilus ducreyi*.

Primary Lesion

Small, superficial, or deep erosions occur with surrounding redness and edema (Fig. 24-11). This is referred to as a "soft

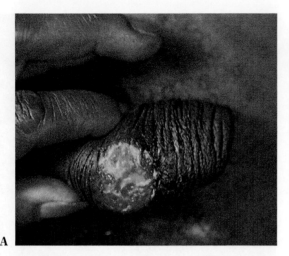
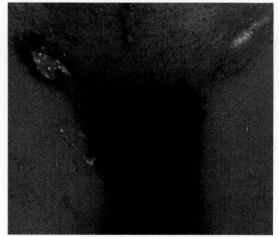

FIGURE 24-11: **A:** Chancroid of the penis. **B:** Chancroid buboes in the inguinal area. (Courtesy of Derm-Arts Laboratories.)

chancre" versus the "hard chancre" of syphilis with an indurated border. Multiple genital or distant lesions can be produced by autoinoculation.

Secondary Lesions

Deep, destructive ulcers form in chronic cases, which may lead to gangrene. Marked regional adenopathy, usually unilateral, is common and eventually suppurates in untreated cases.

Course

Without therapy most cases heal within 1 to 2 weeks. In rare cases, severe local destruction and draining lymph nodes (buboes) result. Early therapy is effective.

Laboratory Findings

The organisms are arranged in "schools of fish" and can often be demonstrated in smears of clean lesions.

Differential Diagnosis

- *Primary or secondary syphilis genital lesions:* Longer incubation period; more induration; *Treponema pallidum* found on darkfield examination; serology positive in late primary and secondary stage (see Chapter 29)
- *Herpes simplex progenitalis:* Recurrent multiple painful blisters or erosions; mild inguinal adenopathy; initial episode may have systemic symptoms (see Chapter 29)
- *Lymphogranuloma venereum:* Primary lesion rare; Frei test positive (see Chapter 29)
- *Granuloma inguinale:* Chronic, red velvety plaque; Donovan bodies seen on tissue smear (see preceding section)

Treatment

The therapy for chancroid is a sulfonamide such as sulfisoxazole, 1 g q.i.d. for 2 weeks, or erythromycin, 2 g/day for 10 to 15 days. Third-generation cephalosporins are also effective. A fluctuant bubo should never be incised but should be aspirated with a large needle.

Tuberculosis

Skin tuberculosis (Fig. 24-12) is rare in the United States. However, a text on dermatology would not be complete without some mention of this infection. Although the incidence has been decreasing in the United States and leveled off worldwide since 1992, it is still a significant disease across the world, and multidrug-resistant tuberculosis (MDR-TB), especially in AIDS patients, is a particularly difficult problem. AIDS and tuberculosis act as synergistic infections. An even more resistant form of tuberculosis is now reported called extensively drug-resistant tuberculosis (XDR-TB). The most common cutaneous tuberculosis infection, lupus vulgaris, is discussed in this chapter. A classification of skin tuberculosis is given in Table 24-2.

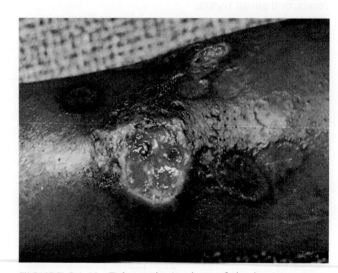

FIGURE 24-12: Tuberculosis ulcer of the leg. (Courtesy of Derm-Arts Laboratories.)

TABLE 24-2 • Classification of Cutaneous Tuberculosis

True Cutaneous Tuberculosis (Lesions Contain Tubercle Bacilli)

1. *Primary tuberculosis* (no previous infection; tuberculin negative in initial stages)
   a. Primary inoculation tuberculosis; Tuberculosis chancre (exogenous implantation into skin producing the primary complex)
   b. Miliary tuberculosis of the skin (hematogenous dispersion)
2. *Secondary tuberculosis* (lesions develop in a person already sensitive to tuberculin as a result of prior tuberculous lesion; tubercle bacilli are difficult or impossible to demonstrate)
   a. Lupus vulgaris (inoculation of tubercle bacilli into the skin from external or internal sources)
   b. Tuberculosis verrucosa cutis (inoculation of tubercle bacilli into the skin from external or internal sources)
   c. Scrofuloderma (extension to the skin from an underlying focus in the bones or glands)
   d. Tuberculosis cutis orificialis (mucous membrane lesions and extension onto the skin near mucocutaneous junctions)

Tuberculids (Allergic Origin; No Tubercle Bacilli in Lesions)

1. *Papular forms*
   a. Lupus miliaris disseminatus faciei (purely papular)
   b. Papulonecrotic tuberculid (papules with necrosis)
   c. Lichen scrofulosorum (follicular papules or lichenoid papules)
2. *Granulomatous, ulceronodular forms*
   a. Erythema induratum (nodules or plaques subsequently ulcerating; may be a nonspecific vasculitis)

Presentation and Characteristics

Lupus vulgaris is a chronic, granulomatous disease characterized by the development of nodules, ulcers, and plaques arranged in any conceivable configuration. In severe, untreated cases, scarring in the center of active lesions or at the edge can lead to atrophy and contraction. This can result in mutilating changes.

Distribution

Facial involvement is most common.

Course

The course is often slow and progressive, in spite of therapy.

Laboratory Findings

The histopathology shows typical tubercle formation with epithelioid cells, giant cells, and a peripheral zone of lymphocytes. The causative organism, *Mycobacterium tuberculosis*, is not abundant in the lesions. The 48-hour tuberculin test is usually positive.

Differential Diagnosis

Other granulomas, such as those associated with syphilis, leprosy, sarcoidosis, deep fungal disease, and neoplasm, are to be ruled out by appropriate studies (see Chapter 18).

Treatment

Early localized lesions can be treated by surgical excision. For more widespread cases, long-term systemic therapy offers high hopes for cure. Isoniazid is usually prescribed along with other antituberculous drugs, such as rifampin and ethambutol (Myambutol). MDR-TB is an increasing problem in AIDS patients.

Leprosy

Leprosy, or Hansen's disease, is to be considered in the differential diagnosis of any skin granulomas. It is endemic in the southern part of the United States and all over the world in semitropical and tropical areas.

Presentation and Characteristics

Two definite types of leprosy are recognized: tuberculoid (Fig. 24-13) and lepromatous (Fig. 24-14). In addition, there are cases, called *dimorphic leprosy* (Fig. 24-15) that cannot presently be classified in either of these two categories. These patients eventually develop either lepromatous or tuberculoid leprosy.

Tuberculoid leprosy is generally benign in its course because of considerable resistance to the disease on the part of the host. This is manifested by a positive lepromin test, histology that is not diagnostic, cutaneous lesions that are frequently erythematous with elevated borders, and minimal effect of the disease on the general health of the patient.

Lepromatous leprosy is the malignant form, and represents minimal resistance to the disease, with a negative lepromin reaction, characteristic histologic appearance, infiltrated cutaneous lesions with ill-defined borders, and unless treated, progression to death, usually from secondary amyloidosis.

Early symptoms of the lepromatous type include reddish macules with an indefinite border, nasal obstruction, and nosebleeds. Erythema nodosum–like lesions commonly occur. The tuberculoid type of leprosy is often first diagnosed in what's called an indeterminant form. The indeterminant form presents as an area of skin with decreased sensation, polyneuritis, and skin lesions with a sharp border and central atrophy.

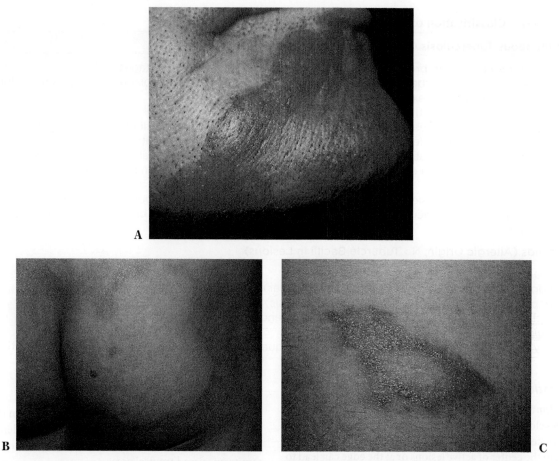

FIGURE 24-13: A: Tuberculoid leprosy of the chin. **B:** Tuberculoid leprosy on the buttocks. (A and B courtesy of Drs. W. Schorr and F. Kerdel-Vegas.) **C:** Tuberculoid leprosy on the chest. (Courtesy of Dr. M. Rico, Durham, NC.)

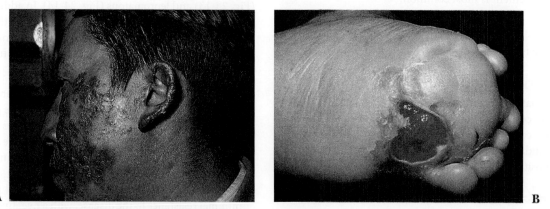

FIGURE 24-14: A: Lepromatous leprosy. (Courtesy of Dr. A. Gongalez-Ochoa, Mexico.) **B:** Lepromatous leprosy on the foot. (Courtesy of Dr. M. Rico, Durham, NC.)

Cause

The causative organism is *Mycobacterium leprae*.

Contagiousness

The source of infection is believed to be from patients with the lepromatous form.

Laboratory Findings

The bacilli are usually discovered in the lepromatous type but seldom in the tuberculoid type. Smears should be obtained from the exposed tissue by a small incision made into the dermis through an infiltrated lesion.

The lepromin reaction, a delayed reaction test similar to the tuberculin test, is of value in differentiating the lepromatous

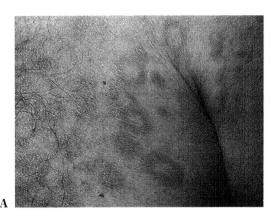 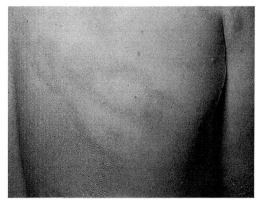

FIGURE 24-15: **A:** Dimorphic leprosy on the chest. (Courtesy of Dr. R. Caputo, Atlanta, GA.) **B:** Dimorphic leprosy on the back. (Courtesy of Dr. M. Rico, Durham, NC.)

form from the tuberculoid form of leprosy, as previously mentioned. False-positive reactions do occur.

Biologic false-positive tests for syphilis are common in patients with the lepromatous type of leprosy.

Differential Diagnosis

Consider any of the granulomatous diseases, such as

- syphilis,
- tuberculosis,
- sarcoidosis, and
- deep fungal infections.

  See also Chapter 16.

Treatment

Dapsone (diaminodiphenylsulfone), rifampin, and isoniazid are all effective.

Other Mycobacterial Dermatoses

Mycobacteria are pathogenic (tuberculosis and leprosy) and saprophytic or environmental (atypical mycobacteria). *Mycobacterium marinum* is the most common saprophytic mycobacteria to cause disease in humans and can cause swimming pool granuloma, granulomas in fishermen, and granulomas in workers or people involved with fish tanks. Minocycline and combinations of either ethambutol, rifampin, clarithromycin, or levofloxacin have been used as treatments.

Mycobacterium avium-intracellulare is seen in patients with AIDS, but skin lesions are rare.

Gonorrhea

Gonorrhea is considerably more prevalent than syphilis. Skin lesions with gonorrheal infection are rare. Untreated or inadequately treated infection caused by *Neisseria gonorrhoeae* can involve the skin through metastatic spread (Fig. 24-16). Primary cutaneous infection with multiple erosions at the site of the purulent discharge is very rare.

Metastatic complications include a bacteremia, in which there is an intermittent high fever, arthralgia, and skin lesions.

The skin lesions are characteristic hemorrhagic vesiculopustules, most commonly seen on the fingers. Arthralgias are common. Treatment with intravenous penicillin for 10 days at 5 to 10 million units per day is indicated.

The rarer septicemic form, with very high fever and meningitis or endocarditis, can have purpuric skin lesions similar to those seen in meningococcemia.

Rickettsial Diseases

The most common rickettsial disease in the United States is Rocky Mountain spotted fever, which is spread by ticks of various types. The skin eruption occurs after 3 to 7 days of fever and other toxic signs. It is characterized by purpuric lesions on the extremities, mainly the wrists and the ankles, which then become generalized. The Weil–Felix test using *Proteus* OX19 and OX2 is positive. Tetracycline and chloramphenicol are effective treatment modalities.

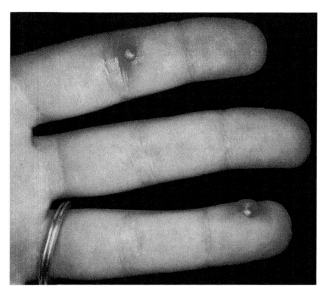

FIGURE 24-16: Gonococcal septicemia with hemorrhagic vesicles. (Courtesy of Derm-Arts Laboratories.)

The typhus group of rickettsial diseases includes epidemic or louse-borne typhus, Brill's disease, and endemic murine or flea-borne typhus. Less common forms include scrub typhus (tsutsugamushi disease), trench fever, and rickettsialpox, which are produced by a mite bite. The mite ordinarily lives on rodents. Approximately 10 days after the bite a primary lesion develops in the form of a papule that becomes vesicular. After a few days of fever and other toxic signs, a generalized eruption that resembles chickenpox appears. The disease subsides without therapy.

Ehrlichiosis is another rickettsial disease well known in dogs and now seen in humans. It is transmitted by a tick bite. The nonspecific symptoms are similar to those of Rocky Mountain spotted fever, but only 20% of the patients have a rash.

Actinomycosis

Actinomycosis is a chronic, granulomatous, suppurative infection that characteristically causes the formation of a draining sinus. The most common location of the draining sinus is in the jaw region, but thoracic and abdominal sinuses can also occur.

Primary Lesion

A red, firm, nontender tumor in the jaw area slowly extends locally to form a "lumpy jaw." It mimics a draining dental sinus from an infected tooth.

Secondary Lesions

Discharging sinuses become infected with other bacteria and, if untreated, may develop into osteomyelitis.

Course

General health is usually unaffected unless extension occurs into bone or deeper neck tissues. Recurrence is unusual if treatment is continued long enough.

Cause

Actinomyces israelii, which is an anaerobic bacterium that lives as a normal inhabitant of the mouth, particularly in persons who have poor dental hygiene, is the causative agent. Injury to the jaw or a tooth extraction usually precedes the development of the infection. Infected cattle are not the source of human infection. The disease is twice as common in men as in women.

Laboratory Findings

Pinpoint-sized "sulfur" granules, which are colonies of the organism, can be seen grossly and microscopically in the draining pus. A Gram stain of the pus shows masses of interlacing, gram-positive fibers with or without club-shaped processes at the tips of these fibers. The organism can be cultured anaerobically on special media.

Differential Diagnosis

- Pyodermas
- Tuberculosis
- Draining dental abscess
- Neoplasm

Treatment

1. Penicillin, 2.4 million units intramuscularly, is given daily, until definite improvement is noted. Then oral penicillin in the same dosage should be continued for 3 weeks after the infection has apparently been cured. In severe cases, 10 million or more units of penicillin given intravenously, daily, may be necessary.
2. Incision and drainage is performed on the lumps in the sinuses.
3. Good oral hygiene is required.
4. In resistant cases, broad-spectrum antibiotics can be used alone or in combination with the penicillin.

Suggested Readings

Aly R, Maibach H. *Atlas of the Infections of the Skin.* Philadelphia, PA: WB Saunders; 1998.

Bailey E, Kroshinsky D. Cellulitis: diagnosis and management. *Dermatologic Therapy.* 2011;24:229–239.

Bhate C, Schwartz RA. Lyme disease. *J Am Acad Dermatol.* 2011;64(4):619–653.

Daum SD. Skin and soft tissue infections caused by methicillin-resistant Staphylococcus aureus. *N Engl J Med.* 2007;357:380–390.

Drugs for sexually transmitted infections. *Med Lett Drugs Ther.* 1999;41:85–90.

Epstein ME, Amodio-Groton M, Sadick NS. Antimicrobial agents for the dermatologist: I. Beta-Lactam antibiotics and related compounds. *J Am Acad Dermatol.* 1997;37(2):149–165.

Epstein ME, Amodio-Groton M, Sadick NS. Antimicrobial agents for the dermatologist: II. Macrolides, fluoroquinolones, rifamycins, tetracyclines, trimethoprim-sulfamethoxazole, and clindamycin. *J Am Acad Dermatol.* 1997;37(3):365–381.

Hansra NK, Shinkai K. Cutaneous community-acquired and hospital-acquired methicillin-resistant Staphylococcus aureus. *Dermatol Ther.* 2011;24: 263–272.

Hirschmann JV, Raugi GJ. Lower limb cellulitis and its mimics: part I and II. *J Am Acad Dermatol.* 2012;67(2):163–185.

Horsburgh CR, Barry CE III, Lange C. Treatment of tuberculosis. *N Eng J Med.* 2015;373(22):2149–2160.

Lesher JL. *An Atlas of Microbiology of the Skin.* London: Parthenon Publishing Group; 2000.

Makdisi J, Friedman A. Bacterial skin and soft tissue infections: a review for the dermatologist. *J Drugs Dermatol.* 2013;12(3):369–373.

Modlin RL, Rea TH. Leprosy: new insight into an ancient disease. *J Am Acad Dermatol.* 1987;17(1):1–13.

Moschella SL. An update on the diagnosis and treatment of leprosy. *J Am Acad Dermatol.* 2004;51:417–426.

Parish LC, Witkowksi JA, Crissey JT. *The Decubitus Ulcer in Clinical Practice.* New York: Springer; 1997.

Sanchez E, Vannier E, Wormser GP, et al. Diagnosis, treatment, and prevention of Lyme disease, human granulocytic anaplasmosis, and babesiosis. *JAMA.* 2016;315(16):1767–1777.

Sanders CV. *Skin and Infection: A Color Atlas and Text.* Baltimore: Williams & Wilkins; 1995.

Sehgal VN, Wagh SA. Cutaneous tuberculosis. *Int J Dermatol.* 1990;29:237–252.

Singer AJ, Talan DA. Management of skin abscesses in the era of methicillin-resistant Staphylococcus aureus. *N Eng J Med.* 2014;370(11):1039–1047.

Spach DH, Liles WC, Campbell GL, et al. Tick-borne diseases in the United States: review article. *N Engl J Med.* 1993;329:936–947.

Treatment of Lyme disease. *Med Lett Drugs Ther.* 2010;52(1342):53–56.

Treatment of Lyme disease. *Med Lett Drugs Ther.* 2016;58:57–58.

Spirochetal Infections

John C. Hall, MD

Two spirochetal diseases are discussed in this chapter: syphilis and Lyme disease.

SYPHILIS

When Gordon C. Sauer was stationed at the West Virginia State Rapid Treatment Center, from 1946 to 1948, the average for patient admittance was 30 a day. Approximately one-third of these patients had infectious syphilis. In 1949, the center was closed because of the patient census. Today, the incidence of reported syphilis has risen again to alarming heights. Many patients with acquired immunodeficiency syndrome (AIDS) also have syphilis. Because of this resurgence, it is imperative that all physicians have a basic understanding of this polymorphous disease.

Cutaneous lesions of syphilis occur in all three stages of the disease. Under what circumstances will the present-day physician be called on to diagnose, evaluate, or manage a patient with syphilis?

1. The cutaneous manifestations, such as a penile lesion or a rash that could be secondary syphilis, may bring a patient into the office.
2. A positive blood test found on a premarital examination or as part of a routine physical examination may be the reason for a patient's visit to the doctor.
3. Syphilis may be seen in conjunction with AIDS. The problem becomes complicated because the serologic test for syphilis (STS) may not be positive in patients with AIDS and routine antibiotic dosage regimens may be ineffective.
4. Cardiac, central nervous system, or other organ disease may be a reason for a patient to consult a physician.

To manage these patients properly, a thorough knowledge of the natural untreated course of the disease is essential.

Primary Syphilis

The first stage of acquired syphilis usually develops within 2 to 6 weeks (average 3 weeks) after exposure. The *primary chancre* most commonly occurs on the genitalia (Figs. 25-1 and 25-2), but extragenital chancres are not rare and are often misdiagnosed. Without treatment, the chancre heals within 1 to 4 weeks but is dependent on the location, the amount of secondary infection, and host resistance.

The blood STS may be negative in the early days of the chancre but eventually becomes positive. The spirochete, *Treponema pallidum*, is readily found with darkfield examination. This test is of limited value because there are few people with the expertise to interpret the test reliably. A cerebrospinal fluid examination by darkfield during the primary stage reveals invasion of the spirochete in approximately 25% of cases.

Clinically, the chancre may vary in appearance from a single small erosion to multiple indurated ulcers of the genitalia. It is usually painless and has an indurated border ("hard chancre"). Primary syphilis commonly goes unnoticed in the female patient because of its intravaginal or rectal location. Men who have sex with men (MSM) may also have hidden rectal chancres. Bilateral or unilateral regional lymphadenopathy is common. Malaise and fever may also be present.

Early Latent Stage

Latency, manifested by positive serologic findings and no other subjective or objective evidence of syphilis, may occur between the primary and secondary stages.

Secondary Syphilis

Early secondary lesions may develop before the primary chancre has healed or after latency of a few weeks (Figs. 25-3 to 25-5). *Late secondary lesions* are more rare and usually are seen after the early secondary lesions have healed. Both types of secondary lesions contain the spirochete *T. pallidum*, which can be easily seen with the darkfield microscope. The STS is positive (an exception is in some patients with AIDS), and approximately 30% of the cases have abnormal cerebrospinal fluid findings.

Clinically, the early secondary rash can consist of macular, papular, pustular, squamous, or eroded lesions or combinations of any of these lesions. Papulosquamous is most common with oval lesions and fine dry adherent scale. This can easily be confused with pityriasis rosea. Palm and sole involvement is characteristic, and there is no herald patch. Secondary syphilis

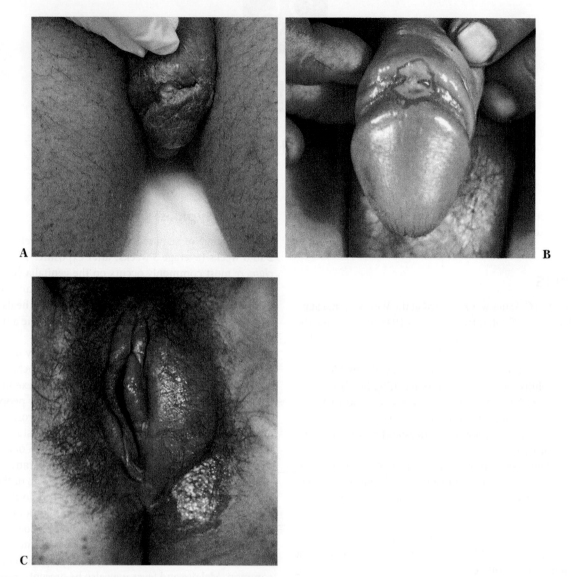

FIGURE 25-1: Primary syphilis with primary chancres of the genitalia. **A:** Chancre of the penis is accompanied by marked edema of the penis. **B:** Penile chancre. **C:** Vulvar chancre with edema of the labia majora. (Courtesy of J.E. Moore and The Upjohn Company.)

can be generalized or localized to the palms and soles, genital area, or mucous membranes. A "moth-eaten" scalp alopecia may develop in the late secondary stage.

Condylomata lata is the name applied to the flat, moist, warty lesions teeming with spirochetes found in the groin and the axillae (Figs. 25-4 and 25-5). Mucous patches are white elevated verrucous skin lesions usually on the oral mucous membranes.

The late secondary lesions are nodular, squamous, and ulcerative and are distinguished from the tertiary lesions only by the time interval after the onset of the infection and by the finding of the spirochete in superficial smears of serum from the lesions. Annular and semiannular configurations of late secondary lesions are common.

Generalized lymphadenopathy, malaise, fever, and arthralgias occur in many patients with secondary syphilis.

Early Latent Stage

Following the secondary stage, many patients with untreated syphilis have only a positive STS. After 4 years of infection, the patient enters the late latent stage.

Late Latent Stage

This time span of 4 years arbitrarily divides the early infectious stages from the later noninfectious stages, which may or may not develop.

Tertiary Syphilis

This late stage is manifested by subjective or objective involvement of any of the organs of the body, including the skin (Figs. 25-6 and 25-7; see also Fig. 3-1). Tertiary changes may be precocious but most often develop 5 to 20 years after

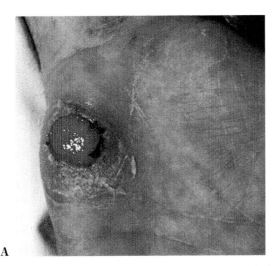
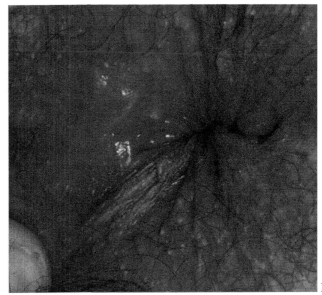

A   **B**

FIGURE 25-2: Primary syphilis with extragenital chancres. **A:** Chancre of the palm. **B:** Chancre over the rectal area. (Courtesy of The Upjohn Company.)

the onset of the primary stage. Clinically, the skin lesions are characterized by nodular and gummatous ulcerations. Solitary multiple annular and nodular lesions are common. Subjective complaints are rare unless considerable secondary bacterial infection is present in a gumma. Scarring is inevitable in the most of the tertiary skin lesions. Larger texts should be consulted for the late changes seen in the central nervous system, the cardiovascular system, the bones, the eyes, and the viscera. Approximately 15% of the patients who acquire syphilis and receive no treatment will die of the disease.

Late Latent Stage

Another latent period may occur after natural healing of some types of benign tertiary syphilis.

Congenital Syphilis

Congenital syphilis is acquired in utero from an infectious mother (Fig. 25-8). The STS required of pregnant women by most states has lowered the incidence of this unfortunate disease. Stillbirths are not uncommon from mothers who are untreated. After the birth of a live infected child, the mortality rate depends on the duration of the infection, the natural host resistance, and the rapidity of initiating treatment. Early and late lesions are seen in these children, similar to those found in the adult cases of acquired syphilis. Blistering can occur.

Laboratory Findings

Darkfield Examination

The etiologic agent, *T. pallidum*, can be found in the serum from the primary or secondary lesions. However, a darkfield microscope is necessary, and very few physicians' offices or laboratories have this instrument. A considerable amount of experience is necessary to distinguish *T. pallidum* from other *Treponema* species.

Serologic Test for Syphilis

The STS is simple, readily available, and has several modifications. The rapid plasma reagin (RPR) test and the Venereal Disease Research Laboratories (VDRL) flocculation test are used most commonly. Treponemal tests such as the fluorescent treponemal antibody absorption (FTA-ABS) test, treponema antibody test (FTA) test among others and modifications are more difficult to perform in the laboratory and are therefore used primarily when the RPR and VDRL tests are "reactive."

When a report is received from the laboratory that the STS is positive (RPR or VDRL reactive), a second blood specimen should be submitted to obtain a quantitative report. In many laboratories, this repeat test is not necessary, because a quantitative test is run routinely on all positive blood specimens. A dilution of 1:2 is only weakly positive and might be a biologic false-positive reaction. A test positive in a dilution of 1:32 is strongly positive. In evaluating the response of the STS to treatment, one must remember that a change in titer from 1:2 to 1:4 to 1:16 to 1:32 to 1:64, or downward in the same gradations in each instance is only a change in one tube. Thus, a change from 1:2 to 1:4 is of the same magnitude as a change from 1:32 to 1:64. Quantitative tests enable the physician to

- evaluate the efficacy of the treatment,
- discover a relapse before it becomes infectious,
- differentiate between a relapse and a reinfection,
- establish a reaction as a seroresistant type, and
- differentiate between true and biologic false-positive serologic reactions.

In most laboratories, it is now routine to do an FTA-ABS test on all patients with reactive RPR and VDRL tests. With rare exceptions, a positive FTA-ABS test means that the patient has or had syphilis and is not a biologic false-positive reactor. The STS may not be positive in patients with AIDS.

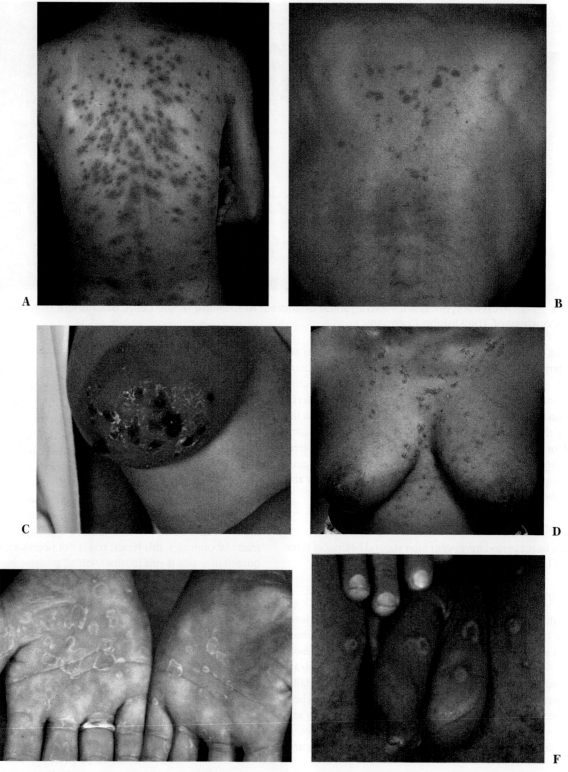

FIGURE 25-3: Secondary syphilis. **A:** Secondary papulosquamous lesions on the back. **B:** Papulosquamous lesions on the back. **C:** Crusted lesions on the breast. **D:** Papular lesions on the chest. **E:** Papulosquamous lesions on the palms. **F:** Late secondary annular lesions on the penis and scrotum. (Courtesy of K.U.M.C.)

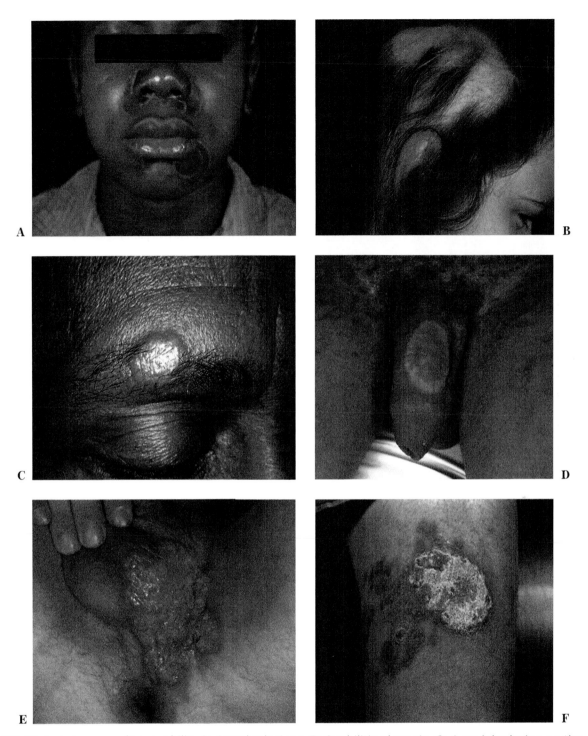

FIGURE 25-4: Late secondary syphilis. **A:** Annular lesions. **B:** Syphilitic alopecia. **C:** A nodular lesion on the eyebrow. **D:** An annular lesion on the penis. **E:** *Condylomata lata* in the groin area. **F:** Psoriatic-type lesion on the leg.

Tissue Examination

A direct fluorescent antibody test for *T. pallidum* can be performed on a lesion exudate or on biopsy tissue.

Cerebrospinal Fluid Test

As has been stated, the cerebrospinal fluid is frequently positive in the primary and secondary stages of the disease. Invasion of the central nervous system is an early manifestation, even though the perceptible clinical effects are a late manifestation. The cerebrospinal fluid should be examined at least once during the course of the disease. However, in actual practice, primary or secondary disease is usually treated without a cerebrospinal fluid exam but with antibiotic doses that are sufficient to eliminate the treponeme from the cerebrospinal fluid. Cerebrospinal fluid examination is appropriate for all

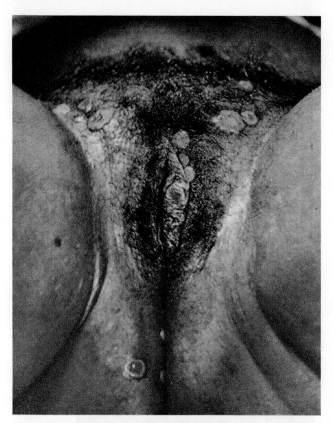

FIGURE 25-5: Secondary syphilis with *condylomata lata* of the vulva. (Courtesy of J.E. Moore and The Upjohn Company.)

patients with syphilis who are at a high risk for human immunodeficiency virus (HIV) infection. The best routine is to perform a cerebrospinal fluid test before treatment is initiated and repeat the test as indicated. If the cerebrospinal fluid is negative in a patient who has had syphilis for 4 years, central nervous system syphilis will not occur, and future cerebrospinal fluid tests are not necessary. If the test is positive, repeat tests should be done every 6 months for 4 years. The following three tests are run on the cerebrospinal fluid:

- *Cell count:* The finding of four or more lymphocytes or polymorphonuclear leukocytes per cubic millimeter is considered positive. The cell count is the most labile of the tests. It increases early in the infection and responds fastest to therapy. Therefore, it is a good index of activity of the disease. The cell count must be done within an hour after the fluid is withdrawn.
- *Total protein:* Measured in milligrams per deciliter, it normally should be below 40.
- *Nontreponemal flocculation test:* Presently, the most common test performed is the qualitative and quantitative VDRL. This test is the last to turn positive and the slowest to return to negativity. In some cases, therapy causes a decrease in the titer, but slight positivity or "fastness" can remain for the lifetime of the patient.

Differential Diagnosis

- *Primary syphilis:* From chancroid, herpes simplex, fusospirochetal balanitis, granuloma inguinale, and any of the *primary chancre-type diseases* (see Dictionary/Index).
- *Secondary syphilis:* From any of the papulosquamous diseases (especially pityriasis rosea), fungal diseases, drug eruption, and alopecia areata.
- *Tertiary skin syphilis:* From any of the granulomatous diseases, particularly tuberculosis, leprosy, sarcoidosis, deep mycoses, and lymphomas.
- *Congenital syphilis:* From atopic eczema, diseases with lymphadenopathy, hepatomegaly, and splenomegaly.

A true-positive syphilitic serology is to be differentiated from a biologic false-positive reaction. This serologic differentiation is accomplished best by using the FTA-ABS test, or one of its modifications, along with a good history and a thorough examination of the patient. Many patients with biologic false-positive reactions develop one of the collagen diseases at a later date.

Treatment

Case Example: A 22-year-old married man presents with a sore 1 cm in diameter on his glans penis of 5 days' duration. Three weeks earlier, he had an extramarital intercourse, and 10 days before this office visit, he had marital intercourse. The patient knows his extramarital sexual contact only as "Jane," and he cannot remember the bar where he met her.

First Visit

1. Perform a darkfield examination of the penile lesion. Treatment can be started if *T. pallidum* is found. If you cannot perform a darkfield examination, refer the patient to the local health department or another facility that can perform a darkfield examination.
2. If a darkfield examination cannot be performed or is negative, obtain a blood specimen for an STS.
3. While waiting for the STS report, advise the patient to soak the site in saline solution for 15 minutes twice a day. The solution is made by placing 1/4 teaspoon of salt in a glass of water.
4. Advise the patient against sexual intercourse until the reports are completed.
5. Explain to the patient the seriousness of treating him for syphilis if he does not have it. The "syphilitic" label is one he should not want, if it is at all possible to avoid it, and allergic reactions to penicillin are not rare and can be serious.

Second Visit

Three days later, the lesion is larger, and the STS report is "nonreactive."

1. Obtain a blood specimen for a second STS.
2. Antibiotic ointment 15.0
   Sig: Apply t.i.d. locally after soaking in saline solution.

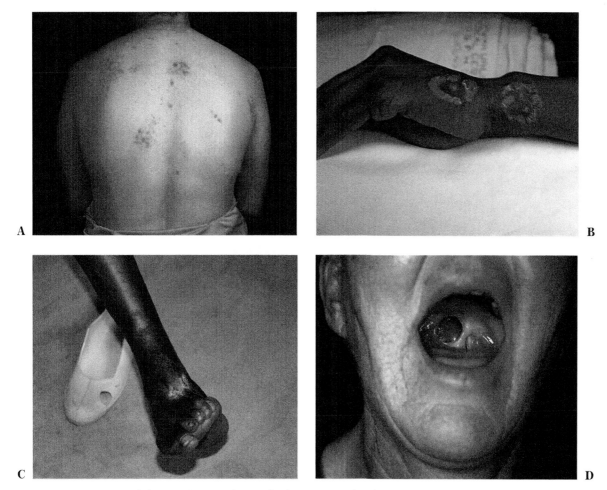

FIGURE 25-6: Tertiary syphilis. **A:** Grouped papular lesions on the back. **B:** Annular nodular lesions on the hand. **C:** Gumma on the leg. **D:** Perforation from an old gumma of the soft palate.

3. Explain again why you are delaying therapy until a definite diagnosis is made.

Third Visit

Three days later, the sore is smaller, but the STS report is "reactive." The diagnosis is now known to be "primary syphilis."

1. The patient is reassured that present-day therapy is highly successful but that he must follow your instructions closely.
2. His wife should be brought in for examination and a blood test. If the blood test is negative, it should be repeated weekly for 1 month. However, some syphilologists believe that therapy is indicated for the marital partner in the presence of a negative STS if the husband has infectious syphilis and is being treated. A single injection of 2.4 million units of a long-acting type of penicillin is used. This prevents "ping-pong" syphilis, which is a cycle of reinfection from one marital partner to another.
3. The patient's contact should be found. The patient's findings, including his contact with an unidentified sexual partner, should be reported to the local health department. This is usually done automatically by the laboratory where the blood tests were done, but this does not relieve the physician of the responsibility of

reporting the patient to the health department. In some local health departments (author's experience), the health officials will give free treatment and follow-up of patient and contacts.

4. A cerebrospinal fluid specimen should be obtained. (The report was returned as normal for all three tests.)
5. Penicillin therapy should be initiated. Here, two factors are important:
    a. The dose must be adequate.
    b. The effective blood levels of medication must be maintained for a period of 10 to 14 days.

Dosage

Primary and Secondary Syphilis

1. Administer 2.4 million units of benzathine penicillin G, half in each buttock, in a single session.
2. Consult larger texts or relevant literature for other treatment modalities.

Latent (Both Early and Late) Syphilis

1. If a spinal tap is not performed, administer 7.2 million units benzathine penicillin G divided into three weekly injections.

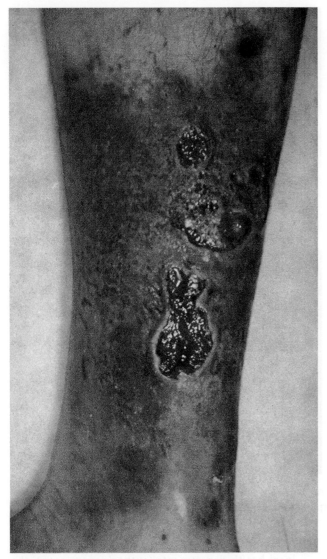

FIGURE 25-7: Tertiary syphilis with a gumma of the leg. This resembles a stasis ulcer. (Courtesy of J.E. Moore and The Upjohn Company.)

2. If cerebrospinal fluid examination is nonreactive, give 2.4 million units in a single dose.

Neurosyphilis or Cardiovascular Syphilis

1. Administer 9 to 12 million units of a long-acting penicillin.
2. For other routines or complicated cases, consult larger texts for therapy and care.
3. HIV-infected patients with neurosyphilis should be treated for 10 days at least with aqueous crystalline penicillin G in a dosage of 2 to 4 million units IV every 4 hours.

Benign Late Syphilis

Treatment is the same as for neurosyphilis.

Congenital Syphilis

1. Early congenital syphilis
   a. *Younger than 6 months of age:* Aqueous procaine penicillin G, 10 daily IM doses totaling 100,000 to 200,000 units/kg.
   b. *Six months to 2 years of age:* As above, or benzathine penicillin G, 100,000 units/kg IM in one single dose.
2. Late congenital syphilis
   a. *Ages 2 to 11 years, or weighing less than 70 pounds:* Same as for 6 months to 2 years.
   b. *Twelve years or older, and weighing more than 70 pounds:* Same treatment as for adult-acquired syphilis, with comparable time and progression of infection.

LYME DISEASE

Originally described as Lyme arthritis, Lyme disease is caused by a spirochete that is transmitted by several species of *Ixodes* tick. Early removal of the tick (<24 hours) usually prevents disease transmission. The disease has been reported from most states and on every continent except Antarctica. Endemic areas include the northeastern United States and the upper

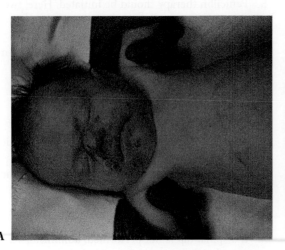
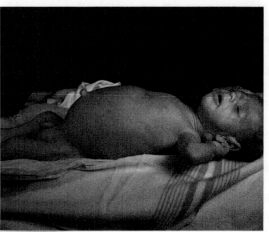

FIGURE 25-8: Congenital syphilis. **A:** Scaly and erosive lesions with a large liver (fatal). **B:** Massively enlarged liver and spleen.

Midwestern states. Clinical manifestations include erythema chronicum migrans (ECM) skin lesions, flulike symptoms, and possible neurologic, cardiac, and rheumatologic involvement.

Late cutaneous manifestations of Lyme disease are borrelia lymphocytoma, acrodermatitis chronica atrophicans and, although controversial, possibly in some cases (especially in Europe) morphea (localized scleroderma).

Presentation and Characteristics

Primary Lesion

The erythematous circular rash appears at the site of the tick bite and enlarges with central clearing, but multiple ECM eruptions can occur. The rash typically develops within 2 to 30 days after the bite. The bite area can become necrotic.

Secondary Lesion

Multiple ECM eruptions can develop.

Distribution

Usually, ECM begins at the site of the tick bite.

Season

The disease occurs from late May through early fall.

Course

In untreated patients, the ECM lesions may last only 10 to 14 days, but they may persist for months, or they may come and go over a year's time. The bite papule and ECM fade rapidly after therapy is begun. Late-stage cutaneous lesions include acrodermatitis chronic atrophicans and borrelia lymphocytoma (see Chapter 42).

SAUER'S NOTES

Syphilis

1. Any patient treated for gonorrhea should have an STS 4 to 6 weeks later.
2. Persons with HIV infection acquired through sexual contact or IV drug abuse should be tested for syphilis.
3. Seventy-five percent of the persons who acquire syphilis suffer no serious manifestations of the disease.
4. Syphilis does not cause vesicular or bullous skin lesions, except in infants with congenital infection.

Primary Stage

1. Syphilis should be ruled in or out in the diagnosis of any penile or vulvar sores.
2. Multiple primary chancres are moderately common.

Secondary Stage

1. The rash of secondary syphilis, except for the rare follicular form, does not usually itch.

2. Secondary syphilis should be ruled in or out in any patient with a generalized, nonpruritic rash, especially when it is papulosquamous. A high index of suspicion is necessary.

Latent Stage

The diagnosis of "latent syphilis" cannot be made for a particular patient unless cerebrospinal fluid tests have been done and are negative for syphilis.

Tertiary Stage

1. Tertiary syphilis should be considered in any patient with a chronic granuloma of the skin, particularly if it has an annular or circular configuration.
2. Invasion of the central nervous system occurs in the primary and secondary stages of the disease. A cerebrospinal fluid test is indicated during these stages.
3. If the cerebrospinal fluid tests for syphilis are negative in a patient who has had syphilis for 4 years, central nervous system syphilis usually will not occur, and future spinal punctures are not necessary.
4. Twenty percent of patients with late asymptomatic neurosyphilis have a negative STS.

Congenital Syphilis

An STS should be done on every pregnant woman to prevent congenital syphilis of the newborn.

Serology

1. The STS may be negative in the early days of the primary chancre. The STS is always positive in the secondary stage. An exception to this rule is in patients with AIDS.
2. A quantitative STS should be done on all syphilitic patients to evaluate the response to treatment or the development of relapse or reinfection.
3. The finding of a low-titer STS in a patient not previously treated for syphilis calls for a careful evaluation to rule out a biologic false-positive reaction.

Subjective Symptoms

Flulike symptoms, with fever, chills, myalgias, and headache, appear with the rash, but in the author's experience, systemic symptoms are not commonly reported. Later, other organs may be affected.

Cause

The spirochete *Borrelia burgdorferi* is transmitted by the Ixodes species of ticks and possibly by the hard-bodied ticks. The white-tailed deer and white-footed mouse are preferred hosts of the tick.

Diagnosis

A high index of suspicion, history of a tick bite (patient is not always aware of the bite), a previous "ringworm-type" rash, and, later, a positive Lyme disease antibody titer may be present (however, these tests are not reliable).

Histologic findings are not specific, and culture of the spirochete is often not practical. Polymerase chain reaction may be helpful on biopsy tissue in a qualified laboratory.

Differential Diagnosis

Cutaneously, the ECM rash can resemble an allergic reaction or tinea. See *figurate erythemas* in the Dictionary/Index. Any patient who presents with fever, myalgia, cardiac, joint, or neurologic manifestations should have a broad differential diagnosis.

ECM is nonspecific and has many mimics (Table 25-1). It is common in skin creases and under clothing straps and tends to be central in location. It may be multiple (90% single), is usually large (mean is 16 cm but can be 5 to 70 cm), and evolves over days to weeks (2 to 3 cm a day) with or without central clearing. It does not have a scale as in erythema annulare centrifugum, and does not have a scaling, vesicular, or elevated border as in tinea corporis. It is not a generalized cutaneous condition, as is erythema gyratum repens. It is asymptomatic but may have mild pain, pruritus, or mild systemic symptoms. These may occur days to weeks after the tick bite (Fig. 25-9).

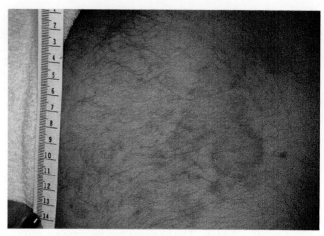

FIGURE 25-9: Erythema chronic migraines with multiple confluent non-scaling pink rings.

Treatment

Because a diagnosis of Lyme disease is difficult, treatment may be indicated, especially in endemic areas, based on history and clinical findings alone. Early therapy for this disease is doxycycline, 100 mg, b.i.d. for 21 days, or amoxicillin, 500 mg, t.i.d. for 21 days. Early tick removal (<24 hours) probably prevents disease transmission. Removing deer and mice habitats such as brush, leaves, stonewalls, and woodpiles may be helpful.

For late stages of the disease with cardiac or neurologic manifestations, treatment is ceftriaxone, 2 to 4 g/day IM or IV for 14 days. Because efficacy of therapy is difficult to evaluate, the literature is replete with other therapeutic regimens. Lyme vaccination is effective and should be considered in people at high risk in endemic areas. It takes 12 months to confer immunity.

Lymephobia is a term coined to describe a common psychological problem owing to the nonspecific nature of symptoms and the lack of specific tests. Well-meaning physicians can fall into the trap of long-term antibiotics for multiple vague systemic complaints.

Permethrin 5% applied to clothing is a helpful tick repellent.

TABLE 25-1 • Mimics of Erythema Chronicum Migrans

1. Tinea-clearing may occur in the center with a peripheral scale or crusts or vesicles. It is usually very pruritic, spreads over days to weeks, and may have satellite lesions.
2. Hypersensitivity to a tick bite is often itchy; the tick is often still attached; small (several centimeters), inflammatory papules rapidly develop without much evolution over days, and will occur at multiple sites of multiple bites.
3. Granuloma annulare—acral, especially over the dorsal hands, feet, knees, and elbows; dull red with central clearing and no scale; chronic over months to years with slow evolution; and asymptomatic.
4. Herald patch of pityriasis rosea—a collarette of scale just inside the pinkish plaque, will be followed usually within 5–7 d with an explosion of similar lesions that line up along Langer lines.
5. Nummular eczema—extremely pruritic with oozing and crusting and does not remain single for long.
6. Cutaneous T-cell lymphoma—chronic rather than sudden in onset, eventually becomes multiple, often asymmetric.

Suggested Readings

Abele DC, Anders KH. The many faces and phases of borreliosis: I. Lyme disease. *J Am Acad Dermatol.* 1990;23:167–186.

Abele DC, Anders KH. The many faces and phases of borreliosis: II. *J Am Acad Dermatol.* 1990;23:401–410.

Anonymous. Drugs for sexually transmitted infections. *Med Lett Drugs Ther.* 1999;41(1062):85–90.

Anonymous. Treatment of Lyme disease. *Med Lett Drugs Ther.* 2007;49:47–51.

Baum EW, Bernhardt M, Sams WM Jr. Secondary syphilis, still the great imitator. *JAMA.* 1983;249:3069–3070.

Bennet ML, Lynn AW, Klein LE. Congenital syphilis: subtle presentation of fulminant disease. *J Am Acad Dermatol.* 1997;36(2):351–354.

Burlington DB. *FDA Public Health Advisory: Assays for Antibodies to Borrelia burgdorferi: Limitations, Use, and Interpretation for Supporting a Clinical Diagnosis of Lyme Disease.* Rockville, MD: FDA; 1997.

Don PC, Rubinstein R, Christie S. Malignant syphilis (lues maligna) and concurrent infection with HIV. *Int J Dermatol.* 1995;34:403–407.

Stere AC, Taylor E, McHugh GL, et al. The overdiagnosis of Lyme disease. *JAMA.* 1993;269:1812–1816.

Trevisan G, Cinco M. Lyme disease. *Int J Dermatol.* 1990;29:1–8.

Dermatologic Virology

Andrew J. Peranteau, MD, Yun Tong, MD, Zeena Y. Nawas, MD, and Stephen K. Tyring, MD, PhD

Viral diseases of the skin are exceedingly common. The various clinical entities are distinct, and because we have no specific antiviral drug for many diseases, the treatment varies for each entity. The following viral diseases are discussed here:

- Herpes simplex virus 1 and 2
- Varicella-zoster virus
- Human herpesvirus 6
- Human herpesvirus 7
- Human herpesvirus 8
- Human papillomaviruses
- Human polyomaviruses
- Molluscum contagiosum virus
- Measles (rubeola)
- German measles (rubella)
- Erythema infectiosum
- Coxsackievirus infections (Herpangina and Hand, foot, and mouth disease)
- Echovirus exanthema

HERPES SIMPLEX VIRUS 1

Herpes simplex virus 1 (HSV-1) is the usual cause of herpes labialis as well as an increasing cause of first-episode genital herpes infections. Recent studies have shown that the rate of primary HSV-1 infection was over twice that of HSV-2 and presented most commonly as genital rather than oral disease. Approximately 80% to 90% of people worldwide have antibodies against HSV-1, with seroprevalence being about 58% in the United States. The primary infection typically occurs early in life, with viral latency established in the neural ganglia. Reactivation can occur because of several different triggers, including immunosuppression, respiratory tract viral infection, or any febrile disease, physical trauma, psychological stress, or sun exposure. Transmission of HSV-1 occurs with viral shedding during the asymptomatic and symptomatic periods through direct contact with infected secretions (i.e., saliva). Additionally, recent research has shown that infected individuals exhibit frequent, brief shedding episodes that are typically asymptomatic. These episodes are much more frequent than previously thought, and data now indicate that most HSV transmission occurs in asymptomatic patients.

Presentation and Characteristics

True primary infection occurs when a patient is seronegative for HSV types 1 and 2 before the episode. Nonprimary initial episodes occur when the first symptomatic episode occurs later than the initial infection, and tend to be less severe. Asymptomatic primary infection is the rule. During symptomatic episodes, 60% of patients experience prodromal symptoms such as burning, itching, or tingling. Systemic symptoms such as fever, chills, fatigue, and muscle aches may also accompany primary infection. The mouth and lips are the most common areas of primary infection (Figs. 26-1 and 26-2). Lesions start as papules on an erythematous base that become vesicular, progress to ulcers, then crust, and eventually heal, generally within 72 to 96 hours. Symptomatic primary episodes tend to be followed by less severe recurrences; however, some patients may never experience a second episode. Recurrent episodes often present as three to five vesicles at the vermilion border of the lip, which last at least 48 hours. Other locations include the palate, chin, or oral mucosa. Recurrent labial herpes affects approximately one-third of the US population, with patients typically experiencing one to six episodes annually.

Treatment

Oral acyclovir, famciclovir, and valacyclovir are effective for the treatment of herpes labialis. Different doses are recommended depending on whether the patient is presenting with a primary episode or a recurrent episode, or for suppressive therapy (Table 26-1). The use of suppressive therapy requires periodic reevaluation, and is generally recommended in those with frequent recurrences (more than 2 in 4 months) or in patients with systemic symptoms. Topical therapies that may be used are acyclovir 5% cream five times daily for 4 days, penciclovir 1% cream every 2 hours (while awake) for 4 days, or OTC docosanol 10% five times daily (Table 26-2). In addition, short-term prophylactic treatment may be helpful in patients who anticipate high-risk activity (i.e., intense sun exposure) along with use of an opaque cream such as zinc oxide or with a sun-blocking agent incorporated into a lip balm.

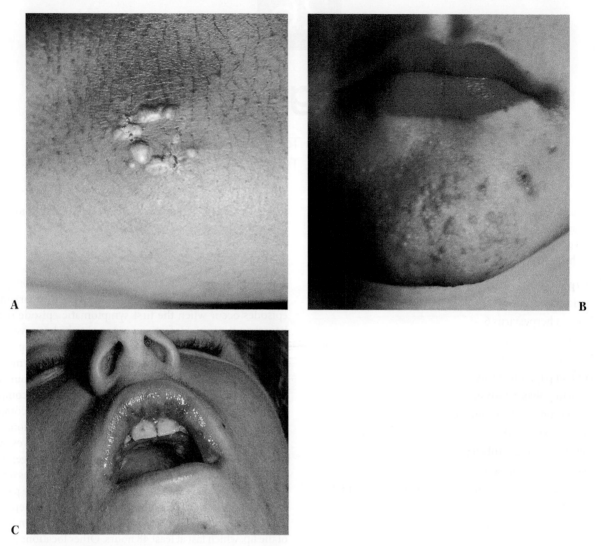

FIGURE 26-1: Herpes simplex on the arm **(A)**, chin **(B)**, and true primary infection on the lips and mouth (interoral) **(C)**. (Courtesy of Dermik Laboratories, Inc.)

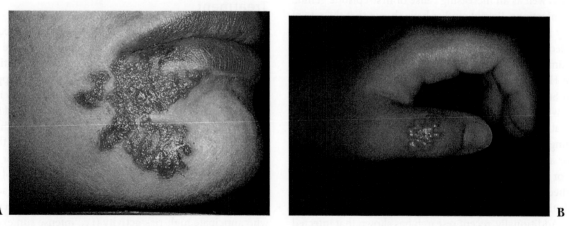

FIGURE 26-2: **A:** Recurrent herpes simplex on the chin with secondary bacterial infection. **B:** Recurrent herpes simplex on the thumb. (Courtesy of Dermik Laboratories, Inc.)

TABLE 26-1 • Treatments for Herpes Labialis

First Clinical Episode of Herpes Labialis	Intermittent Episodic Therapy for Recurrent Herpes Labialis	Suppressive Therapy for Recurrent Herpes Labialis
Acyclovir 400 mg PO 5 times daily for 7–10 d	Acyclovir 400 mg PO 5 times daily for 5 d	Acyclovir 400 mg PO b.i.d.
Famciclovir 500 mg PO b.i.d. for 7 d	Famciclovir 1.5 g PO once	Famciclovir 500 mg PO b.i.d.
Valacyclovir 1 g PO b.i.d. for 1 d	Valacyclovir 1 g PO b.i.d. for 1 d	Valacyclovir 500 mg PO q.d.

TABLE 26-2 • Antiviral Agents for Herpes Labialis: A Comparison

	Drug	Regimen (or Placebo)
Oral	Valacyclovir[a]	2 g twice daily for 1 d
	Acyclovir	400 mg 5 times a day for 5 d
Topical	Penciclovir[a] 1%	Every 2 h during waking hours for 4 d
	Acyclovir 5%	5 times a day for 4 d
	Docosanol[a] 10% (available OTC)	5 times daily

[a]FDA approved.

HERPES SIMPLEX VIRUS 2

Herpes simplex virus 2 (HSV-2) is one of the most widespread sexually transmitted diseases (STDs) in the world. In the United States, 50 million people have genital herpes, and approximately 1 million new infections are diagnosed each year. Approximately 16% of the global population aged 16 to 49 are seropositive for HSV-2. In addition, genital herpes (caused by either HSV-1 or HSV-2) increases the risk of HIV acquisition by two to three-fold. Similar to HSV-1, HSV-2 causes primary, latent, and recurrent infections, and is transmitted during both asymptomatic and symptomatic phases, typically through sexual contact. Genital herpes infections caused by HSV-2 tend to be more severe than those caused by HSV-1, are more likely to have recurrent episodes (median 4 recurrences per year vs. 1.3 per year in HSV-1), and have a greater frequency of subclinical viral shedding. HSV-2 can also cause neonatal herpes, with the highest risk occurring when the mother has primary genital herpes during delivery. In addition to cutaneous lesions, the infected neonate may develop multiorgan involvement, which carries a high mortality rate.

Presentation and Characteristics

Studies have shown that asymptomatic shedding occurs in the genital tract of 80% to 90% of HSV-2 seropositive individuals on approximately 20% of days, which means most of the transmission of genital herpes occurs in asymptomatic individuals. The first clinically recognized lesions of genital herpes may be either true primary or a first-episode nonprimary. True primary genital herpes usually develops 2 to 14 days after HSV exposure. Lesions may be widespread and typically present initially as papules, which then turn into vesicles, which become umbilicated in 2 or 3 days before eroding and forming crusts (Fig. 26-3). Along with lesions on the genitalia, inguinal adenopathy may also be appreciated along with systemic symptoms such as discharge, dysuria, fever, lethargy, myalgias, and photophobia. Women tend to have more severe and extensive disease than men. The most common site of involvement in women is the cervix, although the classic clinical presentation is that of painful vaginal and vulvar lesions.

More than half of patients with the first recognized signs and symptoms of genital herpes have a nonprimary first episode, which occurs when the initial infection is asymptomatic. This may occur weeks, months, or even years after initial HSV infection. A strong immune response may prevent the infection from becoming clinically recognizable. The initial immune response does attenuate the severity of first-episode nonprimary genital herpes. Lesions are often less extensive, and systemic symptoms are less common and severe compared with those of true primary genital herpes.

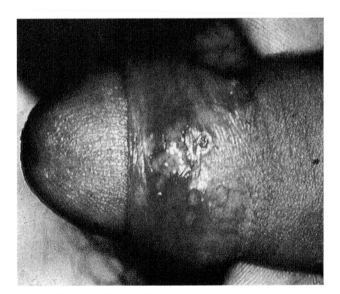

FIGURE 26-3: Genital herpes in an immunocompetent male. (From Fatahzadeh M, Schwartz RA. Human herpes simplex virus infections: epidemiology, pathogenesis, symptomatology, diagnosis, and management. *J Am Acad Dermatol.* 2007;57(5):737-763. Reprinted with permission from *Journal of the American Academy of Dermatology*)

TABLE 26-3 • Treatments for Genital Herpes

First Clinical Episode of Genital Herpes	Intermittent Episodic Therapy for Recurrent Genital Herpes	Suppressive Therapy for Recurrent Genital Herpes
Acyclovir 400 mg PO t.i.d. for 7–10 d	Acyclovir 400 mg PO t.i.d. for 5 d	Acyclovir 400 mg PO b.i.d.
Acyclovir 200 mg PO 5 times a day for 7–10 d	Acyclovir 800 mg PO t.i.d. for 2 d	Famciclovir 250 mg PO b.i.d.
Famciclovir 250 mg PO t.i.d. for 7–10 d	Acyclovir 800 mg PO b.i.d. for 5 d	Valacyclovir 500 mg PO q.d. (≤9 outbreaks/y)
Valacyclovir 1 g PO b.i.d. for 7–10 d	Famciclovir 125 mg PO b.i.d. for 5 d Famciclovir 1 g PO b.i.d. for 1 d	Valacyclovir 1 g PO q.d. (>9 outbreaks/y)
	Valacyclovir 500 mg PO b.i.d. for 3 d	
	Valacyclovir 1 g PO q.d. for 5 d	

Treatment

Although there has been some promising work on therapeutic and prophylactic vaccines, to date there remains no FDA-approved vaccine for genital herpes. Because there is no cure for genital herpes, therapy is aimed at controlling the signs and symptoms of an outbreak. In 2006, the Centers for Disease Control and Prevention (CDC) made therapeutic recommendations for individuals with a first clinical episode of genital herpes; for episodic development of genital herpes; and for suppressive therapy for recurrent genital herpes (Table 26-3). Pharmacologic therapies for genital herpes include

- acyclovir,
- valacyclovir,
- famciclovir,
- cidofovir,
- foscarnet (especially in immunocompromised HIV patients), and
- penciclovir.

VARICELLA-ZOSTER VIRUS

Varicella-zoster virus (VZV) causes primary varicella (chickenpox) and herpes zoster (shingles), which is a reactivation of the primary varicella infection. Primary varicella is usually a self-limited disease in immunocompetent children. Before the varicella vaccine became available, it occurred in 90% of children by 10 years of age and accounted for more than 11,000 hospitalizations each year in the United States owing to complications of the virus in otherwise healthy children. Susceptible adults typically develop more extensive skin lesions, more frequent complications, and more severe constitutional symptoms, such as prolonged fever.

Following primary VZV infection, the virus resides in a latent state in the sensory ganglia. With aging or a weakened immune system, the VZV may reactivate as shingles, which is also known as herpes zoster. Herpes zoster has the highest incidence of all neurologic diseases, its annual incidence in the United States and Europe being 2.5/1,000 persons between the

ages of 20 to 50, 5/1,000 between ages 51 to 79, and 10/1,000 in those more than 80 years of age. There are an estimated 1 million cases of herpes zoster annually in the United States, where almost one out of every three people will develop zoster in their lifetime. Since childhood varicella vaccination was introduced in the United States in 1995, the incidence of shingles has increased. Experts suggested this was attributable to the lack of subclinical immune boosting that generally results from the wild-type virus in the environment. However, two recent CDC studies found that herpes zoster rates started increasing before the vaccine was introduced in the United States and that rates did not accelerate after the routine vaccination program was implemented. In addition, other countries that do not routinely perform varicella vaccination have also observed similar increases in herpes zoster rates.

Presentation and Characteristics

Two weeks after exposure, primary varicella may start with 2 to 3 days of prodromal symptoms such as low-grade fever, chills, headache, malaise, nausea, and vomiting. The rash appears as crops of small red macules and papules on the face and scalp, which then spreads to the trunk and extremities. Sparing of the distal and lower extremities is common. Older lesions evolve to form pustules and crusts and heal within 7 to 10 days. One of the hallmarks of varicella is the presence of lesions in all stages of development (Fig. 26-4).

Reactivation of VZV may occur at any time after the development of varicella. More than 90% of patients with herpes zoster have a prodrome of pruritus, tingling, tenderness, hyperesthesia and/or intense pain in the involved single sensory ganglion (dermatome) preceding the zoster rash. The appearance of the characteristic dermatomal rash (grouped vesicles on an erythematous base with subsequent crusting) is often accompanied by severe pain (Fig. 26-5). Lesions can involve more than one contiguous dermatome, and although less common, will occasionally cross the midline. Although any dermatome can be affected, the most common regions of involvement are the trunk, followed by the face. Older adults and the immunocompromised typically have more severe disease or unusual or disseminated presentations (i.e., verrucous lesions

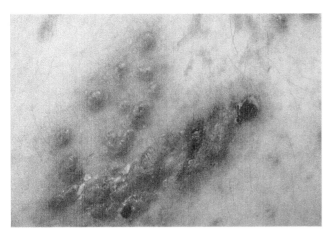

FIGURE 26-4: Herpes zoster lesions in multiple stages of development. (Courtesy of Stephen K. Tyring, MD, PhD.)

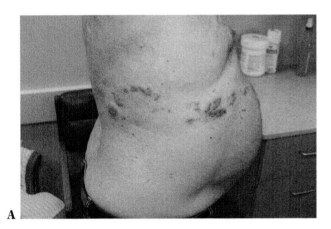

A

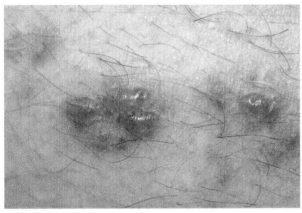

B

FIGURE 26-5: Herpes zoster in a 70-year-old diabetic male in the T7 dermatome area **(A)**, close-up of lesions **(B)** showing classic grouped vesicles on an erythematous base. (Courtesy of Stephen K. Tyring, MD, PhD.)

in HIV-infected patients) along with higher complication rates. The rash typically heals within 2 to 4 weeks, but the pain often persists. Postherpetic neuralgia (PHN) is the most common complication, which is characterized by burning or stabbing sensations and allodynia that persist after the skin lesions are healed. PHN can last for weeks, months, or even years, and

affects 10% to 20% of all herpes zoster patients. Its incidence and severity increase with age. Diagnosis is usually clinical, but Tzanck smears and/or PCR can be helpful to confirm the diagnosis of VZV.

Treatment

Primary varicella in immunocompetent children is self-limited and may be treated symptomatically (i.e., antipyretics, calamine lotion). If started ideally within 24 hours of rash onset, acyclovir 20 mg/kg q.i.d. up to 800 mg/dose for 5 to 7 days has been shown to decrease the severity and duration of varicella. Systemic antiviral treatment (valacyclovir, acyclovir, famciclovir) is recommended for primary varicella in immunocompetent adults, as well as in unvaccinated adolescents (i.e., children ≥13 years of age), adolescents with chronic cutaneous or pulmonary disorders, or in those taking intermittent oral or inhaled steroids. Intravenous acyclovir for 7 to 10 days is indicated in immunocompromised patients. Oral acyclovir is recommended for pregnant women with uncomplicated varicella. Postexposure prophylaxis with varicella-zoster immune globulin is recommended within 96 hours of varicella exposure in nonimmune patients.

Treatment for herpes zoster should optimally begin within 72 hours of development of skin lesions. Although treatment can begin after 72 hours (particularly if new skin lesions are still appearing), antiviral therapy is generally of minimal benefit if lesions have already crusted over. Antiviral therapy is recommended in all immunocompromised patients, even if they present after 72 hours. Acyclovir (800 mg five times daily for 7 days), famciclovir (500 mg three times daily for 7 days), and valacyclovir (1,000 mg three times daily for 7 days) are all FDA-approved treatments of herpes zoster in immunocompetent patients and result in decreased severity and duration of both skin lesions and pain (see Table 26-3). However, in controlled studies, valacyclovir and famciclovir were as effective as (or superior to) acyclovir in treating herpes zoster and are often preferred because of their greater bioavailability and the convenience of their less frequent dosing schedule (although they are more expensive). The most effective therapy for acute herpes zoster to reduce the severity and duration of PHN is the combination of an antiviral drug (i.e., valacyclovir) and gabapentin, and it is now considered the standard of care.

IV administration (10 mg/kg every 8 hours for 10 days) is indicated for the treatment of severe complications in immunocompetent patients and for the treatment of zoster in severely immunosuppressed patients requiring hospitalization. Adverse effects with acyclovir are rare and include headache, nausea, diarrhea, and renal toxicity (especially in dehydrated elderly patients).

Vaccination

Varivax, a live, attenuated varicella vaccine, was approved for use in the United States in 1995. It prevents chicken pox in 70% to 90% of vaccinees, and severe chicken pox in over 95% of vaccinees. The varicella vaccine is recommended in all children ≥12 months of age, and adults without evidence of immunity.

The main contraindications to the vaccine are previous allergic reaction to a component of the vaccine, and pregnancy.

Zostavax, a live, attenuated varicella-zoster vaccine that is greater than 10 times the strength of Varivax, was approved in 2006 for use in individuals aged 60 and older for the prevention of herpes zoster. On the basis of the results of recent clinical trials, the vaccine is now approved by the FDA to prevent herpes zoster in persons 50 years of age or older. In patients who develop herpes zoster despite receiving the vaccination, the incidence of PHN is decreased by 39%. Considering that the greatest risk factor for herpes zoster (other than age and immune status) in VZV-seropositive persons is familial predisposition, persons with a family history of shingles should be urged to receive the vaccine. The vaccine is contraindicated in pregnancy and in those who are highly immunosuppressed, although a recent phase 3 herpes zoster vaccine, which utilizes a single VZV glycoprotein in an adjuvant system, may hold promise for future application. Because this vaccine contains only a single virus protein and therefore cannot replicate, it could prove promising in those with impaired cellular immunity who are at the highest risk for herpes zoster.

HUMAN HERPESVIRUS 6

Human herpesvirus 6 (HHV-6) was first isolated in 1986 and has been found to be associated with roseola infantum (exanthem subitum). HHV-6 infects over 90% of the population by early childhood.

Presentation and Characteristics

Primary infection with HHV-6 usually occurs by 3 years of age and is often accompanied by an indistinctive febrile illness. The characteristic rash is observed either during the illness or after defervescence in approximately 30% of patients experiencing primary HHV-6 infection. Classic presentation is a typically well-appearing infant presenting with a high fever (102° to 105°F; 38.9° to 40.6°C) that lasts for 3 to 5 days, followed by a cutaneous eruption as the fever subsides. The incubation period ranges from 5 to 15 days, and the cutaneous eruption usually lasts for 24 to 48 hours. The lesions typically start on the trunk and later spread to the proximal extremities, neck, and less often the face. Lesions are discrete, circular or elliptical, "rose-red" 2 to 5 mm macules and papules that rarely coalesce and blanche with pressure. Uvulopalatoglossal junctional macules or ulcers (Nagayama spots) are often seen as well and represent a characteristic finding. Main differential diagnoses include, but are not limited to, other viral exanthems (i.e., rubeola, rubella, parvovirus), drug allergy, and Rocky Mountain spotted fever. Diagnosis is usually made clinically. HHV-6 has been implicated in the pathogenesis of other skin conditions including "glove-and-socks" syndrome, hypersensitivity drug reactions, Gianotti–Crosti syndrome, pityriasis rosea, DRESS syndrome, and lymphoproliferative malignancies. In addition, infection with or reactivation of HHV-6 in immunocompromised patients can lead to fever, rash, and more serious complications such as hepatitis, pneumonitis, bone marrow suppression, encephalitis, and transplant rejection.

Treatment

Treatment is symptomatic. Antipyretics may be used to reduce fever and lower the chance of febrile seizures, which occur in 10% to 15% of affected infants and children. For serious complications in the immunosuppressed, no evidence-based treatment regimens are yet available. However, several case reports have noted successful treatment of serious complications with foscarnet and ganciclovir.

HUMAN HERPESVIRUS 7

Human herpesvirus 7 (HHV-7) is very similar to HHV-6 in that it is highly prevalent worldwide, with more than 95% of adults being seropositive. Infections mainly occur during the first 5 years of life and then typically remain latent. The mode of transmission is most likely through salivary fluid.

Presentation and Characteristics

HHV-7 is thought to be the causative agent of pityriasis rosea and has also been associated with exanthem subitum in addition to the more common HHV-6. Isolated cases of encephalitis, hemiconvulsion–hemiplegia syndrome, febrile seizures, and hepatitis have been reported during HHV-7 infection. In addition, although HHV-7 has not been established as a causative factor for clinical disease, it has also been linked to chronic fatigue syndrome, posttransplant skin eruptions, and reactivation of HHV-6 infection.

Differential Diagnosis

Similar to that of exanthem subitum.

Treatment

No clinical settings in which HHV-7 infection warrants treatment have been identified. Several antiviral agents are under investigation.

HUMAN HERPESVIRUS 8

Human herpesvirus 8 (HHV-8) is a latent virus found in all types of Kaposi sarcoma (KS). The disease first associated with HHV-8 was KS; however, HHV-8 is also associated with other cancers in AIDS patients such as Castleman disease and body cavity–based lymphomas. Interestingly, HHV-8 is not evenly distributed globally. Higher rates of classic KS and higher HHV-8 infections prevail in Mediterranean countries such as Italy, Greece, Israel, and Saudi Arabia than in North America and Northern Europe. In parts of Africa, HHV-8 has infected over half the adult population. It is also not known why Kaposi sarcoma is found predominately in males. The exact mode(s) of transmission for HHV-8 remains

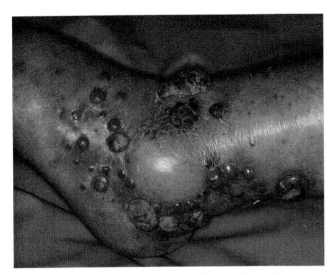

FIGURE 26-6: Advanced stage classic Kaposi sarcoma characterized by multiple nodules of different sizes, partly clustered and eroded, arising on the lower leg. Diffuse edema is also evident. (From Schwartz RA, Micali G, Nasca MR, et al. Kaposi sarcoma: a continuing conundrum. *J Am Acad Dermatol.* 2008;59:179–206. Reprinted with permission from *Journal of the American Academy of Dermatology*)

unclear. Saliva appears to be a source of infectious virus. It has been proposed that saliva may be the main mode of HHV-8 transmission in children and that it could be a source of mother-to-child transmission. Other possible modes of transmission include sexual transmission, blood transfusions, and solid organ transplantation.

Presentation and Characteristics

There are four types of KS (classic, HIV/AIDS related, immunosuppression associated, and African-endemic), which have different presentations and clinical courses, but all typically feature red, brown, or violaceous papules, plaques, and nodules. Edema is a common finding in all types (Fig. 26-6).

- Classic Type: initially develops as purplish-red plaques with multiple nodules with a spongy feel primarily on the lower legs of elderly men of Mediterranean descent; it becomes more firm with time and can become hyperkeratotic and/or eczematous (Fig. 26-7). These lesions progress slowly and respond well to treatment.
- HIV/AIDS related: multifocal and widespread macules, patches, or plaques, which can become ulcerative. Commonly affected areas include face and oral cavity as well as genital mucosa, lungs, and gastrointestinal tract (Fig. 26-8). Course of disease is fulminant, and response to treatment is poor.
- Immunosuppression-associated KS: Similar to AIDS-related KS with rapid progression and dissemination, with lesions regressing with reduction in immunosuppression.

- African-endemic KS: The endemic form of KS is found in all parts of equatorial Africa, affecting both children and adults, particularly in sub-Saharan Africa. It is not typically associated with immune deficiency. Endemic KS is frequently more aggressive than classic KS, and may be accompanied by dissemination to lymph nodes, bone, and skin.

Treatment

Diagnosis of KS is typically made by a skin biopsy of a suspected lesion. Treatment options are numerous and depend on the type of KS, but include immune reconstitution in AIDS-related KS, radiation, cryotherapy, intralesional chemotherapy, and topical retinoids. Other agents such as antiangiogenic agents and valganciclovir (which can inhibit HHV-8 replication) are currently under investigation.

HUMAN PAPILLOMAVIRUS

There are over 120 different genotypes of human papillomavirus (HPV), which are DNA viruses of the family Papillomaviridae that infect the epithelial cells of skin and mucosa and cause warts, benign papillomas, or neoplasias. HPV infection is the most common sexually transmitted infection in the United States, with approximately 75% of sexually active females acquiring the virus during their lifetime. Current prevalence estimates done in conjunction with the CDC showed that 39.8% of sexually active US women between the ages of 14 and 59 were infected with HPV. Over 40 distinct types can infect the genital tract, although most infections remain asymptomatic and resolve spontaneously within 2 years.

The HPVs are commonly categorized as having low or high oncogenic potential. Infections with the high-risk types such as HPV-16 and HPV-18 have been implicated in cervical–anogenital cancer and oral squamous cell carcinomas. In the United States, it has been calculated that 6.2 million new cases of high-risk HPV infections occur each year, close to 20 million Americans are infected, and 1% of sexually active adults have genital warts. It is estimated that >99% of cervical, as well as >70% of anal and vaginal cancers are related to HPV infection (cervical cancer is the second most frequent cause of cancer death among women worldwide). About 30% to 40% of penile, vulvar, and oropharynx cancers are related to HPV-16 and HPV-18. HPV-6 and 11, on the other hand, are responsible for approximately 90% of genital warts.

Presentation and Characteristics

Owing to the number of different subtypes of HPV, warts caused by HPV can have a variety of appearances. Common warts typically have a hard surface, are hyperkeratotic, exophytic, dome-shaped papules most commonly located on the fingers and dorsal surface of the hands. One characteristic feature of common warts is punctate black dots, which are thrombosed capillaries within the wart. Palmar and plantar warts appear

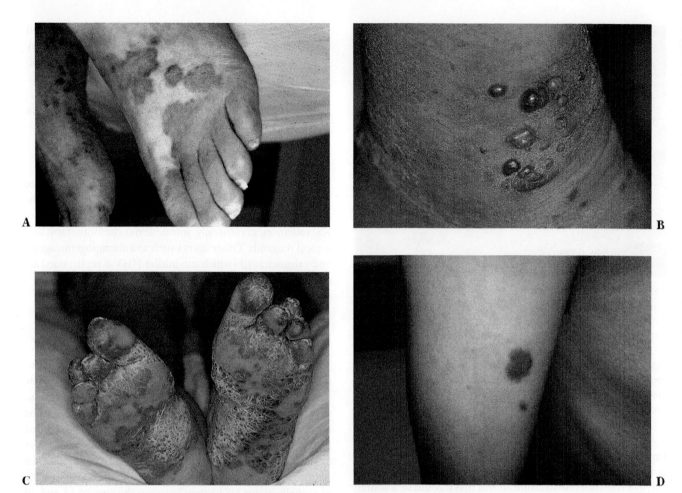

FIGURE 26-7: A: Patch stage classic Kaposi sarcoma characterized by violaceous irregularly shaped macules relentlessly enlarging on the distal upper extremities. **B:** Raised nodules developing within a Kaposi sarcoma plaque on the lower leg. **C:** Advanced stage Kaposi sarcoma showing extensive indurated and hyperkeratotic plaques involving both soles. **D:** Violaceous plaques of classic Kaposi sarcoma on the upper extremity. (Images A–C From Schwartz RA, Micali G, Nasca MR, et al. Kaposi sarcoma: a continuing conundrum. *J Am Acad Dermatol*. 2008;59:179–206. Reprinted with permission from *Journal of the American Academy of Dermatology*. Image D courtesy of Stephen K. Tyring, MD, PhD).

as thick, endophytic papules on the palms, soles, and lateral aspects of the hands and feet. On the feet these can often be painful because of their inward growth. Plantar warts that coalesce into large plaques are known as mosaic warts. HPV-1 and 2 usually cause common palmar, plantar, and mosaic warts, whereas HPV-3 and HPV-10 typically cause flat warts. HPV-6 and HPV-11 are the main causes of anogenital warts, or condyloma acuminatum, which are soft, flesh-colored, and flat, papular, or pedunculated lesions that occur on the genitals or surrounding skin (Fig. 26-9). Cervical warts are common but may be difficult to visualize by examination without application of acetic acid and the use of a colposcope.

Treatment

Currently, there is no curative treatment for HPV infections. The CDC recommendations for therapy of HPV anogenital lesions include:

- podofilox 0.5% solution or gel
- imiquimod 3.75% or 5% cream
- sinecatechins 15% ointment
- cryotherapy
- Electrosurgery, laser removal, or scissor excision
- trichloroacetic acid (TCA) or bichloroacetic acid (BCA) 80% to 90%

Imiquimod stimulates the host's immune response against infected cells and, along with sinecatechins (a green tea extract), have the lowest recurrence rates following a complete response. Sinecatechins have a similar clearance rate as does imiquimod and cause similar local irritation, but results are often not seen until 16 weeks, which can affect patient compliance. Sinecatechins, podofilox, and imiquimod are patient-applied therapies, whereas the other listed therapies must be applied or performed by a health care provider (Table 26-4). Alternative treatments for genital or nongenital warts include:

- laser surgery
- surgical excision
- intralesional interferon

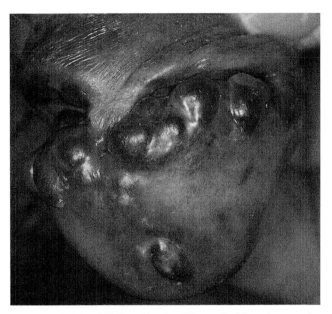

FIGURE 26-8: AIDS patient with genital involvement with multiple nodules arising along the coronal sulcus. (From Schwartz RA, Micali G, Nasca MR, et al. Kaposi sarcoma: A continuing conundrum. *J Am Acad Dermatol.* 2008;59:179–206. Reprinted with permission from *Journal of the American Academy of Dermatology.*)

- 5-fluorouracil
- retinoids
- bleomycin (intralesional and systemic)
- salicylic acid
- cidofovir (topical and intravenous)

Vaccination

Gardasil is a quadrivalent vaccine that is effective against HPV types 6, 11, 16, and 18—the major types causing anogenital warts as well as cervical cancer. It was approved by the FDA for use in the United States in 2006 for females 9 to 26 years of age, and for use in men 9 to 26 years of age in October 2009. In 2014, a 9-valent vaccine (Gardasil 9) was approved that protects against the same four HPV types as does the quadrivalent vaccine, but also protects against oncogenic HPV types 31, 33, 45, 54, and 58. Cervarix, a bivalent vaccine, protects only against HPV types 16 and 18.

HUMAN POLYOMAVIRUSES

Human polyomaviruses (HPyVs) are small, nonenveloped DNA tumor viruses, which are widespread in nature. Today, the HPyV family consists of 10 members, with notable viruses such as BK virus and JC virus discovered over 40 years ago along with the more recently identified Merkel cell polyomavirus (MCPyV) and trichodysplasia spinulosa–associated virus (TSPyV). Serologic studies suggest that HPyVs subclinically infect the general population with rates ranging from 35% to

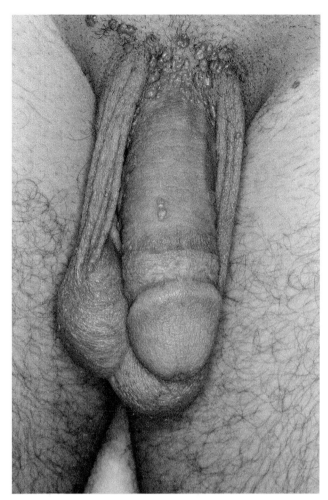

FIGURE 26-9: Numerous small papular warts on the pubis, penile shaft, and scrotum of a young male. (Courtesy of Stephen K. Tyring, MD, PhD.)

90%. However, significant disease is observed only in patients with impaired immune functions or in the elderly.

Presentation and Characteristics

BK virus has been linked to hemorrhagic cystitis (HC) after allogeneic hematopoietic stem cell transplantation, and PyV-associated nephropathy (PyVAN) after kidney transplantation; JC virus is associated with progressive multifocal leukoencephalopathy (PML) in HIV-AIDS, hematologic diseases, and in autoimmune diseases treated with certain lymphocyte-specific antibodies. Merkel cell polyomavirus (MCPyV) has been causally linked to the development of Merkel cell carcinoma (MCC). Numerous studies have shown MCPyV is clonally integrated into the cell genome in approximately 80% of MCCs, with studies showing that one or more viral proteins are key oncogenic drivers. MCC is a rare, aggressive cutaneous malignancy typically affecting older adults with fair skin. MCC has a propensity for local recurrence and regional lymph node metastasis and typically presents on the head, neck, or extremities (sun-exposed areas) as a pink-red or violacious, firm, dome-shaped nodule that has grown rapidly. Ulceration can occur. Diagnosis is made by biopsy and histologic examination.

TABLE 26-4 • Comparison of Treatment Modalities for Genital Warts

Treatment Type	Mechanism of Action	Administered By	Complete Clearance %	Recurrence %	Comments
Topical					
Podophyllotoxin	Antiwart lignans	Patient	45–77	38–65	Cost-effective home treatment
Imiquimod 5% cream	Induces secretion of cytokines that reduce HPV DNA viral load	Patient	35–56	13–15	Lengthy duration and sporadic dosing frequency can affect compliance
Imiquimod 3.75% cream	Induces secretion of cytokines that reduce HPV DNA viral load	Patient	27–33	15	Newer formulation with more intuitive dosing regimens
Sinecatechins	Possess antitumor, antiviral, antioxidant effects	Patient	53–58	6–9	Can often take 16 wk to elicit positive response
Podophyllin	Antiwart lignans	Patient	42–50	46–60	Not generally recommended for EGW treatment
5-FU	Inhibits key enzyme in DNA replication	Physician	10–50	50	Sometimes used for urethral warts
Destructive and Surgical					
TCA	Chemically destructive acids	Physician	70	18	High clearance rates with relatively low morbidity
Cryotherapy	Dermal damage induced by cold temps initiates immune response	Physician	71–88	25–40	Treated areas can take several weeks to heal, requires multiple treatments
Electrosurgery	Thermal coagulation	Physician	94	22	Long-term effectiveness comparable to cryotherapy
Scissor excision	Physical removal of diseased tissue	Physician	72	19–29	Outdated treatment modality, utilized with large lesions causing obstruction
CO_2 Laser	Infrared light energy vaporizes lesions	Physician	26–52	60–77	Treatment of choice in immunocompromised
Systemic					
Interferon	Interferes with viral replication	Physician	17–67	9–69	Topical use has higher clearance rates vs. placebo; systemic use has comparable clearance rates vs. placebo

TSPyV causes trichodysplasia spinulosa, a rare skin disease in immunocompromised hosts (typically solid organ transplant recipients or in patients undergoing chemotherapy for leukemia or lymphoma), characterized by numerous erythematous to skin-colored follicular papules with a central spiny projection on the face (known as keratin spines or spicules) and alopecia (eyebrows and eyelashes > other facial and body hair). Thickening of the skin may also occur, resulting in a leonine appearance. Diagnosis is suggested by typical clinical presentation in an immunosuppressed patient and confirmed by detection of the polyomavirus in a skin biopsy.

Treatment

MCC is usually treated by wide local excision and possibly radiotherapy or chemotherapy depending on whether lymph node involvement or distant metastatic disease is observed. Treatment of trichodysplasia spinulosa generally involves reducing or discontinuing immunosuppressive medications, which results in marked improvement. In addition, successful treatment with topical cidofovir cream or ointment (1% to 3%) and oral valganciclovir has been reported.

MOLLUSCUM CONTAGIOSUM VIRUS

Molluscum contagiosum, caused by the molluscum contagiosum virus of the DNA poxvirus group, is a benign, self-limited skin infection that commonly affects children. It also occurs in adults, usually as an STD, and has been noted with increasing frequency in the immunocompromised, particularly in HIV-positive patients (where prevalence estimates range from 5% to 18%). Because the infection is limited to the epidermis, most lesions regress spontaneously within 9 to 12 months, and molluscum contagiosum has not been reported to progress to malignancy.

Presentation and Characteristics

Molluscum contagiosum lesions present as discrete, umbilicated, flesh-colored, dome-shaped pearly papules, 2 to 5 mm in diameter, with a waxy surface (Fig. 26-10). In sexually active young adults, these lesions are spread through sexual contact and are found primarily on the lower abdomen, inner thighs, genitalia, and pubic areas. In cases of nonsexually transmitted molluscum, spread occurs through skin contact. Lesions are found primarily on the trunk, skin folds (i.e., neck, axillae), and extremities, and are often spread from one area to another on a patient's body via autoinoculation (particularly in atopic patients), scratching, or shaving. The lesions are generally found in groups, but may also be widely disseminated. Widespread, large, and occasionally disfiguring lesions can be seen with HIV infection, and are often a marker of late-stage disease. The differential for molluscum includes warts, herpes simplex, Spitz nevi, and juvenile xanthogranuloma. In AIDS patients, it can mimic cryptococcus, histoplasmosis, and aspergillosis.

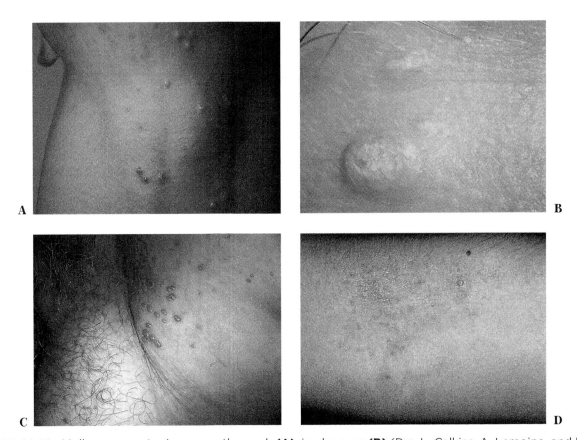

FIGURE 26-10: Molluscum contagiosum on the neck **(A)**, in close-up **(B)** (Drs. L. Calkins, A. Lemoine, and L. Hyde), of vulvar area **(C)**, and with atopic eczema of cubital fossae **(D)**. (Courtesy of Glaxo Dermatology.)

Treatment

Molluscum contagiosum lesions are self-limiting and generally resolve within 6 to 12 months in immunocompetent individuals. However, they may persist for years. Therapeutic modalities are similar to those available for warts, and treatment is generally administered in order to control transmission and for cosmetic reasons. Effective therapies are:

- imiquimod (although some authors question its effectiveness)
- cryotherapy
- cantharidin
- electrosurgery
- curettage

  Less commonly used therapies are:

- topical cidofovir
- lasers
- podofilox
- TCA
- retinoids

MEASLES (RUBEOLA)

Despite the introduction of a live vaccine in 1963, which markedly decreased rates of infection, measles remains a major health burden. Use of the vaccine is estimated to have reduced global measles morbidity and mortality by 74% and 85%, respectively, compared with the prevaccine era. However, outbreaks remain common, and, according to 2011 World Health Organization (WHO) statistics, more than 30 countries in the WHO European Region reported an increase in measles. In addition, despite global vaccination efforts, measles remains common in Europe, Asia, the Pacific, and Africa.

Presentation and Characteristics

Prevaccine, measles was a very common childhood disease in the United States. It is highly contagious and is spread via respiratory droplets. The disease can be spread from 4 days before the onset of the rash to 4 days after onset. The incubation period averages 14 days before the appearance of the rash. Once infected, the virus replicates within the epithelial cells of the respiratory tract, with subsequent spread to lymphoid tissue and blood, resulting in viremia. From there, the virus can disseminate to internal organs such as the lungs, liver, and gastrointestinal tract. The prodromal stage appears around the 9th day after exposure and consists of fever, conjunctivitis, rhinorrhea, and Koplik spots. Koplik spots, which are pathognomonic for measles, occur during the prodrome and are erythematous papules, 1 to 3 mm in diameter, with a bluish-white central discoloration on the buccal mucosa. The characteristic "morbilliform" rash of measles consists of erythematous macules and papules that first appear behind the ears and on the forehead and then spread down over the face, neck, trunk, and extremities. The

fever begins to decrease as the rash develops. The disease may resolve with scaling. Complications include secondary bacterial infection, encephalitis, otitis, pneumonia, and myocarditis. The most serious late complication is subacute sclerosing panencephalitis, which is a delayed neurodegenerative disorder that can occur many years after the acute disease. It is characterized by personality changes, seizures, coma, and death. Diagnosis of measles can be made by detection of measles-specific IgM antibody and measles RNA by real-time polymerase chain reaction (RT-PCR). Health care providers should obtain both a serum sample and a throat swab (or nasopharyngeal swab) from patients suspected to have measles.

Differential Diagnosis

- *Rubella (German measles):* Postauricular lymphadenopathy; milder fever and rash; no Koplik spots (see following section).
- *Scarlet fever:* Circumoral pallor; rash brighter red and confluent (see Chapter 24).
- *Drug eruption:* History of new drugs; usually no fever (see Chapter 8).
- *Kawasaki disease:* fever and mucocutaneous involvement including conjunctivitis, erythema of the lips and oral mucosa (not seen in measles), rash, and cervical lymphadenopathy
- *Infectious mononucleosis:* Rash similar; characteristic hematology; high titer of heterophile antibodies.

Treatment

There is no specific antiviral therapy for measles. Supportive therapy includes treatment of cough, bed rest, antipyretics, fluids, and treatment of any bacterial superinfections. Because low serum vitamin A levels are associated with increased morbidity and mortality, the WHO recommends vitamin A therapy once daily for 2 days for all children with acute measles at the following doses:

- Infants <6 months of age: 50,000 international units
- Infants 6 to 11 months of age: 100,000 international units
- Children ≥12 months: 200,000 international units

Vaccination

A live, attenuated measles vaccine is available for routine childhood immunization in the United States. However, owing to increased global travel from areas where measles is common or because of pockets of people that refuse the vaccine, more cases of measles have been reported in the United States in recent years. According to CDC statistics, there were 644 reported cases of measles in the United States in 2014, which was the highest number of cases in over 20 years. Additionally, 189 cases were reported in 2015, largely because of an outbreak at an amusement park in California. The year 2015 also marked the first death from measles in the United States since 2003. The majority of these cases occurred in unvaccinated individuals.

RUBELLA (GERMAN MEASLES)

Although German measles or rubella is a benign, self-limited disease in children and adults, it can cause serious complications if it develops in utero during the first trimester. Complications can include miscarriage, stillbirth, and severe congenital malformations.

The incubation period is approximately 18 days, and, as in measles, there may be a short prodromal stage of fever and malaise. The rash also resembles measles, because it occurs first on the face, then spreads downward. However, the redness is less intense, and the rash disappears within 2 to 3 days. Enlargement of the cervical and postauricular nodes is a characteristic finding. Arthralgias and arthritis occur in as many as 70% of teenagers and adult women, usually concurrently with the rash, and can persist for months. Serious complications are extremely rare, with encephalitis occurring in about 1 in 6,000 cases and hemorrhagic complications (i.e., hemolytic anemia, thrombocytopenia) occurring in approximately 1 in 3,000 cases.

Differential Diagnosis

- *Measles:* Koplik spots; the fever and the rash are more severe; no postauricular nodes.
- *Scarlet fever:* High fever; perioral pallor; rash may be similar (see Chapter 24).
- *Drug eruption:* New drug history; usually no fever (see Chapter 8).

Treatment

Active treatment is generally unnecessary. Immune globulin given to an exposed pregnant woman in the first trimester of pregnancy may prevent the disease in the fetus. A live, attenuated rubella vaccine is available and is a routine childhood vaccination in the United States.

Congenital Rubella Syndrome

Infants born to mothers who had rubella in the first trimester of pregnancy can have multiple systemic abnormalities including cataracts, deafness, congenital heart defects, and CNS abnormalities. The skin lesions that may be seen include:

- thrombocytopenic purpura
- hyperpigmentation of the navel, forehead, and cheeks
- acne
- seborrhea
- reticulated erythema of the face and extremities

ERYTHEMA INFECTIOSUM

Also known as "fifth disease," erythema infectiosum occurs seasonally, with winter and spring being the peak times. It is caused by parvovirus B19, most commonly affects school-age children, but can also affect adults and the immunocompromised.

Presentation and Characteristics

The incubation period is typically between 4 and 14 days. In children, the prodromal stage lasts from 2 to 4 days and is manifested by low-grade fever, myalgias, and, occasionally, joint pains. The prodromal stage typically occurs 7 to 10 days before the characteristic rash appears. The exanthem begins with bright red macular erythema of the cheeks ("slapped cheek" rash). One to four days later, the second stage of the rash appears, which is characterized by erythematous macules and papules on the extremities and trunk, which eventually progress to a lacy, reticulated pattern. The rash also tends to be more red and confluent on the extensor surfaces of the extremities. A low-grade fever persists for a few days after the onset of the rash, which can last from 1 to 3 weeks. In adults, the rash on the face is less conspicuous, joint complaints are more common, and pruritus is present. Parvovirus infection may also result in the papular–purpuric gloves-and-socks syndrome (PPGSS), which occurs more often in adults and is characterized by petechiae and small purpuric papules on the hands and feet in a gloves-and-socks distribution. In the acropetechial variant of this syndrome, involvement may also be seen in the perioral and chin area and, less commonly, the buttocks, genital, and axillary regions.

Differential Diagnosis

- *Drug eruption:* See Chapter 8.
- *Measles:* Coryza, eruption begins on face and behind ears.
- *Other morbilliform eruptions.*

Treatment

Treatment is generally unnecessary, and only supportive care is needed.

COXSACKIEVIRUS INFECTIONS

Coxsackieviruses are in the genus *Enterovirus.* Coxsackievirus infections are identified by type-specific antigens that appear in the blood 7 days or so after the onset of the disease. It can present with erythematous macules and papules along with a mild prodrome of fever and malaise.

Differential Diagnosis

- measles
- German measles
- scarlet fever
- infectious mononucleosis
- drug eruption

Treatment

Treatment is symptomatic. Antipyretics may be used to reduce the high fever.

HERPANGINA

Herpangina is an acute febrile disease that occurs mainly in children 3 to 10 years of age in the summer months. The first complaints are fever, headache, sore throat, nausea, and stiff neck. Painful vesicles (approximately 2 mm in size) surrounded by an intense erythema are present on the soft palate, uvula, tonsils, pharynx, and buccal mucosa. An exanthema is usually absent. These lesions may coalesce and some may ulcerate. The course of symptomatic infection is usually 7 to 10 days.

The cause of herpangina is primarily coxsackievirus A and B, but echovirus types have also been isolated from sporadic cases.

Differential Diagnosis

- aphthous stomatitis
- drug eruption
- primary herpes gingivostomatitis
- hand–foot–mouth disease

Treatment

Treatment is symptomatic. Soothing mouthwashes and antipyretics may be used.

SAUER'S NOTES

1. Viral diseases are the most adaptable of all infections and the most difficult to treat.
2. There are few cutaneous viral diseases that cannot become a serious systemic disease in the proper setting.
3. Even the lowly human papilloma virus can lead to the most dreaded of all systemic diseases—metastatic cancer.
4. Tremendous progress in therapy and prevention of this group of skin disorders has been made, and recognition of this progress is mandatory in order for good medicine to continue to be practiced.

HAND, FOOT, AND MOUTH DISEASE

Hand, foot, and mouth disease (HFMD) is caused by viruses in the *Enterovirus* genus, most commonly Coxsackievirus A16 and Enterovirus 71. Other coxsackieviruses and other enteroviruses are also associated with HFMD. Infection is spread by direct contact with the virus, which is found in the nasal and pharyngeal secretions, saliva, vesicular fluid, and stool of infected individuals, as well as by fomites. Individuals are most infectious the first week after the onset of symptoms. Generally, the infection begins with constitutional symptoms such as fever, malaise, anorexia, and pharyngitis. One to two days after onset of the fever, painful oral lesions develop on the tongue, gingival, and buccal mucosa that start as erythematous macules, progress to vesicles, and then

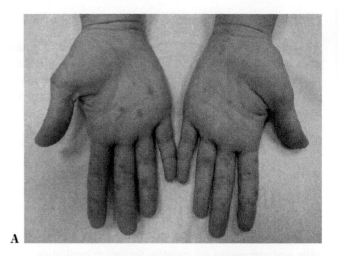

A

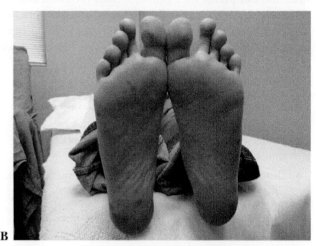

B

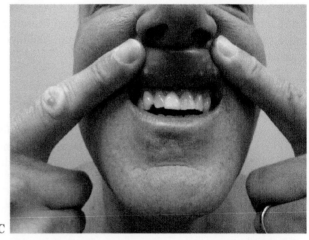

C

FIGURE 26-11: Erythematous macules and papules on the palms **(A)** and soles **(B)** of an adult male with hand, foot, and mouth disease. Multiple aphthaelike erosions in the oral cavity in the same patient **(C)**. (Courtesy of Stephen K. Tyring, MD, PhD.)

eventually ulcerate. Concurrently, a rash also develops on the palms and soles, consisting of erythematous macules and papules as well as vesicles. These lesions may also be present on the buttocks and/or genitalia. HFMD most commonly occurs in children under the age of 10. Recently, however, an increasing number of adults have been affected by HFMD, mostly because of Coxsackievirus A6 (Fig. 26-11). In general, signs and symptoms of HFMD in adults are more severe than in children. Onychomadesis occasionally occurs following resolution of acute HFMD caused by Coxsackievirus A6 as a consequence of temporary nail matrix arrest secondary to the viral infection. The course of HFMD is normally benign and self-limited, but rare complications including meningitis, encephalitis, cardiopulmonary complications, and death have occurred; these complications were caused by a severe strain of Enterovirus 71.

Treatment

Treatment is symptomatic. Mouthwashes, sprays, or analgesics can be used for mouth pain caused by ulcers, and antipyretics may be used for fever.

ECHOVIRUS EXANTHEM

Echoviruses are RNA viruses in the *Enterovirus* genus. Symptoms of infection include fever, nausea, vomiting, diarrhea, sore throat, and cough; rare complications include viral meningitis, encephalitis, myositis, pleurodynia, and myopericarditis. A viral exanthem, which may be maculopapular, morbilliform, macular, petechial, or papulopustular, occurs in one-third of cases. Small erosions may develop on the buccal mucosa. Echoviruses 5, 9, and 25 are most commonly isolated from cases with skin lesions or exanthems. The duration of symptomatic infection is generally 1 to 2 weeks.

Treatment

Treatment is symptomatic. Antipyretics may be used to reduce fever.

Suggested Readings

Ahmed AM, Madkan V, Tyring SK. Human papillomaviruses and genital disease. *Dermatol Clin.* 2006;24:157–165.

Arduino PG, Porter SR. Herpes simplex virus type I infection: overview on relevant clinico-pathological features. *J Oral Pathol Med.* 2008;37:107–121.

Beutner KR. Antivirals in the treatment of pain. *J Geriatr Dermatol.* 1994;6 (suppl 2):23A–28A.

Brown ST, Nalley JF, Kraus SJ. Molluscum contagiosum. *Sex Transm Dis.* 1981;8:227–334.

Brown TJ, Yen-Moore A, Tyring SK. An overview of sexually transmitted disease Part I. *J Am Acad Dermatol.* 1999;41:511–529.

Centers for Disease Control and Prevention. Sexually transmitted diseases treatment guidelines, 2006. *MMWR Recomm Rep.* 2006;55:1–100.

Cernik C, Gallina K, Brodell RT. The treatment of herpes simplex infections: an evidence-based review. *Arch Intern Med.* 2008;168:1137–1144.

Chon T, Nguyen L. What are the best treatments for Herpes Labialis. *J Fam Prac.* 2007;56(7):576–578.

Cohen JI. A new vaccine to prevent herpes zoster. *N Engl J Med.* 2015;372(22):2149–2150.

Dalianis T, Hirsch HH. Human polyomaviruses in disease and cancer. *Virology.* 2012;437(2):63–72.

Donohue JG, Choo PW, Manson JE, et al. The incidence of herpes zoster. *Arch Intern Med.* 1995;155:1605–1609.

Fatahzadeh M, Schwartz RA. Human herpes simplex virus infections: epidemiology, pathogenesis, symptomatology, diagnosis, and management. *J Am Acad Dermatol.* 2007;57(5):737–763.

Genital HSV Infections. Atlanta, GA: Centers for Disease Control and Prevention. http://www.cdc.gov/std/tg2015/herpes.htm. Updated June 08, 2015.

Karnes JB, Usatine RP. Management of external genital warts. *Am Fam Physician.* 2014;90(5):312–318.

Lapolla W, Digiorgio C, Haitz K, et al. Incidence of postherpetic neuralgia after combination treatment with gabapentin and valacyclovir in patients with acute herpes zoster: open-label study. *Arch Dermatol.* 2011;147(8):901–907.

Markowitz, LE, Hariri S, Lin C, et al. Reduction in human papillomavirus (HPV) prevalence among young women following HPV vaccine introduction in the United States, National Health and Nutrition Examination Surveys, 2003–2010. *J Infect Dis.* 2013;208:385–393.

Measles Cases and Outbreaks. Atlanta, GA: Centers for Disease Control and Prevention. http://www.cdc.gov/measles/cases-outbreaks.html. Updated December 16, 2015.

Pereira FA. Herpes simplex: evolving concepts. *J Am Acad Dermatol.* 1996;35:503–520.

Rivera A, Tyring SK. Therapy of cutaneous human Papillomavirus infections. *Dermatol Ther.* 2004;17:441–448.

Schwartz RA, Micali G, Nasca MR, et al. Kaposi sarcoma: a continuing conondrum. *J Am Acad Dermatol.* 2008;59:179–206.

Spruance SL, Stewart JC, Rowe NH, et al. Treatment of recurrent herpes simplex labialis with oral acyclovir. *J Infect Dis.* 1990;161:185–190.

Ting PT, Dytoc MT. Therapy of external anogenital warts and molluscum contagiosum: a literature review. *Dermatol Ther.* 2004;17:68–101.

Tyring SK. Management of herpes zoster and postherpetic neuralgia. *J Am Acad Dermatol.* 2007;57(suppl 6):S136–S142.

Tyring SK, Belanger R, Bezwoda W, et al. A randomized, double-blind trial of famciclovir versus acyclovir for the treatment of localized dermatomal herpes zoster in immunocompromised patients. *Cancer Invest.* 2001;19:13–22.

Tyring SK, Beutner KR, Tucker BA, et al. Antiviral therapy for herpes zoster: randomized, controlled clinical trial of valacyclovir and famciclovir therapy in immunocompetent patients 50 years and older. *Arch Fam Med.* 2000;9:863–869.

Tyring SK, Moore AY, Lupi O, eds. *Mucocutaneous Manifestations of Viral Diseases: An Illustrated Guide to Diagnosis and Management.* London, UK: CRC Press; 2010:586.

White MK, Gordon J, Khalili K. Rapidly expanding family of human polyomaviruses: recent developments in understanding their life cycle and role in human pathology. *PLoS Pathog.* 2013;9(3): e1003206.

Yanofsky VR, Patel RA, Goldenberg G. Genital warts: a comprehensive review. *J Clin Aesthet Dermatol.* 2012;5(6):25–36.

Yeung-Yue KA, Brentjens MH, Lee PC, et al. Herpes simplex viruses 1 and 2. *Dermatol Clin.* 2002;20:249–266.

Cutaneous Diseases Associated With Human Immunodeficiency Virus

Christie Riemer, BS, Annie O. Morrison, MD, Nicole M. Candelario, MD, Clay J. Cockerell, MD, and Antoanella Calame, MD

> **SAUER'S NOTES**
>
> 1. Dermatologists have been at the forefront in diagnosis and therapy during the HIV pandemic.
> 2. The skin can be used as a marker for early diagnosis and follow-up for disease regression or progression.
> 3. Morbidity and, occasionally, mortality from skin diseases underline the importance of dermatology in HIV.

Worldwide, there are an estimated 36.9 million individuals infected with human immunodeficiency virus (HIV), and up to 2 million cases are diagnosed annually. Cutaneous diseases are frequently the initial manifestation of HIV. Knowledge of the most common presentations may aid in the diagnosis of immunodeficiency. The spectrum of HIV-associated cutaneous manifestations is broad and includes infectious diseases, inflammatory disorders, neoplastic conditions, and hypersensitivity reactions, some of which may be related to antiretroviral therapies. The following is an outline of the most commonly encountered skin disorders in the HIV-infected population and the array of cutaneous manifestations associated with each entity.

INFECTIOUS DISEASES

Viral Infections

Acute Retroviral Syndrome

Acute HIV infection, also termed acute retroviral syndrome (ARS), spans the period from primary infection to complete seroconversion and HIV-1 antibody detection. ARS is often subclinical, but may resemble a transient, nonspecific viral infection with fever, malaise, myalgia, headache, pharyngitis, and lymphadenopathy. Early identification and treatment of patients with ARS may help preserve immune function and prevent rapid CD4 cell count decline. Cutaneous manifestations can be seen in up to 75% of symptomatic patients with ARS and appear several days after onset of prodromal symptoms. The most common presentation is a morbilliform eruption on the trunk, face, or extremities that lasts 4 to 5 days. Vesicles, pustules, urticarial lesions, alopecia, and desquamation of the palms and soles have also been reported. In addition, approximately 25% of patients with ARS exhibit painful erosions and shallow ulcerations of the mucous membranes, most commonly in the oral cavity.

Molluscum Contagiosum

Molluscum contagiosum (MC) is a viral infection present in 5% to 20% of HIV-positive patients. The causative virus is a member of the family Poxviridae, transmitted via direct skin-to-skin contact. In adults, the lesions are often sexually transmitted and occur most commonly in the genital region, lower abdomen, and thighs. They appear as solitary or multiple skin-colored, umbilicated papules (1 to 10 mm). Severely immunocompromised patients, particularly those with CD4 cell counts $<200/mm^3$, may exhibit unusual morphologies and growth patterns such as giant lesions (>1 cm), clusters of several hundred papules or extensive facial involvement. Although most lesions are generally self-limited, MC in HIV patients is characteristically difficult to treat and lesions rarely spontaneously regress. Treatment options include cryotherapy, electrocauterization, laser surgery, topical tretinoin, intralesional interferon, or the antiviral agent cidofovir for refractory lesions. Imiquimod has been used to treat MC; however, recent studies show this to be less efficacious than cidofovir in pediatric populations.

Human Papillomavirus

Human papillomavirus (HPV) is a double-stranded DNA virus of the *Papillomaviridae* family that is transmitted via direct skin-to-skin contact. HPV induces hyperproliferative lesions in the skin and mucous membranes. More than 150 types of HPV have been identified, and several strains have been shown to play a role in oncogenesis, particularly HPV types 16 and 18. HPV infections can be subdivided clinically into three categories: cutaneous lesions (e.g., verruca vulgaris), anogenital/mucosal lesions (e.g., condyloma acuminata), and epidermodysplasia verruciformis (EDV). EDV is an inheritable susceptibility to cutaneous HPV infection, thought to result from an autosomal recessive impairment of cell-mediated immunity. Patients present with widespread flat, wart-like papules and hypo- or hyperpigmented macules. Similar cutaneous lesions may appear in AIDS, described as acquired epidermodysplasia verruciformis. HIV patients with cutaneous and/or anogenital HPV infection are at increased risk for recurrence, high-grade anogenital intraepithelial dysplasia, and invasive squamous cell carcinomas (SCCs). Treatment modalities for cutaneous lesions include cryotherapy, podophyllin, salicylic acid, trichloroacetic acid, laser therapy, topical imiquimod, and surgical techniques. Antiretroviral therapy (ART) does not prevent lesions and can paradoxically worsen manifestations as the immune system begins to attack virus-infected cells. HPV vaccines may confer protection; however current studies have not investigated efficacy in HIV patients.

Herpes Simplex Virus

Herpes simplex virus (HSV) infections are common in HIV patients. Approximately 70% are HSV-2 seropositive and 95% are seropositive for either HSV-1 or HSV-2. Historically, HSV-1 was more commonly affiliated with oral lesions, while HSV-2 localized to the anogenital region; however, the crossover rate has become high enough that the association is no longer clinically relevant. Transmission occurs through bodily fluid exchange, as well as direct contact with vesicular fluid of active herpetic lesions. In the early stages of HIV infection, the clinical presentation of HSV infection is similar to that seen in immunocompetent individuals (Fig. 27-1). However,

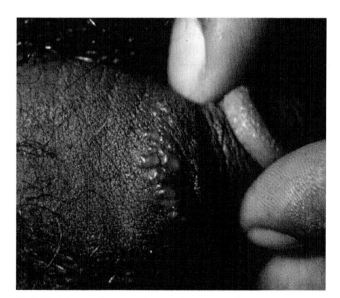

FIGURE 27-1: Grouped vesicles in a posterior auricular location in an AIDS patient. There is nothing characteristic about this clinical presentation to differ from an HIV(−) patient.

an increased incidence of disease manifestation occurs when CD4 cell counts decrease to <100 cells/μL. With advanced immunosuppression, HSV lesions can be atypical and are divided into three clinical forms: chronic ulcerative, generalized acute mucocutaneous, and systemic. Chronic ulcerative HSV presents with recalcitrant ulcerations, most often of the anogenital and perioral regions. Lesions peripherally expand, deepen, and become confluent. Generalized acute mucocutaneous HSV is characterized by disseminated vesicular skin and mucous membrane lesions plus high fever and systemic symptoms. Systemic HSV infection is relatively rare, and most commonly involves the lungs, liver, adrenal glands, pericardium, and brain. Acyclovir remains the intravenous therapy of choice for severe mucocutaneous disease and disseminated infection. However, increasing rates of acyclovir resistance have developed among AIDS patients in whom prolonged, low-dose administration is used for suppressive therapy. IV foscarnet (vidarabine) and cidofovir have been shown to be effective against some acyclovir-resistant strains. Suppressive therapy with oral acyclovir, valacyclovir, or famciclovir remains effective in preventing recurrence.

Varicella-Zoster Virus

Varicella-zoster virus (VZV) infection, transmitted via aerosol droplets, initially manifests as varicella (chickenpox). Reactivation of the disease is termed herpes zoster (shingles), and incidence is >15× higher in HIV patients. In immunocompromised patients, VZV infection is often severe and can generally be categorized clinically as severe and persistent varicella, dermatomal zoster, recurrent zoster, chronic zoster, and disseminated zoster with or without precedent dermatomal lesions. Chronic herpes zoster manifests as hyperkeratotic nodules, verrucous lesions, or ulcerations, most commonly affecting the buttocks and lower extremities. Resolution can take weeks to months. Disseminated zoster is defined as more than 20 lesions outside the originally affected dermatome, greater than three contiguous dermatomes involved, or systemic infections such as pneumonitis, hepatitis, or encephalitis. When HIV-positive individuals are exposed to VZV, varicella-zoster immune globulin (VZIG) should be given as soon as possible. Valacyclovir or famciclovir are the drugs of choice for active disease treatment. Valacyclovir (1,000 mg q8hr) has been shown to speed rates of cutaneous healing in immunocompromised patients. Extensive cutaneous involvement may require IV acyclovir.

Bacterial Infections

Staphylococcus aureus

Staphylococcus is the most common pathogen to infect HIV-positive patients and can cause cellulitis, folliculitis (pustules and papules around hair follicles), furuncles, deep tissue abscesses (red, warm painful nodules), and impetigo (vesiculopustular plaques and erythematous macules with honey colored crust). Infections are often recurrent secondary to nasal colonization. HIV patients are at increased risk for infection with methicillin-resistant *S. aureus* (MRSA). Skin colonization may be controlled with chlorhexidine gluconate and/or bleach baths, and nasal colonization can temporarily be eradicated with mupirocin ointment.

Bacillary Angiomatosis

Bacillary angiomatosis is a rare cutaneous disease caused by *Bartonella* species *B. henselae* and *B. quintana*. Symptomatic disease is common in HIV-positive patients, particularly when CD4 cell counts drop below 200/mm^3. Cutaneous lesions may manifest as tender violaceous papules resembling pyogenic granuloma, ulcerated or crusted nodules similar to Kaposi sarcoma (KS), subcutaneous nodules, or widespread erythematous plaques (Fig. 27-2). While cutaneous manifestations are most common, visceral involvement may also occur, including peliosis hepatis of the liver, lymph node or soft tissue involvement, and lytic bone lesions. Erythromycin and doxycycline are first-line treatments, and should be administered for more than 3 months. Alternative therapies include clarithromycin or azithromycin. Some patients may experience a disseminated inflammatory reaction as the organisms die after antibiotic administration and *Bartonella spp.* antigens are released into the bloodstream (Jarisch–Herxheimer-like reaction). Anti-inflammatory agents can alleviate symptoms.

Syphilis

The spirochete *Treponema pallidum* causes syphilis. Although nearly eradicated in the early to mid-2000s, the prevalence of primary and secondary syphilis has increased in the United States in recent years. Between 2012 and 2013, the rate increased by 10%, with the majority of cases occurring in young men. Syphilis has a higher prevalence among HIV-positive populations. *T. pallidum* is sexually transmitted and initially manifests as a painless, clean-based ulceration (chancre), which is the hallmark of primary syphilis. If left untreated, secondary syphilis develops within 4 to 10 weeks, manifesting as numerous, diffuse erythematous macules and papules on the face, trunk, and genital region. Syphilis has been called the "great masquerader," and may present as mucous membrane ulcerations, palmoplantar eruptions, or alopecia. Latent

syphilis, an asymptomatic period following the resolution of secondary syphilis, may continue indefinitely. However, if untreated, one-third of patients develop tertiary syphilis within 15 years. The cutaneous manifestations of tertiary disease include granuloma formation, psoriasiform plaques, and gummas (painless, indurated nodules, which may ulcerate and become locally destructive). Rare, unusual features may be seen in immunocompromised hosts, including extensive chancres, lues maligna (papulopustular or necrotic lesions, ocular disease, and/or vasculitis), and rapid progression to neurosyphilis despite appropriate treatment. In general, the treatment of syphilis in HIV-positive patients is intramuscular benzathine penicillin G, similar to those without HIV. HIV-positive patients should be followed closely for clinical and serologic evidence of treatment failure.

Mycobacteria

Cutaneous mycobacterial disease is a manifestation of systemic disease, most commonly caused by *Mycobacterium tuberculosis*. Infection may be primary, through direct transmission in broken skin, or secondary via hematogenous spread (miliary tuberculosis). Lesions present as erythematous papules, abscesses, chancres, verrucous plaques, or dermal nodules. Histologically, cutaneous lesions appear as suppurative granulomatous infiltrates in the dermis. Although relatively rare in developed countries, the incidence of cutaneous mycobacteria is higher among HIV patients. There appears to be a synergistic effect between tuberculosis and HIV, wherein each condition becomes more virulent. Multidrug-resistant tuberculosis (MDR-TB) and extensively drug-resistant tuberculosis (EDR-TB) are major problems in the HIV population worldwide. Other mycobacterial species known to cause cutaneous infections include *M. kansasii, M. szulgai, M. marinum M. avium-intracellulare, M. abscessans, M. leprae, and M. ulcerans*. Antitubercular prophylaxis may decrease complications. Treatment includes a four-drug regimen of isoniazid, rifampin, pyrazinamide, and ethambutol for at least 6 months. Concurrent ART may induce paradoxical worsening of cutaneous TB symptoms due to the development of immune reconstitution inflammatory syndrome (IRIS).

Fungal Infections

Dermatophytosis

The incidence of epidermal dermatophytosis in HIV-positive patients is similar to that of immunocompetent individuals. However, the severity and variability of presentation is typically increased in the setting of HIV infection. The most common dermatophytic pathogens seen in this patient population are *Trychophyton rubrum* and *Trichophyton mentagrophytes*. Lesions generally appear as annular erythematous plaques with scale and can present on the extremities or trunk (tinea corporis), feet (tinea pedis), beard (tinea barbae), or head (tinea capitis). Proximal white subungual onychomycosis caused by *Trichophyton rubrum* is commonly seen in HIV patients, as is fungal folliculitis. Patients not receiving antiretroviral or antifungal therapy may develop chronic infections (most

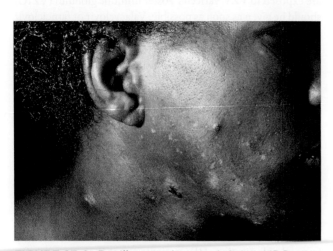

FIGURE 27-2: Bacillary angiomatosis in an AIDS patient showing crusted, pyogenic granuloma-like papules on side of the face and neck.

notably interdigital tinea pedis) that can serve as portals of entry for superinfection, most commonly with *Staphylococcus aureus* or group A *Streptococcus*. Dermatophytosis occurring in HIV disease is best treated with oral antifungal medications, such as oral terbinafine, itraconazole, or griseofulvin. Topical antifungal preparations (terbinafine, miconazole) may serve as useful adjuncts to systemic therapy and may help prevent recurrences.

Candidiasis

The most common form of yeast infection in HIV-positive patients is oral candidiasis, which is caused by numerous *Candida* species, most notably *C. albicans*. In the absence of ART, oropharyngeal candidiasis is a common presenting symptom. Overall, oral candidiasis occurs in 45% to 90% of individuals with AIDS. A major risk factor is a CD4 count <200 cells/mm^3. Esophageal candidiasis is an AIDS-defining lesion, though the incidence has declined in recent years because of highly active antiretroviral therapy (HAART) therapy. Four clinical variations of oral candidiasis have been described in HIV-infected individuals: pseudomembranous candidiasis, erythematous (atrophic) candidiasis, hyperplastic candidiasis, and angular cheilitis. Candida infection may also become disseminated, leading to complications such as urethritis, refractory vaginal candidiasis, or onychodystrophy (nail malformation). Oral fluconazole remains the first-line treatment for oral candidiasis, though systemic antifungal-resistant organisms have emerged. Topical therapies, such as clotrimazole (available as a troche) or nystatin (available as an oral solution) may be used for mild to moderate episodes. Systemic medications include ketoconazole, itraconazole, echinocandins, or amphotericin B.

Cryptococcosis

Cryptococcosis, caused by *Cryptococcus neoformans*, is a life-threatening fungal infection in HIV-positive patients, most commonly seen when the CD4 cell count is below 100/mm^3. Infection with *C. neoformans* occurs via inhalation of organisms found in soil contaminated with bird droppings. Cutaneous manifestations are seen in 10% to 20% of cases of disseminated cryptococcosis, and may present 2 to 6 weeks prior to systemic symptoms. The most common findings of cutaneous cryptococcosis are umbilicated flesh-colored papules or nodules that resemble lesions of MC (Fig. 27-3A and B). Lesions have reportedly been mistaken for basal cell carcinoma (BCC), and may also appear as ulcers, pustules, subcutaneous abscesses, cellulitis, panniculitis, palpable purpura, and plaques. The face is most commonly involved, although lesions may be widespread. Nonmeningeal cryptococcosis should be treated similar to that used for central nervous system (CNS) disease. An induction phase with amphotericin B and flucytosine for a minimum of 2 weeks is followed by 8 weeks of fluconazole therapy. Fluconazole plus flucytosine is an alternative to amphotericin B therapy. Chronic maintenance therapy with lower doses of fluconazole is recommended for at least 1 year. Introduction of ART therapy may induce IRIS, as in treatment of HIV patients with TB. Continuation of ART and antifungal therapy is recommended.

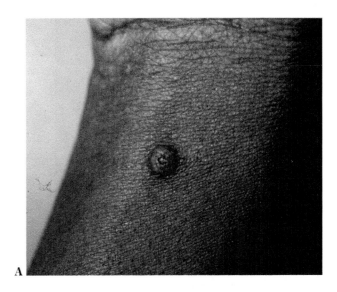

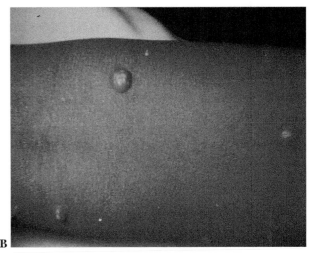

FIGURE 27-3: **A:** Umbilicated papule on the flexor wrist of disseminated cryptococcal infection in an AIDS patient. **B:** Umbilicated papule of MC for comparison.

Histoplasmosis

Histoplasmosis is a granulomatous disease caused by the intracellular fungus *Histoplasma capsulatum*, present in the soil in the vicinity of chicken coops, roosting places of birds, or bat caves. It is an AIDS-defining illness. Disseminated disease is seen in 2% to 5% of HIV-positive individuals, particularly those with CD4 cell counts less than 150/mm^3 who inhabit or have traveled to endemic regions of the United States, South America, or the Caribbean. Cutaneous manifestations, present in less than 10% of cases, most often occur on the face, followed by the extremities and trunk. Lesions appear as macules, papules, pustules, ulcers, subcutaneous nodules, or rosacea-like eruptions (Fig. 27-4). Oropharyngeal plaques, nodules, and ulcers are also common with concurrent skin disease. The treatment of choice in severe cutaneous or disseminated histoplasmosis is amphotericin B (amp B). IV liposomal amp B is more effective than standard IV amp B deoxycholate. Maintenance or

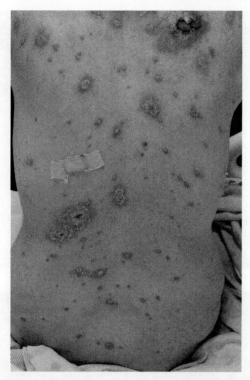

FIGURE 27-4: Disseminated histoplasmosis in an HIV patient with CD4 count of 4/mm². Pustular crusted lesions coalescing into a necrotic plaque with central ulceration and secondary impetiginization. (Photo courtesy of Jeffrey Cizenski, MD & John Griffen, MD.)

prophylactic therapy with itraconazole is recommended for 12 months in patients with CD4 cell counts below 150/mm³.

Coccidioidomycosis

Coccidioidomycosis is caused by *Coccidioides immitis*, a dimorphic fungus present in soil, endemic to the southwestern United States, northern Mexico, and scattered regions of Central and South America. Clinically significant infections occur more frequently in individuals with CD4 cell counts below 250/mm³. Cutaneous lesions are the most common presentation of disseminated coccidioidomycosis, manifesting as papules and verrucous lesions. In some cases, lesions expand and become confluent with the formation of ulcers, abscesses, or sinus tracts. The presence of skin lesions warrants a detailed investigation into other possible sites of dissemination (lungs, CNS, liver). HIV-positive patients with disseminated disease should be treated with amp B until clinically improvement is seen. Oral fluconazole or itraconazole may be added at the initiation of therapy, and should be continued indefinitely.

NEOPLASTIC DISEASES

Kaposi Sarcoma

KS is a common neoplastic disorder occurring in HIV-positive patients and is most prevalent in homosexual or bisexual men. Human herpesvirus type 8 (HHV-8) is present in all lesions.

Primary lesions of KS occur on the face or trunk as unilateral, violaceous to yellowish-green macules or patches. With time, these lesions may progress to bilateral involvement and enlarge to form confluent plaques. In later stages of the disease, patients present with nodules, tumors, and areas of erosion or ulceration. KS may also involve the oral cavity, particularly the hard palate (Fig. 27-5), and its presence indicates CD4 cell counts less than 200/mm³. Extracutaneous KS commonly occurs in the lymph nodes, gastrointestinal tract, and lungs. Treatment of KS in HIV populations is HAART therapy. Additional treatment modalities include localized radiation therapy, cryosurgery, laser surgery, excisional surgery, and electrocauterization. Lesion regression has been documented with systemic ganciclovir or foscarnet therapy. In patients with visceral involvement and life-threatening disease, chemotherapy, radiotherapy, and immunotherapy should be considered.

Lymphomas

The incidence of lymphoma in HIV-positive patients is increased 60 to 200 fold compared to the non–HIV infected population. It is the first AIDS-defining illness in 3% to 5% of patients, presenting mainly as non-Hodgkin lymphoma, predominantly of B-cell origin. Cutaneous lymphomas arising in HIV-positive patients may include mycosis fungoides (MF), CD30+ anaplastic large cell lymphoma, or diffuse large B-cell lymphoma. An association with Epstein–Barr virus has been documented in many cutaneous B-cell lymphomas.

Carcinomas and Melanoma

HIV patients are at increased risk of nonmelanoma skin cancer, including BCC, SCC, and SCC in situ (Bowen disease). Rates of occurrence are three to five times that of HIV-negative individuals, with BCC occurring most frequently. Epithelial neoplasms of oral and anogenital sites are especially increased in HIV patient populations. With the exception of BCC, cutaneous neoplasms that develop in immunosuppressed states are often more aggressive, with higher rates of recurrence and metastases. Adequate surgical margins help with early

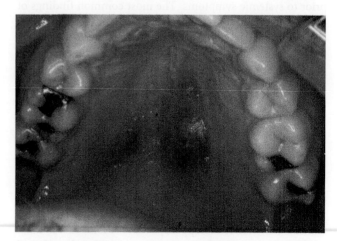

FIGURE 27-5: Asymmetric, purple, plaques of KS on the hard palate in an AIDS patient.

control of carcinomas, and have been shown to be important in reducing morbidity and mortality in HIV-infected patients.

Malignant melanoma may have an increased incidence in HIV patients, although no definitive data exist regarding the relationship. The development of multiple primary melanomas and early nodular lesions in HIV patients has been reported; however, it is uncertain whether this finding is secondary to increased surveillance, detection, and reporting, or an actual increase of melanoma in these patients. HIV-positive patients with melanoma have demonstrated a significantly decreased disease-free survival, with lower CD4 cell counts predictive of a poorer prognosis. Primary prevention, routine skin examinations, and early biopsy of suspicious lesions are essential in this patient population.

INFLAMMATORY DISEASES

Seborrheic Dermatitis

Seborrheic dermatitis is one of the most common cutaneous diseases in the HIV-positive patient population, with a prevalence of approximately 83%. The severity of clinical presentation has been shown to correlate with the higher degrees of immune suppression and lower CD4 cell counts. Clinically, seborrheic dermatitis presents as well-demarcated, erythematous, scaly patches and plaques of the scalp, eyebrows, nasolabial folds, ears, and intertriginous areas. Five features characteristic of AIDS-related seborrheic dermatitis include: a greater degree of inflammation; presence of plaques resembling psoriasis; involvement of atypical areas such as the trunk, groin, and extremities; "cradle cap" of the scalp producing a nonscarring alopecia; and hypo- or hyperpigmentation of affected areas. Recommended treatment consists of the use of topical corticosteroid and antifungal medications (clotrimazole or ketoconazole). Some refractory cases may require adjunctive therapies such as ultraviolet B (UVB) phototherapy, coal tar, sulfur, salicylic acid shampoos, pimecrolimus cream, and oral fluconazole.

Eosinophilic Folliculitis

HIV-associated eosinophilic folliculitis (EF) has an incidence of 5% to 12% and most commonly presents in patients with CD4 cell counts less than 250/mm^3. The etiology of the disease is currently uncertain. However, given the folliculotropic nature of the inflammation, it has been hypothesized that an opportunistic infection (possibly secondary to bacteria, *Pityrosporum*, or *Demodex* mites), or a hypersensitivity response due to HIV-related immune dysregulation may be the cause. Patients with HIV-associated EF classically present with a persistent, erythematous, intensely pruritic, cutaneous eruption on the face, trunk, shoulders, upper arms, and neck (Fig. 27-6). Recommended first-line treatment options include topical corticosteroids, topical tacrolimus, or oral indomethacin. Use of cetirizine, metronidazole, and itraconazole have also been reported in the literature. UVB phototherapy is the gold standard of treatment, and is often curative. Systemic corticosteroids may be necessary to control the intense pruritus.

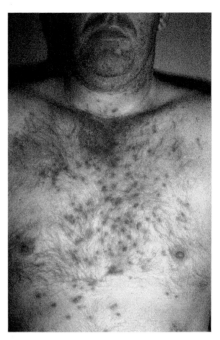

FIGURE 27-6: Inflammatory papules on the chest that were intensely pruritic and persistent, which is typical of EF in AIDS.

HYPERSENSITIVITY DISEASES

Drug Reactions Associated With HAART

The advent of HAART in the mid-1990s produced a dramatic decrease in the morbidity and mortality among patients infected with HIV. However, HAART administration has also been associated with adverse effects, many of which are dermatologic in nature. The drugs that comprise HAART regimens are categorized into four main groups based on their specific mechanism of action: nonnucleoside reverse transcriptase inhibitors (NNRTIs), nucleoside reverse transcriptase inhibitors (NRTIs), protease inhibitors (PIs), and fusion or entry inhibitors (FIs). Side effects associated with NNRTIs (nevirapine, etravirine, and efavirenz), may manifest as urticaria, morbilliform eruptions, leukocytoclastic vasculitis, as well as Stevens–Johnson syndrome or "drug reaction with eosinophilia and systemic symptoms" (DRESS). NRTIs, particularly zidovudine and abacavir, are known for nail and mucocutaneous hyperpigmentation (Fig. 27-7), multisystem hypersensitivity reaction, and lipodystrophy. As a group, PIs are associated with lipodystrophy, morbilliform or urticarial hypersensitivity reactions, acute generalized exanthematous pustulosis, generalized pruritus, xerosis, desquamative cheilitis, striae formation, and angiolipomatosis. Maraviroc and enfuvirtide are FDA-approved FIs for use in HIV-positive patients. Efuviritide subcutaneous administration has been associated with injection site reactions in a significant proportion of patients.

Photosensitivity Reactions

Photoeruptions have become increasingly recognized in the setting of HIV disease and can be classified into the following

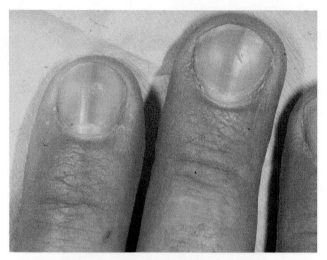

FIGURE 27-7: Hyperpigmented streaks on fingernails, which are seen in patients on NRTI medications for AIDS.

categories: chronic actinic dermatitis (CAD), lichenoid photoeruptions, photosensitive hyperpigmentation, porphyria cutanea tarda, and photosensitive granuloma annulare. Among these, CAD and lichenoid photoeruptions are the two categories most commonly associated with HIV. CAD is characterized by a marked male predominance, and presents as erythematous or lichenified papules and plaques in a photodistributed pattern. An increased incidence of lichenoid photoeruptions is seen in African-American patients infected with HIV, particularly those with CD4 cell counts below 50/mm^3. Eruptions usually last several months and, similar to lichen planus, are characterized by violaceous, flat-topped papules and plaques. Lesions are predominantly on the face, neck, and dorsal forearms and hands. The lack of mucosal involvement, with the exception of the lower lip, can aid in distinguishing these lesions from idiopathic lichen planus.

Suggested Readings

Akgul B, Cooke JC, Storey A. HPV-associated skin disease. *J Pathol.* 2006;208(2):165–175.

Ampel NM, Dols CL, Galgiani JN. Coccidioidomycosis during human immunodeficiency virus infection: results of a prospective study in a coccidioidal endemic area. *Am J Med.* 1993;94(3):235–240.

Aquilina C, Viraben R, Roueire A. Acute generalized exanthematous pustulosis: a cutaneous adverse effect due to prophylactic antiviral therapy with protease inhibitor. *Arch Intern Med.* 1998;158(19):2160–2161.

Bourezane Y, Salard D, Hoen B, et al. DRESS (drug rash with eosinophilia and systemic symptoms) syndrome associated with nevirapine therapy. *Clin Infect Dis.* 1998;27(5):1321–1322.

Buchbinder SP, Katz MH, Hessol NA, et al. Herpes zoster and human immunodeficiency virus infection. *J Infect Dis.* 1992;166(5):1153–1156.

Chatis PA, Crumpacker CS. Resistance of herpesviruses to antiviral drugs. *Antimicrob Agents Chemother.* 1992;36(8):1589–1595.

Chéret A, Bacchus-Souffan C, Avettand-Fenoël V, et al. Combined ART started during acute HIV infection protects central memory CD4+ T cells and can induce remission. *J Antimicrob Chemother.* 2015;70(7):2108–2120.

Cockerell CJ. Cutaneous manifestations of HIV infection other than Kaposi's sarcoma: clinical and histologic aspects. *J Am Acad Dermatol.* 1990;22(6 pt 2):1260–1269.

Cockerell CJ. Seborrheic dermatitis-like and atopic dermatitis-like eruptions in HIV-infected patients. *Clin Dermatol.* 1991;9(1):49–51.

Cockerell CJ. Bacillary angiomatosis and related diseases caused by Rochalimaea. *J Am Acad Dermatol.* 1995;32(5 pt 1):783–790.

Coldiron BM, Bergstresser PR. Prevalence and clinical spectrum of skin disease in patients infected with human immunodeficiency virus. *Arch Dermatol.* 1989;125(3):357–361.

Cooley TP. Non-AIDS-defining cancer in HIV-infected people. *Hematol Oncol Clin North Am.* 2003;17(3):889–899.

Dias M, Filho B. Quaresma M, et al Update on cutaneous tuberculosis. *An Bras Dermatol.* 2014;89(6):925–938.

Ellis E, Scheinfeld N. Eosinophilic pustular folliculitis: a comprehensive review of treatment options. *Am J Clin Dermatol.* 2004;5(3):189–197.

Garcia-Silva J, Almagro M, Juega J, et al. Protease inhibitor-related paronychia, ingrown toenails, desquamative cheilitis and cutaneous xerosis. *AIDS.* 2000;14(9):1289–1291.

Golden MR, Marra CM, Holmes KK. Update on syphilis: resurgence of an old problem. *JAMA.* 2003;290(11):1510–1514.

Grogg K, Miller R, Dogan A. HIV infection and lymphoma. *J Clin Pathol.* 2007;60(12):1365–1372.

Hall JC, Hall BJ, Cockerell CJ. *HIV/AIDS in the Post-HAART Era.* Shelton: People's Medical Publishing House-USA;2011:147–185.

Hetherington S, McGuirk S, Powell G, et al. Hypersensitivity reactions during therapy with the nucleoside reverse transcriptase inhibitor abacavir. *Clin Ther.* 2001;23(10):1603–1614.

Kahn JO, Walker BD. Acute human immunodeficiency virus type 1 infection. *N Engl J Med.* 1998;339(1):33–39.

Nguyen P, Vin-Christian K, Ming ME, et al. Aggressive squamous cell carcinomas in persons infected with the human immunodeficiency virus. *Arch Dermatol.* 2002;138(6):758–763.

Noy A. Update on HIV lymphoma. *Curr Oncol Rep.* 2007;9(5):384–390.

Phelan JA. Oral manifestations of human immunodeficiency virus infection. *Med Clin North Am.* 1997;81(2):511–531.

Sadick NS, McNutt NS, Kaplan MH. Papulosquamous dermatoses of AIDS. *J Am Acad Dermatol.* 1990;22(6 pt 2):1270–1277.

Samaranayake LP, Holmstrup P. Oral candidiasis and human immunodeficiency virus infection. *J Oral Pathol Med.* 1989;18(10):554–564.

Simpson-Dent S, Fearfield LA, Staughton RC. HIV associated eosinophilic folliculitis—differential diagnosis and management. *Sex Transm Infect.* 1999;75(5):291–293.

Wheat J, Sarosi G, McKinsey D, et al. Practice guidelines for the management of patients with histoplasmosis. Infectious Diseases Society of America. *Clin Infect Dis.* 2000;30(4):688–695.

Wilkins K, Turner R, Dolev JC, et al. Cutaneous malignancy and human immunodeficiency virus disease. *J Am Acad Dermatol.* 2006;54(2):189–206; quiz 207–110.

Wilks D, Boyd A, Clutterbuck D, et al. Clinical and pathological review of HIV-associated lymphoma in Edinburgh, United Kingdom. *Eur J Clin Microbiol Infect Dis.* 2001;20(9):603–608.

Zuger A, Louie E, Holzman RS, et al. Cryptococcal disease in patients with the acquired immunodeficiency syndrome. Diagnostic features and outcome of treatment. *Ann Intern Med.* 1986;104(2):234–240.

Dermatologic Mycology

John C. Hall, MD

Fungi can be present as part of the normal flora of the skin or as abnormal inhabitants. Dermatologists are concerned with the abnormal inhabitants, or pathogenic fungi. However, the so-called nonpathogenic fungi can proliferate and infect immunosuppressed persons.

Pathogenic fungi have a predilection for certain body areas; most commonly, they infect the skin, but the lungs, the brain, and other organs can also be infected. Pathogenic fungi can invade the skin *superficially* and *deeply,* and are thus divided into these two groups.

SUPERFICIAL FUNGAL INFECTIONS

The superficial fungi live on the dead horny layer of the skin and elaborate an enzyme that enables them to digest keratin, causing the superficial skin to scale and disintegrate, the nails to crumble, and the hairs to break off. The deeper reactions of vesicles, erythema, and infiltration are presumably due to the fungi liberating an exotoxin. Fungi are also capable of eliciting an allergic or id reaction.

When a skin scraping, a hair, or a culture growth is examined with the microscope in a wet preparation, the three structural elements of the fungi are seen: the spores, the hyphae, and the mycelia.

Spores are the reproducing bodies of the fungi. Sexual and asexual forms occur. Spores are rarely seen in skin scrapings, but they are the identifying structures on microscopic examination of fungal cultures.

Hyphae are threadlike, branching filaments that grow out from the fungus spore. The hyphae are the identifying filaments seen in skin scrapings in potassium hydroxide (KOH) solution.

Mycelia are matted clumps of hyphae that grow on culture plates.

Culture media vary greatly in content, but modifications of Sabouraud dextrose agar are used to grow the superficial fungi. Sabouraud agar and corn meal agar are both used to identify the deep fungi. Hyphae and spores grow on the media, and identification of the species of fungi is established by the gross appearance of the mycelia, the color of the substrate, and the microscopic appearance of the spores and the hyphae when a sample of the growth is placed on a slide. Some media show a color change when pathogenic fungi are isolated.

Classification

Superficial dermatophyte fungi are divided into three genera: *Microsporum, Epidermophyton*, and *Trichophyton*. Species of only two of these invade the hair: *Microsporum* and *Trichophyton*. As seen in a KOH preparation, *Microsporum* species cause an ectothrix infection of the hair shaft, whereas *Trichophyton* species cause either an ectothrix or an endothrix infection. The ectothrix fungi cause the formation of an external spore sheath around the hair, whereas the endothrix fungi do not. The filaments of mycelia penetrate the hair in both types of infection.

The species of fungi is correlated with the clinical diseases in Table 28-1.

Clinical Classifications

Superficial fungal infections of the skin affect various sites of the body. The clinical lesions, the species of fungi, and the therapy vary for these different sites. Therefore, fungal diseases of the skin are classified, for clinical purposes, according to the location of the infection. These clinical types are as follows:

- Tinea of the feet (tinea pedis)
- Tinea of the hands (tinea manus)
- Tinea of the nails (onychomycosis)
- Tinea of the groin (tinea cruris)
- Tinea of the smooth skin (tinea corporis)
- Tinea of the scalp (tinea capitis)
- Tinea of the beard (tinea barbae)
- Dermatophytid (generalized allergic reaction)
- Tinea versicolor
- Tinea of the external ear.

1. Correct diagnosis of a fungal infection is necessary. An oral antifungal drug should not be prescribed for a patient if the diagnosis has not been confirmed. Systemic antifungal agents are of no value in treating atopic eczema, contact dermatitis, psoriasis, pityriasis rosea, and so on.
2. Except for tinea of the scalp and nails, true fungal infections are noticeably improved after only 1 to 2 weeks of oral antifungal therapy. If there is no improvement, the diagnosis of the dermatosis as a fungus disease is erroneous and the therapy should be stopped.

TABLE 28-1 • Relationship of Fungi to Body Areas

Fungus	Feet and Hands	Nails	Groin	Smooth Skin	Scalp	Beard
Microsporum Species						
M. audouini		O	O	Uncommon	Uncommon	O
M. canis	O	O	O	Common	Uncommon	Rare
M. gypseum	O	O	O	Rare	Rare	O
Epidermophyton Species						
E. floccosum	Moderately common	Rare	Common	Moderately common	O	O
Trichophyton Species						
Endothrix Species						
T. schoenleini	O	Rare	O	Rare	(Favus) rare, especially tropics	O
T. violaceum	O	Rare	O	O	Rare	Rare
T. tonsurans	O	Rare	O	Rare	Common	O
Ectothrix Species						
T. mentagrophytes	Common	Moderately common	O	Common	Rare	Moderately common
T. rubrum	Common	Common	Moderately common	Common	O	Rare

3. An adequate dosage is necessary, including (a) the correct daily dose for the particular type of fungal infection and (b) the correct duration of such dosage.

4. In general, systemic antifungal therapy should not be used to treat tinea of the feet. The recurrence rate after completion of therapy is very high.

5. Candidal infections should not be treated with oral griseofulvin. Very commonly, candidal intertrigo of the groin or candidal paronychias are erroneously treated with griseofulvin. Griseofulvin is of no value in these conditions. Because it is a penicillin-related drug, it can cause an allergic reaction in patients with a penicillin sensitivity.

6. Tinea versicolor does not respond to oral griseofulvin therapy.

7. So-called fungal infection of the ear does not respond to oral antifungal therapy. Most external ear diseases are not caused by a fungus.

SAUER'S NOTES

Since the discovery of specific systemic antifungal agents, many physicians have believed that
1. These agents are indicated for every fungus infection.
2. Most skin diseases are caused by a fungus, so they should treat the patient with an antifungal agent and make a diagnosis later.

Both of these assumptions are erroneous.

There is a predilection for certain sites of tinea in which the frequency varies with the age of the patient. This is outlined in Table 28-2.

Tinea of the Feet (Tinea Pedis)

Tinea of the feet (athlete's foot, fungal infection of the feet, and ringworm of the feet) is a very common skin infection. Many persons have the disease and are not even aware of it (Figs. 28-1 to 28-3). The clinical appearance varies.

Primary Lesions

Acute form: Blisters (vesicular tinea pedis) occur on the soles and the sides of feet or between the toes.

TABLE 28-2 • Sites of Tinea in Relationship to Age Groups

Tinea Site	Children (0–16 y)	Adults
Tinea capitis (scalp)	Common	Very rare
Tinea corporis (body)	Common	Fairly common
Tinea cruris (groin)	Rare	Common (esp. males)
Tinea pedis (feet)	Rare (mimics eczema)	Very common
Onychomycosis (nails)	Very rare	Very common

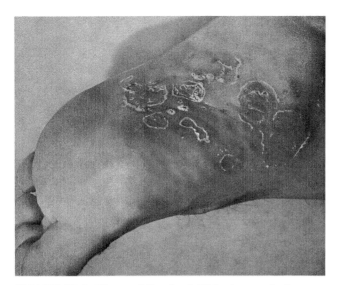

FIGURE 28-1: Tinea of the foot. This dry, scaly form of fungus infection is usually due to *T. rubrum*. (Courtesy of Smith Kline & French Laboratories.)

Chronic form: Lesions are dry and scaly ("moccasin" tinea pedis).
Interdigital form: Macerated skin appears between the toes.

Secondary Lesions

Bacterial infection may occur in the acute and interdigital form. Fissures are not uncommon in the interdigital form.

Course

Recurrent acute infections can lead to a chronic infection. If the toenails become infected, a cure is highly improbable, because this focus is very difficult to eradicate and the fungus is ubiquitous and the patient's susceptibility (almost always lifelong) cannot be decreased.

The species of fungus influences the response to therapy. Most vesicular, acute fungal infections are due to *Trichophyton mentagrophytes* and respond readily to correct treatment. The chronic scaly type of infection is usually due to *Trichophyton rubrum* and is exceedingly difficult, if not impossible, to cure.

Contagiousness

Experiments have shown that there is a susceptibility factor necessary for infection. Males are much more susceptible than are females.

Laboratory Findings

KOH-ink preparations of scrapings and cultures on Sabouraud media serve to demonstrate the presence of fungi and the specific type. A KOH preparation is a very simple office procedure and should be resorted to when the diagnosis is uncertain or the response to therapy is slow.

Differential Diagnosis

Contact dermatitis: Due to shoes, socks, gloves, foot powder usually on dorsum of feet; history of new shoes or new foot powder; fungi not found.
Atopic eczema: Especially on dorsum of toes in children; quite chronic; usually worse in winter; very pruritic; atopic family history; fungi not found.
Psoriasis: Affects soles and palms; pustular, thickened, well-circumscribed lesions; psoriasis elsewhere on body; fungi not found.
Pustular bacterid: Pustular lesions only, especially on palms and soles; chronic; resistant to local therapy; fungi not found. This condition may be associated with a focus of infection, as in tonsil, teeth, or gall bladder.
Hyperhidrosis of feet: Can be severe and cause white, eroded maceration of the soles, accompanied by a foul odor. No fungi found. Zeasorb AF powder is helpful, as is Drysol solution.
Pitted keratolysis (keratolysis plantare sulcatum): Produces circular areas of erosions with a punched-out appearance on the soles of the feet; associated with hyperhidrosis; filamentous, gram-positive, branching microorganisms are found on skin scrapings caused by corynebacterium, actinomyces, *Kytococcus sedentarius* (*Dermatococcus sedentarius*), or *Dermatophilus congolensis*. Topical or systemic erythromycin is usually beneficial.

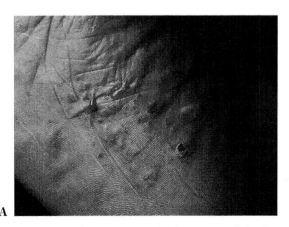

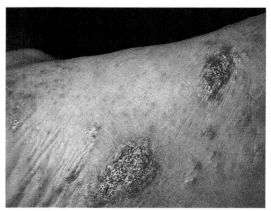

A   **B**

FIGURE 28-2: A and **B**: Acute vesicular tinea of the foot often due to *T. mentagrophytes*. (Courtesy of Schering Corp.)

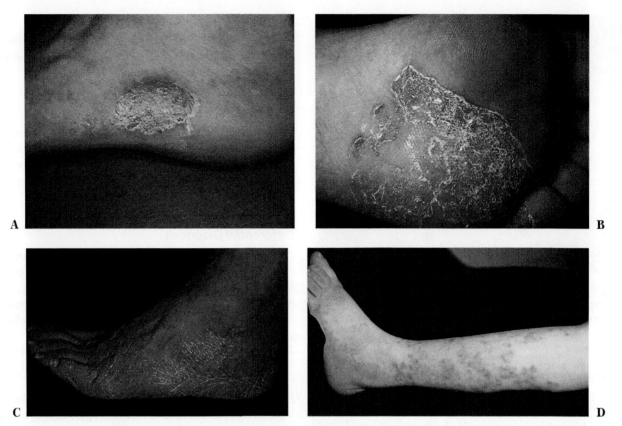

FIGURE 28-3: Tinea of the foot. **A:** Chronic tinea of side of foot. **B:** Chronic tinea of sole due to *T. rubrum*. **C:** Chronic extensive tinea on patient on corticosteroids. **D:** Chronic tinea extending up leg; the fungus was under a leg brace that encouraged a wet warm environment for optimal growth. (Courtesy of Schering Corp.)

Treatment

Case Example: *Acute Infection.* An acute vesicular, pustular fungal infection of 2 weeks duration is present on the soles of the feet and between the toes in a 16-year-old boy. This clinical picture is usually caused by the organism *T. mentagrophytes*.

First Visit

1. The fear of the infectiousness of athlete's foot should be minimized but normal cleanliness emphasized, including the wearing of slippers over bare feet, wiping the feet last after a bath (not the groin last), and changing socks daily (white socks are not necessary).
2. Debridement. The physician or the patient should snip off the tops of the blister with small scissors. This enables the pus to drain out and allows the medication to reach the organisms. The edges of any blister should be kept trimmed, since the fungi spread under these edges. This debridement is followed by a foot soak.
3. Burow solution soak
    Sig: One packet of Domeboro powder to 1 quart of warm water. Soak feet for 10 minutes b.i.d. Dry skin carefully afterward.
4. Antifungal cream 15.0
    Miconazole (Monistat Derm, Micatin), clotrimazole (Lotrimin, Mycelex), econazole (Spectazole), keto-conazole (Nizoral), ciclopirox (Loprox), oxiconazole

(Oxistat), naftifine (Naftin), terbinafine (Lamisil), butenafine (Mentax, Lotrimin AF is over the counter), econazole (Ertaczo), and tolnaftate (Tinactin) (see Table 28-3 for detailed list of antifungal agents).
    Sig: Apply b.i.d. locally to feet after soaking.
    Sig: Apply b.i.d. locally for long-term.
5. Rest at home for 2 to 4 days may be advisable, if severe.
6. Place small pieces of cotton sheeting or cotton between the toes when wearing shoes.
    Five days later, the secondary infection and blisters should have decreased.
7. Oral terbinafine 250 mg once a day for 1 week is safe and very effective.

SAUER'S NOTES

A favorite medication of mine for tinea of the feet and body is

Sulfur, ppt.	5%
Hydrocortisone	1%
Antifungal cream q.s.	30.0

TABLE 28-3 • Antifungal Agents

Antifungal Agents	Route of Administration	Organism Responsive	Side Effects
Allylamines			
Naftifine (Naftin)	Cream (2% higher available), gel	Dermatophytes	Rare
Terbinafine (Lamisil)	Cream, spray, oral	Dermatophytes, tinea versicolor	Oral, rarely liver toxicity
Benzylamines			
Butenafine HCL (Mentax, Lotrimin Ultra Cream)	Cream	Dermatophytes	Rare
-Azoles			
Clotrimazole (Mycelex, Lotrimin cream, solution Troches suppositories)	Cream	Dermatophytes, tinea versicolor, Candida	Rare
Econazole (Spectazole)	Cream	Dermatophytes, tinea versicolor, gram(+) bacteria	Rare
Fluconazole (Diflucan)	Oral	Dermatophytes, tinea versicolor, cryptococcosis, Candida	Rare
Itraconazole (Sporanox)	Oral (with food)	Dermatophytes, tinea versicolor, Candida, sporotrichosis, some deep fungi	Rare liver toxicity
Ketoconazole (Nizoral)	Cream shampoo, oral	Dermatophytes, some deep fungi, Candida, tinea versicolor	Liver toxicity when oral
Miconazole (Micatin, Monistat, Zeasorb AF)	Cream, powder spray, suppositories	Dermatophytes, tinea versicolor, Candida	Rare
Oxiconazole (Oxistat)	Cream	Dermatophytes, tinea versicolor, Candida	Rare
Sertaconazole (ertaczol)	Cream	Dermatophytes, tinea versicolor, Candida	Rare
Polyenes			
Amphotericin B (Fungizone, Abelcet)	Intravenous	Deep fungi sepsis, Candida sepsis	Common renal toxicity thrombophlebitis, hypokalemia
Nystatin (Mycostatin)	Cream, ointment, powder, oral (not absorbed), pastilles, with triamcinolone (Mycolog II cream, ointment)	Candida	Rare
Miscellaneous			
Flucytosine (Ancobon)	Oral, usually given with amphotericin B	Deep fungi sepsis, Candida sepsis	Liver, renal, bone marrow toxicity, gastrointestinal
Ciclopirox (Loprox, Penlac) Penlac Nail Lacquer	Gel, cream, shampoo, suspensions	Dermatophytes, Candida	Rare
Griseofulvin (Gris-Peg), Fulvicin, Grifulvin	Oral (evening with fatty meal) tablets, suspension		Rare

(continued)

TABLE 28-3 • Antifungal Agents (continued)

Antifungal Agents	Route of Administration	Organism Responsive	Side Effects
Selenium sulfide (Selsun, Head & Shoulders Intensive Treatment)	Shampoo (sometimes used as lotion)	Tinea versicolor	Irritation
Saturated solution of potassium iodide (SSKI)	Oral	Sporotrichosis	Gastrointestinal toxicity, bitter taste, goiter if long-term
Tolnaftate (Tinactin)	Cream	Dermatophytes	Rare
Undecylenic acid (Desenex)	Cream	Dermatophytes	Rare
Caspofungin (Candidas)	Intravenous	Candidiasis sepsis, Aspergillosis sepsis	Common, fever, headache thrombophlebitis, rash
Micafungin (Mycoviral)	Intravenous	Candidiasis sepsis, esophagitis	Common, headaches, rash, fever, bone marrow thrombophlebitis
Vericonazole (Ufend)	Intravenous, oral	Candida sepsis, esophageal, Aspergillosis sepsis, Fusariosis sepsis	Visceral impairment, liver toxicity, fever, cardiac toxicity

Subsequent Visits

1. The soaks may be continued for another 3 days or stopped if no marked redness or infection is present.
2. The previously described salve is continued or the following salves are substituted: A combination of an antifungal cream and a corticosteroid, as in Lotrisone cream, is beneficial. Antifungal solutions, such as Lotrimin or Mycelex or Loprox are quite effective. Apply a few drops on affected skin and rub in.
3. Antifungal powder q.s. 45.0.
   Zeasorb AF, Micatin, Tinactin, and Desenex.
   Sig: Supply in powder can. Apply small amount to feet over the salve and to the shoes in the morning.

Case Example: *Chronic Infection.* A patient presents with chronic, scaly, thickened fungal infection of 4 years duration. In the past week, a few small tense blisters on the sole of the feet had developed. This type of clinical picture probably is due to the organism *T. rubrum.*

First Visit

1. The patient is told that the acute flare-up (the blisters) can be cleared but that it will be difficult and time-consuming to cure the chronic infection. If the toenails are found to be infected, the prognosis for cure is even poorer (see Tinea of the Nails section).
2. The blisters are debrided and trimmed with manicure scissors.
3. Any of the antifungal creams,
   Sig: Apply locally to soles b.i.d., or

Antifungal solution 10.0.
Sig: Rub in a few drops b.i.d.

Subsequent Visits

1. Systemic antifungal therapy: This type of oral therapy is not recommended for chronic tinea of the feet. But the patient may have heard or read about the "pill for athlete's feet," so it would be wise for you to discuss this with the patient. If you mention that you cannot guarantee a cure, most patients will be content with keeping the chronic infection in an innocuous state with sporadic local therapy.
2. However, if the patient still wants to try oral therapy, then consider the systemic antifungal agents listed in the following section on Tinea of the Hands and in Table 28-3. Long-term pulse therapy is indicated.

Tinea of the Hands (Tinea Manuum)

A primary fungal infection of the hand or hands is quite rare. In spite of this fact, the diagnosis of "fungal infection of the hand" is commonly applied to cases that are in reality contact dermatitis, atopic eczema, pustular bacterid, or psoriasis. The best differential point is that tinea of the hand usually is seen only on one hand, not bilaterally. It mimics dry skin in the common chronic form and may have fingernail involvement (Fig. 28-4A–E).

Primary Lesions

Acute form: Blisters on the palms and the fingers are seen at the edge of red areas.

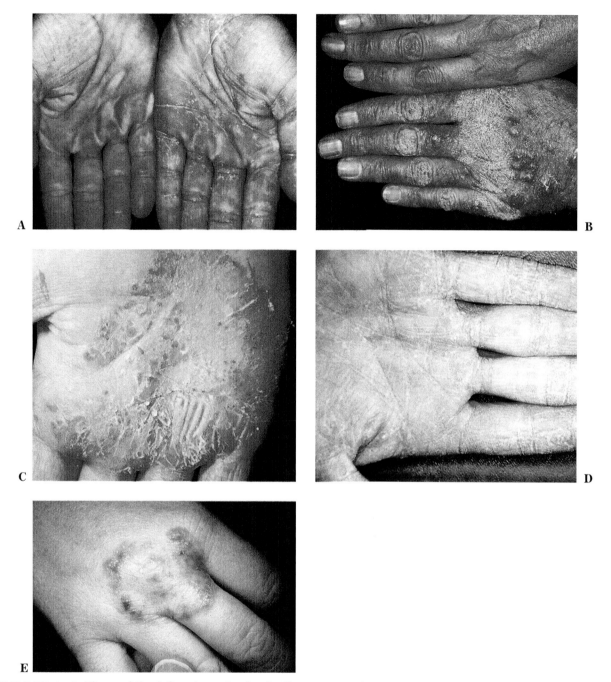

FIGURE 28-4: A: Tinea of the left palm only, due to *T. mentagrophytes*. **B:** Deep tinea of left hand, due to *T. mentagrophytes*. **C:** Tinea of the palm, due to *T. rubrum*. **D:** Tinea of the palm, of dry, scaly type, due to *T. rubrum*. **E:** Tinea on the back of the hand.

Chronic form: Lesions are dry and scaly; usually there is a single patch, not separate patches.

Secondary Lesions

Bacterial infection is rather unusual.

Course

This gradually progressive disease spreads to fingernails. It is usually asymptomatic.

Laboratory Findings

KOH or ink preparations reveal mycelia, or cultures on Sabouraud media grow the fungus.

Differential Diagnosis

Contact dermatitis of hands: Due to soap, detergents, and other irritants; usually bilateral, periodic, more vesicular, and less frequently chronic; fungi not found. Prefers backs of hands to palms.

Atopic eczema: History of atopy in patient or family; bilateral; periodic; fungi not found.

Psoriasis: See thick patch or patches in palms, usually bilateral; occasionally see psoriasis elsewhere; fungi not found. Psoriatic nail involvement may mimic onychomycosis of fingernails.

Pustular bacterid: Pustular lesions only; periodic and chronic; resistant to local therapy; fungi not found.

Dyshidrosis of palms: Recurrent; seasonal incidence; mainly vesicular on the sides of the fingers: not scaly; bilateral; may be related to atopic eczema; fungi not found.

Treatment

Case Example: A man presents with scaly thickening of one palm of 8 years duration. His fingernails are not involved. Itching is noted slightly at times.

1. Antifungal creams, especially naftifine (Naftin pump cream or gel), terbinafine (Lamisil) cream, or butenafine (Mentax) may control or occasionally cure the tinea of the hand.
2. Systemic therapy (Table 28-3). The following medicines are all expensive, especially because therapy must be continued, as for hand tinea, for several months. Appropriate monitoring of the patient during therapy is necessary. There are also drug interactions that can occur.
   a. Griseofulvin (Gris-Peg, 250 mg; Fulvicin P/G, 330 mg; Grisactin, 330 mg; Grifulvin, 330 mg).
      Sig: One tablet t.i.d. after meals for at least 8 weeks, and probably for 4 to 6 months.
      Comment: Griseofulvin commonly causes headaches in the first few days of therapy. It is a penicillin derivative and cross-reactions may occur.
   b. Ketoconazole (Nizoral), 200 mg (rarely 400 mg)
      Sig: One tablet once a day for 3 to 4 months.
      Comment: Hepatotoxicity has been rarely reported with ketoconazole therapy, also impotence.
   c. Itraconazole (Sporanox) capsule, 100 mg. 200 mg b.i.d. for 7 days, repeated once a month for 3 to 4 months. Monitoring for rare liver toxicity must be done. Drug interactions are numerous.
   d. Fluconazole (Diflucan) has not been approved for superficial dermatophyte therapy. It may be effective in doses of 200 mg/week for 1 to 3 months. Drug interactions are numerous.
   e. Terbinafine (Lamisil) 250 mg is the author's choice
      Sig: One tablet each day for 1 week is cheap, safe, and effective. It can be periodically repeated or topical agents can be used once control is achieved.

Tinea of the Nails (Onychomycosis)

Tinea of the toenails is very common, but tinea of the fingernails (Fig. 28-5) is uncommon. Tinea of the toenails is almost inevitable in patients who have recurrent attacks of tinea of the feet. Once developed, the infected nail serves as a resistant focus for future skin infection.

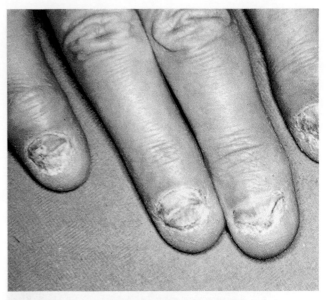

FIGURE 28-5: Tinea of fingernails, due to *T. rubrum.* (Courtesy of Duke Laboratories, Inc.)

Primary Lesions

Distal and lateral detachment of the nail occurs with subsequent thickening, subungual white keratotic debris, and deformity.

Secondary Lesions

Bacterial infection can result. Ingrown toenails are another undesirable consequence.

Dermatophytoma—this is a condition where there is a compacted fungal ball of large spores and fungal filaments under a nail. It manifests as white or yellow nail bands that are subungual and can be associated with total dystrophic onychomycosis. Possibly related to biofilm formation, total dystrophic onychomycosis is difficult to treat, and nail avulsion is necessary as part of the therapeutic regimen along with antifungal medications.

Distribution

The infection usually begins in the fifth toenail and may remain there or spread to involve the other nails.

Course

Tinea of the fingernails can rarely be cured. Aside from the deformity, ingrown toenail (especially in diabetes mellitus and marked vascular or neurologic compromise to the feet) and an occasional mild flare-up of acute tinea, treatment is not necessary. Progression is slow and recurrence is the rule.

Tinea of the fingernails can be treated, but the treatment usually takes months.

Etiology

This type of tinea is usually caused by *T. rubrum* and, less likely, by *T. mentagrophytes.* Approximately 8% of cases are caused by nondermatophyte molds, especially scopulariopsis, scytalidium (treatment by surgery only), fusarium, aspergillosis, and acremonium. These nondermatophyte molds are very difficult to treat. Approximately 1% are yeasts, especially candida species.

Laboratory Findings

These organisms can be found in a KOH preparation of a scraping and can occasionally be grown on culture media. The material should be gathered from the most proximal debris under the nail plate. It is often difficult to obtain a positive test. The author's favorite technique is obtaining the most proximally involved nail and sending it in a dry container for histopathology and PAS staining. I find it greatly decreases false-negative results and has virtually no false-positive results.

Differential Diagnosis

Nail injury: A history of the injury must be obtained (jogger's nails or pseudoonychomycosis), although tinea infection often starts in an injured nail; fungi are absent. If the second toe is longer than pseudoonychomycosis is more common in this digit. Otherwise, the great toe is most often affected.

Psoriasis of fingernails: Pitting, red areas occur under nail with resulting detachment; psoriasis is seen elsewhere, usually; no fungi are found. Appearance is that of an "oil drop" on the nail. Arthritis may be present in fingers.

Psoriasis of toenails: This may be impossible to differentiate from tinea, because many psoriatic nails have some secondary fungal invasion, and they are so similar clinically.

Candidiasis of fingernails: Common in people who frequently wash their hands; paronychial involvement common; *Candida* found (see later in this chapter).

Green nails: This fingernail infection yields *Candida albicans* and *Pseudomonas aeruginosa* most commonly. Clinically, there is a distal detachment of the nail plate, with underlying greenish-black debris. For cure, complete debridement of the detached part of the nail is necessary, plus local or systemic antiyeast therapy.

Treatment

Case Example: *Tinea of the Fingernails.* A young salesman presents with a fungal infection in three fingernails of his left hand of 9 months duration. The surrounding skin shows mild redness and scaling.

1. Griseofulvin therapy (see earlier and Table 28-3). Griseofulvin ultrafine type, 250 to 330 mg or equivalent.
   Sig: One tablet b.i.d. or t.i.d. for 9 months.
   Comment: Therapy is stopped when there is no clinical evidence of infection (crumbling, thickening of nail plate, or subungual debris) and no cultural or KOH or ink mount evidence of fungi.
2. Ketoconazole (Nizoral) therapy. If the patient and the physician are aware of the possibility of liver or other toxicity, then a 200-mg tablet once a day for 9 months might be curative. Close patient monitoring is necessary. Many drug interactions.
3. Itraconazole (Sporanox) therapy has been reported to be curative; 200 mg b.i.d. for 7 days, repeated monthly for 4 to 6 months. Available as a pulse pack. Many drug interactions.
4. Terbinafine (Lamisil) 250 mg. The author's experience is to prescribe terbinafine 250 mg a day for 1 week. This is repeated every 3 months. It is safe, inexpensive ($4 for 30 pills at some discount pharmacies in the United States), and effective. This is referred to as pulse therapy, and there are many other regimens recommended for this drug as well as other oral antifungals.
5. Loprox (ciclopirox) nail lacquer two times a week. It is expensive.

Case Example: *Tinea of the Toenails.* A 45-year-old woman presents with three infected toenails on the right foot and two on the left foot. These are causing mild pain when she wears certain tight-fitting shoes. Scaliness of soles of feet is also evident.

1. Griseofulvin or ketoconazole therapy. This oral therapy is not effective or indicated for tinea of the toenails. Apparently some dermatologists have cured cases after oral therapy was continued for several years or when oral therapy was combined with avulsion of the toenails. The only time such therapy for toenails is prescribed, in our practice, is when the patient understands the problem but still wants to attempt a cure or a cosmetic improvement. At least 12 months of griseofulvin therapy is necessary. Women respond to this therapy better than men.
2. Itraconazole (Sporanox) may be used. A dosage of 200 mg b.i.d. for 7 days, repeated monthly for 4 to 8 months, has been suggested. A pulse pack is available. Watch for drug interactions. Monitoring of the patient is necessary for rare liver toxicity. Very expensive.
3. Terbinafine (Lamisil) 250 mg a day for 1 week every 3 months for 1 year—author's choice since it is inexpensive, safe, and effective.
4. Antifungal solution, 15 mL. For the patient who wants to "do something," applications two times a day for months might help some mild cases. One can combine this therapy with debridement of the nails. These solutions include Fungi-Nail, Fungoid, and Loprox (ciclopirox, also comes as a gel). Penlac (ciclopirox) nail lacquer is expensive but helpful if systemic therapy wants to be avoided. Unlike package insert, I prescribe it only twice weekly and have been successful.
5. Debriding of thick nails by patient, dermatologist, or podiatrist offers obvious relief from discomfort. This can be accomplished by the use of nail clippers, filing, or a motor-driven drill (Dremel).
6. Surgical avulsion of the toenail is rarely curative. As stated previously, this surgical approach can be combined with oral systemic therapy with probable enhancement of the end result. Permanent removal of nail and nail matrix is advocated by some. In the author's experience, occasional regrowth of nail spicules due to incomplete matrix removal has been observed.

Tinea of the Groin

Tinea of the groin is a common, itching, annoying fungal infection appearing usually in men and often concurrently with tinea of the feet. Home remedies often result in a contact dermatitis that adds "fuel to the fire."

Primary Lesions

Bilateral, fan-shaped, red, scaly patches with a sharp, slightly raised border, and central clearing occur. Small vesicles may be seen in the active border. No scrotal involvement.

Secondary Lesions

Oozing, crusting, edema, and secondary bacterial infection. In chronic cases, lichenification may be marked. Lichen simplex chronicus can develop.

Distribution

The infection affects the crural fold, thighs, perianal area, and buttocks.

Course

Factors that affect the course and recurrences are obesity, hot weather, sweating, and chafing garments.

Etiology

Tinea of the groin is commonly caused by the fungi of tinea of the feet, *T. rubrum*, and *T. mentagrophytes*, and also by the fungus *Epidermophyton floccosum*.

Contagiousness

This is minimal, even between husband and wife.

Laboratory Findings

The organism is found in KOH preparations of scrapings and can be grown on culture. Material is taken from the active border.

Differential Diagnosis

Candidiasis: No sharp border; fine scales, oozing, redness, satellite pustule-like lesions at edges; more common in obese females; marked itching and burning; *Candida* found. History of oral antibiotics is common.

Contact dermatitis: Often coexistent, but can be a separate entity; new contactant history; no fungi found; no active border; very pruritic and can be vesicular.

Prickly heat: Pustular, papular; no active border, no fungi; may also be present with tinea.

Lichen simplex chronicus: Unilateral, usually; may have resulted from old chronic tinea; no fungi. Severe paroxysmal pruritis.

Psoriasis: Often unilateral; may or may not have raised border; psoriasis elsewhere; no fungi.

Erythrasma: Faint redness, fine scaling with no elevated border, also seen in axilla and webs of toes; coral reddish fluorescence under Wood light; due to a diphtheroid organism called *Corynebacterium minutissimum*. Responds to topical erythromycin.

Bowen Disease or Extramammary Paget Disease: Consider these diagnoses if unilateral and recalcitrant to therapy. Biopsy is necessary to make these diagnoses.

Treatment

Case Example: Oozing, symmetrical, red dermatitis with sharp border occurring in crural area of young man.

1. Because the infection may come from chronic tinea of the feet, to prevent recurrences, advice the patient to dry the feet last and not the groin area last when taking a bath.
2. Vinegar wet packs
   Sig: Half cup of white vinegar to 1 quart of warm water. Wet the sheeting or thin toweling and apply to area for 15 minutes twice a day.
3. Antifungal cream 15.0.
   Sig: Apply b.i.d. locally (Table 28-3).
4. Griseofulvin oral therapy
   Griseofulvin ultrafine types, 250 to 330 mg
   Sig: One tablet b.i.d. for 6 to 8 weeks for extensive case.
5. Ketoconazole, itraconazole, or terbinafine therapy may also be used.
6. Author uses terbinafine 250 mg daily for 7 days and then a topical for further control.

SAUER'S NOTES

An effective therapy for tinea of the groin is:
Sulfur, ppt. 5%
Hydrocortisone 1%
Antifungal cream q.s. 15.0
Sig: Apply b.i.d. locally and continue for 7 days after apparent clearance ("therapy-plus" routine).

Tinea of the Smooth Skin (Tinea Corporis)

The familiar ringworm of the skin is most common in children, partially because of their intimacy with animals and other children. The lay public believes that *most* skin conditions are "ringworm," and many physicians erroneously agree with them (Fig. 28-6A–D).

Primary Lesions

Round, oval, or semicircular scaly patches have a slightly raised border that commonly is vesicular. Rarely, deep, ulcerated, granulomatous lesions (Majocchi granuloma) are due to superficial dermatophyte fungi.

Secondary Lesions

Bacterial infection, particularly at the advancing border.

Course

Infection is short lived, if treated correctly. It seldom recurs unless treatment is inadequate.

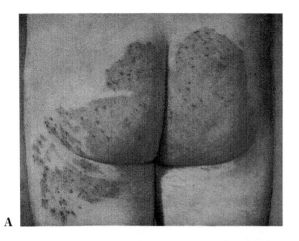
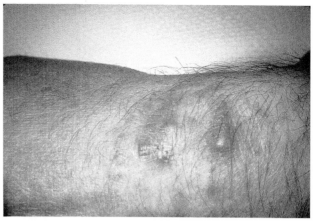
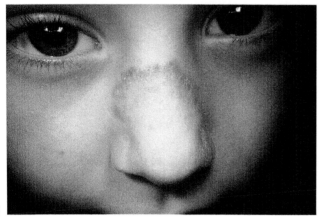
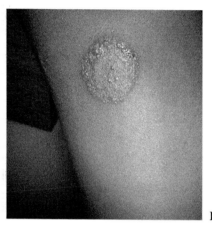

FIGURE 28-6: Tinea of the smooth skin. **A:** This infection on the buttocks had spread from the crural region. **B:** Majocchi granulomas on flexor wrist. **C:** Tinea faciei on young girl, caught from cat. **D:** Tinea corporis on arm. (Courtesy of Smith Kline & French Laboratories.)

Etiology

This disorder is most commonly due to *M. canis* from kittens and puppies and less commonly due to *E. floccosum* and *T. mentagrophytes* from groin and foot infections.

Contagiousness

It is very contagious.

Laboratory Findings

This is the same as for previously discussed fungal diseases.

Differential Diagnosis

Pityriasis rosea: History of herald patch; sudden shower of oval lesions; fungi not found.

Impetigo: Vesicular, honey-colored, crusted; most commonly on face; no fungi found.

Contact dermatitis: No sharp border or central healing; may be coexistent with ringworm, worsened by overtreatment.

Treatment

Case Example: A child has several 2 to 4 cm scaly lesions on his arms of 1 week's duration. He has a new kitten that he holds and plays with.

1. Examine the scalp, preferably with a Wood light, to rule out scalp infection.
2. Advise the mother regarding moderate isolation procedures in relation to the family and others.
3. Antifungal salve q.s. 15.0.
   Sig: Apply b.i.d. locally (Table 28-3).

Subsequent Visit of Resistant Case or a New Widespread Case: Griseofulvin Oral Therapy: Griseofulvin (ultrafine types) can be given in tablet or oral suspension form. The usual dose for children is 165 mg b.i.d., but the pharmaceutical company's product information sheet should be consulted. Therapy should be maintained for 3 to 6 weeks or until lesions are gone. Occasionally, a higher dose is needed in deeper forms of infection. Terbinafine (author's choice) 250 mg daily for 2 weeks.

Tinea of the Scalp (Tinea Capitis)

Tinea of the scalp (Fig. 28-7A–D) is the most common cause of patchy hair loss in children (Fig. 28-10). Endemic cases are with us always, but epidemics, usually due to the human type, were, until the discovery of griseofulvin, the real therapeutic problem. Griseofulvin orally finds its greatest therapeutic usefulness and triumph in the management of tinea of the scalp. Before griseofulvin, children with the human type of scalp

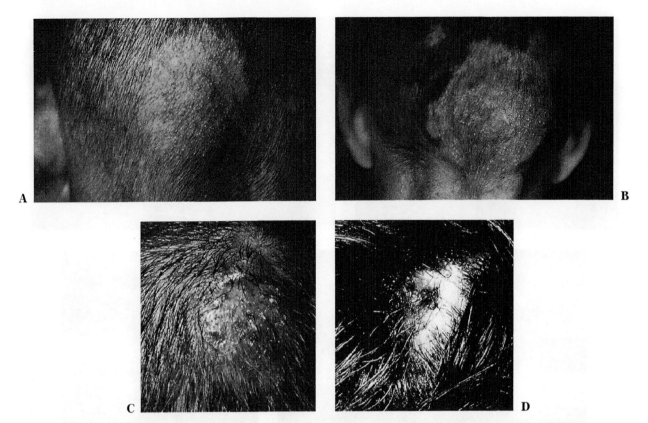

FIGURE 28-7: Tinea of the scalp. **A:** Due to *M. audouini*. Note absence of visible inflammation. **B:** Due to *T. tonsurans*. Wood light examination revealed no fluorescence. **C:** Due to *T. mentagrophytes*. Note inflammation, **D:** Favus, due to *T. shoenleini*, of 11 years' duration. (Courtesy of Ortho Pharmaceutical Corp.)

tinea had to be subjected to traumatic shampoos and salves for weeks or months, or they had to be epilated by x-ray. Often, they were kept out of school for this entire period of therapy.

Ketoconazole, terbinafine (author's choice), or itraconazole systemic therapy is available for griseofulvin-resistant cases, if these truly occur in tinea of the scalp.

Tinea capitis infections can be divided into two clinical types: (1) *noninflammatory* and (2) *inflammatory*. The treatment, the cause, and the course vary for these two types.

Noninflammatory Type

Primary Lesions: Grayish, scaly, round patches with broken-off hairs are seen, causing balding areas. The size of the areas varies.

Secondary Lesions: Bacterial infection and id reactions are rare. A noninflammatory patch can become inflamed spontaneously or as the result of strong local treatment. Scarring almost never occurs. "Black dot" hairs (short broken-off hairs) are seen with *Trichophyton tonsurans* on culture.

Distribution: The infection is most common in the posterior scalp region. Body ringworm from the scalp lesions is common, particularly on the neck and the shoulders.

Course: Incubation period is usually 3 or more weeks after exposure. Parents often do not notice the infection for another 3 weeks to several months, particularly in girls. Spontaneous cures are rare in the first 2 to 6 months, but after that time occur with greater frequency. Some cases last for years, if untreated. Recurrence of the infection after the cure of a previous episode is possible because adequate immunity does not develop.

Age Group: Infection of the noninflammatory type is most common between the ages of 3 and 8 years and is rare after puberty. This adult resistance to infection is attributed in part to the higher content of fungistatic fatty acids in the sebum after puberty.

T. tonsurans infection is seen mainly in African-American urban preadolescent children (often females who braid their hair). It is endemic in this population and may go unnoticed.

Spontaneous cures at puberty, particularly for girls, do not always occur.

Etiology: The noninflammatory type of scalp ringworm is caused most frequently by *T. tonsurans* and occasionally by *Microsporum canis* and *Microsporum audouini*. *M. audouini* and *T. tonsurans* are anthropophilic fungi (human-to-human passage only), whereas *M. canis* is a zoophilic fungus (animals are the original source, mainly kittens and puppies).

Contagiousness: This can be a part of a large urban epidemic.

Laboratory Findings: *Wood light examination of the scalp hair* is an important diagnostic test, but hairs infected with *T. tonsurans* do not fluoresce. The Wood light is a specially filtered long-wavelength ultraviolet light. The hairs infected with *M. audouini* and *M. canis* fluoresce with a bright yellowish-green color. The bright fluorescence of fungus-infected hairs is not to be confused with the white or dull yellow color emitted by lint particles or sulfur-laden scales.

Microscopic examination of the infected hairs in 20% KOH solution shows an ectothrix arrangement of the spores when the causative agent is *Microsporum* species and endothrix spores when it is *T. tonsurans*. Culture is necessary for species identification. The cultural characteristics of the various fungi can be found in many larger dermatologic or mycologic texts, and so are not presented here.

Treatment
Prophylactic

1. Hair is washed with Loprox (ciclopirox) shampoo or Nizoral (ketoconazole) shampoo after every haircut by a barber, beautician, or parent.
2. Parents and teachers should be educated on methods of spread of disease, particularly during an epidemic.
3. Suggestions should be given for provision for individual storage of clothing, particularly caps, combs, barrettes, and other hair styling products, in school and at home.

Active

1. Griseofulvin oral therapy. The ultrafine types of griseofulvin (Fulvicin U/F, Fulvicin P/G, Gris-Peg, Grifulvin V, and Grisactin) can be administered in tablet form or liquid suspension (not all brands available in liquid form). The usual dose for a child aged 4 to 8 years is 250 mg b.i.d., but some require a larger dose. The duration of therapy is usually 6 to 8 weeks. Both dose and duration have to be individualized and based on clinical, Wood light, or culture response.
2. Ketoconazole, terbinafine, itriconazole, or fluconazole oral therapy. This type of therapy is usually not indicated or necessary, but regimens are effective and preferred by some.
3. Selenium sulfide (Selsun, Head & Shoulders Intensive Treatment) shampoo is sporicidal and may help decrease the spread of infection.

4. Manual epilation of hairs. Near the end of therapy, the remaining infected and fluorescent hairs can be plucked out, or the involved area can be shaved closely. This will eliminate the infected distal end of the growing hair.

Inflammatory Type

Primary Lesions: Pustular, scaly, round patches with broken-off hairs are found, resulting in bald areas.

Secondary Lesions: Bacterial infection may occur. When the secondary reaction is marked, the area becomes swollen and tender. This inflammation is called a *kerion*. Minimal scarring sometimes remains.

Distribution: Any scalp area is involved. Concurrent body ringworm infection is common.

Course: Duration is much shorter than the noninflammatory type of infection. Spontaneous cures will result after 2 to 4 months in many cases, even if untreated, except for the *T. tonsurans* type.

Etiology: The inflammatory type of scalp ringworm is most commonly caused by *T. tonsurans* and *M. canis,* and rarely by *M. audouini, M. gypseum, T. mentagrophytes,* and *T. verrucosum. T. tonsurans, M. audouini,* and *T. mentagrophytes* are anthropophilic (coming from humans); *M. canis* and *T. verrucosum* are zoophilic (passed from infected animals); and *M. gypseum* is geophilic (coming from the soil).

Contagiousness: Contagiousness is high in children. It is mainly endemic, except for cases caused by *M. audouini*.

Laboratory Findings: Microscopic examination of the infected hairs in 20% KOH solution shows an ectothrix arrangement of the spores, but *T. tonsurans* shows endothrix spores. The hairs infected with *M. canis* and *M. audouini* fluoresce with a bright yellowish-green color under the Wood light.

Differential Diagnosis: See Table 28-4.

Treatment
Prophylactic
This is the same as for noninflammatory cases.
Active

1. Griseofulvin oral therapy (as under noninflammatory type).
2. If kerion is severe, with or without oral terbinafine or griseofulvin therapy:
   a. Burow solution wet packs.
      Sig: One Domeboro packet to 1 pint of warm water. Apply soaked cloths for 15 minutes twice a day.
   b. Antibiotic therapy orally helps to eliminate secondary bacterial infection.

TABLE 28-4 • Differential Diagnosis of Scalp Dermatoses

Dermatosis	Wood Light	Scales	Redness	Hair Loss	Remarks
Tinea capitis	Pos	Dry or crusted	Uncommon	Yes	Back of scalp, children
Alopecia areata	Neg	None	No	Yes	Exclamation point hairs at edges
Seborrheic dermatitis	Neg	Greasy	Yes	No	Diffuse scaling
Psoriasis	Neg	Thick and dry	Yes	No	Look at elbows, knees, and nails
Trichotillomania	Neg	None	No	Yes	Psychoneurotic child
Pyoderma	Neg	Crusted	Yes	Occasional	Poor hygiene

3. Some authors advocate a 1- to 2-week course of systemic corticosteroids to decrease inflammation.

Tinea of the Beard (Tinea Barbae)

Fungal infection is a rare cause of dermatitis in the beard area (Fig. 28-8). Farmers occasionally contract it from infected cattle. Any presumed bacterial infection of the beard that does not respond readily to proper treatment should be examined for fungi.

Primary Lesions

Follicular, pustular, or sharp-bordered ringworm-type lesions or deep, boggy, inflammatory masses are seen.

Secondary Lesions

Bacterial infection is common. Scarring is unusual.

Etiology

See Table 28-1.

Differential Diagnosis

Bacterial folliculitis: Acute onset, rapid spread; no definite border; responds rather rapidly to antibiotic therapy; no fungi found on examination of hairs or culture.

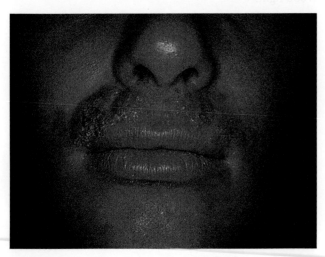

FIGURE 28-8: Tinea of the beard, due to *T. mentagrophytes.*

Treatment

A farmer presents with a quarter-sized, boggy, inflammatory, pustular mass on his chin of 3 weeks' duration.

1. Have veterinarian inspect cattle if farmer is not aware of source of infection.
2. Burow's solution wet packs.
   Sig: One Domeboro packet to 1 pint of hot water. Apply wet cloths to area for 15 minutes t.i.d.
3. Antifungal cream q.s. 15.0
   Sig: Apply locally b.i.d.
4. Griseofulvin oral therapy. The usual dose of griseofulvin, ultrafine type, for an adult is 250 to 330 mg b.i.d. for 6 to 8 weeks or longer, depending on clinical response or negative Sabouraud culture.
5. Other oral antifungals can be used.

Dermatophytid

During an acute episode of any fungal infection, an id eruption can develop over the body. This is a manifestation of an allergic reaction to the fungal infection. The most common id reaction occurs on the hands during an acute tinea infection on the feet. To assume a diagnosis of an id reaction, the following criteria should be followed: (1) The primary focus should be acutely inflamed or infected with fungi, not chronically infected; (2) the id lesions must not contain fungi; and (3) the id eruption should disappear or wane after adequate treatment of the acute focus.

Primary Lesions

Vesicular eruption of the hands (primary lesion on the feet) and papulofollicular eruption on body (primary lesion commonly is scalp kerion) are found; pityriasis rosea–like id eruptions and others are seen less commonly.

Secondary Lesions

Excoriation and infection occur, when itching is severe, which is unusual.

Treatment

1. Treat the primary focus of infection.
2. For a vesicular id reaction on the *hands:*
   Burow's solution soaks.

Sig: One Domeboro packet to 1 quart of cool water. Soak hands for 15 minutes b.i.d.

3. For an id reaction on the *body* that is moderately pruritic: Aveeno oatmeal bath.

   Sig: One packet of Aveeno to 6 to 8 inches of cool water in a tub, once daily.

   Hydrocortisone 1% lotion 120.0

   Sig: Apply locally b.i.d.

   Comment: Menthol 0.25%, phenol 0.5%, or camphor 2% could be added to this lotion.

4. For a severely-itching, *generalized* id eruption: Prednisone, 10 mg, or related corticosteroid tablets #30

   Sig: Five tablets each morning with food for 2 days and decrease by one tablet every 2 days (10 day course).

DEEP FUNGAL INFECTIONS

Those fungi that invade the skin deeply and go into living tissue are also capable of involving other organs. Only the skin manifestations of these deeply invading fungi are discussed here. These fungi are compared in Fig. 28-3.

The following diseases are included in this group of deep fungal infections:

Blastomycosis
Coccidioidomycosis
Paracoccidioidomycosis
Histoplasmosis

Deep fungal infections that were rare are now being seen more frequently in patients who are immunocompromised, such as patients on chemotherapy, organ transplant recipients, and those with AIDS.

Differential Diagnosis

Consider any of the following granuloma-producing disease for all four deep fungal infections:

Anthrax
Insect bite
Iodide or bromide ingestion
Leprosy
Leishmaniasis
Neoplasm
Pyoderma
Sarcoidosis
Sporotrichosis
Syphilis
Tularemia
Tuberculosis

Blastomycosis (North American Blastomycosis)

Two cutaneous forms of the disease are seen: primary cutaneous blastomycosis and secondary localized cutaneous blastomycosis.

Primary cutaneous blastomycosis (Fig. 28-9A and B) occurs in laboratory workers and physicians after accidental inoculation. A primary chancre develops at the site of innoculation and the regional lymph nodes enlarge. In a short time, the primary lesion and lymph nodes heal spontaneously, and the patient is completely cured.

The following discussion is confined to the secondary cutaneous form. Systemic blastomycosis is rarer than the cutaneous form but is seen occasionally in immunosuppressed patients.

Primary Lesion (Secondary, Localized, Cutaneous Form)

The lesion begins as a papule that ulcerates and slowly spreads peripherally with a warty, pustular, raised border. The face, hands, and feet are involved most commonly.

Secondary Lesion

Central healing of the ulcer occurs gradually with a resultant thick scar.

Course

A large lesion develops over several months. Therapy is moderately effective on a long-term basis. Relapses are common.

Cause

The fungus *Blastomyces dermatitidis* is believed to invade the lungs primarily and the skin is secondarily as a metastatic lesion. High native immunity prevents the development of more than one skin lesion. This immunity is low in the rare systemic form of blastomycosis in which multiple lesions occur in the skin, bones, and other organs.

Laboratory Findings

The material for a 20% KOH solution mount is collected from the pustules at the border. Round, budding organisms can be found in this manner or in a histopathology specimen. A chest x-ray is indicated in every case.

Treatment

Surgical excision and plastic repair of early lesions is effective.

Amphotericin B suppresses the chronic lesion more effectively than any other drug. It is administered by IV infusion daily in varying schedules, which are best described in larger texts or reviews. AmBisome (liposomal amphotericin B) is a safer, expensive form of amphotericin B.

Ketoconazole or itraconazole therapy on a long-term basis is also beneficial. Higher-than-normal dosages for a longer period of time are necessary for immunosuppressed patients.

Coccidioidomycosis (San Joaquin Valley Fever)

There are three cutaneous types. The skin has a cutaneous form mainly in farmers and laboratory workers who become accidentally inoculated. There is a sporotrichoid form that mimics sporotrichosis with a chancre and nodules that spread up a lymphatic channel. The most severe and common form

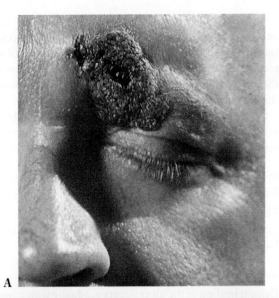
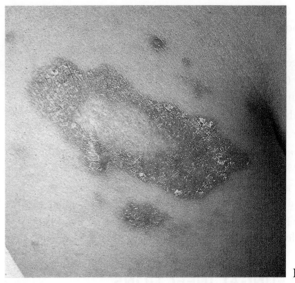
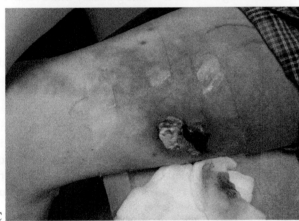

FIGURE 28-9: Deep fungus infections.
A: Blastomycotic primary lesion of eyebrow.
B: Blastomycotic primary lesion on scapular area.
C: Hemorrhagic, necrotic area with a background or red indurated cellulitis on the inner thigh. This patient had been treated with very high doses of systemic corticosteroids for years for lupus erythematousus. (Courtesy of Stiefel Laboratories.)

is a disseminated form from the lungs seen mainly in immunocompromised patients.

Primary Lesion

In the disseminated form, nodules, papules, or plaques appear on a dusky red indurated border.

Secondary Lesion

Sinuses, ulcers, and cold abscesses may appear. Healing occurs with a scar. Erythema multiforme and erythema nodosum may occur as immune responses.

Course

The severity of the disseminated form depends on the immune status of the patient and the amount of inoculum inhaled.

Cause

Coccidioides immitis is a dimorphic fungus seen endemically in the United States (southwestern areas, "San Joaquin Valley Fever"), South and Central America, and Mexico. Blood types A and AB are more frequently pathogenic. It is common in Filipino immigrants to the United States.

Laboratory Findings

Tissue examination shows brown yeast organisms called Medlar bodies within giant cells, pseudoepitheliomatous hyperplasia, and granulomas. Fungal culture on Sabouraud agar shows aerial hyphae grossly and branched septate hyphae with arthrospores microscopically.

Treatment

Surgical excision or incision and drainage along with IV amphotericin B, or oral ketoconazole or itriconazole as second choices.

Paracoccidioidomycosis (South American Blastomycosis)

Chronic disease is seen mainly in the lungs and lymph nodes, with occasional spread to the skin and mucous membranes. It can be latent for decades, only to show up after immunosuppression. It is dimorphic and seen only in the yeast phase in humans. Primary infection is in the lung where it is often asymptomatic and not contagious. It may rarely be directly inoculated in the skin. Seen in AIDS patients who have traveled to an endemic area.

Primary Lesion

Oral disease is seen commonly as granulomas (punctate vessels over a fungating base give a mulberry appearance) and crusts of the mouth, throat, larynx, and nasal cavities. Crusts, papules nodules, and verrucous plaques prefer a central facial location.

Secondary Lesion

Hoarseness, dysphagia, destruction of the uvula, and perforation of the hard palate may occur. Disfiguring scars occur, especially over the face.

Course

Response to therapy is variable since most patients are immunocompromised. Pulmonary fibrosis, adrenal, and central nervous system (CNS) disease are sequelae.

Cause

Paracoccidioides brasiliensis is found in the soil mainly between latitudes 23 to 34 degrees in Mexico, Latin America, and South America. The exact natural history is not completely understood.

Laboratory Findings

Histologic examination of tissue reveals a mother cell with yeasts forming from the cell wall, giving the look of a "pilot's wheel." Culture at 19°C to 28°C grows slowly, producing thin septate hyphae with chlamydospores. Serology is helpful in diagnosis.

Treatment

Sulfamethoxazole/trimethoprim for at least 30 days by mouth. Amphotericin B for more severe disease, with ketoconazole and itraconazole as second choices.

Histoplasmosis

Mainly an asymptomatic lung infection. It can spread from the lung to the skin or rarely be primarily inoculated into the skin. AIDS is particularly a commonly associated underlying illness.

Primary Lesion

Papules (mimicking molluscum contagiosum) and hemorrhagic necrotic areas (Fig. 28-9C).

Secondary Lesion

Ulcers and scars.

Course

Immunocompetent patients usually recover without treatment, but in AIDS patients therapy must be given or CNS disease will ensue and become serious. Serology can be helpful. Culture on Sabouraud agar reveals white colonies at 30°C that microscopically show tuberculate macroconidia.

Treatment

Amphotericin B in AIDS patients with concomitant azoles (itriconazole, fluconazole). The azoles are also often used as maintenance therapy.

Candidiasis

Candidiasis (moniliasis) (Fig. 28-10A–H) is a fungal infection caused by *Candida albicans* that produces lesions in the mouth, the vagina, the skin, the nails, the lungs, or the gastrointestinal tract and occasionally results in sepsis. The latter condition is seen in patients who are on long-term, high-dose antibiotic therapy and in those who are immunosuppressed. Because *C. albicans* exists commonly as a harmless skin inhabitant, the laboratory findings of this organism are not adequate proof of its pathogenicity and etiologic role. *Candida* organisms commonly seed preexisting skin conditions. Concern here is with the *cutaneous* and the *mucocutaneous* candidal diseases. The following classification is helpful.

Cutaneous Candidiasis

1. Localized diseases
   a. Candidal paronychia (Fig. 28-10J). This common candidal infection is characterized by the development of painful, red swellings of the skin around the nail plate. In chronic infections the nail becomes secondarily thickened and hardened. Candidal paronychia is commonly seen in housewives and those persons whose occupations predispose them to frequent immersion of the hands in water. Terms such a "housewife's nail" or "barmaid's nail" relate to this water exposure.

      This nail involvement is to be differentiated from *superficial tinea of the nails* (the candidal infection usually does not cause the nail to lose its luster or to become crumbly, and debris does not accumulate beneath the nail, except in chronic mucocutaneous candidiasis) and from *bacterial paronychia* (this is more acute in onset and throbs with pain and may drain pus).
   b. Candidal intertrigo. This moderately common condition is characterized by red, eroded patches, with scaly, pustular or pustulovesicular lesions, with an indefinite border of satellite papules or pustules. The most common sites are axillae, inframammary areas, umbilicus, genital area, anal area, and webs of toes and fingers. Obesity, diabetes, and systemic antibiotics predispose to the development of this infection.

      Candidal intertrigo is to be differentiated from *superficial tinea infections*, which are not as red and eroded, and from *seborrheic dermatitis* or *psoriasis,* both of which may show signs of disease elsewhere.
2. Generalized mucocutaneous candidiasis. This rare infection involves the smooth skin, mucocutaneous orifices, and intertriginous areas. It follows in the wake of general debility, as seen in immunosuppressed patients, and was very resistant to treatment before the discovery of ketoconazole and, more recently, fluconazole and itraconazole. Thickened toenails and fingernails mimic onychomycosis. It can be associated with multiple endocrinopathies and thymoma.

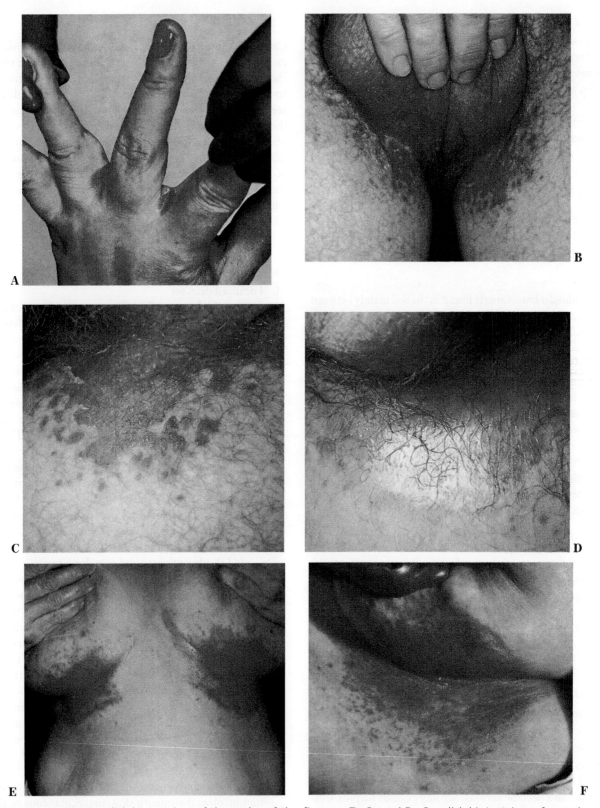

FIGURE 28-10: **A:** Candidal intertrigo of the webs of the fingers. **B, C,** and **D:** Candidal intertrigo of crural area and close-up showing satellite lesions without the sharp border as seen in tinea cruris. **E:** Candida intertrigo under breasts. **F:** Note the lack of a definite border to the eruption, which distinguishes it from a tinea infection. **G:** Extensive candidiasis around the mouth. **H:** Candida on the dorsum of the hand in a child with Addison's disease. **I:** Severe candida albicans thrush in an adult patients. Thick white adherent coating of tongue. This was the first sign of AIDS in this patient. **J:** Paronychia of forth finger with loss of cuticle, red swollen proximal nail fold and nail dystrophy with a deep Beau's line indicating severe infection in the past. (Courtesy of Smith Kline & French Laboratories; Herbert Laboratories.)

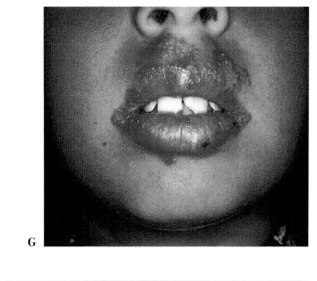
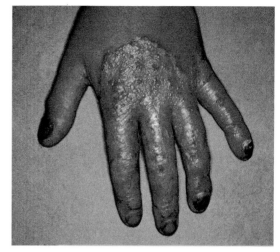
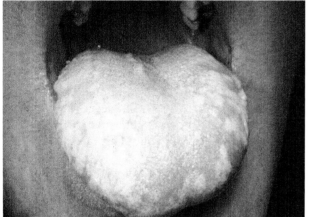
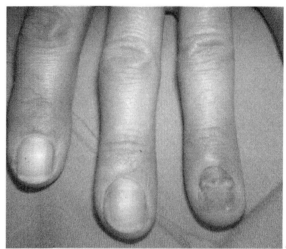

FIGURE 28-10: (continued)

Mucous Membrane Candidiasis

Oral candidiasis (thrush and perlèche): Thrush is characterized by creamy white flakes on a red, inflamed mucous membrane. The tongue may be smooth and atrophic, or the papillae may be hypertrophic, as in the condition labeled "hairy tongue." Therapy with Mycostatin pastilles (lozenges) or Mycelex troches is effective. Perlèche is seen as cracks or fissures at the corners of the mouth and is usually associated with candidal disease elsewhere, ill-fitting dental appliances, any alteration in a patient's bite that allows for collection of saliva at the corner of the mouth, and rarely a dietary deficiency (usually vitamin B complex or iron deficiency). Thrush is seen commonly in immunosuppressed patients (Fig. 28-10I).

Oral candidiasis is to be differentiated from allergic conditions, such as those due to toothpaste or mouthwash and leukoplakia.

Candidal vulvovaginitis: The clinical picture is an oozing, red, sharply bordered skin infection surrounding an inflamed vagina that contains a buttermilk-like discharge. This type of candidal infection is frequently seen in pregnant women, diabetics, and those who have been on antibiotics systemically.

It is to be differentiated from *allergic contact dermatitis, bacillary vaginosis, trichomonas infection,* or *chlamydial vaginitis.*

Laboratory Findings: Skin or mucous-membrane scrapings placed in 20% KOH solution and examined with a high-power microscope lens reveal small, oval, budding, thin-walled, yeast-like cells with occasional mycelia. Culture on Sabouraud media produces creamy dull-white colonies in 4 to 5 days. Further cultural studies on corn meal agar are necessary to identify the species as *C. albicans.*

Treatment
Case 1

Candidal paronychia of two fingers is seen in a 37-year-old male bartender.

1. Advise the patient to avoid exposure of his hands to soap and water by wearing cotton gloves under rubber gloves, hiring a dishwasher, and so on.
2. Antifungal imidazole-type solution (Lotrimin or Mycelex solution 1%) 15.0
   or Fungi-nail 15.0

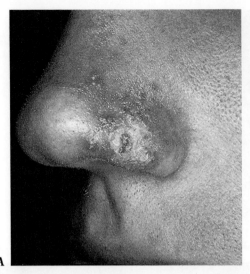 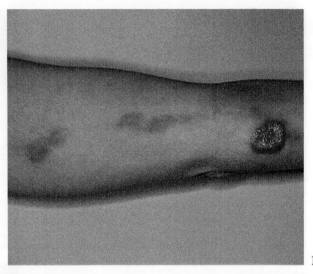

FIGURE 28-11: A: Sporotrichotic primary lesion on the nose. **B:** Sporotrichotic chancre on arm with subcutaneous nodules. (Courtesy of Stiefel Laboratories.)

or Mycolog II (generic) cream or ointment (nystatin and triamcinolone) 15.0

Sig: Apply to base of nail q.i.d. especially after hand washing. Continue treatment for several weeks.

3. Consider, if severe, a brief course of fluconazole such as 200 mg a week for 1 month.

Case 2

Candidal intertrigo of inframammary and crural region is seen in an elderly obese woman.

1. Advise the patient to wear pieces of cotton sheeting under breasts to keep the apposing tissues drier. Frequent bathing with thorough drying is helpful. Use of antibacterial soap should be avoided.

2. Sulfur, ppt. 5%
   Hydrocortisone 1%
   Mycostatin cream q.s. 30.0
   Sig: Apply locally t.i.d.

3. Powder can be used over cream:
   Mycostatin dusting powder q.s. 15.0
   Sig: Apply locally t.i.d.

Case 3

Candidal vulvovaginitis is found in a woman who is 6 months pregnant.

1. Mycostatin vaginal tablets, 100,000 units #20
   Sig: Insert one tablet b.i.d. in vagina.

2. Monistat-Derm lotion, or
   Sulfur, ppt. 5%
   Hydrocortisone 1%
   Mycostatin cream q.s. 30.0
   Sig: Apply locally b.i.d. to vulvar skin.

3. Diflucan (fluconazole)
   150 mg tablet. Single dose p.o. Can repeat for resistant cases.

Ketaconazole (Nizoral), itraconazole (Sporanox), or fluconazole (Difulcan) systemic therapy is rarely indicated for routine candidal infections. For chronic mucocutaneous candidiasis, ketoconazole and fluconazole can help the healing process significantly. Dosage information is provided in the package insert. The patient must be monitored carefully.

Sporotrichosis

Sporotrichosis (Fig. 28-11A and B) is a granulomatous fungal infection of the skin and the subcutaneous tissues. Characteristically, a primary chancre precedes more extensive skin involvement. Invasion of the internal viscera is rare.

Primary Lesion

A sporotrichositic chancre develops at the site of skin inoculation, which is commonly the hand and less commonly the face or the feet. The chancre begins as a painless, movable, subcutaneous nodule that eventually softens and breaks down to form an ulcer.

Secondary Lesions

Within a few weeks, subcutaneous nodules arise along the course of the draining lymphatics and form a chain of tumors that develop into ulcers. This is the classic clinical picture, of which there are variations.

Course

The development of the skin lesions is slow and rarely affects the general health.

Etiology

The causative agent is *Sporothrix schenckii*, a fungus that grows on wood, sphagnum moss, and in the soil. It invades open wounds and is an occupational hazard of farmers (especially sphagnum moss), gardeners (especially roses), laborers, and miners.

Laboratory Findings

Cultures of the purulent material from unopened lesions readily grow on Sabouraud media. The organism is difficult to see, even with special stains or tissue examination from a biopsy.

Differential Diagnosis

Any of the skin granulomas should be considered, such as *pyodermas, syphilis, tuberculosis, sarcoidosis,* and *leprosy.* An *ioderma* or *bromoderma* can cause a similar clinical picture.

Treatment

1. Saturated solution of potassium iodide, 60.0 mL.

   Sig: On the first day, 10 drops t.i.d., p.c., added to milk or water; second day, 15 drops t.i.d.; third day, 20 drops t.i.d., and increase until 30 to 40 drops t.i.d. is given.

   Comment: The initial doses may be smaller and the increase more gradual if one is concerned about tolerance. Gastric irritation and ioderma should be watched for. There is a very bitter taste. This very specific treatment must be continued for 1 month after apparent cure.

2. Ketoconazole (Nizoral), 200 mg.

   Sig: Two tablets a day for 8 weeks.

   Comment: Not effective in some cases. The patient must be monitored closely.

3. Itraconazole (Sporanox), 100 mg.

   Sig: One tablet daily for 4 to 6 weeks.

   Comment: Patient should be monitored for rare liver toxicity.

Suggested Readings

Baran R, Hay R, Haneke E, et al. *Onychomycosis the Current Approach to Diagnosis and Therapy.* 2nd ed. Boca Raton, FL: Taylor and Francis; 2006.

Carpenter MD, Feldman JS, Leyva WH, et al. Clinical and pathologic characteristics of disseminated cutaneous coccidioidomycosis. *J Am Acad Dermatol.* 2010;62(5):831–837.

Drake LA, Dinehart SM, Farmer ER, et al. Guidelines of care for superficial mycotic infections of the skin: Mucocutaneous candidiasis. *J Am Acad Dermatol.* 1996; 34:287.

Ellis D. Systemic antifungal agents for cutaneous fungal infections. *Aust Prescr.* 1996;19:72–75.

Gupta AK, Hofstader SLR, Adam P, et al. Tinea capitis: an overview with emphasis on management. *Pediatr Dermatol.* 1999;16(3):171–189.

Gupta AK, Uro M, Cooper E. Onychomycosis therapy: past, present, future. *J Drugs Dermatol.* 2010;9(9):1109–1113.

Hart R, Bell-Syer SE, Crawford F, et al. Systematic review of topcial treatments for fungal infections of the skin and nails of the feet. *BMJ.* 1999;319:79–82.

Mooney MA, Thomas I, Sirois D. Oral candidosis. *Int J Dermatol.* 1995;34:759–765.

Odom R. Pathophysiology of dermatophyte infections. *J Am Acad Dermatol.* 1993;28:S2–S7.

Onychomycosis: art and science. *J Drugs Dermatol.* 2013;12(7):S96–S103.

Pariser D, Elewski B, Rich P, et al. Update on onychomycosis: effective strategies for diagnosis and treatment. *Skin & Allergy News.* June, 2013.

Peikert JM. Prospective trial of curettage and cryosurgery in the management of non-facial, superficial, and minimally invasive basal and squamous cell carcinoma. *Int J Dermatol.* 2011;50:1135–1138.

Proceedings of a Symposium. Onychomycosis: Issues and Observations, Chicago, IL. *J Am Acad Dermatol Suppl.* 1995;35(3):S13–S16.

Proceedings of the International Summit on Cutaneous Antifungal Therapy and Mycology Workshop, San Francisco, California, October 21–24, 1993. *J Am Acad Dermatol Suppl.* 1994;31:S1–S116.

Radentz WH. Opportunistic fungal infections in immunocompromised hosts. *J Am Acad Dermatol.* 1989; 20:989–1003.

Rand S. Overview: The treatment of dermatophytosis. *J Am Acad Dermatol.* 2000;43(5, suppl):S104–S112.

Sehgal VN, Jain S. Onychomycosis: clinical perspective. *Int J Dermatol.* 2000;39:241–249.

Smith EB. Topical antifungal drugs in the treatment of tinea pedis, tinea cruris, and tinea corporis. *J Am Acad Dermatol.* 1993;28:S24–S28.

Sugar AM, Lyman CA. *A Practical Guide to Medically Important Fungi and the Diseases They Cause.* Philadelphia, PA: Lippincott–Raven Publishers; 1997.

Suhonen RE, Ellis DH, Dawber RPR. *Fungal Infections of the Skin Hair and Nails.* London: Informa Health Care; 1999.

Sexually Transmitted Infections

Gabriela Soza, MD, Kellie E. Reed, MD, and Dayna G. Diven, MD

Sexually transmitted infections (STIs) pose a serious public health concern in both resource-rich and limited settings throughout the world. Although all sexual activity comes with some risk of STIs, it is up to clinicians to determine which individuals are at high risk and require additional screening. Significant risk factors include both risky sexual behavior and high-risk demographic groups. High-risk behavior includes a history of multiple sex partners, a new sex partner in the past 60 days, anal intercourse, the exchange of sex for money or goods, and meeting partners on the Internet. Specific groups, such as men who have sex with men (MSM), those with a history of a prior STI, unmarried marital status, lower socioeconomic status and illicit drug use are associated with a higher prevalence of STIs.

The CDC estimates there are nearly 20 million new STIs in the United States each year. Half of those cases occur in youth ages 15 to 24, although that group accounts for only 25% of the sexually experienced population. Nationwide, there are estimated to be more than 110 million cases of both new and existing infections.

There are at least 20 different types of STIs. Carriers of STIs are often asymptomatic, and thereby remain undiagnosed and untreated, spreading the disease unknowingly. A skin examination is helpful; however, some STIs present with erosions and ulcers on the genitalia, abnormal discharge, or inguinal lymphadenopathy (Table 29-1).

In this chapter, STIs have been grouped into four categories: viruses, bacteria, parasites, and fungi.

TABLE 29-1 • STIs With Genital Ulcers

STI	Skin Lesion	Painful	Incubation	Inguinal Lymphadenopathy	Diagnosis	Organism
Herpes	Groups of vesicles, erosions, and ulcers on a red base	Yes	3-14 d	Bilateral, tender, discrete, non-suppurative, and nonindurated	Clinical, PCR, Tzanck, culture	HSV-2>HSV-1
LGV	Vesicle or shallow ulcer that heals rapidly	No	3-20 d	Mostly unilateral, becomes violaceous and tender before fistula formation	PCR	*Chlamydia trachomatis* serovariants L_1, L_2, and L_3
Granuloma inguinale	Papule that ulcerates with overhanging edges	No	2-3 wk	Not typical	Giemsa stain of smear	*Calymmatobacterium granulomatis*
Primary syphilis	Ulcer with firm indurated border	No	3 wk	Painless, regional, nonsuppurative, and rubbery	Serology, dark field microscopy	*Treponema pallidum*
Chancroid	Papule that becomes a friable, shallow, nonindurated ulcer	Yes	1-5 d	Mostly unilateral, painful, and suppurative	Culture, rule out other causes of ulcers	*Haemophilus ducreyi*

VIRUSES

Genital Herpes

Herpes simplex virus (HSV) is a chronic, lifelong disease. There are two serotypes, HSV-1 and HSV-2, and both can cause genital herpes. HSV-2 is the most common culprit, affecting an estimated 50 million Americans with recurrent genital herpes. HSV-1, historically the cause of oral lesions, is increasingly more common as the etiologic agent behind anogenital herpes, especially in young women and MSM. Transmission via oral–genital sex is often implicated in these cases. The virus initially infects the contacted area, and then travels to the sensory root ganglia, where it lies dormant. Recurrence, much more common in HSV-2, occurs when the virus dormant in the ganglia travels back down the nerve to the skin.

Skin Manifestations

HSV lesions present as grouped (herpetiform) discrete vesicles of clear fluid on an erythematous base that develop into erosions and then crust over time (Fig. 29-1). The lesions are painful because there is inflammation of the affected nerves. The lesions are neither suppurative nor indurated.

Course

Clinical manifestations of genital herpes vary between the primary and recurrent outbreaks of the disease. The primary herpes outbreak occurs after an average 4-day incubation period (range, 2 to 12). The vesicular lesions of primary herpes last 10 to 14 days, and new vesicles will continue to form over a 1- or 2-week period. Associated systemic symptoms include fever, headache, body aches, or extensive bilateral inguinal lymphadenopathy.

A recurrent episode of herpes will usually be preceded by a prodrome of burning, itching, or tingling in the affected area. Usually, herpetic vesicles follow in less than 24 hours. The duration of recurrent herpes is much shorter, and the outbreak less severe than that of the primary outbreak. Herpes can remain in the body for life, but the number of outbreaks usually becomes less frequent over time.

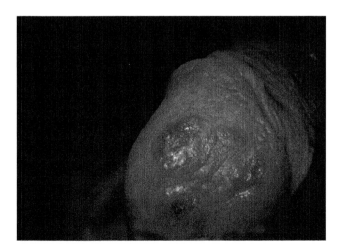

FIGURE 29-1: Genital herpes erosions and crusts.

Most infected with HSV-2 are asymptomatic. The CDC reports that of Americans infected with HSV-2, 87.4% of those aged 14 to 49 years will never receive a clinical diagnosis. With so many asymptomatic primary infections, an outbreak of recurrent herpes may often be confused with a primary infection.

Communicability

Genital herpes is spread by direct physical contact from lesions, skin or mucosal surfaces, or secretions infected with the virus. The virus is fragile and does not survive long outside of its host. Active vesicles and erosions have high viral titers and are the most contagious. However, asymptomatic viral shedding and transmission is extremely common because many patients have none to very mild symptoms. As a result, patients who have asymptomatic primary or recurrent infections may unknowingly transmit the virus to others. Among monogamous couples, an uninfected partner will acquire the virus at a rate of 5% to 10% annually. To decrease rates of HSV transmission, discordant, heterosexual couples may be counseled on options such as consistent condom use, the avoidance of sexual activity as well as intimate contact during outbreaks (however, the virus can be transferred in the asymptomatic state), and/or implementing a suppressive antiviral therapy.

Diagnosis

The diagnosis is based on the characteristic lesions and/or the history of recurrent vesicles and erosions in the anogenital area. There are two gold standard methods of virologic testing, the viral cell culture and polymerase chain reaction (PCR), both of which can be typed to determine the type of active HSV. The viral culture, from a vesicle or moist erosion, has low sensitivity that is further decreased as the lesion heals. PCR assays offer a higher sensitivity. A negative cell culture or PCR does not necessarily imply the absence of an HSV infection due to intermittent viral shedding. A direct fluorescent antibody test is also available and differentiates between HSV-1, HSV-2, and varicella zoster. The Tzanck smear is a rapid diagnostic test, where the base of a vesicle is gently scraped with a scalpel, smeared onto a glass slide, and stained with Wright or Giemsa stain. A positive Tzanck has large, multinucleated keratinocytes (Fig. 29-2). A positive result, however, cannot distinguish between HSV-1, HSV-2, or varicella-zoster virus. Serologic testing for antibodies can be done; however, 50% to 90% of individuals 20 to 40 years old are seropositive for HSV-1 antibodies, and 16% of individuals 14 to 49 years old are seropositive for HSV-2 antibodies, according to a survey performed by the CDC. HSV-2 seropositivity was higher in some subgroups. Eighty percent of those with a positive serology for HSV-2 did not have any clinical symptoms or a previous diagnosis of a genital HSV infection. Screening for HSV-1 and HSV-2 is not indicated in the general population.

Treatment

Currently, there is no cure for genital herpes. The goal of treatment is to decrease the frequency, duration, and severity of outbreaks. Treatment can also decrease, but not eliminate,

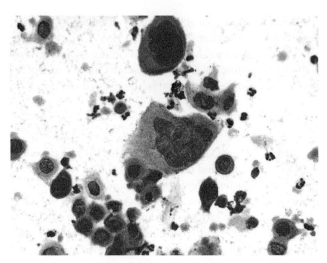

FIGURE 29-2: Positive Tzanck smear with Giemsa stain demonstrates giant multinucleated keratinocytes.

asymptomatic shedding. To decrease transmission of the virus, sexual activity and intimate contact should be avoided when there are vesicles, erosions, or fissures. Also, condoms should be used to decrease transmission during asymptomatic shedding. The antiviral medications currently available to treat herpes are acyclovir, famciclovir, and valacyclovir. These medications are relatively safe and are preferentially absorbed by infected cells. Valacyclovir and famciclovir offer the advantage of less frequent dosing and enhanced systemic absorption.

Patients with a primary genital herpes eruption should be treated to decrease the risk of severe or prolonged symptoms. Patients can be treated with any of the following: acyclovir 400 mg orally three times a day, acyclovir 200 mg orally five times a day, famciclovir 250 mg orally three times a day, or valacyclovir 1 g orally twice a day. These treatment regimens are 7 to 10 days, but can be extended if the lesions are not completely healed by day 10 of therapy.

Patients with recurrent genital herpes can be treated either episodically or continually for suppressive therapy. Episodic treatment of recurrent genital herpes entails that the patient start treatment as soon as prodromal symptoms are noticed, in order to obtain maximum benefit. Once a skin eruption begins, only mild symptomatic improvement occurs. The dosage for episodic treatment is usually a 5-day course of acyclovir 400 mg three times a day or 800 mg twice a day; famciclovir 125 mg twice a day; or valacyclovir 1 g once a day. Shorter treatment durations include acyclovir 800 mg for 2 days, famciclovir 1,000 mg twice daily for 1 day, or valacyclovir 500 mg twice daily for 3 days.

Chronic suppressive therapy is generally used in patients with greater than six outbreaks a year or for those with symptomatically severe outbreaks. Suppressive therapy can reduce outbreaks by 70% to 80%. Twenty percent of suppressed patients have no visible outbreaks. Perhaps the greatest benefit of suppressive therapy comes from the added advantage of decreasing viral shedding, thereby decreasing the risk for genital herpes infection to HSV-negative partners. As the frequency

of recurrences decreases with time, a "drug holiday" can be tried every year to assess whether the patient still requires suppressive therapy. The recommended dosages for suppressive therapy are acyclovir 400 mg orally twice a day, famciclovir 250 mg orally twice a day, valacyclovir 500 mg orally once a day, or valacyclovir 1 g orally once a day. Valacyclovir 500 mg may be less effective in those with 10 or more episodes a year. Minimal clinical benefit is seen with topical antiviral therapy.

Venereal Warts (Condylomata Acuminata)

Human Papilloma Virus (HPV) is the most common STI in the world. HPV can lead to venereal warts or certain types of cancer. According to the CDC, "most sexually active men and women will get HPV at some point in their lives." About 14 million Americans become infected with HPV every year. In total, there are more than 79 million Americans currently infected with HPV. HPV is a circular, double-stranded DNA virus. There are greater than 100 different types of HPV. The HPV types can be grouped as either low risk or high risk, depending on their risk for causing cervical cancer. The most common types, HPV-6 and HPV-11, are low risk for cancer, but do cause genital warts. The most common high-risk types are 16, 18, 31, and 33. High-risk HPV types can not only lead to cervical cancer, but also increase the risk of developing cancers of the vulva, vagina, glans penis, anus, and oropharynx.

Skin Manifestations

Venereal warts, also known as condylomata acuminata, are multiple, painless, cauliflower-shaped, soft, lobulated papules located in moist anogenital regions (Fig. 29-3). In females, they are typically found on the vulva, cervix, perineum, or anus. In males, they are usually on the penis or perianal area. Warts are less common on the scrotum, unless the immune system is deficient. Bowenoid papulosis is a rare phenotype of venereal wart that is most often associated with the high-risk HPV-16. Bowenoid warts are less prominent flat papules that may have hyperpigmentation.

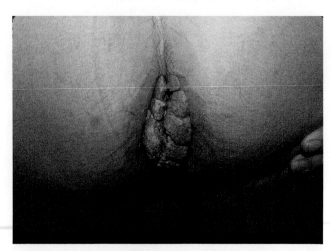

FIGURE 29-3: Large perianal condylomata acuminata.

Course

The incubation period can vary; it is usually 2 to 3 months, but can be longer, making it difficult to pinpoint the source of infection. Most infections are transient, lasting 1 to 2 years on average, before spontaneous regression. Twelve months after detection of HPV infection, an estimated 70% of females have undetectable levels of HPV DNA. After 18 months, more than 80% are clear of HPV infection. "Recurrent" warts may be areas that were subclinical at the time of treatment or new infections.

Communicability

HPV spreads via direct skin-to-skin contact, including oral, anal, or vaginal sex. Risk factors include the number of lifetime sexual partners and frequency of intimate episodes and sexual contact with a partner with active warts. As with genital herpes, HPV can be passed when genital warts are not present on the infected, asymptomatic individual. Genital warts in children less than 2 years old do not necessarily signify abuse, as warts can spread during delivery, from autoinoculation, and from nonsexual contact. The possibility of abuse can be considered if the situation warrants. Men who are circumcised are less likely to carry and transmit HPV infection. Anal HPV infection is prevalent (up to 75%) in MSM.

Diagnosis

The diagnosis of venereal warts is usually clinical. Flat or sessile warts may occasionally warrant a biopsy for bowenoid papulosis given its higher association with cancer. In the case of an abnormal Papanicolaou (Pap) test, PCR and in situ hybridization tests are used to type the HPV infection. These tests can differentiate the low-risk HPV types (6, 11) from the high-risk (16, 18, 31, 33), which may require further workup.

Treatment

There are a large number of treatment options for genital warts. These treatments can be grouped into those that physically destroy the wart, those that kill infected cells, and those that stimulate the immune system to destroy the wart. There is a high recurrence rate of 20% to 50% for genital condylomata.

Liquid nitrogen cryotherapy is the most commonly used in-office destructive method because it is quick, effective, and inexpensive. The wart and a 2 mm ring of surrounding skin are frozen white once or twice with a liquid nitrogen dispenser or cotton swab. Reevaluate the lesions about every 4 weeks until there are no remaining lesions. Trichloroacetic acid can be used to destroy small warts in a moist region.

Prescription imiquimod 3.75% or 5% cream (~50% efficacious) has a low recurrence rate and its application is recommended three times a week nightly until total clearance or up to 16 weeks. The authors find that some patients tolerate nightly application, or 5 consecutive days weekly, as well. The cream, which has an immunomodulatory effect, can lead to mild to moderate irritation, and has also been reported to flare concomitant psoriasis.

5-Fluorouracil (5-FU) 5% cream applied twice a day can be effective and should be considered when all other treatment options fail to clear recalcitrant warts. This is because of the severe irritation. 5-FU works well for intraurethral warts, but it can cause inflammation and painful scrotal erosions.

Electrofulguration and electrocautery are effective; however, this method has fallen out of favor because the smoke plume can, theoretically, cause warts in the respiratory tract. In response to this theory, many wear masks or use smoke evacuators during the treatment of warts.

Podophyllotoxin 0.5% solution (the most active constituent of podophyllin) can be applied by the patient at home twice daily for 3 days repeated in weekly cycles. Podophyllotoxin and podophyllin are contraindicated in pregnancy. Podophyllin is no longer recommended because of low efficacy and potential toxicity.

Veregen 15% (sinecatechin) is a botanical topical agent applied each night or three times a week and can sometimes cause irritation.

There are currently three HPV vaccines used for routine vaccination. Gardasil, a quadrivalent vaccine against HPV types 6, 11, 16, and 18; Cervarix, a bivalent vaccine against HPV-16 and HPV-18; and the newest Gardasil 9, which offers added protection against five more of the most cancer-causing strains (31, 33, 45, 52, and 58). These vaccines are very effective at preventing warts, cervical cancer, and other cancers caused by the nine most common high- and low-risk HPV types. HPV 6 and 11 cause 90% of genital warts. Vaccination is currently recommended for females aged 11 to 26 years old and males aged 11 to 21 years old. MSM and the immunocompromised (such as those with HIV) may receive the vaccine up to age 26. No therapeutic vaccine currently exists.

Hepatitis B Virus

Hepatitis B virus (HBV) is a small enveloped, circular, partially double-stranded DNA virus of the hepadnaviridae family. The virus can cause a self-limited or chronic infection. Approximately 240 million people worldwide have chronic HBV, a number of which are found in the Far East. In the United States, half of all cases arise from sexual contact.

Skin Manifestations

HBV does not produce any genital lesions. Nevertheless, HBV can cause jaundice, urticaria, and vasculitis. Extrahepatic manifestations are seen in 10% to 20% of patients. Some acutely infected patients will develop a transient serum sickness–like infection 1 to 6 weeks before the onset of jaundice. These patients typically have fever, urticaria, and polyarthritis. This sickness gradually resolves spontaneously. Polyarteritis nodosa, also known as acute necrotizing vasculitis, develops in 7% to 8% of cases, most commonly within the first 6 months. Membranous glomerulonephritis occurs in children and adults and usually clears when the active infection clears.

Course

HBV has an incubation time of 6 weeks to 6 months, with the average being 10 weeks before an acute infection becomes clinically apparent. Patients complain of fevers, anorexia, nausea, diarrhea, right upper quadrant pain, and general malaise. Very few (<1%) acute infections go on to fulminant hepatitis, or liver failure. The risk of chronicity is inversely related to age at acquisition; 90% of infected infants suffer from chronic infection versus only 2% to 6% of newly infected adults. Up to a quarter of the chronically affected go on to develop cirrhosis and/or hepatocellular carcinoma.

Communicability

The virus is found in body fluids such as blood, saliva, semen, and cervical fluid. The disease typically spreads by percutaneous or mucous membrane exposure via intimate contact, intravenous drug use, perinatally from mother to baby, and from accidental exposures in the health care field.

Diagnosis

The diagnosis of an HBV infection is made serologically. Acute infections are diagnosed with the presence of IgM antibody against hepatitis B core antigen (IgM anti-HBc), which is almost always positive when jaundice is present. Chronic infections are diagnosed by finding both the HBV surface antigen (HBsAg) and total anti-HBc, with the lack of the IgM anti-HBc in the blood. If antibody to the surface antigen is present (anti-HBs), the patient is protected against the virus and has either a resolved HBV infection or has been previously vaccinated against the virus.

Treatment

Acute infections are treated with supportive care, as no medication is available. Chronic infections can be treated with α_{2b}-interferon, lamivudine, entecavir, telbivudine, or adefovir dipivoxil. HBV-associated polyarteritis nodosa is typically treated with systemic steroids, lamivudine, and rarely with plasma exchange. A vaccine is available to prevent infections, and it is recommended for many categories of persons including health care workers, infants, children, MSM, HIV-positive patients, injection drug users, and certain high-risk sexually active individuals.

Hepatitis C Virus

Hepatitis C virus (HCV) is an enveloped, positive-sense single-stranded RNA virus of the Flaviviridae family. The CDC estimates "approximately 29,718 cases (of acute hepatitis C) occurred in 2013" in the United States. Approximately 2.7 million Americans have chronic hepatitis C infection, the most common cause of cirrhosis in the United States.

Skin Manifestations

There are no acute genital lesions. The stigmata of liver cirrhosis, such as jaundice, caput medusa, palmar erythema, and telangiectasias develop with chronic infections.

Course

Most acute infections are asymptomatic; however, 20% to 30% of individuals may develop jaundice, fatigue, abdominal pain, or anorexia. In those individuals, there is a 4 to 12 week incubation period after exposure before the onset of symptoms. Of those infected, 75% to 85% of those will develop a chronic infection that can lead to liver cirrhosis. Chronic HCV has also been associated with polyarteritis nodosa, sporadic porphyria cutanea tarda, lichen planus, necrolytic acral erythema, essential mixed cryoglobulinemia, and cutaneous necrotizing vasculitis.

Communicability

Although sexual transmission of HCV is uncommon, it is of concern in the HIV-positive and MSM populations. Most of the cases in developed nations are now acquired from intravenous drug abuse and not blood transfusions because the screening of blood and blood products for HCV has been available in the United States since 1992.

Diagnosis

Several blood tests are available to diagnose HCV infection. An enzyme immunoassay (EIA) screening test looks for antibodies to HCV. Qualitative tests detect the presence or absence of HCV RNA PCR, whereas quantitative tests detect the amount of virus via PCR for HCV RNA.

Treatment

Treatment is similar for both acute and chronic HCV infections. Until very recently, a combination of interferon-α and ribavirin was the standard treatment regimen. Two new options exist for a 12-week treatment regimen offering a greater than 95% sustained virologic response rate. Treatment can be either a combination of daily daclatasvir and sofosbuvir or a once-daily pill containing ledipasvir and sofosbuvir.

HIV/AIDS

The human immunodeficiency virus (HIV) was first recognized in the United States in 1981, but it is thought to have been present in Africa since the early 20th century. HIV causes an immunodeficient state principally by depleting the body of $CD4^+$ helper T cells. Acquired immunodeficiency syndrome (AIDS) is a term used to describe the later stages of HIV infection, defined by CD4 count below 200 cells/mL. Approximately 50,000 people in the United States are infected with HIV each year. Patients with AIDS usually present with an opportunistic infection (characteristic viral or fungal pneumonia), malignancy (Kaposi sarcoma or one of several lymphomas), or chronic fatigue syndrome (encephalopathy, wasting). Most HIV-infected individuals develop skin disorders related to their immunocompromised status.

Skin Manifestations

Acute HIV infections are not associated with specific genital lesions. Most initial infections are asymptomatic, but some present with a mononucleosis-like illness 2 to 4 weeks after exposure. This illness consists of a nonspecific rash with discrete, erythematous macules and papules primarily on the trunk but occasionally involving the palms or soles. Systemic symptoms include fevers, pharyngitis, cervical lymphadenopathy, arthralgias, and oral and genital ulcers.

Patients with HIV can manifest other skin disorders such as refractory psoriasis, severe seborrheic dermatitis, and xerotic skin. Once HIV has developed into AIDS, the clinician may note stigmata of disease, such as the reddish-brown plaques of Kaposi sarcoma, the whitish plaques of oral candidiasis, or cutaneous nodules caused by tuberculosis or disseminated fungal infections such as cryptococcus, histoplasmosis, or coccidioides.

Course

After the initial infection, many years can pass before symptoms appear. The virus can directly cause muscle wasting, neurologic degeneration, diarrhea, and increase the risk of malignancies. The immunodeficient status leads to opportunistic infections and severe manifestations of common infections. Syphilis can be accelerated to tertiary syphilis, chancres can become uncharacteristically painful from coinfection, and syphilitic serologic tests can be falsely negative. Genital warts, HSV lesions, and molluscum contagiosum can be diffusely spread, larger in size, and more resistant to treatment. Also, patients are more likely to have candidiasis, tinea ("ringworm"), and staphylococcal infections.

Communicability

HIV is spread through exposure to infected fluids, often via sexual contact. The probability of transmission per sexual act is actually low (0.0003 to 0.0015). Male-to-female transmission rates are much greater than female-to-male rates. Having a sore, such as a syphilitic chancre, herpetic ulcer, or chancroid can increase the risk of transmission. HIV can also be spread from blood transfusions (uncommon in the United States since the universal screening of all donated blood in the mid-1980s), sharing of contaminated needles during intravenous drug use, and from mother to child either transplacentally, perinatally, or via breast-feeding.

Diagnosis

HIV is typically screened for using a highly sensitive serologic screening test, usually a combination antigen/antibody or antibody immunoassay (IA). Although results can be received within 30 minutes, this rapid test can provide falsely negative results in recently infected patients. This serologic screening test is then followed by a confirmation test performed by antigen-antibody differentiation assay, indirect immunofluorescence assay, or Western blot test. In addition, HIV RNA testing is performed on all persons with a reactive immunoassay and negative confirmation test because these discordant results can be caused by an acute HIV infection.

Treatment

HIV is treated with highly active antiretroviral therapy (HAART), a cocktail of drugs, including antiviral proteases and reverse transcriptase inhibitors. Most of the opportunistic infections and malignancies associated with HIV infection will resolve with HAART therapy. Extensive molluscum contagiosum cases in HIV patients have decreased because of the increasing use of HAART. The immune reconstitution inflammatory syndrome can sometimes occur after starting HAART, and exacerbations of herpes zoster, leprosy, CMV infections, and *Mycobacterium avium* complex, among other cutaneous diseases, can flare. Daily oral antiretroviral preexposure prophylaxis is a prevention option being offered by clinicians to male and female patients whose sexual or injection behaviors place them at substantial risk of acquiring an HIV infection.

Molluscum Contagiosum

Molluscum contagiosum is a common nonsexually acquired infection in young children, but it can also be found among sexually active young adults and among immunocompromised patients. The infection is caused by a poxvirus.

Skin Manifestations

The primary lesion is a small, firm, shiny, smooth-surfaced, dome-shaped, flesh-colored papule with a central umbilication (Fig. 29-4). Papules that are scratched or irritated can become crusted or pustular. Genital papules can occur in children as part of a more widespread infection. Adults typically have fewer papules that are located in the genital region, upper thighs, and lower abdomen.

Course

Molluscum contagiosum frequently resolves spontaneously within a year in healthy individuals, but may take longer. Treatment can expedite the resolution.

Communicability

The disease typically spreads from skin-to-skin contact, which is amplified in wet environments, such as bathtubs or swimming pools.

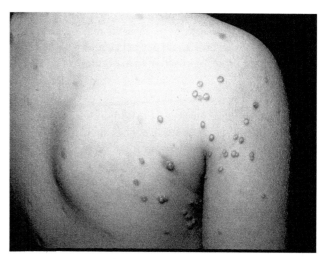

FIGURE 29-4: Molluscum contagiosum demonstrates classic umbilicated papules.

Diagnosis

The diagnosis is made clinically with identification of the distinctive umbilicated papules. Light cryotherapy can aid in the diagnosis by making the umbilication more apparent. When necessary, a technique similar to a Tzanck smear will demonstrate characteristic "molluscum bodies." These intracytoplasmic inclusion bodies can also be seen on a skin biopsy as Henderson–Patterson bodies.

Treatment

Many modalities can be used to physically destroy the papules. Education on the risks, benefits, and adverse events of treatment versus nonintervention should be communicated to the patient and caregiver. Commonly used treatments include cryotherapy with liquid nitrogen, topical imiquimod (some authors do not think this is efficacious), and curettage. Curettage is efficacious and offers the least amount of adverse effects. However, considerations of anesthesia and time consumption often defer this form of treatment in children. Chemical removal with topical cantharidin, KOH, or tretinoin can be used to avoid the pain of the aforementioned treatment modalities. In office, plucking out or expressing the contents of the core of the papules can also help. Suggested follow-up is about 1 month to evaluate and treat any remaining lesions should the patient desire.

PARASITES

Pubic Lice

Pubic lice, also known as crabs or pediculosis pubis, is caused by the crab louse, *Phthirus pubis*. Lice have three pairs of legs and attach their eggs, called nits, to hair shafts. More than half of the time, pubic lice can also infest a second hair-bearing area such as the eyelashes, eyebrows, axilla, or the scalp.

Skin Manifestations

On exam, tiny crab lice and nits attached to the base of hairs can be seen with the naked eye. Pruritus may be present as well as excoriations, crusts, and perifollicular erythema. Sores and secondary bacterial infections can occur.

Course

The adult crab louse survives 24 to 48 hours from the host, requiring human blood to survive. Eggs are laid on the hair shaft, and they are viable for up to 10 days. Of note, lice that survive shaving or treatment can find refuge in other hair-bearing areas of the body.

Communicability

Pubic lice more commonly infest those with ample amounts of pubic hair. Most commonly transmitted via sexual contact, pubic lice can be spread from infested fomites such as sheets and clothing.

Diagnosis

The infestation is clinically diagnosed by finding the crabs (Fig. 29-5) and nits. Persons diagnosed with pubic lice should also be worked up for other STIs.

Treatment

The recommended regimen is topical treatment with either permethrin 1% cream rinse or pyrethrin with piperonyl butoxide applied to affected areas and washed off after 10 minutes. There is increasing resistance to these two drugs, also called pediculicides. Therapy with malathion 0.5% lotion applied to the affected areas and washed off after 8 to 12 hours is used in cases of treatment failure thought to be caused by pediculicide resistance. An alternative option is ivermectin 250 μg/kg orally, repeated in 14 days. If the eyelashes are involved, occlusive erythromycin ophthalmic ointment or simple petroleum jelly can be applied twice a day to the eyelid margin for 10 days. All topical insecticides should be applied twice, 1 week apart. This ensures proper therapy because of hatched eggs. Partners and close contacts should be treated, and the presence of additional STIs should be considered, including HIV.

Scabies

Scabies is caused by infestation of the skin by the human itch mite, *Sarcoptes scabiei* var. *hominis*. This common condition is spread by humans only and is found worldwide. The female burrows into the upper epidermis, lays her eggs, and lives for a month feeding and defecating within her burrow.

Skin Manifestations

Pruritus is the chief symptom of scabies. Severe itching that worsens at night and after hot showers is a typical pattern seen in the first manifestation of scabies. The most common lesions are small, erythematous, pruritic papules. Papules and indurated nodules can be found on the scrotum and shaft and glans of the penis (Fig. 29-6). The pathognomonic sign is the serpentine linear burrow, which is skin-colored or tinted gray, with or without fine scale, and can be more than a centimeter in length. These burrows are most often seen in the

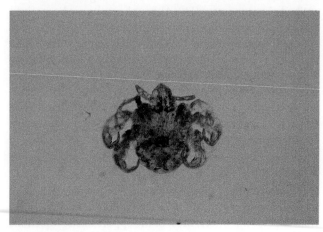

FIGURE 29-5: Microscopic view of a pubic louse.

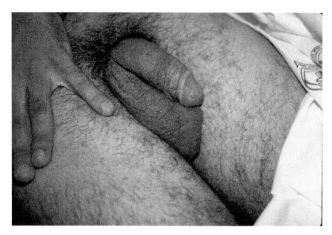

FIGURE 29-6: Scabies-induced pruritic papules.

interdigital web spaces and volar wrist. Other infected areas may include the elbows, axillae, central abdomen, buttocks, and anterior thighs.

Course

After the initial infestation with *S. scabiei*, sensitization must occur before itching commences. This may take weeks to months to develop after the first infestation, and as a result, many asymptomatic carriers exist. Subsequent infestations may become symptomatic in less than 24 hours owing to previous sensitization of the host to the mite antigens. Those who are immunosuppressed or who are unable to sense itching or scratch themselves adequately are at risk for developing a severe form of the scabies, also known as crusted scabies. Crusted scabies is a massive infestation of mites and eggs, highly contagious to others. The gigantic numbers of mites residing in the thickened, crusted epidermis set the stage for a potential scabies outbreak. In this situation, aggressive treatment should be swiftly delivered.

Communicability

The mite is spread by close physical contact, most often with children, family members, and by fomites such as clothing, bedding, or even furniture. It can also be transmitted by sexual contact.

Diagnosis

In the clinic, a diagnosis can be made by using scalpel blade to scrape the infested areas or serpiginous burrows onto a glass slide topped with a drop of mineral oil. Under light microscopy, visualization of mites, eggs, or scybala (fecal material) confirms the diagnosis (Figs. 29-7 and 29-8). Most patients will have only a few mites, which can make it difficult to get a positive scraping. Mites are particularly hard to find in excessively clean, easily scratched, or partially treated areas.

Treatment

Permethrin 5% cream should be applied overnight from the neck down (head to toe if crusted scabies or an infant) with

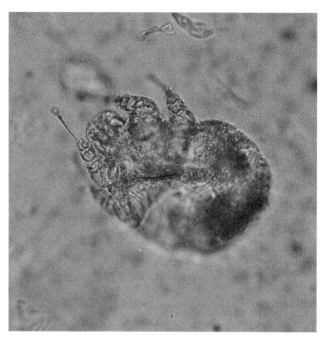

FIGURE 29-7: Mineral oil smear demonstrating a scabies mite at 40×.

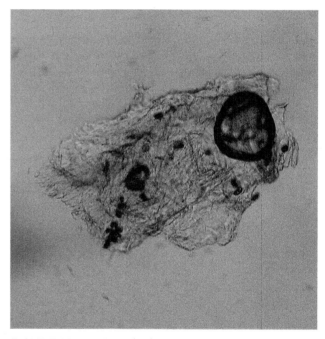

FIGURE 29-8: Mineral oil smear of an epidermal scale containing brown scybala at 10×.

particular attention paid to covering the subungual, genital, and waistline areas. The cream is washed off after 8 to 14 hours, and treatment is repeated in 7 days. A second recommended regimen consists of two doses of oral ivermectin at 200 μg/kg, with the second dose given 14 days after the initial.

For crusted scabies, there is no ideal recommended treatment per the CDC. Combination therapy with topical scabicide and oral ivermectin is recommended. Of note, ivermectin should be avoided in pregnant women, nursing mothers, and children less than 15 kg. It is common for itching and lesions to last 2 to 4 weeks even following adequate treatment. To prevent reinfection, the entire household and close contacts should be treated because asymptomatic carriers are common. Following each treatment, pajamas, bedding, and towels should be sterilized with hot water and a hot dryer or stored in an airtight bag for 10 days to kill the mites.

Trichomoniasis

It is estimated that 3.7 million persons in the United States are infected with the protozoan trophozoite *Trichomonas vaginalis*. A quarter of all sexually active women will acquire the disease, also known as "trich," usually between the ages of 16 and 35.

Skin Manifestations

There are typically no skin manifestations. Erythema can often be found in the vagina or on the cervix. In severe cases, erosions and petechial hemorrhages may be seen. The association with a red, friable endocervix ("strawberry cervix") is well known, but is uncommonly found. Vaginal discharge is classically thin, yellow to green, and frothy, but in practice, these characteristics vary widely.

Course

Trichomonas causes a chronic vaginitis that lasts for months to years until treated. Symptoms wax and wane, and can worsen with menses or pregnancy. Approximately 30% of those infected are symptomatic with symptoms ranging from mild to severe. Common symptoms are discharge, itching, burning, dyspareunia, dysuria, and foul odor. Men typically are asymptomatic, but can complain of dysuria and scant discharge. Clinically significant immunity does not develop.

Communicability

The disease is mostly linked to sexual contact. However, trichomonads can survive 1 to 2 hours on moist surfaces and for 24 hours in urine, semen, and water. Very rarely does the disease transmit via fomites even in places where washcloths are shared.

Diagnosis

Historically, a wet mount of genital discharge was performed to make the diagnosis in-house. The secretions are placed on a glass side and visualized under light microscopy, a positive test consisting of visualized trichomonads, with their jerky movements and five flagella. However, wet mounts are only 51% to 65% sensitive in females, with even decreased sensitivity in men. Culture is slow, and previously was the gold standard for diagnosis. 2015 guidelines from the CDC recommend highly sensitive and specific molecular detection methods, such as nucleic acid amplification testing (NAAT). DNA and RNA probes are now readily available. In addition, a FDA-cleared rapid hybridization probe point of care test exists for *T. vaginalis*, *G. vaginalis*, and *C. albicans* infections.

Treatment

Oral metronidazole is the most commonly used treatment resulting in a cure rate of more than 90%. Metronidazole is recommended as a single 2,000 mg dose or, alternatively, given in a 7-day regimen of 500 mg twice a day. Also recommended is tinidazole 2 g orally in a single dose. Owing to the possibility of a disulfiram-like reaction, these drugs should not be taken concomitantly with alcoholic beverages. These drugs are contraindicated in pregnant women during their first trimester.

BACTERIA

Chlamydia

Chlamydia trachomatis causes the most frequent reportable infectious disease in the United States, according to the CDC, with the highest prevalence in persons 24 years of age and younger. Serovariants B, D, E, F, G, H, I, J, and K frequently cause genital infections and will be discussed in this section. Serovariants L_1, L_2, and L_3 produce a clinically distinct variant known as lymphogranuloma venereum, which is discussed in the section following this one. Serovariants A, B, and C are associated with trachoma, a chronic follicular conjunctivitis that can lead to blindness.

Skin Manifestations

Most infections are asymptomatic. Symptoms include dysuria and an abnormal discharge from the penile urethra or vagina. Chlamydia is the most common cause of epididymitis in young men, which presents with pain and swelling in one or both testicles.

Course

Urethritis in men usually develops after a 2- to 6-week incubation period. Symptomatic women may develop cervicitis or vaginitis. With decreasing rates of gonorrhea, chlamydial infections are the most common cause of pelvic inflammatory disease (PID) and preventable infertility. PID can cause infertility by scarring the reproductive tract.

Infected males with the HLA-B27 genotype are most at risk for developing reactive arthritis. Also known as Reiter syndrome, it may consist of the triad of arthritis, urethritis, and conjunctivitis. Painless oral erosions also occur. Reactive arthritis patients can develop small, scattered, thick, or pustular lesions on their genitals, palms, and soles. This condition is called balanitis circinata when on the glans penis, and keratoderma blennorrhagicum when located on the plantar feet. Reactive arthritis is a rare complication and typically develops 1 to 3 weeks after infection by *Chlamydia*.

Communicability

Chlamydial genital infections are typically transmitted via sexual contact. Chlamydia transmission rates are quite high, with approximately one-third of exposed males developing urethritis. Reinfection is common, particularly after exposure to an untreated sexual partner.

Diagnosis

As most of the clinical findings are nonspecific, laboratory testing is required to make the diagnosis. NAATs are the gold standard diagnostic tests. In women, urogenital testing can be performed on first-catch urine or by swabbing the endocervix or vagina. In men, urethral testing consists of swabbing the urethra, or by testing a first-catch urine specimen. NAATs are more sensitive than cell cultures and can be used on self-collected vaginal swabs or urine samples. Annual screening of all sexually active women aged <25 years and older women who are at increased risk for infection is recommended.

Treatment

Recommended regimens include treatment with azithromycin 1 g orally once or with doxycycline 100 mg orally twice a day for 7 days. Alternative regimens include oral treatment with erythromycin, levofloxacin, or ofloxacin.

Lymphogranuloma venereum

Lymphogranuloma venereum (LGV) is a rare STI caused by *C. trachomatis* serovariants L_1, L_2, and L_3. Although most cases are found in Africa, India, Southeast Asia, and South America, there are occasional outbreaks elsewhere.

Skin Manifestations

At the primary site of infection, a 2 to 3 mm painless genital vesicle or shallow erosion appears, which then spontaneously resolves shortly thereafter. Urethritis may also occur. Two weeks after the primary infection, the inguinal and/or femoral lymph nodes enlarge, typically unilaterally, although occasionally bilaterally. The chain of enlarging inguinal nodes, called buboes, fuse, and the overlying skin becomes red and tender. A characteristic groove (the "groove sign") can be seen as lymph nodes both above and below the inguinal ligament become swollen. The firm buboes spontaneously ulcerate, drain pus, and then involute. An alternative site of infection is the rectum, where a proctocolitis with mucopurulent discharge can progress to rectal strictures. In the United States, the rectal presentation is more common in MSM, and also in women who engage in receptive anal intercourse.

Course

There is a 3- to 20-day incubation period after exposure before manifestation of the primary infection. In addition to the cutaneous presentation, infected individuals may complain of malaise, arthritis, conjunctivitis, fever, weight loss, and a poor appetite. Additional complications include hepatosplenomegaly, encephalitis, and chronic genital swelling (elephantiasis) secondary to scarring of the lymphatic system (Fig. 29-9). Untreated infections recur one-fifth of the time.

Communicability

The disease is spread through sexual contact. Men are more commonly symptomatic. Symptomatic women rarely have an observed primary lesion and have fewer buboes; however, they

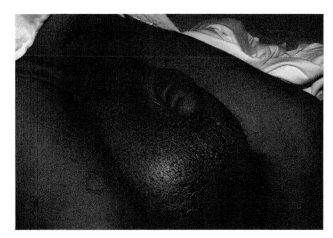

FIGURE 29-9: Lymphogranuloma venereum—induced genital elephantiasis.

are more likely to present at a later stage with rectal strictures or genital elephantiasis.

Diagnosis

Culture, direct immunofluorescence, or NAAT can be performed on lesional tissue from the genitalia, rectum, and lymph node specimens to identify *Chlamydial* DNA. Although the FDA has not cleared NAAT use on rectal specimens, the CDC still recommends this method as the preferred diagnostic tool when approaching a MSM with proctocolitis. A complement fixation test can be used in conjunction with the PCR to identify serovariant-specific antibodies, although the diagnostic utility of this test is unknown.

Treatment

The first-line treatment is doxycycline 100 mg orally twice a day for 21 days, with erythromycin 500 mg orally four times a day for 21 days as the second-line regimen. Aspiration or incision and drainage may need to be performed on the large fluctuant buboes to prevent development of inguinal or femoral ulcerations, prevent rupture, and to help clear the infection. All sexual contacts 60 days before the onset of the patient's symptoms should be evaluated and empirically treated with a recommended chlamydia regimen noted above (azithromycin 1 g orally once or with doxycycline 100 mg orally twice a day for 7 days).

Granuloma Inguinale

Granuloma inguinale, also known as donovanosis or granuloma venereum, is a rare, locally destructive disease caused by the encapsulated gram-negative bacillus *Calymmatobacterium (Donovania) granulomatis,* now known as *Klebsiella granulomatis.* The disease is endemic in tropical developing countries such as India, southern Africa, New Guinea, the Caribbean, and central Australia.

Skin Manifestations

The first manifestation of the disease is painless or mildly painful papules or nodules that slowly enlarge and erode through the skin to produce clean, well-defined ulcers with overhanging edges. The highly vascular ulcers are composed of a beefy-red base of friable hypertrophic granulation tissue. Most of the lesions are found on the genitals, the most common sites being the prepuce, glans, and labia majora. However, the lesions can also be found in the perineal areas, or the inguinal folds, extending to more distant locations of the lower abdomen and thighs. Lymphadenopathy is not a typical feature.

Course

The incubation period varies from 1 to 12 weeks, but signs usually appear in 2 to 3 weeks. The disease progresses slowly and spreads by both peripheral extension and autoinoculation. Secondary bacterial infection of the lesions may occur, as can lesional coinfection with a second STI. Ulcers can lead to persistent draining sinuses and depigmented scars. Long-standing disease can occasionally scar the local lymphatic channels causing pseudoelephantiasis (swelling).

Communicability

Sexual transmission is considered the most likely manner of transmission. The disease is only mildly contagious and likely needs to be inoculated through broken skin.

Diagnosis

As no reliable serologic tests or cultures exist, clinical suspicion and smears of active lesions demonstrating Donovan bodies are required to diagnose the disease. To perform a smear, an ulcer is scraped and smeared onto a glass slide, air-dried, and then stained with either a Wright or a Giemsa stain. A smear can also be taken from tissue preparations or biopsy site histologic sections. Donovan bodies are darkly staining clusters of encapsulated bacilli within the cytoplasm of mononuclear cells. HIV should be tested in those diagnosed with granuloma inguinale.

Treatment

The first-line treatment is azithromycin 1 g orally once per week or 500 mg daily for a minimum of 3 weeks and until all the lesions are completely healed. Alternative medications include erythromycin 500 mg four times daily, trimethoprim/sulfamethoxazole 160 mg/800 mg tablet twice daily, doxycycline 100 mg orally twice a day, or ciprofloxacin 750 mg twice daily. All alternative treatments also require treatment for at least 3 weeks and until all the lesions are completely healed. Relapses are common, and can occur 6 to 18 months after a seemingly successful treatment.

Gonorrhea

Gonorrhea, also known as GC or "the clap," is a common STI that has been with humans for millennia. Galen, the Roman physician, named it gonorrhea or "flowing seed" because of the disease's characteristic purulent urethral discharge. Caused by the gram-negative diplococcus *Neisseria gonorrhoeae*, the infection is most commonly found among young adults between the ages of 15 and 24 years. Both gonorrhea and chlamydia infections can cause PID, the most common preventable cause of infertility.

Skin Manifestations

The primary symptoms include dysuria and a white, green, or yellow penile or vaginal discharge. Rarely, a gonococcal dermatitis may occur on the median raphe of the penis. Just like the other STIs, many of those infected have no symptoms at all.

Course

Symptoms of gonorrhea usually develop within 1 to 2 weeks after exposure. Compared with other infectious causes of urethritis, many men with gonococcal urethral infections develop symptoms, whereas most infected women do not. Untreated symptomatic individuals often become asymptomatic carriers, a state that can last for months. Occasionally, certain strains of gonorrhea disseminate hematogenously. This disseminated gonococcal infection (DGI) causes fevers, asymmetric polyarthralgias, tenosynovitis, oligoarticular septic arthritis, and hemorrhagic vesiculopustules on the skin (Fig. 29-10). The vesiculopustules are tender, sparse, and occur usually on the palms, soles, or over joints. Initially tiny erythematous macules, they become vesiculopustules on a deeply erythematous or hemorrhagic base. The macules can also enlarge to purpuric patches up to 2 cm in diameter. In females, DGI often occurs during pregnancy or menstruation. Rarely, DGI leads to perihepatitis, endocarditis, or meningitis. Other complications of untreated gonorrhea infection include PID, sterility, epididymitis, and proctitis.

Communicability

The disease is highly contagious, with a 20% to 50% transmission rate per episode of intercourse. Because a large reservoir of asymptomatic carriers exists, controlling the spread of the disease has been difficult. The bacteria can also infect the anorectal, oropharynx, and conjunctival areas. Nonsexual transmission is rare, so sexual abuse should be considered in all infected children.

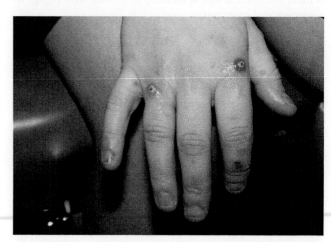

FIGURE 29-10: Disseminated gonorrhea with hemorrhagic vesiculopustules.

Diagnosis

A Gram-stained smear of urethral discharge is over 95% sensitive and specific in symptomatic men. A positive smear demonstrates gram-negative diplococci within neutrophils. However, a negative Gram stain is not enough to rule out disease in asymptomatic men. In addition, the use of Gram stains with endocervical, rectal, or pharyngeal specimens is not recommended. Cultures can also be obtained from the endocervix or male urethra. The use of culture to diagnose rectal, oropharyngeal, and conjunctival infections is FDA approved, whereas the use of NAAT in these scenarios is not. NAAT is widely popular owing to the high sensitivity and specificity, the rapid results, and the fact that it can be used on noninvasively obtained urine samples, in addition to swabs of the vagina, endocervix, or male urethra. Annual screening of all sexually active women aged <25 years and older women who are at increased risk for infection is recommended. Those who test positive for gonorrhea should be tested for other STIs.

Treatment

Dual therapy is the recommended plan of action with gonococcal infections with a cephalosporin plus azithromycin, even if NAAT for *C. trachomatis* is negative at the time of treatment. According to the CDC, there is a theoretical basis for a second antibiotic to improve treatment efficacy, while also delaying cephalosporin resistance. The first-line treatment of an uncomplicated infection of the cervix, urethra, rectum, or pharynx is a single intramuscular (IM) dose of ceftriaxone 250 mg plus a single dose of azithromycin 1 g orally. Conjunctivitis is treated with 1 g of IM ceftriaxone plus 1 g of oral azithromycin in a single dose. Disseminated gonococcal infections should receive ceftriaxone 1 g IM or IV each day until they have shown 1 to 2 days of clinical improvement plus azithromycin 1 g orally in a single dose. In all cases, intimate partners in the previous 60 days should be evaluated, tested, and offered treatment.

Syphilis

Syphilis, caused by the spirochete *Treponema pallidum*, subspecies *pallidum*, has been present for centuries, with early references in the works of Shakespeare and Voltaire. Some historians believe that it may have originated in the New World and traveled to Europe via Christopher Columbus' crew, where it became known as the Great Pox. In recent times within the United States, the incidence of syphilis decreased dramatically throughout the 1990s, but since 2000 the incidence has slowly increased. Currently, 75% of cases of syphilis in the United States are among MSM. Syphilis infections are divided into four stages: the initial infection (primary syphilis), the disseminated stage (secondary syphilis), the clinically asymptomatic stage (latent syphilis), and the late stage infection (tertiary syphilis).

Skin Manifestations

The classic primary lesion is the chancre, a single, nonpainful ulcer with a firm, indurated border. Most commonly found on the genitalia, the sores can also appear on the anus, lips, or inside the mouth. Half of all chancres do not meet the "classical" description, in that they can be nonindurated, painful, or multiple in number. A week after a chancre appears, a painless, regional, nonsuppurative, rubbery lymphadenopathy can develop.

A secondary syphilis infection can mimic many diseases and has a large number of possible skin findings. The most common finding is a widespread, symmetric, nonpruritic, papulosquamous eruption, classically affecting the palms and soles (Fig. 29-11). Moist areas, such as the anus, penis, labia, and inner thighs, may grow wartlike condyloma lata, whitish or grayish flat papules (Fig. 29-12). Painful shallow erosions, also known as mucous patches, may affect the mucous membranes. A diffuse, nonscarring alopecia may affect the scalp and eyebrows. The classic moth-eaten patchy alopecia of syphilis is uncommon.

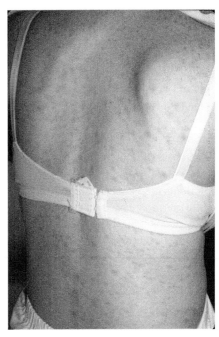

FIGURE 29-11: Secondary syphilis papulosquamous eruption.

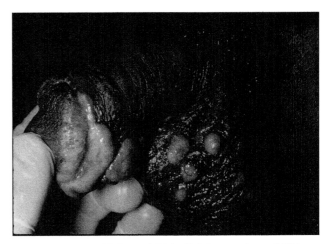

FIGURE 29-12: Moist, whitish, flat-topped, syphilitic papules of condylomata lata.

The principal skin manifestation of tertiary syphilis is the gumma. The gumma is a scarring, locally destructive plaque, nodule, or ulcer, which is sometimes arcuate. Ulcerative gummas, particularly on the chest and calves, may appear "punched out." Gummas are not limited to the skin and can be found on the nasal septum, palate, bones, and internal organs.

Course

The primary chancre develops after an average incubation of 3 weeks and lasts for 2 to 8 weeks. Secondary syphilis develops about 6 weeks after the primary chancre appears (the chancre may still be present at this time). Secondary syphilis is the result of a disseminated infection, and, as such, it typically has systemic symptoms such as headaches, low-grade fevers, generalized lymphadenopathy, malaise, anorexia, hepatosplenomegaly, pharyngitis, and myalgias. This stage, if left untreated, spontaneously resolves in 2 to 10 weeks. Latent syphilis follows. Tertiary syphilis appears an average of 3 to 10 years after secondary syphilis in about a quarter of untreated patients, but its onset may be accelerated in immunocompromised individuals. Besides gummas, tertiary syphilis can affect the neurologic and cardiovascular systems. Neurosyphilis can occur at any stage of syphilis.

Communicability

Syphilis is primarily transmitted via direct sexual contact with a primary or secondary syphilitic lesion. Much less commonly, it spreads via nongenital contact, intravenous drug use, or transplacentally from an infected mother to her unborn child. Fomite transmission is unlikely because T. pallidum is easily killed outside of its host environment.

Diagnosis

Most cases of syphilis are diagnosed via clinical suspicion and positive serologic testing. Suspected patients are typically screened with the sensitive, but not specific, rapid plasma reagin (RPR) or Venereal Disease Research Laboratory (VDRL) tests. The RPR and VDRL tests can be negative early in a primary infection. Thus, if syphilis is suspected, these tests should be repeated weekly for a month to rule out syphilis. These tests can be falsely positive from many things including autoimmune diseases, hyperlipidemia, and pregnancy. As a result, a specific serologic test that targets treponemal antigens is used to confirm the infection. The fluorescent treponemal antibody-absorption test (FTA-ABS) and the microhemagglutination test for T. pallidum (MHA-TP) are two such tests. These specific tests, unlike the RPR and VDRL, remain positive after effective syphilis treatment. Syphilis can be diagnosed microscopically from primary and secondary syphilitic lesions, using dark field microscopy (seldom done anymore) to visualize the corkscrew-shaped organisms.

Treatment

Slow-release penicillin, penicillin G benzathine, is the treatment of choice for syphilis. Primary and secondary syphilis can be treated with a single intramuscular injection of 2.4 million units of benzathine penicillin G. Those allergic to penicillin can be treated with doxycycline 100 mg twice a day orally for 14 days, or tetracycline 500 mg orally four times daily for 14 days. An acute febrile reaction, the Jarisch–Herxheimer reaction, with chills, myalgias, increased lesional inflammation, pharyngitis, and headaches can occur within a day of starting penicillin or occasionally after other antibiotic treatments. To ensure clearance of the infection, RPR or VDRL titers should be drawn at 6 and 12 months posttreatment to document a fourfold titer decrease. Sexual partners of the patient should also be treated.

Chancroid

Chancroid is an ulcerative STI caused by the gram-negative bacterium *Haemophilus ducreyi*. Chancroid is very common in developing regions of Africa and the Caribbean. It is rare in industrialized nations, but periodic outbreaks do occur. Men are much more likely to be affected by the disease than women, by a factor of 10 to 1.

Skin Manifestations

The primary lesion is an erythematous papule, which progresses to a pustule, and then ruptures to form an ulcer. The ulcer has a friable base, serpiginous border, and a well-demarcated, undermined, hyperemic edge (Fig. 29-13). It is very painful, nonindurated, and is covered with a necrotic, typically purulent exudate. Commonly found on the prepuce and frenulum of the penis, or the vulva or cervix in women, chancroid ulcers are also found on the perineum. "Kissing lesions" can be present from autoinoculation of opposing skin surfaces. Almost half of patients develop a painful, usually unilateral, suppurative lymphadenitis (bubo) that may rupture and produce a chancrous-appearing lesion.

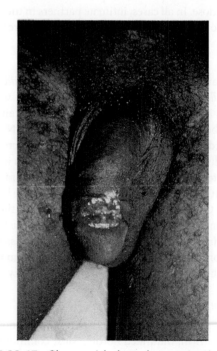

FIGURE 29-13: Chancroid ulcer demonstrating a purulent base with well-demarcated, undermined edges.

Course

The primary lesion usually appears after a 1- to 5-day incubation period. The disease is rarely asymptomatic.

Communicability

Chancroid is spread via sexual contact.

Diagnosis

There is no perfect test to diagnose chancroid; even bacterial culture on special media is only 80% sensitive. Most often, a diagnosis is made with the clinical presentation combined with the ruling out of other causes of genital ulcers, such as syphilis, herpes, and LGV. Smears of chancroid ulcers may reveal the characteristic gram-negative rods in chains, but this finding is neither specific nor sensitive. If a diagnosis of chancroid is made by culture, syphilis should still be ruled out as syphilis often coinfects chancroid ulcers.

Treatment

A single 1 g oral dose of azithromycin is the first-line treatment. Other recommended treatment options include erythromycin 500 mg orally three times daily for 7 days, ceftriaxone 250 mg IM once, or ciprofloxacin 500 mg orally twice daily for 3 days. Ciprofloxacin should be avoided in pregnant or lactating women and in children. Despite successful treatment, scarring can occur in patients with advanced disease. Sexual partners from the 10 days prior to symptom onset should be treated.

FUNGI

Candidiasis

Candida albicans is a common inhabitant of the oropharynx, the gastrointestinal tract, and the female genitalia. Vaginal candidiasis can occur following changes in the vaginal pH or weakening of the immune system. Risk factors associated with vulvovaginal candidiasis include pregnancy, diabetes, long-term use of broad-spectrum antibiotics, and use of corticosteroid medications.

Skin Manifestations

Candida spp. can cause a vulvovaginitis in females and a balanitis in uncircumcised males. Commonly, external dysuria and pruritus occur. The vulva can be erythematous, swollen, and macerated. There can be a watery to thick, cottage cheese–like vaginal discharge. The cervix can be hyperemic, swollen, and covered with small erosions and small vesicles.

Course

The lifetime prevalence of candidiasis is 75%, with over 40% of women having more than one episode. Symptoms typically worsen a week before menses. Less than 5% of women develop recurrent vulvovaginal candidiasis (RVVC), which is classified as greater than three episodes per year. Usually there are no apparent predisposing or underlying conditions for those patients who develop RVVC, but consider *Candida*

glabrata and other nonalbicans *Candida spp.* because this can be observed in 10% to 20% with RVVC.

Communicability

Most infections are merely an overgrowth of endogenous Candida, but some cases can be caused by direct mucosal contact, as in sexual intercourse.

Diagnosis

The diagnosis is made clinically with a KOH or Gram stain smear of vaginal discharge positive for budding yeast, hyphae, or pseudohyphae.

Treatment

Commonly, over-the-counter topical medications such as miconazole, nystatin, clotrimazole, and terconazole can be used as first-line agents. They are used once daily for 1 to 7 days, and it is important to note that these creams and suppositories may interfere with the effectiveness of condoms. Only topical, not oral, azoles should be used to treat pregnant women. The recommended oral option is a single 150 mg dose of fluconazole. This can be repeated in 72 hours if symptoms persist. If the patient is immunosuppressed, diabetic, or possesses other predisposing factors, a more prolonged course of fluconazole is necessary. The antifungals griseofulvin, terbinafine, and naftifine are not effective treatment options.

SAUER'S NOTES

The field of dermatology has long been considered the specialty most expert in the diagnosis of sexually transmitted diseases. In fact, the American Academy of Dermatology was formerly called "American Academy of Dermatology and Syphilology." As the cosmetic aspects of skin care have begun to replace the medical aspects, the expertise of the doctor has been waning. It is imperative that this trend be reversed for the sake of the specialty and, more importantly, for the sake of patients.

Suggested Readings

Bolognia JL, Jorizzo JL, Rapini RP. *Dermatology.* 3rd ed. Philadelphia: Elsevier Inc; 2012.

Division of Viral Hepatitis. Centers for Disease Control and Prevention. Web. Updated May 31, 2015. Accessed October, 2015.

James WD, Berger TG, Elston DM. *Andrews' Diseases of the Skin.* 10th ed. Philadelphia: Elsevier Inc; 2006.

Preexposure prophylaxis for the prevention of HIV infection in the United States – 2014. http://www.cdc.gov/hiv/pdf/prepguidelines2014.pdf. Accessed December, 2015.

Ryan KJ, Ray CG. *Sherris Medical Microbiology: An Introduction to Infectious Diseases.* 4th ed. New York: McGraw-Hill; 2004.

Sexually Transmitted Diseases. Centers for Disease Control and Prevention. Web. Updated October 28, 2015. Accessed October, 2015.

Sobel JD. Vulvovaginal candidosis. *Lancet.* 2007;369:1961–1971.

2015 Sexually Transmitted Diseases Treatment Guidelines. Centers for Disease Control and Prevention. Web. Updated October 21, 2015. Accessed October, 2015.

Tumors of the Skin

John C. Hall, MD

CLASSIFICATION

A patient comes into your office for care of a tumor on his skin. What kind is it? What is the best treatment? This complex process of diagnosing and managing skin tumors is not learned easily. As an aid to the establishment of the correct diagnosis, all skin tumors (excluding warts, which are caused by a virus) are classified

1. as to their histologic origin (Table 30-1),
2. according to the patient's age group (Table 30-2),
3. by location (Table 30-3), and
4. on the basis of clinical appearance (Table 30-4).

A complete histologic classification is found at the end of this chapter; only the more common tumors are classified and discussed here. This histologic classification is divided into

---

TABLE 30-1 • Histologic Classification of Tumors of the Skin

Epidermal Tumors

Tumors of the surface epidermis

1. *Benign tumors:* Defined as neoplasms that probably arise from arrested embryonal cells
   a. Seborrheic keratosis
   b. Pedunculated fibroma (skin tag, fibroepithelial polyp, acrochordon)
   c. Cysts
      - Epidermal cyst
      - Trichilemmal (pilar or sebaceous cyst)
      - Milium
      - Dermoid cyst
      - Mucous cyst
2. Precancerous tumors
   a. Actinic keratosis and cutaneous horn
   b. Arsenical keratosis
   c. Leukoplakia
   d. Porokeratosis
3. *Carcinoma:* squamous cell carcinoma

Tumors of the epidermal appendages

1. Basal cell carcinoma
2. Sebaceous gland hyperplasia
3. Numerous other types benign and malignant, usually classified by appendage of origin

---

Mesodermal Tumors

Tumors of fibrous tissue

1. Histiocytoma and dermatofibroma
2. Keloid

Tumors of vascular tissue

1. Hemangiomas

Nevus Cell Tumors

Nevi

1. Junctional (active) nevus
2. Intradermal (resting) nevus
3. Dysplastic nevus syndrome (familial atypical mole–melanoma syndrome or sporadic atypical mole–melanoma syndrome)

Malignant melanoma

Lymphoma and Myelosis

Monomorphous group

Polymorphous group

1. Mycosis fungoides (cutaneous T-cell lymphoma)

Source: Modified from Lever WF, Schaumberg-Lever G. *Histopathology of the Skin.* 8th ed. Philadelphia: Lippincott; 1997.

TABLE 30-2 • Age-Based Classification of Tumors of the Skin

Age Group	Possible Tumor Types[a]
Children	1. Warts (viral), very common
	2. Nevi, junctional type, common
	3. Molluscum contagiosum (viral)
	4. Hemangiomas
	5. Café-au-lait spot
	6. Granuloma pyogenicum
	7. Mongolian spot
	8. Xanthogranulomas

TABLE 30-2 • Age-Based Classification of Tumors of the Skin (continued)

Age Group	Possible Tumor Types[a]
Adults	1. Warts (viral), plantar-type common 2. Nevi 3. Cysts 4. Pedunculated fibromas (skin tags, acrochordons) 5. Sebaceous gland hyperplasias 6. Histiocytomas (dermatofibromas, sclerosing hemangiomas) 7. Keloids 8. Lipomas 9. Granuloma pyogenicum
Older Adults[b]	1. Seborrheic keratoses 2. Actinic keratoses 3. Capillary hemangiomas (cherry angiomas, senile angiomas) 4. Basal cell carcinomas 5. Squamous cell carcinomas 6. Leukoplakia

[a]The most common tumors are listed first.
[b]In addition to tumors of adults.

TABLE 30-3 • Classification of Tumors Based on Location

Location	Possible Tumor Type
Scalp	Seborrheic keratosis Epidermal cyst (pilar cyst) Nevus Actinic keratosis (bald males) Wart Trichilemmal cyst Basal cell carcinoma Squamous cell carcinoma Nevus sebaceous Proliferating trichilemmal tumor Cylindroma Syringocystadenoma papilliferum Seborrheic keratosis
Ear	Actinic keratoses Basal cell carcinoma Nevus Squamous cell carcinoma Keloid Epidermal cyst Chondrodermatitis nodularis helices Venous lakes (varix) Gouty tophus
Face	Seborrheic keratosis Sebaceous gland hyperplasia Actinic keratosis Lentigo Milium Nevi Basal cell carcinoma Squamous cell carcinoma Lentigo maligna melanoma Flat wart Trichoepithelioma Dermatosis papulosa nigra (African American women) Fibrous papule of the nose Colloid milium Dilated pore of Winer Keratoacanthoma Pyogenic granuloma Spitz nevus Ephelides Hemangioma Adenoma sebaceum Apocrine hidrocystoma Eccrine hidrocystoma Trichilemmoma Trichofolliculoma Merkel cell carcinoma Angiosarcoma (elderly men) Nevus of Ota Warty dyskeratoma Atypical fibroxanthoma Angiolymphoid hyperplasia with eosinophilia Blue nevus Pedunculated fibroma
Eyelids	Seborrheic keratosis Milium Syringomas Basal cell carcinoma Xanthoma Pedunculated fibroma
Neck	Seborrheic keratosis Epidermal cyst Keloid
Lip and Mouth	Fordyce disease Lentigo Venous lake (varix) Mucous retention cyst Leukoplakia Pyogenic granuloma Squamous cell carcinoma Granular cell tumor (tongue) Giant cell epulis (gingivae) Verrucous carcinoma White sponge nevus Acral lentiginous melanoma Pedunculated fibroma

(continued)

TABLE 30-3 • Classification of Tumors Based on Location (*continued*)

Location	Possible Tumor Type
Axilla	Epidermal cyst Molluscum contagiosum Lentigo (multiple lentigo in the axillae neurofibromatosis called Crowe sign) Seborrheic keratosis
Chest and Back	Angioma Nevi Ephelides Actinic keratosis Lipoma Basal cell carcinoma Epidermal cyst Keloid Lentigo Café-au-lait spot Squamous cell carcinoma Melanoma Hemangioma Histiocytoma Steatocystoma multiplex Eruptive vellus hair cyst Blue nevus Nevus of Ito Becker nevus Pedunculated fibroma
Groin and Crural Areas	Seborrheic keratosis Molluscum contagiosum Wart Bowen disease Extramammary Paget disease Wart
Genitalia	Molluscum contagiosum Squamous intraepithelial lesions Epidermal cyst Angiokeratoma (scrotum) Pearly penile papules (around edge of glans) Squamous cell carcinoma Seborrheic keratosis Erythroplasia of Queyrat Bowen disease Median raphe cyst of penis Verrucous carcinoma Hidradenoma papilliferum (labia majora) Wart
Hands	Seborrheic keratosis Actinic keratosis Lentigo Myxoid cyst (proximal nail fold) Squamous cell carcinoma Glomus tumor (nail bed) Ganglion

Location	Possible Tumor Type
	Common blue nevus Acral lentigines melanoma Giant cell tumor of tendon sheath Pyogenic granuloma Acquired digital fibrokeratoma Recurrent infantile digital fibroma Traumatic fibroma Xanthoma Dupuytren contracture Wart
Feet	Nevi Blue nevus Acral lentigines melanoma Seborrheic keratosis Verrucous carcinoma Eccrine poroma Seborrheic keratosis
Arms and Legs	Lentigo *Wart* *Histiocytoma* *Actinic keratosis* *Squamous cell carcinoma* *Melanoma* *Lipoma* *Xanthoma* *Clear cell acanthoma (legs)* *Kaposi sarcoma (legs, classic type)*

TABLE 30-4 • Classification of Skin Tumors Based on Clinical Appearance

Appearance	Possible Tumor Type
Flat, skin-colored tumors	1. Flat warts (viral) 2. Histiocytomas 3. Leukoplakia
Flat, pigmented tumors	1. Nevi, usually junctional type 2. Lentigo 3. Café-au-lait spot 4. Histiocytomas 5. Mongolian spot 6. Melanoma (superficial spreading type)
Raised, skin-colored tumors	1. Warts (viral) 2. Pedunculated fibromas (skin tags) 3. Nevi, usually intradermal type 4. Cysts 5. Lipomas 6. Keloids 7. Basal cell carcinomas 8. Squamous cell carcinoma 9. Molluscum contagiosum (viral) 10. Xanthogranuloma (yellowish, usually children)

TABLE 30-4 • Classification of Skin Tumors Based on Clinical Appearance (*continued*)

Appearance	Possible Tumor Type
Raised, brownish tumors	1. Warts (viral) 2. Nevi, usually compound type 3. Actinic keratoses 4. Seborrheic keratoses 5. Pedunculated fibromas (skin tags) 6. Basal cell epitheliomas 7. Squamous cell carcinoma 8. Malignant melanoma 9. Granuloma pyogenicum 10. Keratoacanthomas
Raised, reddish tumors	1. Hemangiomas 2. Actinic keratoses 3. Granuloma pyogenicum 4. Glomus tumors 5. Senile or cherry angiomas
Raised, blackish tumors	1. Seborrheic keratosis 2. Nevi 3. Granuloma pyogenicum 4. Malignant melanomas 5. Blue nevi 6. Thrombosed angiomas or hemangiomas

epidermal tumors, mesodermal tumors, nevus cell tumors, lymphomas, and myeloses. In making a clinical diagnosis of any skin tumor, one should apply a histopathologic label if possible. Whether the label is correct or not depends on the clinical acumen of the physician and on whether the tumor, or a part of it, has been examined microscopically.

An age-group classification is helpful from a differential diagnostic viewpoint. Viral warts are considered in this classification because of the frequent necessity of differentiating them from other skin tumors.

The clinical appearance of any tumor is the most important diagnostic factor. Some tumors have a characteristic color and growth that is readily distinguishable from any other tumor, but a large number, unfortunately, have clinical characteristics common to several similar tumors or are nonspecific in appearance even to the most trained observer. A further hindrance to making a correct diagnosis is that the same histopathologic lesion may vary in clinical appearance. The following generalizing classification should be helpful, but if in doubt, the lesion should be examined histologically.

SAUER'S NOTES

1. A histologic examination should be performed on every malignant skin tumor.
2. Similarly, a biopsy should be performed on any tumor when clinically a malignancy cannot be definitely ruled out.

SEBORRHEIC KERATOSES

It is a rare elderly patient who does not have any seborrheic keratoses. These are the unattractive "moles" or "warts" that perturb the elderly patient, and occasionally become irritating, but are benign (Fig. 30-1).

Dermatosis papulosa nigra is a form of seborrheic keratosis of African Americans that occurs on the face, mainly in women. These small, black, multiple tumors can be removed, but there is a possibility of causing keloids or hypopigmentation. Stucco keratoses are numerous white 1- to 3-mm seborrheic keratoses that occur mainly over the feet, ankles, and lower legs. A very large seborrheic keratosis is sometimes referred to as a *melanoacanthoma*.

Presentation and Characteristics

Description

The size of the seborrheic keratoses varies up to 3 cm for the largest, but the average diameter is 1 cm. The color may be flesh-colored, tan, brown, or coal black. They are usually oval in shape, elevated, and have a greasy, warty sensation to the touch. White, brown, or black pinhead-sized keratotic areas called *pseudohorn cysts* are commonly seen within this tumor. They have the appearance of being superficial and "stuck on" the skin. Markings on the skin may be accentuated in superficial seborrheic keratoses. Pruritus is common, and sudden appearance may occur. Numerous lesions coming on rapidly can be a marker of underlying cancer (sign of Leser–Trélat). They can suddenly appear at the site of inflamed skin (Meyerson phenomenon) and may dissipate as the inflammation is brought under control.

Distribution

The lesions appear on the face, neck, scalp, back, and upper chest, and less frequently on the arms, legs, and the lower part of the trunk. Mucous membranes, palms, and soles are spared.

Course

Lesions become darker and enlarge slowly. However, sometimes they can enlarge rapidly, and this can be accompanied by bleeding and inflammation, which can be very frightening to the patient. Trauma from clothing occasionally results in infection and bleeding, and this prompts the patient to seek medical care. Any inflammatory dermatitis around these lesions causes them to enlarge temporarily and become more evident, so much so that many patients suddenly note them for the first time. After the inflammation subsides, the seborrheic keratosis may dissipate. Malignant degeneration of seborrheic keratoses does not occur.

Cause

Heredity is the biggest factor, along with old age.

Differential Diagnosis

- *Actinic keratoses:* See Table 30-5
- *Pigmented nevi:* Longer duration, smoother surface, softer to the touch; may not be able to differentiate clinically

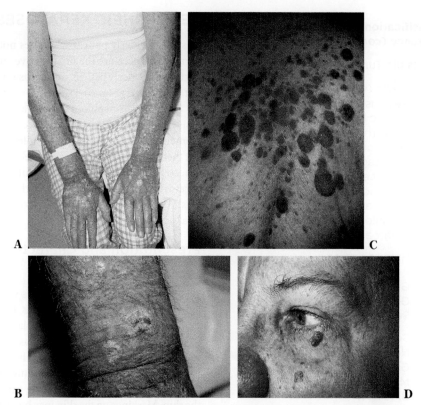

FIGURE 30-1: **A:** Actinic keratoses in an oil refinery worker. **B:** Hyperkeratotic actinic keratoses. **C:** Seborrheic keratoses on the back. **D:** Pedunculated seborrheic keratosis of the eyelid. (Courtesy of Stiefel Laboratories, Inc.)

TABLE 30-5 • Differential Diagnosis of Keratoses

Parameter	Actinic or Senile Keratosis	Seborrheic Keratosis
Appearance	Flat, brownish, reddish, or tan scale firmly attached to the skin, poorly demarcated	Greasy, elevated, brown, black, flesh-colored, warty scale and can be easily scratched away at times, "stuck on," well demarcated
Location	Sun-exposed areas	Face, back
Complexion	Blue eyes, light hair, dry skin	Brown eyes, dark hair, oily skin
Symptoms	Some burning and stinging	Occasional itching
Precancerous	Yes	No
Cause	Sun	Inherited

- *Flat warts:* In younger patients; acute onset, with rapid development of new lesions, colorless, and flat topped without pseudohorned cysts; tiny black thrombosed capillaries may be seen, usually smaller; may koebnerize (see Chapter 26)
- *Malignant melanoma:* Less common, usually with rapid growth, indurated; histologic examination with biopsy may be necessary

Treatment

Case Example: A 58-year-old woman requests the removal of a warty, tannish, slightly elevated 2 × 2 cm lesion on the right side of her forehead.

1. The lesion should be examined carefully. The diagnosis usually can be made clinically, but if there is any question, a scissor biopsy (see Chapter 2) can be performed. It would be ideal if all of these seborrheic keratoses could be examined histologically, but this is not economically feasible or necessary. If in doubt, always send for histologic examination.
2. An adequate form of therapy is curettement, with or without local anesthesia, followed by a light application of trichloroacetic acid, Monsel solution, or aluminum chloride. The resulting fine atrophic scar will hardly be noticeable in several months.
3. Electrosurgery can be used, but this usually requires anesthesia, and if the physician is not careful, it may scar.

4. If available, liquid nitrogen freezing therapy works well. It is the therapy of choice of most doctors. Do not freeze excessively.
5. Laser therapy has been used recently by some authors.
6. Surgical excision is an unnecessary and more expensive form of removal.

> ### SAUER'S NOTES
>
> 1. For many benign lesions, it often is best cosmetically to err on the side of surgical under-treatment rather than overtreatment. You can always remove any remaining growth later, but you cannot put back what you took off.
> 2. Scarring should be kept to a minimum.
> 3. After any surgical procedure, I hand out a "Surgical Notes" sheet that indicates postoperative care. Skin surgery sites usually heal without any complication. However, there are always questions and concerns from the patient about aftercare.

PEDUNCULATED FIBROMAS (SKIN TAGS, ACROCHORDONS)

Multiple skin tags are common on the neck and the axillae of middle-aged, usually obese, men and women (Fig. 30-2). The indications for removal are twofold: cosmetic, as desired and requested by the patient, and to prevent the irritation and the secondary infection of the pedicle that frequently develops from trauma of a collar, necklace, or other article of clothing. These are often inherited and may be part of the metabolic syndrome.

Presentation and Characteristics

Description

Pedunculated pinhead-sized to pea-sized soft tumors of normal skin color or light brown color are seen. The base may be inflamed from injury, and the lesion may thrombose and turn black if twisted. This can cause alarm in the patient.

Distribution

The lesions occur on the neck, axillae, submammary, or groin, or less frequently on any other area.

Course

These fibromas grow very slowly. They may increase in size during pregnancy. Some become infected or thrombosed and drop off.

Differential Diagnosis

- *Filiform wart:* Digitate projections, more horny; also seen on the chin area
- *Pedunculated seborrheic keratosis:* Larger lesion, darker color, warty, or velvety appearance (see preceding section)
- *Neurofibromatosis:* Lesions seen elsewhere; larger; can be pushed back into the skin; also café-au-lait spots; hereditary; single lesions do not indicate systemic disease (see Chapters 42 and 44)

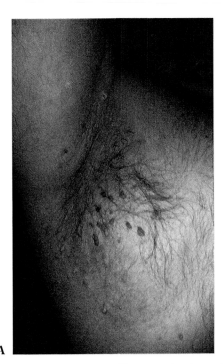
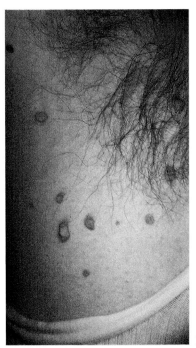

FIGURE 30-2: **A and B:** Pedunculated fibromas in the axilla. (Courtesy of Stiefel Laboratories, Inc.)

Treatment

Case Example: A 42-year-old woman has 20 small pedunculated fibromas on her neck and axillae that she wants removed. This could be done by electrosurgery. Without anesthesia, gently grab the small tumor in a thumb forceps and stretch the pedicle. Touch this pedicle with the electrosurgery needle, and turn on the current for a split second. The tumor separates from the skin and no bleeding occurs. The site heals in 4 to 7 days.

SURGICAL NOTES FOR THE PATIENT

Minor surgery has been performed for the removal or biopsy of a skin lesion.

If liquid nitrogen was used to remove the growth, a blister or peeling at the growth site will develop in 24 hours; if electrosurgery, laser, or burning was used, a crust and scab will form; if a biopsy was made, there will be a crust or suture(s).

The treated sites heal better if they are covered with a dressing with polysporin ointment underneath during the day for 5 to 7 days and left uncovered at night and while bathing. Do not pick at the spot, and try to avoid accidentally hitting the area.

You can wash over the area lightly.

A certain amount of redness and swelling around the surgery site is to be expected. Moreover, you might have a small amount of drainage and crusting. A mild amount of redness and infection can be treated with polysporin ointment locally three times a day.

If more drainage or infection develops, apply a wet dressing with sheeting, or soak the area. Oral antibiotics can be given. Use a solution made with 1 teaspoon of salt to 1 pint of cool water or Domeboro compresses, and apply for 20 minutes three times a day. Make a fresh solution every day.

If the infection becomes excessive, call the office or go to a hospital emergency department.

If the scab is knocked off prematurely, bleeding may occur. This can be stopped by applying firm pressure with gauze or cotton for 10 minutes by the clock, and then releasing pressure gradually.

Depending on the size of the surgery site, healing takes from 1 to 8 weeks. Some scarring or loss of pigment at the surgery site is possible. A few individuals have a tendency to form thick or keloidal scars, which is not predictable.

If a biopsy was done, you may receive a separate bill for the pathology study from the laboratory. Call the office in 7 days for this report.

Return to the office for further care or follow-up as directed.

For very small lesions, a short spark with the electrosurgical needle suffices. Scissor excision with or without local anesthetic is commonly done.

CYSTS

The three common types are

- epidermoid (epidermal inclusion) cyst,
- trichilemmal (pilar) or sebaceous cyst, and
- milium.

An *epidermal cyst* (Fig. 30-3A and B) has a wall composed of true epidermis and probably originates from an invagination of the epidermis into the dermis and subsequent detachment from the epidermis, or it can originate spontaneously. The most common locations for epidermal cysts are the face, ears, neck, back, and scalp, where tumors of varying size can be found. A central pore may be seen over the surface. There may be a history of drainage of foul-smelling, cheesy debris.

Trichilemmal cysts, formerly known as *wens* and *pilar* or *sebaceous cysts* (Fig. 30-3C), are less common than epidermal cysts, occur mainly on the scalp, usually are multiple, and show an autosomal dominant inheritance. The sac wall is thick, smooth, and whitish and can be quite easily enucleated.

Milia (Fig. 30-3D) are very common, white, pinhead-sized, firm lesions that are seen on the face. They are formed by proliferation of epithelial buds following trauma to the skin (dermabrasion for acne scars), following certain dermatoses (pemphigus, epidermolysis bullosa, and acute contact dermatitis), or from no apparent cause. Occurrences with porphyria cutanea tarda, after 5-fluorouracil therapy, in areas of corticosteroid-induced atrophy, after burns, and after radiation therapy are other causes.

They can occur spontaneously at any age including newborns where they may dissipate. Treatment consists of opening the lesion with a No. 11 Bard Parker blade and expression with a comedone extractor. This is done for cosmetic reasons only.

Differential Diagnosis of Epidermal and Trichilemmal Cysts

- *Lipoma:* Difficult to differentiate clinically; more firm, no central pore, lobulated; no cheesy material extrudes on incision; removal is by complete excision or by liposuction; clinically similar to hibernoma
- *Dermoid cyst:* Clinically similar; can also be found internally; usually a solitary skin tumor; histologically, contains hairs, eccrine glands, and sebaceous glands
- *Mucous cysts* (Fig. 30-4): Translucent pea-sized or smaller lesions on the lips, treated by cutting off the top of the lesion and carefully, lightly cauterizing the base with a silver nitrate stick or light electrosurgery; laser therapy can also be used
- *Synovial cysts (myxoid cysts) of the skin* (Fig. 30-5): Globoid, translucent, pea-sized swellings around the joints of fingers and toes that drain a syrupy clear liquid and are most common at the base of the nail on the proximal nail fold

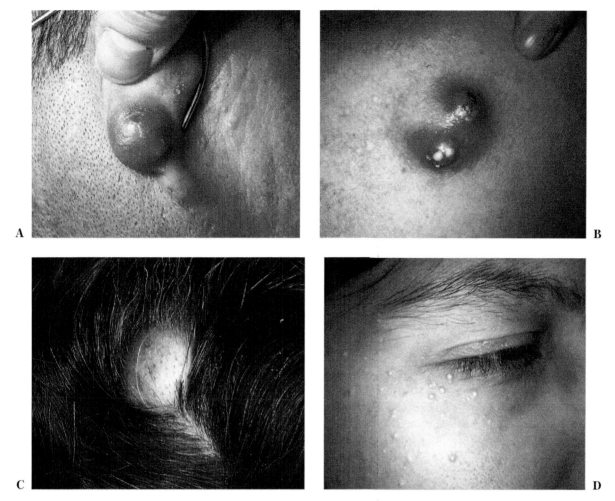

FIGURE 30-3: **A:** Epidermal cyst of the earlobe. **B:** Infected epidermal cyst on the shoulder. **C:** Pilar or sebaceous cyst of the scalp. **D:** Milia on the upper cheek of a 21-year-old woman. (Courtesy of Texas Pharmacal.)

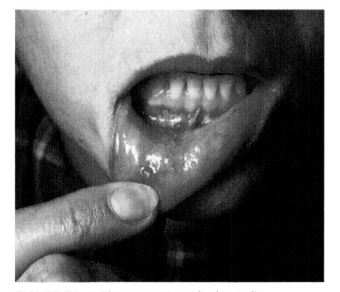

FIGURE 30-4: Mucous cyst on the lower lip. (Courtesy of Texas Pharmacal)

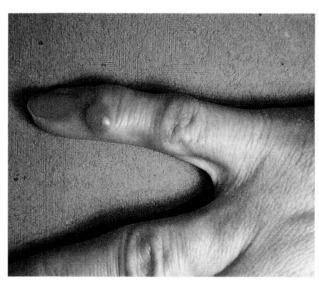

FIGURE 30-5: Synovial cyst on the finger. (Courtesy of Texas Pharmacal)

Treatment of Epidermal and Trichilemmal Cysts

Several methods can be used with success. The choice depends on the ability of the operator, the site, and the number of cysts. Cysts can regrow after even the best surgical care because of incomplete removal of the sac.

1. A single 3-cm cyst on the back should be removed by surgical excision and suturing. This can be done in two ways: either by incising the skin and skillfully removing the intact cyst sac with an ellipse excision or by cutting straight into the sac with a small incision, shelling out the evacuated lining by applying strong pressure to the sides of the incision, and suturing the skin. The latter procedure is simpler, requires a smaller incision, and is quite successful.
2. A patient with several cysts on the scalp can be treated in another simple way. A 3- to 4-mm incision can be made directly over and into the cyst. The cheesy, foul-smelling contents can be evacuated by pressure and the use of a small curette. The sac can then be popped out of the hole with very firm pressure, or the sac can be grasped with a small hemostat and pulled out of the opening. No suturing, or only a single suture, is necessary. The resulting scar is imperceptible after a short time.
3. If, during incision by any technique, a solid tumor is found instead of a cyst, the lesion should be excised completely and the material studied histologically. This diagnostic error is common because of the clinical similarity of cysts, lipomas, and other related tumors.

Treatment of Milia

1. Simple incision of the small tumors with a scalpel or a Hagedorn needle and expression of the contents by a comedone extractor is sufficient.
2. Another procedure is to remove the top of the milia lightly with electrodesiccation.
3. An 11 Bard Parker blade can be used to open the top, and then an acne stylette can be used to express the contents.

PRECANCEROUS TUMORS

Precancerous types of tumors include actinic keratoses, cutaneous horns, arsenical keratoses, and leukoplakia.

> **SAUER'S NOTES**
>
> 1. Patients with actinic keratoses should be advised to return every 6 to 12 months for examination; this is especially important if they have extensive actinic damage.
> 2. All patients with actinic keratoses should be told to use a sunscreen lotion or cream to lessen the occurrence of future keratoses. Patients should be advised to wear protective clothing and to avoid exposure to sun between 10:00 AM and 4:00 PM.

Actinic Keratosis

Actinic keratosis is a common skin lesion of light-complexioned older persons that occurs on the skin surfaces exposed to sunlight (Fig. 30-6). A small percentage of these lesions develop into squamous cell carcinomas (approximately 5% to 10%). Because of the popularity of sunbathing and the use of sun-tanning salons, these lesions (probably 5% to 10%) are also seen in persons in the 30- to 50-year-old age group.

Description

Lesions are usually multiple, flat or slightly elevated, pink, brownish or tan colored, scaly and adherent, measuring up to 1.5 cm in diameter, and often arising on an ill-defined pink base (Fig. 30-7). There is a dark variant called a superficial pigmented actinic keratosis (SPAK). Individual lesions may become confluent. A *cutaneous horn* may be a proliferative, hyperkeratotic form of actinic keratosis that resembles a horn (Fig. 30-8). A cutaneous horn can also originate from a seborrheic keratosis, wart, squamous cell carcinoma, keratotic basal cell carcinoma, keratoacanthoma, and, most commonly, an actinic keratosis. If a biopsy is done, enough of the base of the lesion must be removed to obtain an accurate histologic diagnosis.

Distribution

Areas of skin exposed to sunlight, such as the face, ears, neck, extensor forearms, lower legs distal to the knees, and dorsum of the hands, are involved.

Course

The lesion begins as a faint red, slightly scaly patch that enlarges slowly, peripherally, and deeply, over many years. Early actinic keratoses may come and go but do not dissipate completely. A sudden spurt of growth, increased thickness, or surrounding induration could indicate a change to a squamous cell carcinoma.

Subjective Symptoms

Patients often complain that these lesions are sensitive or that they burn and sting.

Cause

Heredity and sun exposure are the two main causative factors. The blue-eyed, thin-skinned, light-haired person with a family history of such lesions is the best subject for multiple actinic keratoses.

Sex Incidence

The disorder is most commonly seen in men.

Differential Diagnosis

- *Seborrheic keratosis:* See Table 30-5
- *Squamous cell carcinoma:* Any thickened lesion that has grown rapidly should undergo biopsy. This needs to be done since squamous cell cancers are protean in clinical appearance and the only change may be the increase in size.

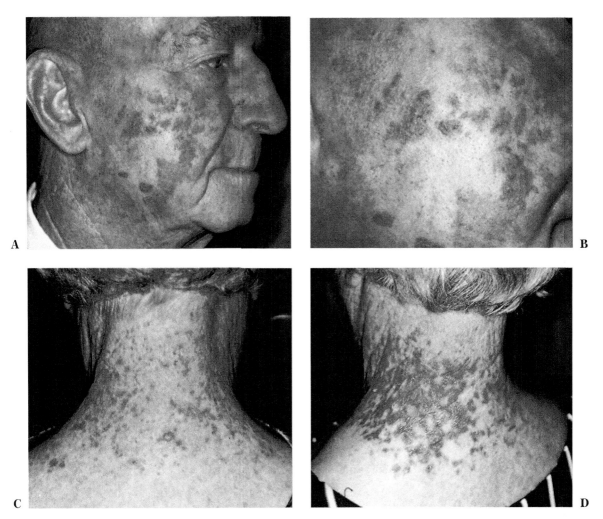

FIGURE 30-6: Actinic keratoses. **A:** Multiple actinic keratoses on the face of an 80-year-old, fair-complexioned farmer. **B:** Closeup. **C:** Actinic keratoses of the back of the neck showing lesions before therapy. **D:** Normal accentuation after therapy with 5-fluorouracil for 2 weeks. (Courtesy of Dermik Laboratories, Inc., and Owen Laboratories, Inc.)

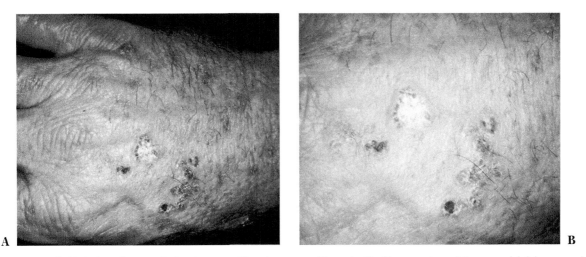

FIGURE 30-7: Actinic keratoses. **A:** Lesions on the dorsum of hands. **B:** Closeup in a 44-year-old, blue-eyed outdoor worker. (Courtesy of Dermik Laboratories, Inc. and Owen Laboratories, Inc.)

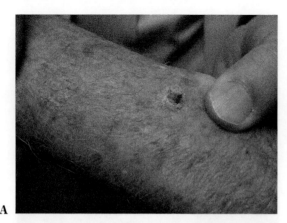
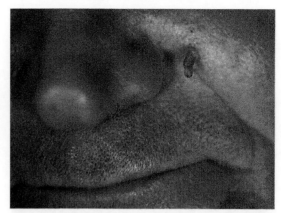

A   B

FIGURE 30-8: A: Cutaneous horn on sun-damaged forearm. A deep biopsy under the horn showed a squamous cell cancer. Notice the spread of scale at the base of tumor. **B:** Cutaneous horn on the left nasolabial area with some surrounding erythema that indicates an underlying basal cancer on biopsy. (Courtesy of Texas Pharmacal and Syntex Laboratories, Inc.)

- *Arsenical keratosis:* Mainly on the palms and soles; history of arsenic ingestion
- *Porokeratosis:* Mainly on the legs in women; threadlike keratotic border (cornoid lamellae) that sharply demarcates tumor from surrounding skin

Treatment

Case Example: A 60-year-old farmer has three small actinic keratoses on his face. The lesions should be examined carefully. If there is any evidence of induration or marked inflammation, the lesion should undergo biopsy (see Chapter 2). There are two methods of removal of these keratoses. For a single lesion, or only three or four lesions, a one-visit surgical treatment is usually preferable, especially if the lesion is relatively thick.

Surgical Method: Liquid nitrogen, if available, applied very lightly to the lesion is an effective and rapid method of removal. This is the therapy of choice of doctors.

Curettement, followed by destruction of the base by acid or electrosurgery, is satisfactory. Local anesthesia is usually necessary. Firmly scrape the lesion with the dermal curette, which removes the mushy, scaly keratosis and exposes the more fibrous normal skin. Experience provides the necessary "feel" of abnormal versus normal tissue. Some of the bleeding can be controlled by pressure or use of either one of the two following procedures:

1. Application with a cotton-tipped applicator of a saturated solution of trichloroacetic acid, aluminum chloride solution, or Monsel solution cautiously to the bleeding site; or
2. Electrocoagulation of the bleeding base.

Small lesions heal in 7 to 14 days. No bandage is required. Laser is also an acceptable form of therapy used by some doctors.

Solareze Method: Apply a thin coat over the area of involvement twice a day for 3 months. There is not as much irritation as fluorouracil and imiquimod.

Fluorouracil Method: For the patient with multiple superficial actinic keratoses, fluorouracil therapy is effective and eliminates for some months or years the early damaged epidermal cells. Thus, this fluorouracil therapy is really a cancer-prevention routine.

Three preparations available are as follows:

Fluoroplex 1% solution, or cream 30.0 used as below for Efudex
Efudex 2% solution or Efudex 5% cream 10.0

    Sig: Apply with fingers twice a day to the area to be treated

    Comment: It is wise to treat only a small area on the face at a time. Give instructions carefully, and warn the patient that it is natural for the skin to get quite red and irritated and sore after 4 to 5 days. The most common method of therapy in the past was a thin coat twice a day for 2 weeks. Some patients must stop therapy sooner, and some need more time to get the desired effect.

After completion of the course of therapy, the skin usually heals rapidly. A corticosteroid cream may be prescribed to hasten healing.

Another form of administration of fluorouracil is the pulse method. Here, the medication is applied twice a day for only 2 to 4 consecutive days of each week, for a total duration of 3 or 4 months of therapy; or another example is each night Mon–Wed–Fri for approximately 3 months.

This therapy may have to be repeated in several months or years. If some keratoses are too thick to be removed by this fluorouracil method, then the liquid nitrogen or surgical method, as described, is indicated for these lesions.

Carac (0.5%) Cream used as described previously for Efudex.

Aldara (Imiquimod) Method: This can be used twice a day for 2 weeks or as a pulse therapy three times a week for 3 months. Unlike fluorouracil therapy, it does not cause a more severe reaction in the sun, but topical steroids probably should not be used to lessen the reaction because they may decrease the benefit. Basal cancers and superficial squamous cell carcinomas can also be destroyed with imiquimod.

Retinoic Acid Preparations: These may treat early actinic keratoses, but their main efficacy has been shown to be as a preventative in a thin coat at night. There are many preparations that can be applied as a thin coat each night. Irritation can be a problem, but with time the skin may become more tolerant. Tazorac (tazarotene) is a similar topical retinoid preparation that may be even more effective, but irritation may be more severe.

Photodynamic therapy (PDT): PDT is very effective and is done in the office, so worry about patient compliance is not a problem. The skin is painted with a photosensitizer and light of appropriate wavelength is used to activate the photosensitized. The reaction can be moderately severe. It helps to treat basal cell cancers and squamous cell cancers as well as actinic keratosis.

Treatment of a Cutaneous Horn

The same surgical technique as for actinic keratosis is used. To rule out cancer, most cutaneous horns should be sent with an intact base for histopathologic examination.

Arsenical Keratosis

Prolonged ingestion of inorganic arsenic (e.g., Fowler solution, Asiatic pills, well water that is high in arsenic) can result, many years later, in the formation of small, punctate keratotic lesions, mainly seen on the palms and the soles. Progression to a squamous cell carcinoma can occur but is unusual. These patients have an increased risk of underlying solid tumor malignancies.

Treatment

Small arsenical keratoses can be removed by electrosurgery; larger lesions can be excised and skin grafted if necessary.

Leukoplakia

Leukoplakia is an actinic keratosis of the mucous membrane (Fig. 30-9). A more general use of the term leukoplakia is any white mucous membrane plaque.

Description

A flat, whitish plaque occurs localized to the mucous membranes of the lips, mouth, vulva, and vagina. Single or multiple lesions may be present.

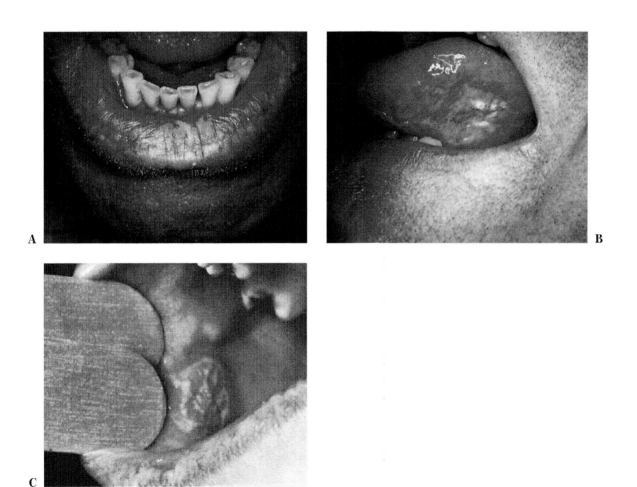

FIGURE 30-9: **A:** Leukoplakia on the lower lip, mild. **B:** Leukoplakia on the tongue, from chronic biting. **C:** Biopsy-proven leukoplakia on the mucous membrane of the cheek. This was erroneously diagnosed, clinically, as lichen planus. (Courtesy of Westwood Pharmaceuticals.)

Course

Progression to squamous cell carcinoma occurs in 20% to 30% of chronic cases. Squamous cell cancer of the mucous membrane is more aggressive with 40% to 50% metastasis versus only 4% to 5% on the skin.

Cause

Smoking, sunlight, ethanol ingestion, chewing tobacco, snuff, and chronic irritation are the important factors in the development of leukoplakia. Recurrent actinic cheilitis may precede leukoplakia of the lips. The vulvar form may develop from presenile or senile atrophy of this area.

Differential Diagnosis

- *Lichen planus:* A lacy network of whitish lesions, mainly on the sides of the buccal cavity; when on lips, it may clinically resemble leukoplakia; lichen planus elsewhere on the body (see Chapter 17); biopsy is often indicated; ulcerative lichen planus in the oral mucous membranes may have an increased risk of squamous cell carcinoma
- *Pressure calluses* from teeth or dentures: Evidence of irritation; differentiation may be possible only by biopsy
- On the vulva, *lichen sclerosus et atrophicus* or *kraurosis vulvae:* No induration, as in leukoplakia of this area; can extend onto skin of the inguinal folds and perianal region; pruritus may or may not be present and can be severe with dyspareunia; biopsy is helpful; up to 5% of lichen sclerosis et atrophicus may develop a squamous cell cancer
- Oral lichen simplex chronicus (benign alveolar ridge keratosis) is believed by some authors to be a distinct clinicopathologic entity, which, unlike leukoplakia, is without cancer potential. It occurs more commonly in males on the attached gingival mucosa, especially retromolar and on the alveolar ridge. Histologically and clinically, it mimics lichen simplex chronicus in the skin.

Treatment

Case Example: Small patch of leukoplakia is seen on the lower lip of a man who smokes considerably.

1. The lesion should be examined carefully. A biopsy should be performed on any questionable area that shows inflammation and induration. If a squamous cell carcinoma is present, the patient should receive surgical or radiation therapy by a physician who is an expert in this form of treatment.
2. The patient should be advised against use of tobacco products. The seriousness of continued smoking or other use of tobacco must be pointed out to the patient. Many early cases of leukoplakia disappear when smoking is stopped.
3. Any chronic irritation from teeth or dentures should be eliminated.
4. The lips must be protected from sunlight with a sunscreen stick.
5. Electrosurgery, preceded by local anesthesia, is excellent for small, persistent areas of leukoplakia. The coagulating current is effective. Healing is usually rapid. Laser therapy or a surgical lip shave are used by some doctors.
6. Liquid nitrogen freezing is also effective.

EPITHELIOMAS AND CARCINOMAS

Basal Cell Carcinoma

See Chapter 31 for discussion.

Squamous Cell Carcinoma

See Chapter 31 for discussion.

HISTIOCYTOMA AND DERMATOFIBROMA

Histiocytomas and dermatofibromas are common, usually single, flat, or only slightly elevated, tannish, reddish, or brownish nodules, less than l cm in size that occur mainly on the extremities (Fig. 30-10). These tumors have a characteristic clinical appearance and firm buttonlike feel that establishes the diagnosis. They often dimple when firm pressure is applied from both sides. They occur in adults and are usually asymptomatic and unchanging.

The histologic picture varies with the age of the lesion. The younger lesions are called *histiocytomas and are quite cellular;* the older ones *dermatofibromas and are more fibrous.* If the nodule contains many blood vessels, it is histologically labeled as a *sclerosing hemangioma.* It is thought to possibly be a scarlike reaction to an insect bite.

Differential Diagnosis

Fibrosarcoma: Active growth with invasion of subcutaneous fat; any questionable lesions should be excised and examined histologically

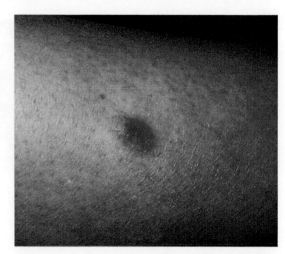

FIGURE 30-10: Histiocytoma, on the leg. Very firm and indents upon squeezing. (Courtesy of Syntex Laboratories, Inc.)

Treatment

No treatment is indicated. If there is any doubt as to the diagnosis, surgical excision and histologic examination are indicated.

For the female patient who shaves her legs and hits this lesion, liquid nitrogen applied to the papule flattens it, and excision with an ellipse or a punch eliminates it.

KELOID

A keloid is a tumor resulting from an abnormal overgrowth of fibrous tissue following injury in certain predisposed persons (Fig. 30-11). Unusual configurations can occur, depending on the site, extent, and variety of the trauma. This tendency occurs so commonly in African Americans that one should think twice before attempting a cosmetic procedure on a dark-skinned person or on any other person with a history of keloids. The back and the upper chest areas are especially prone to this proliferation. They may be tender and painful, especially on the chest after coronary artery bypass surgery.

Differential Diagnosis

- *Hypertrophic scar:* Initially, the same clinically and histologically as a keloid; flattens spontaneously in most cases after one or several years and does not extend beyond the original site of trauma

Treatment

Therapy is unsatisfactory. Intralesional corticosteroids after cryospray or massaging with a corticosteroid ointment for 60 seconds daily after bath or shower can be tried. Occasionally, combined procedures using excision or laser and intralesional corticosteroid injections or interferon α-2b (Intron A) injections have been successful. Silicone sheeting therapy has its advocates. Excision should be done cautiously because recurrence of a larger tumor may occur. If removal is done, intralesional corticosteroids should be used to attempt to prevent a recurrence. Radiation therapy has its proponents.

> **SAUER'S NOTES**
>
> Before any surgical procedure, the patient should be warned that a hypertrophic scar or keloid could follow the procedure. This is especially frequent following surgery on the chest or upper back.

HEMANGIOMAS

Spider Hemangioma

A spider hemangioma consists of a small pinpoint- to pinhead-sized central red arteriole with radiating smaller vessels like the spokes of a wheel or the legs of a spider (Fig. 30-12). On diascopy, they dissipate and rapidly refill from the center. These lesions develop for no apparent reason or may develop in association with pregnancy or in chronic liver disease when very numerous on the upper trunk. The most common location is on the face. The reason for removal is cosmetic. In younger children, they may spontaneously disappear.

Differential Diagnosis

- *Venous stars:* Small, bluish, telangiectatic veins, usually seen on the legs and the face but may appear anywhere on the body; these can be removed, if desired, by the same method as for spider hemangioma
- *Hereditary hemorrhagic telangiectasis* (Osler–Weber–Rendu disease): Small, red lesions on any organ of the body that can hemorrhage and are numerous on the lips and oral mucous membranes as well as far into the gastrointestinal tract; family history should be obtained

Treatment

Case Example: A spider hemangioma is present on the cheek of a young woman who is 6 months postpartum. This lesion developed during her pregnancy and has persisted unchanged.

Electrosurgery or laser is the treatment of choice. The fine epilating needle is used with either a very low coagulating

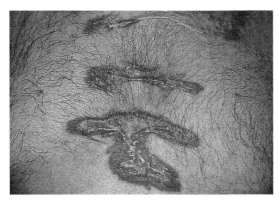

FIGURE 30-11: Keloids on the chest (common).

FIGURE 30-12: Two spider hemangiomas on the arm of a pregnant woman.

sparking current or a low cutting current. The needle is stuck into the central vessel and the current turned on for 1 or 2 seconds until the vessel blanches. No anesthetic is necessary in most patients. The area forms a scab and heals in about 4 days, leaving an imperceptible scar. Rarely, a second treatment is necessary to eliminate the central vessel. If the radiating vessels are large and persistent, they can be treated in the same manner as the central vessel. For laser therapy, see Chapter 5.

Venous Lake (Varix)

Another vascular lesion that occurs in older persons is a *venous lake*. Clinically, it is a soft, compressible, flat or slightly elevated, bluish-red, 3- to 6-mm lesion, usually located on the lips or the ears. The color decreases on diascopy. Lack of induration and rapid growth distinguish it from a melanoma. Lack of pulsation distinguishes a venous lake on the lower lip from a tortuous segment of the inferior labial artery.

Treatment is usually not desired, only reassurance concerning its nonmalignant nature.

Angiokeratomas

Three forms of angiokeratoma are known:

The Mibelli form occurs on the dorsa of the fingers, the toes, and the knees;
The Fabry form occurs over the entire trunk in an extensive pattern; and
the Fordyce form occurs on the scrotum.

The lesions are dark-red, pinhead-sized papules with a somewhat warty appearance. Treatment or further workup is not indicated for the Mibelli form and the Fordyce form. The Fabry form (angiokeratoma corporis diffusum), however, is the cutaneous manifestation of a systemic phospholipid storage disease (fucosidosis) in which phospholipids are deposited in the skin, as well as in various internal organs. Death usually occurs in the fifth decade as a result of such deposits in the smooth muscles of the blood vessels, in the heart, and in the kidneys (see Chapter 42). Renal transplantation may be curative.

NEVUS CELL TUMORS

Nevus cell tumors can be classified as melanocytic nevi or as malignant melanoma. Nevi, in turn, are classified as

- Junctional or active nevus
- Intradermal or resting nevus
- Compound nevus (components of both junctional nevus manifested by color and intradermal nevus manifested by elevation)
- Dysplastic nevus syndrome (BK mole syndrome, FAMM [familial atypical malignant melanoma mole syndrome], SAMM [sporadic atypical malignant melanoma mole syndrome])

Nevi are discussed here, but malignant melanoma is discussed separately in Chapter 32.

Melanocytic Nevi

Nevi are pigmented or nonpigmented tumors of the skin that contain nevus cells (Fig. 30-13). Nevi are present on every adult, but some persons have more than others. There are two main questions concerning nevi or moles: When and how should they be removed, and what is the relationship between nevi and malignant melanomas?

Histologically, it is possible to divide benign nevi into *junctional (active nevi)* and *intradermal (resting nevi)*. Combinations of these two forms commonly exist and are labeled as *compound nevi*.

In the dysplastic nevus syndrome (FAMM when a positive family history and SAMM when no family history), the nevi are more numerous and larger than ordinary (usually 5 to 15 mm in size), have an irregular border, and show a haphazard mixture of tan, brown, pink, and black. There is a propensity when this type of nevus is present, especially when familial, for these patients to develop a malignant melanoma.

Clinically, one can never be certain with which histopathologic type of nevus one is dealing, but certain criteria are helpful in establishing a differentiation between the forms.

Description

Clinically, nevi can be pigmented or nonpigmented, flat or elevated, hairy or nonhairy, warty, papillomatous, or pedunculated. They can have a small or a wide base. The brown- or black-pigmented, flat or slightly elevated, nonhairy nevi are usually junctional nevi. The nonpigmented or pigmented, elevated, hairy nevi are more likely to be the intradermal nevi.

A nevus with a depigmented area surrounding it is called a *halo nevus, Sutton nevus,* or *leukoderma acquisitum centrifugum.* The nevus in the center of the halo that histologically has an inflammatory infiltrate around it usually involutes in several months in contradistinction to the rarer noninflammatory halo nevus, which may not involute. Excision of the halo nevus is usually not indicated unless the central nevus has the appearance of melanoma.

Distribution

Nevi are very prevalent on the head and the neck but may appear on any part of the body. The nevi on the palms, the soles, and the genitalia are usually junctional nevi.

Course

A child is born with no, or relatively few, nevi, but with increasing age, particularly after puberty, nevi slowly become larger, can remain flat or become elevated, and may become hairy and darker. A change is also seen histologically with age. A junctional type active nevus, although it may remain as such throughout the life of the person, more commonly changes slowly into an intradermal or resting nevus. Some nevi do not appear until adult or later life, but the precursor cells for the nevus were present at birth. A malignant melanoma can originate from a junctional nevus, compound nevus, very rarely an intradermal nevus, and from dysplastic

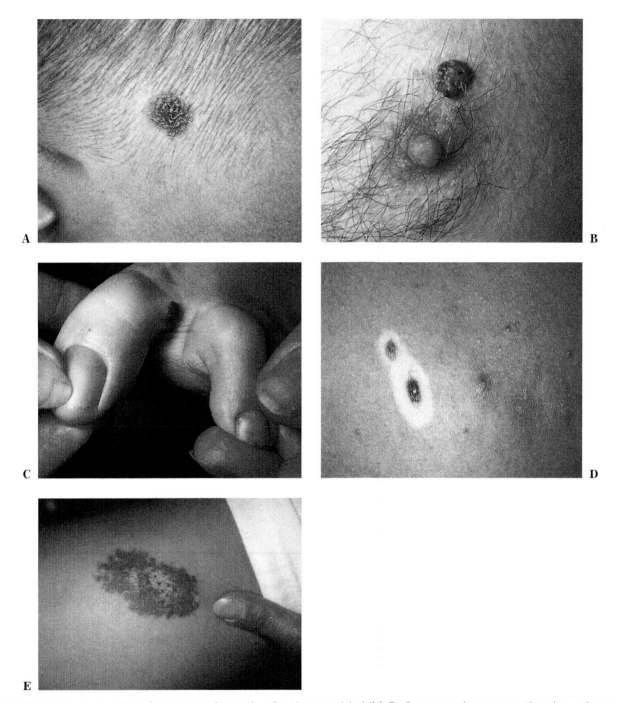

FIGURE 30-13: **A:** Junctional nevus on the scalp of a 12-year-old child. **B:** Compound nevus, on the chest above the nipple. **C:** Junctional nevus on the web of the toe of an 8-year-old child. **D:** Halo nevus, or leukoderma acquisitum centrifugum, on the back. **E:** Giant pigmented nevus on the thigh. (Courtesy of the Upjohn Company.)

nevi, particularly in relationship to ultraviolet exposure. Most melanomas arise de novo. A benign junctional nevus in a child can histologically look like a malignant melanoma. Known as a *Spitz nevus (spindle cell nevus)*, this poses a difficult diagnostic and management problem. It is usually a dome-shaped, reddish-brown tumor and rarely can occur in adults. It is histologically very difficult to distinguish from a melanoma. It is good to consult a dermatopathologist for a first or second opinion and always consider a second opinion.

Strong p16 staining seen in Spitz nevi as well as lack of mitoses and low Ki-67 index may also help in differentiating a Spitz nevus from a spitzoid melanoma. They can sometime fall into a group of tumors called METLUMP (melanocytic tumors of uncertain malignant potential). This group of tumors causes an upset stomach and headache in dermatopathologists due to difficulty to determine cancer risk.

There are three rare forms: zosteriform, agminated, and eruptive disseminated.

Some experts believe there is a subgroup of Spitz nevi that can metastasize locally to lymph node basins, although they do not extend beyond the regional lymph node basin and do not prove fatal. These are sometimes referred to as atypical Spitz tumors.

In the following patients with nevi, the most important group to follow is those who are over 50 years of age with a personal history of skin cancer or a family history of melanoma. This group of patients is most likely to have a melanoma diagnosed by physician surveillance.

Histogenesis

The origin of the nevus cell is disputed, but the most commonly accepted theory is that it originates from melanocytes.

Differential Diagnosis

In Childhood

- *Warts:* Flat or common warts not on the hands or the feet may be difficult to differentiate clinically; should see warty growth with black "seeds" (clotted capillary loops), rather acute onset, and rapid growth (see Chapter 26)
- *Freckles:* On exposed areas of the body; many lesions; fade in winter; not raised
- *Blue nevus:* Flat or elevated, soft, dark bluish, steel gray or black nodule; usually solitary but may be multiple and eruptive in nature in response to puberty, pregnancy, or sunburn
- *Granuloma pyogenicum:* Rapid onset of reddish or blackish vascular tumor, usually at the site of an injury and often with a history of bleeding
- *Molluscum contagiosum:* One, or usually more, crater-shaped, waxy tumors (see Chapter 26)
- *Urticaria pigmentosa:* Single, or multiple slightly elevated, yellowish to brown papules that urticate with trauma (Darier sign) (see Chapter 45)

In Adulthood

- *Warts:* Usually rather obvious; black "seeds"
- *Pedunculated fibromas:* On the neck and axillae
- *Histiocytoma* (sclerosing hemangioma and dermatofibroma are other names used) (see Fig. 30-10): On the extremities; flat, buttonlike in consistency (see earlier in this chapter) that indents upon squeezing

Other epidermal and mesodermal tumors are differentiated histologically.

In Older Adults

- *Actinic or senile keratosis:* On exposed areas; scaly surrounding pink skin usually thin and dry; not a sharply demarcated lesion (see earlier in this chapter)
- *Seborrheic keratosis:* Greasy, waxy, warty tumor, "stuck on" the skin; white, brown, or black dots (pseudo-horned cysts); however, some are difficult to differentiate clinically from nevus or malignant melanoma (see earlier in this chapter)

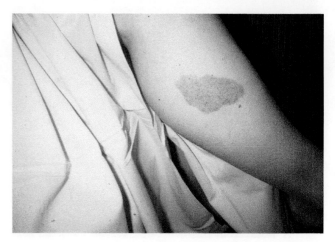

FIGURE 30-14: See dictionary index. Macular hyperpigmentation on the calf studded with darker small macules is typical for a nevus spilus (speckled lentiginous nevus).

- *Nevus spilus* (speckled lentiginous nevus): A light brownish gray oval lentigo 2 to 6 cm in size is speckled with nevi. Not present at birth. Malignant melanoma formation is very rare but has been reported. Attempt to evaluate each nevi individually and watch for any changes (see Fig 30-14)
- *Lentigo:* Flat, tan, or brown spot, usually on exposed skin surface, sometimes appears as a small splotchy splash of flat black color (solar ink-spot lentigo)
- *Malignant melanoma:* Seen at the site of a junction nevus or can arise from skin that appears normal, shows a change in pigmentation either by spreading, becoming spotty, or turning darker; may bleed, form a crust, or ulcerate (see Chapter 32)
- *Basal cell and squamous cell carcinomas:* If there is any doubt of malignancy, a biopsy is indicated (see earlier in this chapter)

Treatment

Case Example 1: A mother comes into your office with her 5-year-old son, who has an 8 × 8-mm flat, brown nevus on the forehead. She wants to know if this "mole" is dangerous and if it should be removed.

1. Examine the lesion carefully. This lesion shows no sign of recent growth or change in pigmentation. (If it did, it should be excised and examined histologically.)
2. Reassure the mother that this mole does not appear to be dangerous and that it would be unusual for it to become dangerous. If any change in the color or growth appears, the lesion should be examined again.
3. Tell the mother that it is best to leave the nevus alone at this time. The only treatment would be surgical excision, and you are quite sure that her boy would not sit still for this procedure unless he was given a general anesthetic. When the boy is 10 years of age or older, the lesion can

be examined again and possibly removed at that time by a simpler method under local anesthesia.

Case Example 2: A 25-year-old woman desires a brown, raised, hairy nevus on her upper lip removed. There has been no recent change in the tumor.

1. Examine the lesion carefully for induration, scaling, ulceration, and bleeding. None of these signs are present. (If the diagnosis is not definite, a scissor biopsy may be performed safely and the base gently coagulated by electrosurgery or Monsel solution applied. Further treatment depends on the biopsy report.)
2. Tell the patient that you can perform a biopsy and remove the mole safely but that there will be a residual, very slightly depressed scar and that probably the hairs will have to be removed separately after the first surgery has healed.
3. Surgical excision with tissue examination is the best method of removal. However, hairy, raised, pigmented nevi have been removed by shave excision with biopsy for years with no proof that this form of removal has caused a malignant melanoma.
4. First, following local anesthesia, perform a shave biopsy. Then electrosurgery can be done with the coagulating or cutting current or with cautery or applying aluminum chloride or Monsel solution. The site should not be covered and will heal in 7 to 14 days, depending on the size. If the hairs regrow, they can be removed later by electrosurgical epilation or laser (see Chapter 6).

SAUER'S NOTES

Dos and Don'ts Regarding Nevi

1. Do not remove a nevus in a child by destructive methods. Remove only by surgical excision and submit nevus for histopathologic examination.
2. Do remember that in a child a benign junctional nevus may resemble a malignant melanoma histologically (Spitz nevus). Do not alarm the parents unnecessarily, because these nevi are no threat to life. A second pathology opinion can be helpful in equivocal cases.
3. Do not perform a radical deforming surgical procedure on a possible malignant melanoma until the biopsy report has been returned. Many of these tumors can turn out to be seborrheic keratoses, granuloma pyogenicum, and so on.

MALIGNANT MELANOMA

See Chapter 32 for discussion.

LYMPHOMAS

See Table 30-6. Also see Chapter 34 for discussion.

TABLE 30-6 • WHO-EORTC Classification

Cutaneous T-cell lymphoma
  Indolent clinical behavior
        Mycosis fungoides
        Folliculotropic MF
        Pagetoid reticulosis
        Granulomatous slack skin
        Primary cutaneous anaplastic large cell lymphoma
        Lymphomatoid papulosis
        Subcutaneous panniculitis-like T-cell lymphoma
        Primary cutaneous CD4$^+$ small/medium pleomorphic T-cell lymphoma
  Aggressive clinical behavior
        Sézary syndrome
        Primary cutaneous NK/T-cell lymphoma, nasal-type
        Primary cutaneous aggressive CD8$^+$ T-cell lymphoma
        Primary cutaneous/T-cell lymphoma
        Primary cutaneous peripheral T-cell lymphoma, unspecified
Cutaneous B-cell lymphoma
  Indolent clinical behavior
        Primary cutaneous marginal zone B-cell lymphoma
        Primary cutaneous follicle center lymphoma
  Intermediate clinical behavior
        Primary cutaneous diffuse large B-cell lymphoma, leg type
        Primary cutaneous diffuse large B-cell lymphoma, other
        Primary cutaneous intravascular large B-cell lymphoma

Source: This research was originally published in Blood. Willemze R, Jaffe ES, Burg G, et al. WHO-EORTC classification for cutaneous lymphomas. *Blood.* 2005;105(10):3768-3785.

COMPLETE HISTOLOGIC CLASSIFICATION

A histologic classification of tumors of the skin is listed here. Those tumors discussed in the first part of this chapter are marked with an asterisk. The rarer tumors listed are defined or can be found in the Dictionary–Index. This classification is modified from Lever and Schaumberg–Lever (1997).

I. Epidermal Tumors

A. Tumors of the surface epidermis
   1. Benign tumors
      a. Linear epidermal nevus (Fig. 30-15): A rather common tumor usually present at birth, consisting of single or multiple lesions in various forms that give rise to several clinical designations, such as hard nevus, nevus verrucous, nevus unius lateris, and, when systematized

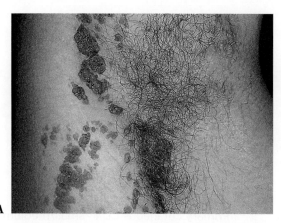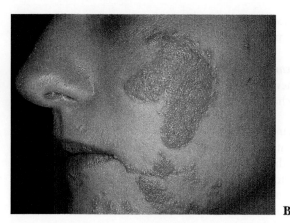

FIGURE 30-15: A: Linear epidermal nevus in the axilla. **B:** Nevus unius lateris of the face. (Courtesy of Owen/ Galderma.)

(more generalized), ichthyosis hystrix. No nevus cells are present, but there is verrucous overgrowth of epidermal tissue. There is epidermal nevus syndrome with multiple underlying abnormalities.

    b. Seborrheic keratosis and dermatosis papulosa nigra

    c. Fibroma

    d. Cysts

       1. Epidermal cyst

       2. Trichilemmal, pilar, or sebaceous cyst

       3. Steatocystoma multiplex: A dominantly inherited condition with small, moderately firm, cystic nodules adherent to the overlying skin, which on incision yield an oily fluid.

       4. Milium

       5. Dermoid cyst

       6. Mucous retention cyst

    e. Clear cell acanthoma: A rare, usually single, slightly elevated, flat, pale red, scaling nodule less than 2 cm in diameter, nearly always located on the lower extremities.

    f. Warty dyskeratoma: A solitary warty lesion with a central keratotic plug, most commonly seen on the scalp, face, and neck. Histology is characteristic.

    g. Keratoacanthoma (see Chapter 31)

  2. Precancerous tumors

    a. Senile or actinic keratosis and cutaneous horn

    b. Arsenical keratosis

    c. Leukoplakia

  3. Epitheliomas and carcinomas

    a. Basal cell cancer (see Chapter 31)

    b. Squamous cell cancer (see Chapter 31)

    c. Bowen disease and erythroplasia of Queyrat: Bowen disease is a single red scaly lesion with a sharp but irregular border that grows slowly by peripheral extension. Histologically, it is an intraepidermal squamous cell carcinoma (Fig. 30-16). Erythroplasia of Queyrat represents Bowen disease of the mucous membranes and occurs on the glans penis and rarely on the vulva. The lesion has a bright red, velvety surface.

    d. Paget disease: A unilateral scaly red lesion resembling dermatitis, usually present on the female nipple,

but the lesion can be extramammary. The early lesion on the nipple is an intraductal carcinoma that also involves the mammary ducts and deeper connective tissue. In the perirectal area, it can be associated with underlying bowel cancer.

    e. Merkel cell carcinoma (neuroendocrine carcinoma) (Fig. 30-20G): Aggressive often fatal tumor arising from the light touch sensors in the skin. Clinical diagnosis is difficult but a phemonic used is AEIOU: A is for asymptomatic, E is for expanding rapidly, I is for immunosuppressed patine, O is for older than 50, and U is for ultraviolet exposed site in a fair skinned person.

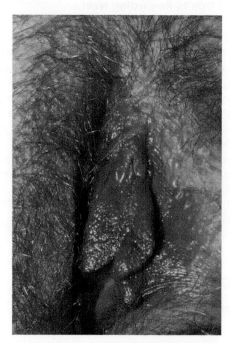

FIGURE 30-16: Bowen disease represented by an innocuous-appearing red patch near the right side of the slide near the labia minora.

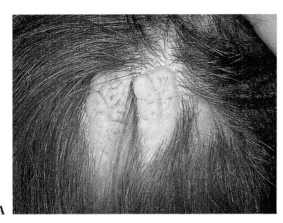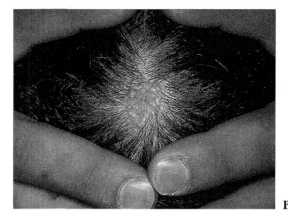

A   B

FIGURE 30-17: **A:** Nevus sebaceous of Jadassohn on the scalp. **B:** Nevus sebaceous on the scalp. (Courtesy of Owen/Galderma.)

B. Tumors of the epidermal appendages
   1. Nevoid tumors
      a. Organic nevi or hamartomas
         1. Sebaceous nevi
            a. Nevus sebaceous (Jadassohn) (Fig. 30-17): Seen on the scalp or face as a single lesion present from birth, slightly raised, firm, hairless, yellowish, with furrowed surface. Large examples may be associated with a "neurocutaneous syndrome" of epilepsy and mental retardation. Basal cells and squamous cell carcinomas can develop with these tumors in less than 1% of cases.
            b. Adenoma sebaceum (Pringle disease): Part of a triad of epilepsy, mental deficiency, and the skin lesions of adenoma sebaceum. This is called *tuberous sclerosis.* The skin lesions occur on the face and consist of yellowish brown, papular, nodular lesions with telangiectasias. Histopathology shows an angiofibroma (see Chapter 42).
            c. Sebaceous hyperplasia (Fig. 30-18): Very common on the face in older persons and consists of one or several small, yellowish, translucent, slightly umbilicated nodules. It may be the most common tumor to be confused clinically with a basal cell cancer.
            d. Fordyce disease (see Chapter 37): A rather common condition of pinpoint-sized yellowish lesions of the vermilion border of the lips or the oral mucosa that represent ectopic sebaceous glands.
      b. Adenomas or organoid hamartomas
         1. Sebaceous adenoma: A very rare solitary tumor of the face or the scalp, smooth, firm, elevated, often slightly pedunculated, and measuring less than 1 cm in diameter; may be associated with an adenocarcinoma of the bowel (Muir–Torre syndrome).

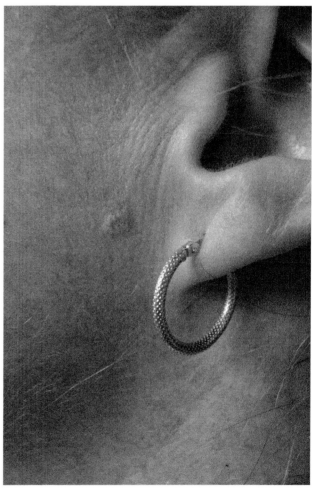

FIGURE 30-18: Sebaceous hyperplasia is most common on the forehead but is seen here in the preauricular area. Note orange color, sebaceous lobules seen through the skin, fine telangiectasis, and central dell. A basal cell cancer when stretched appears more translucent, and the edge is more distinctive, whereas in sebaceous hyperplasia, when stretched there is no change.

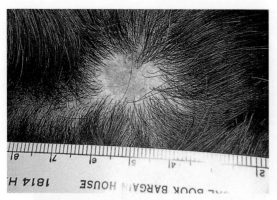

FIGURE 30-19: Syringocystadenoma papilliferum. (Courtesy of Owen/Galderma.)

2. Apocrine adenomas
   a. Syringocystadenoma papilliferum (Fig. 30-19): This adenoma of the apocrine ducts appears as a single verrucous plaque, usually seen on the scalp. Basal cell epitheliomatous change occasionally does occur and may arise in sebaceous nevi.
   b. Hidradenoma papilliferum: This adenoma of the apocrine glands occurs almost exclusively on the labia majora and the perineum of women as a single, intracutaneous, benign tumor covered by normal epidermis.

3. Eccrine syringofibroadenoma (ESFA): Solitary or multiple nodules with the following subtypes:
   a. Solitary ESFA
   b. Multiple ESFAs with hidrotic ectodermal dysplasia
   c. Multiple ESFA
   d. Nonfamilial linear ESFA
   e. Reactive ESFA associated with inflammatory or neoplastic dermatoses usually seen on the lower extremities and easily confused with squamous cell carcinoma
c. Benign epitheliomas or suborganoid hamartomas
   1. Apocrine epitheliomas
      a. Syringoma (Fig. 30-20B): This is characterized by the appearance of pinhead-sized, soft, yellowish nodules at the age of puberty in women, developing around the eyelids, the chest, the abdomen, and the anterior aspects of the thighs.
      b. Cylindroma (Fig. 30-21): These appear as numerous smooth, rounded tumors of various sizes on the scalp in adults, and resemble bunches of grapes or tomatoes. These tumors may cover the entire scalp like a turban and are then referred to as *turban tumors*. It can be multiple and autosomal dominant with associated trichoepitheliomas and eccrine spiradenomas.

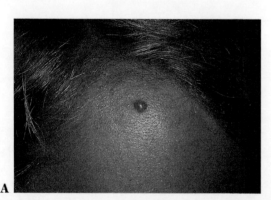

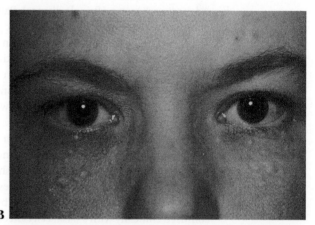

FIGURE 30-20: **A:** Eccrine spiradenoma of the forehead. **B:** Benign, soft, yellowish papules seen most often symmetrically on the lower eyelids make the diagnosis of syringomas. **C:** Deep-seated, soft, asymptomatic, subcutaneous tumors freely movable over underlying skin are indicative of lipomas. If the tumors are bound down to underlying skin, then a biopsy is indicated to rule out a malignancy. **D:** Lymphangioma circumscriptum superior to the umbilicus showing frog-spawn, clear papules, and some hemorrhage. A deep-seated lymphatic cistern often lies underneath. **E:** White keratotic papule with some surrounding erythema and slight indentation on the cartilage of superior helix, which is the commonest site for chondrodermatitis nodularis helicis chronicus. It may occur on the antihelix. Very painful and thought to be trauma related. This patient had slept mainly on this side of his body, but now he wakes at night because of pain. **F:** Near the inner canthus on the upper eyelid is a clear cystic papule indicative of an apocrine hidrocystoma. **G:** Merkel carcinoma on the leg anterior to the knee in a lady. She was fair-skinned and had a large amount of sun exposure. She was not immunosuppressed but was over 50 years of age. The pink nodule shown here is very nonspecific, which makes early diagnosis difficult.

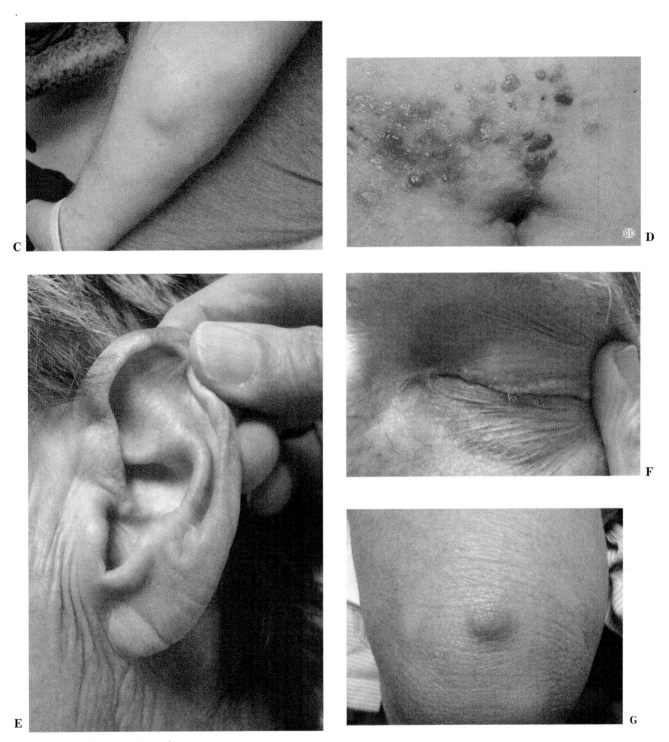

FIGURE 30-20: (continued)

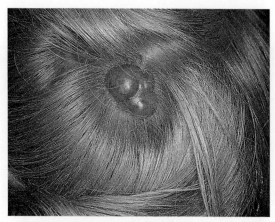

FIGURE 30-21: Cylindroma of the scalp.

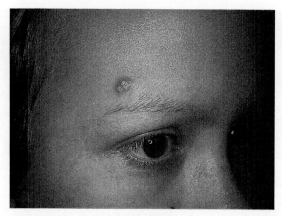

FIGURE 30-23: Eccrine spiradenoma of the forehead. (Courtesy of Owen/Galderma.)

c. Apocrine hidrocystom (Fig. 30-20F): Benign cystic clear tumor. May have a bluish tint. Usually on or near the eyelid. A similar eccrine tumor is called an eccrine hidrocystoma and it will swell when exposed to heat.

2. Hair epitheliomas
a. Trichoepithelioma (Fig. 30-22): Also known as epithelioma adenoides cysticum and multiple benign cystic epithelioma when multiple. This begins at the age of puberty, frequently on a hereditary basis, and is characterized by the presence of numerous pinhead- to pea-sized, rounded, yellowish or pink nodules on the face and occasionally on the upper trunk. This may also appear as a single lesion that can be confused with a basal cell cancer histologically.
b. Calcifying epithelioma of Malherbe (Fig. 30-23) or pilomatrixoma: Hard, nodular, nondescript 0.5 to 1.0 cm tumors, especially on the scalp and face. Malignant degeneration is very rare. There is a perforating form.
c. Microcystic adnexal carcinoma: Relatively rare, often extensive and invasive with perineural invasion. Up to 25% misdiagnosed

on initial biopsy. It is slow growing, and 5- to 10-year follow-up is needed. Mohs surgery may be the best therapy.

3. Eccrine epitheliomas
a. Eccrine spiradenoma (Fig. 30-20): A rare, usually solitary, intradermal, firm, tender nodule
b. Clear cell hidradenoma: A rare, well-circumscribed, often encapsulated tumor of dermis and subcutaneous tissue.
c. Eccrine poroma (Fig. 30-24): This occurs as an asymptomatic solitary tumor on the soles and the palms. There is a rare malignant eccrine poroma
2. Carcinomas of sebaceous glands and eccrine and apocrine sweat glands (rare)
C. Metastatic carcinoma of the skin
This occurs frequently from carcinoma of the breast and melanoma but rarely from other internal carcinomas. Metastatic carcinoid nodules may appear in the skin, as well as in lymph nodes and the liver. The primary tumor and the metastases produce excess 5-hydroxytryptamine (serotonin), which in turn produces attacks of flushing of the skin.

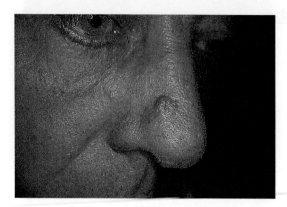

FIGURE 30-22: Trichoepithelioma on the nose.

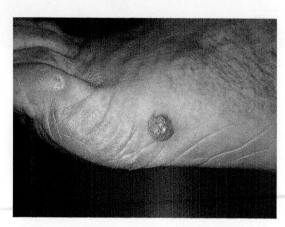

FIGURE 30-24: Eccrine poroma on the foot.

II. Mesodermal Tumors

A. Tumors of fibrous tissue
1. Histiocytoma and dermatofibroma
2. Keloid
3. Fibrosarcomas
   a. True fibrosarcoma: A rare tumor that starts most commonly in the subcutaneous fat, grows rapidly, causes the overlying skin to appear purplish, and finally ulcerates.
   b. Dermatofibrosarcoma protuberans: A tumor that grows slowly in the corium and spreads by the development of adjoining reddish or bluish nodules that may coalesce to form a plaque that can eventually ulcerate. Margins are very difficult to evaluate, making recurrence common. Mohs surgery and positive CD34 immunohistochemical staining are helpful.
B. Tumors of mucoid tissue
1. Myxoma: Clinically seen as fairly well-circumscribed, rather soft intracutaneous tumors with normal overlying epidermis
2. Myxofibrosarcoma: Subcutaneous tumors that may eventually ulcerate the skin
3. Synovial cyst of the skin
C. Tumors of fatty tissue
1. Nevus lipomatosus superficialis: A rare, circumscribed nodular lesion, usually in the gluteal area
2. Lipoma (Fig. 30-20C): A rather common tumor that can be multiple or single, lobulated, of varying size, and in the subcutaneous tissue
3. Hibernoma: A form of lipoma composed of embryonic type of fat cells
4. Liposarcoma
5. Malignant hibernoma
D. Tumors of nerve tissue and mesodermal nerve sheath cells
1. Neuroma: Rare, single, or multiple small reddish or brown nodules that are usually tender as well as painful.
2. Neurofibroma: Benign flesh-colored soft tumor that is frequently single, but when multiple it is associated with neurofibromatosis; when very large, it is called a plexiform neuroma; can have sarcomatous degeneration
3. Neurofibromatosis: Also known as von Recklinghausen disease, this hereditary disease classically consists of pigmented patches (café-au-lait spots), pedunculated skin tumors, and nerve tumors. All of these lesions may not be present in a particular case.
4. Schwannoma (neurilemmoma)
5. Granular cell schwannoma (granular cell tumor) or myoblastoma: From neural sheath cells, this appears usually as a solitary tumor of the tongue, the skin, or the subcutaneous tissue. Also, multiple, nodular, or plaquelike.
6. Malignant granular cell schwannoma or myoblastoma
E. Tumors of vascular tissue
1. Hemangioma: See Chapter 33.
2. Granuloma pyogenicum (Fig. 30-25): This is a rather common (especially in pregnancy on the gums) end

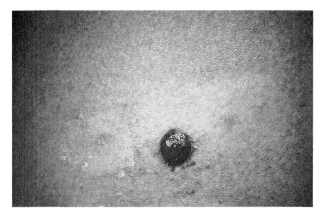

FIGURE 30-25: Pyogenic granuloma of 0.75 cm size on the back. (Courtesy of Syntex Laboratories, Inc.)

result of an injury to the skin that may or may not have been apparent. Vascular proliferation, with or without infection, produces a small red tumor that bleeds easily. It is to be differentiated from a malignant melanoma. Biopsy and mild electrocoagulation are curative.
3. Osler disease: See Osler-Weber-Rendu disease in the Dictionary–Index.
4. Lymphangioma: A superficial form, lymphangioma circumscriptum (Fig. 30-20D) appears as a group of thin-walled vesicles on the skin surface, whereas the deeper variety, lymphangioma cavernosum, causes a poorly defined enlargement of the affected area, such as the lip or the tongue. Large lymphatic cisternae may underlie apparently superficial tumors.
5. Glomus tumor: A rather unusual small, deep-seated, red or purplish nodule that is tender and may produce severe paroxysmal pains. The solitary lesion is usually seen under a nail plate, on the fingertips, or elsewhere on the body and may erode underlying bone.
6. Hemangiopericytoma
7. Kaposi sarcoma (KS; multiple idiopathic hemorrhagic sarcoma) (Fig. 30-26: KS-associated herpes virus [HHV-8] is associated with all forms): Most commonly seen on the feet and the ankles as multiple bluish-red or dark brown nodules and plaques associated with visceral lesions. It is most prevalent in elderly men of Mediterranean or Jewish origin. Sarcomatous malignant degeneration can occur.
   a. KS is also seen as part of the acquired immunodeficiency syndrome (see Chapter 27). In this complex, the sarcoma lesions are small, oval, red, or pink papules that occur on any area of the body. If HIV is not treated aggressively, KS can rapidly grow into tumors, spreading internally (especially to the gastrointestinal tract) and become fatal from bleeding or general debility.
   b. There is an endemic African form often associated with reticuloendothelial cancer.
   c. An immunosuppressive drug-related form is often seen in transplant patients that may dissipate after immunosuppression is decreased.

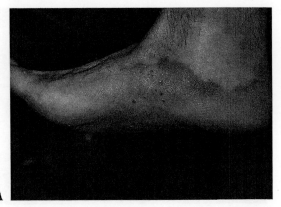
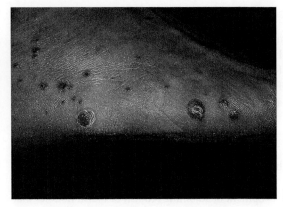

FIGURE 30-26: A: Kaposi sarcoma of the foot. **B:** Kaposi sarcoma of the foot. (Courtesy of Syntex Laboratories, Inc.)

8. Hemangioendothelioma
9. Postmastectomy lymphangiosarcoma (Stewart–Treves syndrome)
10. Glomangiomas: Large dilated vessels lined with glomus cells as in a glomus tumor but are larger tumors that mimic large venous malformations clinically. Some authors prefer the term glomuvenous malformations to indicate they are not true tumors. The rare congenital plaque type is extensively distributed, difficult to diagnose, and progressive. Deep blue or purple, poorly compressible, and usually on the face. They can be large, disfiguring, and inherited in an autosomal dominant manner.

F. Tumors of muscular tissue
1. Leiomyoma: Solitary leiomyomas may be found on the extremities and on the scrotum, whereas multiple leiomyomas can occur on the back and elsewhere as pinhead- to pea-sized, brown or bluish, firm, elevated nodules. Both forms are painful and sensitive to pressure, particularly as they enlarge. They may have a butterfly shape.
2. Leiomyosarcoma: Very rare
3. Multiple leiomyomas may be associated with uterine leiomyomas and renal cancer as a familial syndrome.

G. Tumors of osseous tissue
1. Osteoma cutis
   a. Primary: The primary form of osteoma cutis develops from embryonal cell rests; these may be single or multiple.
   b. Secondary: Secondary bone formation may occur as a form of tissue degeneration in tumors, in scar tissue (such as acne), in scleroderma lesions (see CREST syndrome), and in various granulomas.

H. Tumors of cartilaginous tissue
   a. Nodular chondrodermatitis (Fig. 30-20E) of the ear: A painful, benign, hyperkeratotic nodule, usually on the inner rim of the helix of the ear of elderly men; trauma may be the inciting cause; often awakens the patient at night when pressure is applied; can be treated by excision or sometimes with intralesional corticosteroids

III. Nevus Cell Tumors

A. Melanocytic nevi
1. Junctional (active) nevus
2. Intradermal (resting) nevus
3. Dysplastic nevus syndrome
4. Lentigines: These are to be differentiated from freckles (ephelides). A freckle histologically shows hyperpigmentation of the basal layer but no elongation of the rete pegs and no increase in the number of clear cells and dendritic cells. Juvenile lentigines (lentigo simplex) begin to appear in childhood and occur on all parts of the body. Senile lentigines (solar lentigo), also known as "liver spots," occur in elderly persons on the dorsa of the hands, the forearms, and the face and are related to sun exposure. Solar ink-spot lentigo is commonly seen on sun-exposed areas and has a characteristic black, splotchy, reticulated pattern. Lentigo maligna melanoma (Hutchinson Freckle) is a dark brown or black macular, malignant lesion, usually on the face or arms of elderly persons, and has a slow peripheral growth (see Chapter 32). Lentigines can be caused by ionizing radiation, a tanning bed, a sunlamp, PUVA therapy, and, most commonly, from sun exposure.
5. Mongolian spots: These are seen chiefly in Asian or African American infants, usually around the buttocks. They disappear spontaneously during childhood. Related bluish patchy lesions are the nevus of Ota, seen on the side of the face (may have scleral pigment), and the nevus of Ito, located in the supraclavicular, scapular, and deltoid regions. Laser therapy may be beneficial.
6. Blue nevus: Clinically, the blue nevus appears as a slate blue or bluish black, sharply circumscribed, flat or slightly elevated nodule, occurring on any area of the body. It originates from mesodermal cells. The common blue nevus is always benign. Cellular blue nevus is larger, especially on buttocks.

B. Malignant melanoma

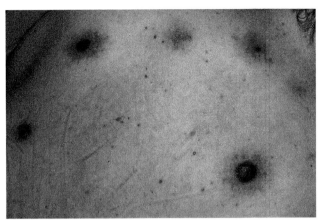

FIGURE 30-27: Nodular multicolored tumors scattered over the back. The biopsy showed leukemia cutis. The color variation is characteristic metastatic myeloproliferative disease of the skin.

IV. Lymphomas (see Chapter 34)

A. Monomorphous group

B. The non-Hodgkin lymphomas are referred to as monomorphous lymphomas because, in contrast to Hodgkin disease, they lack a significant admixture of inflammatory cells and are composed almost entirely of lymphoma cells largely derived from B or T lymphocytes.

C. Lymphomas may have specific skin lesions containing the lymphomatous infiltrate, or nonspecific lesions may be seen. These latter consist of macules, papules, tumors, purpuric lesions, blisters, eczematous lesions, exfoliative dermatitis, and secondarily infected excoriations.

D. Polymorphous group

    1. Hodgkin disease: Specific lesions are very rare, but nonspecific dermatoses are commonly seen.

    2. Mycosis fungoides

       a. Sézary syndrome: This is a very rare form of exfoliative dermatitis (see Chapter 19) that occurs at an early leukemic stage of a cutaneous T-cell lymphoma (CTCL). It is diagnosed by finding unusually large monocytoid cells (so-called Sézary cells) in the blood and in the skin. This cell is indistinguishable from the mycosis cell, both of which are derived from the T cell.

SAUER'S NOTES

Sun tanning salons should be strongly discouraged. They are associated with increased risk of malignant melanoma, squamous cell cancer, and basal cell cancer. All aspects of photoaging are increased. Lupus erythematosus, various porphyrias, photo drug reactions, dermatomyositis, actinic keratoses, and solar urticaria are all caused by or worsened by sun tanning salon usage. The false tan or immediate pigment darkening of high-dose UVA given by most sun tanning salons does not protect from future sunburning as the sun-induced tan does.

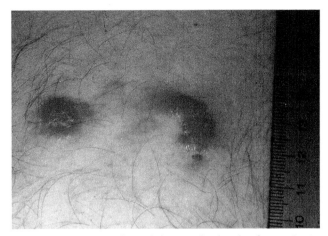

FIGURE 30-28: Pink nodules on the back of a patient with pseudolymphoma. This mimics a true cutaneous lymphoma as well as cutaneous sarcoidosis. A biopsy is necessary for the correct diagnosis and therapy that could be conservative since it is benign. Occasionally, a misdiagnosis or an honest mistake will cause these tumors to be diagnosed in the future as lymphoma.

V. Myelosis (Fig. 30-27)

A. Leukemia: Refers to circulating abnormal blood cells; may be seen along with lymphomas, but in skin almost always associated with myelosis, such as myeloid leukemia. Cutaneous lesions are quite uncommon but may be specific or nonspecific

VI. Pseudolymphoma of Spiegler–Fendt (Fig. 30-28)

A benign, localized, erythematous, nodular dermatosis usually on the face, with clinical and histologic features that make a distinction from lymphoma difficult. Some cases may eventually be diagnosed as a lymphoma.

Suggested Readings

Barnhill RL. *Color Atlas and Synopsis of Pigmented Lesions*. New York: McGraw-Hill; 1995.

Blake PW, Bradford PT, Devesa SS, et al. Cutaneous appendageal carcinoma incidence and survival patterns in the United States. *Arch Dermatol*. 2010;146(6):625–632.

Drake LA, Ceilley RI, Cornelison RL, et al. Guidelines of care for actinic keratoses. *J Am Acad Dermatol*. 1995;32(1):95–98.

Drake LA, Ceilley RI, Cornelison RL, et al. Guidelines of care for nevi: II. Nonmelanocytic nevi, hamartomas, neoplasms, and potentially malignant lesions. *J Am Acad Dermatol*. 1995;32(1):104–108.

Drake LA, Salasche S, Ceilley RI, et al. Guidelines of care for cutaneous squamous cell carcinoma. *J Am Acad Dermatol*. 1993;28:628–631.

Duffy K, Grossman D. The dysplastic nevus: from historical perspective to management in the modern era part I and II. *J Am Acad Dermatol*. 2012;67(1):1–30.

Glick ZR, Frieden IJ, Garzon MC, et al. Diffuse neonatal hemangiomatosis: an evidence-based review of case reports in the literature. *J Am Acad Dermatol*. 2012;67(5):898–903.

Lever WF, Schaumburg-Lever G. *Histopathology of the Skin*. 8th ed. Philadelphia, PA: JB Lippincott; 1997.

Spencer J. Understanding actinic keratosis: Epidemiology, biology, and management of the disease. J Am Acad Dermatol. 2013;68(1):S1–S48.

31

Common Nonmelanoma Skin Cancers

Christopher L. Wilson, MD, Nita Kohli, MD, and Nicholas Golda, MD

BACKGROUND AND EPIDEMIOLOGY

The most common forms of nonmelanoma skin cancer (NMSC) are basal cell carcinoma (BCC) and squamous cell carcinoma (SCC). The cells of origin for BCC and SCC are keratinocytes, the cells that make up the epidermal layer of the skin. BCC is the most common human malignancy, representing about 7 out of 10 diagnosed skin cancers. SCC, the second most common skin malignancy, represents about 2 out of 10 newly diagnosed skin cancers. While nonmelanoma skin cancers are the most common malignancy in the United States, they are generally not reported to national cancer registries, making the exact incidence of NMSC difficult to state. By most recent estimates, 5.4 million NMSCs were treated in 2012, involving 3.3 million people. Other less common skin cancers such as Merkel cell carcinoma, one of the most lethal forms of skin cancer, adnexal tumors, some sarcomas, and others fall into the category of nonmelanoma skin cancers, but will not be individually addressed as they are beyond the scope of this chapter.

Ultraviolet Light Exposure and Risk Factors

Unequivocally, ultraviolet (UV) radiation plays a significant and primary role in inducing NMSC. UV light induces covalent bonding between nucleotide bases, called pyrimidine dimers, resulting in the loss of function of tumor suppressor genes. Such genetic alterations have been demonstrated in chronically sun-exposed skin. Those at greatest risk for development of NMSC have a history of chronic UV exposure—the cumulative effect of which plays a definitive role in the development of NMSC. UV radiation may be obtained from sun exposure or artificial sources of UV light, such as tanning beds, clinical UV therapy lamps, UV lamps at nail salons, and welding. Individuals with light-colored eyes, fair skin that burns easily and tans poorly, and light-colored hair are at greater risk for NMSC development, whereas darkly pigmented individuals develop NMSC much less commonly because of the protective effect of increased melanin in their skin.

Of particular concern is the alarming increase in NMSC cases in young adults, with a very significant increase in the age group from 20 to 40 years. Studies in this population suggest a causal link between tanning bed usage and NMSC,

a significant modifiable risk factor that accounts for hundreds of thousands of new cancer cases annually in the United States. Indoor tanning use has been shown to be associated with a 29% higher risk for BCC as well as a 67% higher risk for SCC.

BASAL CELL CARCINOMA

Clinical

Basal cell carcinoma generally presents innocuously as a pearly, telangiectatic papule or small, crusted area that tends to bleed and become a nonhealing sore. Most BCCs occur on sun-exposed areas, such as the head and neck, but they may develop on any skin surface, including seemingly sun-protected areas such as the genitalia and perineum. Often, they are mistaken by the patient for a nonhealing pimple or other benign entity, leading to delays in diagnosis. Basal cell carcinomas may frequently, but not always, develop a crusted, ulcerated appearance owing to their friable and easily traumatized nature. Ulceration is sufficiently uncommon in the early stages of BCC that its absence should not dissuade the provider from seeking a biopsy of an otherwise concerning lesion. Given their slow growth, it may be months before a patient seeks attention for the area of concern.

Clinically and histologically, there are many different variants of BCC, which are all characterized by relatively slow growth and a rare rate of metastasis of approximately 0.0028% to 0.55%. Nodular BCC is the most commonly encountered form of BCC. It typically grows as a pearly papule, frequently covered by thin, superficial blood vessels called telangiectasias

(Figs. 31-1 to 31-4). The clinical presentation of nodular BCC often described in textbooks as the "rodent ulcer" with a ragged, central ulcer and smooth, elevated borders. It is important to note that this presentation is a later manifestation of BCC, and small, earlier-diagnosed, nodular BCCs often do not have a clinically hemorrhagic crust or ulceration. These will commonly manifest as a small sore or a bleeding lesion recurring at the same site following minor manipulation of the skin, such as face washing or shaving. In some cases, the papule may be completely asymptomatic and remain unnoticed by the patient. The physician should be alert to the possibility of an underlying BCC, even in the absence of classical morphology.

Superficial BCC has a scaly, red, sometimes shiny appearance that is commonly mistaken for a plaque of eczema. It is eventually recognized as BCC owing to its lack of response to typical topical treatments for a presumed inflammatory skin

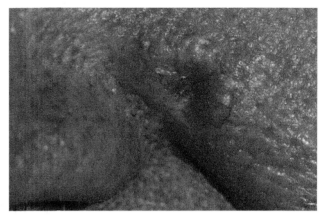

FIGURE 31-3: Basal cell cancer at the nasolabial border with a central dell, a translucent edge that may be seen better with stretching of the skin, and telangiectasia.

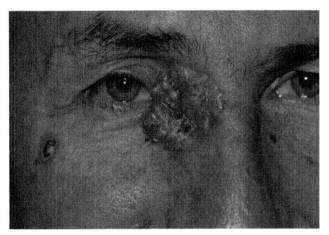

FIGURE 31-1: Basal cell cancer with telangiectasias and a pearly edge.

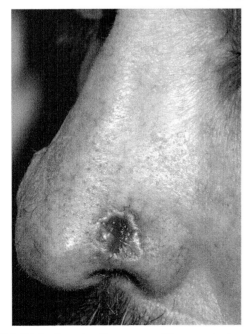

FIGURE 31-2: Basal cell cancer with a central hemorrhagic crust.

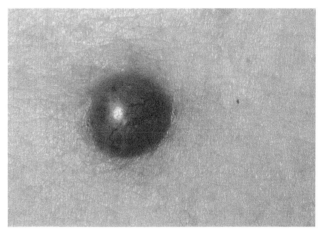

FIGURE 31-4: Nodular basal cell cancer with a translucent, telangiectatic, domed appearance. It mimics an intradermal nevus.

disease, if not detected earlier by a trained eye (Figs. 31-5 and 31-6). Aggressive forms of BCC include morpheaform, sclerosing, micronodular, and infiltrative subtypes. These often have clinical similarity to scars or scar-like plaques and have a tendency to grow subtly and escape clinical detection for a prolonged period of time. Because of this, these subtypes are often larger than they appear clinically and may require special treatment.

Although BCC rarely metastasizes, it can be very destructive locally, invading neighboring skin, muscle, cartilage, bone, and may adversely affect functionally important structures such as the eyelid and lip (Figs. 31-7 to 31-10). The clinical differential diagnosis of BCC includes SCC, melanoma (especially in the case of pigmented BCC or amelanotic melanoma), adnexal or follicular neoplasms, benign fibrous growths, scars, and other lesions.

Pathogenesis

The most common site of presentation of BCC is on the head and neck—areas that are exposed to the most UV radiation

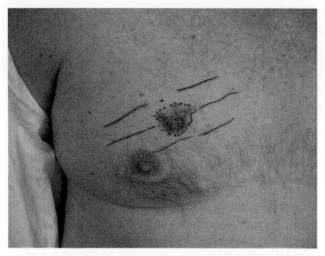

FIGURE 31-5: Superficial basal cell cancer mimicking a dermatitis.

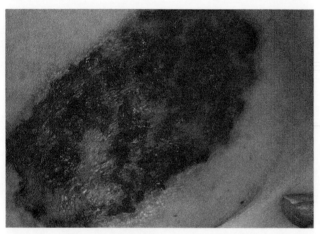

FIGURE 31-6: Large eroded basal cell cancer with a thin pearly edge.

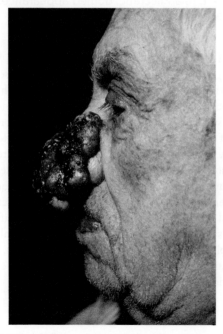

FIGURE 31-7: Large neglected basal cell cancer that mimics rhinophyma.

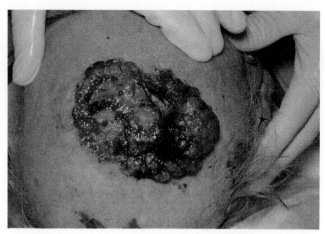

FIGURE 31-8: A neglected exophytic scalp basal cell cancer.

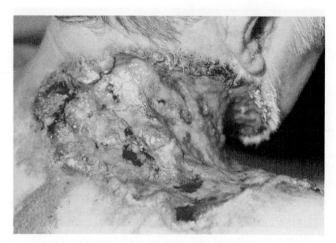

FIGURE 31-9: A very large basal cell cancer. Even though metastasis of these tumors is very uncommon, the size of this tumor would necessitate a consideration of metastatic disease.

over an individual's lifetime. However, as noted previously, BCC may occur on any skin surface, including areas with minimal sun exposure.

Along with UV light exposure, another common and clinically important risk factor for BCC development is exposure to ionizing radiation. Exposure may be occupational, but it most commonly develops in patients who have been irradiated for clinical purposes, such as following treatment of internal malignancies. An increased risk of basal cell carcinoma has been shown to be associated with doses of radiation equaling 1 Gy or more. BCC developing in this setting most commonly occurs approximately 20 years following irradiation. Numerous BCCs can develop in irradiated fields, causing troublesome management issues complicated by poor wound healing.

Several genetic syndromes predispose to the formation of BCC. The most common of these is nevoid basal cell carcinoma syndrome. Immunosuppression owing to organ transplantation seems to play a role in the development of BCC, resulting in an approximately 10-fold increased risk of BCC compared with the immunocompetent. Risk is shown to be highest in heart,

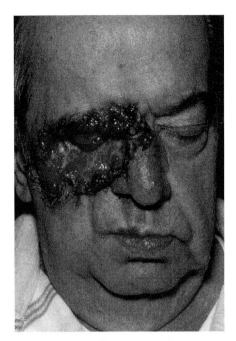

FIGURE 31-10: Basal cell cancer with eye involvement. Radiation or hedgehog-inhibitor therapy might be considered as palliative or potentially curative therapy.

lung, and kidney transplant patients and increases with the duration and level of immunosuppression.

Treatment

Treatment for BCC depends a great deal on the histologic subtype, size, and location of the tumor. The most common treatments for BCC are malignant destruction with electrodesiccation and curettage, curettage and cryotherapy, and excision with 4 mm margins around the clinically evident tumor. Mohs micrographic surgery (MMS) is another procedure used to treat BCC. MMS offers the highest cure rate of any treatment, and is the most tissue-sparing of the surgical treatments for BCC because complete histologic examination of the tumor margins is done by specialized tissue processing intraoperatively (Table 31-1). MMS is used for aggressive histologic subtypes, tumors in functionally or cosmetically sensitive areas, recurrent tumors or tumors with positive margins following prior excisional therapy, large tumors greater than 2 cm, and tumors arising in irradiated skin. Appropriate use criteria have been developed by the American Academy of Dermatology to help providers determine if a tumor warrants treatment with MMS. Radiation therapy, cryosurgery and topical therapies are less commonly used. Systemic oral therapy with the hedgehog-inhibitor class of drugs is available for the rare metastatic or inoperable local BCC. Regardless of the treatment selected, it is important to monitor the patient for recurrence or new cancers through routine skin checks.

Aggressive surgical treatment (i.e., MMS) for BCC in patients with limited life expectancies should be weighed against the possible increased rate of complications in these patients. The issue of wound care is also important, as it may be more difficult for this particular patient population. Quality of life and the increased rate of complications in this patient population should be considered and less invasive treatments may be prudent depending on the patient. Exceptions to this, of course, include symptomatic BCCs or BCCs that may be medically dangerous (such as ones that may erode into any vital structures).

Prevention

In almost all cases, BCC is a UV light–induced malignancy, and as such, the most effective means of preventing BCC involves limiting exposure to UV light. Healthcare workers have an important role in educating the public about the role of UV light in skin cancer development, methods for sun protection, and UV light avoidance. Appropriate use of broad-spectrum (UVA and UVB-blocking) sunscreen with an SPF of at least 30 will significantly reduce the risk for development of BCC. Additionally, it is important to educate patients about wearing wide-brimmed hats and long-sleeved clothing, as well as avoiding peak UV hours (10:00 AM to 4:00 PM). Wearing tightly woven protective clothing with a labeled Ultraviolet Protection Factor (UPF) provides appropriate sun protection and is more reliable than using sunscreen alone. A summer-weight cotton shirt provides an SPF range of 6 to 10 and a wet t-shirt an SPF of only 3. Young patients particularly benefit from early education and intervention because the damaging effect of

TABLE 31-1 • Five-Year Cure Rates for BCC and SCC With Various Treatment Modalities

Technique	Basal Cell Carcinoma (BCC) %		Squamous Cell Carcinoma (SCC) %	
	Primary	Recurrent	Primary	Recurrent
Mohs Micrographic Surgery (MMS)	99.0	94.4	97	90–93.3
Surgical Excision	89.9	82.6	95	76.7
Radiotherapy	91.3	90.2	80	—[b]
Cryosurgery	92.5	87.0	97.3[a]	—[b]
Electrodesiccation and Curettage	92.3	60.0	96	—[b]

[a]For low-risk, small tumors less than 1 cm.
[b]These treatment modalities are generally not considered appropriate for treating recurrent SCC; radiotherapy may be used adjunctively or as a palliative measure.

cumulative UV exposure may not be evident for many years. For this reason, education on avoidance of tanning beds is particularly important in this population.

SQUAMOUS CELL CARCINOMA

Clinical

SCC is often a more rapidly growing malignancy. It generally starts as a scaly papule that can become indurated and "heaped up" with mounds of scale on its surface (Fig. 31-11). SCC may or may not bleed depending on the clinical nature of the lesion and typically does not bleed as readily as an equally sized BCC.

The clinical appearance and location of these tumors vary based on etiology. Many SCCs arise from premalignant lesions, known as actinic keratoses. These appear as red, scaly patches or papules on sun-exposed skin that may be more readily felt with the fingertips than seen. Their texture has been likened to that of a cat's tongue. Induration to the base of such precursor lesions often signals malignant degeneration and should prompt a biopsy. Some SCCs present as volcano-like lesions, especially keratoacanthoma variants, with a central crater and sharply demarcated edges (Figs. 31-12 and 31-13). SCC in situ presents as a flat pink-to-red, often scaling plaque, resembling eczema, psoriasis, or superficial BCC (Figs. 31-14 and 31-15) and can occur on sun-exposed or sun-protected skin (Figs. 31-16 to 31-18). SCC on the genitalia can present as an erosion, ulceration, or as a sessile papule resembling a seborrheic keratosis. Many genital tumors are related to infection with human papilloma virus (HPV), particularly types 16 and 18 (Fig. 31-19). Immunosuppressed patients are at particularly

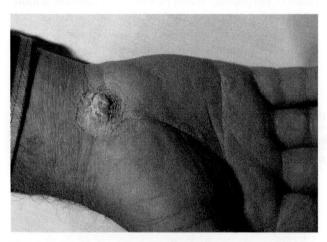

FIGURE 31-11: Squamous cell cancer on the palm that is quite symmetric indicating it may be of the keratoacanthoma type, especially if it grew quickly over weeks to months. Keratoacanthomas seldom metastasize.

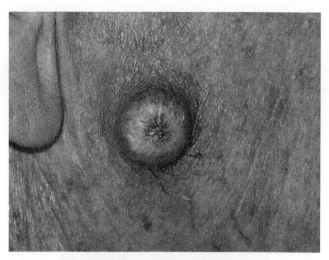

FIGURE 31-12: Preauricular squamous cell cancer, most likely of the keratoacanthoma type considering the marked symmetry of the lesion.

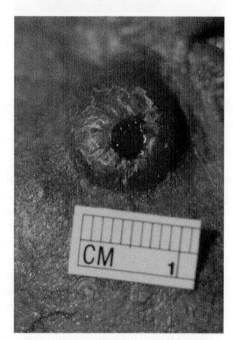

FIGURE 31-13: Squamous cell cancer with eye involvement.

high risk for developing SCC. Cumulative lifetime UV exposure, Fitzpatrick skin type I or II, and HPV viral infection are factors in the development of SCC in such patients, who have a 64- to 250-fold increased risk of developing SCC compared with immunocompetent individuals. Organ transplant patients and those with chronic lymphocytic leukemia (CLL) are at greatest risk of developing numerous and more severe SCC. Verrucous carcinoma, a type of well-differentiated SCC with variants that occur on the foot, hand, and genitals, clinically has a warty appearance and can be related to more common genital wart subtypes such as HPV-6 and HPV-11. SCC sometimes occurs in areas of chronic scarring, such as burns (Marjolin ulcer), irradiated skin, ulcers, and in scarring of chronic inflammatory skin diseases such as

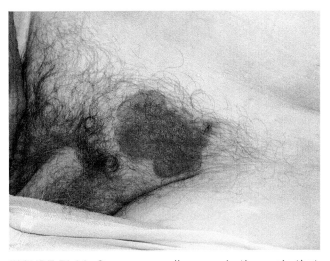

FIGURE 31-14: Squamous cell cancer in the groin that may well have begun as Bowen disease. Dermatitis and extramammary Paget disease, and condyloma acuminata are also diagnostic considerations.

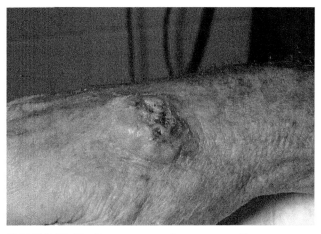

FIGURE 31-17: Squamous cell cancer on the dorsal wrist. Excision with adequate margins is the treatment of choice.

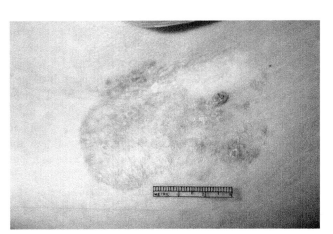

FIGURE 31-15: Superficial squamous cell cancer.

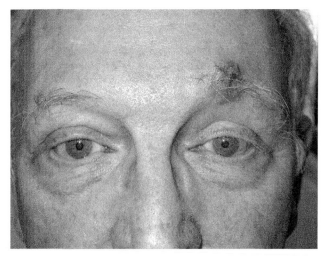

FIGURE 31-18: Squamous cell cancer on a chronic sun-exposed site. Only a biopsy can distinguish a benign tumor from a basal cell cancer. Squamous cell cancers often have a nonspecific clinical appearance.

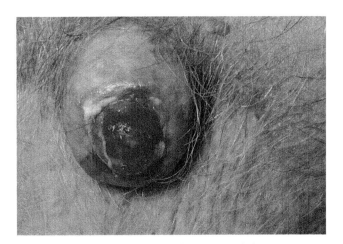

FIGURE 31-16: Squamous cell cancer of the penis. Buschke–Lowenstein tumor (an HPV-induced verrucous carcinoma) may have preceded this malignancy considering its location.

lichen sclerosus, epidermolysis bullosa, and chronic cutaneous lupus. SCC occurring in these settings can be more aggressive than other variants of SCC and have a higher risk of metastasis.

Histologically, SCCs can be quite variable, ranging from well-differentiated lesions that are well-circumscribed and localized to those that are poorly differentiated, ill-defined, and deeply invasive. The occasional tumor is so poorly differentiated that it requires special histopathologic staining to identify it as SCC.

Pathogenesis

Similar to BCC, SCC is unequivocally linked pathogenically to UV light exposure. Darkly pigmented patients are more likely to develop SCC rather than BCC. The development of SCC in races with darker pigment is usually related to an underlying, chronic, scarring condition or ulcer, occurs in less pigmented

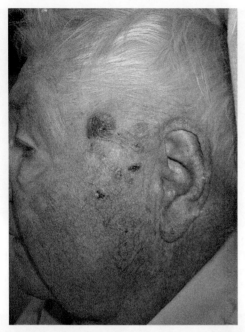

FIGURE 31-19: Large flat squamous cell cancer on a sun-exposed area. History of radiation damage from acne therapy as a teenager is a historical fact of importance. Thyroid cancer is also more common in patients who have had x-ray therapy for acne.

skin of the digits, or is related to immunosuppression or HPV infection. It has been hypothesized that the underlying pathogenesis for tumors of chronic inflammation relates to the induction of mutations in highly proliferative tissue.

Other risk factors for the development of SCC include a history of x-ray exposure, exposure to arsenic, and rare, inherited, skin disorders such as xeroderma pigmentosum and DOCK-8 deficiency.

Treatment

Treatment of SCC is similar to that of BCC, with the caveat that SCC has a much higher risk of metastasis than BCC. For SCC less than 2 cm in diameter, excision with 4- to 6-mm margins offers a 95% cure rate, depending on location and type of tumor. For SCC in situ, curettage and topical modalities, such as 5-fluorouracil or imiquimod, are viable options. The cure rate for SCC in situ with these topical therapies can range from 48% to 87.5%. Recurrent, large, and aggressive histologic subtype tumors (i.e., poorly differentiated SCC), tumors involving critical structures such as the face, ears, genitalia, and acral surfaces, and ill-defined tumors are best managed by MMS, which offers 5-year cure rates in the 97% range for primary tumors, and cure rates approaching 90% for recurrent SCC. Radiation therapy has been shown to have acceptable cure rates but is costly and labor intensive for the patient. Radiation is used when the patient refuses therapy, palliation when the cancer is deemed inoperable, or as adjunctive therapy after surgery when the cancer has a high risk of metastasis. After treatment of cutaneous SCC, patients should undergo regular follow-up visits owing to an increased risk

of developing malignant melanoma and a 30% to 50% risk of developing another NMSC after a 5-year period.

Prevention

Appropriate sun protection and sun avoidance are the keys to preventing SCC. The same precautions as for BCC should be followed. Immunosuppressed patients particularly need to be educated on strict sun protection with broad-spectrum UVA and UVB sunscreens, sun avoidance during peak UV hours, and regular dermatologic examination. These patients are at high risk for the development of aggressive and potentially life-threatening tumors and many die from metastasis of skin cancer. It is recommended that immunosuppressed patients be examined and educated by a doctor soon after their immunosuppression begins owing to an increased risk of SCC development. Rapid referral and timely treatment are important measures for any patient presenting with a lesion suspicious for SCC.

PROGNOSIS AND STAGING

Several factors indicate a greater risk for recurrence or metastasis. These include: a tumor diameter greater than 2 cm, a tumor depth of invasion greater than 4 mm or deeper than the subcutaneous fat, the presence of perineural invasion, particularly invasion of nerves greater than 0.1 mm in diameter, poor histologic differentiation and location on the lip, ear, or scalp. Lip, ear, and scalp SCCs may carry a metastatic risk of 10% or more. (Figs. 31-20 to 31-22). Physical examination of any patient with SCC should include palpation of the regional draining lymph nodes. Metastasis usually occurs first to the regional lymph node basin, but then may proceed to the lungs and other organs. High-risk SCC requires evaluation and management by a cutaneous oncologist and may require multidisciplinary care.

The American Joint Commission on Cancer (AJCC) TNM system is most often used to stage NMSC, and is based upon three main factors: tumor characteristics, lymph node involvement, and metastasis. (Tables 31-2 and 31-3)

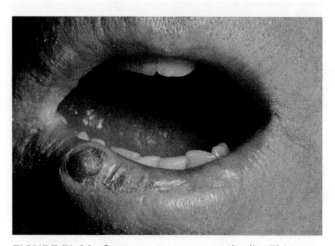

FIGURE 31-20: Squamous cancer on the lip. This can be associated with tobacco abuse, alcohol abuse, and especially chronic sun exposure.

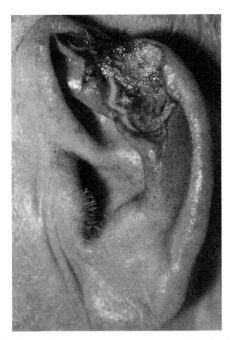

FIGURE 31-21: Squamous cell cancer with destruction of the ear.

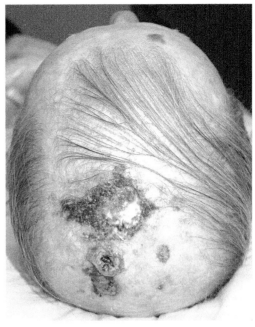

FIGURE 31-22: Extensive squamous cell cancer that will require extensive surgery, most likely with Mohs therapy and skin grafting.

TABLE 31-2 • American Joint Committee on Cancer TNM System Criteria for CSCC

Definition of Primary Tumor (T)	Definition of Regional Lymph Node (N)	Definition of Distant Metastases (M)
TX: Primary tumor cannot be identified	NX: Regional lymph nodes cannot be assessed	M0: No distant metastasis
Tis: Carcinoma in situ	N0: No regional lymph node metastasis	M1: Distant metastasis
T1: Tumor smaller than 2 cm in greatest dimension	N1: Metastasis in a single ipsilateral lymph node, 3 cm or smaller in greatest dimension and ENE(−)	
T2: Tumor 2 cm or larger, but smaller than 4 cm in greatest dimension	N2: Metastasis in a single ipsilateral node larger than 3 cm but not larger than 6 cm in greatest dimension and ENE(−); or metastases in multiple ipsilateral lymph nodes, none larger than 6 cm in greatest dimension and ENE(−); or in bilateral or contralateral lymph nodes, none larger than 6 cm in greatest dimension and ENE(−)	
T3: Tumor 4 cm or larger in maximum dimension or minor bone erosion or perineural invasion or deep invasion[a]	N2a: Metastasis in a single ipsilateral node larger than 3 cm but not larger than 6 cm in greatest dimension and ENE(−)	
T4: Tumor with gross cortical bone/marrow, skull base invasion and/or skull base foramen invasion	N2b: Metastasis in multiple ipsilateral nodes, none larger than 6 cm in greatest dimension and ENE (−)	

(continued)

TABLE 31-2 • American Joint Committee on Cancer TNM System Criteria for CSCC (*continued*)

Definition of Primary Tumor (T)	Definition of Regional Lymph Node (N)	Definition of Distant Metastases (M)
T4a: Tumor with gross cortical bone/marrow invasion	N2c: Metastasis in bilateral or contralateral lymph nodes, none larger than 6 cm in greatest dimension and ENE(−)	
T4b: Tumor with skull base invasion and/or skull base foramen involvement	N3: Metastasis in a lymph node larger than 6 cm in greatest dimension and ENE(−); or metastasis in any node(s) and clinically overt ENE [ENE(+)]	
	N3a: Metastasis in a lymph node larger than 6 cm in greatest dimension and ENE(−)	
	N3b: Metastasis in any node(s) and ENE(+)	

[a]Deep invasion is defined as invasion beyond the subcutaneous fat or >6 mm (as measured from the granular layer of adjacent normal epidermis to the base of the tumor); perineural invasion for T3 classification is defined as tumor cells within the nerve sheath of a nerve lying deeper than the dermis or measuring 0.1 mm or larger in caliber, or presenting with clinical or radiographic involvement of named nerves without skull base invasion or transgression.
Source: From Amin MB, Edge SB, Greene FL, et al, eds. *AJCC Cancer Staging Manual.* 8th ed. New York: Springer; 2017. Used with the permission of the American Joint Committee on Cancer (AJCC), Chicago, Illinois.

TABLE 31-3 • Stage Grouping for CSCC

Stage 0	Tis, N0, M0
Stage I	T1, N0, M0
Stage II	T2, N0, M0
Stage III	T3, N0, M0
	T1-T3, N1, M0
Stage IV	T1-T3, N2, M0
	Any T, N3, M0
	T4, any N, M0
	Any T, any N, M1

Source: From Amin MB, Edge SB, Greene FL, et al, eds. *AJCC Cancer Staging Manual.* 8th ed. New York: Springer; 2017. Used with the permission of the American Joint Committee on Cancer (AJCC), Chicago, Illinois.

WHEN TO REFER TO DERMATOLOGY

After evaluating a patient for a possible NMSC, most primary care physicians may decide to treat the underlying skin cancer on their own. Such a decision is governed by the provider's comfort with dermatologic procedures. In some circumstances, patients may display an aggressive tumor, in which case referral to a doctor is recommended. Patients who fail initial treatment, whether surgical or topical, or have recurrent tumors should also be considered for referral. Evaluating the patient's lesion for speed of growth, site, and type of lesion is of utmost importance in determining if the patient should be referred, as well as if the patient is a candidate for Mohs surgery.

Suggested Readings

Alam M, Ratner D. Cutaneous squamous cell carcinoma. *N Eng J Med.* 2001;344:975–983.

Brenner M, Hearing VJ. The protective role of melanin against UV damage in human skin. *Photochem Photobiol.* 2008;84:539–549.

Connolly SM, Baker DR, Coldiron BM, et al. AAD/ACMS/ASDSA/ASMS 2012 appropriate use criteria for Mohs micrographic surgery: a report of the American Academy of Dermatology, American College of Mohs Surgery, American Society for Dermatologic Surgery Association, and the American Society for Mohs Surgery. *J Am Acad Dermatol.* 2012;67:531–550.

Dinehart SM, Pollack SV. Metastases from squamous cell carcinoma of the skin and lip. *J Am Acad Dermatol.* 1989;21:242–248.

Ganti AK, Kessinger A. Systemic therapy for disseminated basal cell carcinoma: an uncommon manifestation of a common cancer. *Cancer Treat Rev.* 2011;37:440–443.

Karagas MR, Stannard VA, Mott LA, et al. Use of tanning devices and risk of basal cell and squamous cell skin cancers. *J Natl Cancer Inst.* 2002;94(3):224–226.

Kauvar ANB, Arpey CJ, Hruza G, et al. Consensus for nonmelanoma skin cancert, part II: squamous cell carcinoma, including a cost analysis of treatment methods. *Dermatol Surg.* 2015;41:1214–1240.

Kopf W, Bart RS, Schrager D, et al. Curettage-electrodesiccation treatment of basal cell carcinomas. *Arch Dermatol.* 1977;113:439–443.

Kraemer KH. Heritable diseases with increased sensitivity to cellular injury. In: Freedberg IM, Elsen AZ, Wolff K, et al, eds. *Fitzpatrick's Dermatology in General Medicine.* Vol 2. 5th ed. New York, NY: McGraw-Hill; 1999:1848–1862.

Lang PG, Maize JC. Basal cell carcinoma. In: Rigel DS, Friedberg RJ, Dzubow LM, et al, eds. *Cancer of the Skin.* Philadelphia, PA: Elsevier-Saunders; 2005:101–132.

Linos E, Keiser E, Fu T, et al. Hat, shade, long sleeves, or sunscreen? Rethinking US sun protection messages based on their relative effectiveness. *Cancer Causes Control.* 2011;22:1067–1071.

Linos E, Parvataneni R, Stuart SE, et al. Treatment of nonfatal conditions at the end of life: nonmelanoma skin cancer. *JAMA Intern Med.* 2013;173(11):1006–1012.

Mohs FE. Carcinoma of the skin. A summary of therapeutic results. In: *Chemosurgery: Microscopically Controlled Surgery for Skin Cancer.* Springfield, IL: Charles C Thomas; 1978:153.

Robins P. Chemosurgery: my 15 years of experience. *J Dermatol Surg Oncol.* 1981;7:779–789.

Rogers HW, Weinstock MA, Feldman SR, et al. Incidence estimate of nonmelanoma skin cancer (Keratinocyte Carcinomas) in the US population. *JAMA Dermatol.* 2015;151:1081–1086.

Rowe DE, Carroll RJ, Day CL Jr. Prognostic factors for local recurrence, metastasis, and survival rates in squamous cell carcinoma of the skin, ear, and lip: implications for treatment modality selection. *J Am Acad Dermatol.* 1992;26:976–990.

Sarasin A, Giglia-Maria G. *p53* gene mutations in human skin cancers. *Exp Dermatol.* 2002;11:44–47.

Schwartz RA, Nychay SG, Lyons M, et al. Buschke-Lowenstein tumor: verrucous carcinoma of the anogenitalia. *Cutis.* 1991;47:263–266.

Setlow RB, Carrie WL. Pyrimidine dimmers in ultraviolet-irradiated DNAs. *J Mol Biol.* 1966;17:237–254.

Swanson NA, Taylor SB, Tromovitch TA. The evolution of Mohs surgery. *J Dermatol Surg Oncol.* 1982;8:650–654.

Tromovitch TA, Stegman SJ. Microscopic-controlled excision of cutaneous tumors. Chemosurgery fresh tissue technique. *Cancer.* 1978;41:653–658.

Watt TC, Inskip PD, Stratton K, et al. Radiation-related risk of basal cell carcinoma: a report from the Childhood Cancer Survivor Study. *J Natl Cancer Inst.* 2012;104:1240–1250.

Wehner MR, Shive ML, Chren M, et al. Indoor tanning and non-melanoma skin cancer: systematic review and meta-analysis. *BMJ.* 2012;345:e5909.

Zwald FO, Brown M. Skin cancer in solid organ transplant patients: advances in therapy and management: part I. Epidemiology of skin cancer in solid organ transplant patients. *J Am Acad Dermatol.* 2011;65:253–261.

Melanoma

Tiffany J. Herd, MD, Robin S. Weiner, MD, Jaeyoung Yoon, MD, PhD
and Ting Wang, MD, PhD

Melanoma is defined as a malignant tumor arising from melanocytes, and although it may develop in a preexisting nevus, more than 50% of cases are believed to arise de novo without a preexisting lesion. Melanomas lacking pigment are termed *amelanotic melanomas*.

EPIDEMIOLOGY

The incidence of melanoma is rising at a faster rate than any other potentially preventable cancer in the United States. The American Cancer Society estimates that in 2014 there were 76,100 new cases of melanoma in this country, with 9,710 deaths from this disease. Incidence rates for melanoma have increased steadily over the past several decades, currently rising at a rate of approximately 3.1% per year. It is unclear whether this increased incidence is because of better and earlier detection and/or increased public awareness of melanoma or whether it is owing to a change in sun-seeking behavior, or a combination of the aforementioned. The estimated lifetime risk of developing melanoma for a person born in 2010 in the United States is 1 in 39 for Caucasian men and 1 in 58 for Caucasian women.

RISK FACTORS

Several risk factors have been identified for the development of melanoma.

- *Ultraviolet irradiation*: there may be a stronger association between intermittent exposure and sunburn in adolescence and childhood with development of melanoma. Melanoma risk is also increased by ultraviolet irradiation from tanning beds.
- *Atypical nevi*: patients with more than five atypical nevi are at higher risk.
- *Increased numbers of benign nevi*, with those having greater than 100 nevi being at higher risk of developing melanoma.
- *Large and Giant congenital melanocytic nevi*, defined as greater than 20 cm and 40 cm, respectively, have an estimated <5% increased risk of melanoma.
- *Phenotypic features*, including pale or light skin, blonde or red hair, blue or green eyes, a tendency toward freckling, and poor tanning ability.
- *Family history of melanoma*.
- *Host immunosuppression*, which includes transplant patients and patients on chronic immunosuppression for autoimmune diseases.
- *Genetic predisposition*, including defects in the *CDKN2A* gene and/or the *CDK4* gene, and genodermatoses such as xeroderma pigmentosum.

TYPES OF PRIMARY MELANOMA

Superficial spreading melanoma (Fig. 32-1) represents the most common clinical subtype, accounting for approximately 75% of cutaneous melanomas. While the majority arise de novo,

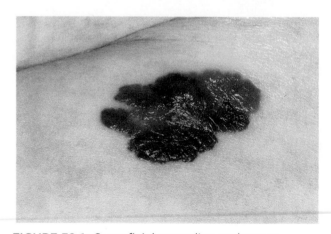

FIGURE 32-1: Superficial spreading melanoma.

about 25% associates with a preexisting nevus. These tumors typically experience a slow horizontal growth phase but can be followed by a rapid vertical growth phase, which may be evident by the development of a papule or nodule. Sites of predilection include the backs of men and the legs of women, although they can occur at any site.

Nodular melanoma accounts for approximately 15% to 30% of cutaneous melanomas and by definition has a vertical growth phase, accounting for its rapid invasion. It quickly enters the vertical growth phase. It is seen more frequently in men, and sites of predilection include the trunk, head, and neck. It typically appears as a dark blue-black papule or nodule that develops rapidly and may include a history of ulceration or bleeding.

Lentigo maligna melanoma is a less common clinical subtype, comprising approximately 10% to 15% of cutaneous melanomas, although the incidence is rising in the United States. This lesion arises from a lentigo maligna (melanoma in situ of sun-exposed skin) and involves dermal invasion. Tumors typically occur in the elderly and arise on sun-damaged skin, including the forearms and the face. These lesions present as large, irregularly asymmetric-shaped macules or patches with variations of tan, brown, or black pigment, and they may eventually develop a papular or nodular component.

Acral lentiginous melanoma (Fig. 32-2) represents approximately 5% of cutaneous melanomas but is the most common type found in darker-complexioned individuals. Most frequent sites include the palms, soles, or beneath the nail plate. Lesions frequently present as brown-to-black macules with irregular borders and variations in color, although papules and nodules may be present. This subtype typically has a poor prognosis, which may be related to delayed diagnosis. Therefore, early biopsy of suspected lesions is critical.

Other Variants

Amelanotic melanoma represents 2% to 8% of all melanomas. Lesions may present as pink macules, plaques, or nodules and are often clinically mistaken for benign lesions. Thus, although uncommon, it often poses serious diagnostic challenges and delay in diagnosis.

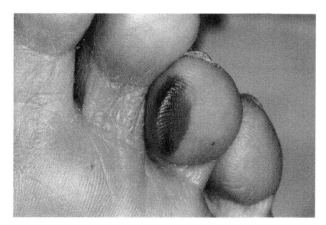

FIGURE 32-2: Acral lentiginous melanoma.

Desmoplastic melanoma is rare. It commonly presents as a pale nodule or plaque located in sun-exposed areas of the head, neck, or upper back of older patients; and thus is clinically confused for a scar or nonmelanoma skin cancer. A helpful clue is the presence of pigmentation over a dermal nodule.

Spitzoid melanoma is a subset of melanoma that morphologically resembles Spitz tumors. They commonly present as enlarging papules, plaques, or nodules, either amelanotic or with brown or blue color.

DIAGNOSIS

Early identification and treatment of melanomas are essential as prognosis depends on the stage of disease at diagnosis. Pertinent data should be gathered from the medical history, including personal or family history of melanoma, any change in existing skin lesions including changes in size, shape, or pigmentation, as well as any history of bleeding or ulceration.

Physical examination should include evaluation of all skin, including scalp and mucous membranes, using the American Cancer Society's ABCDE mnemonic to identify suspicious lesions. *A* is for asymmetry, *B* for irregular borders, *C* for irregular color, *D* for diameter, with size greater than 6 mm, and E for evolution typically considered suspicious. Dermatoscopy, also known as *epiluminescence microscopy*, is a noninvasive tool used for magnification and may contribute to diagnosis.

Once identified, suspicious lesions should be evaluated with full-thickness biopsy and 1 to 2 mm margin along with subcutaneous fat to allow assessment of lesion thickness. Excisional biopsy should be performed when possible to evaluate the entire lesion; prognosis and treatment are determined by tumor thickness. When excisional biopsy is impractical, such as extensive lesions of lentigo maligna on the face or acral melanoma, shave biopsy or punch biopsy may be acceptable, but should be aimed at getting a representative portion of the lesion. Punching a small area of a larger lesion that looks suspicious clinically is an antiquated teaching model and is strongly discouraged except for extensive lesions of lentigo maligna on the face or acral melanomas. Punch biopsies or superficial shave biopsies of a suspected lesion of melanoma can lead to errant histopathologic diagnoses or improper staging of melanoma lesions and are not recommended.

Also remember that in congenital nevi that develop a melanoma, they can do so at a deep location in the dermis or even subcutaneous tissue.

SAUER'S NOTES

1. Any tumor suspicious for melanoma should be biopsied or removed in its entirety whenever possible. This will give the pathologist the best chance at rendering the correct diagnosis, as well as staging and prognostic information.

2. If clinical suspicion for a melanoma is extremely high and the pathology report does not seem to fit with what you are seeing clinically, do not

be afraid to have the pathologist take a second look at the biopsy specimen. There could possibly be a sampling issue where a benign portion of the lesion was sampled in an otherwise malignant lesion, there could have been a specimen mix-up in the lab or in clinic, the malignant portion of the lesion may be deeper in the block of tissue (i.e., it was not cut into deep enough), or it could just be a very tough case. As a clinician, you cannot always think of every pathology report as a "black box" where the correct answer always comes out. Everyone makes mistakes and pathologists are not immune to making them as well.

3. If you still do not feel that the pathology fits with the clinical suspicion, you can also send the pathologist a clinical photo of the lesion and/or ask the pathologist to send out the case for an expert opinion. Trust your clinical instincts/suspicion. It may be a pain for the pathologist, but at the end of the day it is your patient you are caring for. No pathologist will be unhappy if the melanocytic lesion is diagnosed and treated correctly even if their original diagnosis is changed.

STAGING AND PROGNOSIS

The Seventh Edition of the *American Joint Committee on Cancer's Cancer Staging Manual* establishes the TNM staging system for melanoma given in Table 32-1. Stages I and II represent local disease, stage III represents regional involvement, and stage IV represents distant metastases (Table 32-2).

Important negative prognostic factors include increased tumor thickness, mitotic rate, ulceration, and nodal involvement. Tumor thickness is known as *Breslow depth*, which is defined as the distance from the top of the granular cell layer or base of ulceration to the deepest point of tumor invasion. Increased tumor thickness correlates with poorer prognosis and is the most important determinant. *Clark's level of invasion* may also be described:

- Level 1 involves only the epidermis
- Level 2 invades the papillary dermis
- Level 3 fills the papillary dermis
- Level 4 invades the reticular dermis
- Level 5 involves the subcutaneous fat

Other unfavorable prognostic factors include older age, male sex, anatomic location on the head, neck, trunk and/or acral, pathologic features such as tumor burden, growth pattern, lymphatic invasion, and/or desmoplastic melanoma.

TABLE 32-1 • TNM Staging System for Melanoma

T Category	Thickness	Ulceration Status
TX: primary tumor thickness cannot be assessed (e.g., diagnosis by curettage)	Not applicable	Not applicable
T0: no evidence of primary tumor (e.g., unknown primary or completely regressed melanoma)	Not applicable	Not applicable
Tis (melanoma in situ)	Not applicable	Not applicable
T1	≤1.0 mm	Unknown or unspecified
T1a	<0.8 mm	Without ulceration
T1b	<0.8 mm	With ulceration
T2	>1.0–2.0 mm	Unknown or unspecified
T2a	>1.0–2.0 mm	Without ulceration
T2b	>1.0–2.0 mm	With ulceration
T3	>2.0–4.0 mm	Unknown or unspecified
T3a	>2.0–4.0 mm	Without ulceration
T3b	>2.0–4.0 mm	With ulceration
T4	>4.0 mm	Unknown or unspecified
T4a	>4.0 mm	Without ulceration
T4b	>4.0 mm	With ulceration

N Category	Number of Tumor-Involved Regional Lymph Node	Presence of In-Transit, Satellite, and/or Microsatellite Metastases
NX	Regional nodes not assessed (e.g., SLN biopsy not performed, regional nodes previously removed for another reason) **Exception**: pathologic N category is not required for T1 melanomas, use cN.	No
N0	No regional metastases detected	No
N1	One tumor-involved node or in-transit, satellite, and/or microsatellite metastases with no tumor-involved nodes	
N1a	One clinically occult (i.e., detected by SLN biopsy)	No
N1b	One clinically detected	No
N1c	No regional lymph node disease	Yes
N2	Two or three tumor-involved nodes or in-transit, satellite, and/or microsatellite metastases with one tumor-involved node	
N2a	Two or three clinically occult (i.e., detected by SLN biopsy)	No
N2b	Two or three, at least one of which was clinically detected	No
N2c	One clinically occult or clinically detected	Yes
N3	Four or more tumor-involved nodes or in-transit, satellite, and/or microsatellite metastases with two or more tumor-involved nodes, or any number of matted nodes without or with in-transit, satellite, and/or microsatellite metastases	
N3a	Four or more clinically occult (i.e., detected by SLN biopsy)	No
N3b	Four or more, at least one of which was clinically detected, or presence of any number of matted nodes	No
N3c	Two or more clinically occult or clinically detected and/or presence of any number of matted nodes	Yes

M Category	Anatomic Site	LDH Level
M0	No evidence of distant metastasis	Not applicable
M1	Evidence of distant metastasis	See below
M1a	Distant metastasis to skin, soft tissue including muscle, and/or nonregional lymph node	Not recorded or unspecified
M1a(0)		Not elevated
M1a(1)		Elevated

(continued)

TABLE 32-1 • TNM Staging System for Melanoma (*continued*)

N Category	Number of Tumor-Involved Regional Lymph Node	Presence of In-Transit, Satellite, and/or Microsatellite Metastases
M1b	Distant metastasis to lung with or without M1a sites of disease	Not recorded or unspecified
M1b(0)		Not elevated
M1b(1)		Elevated
M1c	Distant metastasis to non-CNS visceral sites with or without M1a or M1b sites of disease	Not recorded or unspecified
M1c(0)		Not elevated
M1c(1)		Elevated
M1d	Distant metastasis to CNS with or without M1a, M1b, or M1c sites of disease	Not recorded or unspecified
M1d(0)		Normal
M1d(1)		Elevated

Source: From Amin MB, Edge SB, Greene FL, et al, eds. *AJCC Cancer Staging Manual.* 8th ed. New York: Springer; 2017. Used with the permission of the American Joint Committee on Cancer (AJCC), Chicago, Illinois.

TABLE 32-2 • Clinical Stage Grouping (AJCC) for Melanoma

Stage 0	Tis	N0	M0
Stage IA	T1a	N0	M0
Stage IB	T1b	N0	M0
	T2a	N0	M0
Stage IIA	T2b	N0	M0
	T3a	N0	M0
Stage IIB	T3b	N0	M0
	T4a	N0	M0
Stage IIC	T4b	N0	M0
Stage III	Any T, Tis	≥N1	M0
Stage IV	Any T	Any N	M1

Source: From Amin MB, Edge SB, Greene FL, et al, eds. *AJCC Cancer Staging Manual.* 8th ed. New York: Springer; 2017. Used with the permission of the American Joint Committee on Cancer (AJCC), Chicago, Illinois.

TABLE 32-3 • Surgical Management of Primary Cutaneous Melanoma

Tumor Thickness	Recommended Surgical Excision Margin
In situ	0.5–1 cm
≤1 mm	1 cm
1.01–2 mm	1–2 cm
2–4 mm	2 cm
>4 mm	At least 2 cm

Despite rising incidence, the overall 5-year survival rate of melanoma has improved from 81.8% in 1975 to 92.8% in 2006, which may be attributed to increased surveillance and early detection. For early stage IA disease, the 5-year survival rate is approximately 97%. However, with advanced stage IV melanoma, the 5-year survival rate ranges from 3% to 14%. Median survival is approximately 7 months.

TREATMENT

Once the diagnosis of melanoma is confirmed, complete excision of the tumor site is performed. Excisional margins are based on Breslow tumor thickness and must take anatomic site and functionality into account. The recommended surgical margins by the American Academy of Dermatology task force are listed in Table 32-3.

Lymphatic mapping and sentinel lymph node (SLN) biopsy can be performed as a staging tool for melanoma. Further studies are warranted, as prognostic implications for overall survival remain unclear. It should also be noted that sentinel lymph node biopsy or complete lymph node dissection are not without possible complications although they are usually rare. Current recommendations are to proceed with sentinel lymph node biopsy for melanomas ≥1 mm Breslow thickness. Complete lymph node dissection should be performed if a positive lymph node is identified. There is insufficient evidence to advocate routine SLN for thin melanomas (<1 mm Breslow depth). However, it can be considered in cases with poor prognostic features such as ≥1/mm^2 mitotic rate, ulceration, especially when the Breslow depth is between 0.75 and 0.99 mm.

For low-risk melanomas such as those at stages I and IIA, surgery is usually sufficient and no adjuvant therapy is indicated. For advanced disease, treatments may include medical management, surgery, and/or radiation therapy. There are three major types of medications: immunotherapy, target therapy, and chemotherapy. Several types of immunotherapy have emerged recently and largely replaced high-dose interferon.

These include anti-PD-1 checkpoint inhibitors (nivolumab, pembrolizumab) and CTLA-4 checkpoint inhibitor (ipilimumab). Target therapy drugs (vemurafenib, dabrafenib, and trametinib) have been developed to block BRAF pathway and improve survival as about one-half of all melanomas carry a mutation in the *BRAF* gene. For those who are not candidates for immunotherapy or target therapy, biochemotherapy is an alternative although this has not been shown to increase survival.

Suggested Readings

Balch CM, Gershenwald JE, Soong SJ, et al. Final version of 2009 AJCC melanoma staging and classification. *J Clin Oncol.* 2009;27(36):6199–6206.

Coit DG, Thompson JA, Andtbacka R, et al; National Comprehensive Cancer Network. Melanoma, version 4.2014. *J Natl Compr Canc Netw.* 2014;12(5):621–629.

Erdei E, Torres SM. A new understanding in the epidemiology of melanoma. *Expert Rev Anticancer Ther.* 2010;10(11):1811–1823.

Ethun CG. Delman KA. The importance of surgical margins in melanoma *J Surg Oncol.* 2015;113(3):339–345.

Fox MC, Lao CD, Schwartz JL, et al. Management options for metastatic melanoma in the era of novel therapies: a primer for the practicing dermatologist: part I: management of stage III disease. *J Am Acad Dermatol.* 2013;68(1):1.e1–1.e9.

Fox MC, Lao CD, Schwartz JL, et al. Management options for metastatic melanoma in the era of novel therapies: a primer for the practicing dermatologist: part II: management of stage IV disease. *J Am Acad Dermatol.* 2013;68(1):13.e1–13.e13.

Higgins HW 2nd, Lee KC, Galan A, et al. Melanoma in situ: part I. Epidemiology, screening, and clinical features. *J Am Acad Dermatol.* 2015;73(2):181–190.

Higgins HW 2nd, Lee KC, Galan A, et al. Melanoma in situ: part II. Histopathology, treatment, and clinical management. *J Am Acad Dermatol.* 2015;73(2):193–203.

Schaffer JV. Update on melanocytic nevi in children. *Clin Dermatol.* 2015;33(3):368–386.

Wong SL, Balch CM, Hurley P, et al. Sentinel lymph node biopsy for melanoma: American Society of Clinical Oncology and Society of Surgical Oncology joint clinical guideline. *J Clin Oncol.* 2012;30(23):2912–2918.

Vascular Tumors

Johanna S. Song, MD, MS and Marilyn G. Liang, MD

CLASSIFICATION

Vascular tumors can be characterized by:

- History
- Physical examination
- Radiologic studies
- Histology

In most cases, vascular tumors can be diagnosed using only history and physical examination. In this chapter, we will discuss the most common and most concerning vascular tumors: infantile hemangioma (IH), congenital hemangiomas, pyogenic granuloma (PG), kaposiform hemangioendothelioma (KHE), tufted angioma (TA), Kaposi sarcoma (KS), and angiosarcoma.

TUMORS VERSUS MALFORMATIONS

It is important to differentiate between *tumors* and *malformations*. In the past, vascular lesions were not well understood and were all called *hemangiomas* or some derivative with the suffix *oma*. These terms continue to be used incorrectly in the current literature. Mulliken and Glowacki proposed a new classification system for vascular anomalies in 1982 based on histologic and pathophysiologic features. *Tumors* are cellular masses with postnatal endothelial proliferative potential. *Malformations* are owing to abnormal vasculogenesis during fetal development. They enlarge over time predominantly through distention of congenitally malformed vessels rather than true endothelial cell proliferation as in an infantile hemangioma. These definitions have remained the same, with revisions (1996, 2014) to sub-categories.

BENIGN TUMORS

Infantile Hemangioma

The most common vascular tumor is the benign infantile hemangioma (IH). These tumors are unique in that they eventually involute over years without treatment, sometimes leaving no trace on the skin surface.

Presentation and Characteristics

Demographics: Of all newborns, 2% present with an IH. The prevalence of IH is about 10% of all Caucasian children. Less than 2% of Black and Asian infants are affected. There is a clear female majority of about 3–5:1. IH are much more common in premature infants, twin/multiple gestations, infants of older mothers, and infants whose mothers undergo chorionic villus sampling.

Description: Most lesions are present at birth or appear within the first week of life, often as a precursor lesion that looks like a telangiectasia or "bruise like" macule. The final size of IH ranges tremendously, from macules or papules a few millimeters in diameter to extensive plaques encompassing several developmental regions. IH can be described as superficial, deep, or mixed. Superficial IH are well-demarcated papules or plaques raised above the skin surface, with a bright red color during the proliferative and early plateau phases (Fig. 33-1). Deep IH are visible through the skin surface as a bluish-purple nodule and often seem softer and more compressible than superficial plaques (Fig. 33-2). Mixed superficial and deep IH combine a bright red superficial lesion overlying a deep component. Reticular IH are thinner, telangiectatic lesions (Fig. 33-3).

Distribution: IH are most commonly found on the head and neck (up to 85%). However, they can present on any part of the body. A patient may have several lesions. IH can be described as focal, multifocal, or regional:

- Focal: a solitary lesion

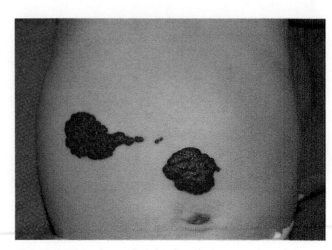

FIGURE 33-1: Superficial infantile hemangioma.

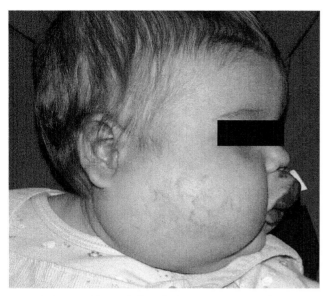

FIGURE 33-2: Deep infantile hemangioma. Also note mixed superficial and deep infantile hemangioma on the lip.

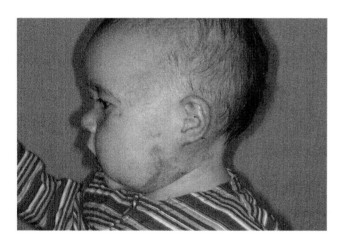

FIGURE 33-3: Reticular infantile hemangioma.

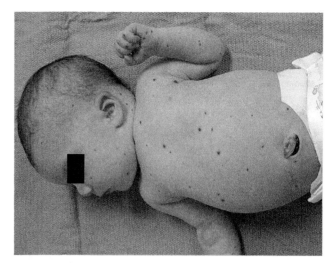

FIGURE 33-4: Multifocal infantile hemangioma.

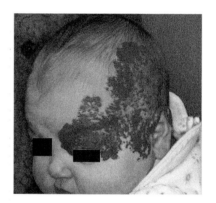

FIGURE 33-5: Regional infantile hemangioma.

- Multifocal: multiple lesions involving different anatomical regions (Fig. 33-4)
- Regional: a lesion encompassing a large surface area but limited to one anatomical or developmental region (also termed segmental) (Fig. 33-5)

Course: At birth, one-third of IH are present; the rest become apparent within the first few weeks of life. The clinical course of IH includes a proliferative, plateau, and involution phase. Superficial IH quickly become bright red over the first month of life, with the most rapid growth between 5.5 and 7.5 weeks of life. Deep IH have a more delayed onset of growth and may not become evident until 2 to 4 months of life. The proliferative phase typically lasts for 6 to 10 months, although small IH may not proliferate much and can involute within the first year or two of life. IH become softer and grayer/paler in color as they plateau in size, then involute (Fig. 33-6). At the end of involution, the lesions may look like scattered telangiectasias;

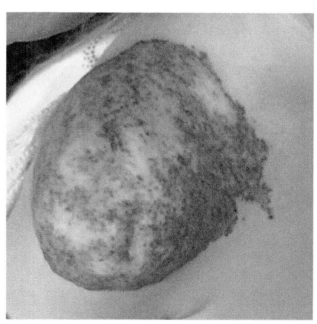

FIGURE 33-6: Involuting infantile hemangioma.

pale, fibrofatty, baggy outpouchings; soft, irregular plaques (Fig. 33-7); or may not be visible at all. Reticulate IH involute leaving only telangiectasias.

Involution time is often proportionate to the size of the lesion; larger and thicker lesions require more time to involute. A general rule in counseling parents is that 50% of all IH stop involuting by the time a child is 5 years old. IH may continue to involute until age 10.

The most common complication of IH is ulceration, usually in patients under 4 months of age. This can occur owing to rapid tumor proliferation, friction/trauma, or infection. The most common sites for ulceration are the lip and intertriginous sites, especially the perineum (Fig. 33-8). Other complications include impingement upon vital structures, such as the airway or visual axis and deformation of structures such as the nose (Fig. 33-9) and lips. IH in the "beard" distribution correlates with risk of airway involvement and respiratory distress; the larger the IH, the greater the risk of airway obstruction (Fig. 33-10). If an IH is large enough (e.g., in the liver), it can overburden the circulatory system, causing cardiac failure.

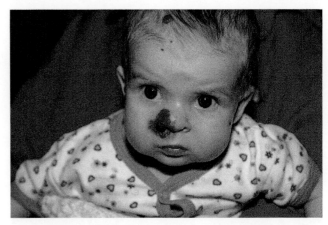

FIGURE 33-9: Nasal deformation risk in infantile hemangioma.

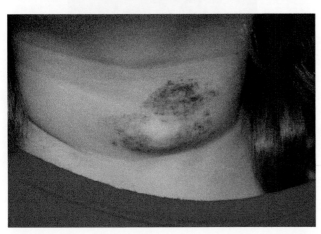

FIGURE 33-7: Residual fibrofatty infantile hemangioma.

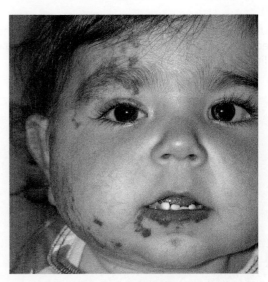

FIGURE 33-10: "Beard" distribution infantile hemangioma with airway obstruction.

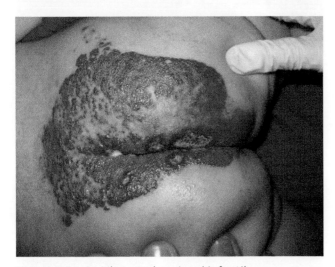

FIGURE 33-8: Ulcerated perineal infantile hemangioma.

Cause: We do not fully understand what causes IH. Evidence supports the existence of an IH endothelial stem cell that drives the proliferative potential of these tumors. A hypothesized source of these stem cells is from embolization of placental cells to the developing fetus. Support for this lies in the increased incidence of IH in infants whose mothers undergo chorionic villus sampling during pregnancy and mothers with placental complications during pregnancy (such as pre-eclampsia). In the fetal or postnatal tissue environment, these stem cells may proliferate owing to an angiogenic milieu as compared to that in placental tissues.

Radiologic Studies

Imaging is usually not necessary. Doppler ultrasound can be helpful in differentiating a bluish, deep IH from a venous malformation. IH are fast-flow lesions whereas venous malformations and other tumors are slow-flow lesions. Ultrasound can be used to screen for spinal dysraphism in young infants with sacral IH or for liver IH in patients with multifocal cutaneous hemangiomas. MRI (with and without contrast) is important to help identify and characterize abnormalities associated with regional IH.

Histology

On hematoxylin and eosin (H&E) preparations, proliferating IH are composed of a dense collection of endothelial cells and pericytes forming many capillary vascular channels arranged in lobules. These lobules are fed and drained by larger vessels. IH are characterized by positive erythrocyte type glucose transporter-1 (GLUT-1) staining, which is also expressed by placental endothelial cells. Sometimes, normal appendageal structures, such as hair follicles and nerves, may be found within the capillary lobules. During involution, there is a steady increase in fibrofatty tissue replacing the endothelial and stromal cells and vascular channels. Persistence of some of the afferent and efferent vessels may correlate with grossly visible remnant telangiectasias.

Associations to Consider

PHACE Association (Posterior fossa malformations, Hemangioma, Arterial anomalies, Coarctation of the aorta and Cardiac anomalies, Eye anomalies, Sternal clefting) should be considered and evaluated for in patients with an IH encompassing one or more developmental regions on the head and neck. This condition is much more common in females. It is not necessary to have more than one or two of the additional associations to carry a diagnosis of PHACE (Fig. 33-11).

Reticular Infantile Hemangioma of Perineum and/or Limb: These IH can be associated with chronic ulceration and ventral caudal anomalies such as omphalocele or genital anatomical defects (e.g., fistulas, ambiguous genitalia, imperforate anus). Renal anomalies have also been described.

Tethered Cord or Other Spinal Abnormalities: IH overlying the lower spine should be investigated radiologically to rule out spinal dysraphism (Fig. 33-12) or extension of IH into the spine.

Multifocal with Visceral Infantile Hemangiomas: Patients who present with five or more superficial IH scattered over the body should be evaluated for liver IH. Ultrasonography can rule out liver lesions, the most common visceral site of involvement. Large liver IH can cause profound hypothyroidism because IH produce type 3 iodothyronine deiodinase, which inactivates thyroxine and triiodothyronine causing a consumptive hypothyroidism. Liver IH can potentially lead to cardiac failure and abdominal compartment syndrome.

Differential Diagnosis

Usually, IH are clinically apparent by the first month of life. If there is ambiguity, Doppler investigation can detect an arterial signal (fast-flow) to confirm this diagnosis.
Precursor lesion differential diagnosis:

- *Ecchymosis/birth trauma:* Observation can clarify the difference, as true ecchymoses will resolve within a week.
- Kaposiform hemangioendothelioma
- Tufted angioma

Superficial hemangiomas differential diagnosis:

- *Capillary malformation (CM):* A very early superficial IH may be macular and confused with a CM. However, observation will show relatively rapid evolution from patch to papule or plaque. In addition, Doppler will demonstrate that CMs are slow-flow lesions.

Deep hemangioma differential diagnosis:

- *Cyst or cyst-like lesions (e.g., dermoid cyst, pilomatrixoma):* Ultrasound is indicated if there is insufficient or inconsistent information supporting a clinical diagnosis of IH.

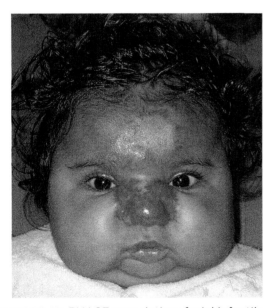

FIGURE 33-11: PHACE association: facial infantile hemangioma and absent corpus callosum.

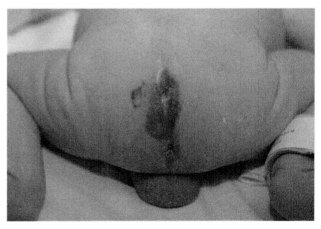

FIGURE 33-12: Sacral infantile hemangioma associated with tethered cord.

- *Congenital hemangiomas:* These are fully formed at birth and involute much more rapidly than IH or do not involute.
- *Soft tissue sarcomas (e.g., fibrosarcoma, rhabdomyosarcoma):* These are less vascularized than IH and do not exhibit a fast-flow signal via Doppler. Computed tomography (CT) and magnetic resonance imaging (MRI) also appear distinct from IH. A tumor that appears later than 4 months of age, displays an unusual proliferation pattern, or lacks fast-flow Doppler signal should be biopsied or excised to rule out malignancy.

Treatment

Most IH do not require any intervention other than bland emollients to reduce risk of frictional breakdown and ulceration. Treatment may depend on the IH location, IH characteristics, and medication complications.

- Local treatment for ulceration (emollients, antibiotics with wound care, laser)
- Topical corticosteroids
- Topical β-blockers (most commonly timolol)
- Intralesional corticosteroid
- Systemic β-blockers (most commonly propranolol; nadalol does not cross the blood–brain barrier)
- Systemic corticosteroid
- Vincristine
- Laser
- Excision

Most patients with involuting hemangiomas are treated before kindergarten, when children become more conscious of social relationships and physical differences.

Congenital Hemangiomas

Congenital hemangiomas are distinct from IH, even though many IH are also visible at birth. Congenital hemangiomas have no postnatal proliferation, and the gross clinical appearance is different from that of IH. The two categories of congenital hemangiomas include *rapidly involuting congenital hemangioma* (RICH) and *noninvoluting congenital hemangioma* (NICH).

Presentation and Characteristics

Demographics: Unlike IH, RICH and NICH occur equally in males and females.

Description: RICH and NICH can be indistinguishable from one another in appearance, especially at birth or early infancy. A pale halo around a congenital hemangioma is characteristic (Fig. 33-13). While most RICH and NICH are smooth, domed, or slightly flat-topped tumors similar to IH (Fig. 33-14), they are often more blue-gray in color. Many congenital hemangiomas exhibit large telangiectasias or coarse hairs. As a RICH involutes, it may become depressed or atrophic (Fig. 33-15).

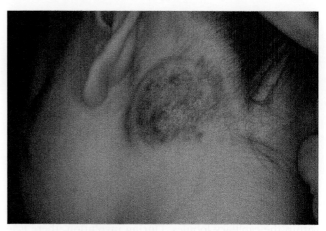

FIGURE 33-13: Noninvoluting congenital hemangioma with characteristic halo.

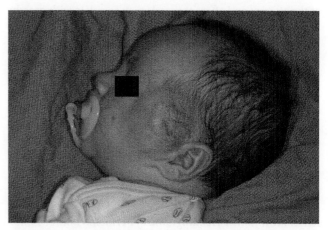

FIGURE 33-14: Rapidly involuting congenital hemangioma before involution.

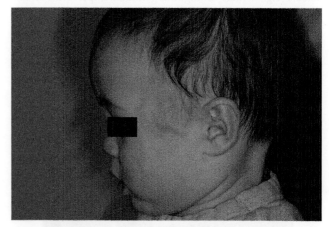

FIGURE 33-15: Rapidly involuting congenital hemangioma after involution (same patient as in Fig. 33-14).

Distribution: Both RICH and NICH tend to be found on the head and neck or extremities. Lesions on the torso are less common.

Course: As the name implies, RICH rapidly decrease in size over the first 6 to 14 months of life. There may be an atrophic plaque or even a partial regression leaving an NICH-like plaque. NICH do not change significantly with time.

Cause: Similar to IH, the cause of congenital hemangiomas is unknown.

Radiologic Studies

RICH may be detected during prenatal ultrasonography as uniformly hypoechoic masses. On MRI, they are characterized by high flow. There are large flow voids mixed with areas that are much less homogeneous than IH, as they may include arteriovenous fistulas, arterial aneurysms, thrombi, cysts, and calcifications. Ultrasonography of NICH often reveals arteriovenous fistulas. MRI and angiography of NICH is very similar to that of IH; uniform hyperintensity is seen on T2 imaging and with gadolinium.

Histology

On H&E staining, RICH display moderately prominent endothelium with rare hobnailing, interlobular fibrous tissue with zonation, and are GLUT-1 negative. As they involute, they may develop thrombi, infarctions, calcification, cysts, aneurysms, and extramedullary hematopoiesis. NICH tend to have endothelial hobnailing, dense fibrous tissue between lobules, no zonation, and are always GLUT-1 negative.

Differential Diagnosis

RICH and NICH are the main entities serving as differential diagnoses for each other. Clinical behavior over time differentiates the two.

Treatment

Many RICH are left to involute on their own. However, if there is risk of significant ulceration or bleeding, these may be excised. NICH may be excised, often after embolization of the largest vessels. Neither lesion recurs after excision.

Pyogenic Granuloma

Pyogenic granuloma (PG) is one of the persisting misnomers in dermatologic nomenclature. It is neither pyogenic (generating pus) nor a granuloma (inflammatory collection of immune cells). It is a highly vascular tumor common in infants and children, often following minor trauma. Another name used by pathologists is *lobular capillary hemangioma*.

Presentation and Characteristics

Demographics: The estimated prevalence of PG is 0.5% to 1%. The male-to-female ratio is 3:2. Half of cases occur in children younger than 5 years of age; the mean age is 6.7 years. Adults with PG are most often pregnant women.

Description: Most PG are friable, exophytic, or pedunculated red papules, which bleed easily with contact. Those that are not friable have a thicker surface that may or may not be lobulated (Fig. 33-16).

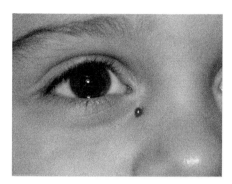

FIGURE 33-16: Pyogenic granuloma.

Distribution: The most common locations for PG are acral sites, such as the face and fingers. They may also appear on the gingiva and intraoral mucous membranes. PG may also arise within capillary malformations.

Course: PG frequently come to attention owing to the tendency to bleed as they enlarge over time, which can be rapid. At times, a pedunculated lesion may fall off at the stalk. Spontaneous regression is possible, but rare.

Cause: The cause of PG is unknown. Preceding trauma was associated in 7% of cases in one series.

Radiologic Studies

These lesions are too small and superficial to be studied radiologically.

Histology

On H&E staining, PG are dome-shaped papules with a feeder vessel giving rise to many capillary vascular spaces and fibrotic stroma. The loose proliferation of vessels simulates granulation tissue. A collarette of epithelium encircles the base of the papule. There is often an area of ulceration from which the lesion bleeds easily.

Differential Diagnosis

- Spitz nevus
- Bacillary angiomatosis (multiple lesions, immunosuppression)
- Well-differentiated angiosarcoma
- Nodular Kaposi sarcoma
- Squamous cell carcinoma
- Amelanotic melanoma
- Peripheral giant cell granuloma
- Peripheral ossifying granuloma
- Oral verrucous carcinoma

Treatment

- Direct pressure usually stops bleeding before medical attention
- Topical corticosteroids

- Topical *β*-blockers (most commonly timolol)
- Pulsed dye laser
- Electrodesiccation, surgical excision, curettage, chemical cauterization
- Imiquimod

Kaposiform Hemangioendothelioma and Tufted Angioma

Kaposiform hemangioendothelioma (KHE) and tufted angioma (TA) are important entities because they are associated with the potentially fatal Kasabach–Merritt phenomenon (KMP). Some consider KHE a low-grade malignant neoplasm because the clinical course can be aggressive and deadly owing to complications. TA is also known as *angioblastoma of Nakagawa*. KHE and TA may be on a spectrum as some vascular lesions have features of both KHE and TA. The incidence of KMP in these two lesions also supports the possibility of a pathophysiologic and histologic overlap.

Presentation and Characteristics

Demographics: KHE and TA are usually congenital lesions but later onset in childhood has been observed.

Description: KHE are classically violaceous or brawny-colored, indurated, highly infiltrative plaques, sometimes with overlying papules or nodules. Lesions are poorly defined at the borders, unlike IHs (Fig. 33-17). Skin is less commonly involved than internal organs. KHE can extend through soft tissue, muscle, and bone.

TA tend to be ruddier than KHE but often cannot be distinguished from them without a biopsy. They may be pink, red, brown, or a combination thereof. Lesion morphology can vary widely, from macules to papules/plaques (Fig. 33-18).

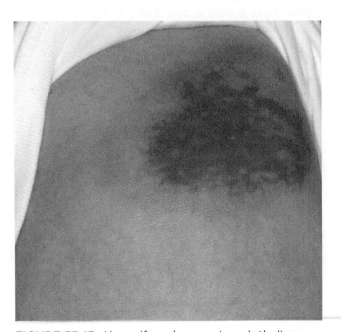

FIGURE 33-17: Kaposiform hemangioendothelioma.

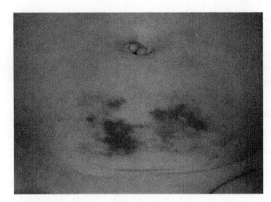

FIGURE 33-18: Tufted angioma.

Some lesions display hypertrichosis or hyperhidrosis. They can be tender to palpation. Occasionally, TA can present as a dermal tumor with a blanching halo, mimicking a rapidly involuting congenital hemangioma (RICH). TA lesions are less well defined than IH.

Distribution: The most common location for KHE is head and neck, mediastinum, and retroperitoneum. On the skin, it is typical to see a neck/shoulder/arm or hip/buttock/thigh distribution. TA are more common on the limbs but can be found anywhere on the body. There is no known metastatic potential but lesions can be locally aggressive and infiltrative.

Course: KHE rarely involutes, whereas TA may spontaneously regress by 2 years of age. However, most persist and remain painful to varying degrees. KHE and TA may increase in size and change shape slowly over time. In cases where the lesion responds to therapy, there is almost always residual tumor, fibrotic plaques, that remains.

Cause: Pathophysiology is not yet understood.

Radiologic Studies

Useful imaging modalities include MRI with and without contrast. KHE and TA may be highly infiltrative, potentially involving skin, muscle, viscera, and bone.

Histology

On H&E staining, KHE demonstrate infiltrating lobules of monomorphous spindled cells arranged in fascicles separated by fibrous septae and slit-like vascular spaces. Lymphatic channels and nests of epithelioid cells can also be seen. Microthrombi can be seen at the periphery of the lesion. Both KHE and TA stain positively for the lymphatic marker D2-40.

On H&E staining, TA demonstrate "tufts of cannonball-like aggregates" of hypertrophied endothelial cells in the middle and lower dermis. They may extend deeply into subcutaneous fat. Surrounding dermis may be fibrotic. These endothelial cells have scant cytoplasm. Vascular spaces are slit-like. There may be lymphatic channels interspersed among the "cannonballs." The epidermis may be unaffected, or there may be some degree of acanthosis and papillomatosis.

Differential Diagnosis

- Kaposiform hemangioendothelioma (KHE)
- Tufted angioma (TA)
- Kaposi sarcoma (KS)
- Spindle-cell hemangioma
- Infantile hemangioma (IH)

Treatment

There is no definitive therapy for KHE or TA. For small lesions, active nonintervention for spontaneous involution is reasonable. Treatment aims to decrease tumor size, reduce or correct coagulopathy, and decrease future sequelae. Corticosteroids, vincristine, excision, systemic β-blockers (propranolol), and sirolimus are most commonly used. Other treatments often used adjunctively may include aspirin, antiplatelet, or antifibrinolytic agents.

Kasabach–Merritt Phenomenon

Kasabach–Merritt phenomenon (KMP) has a high morbidity/mortality potential. It was first described in 1940 by Kasabach and Merritt as a consumptive thrombocytopenia occurring in association with a violaceous, indurated skin lesion. KMP is a consumptive coagulopathy with a mortality rate of 10% to 37%. KMP is typically associated with KHE; TA is less often so, and IH is not. It is not known why KHE and TA are associated with KMP while other vascular tumors are not.

Presentation and Characteristics

Demographics: Mortality is estimated to be between 10% and 40% and occurs in the context of aggressive visceral disease, profound thrombocytopenia, and infection or treatment complications.

Description: Profound thrombocytopenia observed in a patient with a vascular anomaly should immediately raise concern for KMP. Thrombosis and platelet trapping occurs within the vascular spaces of KHE and TA. The lesion becomes engorged and increasingly violaceous as the condition progresses (Fig. 33-19). The most common presenting feature in infancy is an enlarging cutaneous lesion greater than 5 to 8 cm.

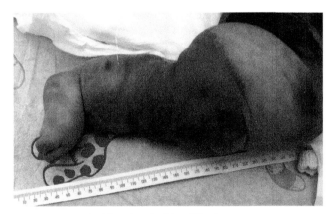

FIGURE 33-19: Kasabach–Merritt phenomenon associated with kaposiform hemangioendothelioma.

Ulceration and hemorrhage may occur. There is consumption of coagulation factors such as fibrinogen, with formation of D-dimers. Laboratory studies to confirm KMP include complete blood count to assess for thrombocytopenia and anemia, decreased fibrinogen level, increased fibrin split products, and elevated D-dimers. Platelet counts fall rapidly and may fall to below 10,000/mm^3. The risk of KMP increases significantly with depth of tumor infiltration or when the KHE or TA arise in the retroperitoneum or mediastinum.

Course: KMP manifests early, at birth or within the first few months of life. Onset in utero and in adulthood is also reported.

Cause: The initial trigger for KMP is unknown. However, there is some correlation of KMP with larger-sized tumors.

Treatment

As KMP is associated with KHE and TA, treatment is similar to that of KHE and TA. Platelet transfusion does not correct the problem and therefore is reserved for hemorrhage owing to the thrombocytopenia and just prior to surgical procedures.

> **SAUER'S NOTES**
>
> Differentiation of vascular tumors is important owing to different prognosis and different therapy. Special stains, Doppler studies, radiographic studies, histopathology, clinical appearance, and clinical course all help in obtaining the correct diagnosis.

MALIGNANT TUMORS

Kaposi Sarcoma

Kaposi sarcoma (KS) is a spindle-cell tumor derived from endothelial cells. It is uncertain if it is a malignancy or a benign vascular tumor with multiple sites of origin. This tumor became a recognizable sign of the AIDS epidemic in the 1970s before effective antiretroviral therapy was developed. Now its appearance is much less common in the HIV/AIDS population but remains a sign of inadequate therapy or noncompliance. There are four subtypes of KS: classical/sporadic, immunocompromised, AIDS-related, and endemic (African).

Presentation and Characteristics

Demographics

Classical: This subtype typically presents in elderly men of Mediterranean and Eastern European descent. The male-to-female ratio is 10–15:1.

Immunocompromised: This subtype typically presents in the organ transplant population, with an equal male-to-female ratio. The incidence of KS is 100-fold more common in transplant patients than other populations at risk. Immunocompromised patients at risk for classical KS have an even higher risk of disease. Reducing the degree of immunosuppression usually causes regression of the disease.

AIDS-related: In the United States, KS is more commonly seen in homosexual men, bisexual men, and the female partners of bisexual men. In Africa, KS is common in both the heterosexual and homosexual population. Nonsexual transmission occurs among intravenous drug abusers and those who received unscreened blood transfusions.

Endemic (African): Heterosexual HIV-seronegative men and women are affected equally and children less so. HIV-negative children are more likely to develop a lymphadenopathic subtype that, if generalized with visceral involvement, is often fatal by 3 years of age.

Description: KS skin lesions are classically dusky or violaceous, red-purple lesions. In darker-skinned patients, they may appear brown or bruise-like, and early lesions may not be appreciated without a high index of suspicion (Fig. 33-20). They evolve from a patch stage to a plaque stage, and in very advanced/aggressive cases, to nodules (Fig. 33-21). They have poorly defined borders. It is common to form more than one lesion. They occur not only in mucocutaneous locations but also in lymph nodes and viscera, potentially impairing organ function.

Distribution: Lesions are more common on the lower extremities and head/neck, including oral mucosa, but they can form anywhere on the body. It is typical to form linear lesions along skin lines in a bilateral, symmetrical distribution. The most common mucous membranes affected are the palate, gingiva, and conjunctivae (Fig. 33-22).

Course: Classical and endemic KS is an indolent disease. AIDS-associated KS is much more aggressive. Nodular KS lesions are typically seen in this latter subtype in resistant strains of HIV or in patients noncompliant with therapy.

Cause: There is an association between human herpes virus 8 (HHV-8) and low CD4 count. Restoration of natural killer (NK) cytotoxic effect and CD4 counts above 200 to 300/mL is associated with regression or indolence.

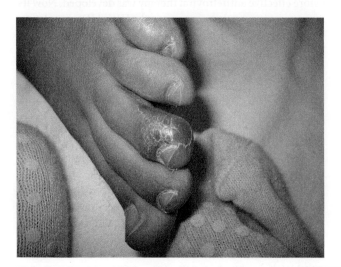

FIGURE 33-20: AIDS-related macular Kaposi sarcoma.

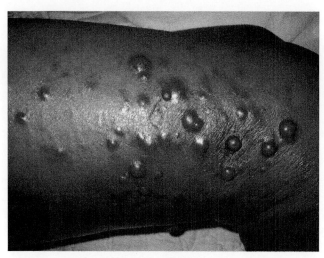

FIGURE 33-21: AIDS-related nodular Kaposi sarcoma.

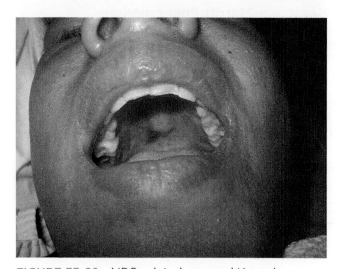

FIGURE 33-22: AIDS-related mucosal Kaposi sarcoma.

Radiologic Studies

CT or MRI should be employed in AIDS-related KS to assess for lymphatic and visceral involvement, especially hepato-splenic disease. Endoscopy, CT, and angiography may be used to assess gastrointestinal involvement. In pulmonary KS, chest radiographs show perihilar and lower lobe involvement, and sometimes pleural effusions.

Histology

KS presents with dermal slit-like vascular spaces and a proliferation of spindle cells, endothelial cells, extravasated erythrocytes, and hemosiderin-laden macrophages. Nuclear pleomorphism and many mitoses are seen. Iron, HHV-8, and CD34 or other vascular immunohistochemical stains are positive.

Differential Diagnosis

- Bacillary angiomatosis
- Ecchymosis (early macular lesions)
- Angiokeratoma

- Pyogenic granuloma
- Pseudokaposiform angiomatosis in arteriovenous malformations
- Reactive angioendotheliomatosis

Treatment

Therapy is dependent on the subtype of KS. For AIDS-related KS, highly active antiretroviral therapy (HAART) is required and may be sufficient for regression of lesions. Other therapy includes anti-HHV-8 agents (e.g., foscarnet, ganciclovir), antiangiogenesis agents (e.g., SU-5416 a VEGF inhibitor), and cytokine inhibitors. Chemotherapy (e.g., vincristine, vinblastine, bleomycin) is used for symptomatic visceral disease or rapidly progressive, severe, and widespread mucocutaneous disease. Antiangiogenic agents (e.g., thalidomide) have shown efficacy and may be combined with cytotoxic chemotherapy agents. Topical retinoids may be helpful for facial lesions.

Cryotherapy may be used for small, superficial lesions such as those on the face. Laser photocoagulation is appropriate for smaller focal lesions and palliation. Radiation therapy may be used for focal disease causing bleeding, pain, or functional impairment (e.g., oral mucosal involvement impeding speech or swallowing) or cosmetically distressful lesions. Extended-field electron beam radiation therapy may be helpful for widespread skin disease. Surgical excision may be required for visceral obstruction, lymphedema, and severe bleeding.

Angiosarcoma

Angiosarcoma is an uncommon but aggressive vascular tumor with high morbidity and mortality. Prompt workup and intervention is very important, but early diagnosis is often difficult. Stewart–Treves syndrome is angiosarcoma arising in areas of chronic lymphedema from congenital or secondary lymphedema owing to disease or surgical complications.

Presentation and Characteristics

Demographics: Cutaneous disease is more common in males, with a male-to-female ratio of 2:1. Bone and soft tissue disease is also more common in males. Caucasians are affected more than other races. Head-and-neck cutaneous disease is classically seen in elderly patients. Soft tissue angiosarcoma has a peak incidence in the seventh decade of life, but can occur even in children. Bone angiosarcoma tends to occur in adults aged 20 years and older. Immunosuppressed patients such as those with AIDS are at higher risk. Stewart–Treves syndrome is most commonly seen in patients following radical mastectomy for breast cancer. While it classically follows chronic lymphedema for many years, it can occur as soon as 1 year after mastectomy, with a median interval of 11 years.

Description: There are four variants of cutaneous angiosarcoma recognized:

- Angiosarcoma of the scalp or face (or head/neck, also known as Wilson–Jones angiosarcoma)—most common form

- Stewart–Treves syndrome
- Radiation-induced angiosarcoma
- Epithelioid angiosarcoma—rare, highly aggressive variant leading to death within 5 years of presentation

Lesions are commonly red or purple vascular papules and plaques (Fig. 33-23). They may be multifocal, arising as multiple lesions or forming satellites around a central focus with eventual coalescence of tumor cells. Early lesions may be macular and dusky, mimicking ecchymoses or radiation dermatitis, thus evading prompt diagnosis. Subcutaneous masses and necrotic, oozing, or bleeding lesions are also reported. In the setting of chronic lymphedema with chronic skin infections and poor wound healing, it can also be difficult to identify a tumor. Rapid and steady progression in tumor size is a clue to diagnosis. Metastasis to nodes occurs in 45% of cases.

Distribution: Skin and soft tissues are most commonly affected, but angiosarcoma can occur anywhere. Lesions are most commonly found on the head and neck.

Course: This is an aggressive tumor with high potential for local recurrence and metastasis regardless of the time of intervention and even with aggressive surgical treatment. Since Stewart–Treves syndrome is most commonly seen in patients following radical mastectomy for breast cancer, the most common cause of death in Stewart–Treves syndrome is metastasis to the chest wall and lungs.

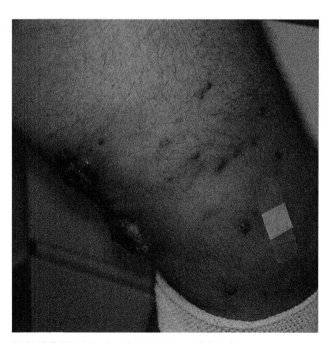

FIGURE 33-23: Angiosarcoma arising in a lymphedematous lower extremity. (Courtesy John B. Mulliken, MD.)

Cause: While it is not known what molecular stimuli trigger angiosarcoma, a high index of suspicion should be maintained in the following clinical scenarios:

- Primary lymphedema (e.g., congenital Milroy disease, idiopathic disease)
- Postsurgical lymphedema
- Secondary lymphedema owing to filariasis, trauma, or other obstructive chronic lymphedema
- Elderly patients with new head/neck vascular lesions
- History of exposure to radiation or chemical carcinogens, foreign materials such as shrapnel, implanted plastic grafts, surgical sponges, and bone wax

Local and systemic immunodeficiency has been considered as an underlying cause of malignant transformation in vascular cells. Radiation may or may not play a direct role in the specific pathophysiology of angiosarcoma.

Radiologic Studies

MRI or CT scans are used for delineating the extent of involvement into deeper tissues, involvement of cervical lymph nodes and response to therapy in head-and-neck angiosarcoma. Chest CT is used for assessment of lung, pleural, and mediastinal metastases. MRI with contrast is recommended for assessing extent of involvement in most soft tissues.

Histology

On histology, angiosarcoma show vascular spaces lined by and later invaded by atypical neoplastic endothelial cells. Higher-grade lesions are more cellular and display more mitoses. Low-grade tumors can be confused with more benign vascular lesions such as hemangioendotheliomas. High-grade, aggressive tumors display sheets of anaplastic cells that can be confused with melanomas and carcinomas. Immunohistochemical staining is positive for CD34, vimentin, factor VIII–related antigen, and cytokeratins.

Differential Diagnosis

- Cellulitis
- Ecchymosis
- Stasis changes owing to lymphedema
- Pyogenic granuloma
- Kaposi sarcoma
- Metastasis from other neoplasms (e.g., breast carcinoma)
- Amelanotic melanoma

- Leiomyosarcoma
- Fibrosarcoma
- Liposarcoma

Treatment

Prompt surgical excision is the primary intervention. Wide local excision (at least 5 cm) is performed, but is often insufficient. Large lesions require amputation of limbs and/or wide regional resection of affected areas. Adjuvant chemotherapy or radiotherapy generally does not confer added survival but excision followed by radiotherapy helps with local disease control, and in focal cutaneous angiosarcoma may prolong survival.

Chemotherapy and/or radiation therapy alone may be attempted if a patient refuses surgical intervention or is a poor candidate for surgical intervention, but this is typically unsuccessful. Surgical intervention is impractical if there is extension into vital structures, if the lesion is very extensive, or for large multifocal lesions. Doxorubicin and actinomycin D are the most commonly used chemotherapeutic agents. Other agents being investigated (e.g., paclitaxel, targeted immunotherapies) may also be beneficial.

Suggested Readings

Antman K, Chang Y. Kaposi's sarcoma. *N Engl J Med.* 2000;342:1027–1038.

Croteau SE, Liang MG, Kozakewich HP, et al. Kaposiform hemangioendothelioma: atypical features and risks of Kasabach-Merritt phenomenon in 107 referrals. *J Pediatr.* 2013;162:142–147.

Drolet BA, Frommelt PC, Chamlin SL, et al. Initiation and use of propranolol for infantile hemangioma: report of a consensus conference. *Pediatrics.* 2013;131:128–140.

Drolet BA, Trenor CC 3rd, Brandão LR, et al. Consensus-derived practice standards plan for complicated Kaposiform hemangioendothelioma. *J Pediatr.* 2013;163:285–291.

Hemangioma Investigator Group, Haggstrom AN, Drolet BA, et al. Prospective study of infantile hemangiomas: demographic, prenatal, and perinatal characteristics. *J Pediatr.* 2007;150:291–294.

Huang SA, Tu HM, Harney JW, et al. Severe hypothyroidism caused by type 3 iodothyronine deiodinase in infantile hemangiomas. *N Engl J Med.* 2000;343:185–189.

Liang MG, Frieden IJ. Infantile and congenital hemangiomas. *Semin Pediatr Surg.* 2014;23:162–167.

Mendenhall WM, Mendenhall CM, Werning JW, et al. Cutaneous angiosarcoma. *Am J Clin Oncol.* 2006;29:524–528.

Metry DW, Garzon MC, Drolet BA, et al. PHACE syndrome: current knowledge, future directions. *Pediatr Dermatol.* 2009;26:381–398.

Mulliken JB, Fishman SJ, Burrows PE. Vascular anomalies. *Curr Probl Surg.* 2000;37:517–584.

Wassef M, Blei F, Adams D, et al. Vascular anomalies classification: recommendations from the International Society for the Study of Vascular Anomalies. *Pediatrics.* 2015;136:e203–e214.

Cutaneous T-cell Lymphoma

Steven E. Eilers, MD, W. Clark Lambert, MD, PhD,
and Robert A. Schwartz, MD, MPH, DSc (Hon), FAAD, FRCP (Edin)

The diagnosis of cutaneous lymphoma mandates consideration of a large and diverse group of malignant B-cell or T-cell lymphocytes in various stages of differentiation. In this chapter, we focus on skin, the primary site of cutaneous lymphoma. Historically, primary cutaneous lymphomas were thought to be of T-cell origin; cutaneous B-cell lymphomas (CBCLs) were assumed to be secondary, or a dissemination of a nodal B-cell lymphoma. With the advent of immunohistochemical and molecular genetic modalities, it has become clear that B-cell cutaneous lymphomas are, in fact, a distinct and important group of primary cutaneous lymphomas. The majority are low-grade malignancies that have a good prognosis and slow course. This chapter will focus on primary cutaneous T-cell lymphomas (CTCLs).

CTCLs are the largest group of cutaneous lymphomas, accounting for 65% to 80% of all cases. They are classified by the World Health Organization (WHO)/European Organization for Research and Treatment of Cancer (EORTC) classification (WHO–EORTC classification) as follows:

Indolent clinical behavior:

- Mycosis fungoides (MF)
- MF variants: Pagetoid reticulosis (localized), follicular, syringotropic, granulomatous, and granulomatous slack skin (GSS) syndrome
- CD30$^+$ T-cell lymphoproliferative disorders of the skin
  - Lymphomatoid papulosis
  - Primary cutaneous anaplastic large cell lymphoma
- Subcutaneous panniculitis-like T-cell lymphoma (SPTL)
- Primary cutaneous CD4$^+$ small/medium-sized pleomorphic T-cell lymphoma

Aggressive clinical behavior:

- Sézary syndrome (SS)
- Primary cutaneous peripheral T-cell lymphoma (PTL), unspecified
  - PTL subtypes: Primary cutaneous aggressive epidermotropic CD8$^+$ T-cell lymphoma
- Cutaneous $\gamma\Delta^+$ T-cell lymphoma (CGD-TCL) Extranodal NK/T-cell lymphoma, nasal type
  - Variant—Hydroa vacciniforme-like lymphoma
- Adult T-cell leukemia/lymphoma (ATLL)
- Angioimmunoblastic T-cell lymphoma

CTCL, most commonly evident as MF, is typically a clonal expansion of T-helper cells, less often of T suppressor/killer cells or NK cells, manifesting as a widespread and long-standing cutaneous eruption. MF is characterized by the relatively predictable and often gradual evolution of patches into plaques and tumors composed of skin-targeting malignant T cells. This progression may be gradual; the patient may outlive the disease.

Pagetoid reticulosis is a noteworthy variant of MF characterized by the presence of localized discrete cutaneous patches or plaques with an intraepidermal proliferation of neoplastic T cells. The term *pagetoid reticulosis* should be restricted to the localized type (Woringer–Kolopp type) and should not be used to describe the disseminated form (Ketron–Goodman type). Generalized cases should probably be classified as aggressive epidermotropic CD8$^+$ CTCL, CGD-TCL, or tumor-stage MF.

GSS syndrome is a rare subtype of CTCL characterized by the development of folds of loose or "slack" skin in the major skin folds and, histologically, by an infiltrate of clonal T cells, with exceptionally large multinucleated giant cells sometimes showing inclusion of fragmented elastic fibers.

SS has been defined historically by the triad of erythroderma, generalized lymphadenopathy, and the presence of neoplastic T cells (Sézary cells) in skin, lymph nodes, and peripheral blood, respectively. Others assert that the definition of SS should include one or more of the following:

- An absolute Sézary cell count of at least $1,000/\mu L$
- Demonstration of immunophenotypical abnormalities (an expanded CD4$^+$ T-cell population resulting in a CD4/CD8 ratio of more than 10:1; loss of any or all of the T-cell antigens CD2, CD3, CD4, CD5; or loss of both CD4 and CD5)
- Demonstration of a T-cell clone in the peripheral blood by molecular or cytogenetic methods

ATLL is an aggressive T-cell neoplasm associated with human T-cell leukemia virus 1 (HTLV-1). Although an indolent form involving the skin may occur, cutaneous findings are usually a manifestation of widely disseminated disease.

SPTL is a type of T-cell lymphoma characterized by the presence of primarily subcutaneous infiltrates of neoplastic T cells and macrophages, predominantly affecting the legs and often complicated by a hemophagocytic syndrome. There are at least two groups of SPTL with different histologies, phenotypes, and prognoses. Cases with an α/β^+ T-cell phenotype are usually CD8$^+$, are restricted to the subcutaneous tissue (with no dermal or epidermal involvement), and tend to run an indolent course. The SPTL designation is used only for patients with an α/β^+ T-cell phenotype, whereas those with a γ/Δ T-cell phenotype are now categorized as having CGD-TCL.

Extranodal NK/T-cell lymphoma is an Epstein–Barr virus (EBV)–associated lymphoma usually with an NK cell, or, less commonly, a cytotoxic T-cell phenotype. The nasal cavity or nasopharynx is the most common site of involvement, and the skin is the second most common site. Cutaneous involvement may be primary or secondary; however, because both primary and secondary involvement are clinically aggressive and require the same type of treatment, distinction between the two cutaneous forms is largely academic.

Primary cutaneous PTL, type unspecified, encompasses those CTCLs that do not fit into any of the subtypes of CTCLs. These include the provisional entities described later, because primary cutaneous aggressive epidermotropic CD8$^+$ cytotoxic T-cell lymphoma, CGD-TCL, and primary cutaneous small/medium CD4$^+$ T-cell lymphoma are sufficiently characteristic that they can be separated as provisional entities:

- Primary cutaneous aggressive epidermotropic CD8$^+$ cytotoxic T-cell lymphoma, a provisional entity, is characterized by a proliferation of epidermotropic CD8$^+$ cytotoxic T cells and aggressive clinical behavior.
- CGD-TCL is composed of a clonal proliferation of mature, activated γ/Δ T cells with a cytotoxic phenotype. It may be a primary or secondary cutaneous lymphoma.
- Primary cutaneous CD4$^+$ small/medium-sized pleomorphic T-cell lymphoma is the diagnosis used when a predominance of small- to medium-sized CD4$^+$ pleomorphic T cells are present without a history of patches and plaques typical of MF. Clinical course is typically indolent, and some newer studies have questioned its

classification as a true lymphoma or simply a lymphoproliferative disorder.

PATHOPHYSIOLOGY

The primary pathophysiologic mechanisms for the development of CTCL (i.e., MF) have not been elucidated. Genetic, genotraumatic, immunologic, and environmental etiologies have all been considered. Chronic exposure to various irritants has been considered in the pathogenesis of CTCL, but evidence thus far is not conclusive. A persistent antigen that over time leads to an accumulation of mutations in oncogenes, suppressor genes, and signal-transducing genes has been suggested. One of us (WCL) has proposed the thymus-bypass hypothesis that aberrant differentiation, in which T cells differentiate in the skin (rather than thymus), may be a cause.

EPIDEMIOLOGY

In the United States, the incidence of CTCL is approximately five cases per million people per year. It is assumed that there is a similar worldwide incidence with some possible increases among workers using machine cutting oils. Areas where HTLV-1 is endemic, such as certain Caribbean Islands, parts of South America, Central Africa, and southwest Japan, have a higher incidence of ATLL. In Jamaica and selected other Caribbean Islands, childhood-infective dermatitis is viewed as a marker of HTLV-1 infection. CTCL is more common in men than women with an approximate ratio of 2:1. Most patients with CTCL are middle aged or elderly. Peak incidence is during the fifth decade, although it may rarely occur in children. Children with CTCL usually have a mild course and excellent prognosis, although progression to tumor stage and death may occur. There does not seem to be a male predominance in children, with one series observing a female predominance. As CTCL in its incipient stage may present as a chronic, poorly defined dermatitis, the average duration from onset to diagnosis of CTCL is 4 to 6 years. Most cases are treated with myriad topical agents preceding biopsy that obscure histologic diagnosis.

HISTORY AND STAGING

Classic MF

MF is divided into three stages: patch, plaque, and tumor (Figs. 34-1 to 34-3). The patch stage may persist for many years and is characterized by a nonspecific dermatitis usually consisting of patches most commonly centrally located on the lower trunk and buttocks. Sometimes, these patches have a thin, wrinkled quality, often with reticulated pigmentation. In this stage, pruritus is usually minimal or absent. Classic MF is usually preceded by a nonspecific indolent inflammatory process, manifesting as atopic dermatitis, nonspecific chronic dermatitis, or parapsoriasis (most commonly, large-plaque parapsoriasis), which may progress over years to decades to

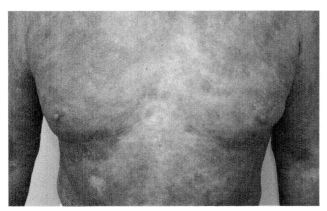

FIGURE 34-1: Plaque-stage CTCL on the anterior trunk.

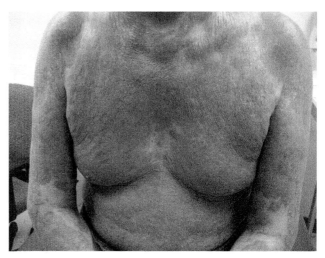

FIGURE 34-3: Mycosis fungoides with partially confluent erythematous plaques.

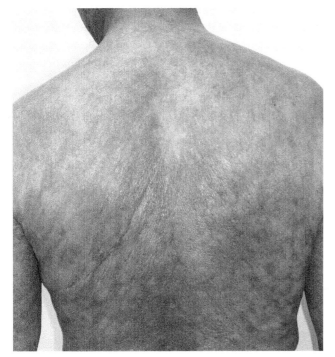

FIGURE 34-2: Patch-stage CTCL with cigarette paper wrinkling atrophy and hyperpigmentation. Some areas are already forming plaques over the left lower back.

Stages IA and IIA

The stage of disease determines the prognosis for most cases of CTCL, particularly MF and SS. Stage IA consists of patches and/or plaques affecting less than 10% of the total body surface without erythroderma, lymph node, or visceral involvement. Stage IB is defined by involvement of 10% or more of the total body surface.

Stages IIA and IIB

CTCL is stage IIA if there are clinically enlarged lymph nodes that histologically do not show evidence of CTCL tumor cells. If skin tumors of CTCL are present with no visceral involvement or erythroderma, the disease is in stage IIB, regardless of lymph node involvement. Either process usually takes years or even decades to develop. Tumors once formed are prone to ulceration.

Stages III, IVA, and IVB

The disease is classified as stage III if erythroderma is present, but neither circulating lymphoma cells nor histologically proven involvement of lymph nodes or viscera is present, regardless of whether lymphadenopathy is noted. If lymph nodes are histologically involved with the lymphomatous process, the disease is in stage IVA. Visceral involvement with histologically proven lymphoma denotes stage IVB.

D'emblee MF

MF usually progresses sequentially through its stages. However, rarely the development of apparent MF tumors may occur without preceding patches or plaques. Most, if not all, such cases may represent primary cutaneous CD30[+] pleomorphic, medium or large cell T-cell lymphomas.

Transformation of MF

MF in any stage may suddenly accelerate or become much more aggressive, progressing rapidly to more advanced stages. This is associated with the histologic appearance of large atypical

early plaque-stage MF. Some authorities regard large-plaque parapsoriasis as patch-stage MF. In many cases, the disease does not progress beyond this stage, and the diagnosis of MF is never confirmed. In other cases, the disease appears from the beginning as rather well-defined superficial plaques that range from 2 cm to more than 20 cm in diameter.

Although well-developed plaques that are clinically diagnostic for MF are usually intensely pruritic, less characteristic ones typically are not. The development of pruritus in such lesions is a sign of progression toward MF. Many cases remain at these stages for many years or decades without further progression.

cells. Often, these are CD30$^+$, and the process is termed large cell transformation.

Pagetoid Reticulosis, Localized (Woringer–Kolopp) Type

Patients with this slowly progressive subtype are usually first seen with a solitary psoriasiform or hyperkeratotic patch or plaque most commonly located on the extremities. Extracutaneous dissemination or disease-related deaths rarely occur. In contrast, multilesional pagetoid reticulosis (Ketron–Goodman disease) has a clinical course similar to MF and is regarded as a variant of MF. Some cases may actually represent primary cutaneous epidermotropic CD8$^+$ (cytotoxic) T-cell lymphoma.

These definitions are depicted in Table 34-1. Table 34-2 lists the TNMB (tumor, node, metastasis, blood) stage definitions. Table 34-3 shows a comparison of the two systems.

Variants of MF

- Folliculotropic MF (FMF) presents commonly with alopecia, follicular cysts, or comedo-like lesions and is usually associated with follicular mucinosis and strong epidermotropism. This variant may also be called alopecia mucinosa when mucin is present. However, the benign form of alopecia mucinosa, not associated with MF, must

be distinguished from MF associated with mucinosis. The most relevant feature, with and without associated follicular mucinosis, is the deep follicular and perifollicular localization of the neoplastic infiltrates, which makes them less accessible to skin-targeted therapies.

- Hypopigmented MF tends to occur in young people of Indian, Latin American, or sub-Saharan African American heritage. It manifests as irregular but fairly well-demarcated hypopigmented or white patches. They are either asymptomatic or slightly pruritic and may appear with or without other more characteristic MF lesions.
- MF may demonstrate a granulomatous reaction pattern.
- Bullous MF may present with flaccid or tense bullae arising on normal skin, an erythematous base, or within typical patch- or plaque-stage lesions of MF. It is most commonly found on the trunk and extremities. Rarely, it may clinically resemble pemphigus foliaceous, pemphigus vulgaris, or erythema multiforme.
- Pustular MF is most often found on the palms but may occur anywhere.
- Hyperpigmented MF is a diffuse macular hyperpigmentation accompanied by typical MF, or, more rarely, as the sole manifestation of the disease. These lesions

---

TABLE 34-1 • Staging of CTCL

Stage	Patches <10%	Plaques ≥10%	Tumors	Lymphadenopathy	Erythroderma	Lymph Nodes	Viscera
	Skin Lesions					**Histologic Lymphoma**	
IA	+	−	−	−	−	−	−
IB	+ or −	+	−	−	−	−	−
IIA	+ or −	+ or −	+ or −	+	−	−	−
IIB	+ or −	+ or −	+	+ or −	−	−	−
III	+ or −	+ or −	+ or −	+ or −	+	−	−
IVA	+ or −	+ or −	+ or −	+ or −	+ or −	+	−
IVB	+ or −	+ or −	+ or −	+ or −	+ or −	+ or −	+

TABLE 34-2 • TNMB Staging of CTCL

T Category	T Criteria
T1	Limited patches, ^{a}papules, and/or plaques^b covering <10% of the skin surface
T1a	T1a (patch only)
T1b	T1b (plaque ± patch)
T2	Patches, papules, or plaques covering ≥10% of the skin surface
T2a	T2a (patch only)
T2b	T2b (plaque ± patch)
T3	One or more tumors^c (≥ cm in diameter)
T4	Confluence of erythema covering ≥80% of body surface area

TABLE 34-2 • TNMB Staging of CTCL (*continued*)

N Category	N Criteria
NX	Clinically abnormal peripheral lymph nodes; no histologic confirmation
N0	No clinically abnormal peripheral lymph nodes[d]; biopsy not required
N1	Clinically abnormal peripheral lymph nodes; histopathology Dutch grade 1 or National Cancer Institute (NCI) LN0–2
N1a	Clone negative[e]
N1b	Clone positive[e]
N2	Clinically abnormal peripheral lymph nodes; histopathology Dutch grade 2 or NCI LN3
N2a	Clone negative[e]
N2b	Clone positive[e]
N3	Clinically abnormal peripheral lymph nodes; Histopathology Dutch grades 3–4 or NCI LN4; clone positive or negative

Definition of Distant Metastasis (M)—Visceral

M Category	M Criteria
M0	No visceral organ involvement
M1	Visceral involvement (must have pathology confirmation, [f]and organ involved should be specified)

Peripheral Blood Involvement (B)

B Category	B Criteria
B0	Absence of significant blood involvement: ≥5% of peripheral blood lymphocytes are atypical (Sézary) cells[g]
B0a	Clone negative[h]
B0b	Clone positive[h]
B1	Low blood tumor burden:>5% of peripheral blood lymphocytes are atypical (Sézary) cells, but does not meet the criteria of B2
B1a	Clone negative[h]
B1b	Clone positive[h]
B2	High blood tumor burden: ≥1,000/μL Sézary cells[g] with positive clone[h]

[a]For skin, *patch* indicates any size skin lesion without significant elevation or induration. Presence/absence of hypo- or hyperpigmentation, scale, crusting, and/or poikiloderma should be noted.

[b]For skin, *plaque* indicates any size skin lesion that is elevated or indurated. Presence/absence of scale, crusting, and/or poikiloderma should be noted. Histologic features such as folliculotropism, large cell transformation (>25% large cells), and CD30 positivity or negativity, as well as clinical features such as ulceration, are important to document.

[c]For skin, *tumor* indicates at least one 1-cm diameter solid or nodular lesion with evidence of depth and/or vertical growth. Note the total number of lesions, total volume of lesions, largest size lesion, and region of body involved. Also note whether there is histologic evidence of large cell transformation. Phenotyping for CD30 is encouraged.

[d]For node, *abnormal peripheral lymph node(s)* indicates any palpable peripheral node that on physical examination is firm, irregular, clustered, fixed or ≥1.5 cm in diameter. Node groups examined on physical examination include cervical, supraclavicular, epitrochlear, axillary, and inguinal. Central nodes, which generally are not amenable to pathologic assessment, currently are not considered in the nodal classification unless used to establish N3 histopathologically.

[e]A T-cell clone is defined by polymerase chain reaction (PCR) or Southern blot analysis of the TCR gene.

[f]For viscera, spleen and liver may be diagnosed by imaging criteria.

[g]For blood, Sézary cells are defined as lymphocytes with hyperconvoluted cerebriform nuclei. If Sézary cells cannot be used to determine tumor burden for B2, then one of the following modified ISCL criteria, along with a positive clonal rearrangement of the TCR, may be used instead: (1) expanded CD4[+] or CD3[+] cells with a CD4/CD8 ratio of ≥10, or (2) expanded CD4[+] cells with abnormal immunophenotype, including loss of CD7 or CD26.

[h]A T-cell clone is defined by PCR or Southern blot analysis of the TCR gene.

Source: From Olsen et al., with permission from the American Society of Hematology; Amin MB, Edge SB, Greene FL, et al, eds. *AJCC Cancer Staging Manual.* 8th ed. New York: Springer; 2017. Used with the permission of the American Joint Committee on Cancer (AJCC), Chicago, Illinois.

TABLE 34-3 • Comparison of Staging Systems for CTCL

When T Is...	And N Is...	And M Is...	And Peripheral Blood Involvement (B) Is...	Then the Stage Group Is...
T1	N0	M0	B0,1	IA
T2	N0	M0	B0,1	IB
T1,2	N1,2	M0	B0,1	IIA
T3	N0-2	M0	B0,1	IIB
T4	N0-2	M0	B0,1	III
T4	N0-2	M0	B0	IIIA
T4	N0-2	M0	B1	IIIB
T1-4	N0-2	M0	B2	IVA1
T1-4	N3	M0	B0-2	IVA2
T1-4	N0-3	M1	B0-2	IVB

Source: From Olsen et al., with permission from the American Society of Hematology; Amin MB, Edge SB, Greene FL, et al, eds. *AJCC Cancer Staging Manual.* 8th ed. New York: Springer; 2017. Used with the permission of the American Joint Committee on Cancer (AJCC), Chicago, Illinois.

may resemble ashy dermatosis or postinflammatory hyperpigmentation.

■ Unilesional MF shows histologic changes that are identical to those that occur with multiple disseminated lesions of MF. The prognosis is excellent following treatment including excision or radiotherapy, although it may recur.

■ In addition to hair follicles (folliculotropism), MF cells may be seen in eccrine glands. Rarely, this may be the only manifestation of MF, designated as syringotropic MF (syringolymphoid hyperplasia). Both the eccrine duct and the eccrine gland may be affected and may mimic eccrine carcinoma. Lesions manifest as flesh-colored, brown, or red papules; patches; and/or scaly plaques. Hair loss without mucinous degeneration in the affected areas is common. All reported cases have occurred in men.

■ Pagetoid reticulosis (Woringer–Kolopp disease) arises preferentially on acral skin as a single, slowly growing psoriasiform plaque. Dissemination or extracutaneous manifestation does not occur. The classic histologic finding is the pagetoid spread of haloed lymphoid cells in the epidermis.

■ Poikilodermic MF, often evident as poikiloderma vasculare atrophicans, represents a combination of atrophic, dry, reticulated dyspigmented skin with telangiectasia developing in cases of otherwise typical MF. It can involve the entire body surface. On occasion, it may be the only presenting manifestation of the disease.

■ Other variants of MF include hyperkeratotic/verrucous and vegetating/papillomatous MF, typically arising in the cervical neck, axillae, perineum, and sometimes on

the breasts near the areolae, resembling acanthosis nigricans or multiple seborrheic keratoses.

■ Persistent pigmented purpura or lichenoid processes also may be manifestations of MF.

■ Mucosal involvement by MF is rare and may occur as part of a more generalized involvement in cases with extensive disease, particularly those that have undergone large cell transformation. It is a poor prognostic sign.

■ GSS syndrome, as described above, affects intertriginous skin, particularly axilla and groin.

PHYSICAL

■ Initially, MF has a predilection for central sun-protected areas such as the proximal lower extremities and buttocks. In tumor-stage MF, the usual presentation is a combination of patches, plaques, and tumors. The tumors are prone to ulceration. However, if only tumors are present, without preceding or concurrent patches or plaques, a diagnosis of MF is highly unlikely and another type of CTCL or CBCL should be considered. In the rare case where MF begins in the tumor stage, it is referred to as the tumor de'emble type of MF, and the prognosis tends to be poor.

■ SS occurs almost exclusively in adults. It is characterized by erythroderma, often associated with marked pruritus and exfoliative dermatitis, edema, and lichenification. Lymphadenopathy, alopecia, onychodystrophy, and palmoplantar hyperkeratosis are also associated.

- GSS syndrome shows circumscribed areas of pendulous loose or slack skin with a predilection for the axillae and groin. An association with Hodgkin lymphoma may exist. Most patients experience an indolent course of disease.
- Acute ATLL manifests with skin lesions in about 50% of cases. It is also characterized by the presence of leukemia, lymphadenopathy, organomegaly, and hypercalcemia. Skin lesions most commonly include nodules or tumors (33%), generalized papules (22%), or plaques (19%).
- SPTL is a rare form of CTCL. Patients usually present with single or multiple nodules and/or plaques, mainly involving the legs. Ulceration is rare, but constitutional symptoms may be present. Visceral or lymph node involvement is rare. SPTL may be preceded for years or decades by a seemingly benign panniculitis suggestive of chronic erythema nodosum or scalp alopecia.
- Primary cutaneous PTL, unspecified, is a heterogeneous group of diseases for which the common characteristic is a lack of typical physical features of MF.
- Cutaneous $\gamma\Delta$ T-cell lymphoma lies within the PTL subset. It is usually aggressive and manifests with disseminated plaques or ulceronecrotic nodules or tumors, particularly on the extremities.
- Primary cutaneous aggressive epidermotropic CD8$^+$ cytotoxic T-cell lymphoma (provisional) manifests localized or disseminated eruptive papules, nodules, and tumors that show central ulceration and necrosis or superficial, hyperkeratotic patches and plaques.
- Primary cutaneous CD4$^+$ small/medium-sized pleomorphic T-cell lymphoma tends to be first apparent as a solitary plaque or tumor, generally on the head/neck, or upper trunk, although it may less commonly appear as one or several papules, nodules, or tumors.
- Extranodal NK/T-cell lymphoma, nasal type, usually appears as a midfacial destructive tumor or multiple plaques or tumors, often with ulceration. It preferentially occurs on the trunk and extremities. This was formerly termed *lethal midline granuloma* and was considered a destructive form of vasculitis. Constitutional symptoms may be present. Extranodal NK/T-cell lymphoma, nasal type, has a variant that resembles hydroa vacciniforme. It occurs in children, mainly in Latin America and Asia, and has a papulovesicular eruption that typically occurs on sun-exposed areas.

DIFFERENTIAL DIAGNOSIS

Differential diagnosis includes atopic dermatitis, psoriasis, sarcoidosis, histoplasmosis, coccidioidomycosis, cutaneous metastatic disease, leukemia cutis, contact dermatitis, dermatophytosis, erythroderma, lichen planus, and pemphigus foliaceous.

LAB STUDIES

- CTCL is a clinical and histologic diagnosis. The use of a molecular assay such as Southern blot or PCR may aid in identifying a dominant lymphocyte clone in skin biopsy specimens and deciphering the T-cell subtype.
- MicroRNA (miRNA) profiling has been demonstrated to help separate benign inflammation from CTCL. A quantitative reverse transcription-PCR–based (qRT-PCR) "minimal" miRNA classifier with miR-155, miR-203, and miR-205 demonstrated 95% classification accuracy for CTCL versus benign disease and 91% sensitivity and 97% sensitivity. mi-R155 expression is increased in CTCL, whereas miR-203 and miR-205 are decreased in CTCL.
- A qRT-PCR–based classifier consisting of miR-155, miR-203, and miR-205 distinguishes CTCL from benign disorders with a high specificity and sensitivity, and with a classification accuracy of 95%.
- CBC with differential, buffy coat smear for Sézary cells, HIV, HTLV-1, uric acid, and lactate dehydrogenase levels; LFTs help identify systemic disease progression and narrow subtypes of CTCL.
- Imaging including a chest radiograph for lung involvement and CT abdomen/pelvis is indicated in Stage IIB–IVB or suspicion of visceral disease.
- The neoplastic MF cells have a mature CD3$^+$, CD4$^+$, CD45RO$^+$, CD8$^-$ memory T-cell phenotype. Rarely, MF may have a CD4$^-$, CD8$^+$ mature T-cell phenotype. An aberrant phenotype, such as a loss of pan–T-cell antigens (e.g., CD2, CD3, CD5) is not unusual and is diagnostically helpful.

HISTOLOGIC FINDINGS

The histopathology is nonspecific in early CTCL/MF. Thus, the condition is often misdiagnosed as a chronic inflammatory disorder. Early patches of MF show a superficial lichenoid lymphohistiocytic infiltrate. Scattered atypical lymphocytes with indented (cerebriform) and occasionally hyperchromatic nuclei are present. They are mostly confined to the epidermis. They usually are located in the basal layer of the epidermis either as single, often-haloed cells or in a linear configuration.

In MF plaques, the histologic changes are more clearly diagnostic. Epidermotropism is generally more pronounced. The presence of intraepidermal collections of atypical cells (Figs. 34-4 and 34-5) (Pautrier microabscesses) is a highly characteristic feature observed in only a minority of patients. In the tumor stage, the infiltrates become more diffuse, and epidermotropism is less apparent. The tumor cells increase in number and size, demonstrating variable proportions of small, medium, and large cerebriform blast cells with prominent nuclei and intermediate forms. Transformation to a diffuse large cell lymphoma of either CD30$^-$ or CD30$^+$ phenotype may occur, which is a harbinger of a poor prognosis.

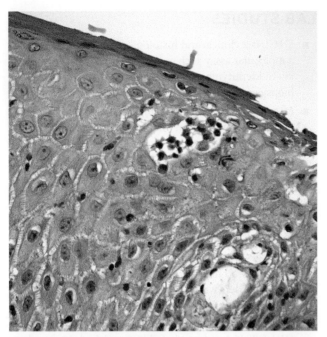

FIGURE 34-4: Five or more atypical cells surrounded by a clear space in the epidermis. This is a Pautrier microabscess in a CTCL patient.

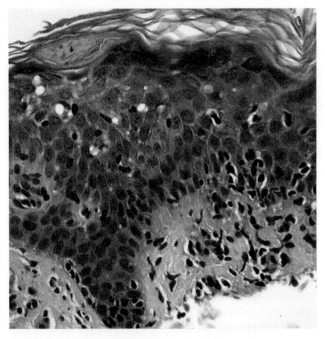

FIGURE 34-5: Atypical clusters of cells in the dermis and dermal–epidermal junction in CTCL.

MEDICAL CARE

SAUER'S NOTES

Aggressive therapy for mild disease has not been shown to be beneficial and may actually worsen the natural history of the disease.

- CTCL/MF that is limited to the skin is often managed with skin-targeted therapies such as topical corticosteroids, photochemotherapy (e.g., psoralen plus UV-A [PUVA]), topical application of cytotoxic agents such as nitrogen mustard (mechlorethamine, Valchlor in 2013) and carmustine (BCNU), or radiotherapy, including total skin electron beam irradiation. Most cases of patch or plaque-stage disease will respond to PUVA, with 76% to 90% complete response. Bexarotene, a third-generation retinoid, is also sometimes used for limited disease. Methotrexate (MTX) has been used, but some concern exists relating to large cell transformation. Tazarotene, long-term low-dose oral etoposide, and imiquimod may be of some value in the treatment of early CTCL. Patients with early stages of CTCL/MF should be treated relatively aggressively to avoid progression of the disease.

- Valchlor was approved in 2013 as the first FDA-approved topical mechlorethamine product and demonstrated noninferiority to compounded formulation. It is approved for stage IA–IIA MF-type CTCL.

- Electron beam irradiation can be used only a limited number of times because of bone marrow toxicity and skin tolerance. A retrospective review found that a single dose of radiation (700 to 800 cGy) in place of multiple-fraction radiation treatment still resulted in excellent palliation. The cost is also 200% less for single-fraction therapy.

- Biologic agents such as interferon-α and other cytokines (e.g., interleukin-2 [IL-2]), retinoids, and receptor-targeted cytotoxic fusion proteins (e.g., DAB389I-2) are being used increasingly. Denileukin diftitox (Ontak), the IL-2 fusion protein, was discontinued in January 2014. IL-12, pentostatin (a potent adenosine deaminase inhibitor), NF-κB inhibitors (bortezomib), cytokine receptor antagonists, immunomodulatory therapies, and allogeneic stem cell therapy can be employed. Combination therapy with bexarotene and PUVA should be considered for patients with treatment-resistant CTCL refractory to monotherapy. The precise use of these new treatments is yet to be established. Various regimens may be palliative, but may not have an impact on prolonging overall survival.

- Histone Deacetylase (HDAC) Inhibitors have become critical in treating CTCL in the relapsed/refractory setting. Most of these are pan-HDAC inhibitors, such as vorinostat, romidepsin, depsipeptide, panobinostat. These are preferred to be used before chemotherapy agents owing to high efficacy and accepted tolerability by most physicians.

- Multiagent chemotherapy is used when lymph node or systemic involvement is present or in cases with widespread tumor-stage MF that is refractory to skin-targeted therapies.

- Perifollicular disease in FMF is often less responsive to skin-targeted therapies than classic plaque-stage MF. In these cases, total skin electron beam irradiation is superior. However, because sustained complete remissions are rarely achieved with electron beam therapy, PUVA combined with retinoids or interferon-α may be used. Cysts and comedones found in follicular CTCL may benefit from isotretinoin therapy.

- Extracorporeal photopheresis, either alone or in combination with other treatment modalities (e.g., interferon-α), is useful for SS and erythrodermic MF, with overall response rates of 30% to 80% and complete response rates of 14% to 25%. Beneficial results have also been described with interferon-α, either alone or in combination with PUVA therapy, prolonged treatment with a combination of low-dose chlorambucil (2 to 4 mg/day) and prednisone (10 to 20 mg/day), or with MTX (5 to 25 mg/week), but complete responses are rare. Skin-directed therapies such as PUVA or potent topical steroids are good adjuvant therapies.

- Cord blood transplantation is another possible therapeutic option.

- Allogeneic stem-cell transplantation has promise in selected patients.

- Alemtuzumab (anti-CD52) has been shown to be effective in treating leukemic CTCL, which is a malignancy of central memory T cells, but not MF, which is a malignancy of skin resident effector memory T cells. Alemtuzumab depletes benign and malignant central memory T cells but spares effector memory T cells in the skin. Alemtuzumab is not associated with increased infections of the skin.

- IL-31 may be considered in the future as a target for pharmacologic therapy to reduce the intense pruritus patients with CTCL may experience. IL-31 was statistically significantly elevated in patients with CTCL and correlates with CTCL pruritus, alopecia, and dermatitis, which can cause significant morbidity and decreased quality of life.

- Simultaneous inhibition of mTOR-containing complex 1 (mTORC1) and MNK resulted in apoptosis of CTCL cells, which may be a future direction for drug therapy.

PROGNOSIS

- As previously noted, the prognosis for CBCLs is generally good to excellent. The prognosis for CTCL/MF is dependent on stage and, in particular, the type and extent of skin lesions and the presence of visceral or lymph node involvement. Patients with limited patch/plaque-stage MF have similar life expectancies to age-, sex-, and race-matched control populations. The 10-year disease-specific survival rates were 97% to 98% for patients with limited patch/plaque disease (covering < 10% of the skin surface), 83% for patients with generalized patch/plaque disease (covering > 10% of the skin surface), 42% for patients with tumor-stage

disease, and approximately 20% for patients with histologically documented lymph node involvement. Patients with effaced lymph nodes, visceral involvement, and transformation to large T-cell lymphoma have an aggressive clinical course and usually die of systemic involvement or infections. Blood eosinophilia may also serve as a poor prognostic indicator.

- The prognosis associated with FMF is worse than that for classic patch- and plaque-stage MF, and corresponds more closely with tumor-stage disease (stage IIB). FMF has a 5-year survival rate of approximately 70% to 80%.

- Increased age, male sex, and increased serum lactate dehydrogenase have been associated with reduced survival and increased risk of disease progression.

- Overall mortality rate is 0.064 per 100,000 persons in the United States. The incidence and associated mortality have shown a decline in patients with MF. This may be because of increased recognition and/or earlier diagnosis of the disease.

- In SS, the prognosis is poor, with a median survival of 2 to 4 years. The 5-year survival rate has been reported to be 24%, with most patients dying of infection from immunosuppression. Patients are especially at risk for fatal *Staphylococcus aureus* or *Pseudomonas aeruginosa* infections.

- Mycosis Fungoides patients may suffer from complications including high-output cardiac failure, anemia of chronic disease, edema, and secondary malignancies.

- In patients with ATLL, the clinical subtype is the main prognostic factor. Survival in persons with acute or lymphomatous variants is poor, ranging from 2 weeks to over 1 year. Chronic and smoldering forms have a more protracted clinical course and a longer survival, but transformation into an acute phase with an aggressive course can develop.

- SPTL (with a CD8$^+$, α/β^+ T-cell phenotype) tends to have a protracted clinical course with recurrent subcutaneous nodules but without extracutaneous spread. The 5-year survival rate of such patients may be greater than 80%.

- Unilesional pagetoid reticulosis (Woringer–Kolopp disease) has an excellent prognosis because of its slow progression.

- Primary cutaneous PTL, type unspecified, is also associated with a poor prognosis, with 5-year survival rates of less than 20%.

- Primary cutaneous CD4$^+$ small/medium pleomorphic T-cell lymphoma (provisional entity) is associated with a more favorable prognosis, with an estimated 5-year survival of approximately 60% to 80%. Patients with solitary or localized skin lesions usually have an excellent prognosis.

- Primary cutaneous aggressive epidermotropic CD8$^+$ cytotoxic T-cell lymphoma often has an aggressive clinical course, and patients have a median survival of 32 months.

- CGD-TCL patients tend to have aggressive disease recalcitrant to both multiagent chemotherapy and radiation, with a median survival in one study of 15 months. Subcutaneous fat involvement is a poor prognostic indicator.

- Nasal-type NK/T-cell lymphoma manifesting in the skin is highly aggressive; patients have a median survival of less than 1 year. The most important factor predicting a poor outcome is the presence of extracutaneous involvement at baseline or initial presentation. CD30[+] and CD56[+] tumor cells may indicate a better prognosis, possibly identifying examples of cutaneous anaplastic large cell lymphoma with co-expression of CD56.

Suggested Readings

Agar NS, Wedgeworth E, Crichton S, et al. Survival outcomes and prognostic factors in mycosis fungoides/Sézary syndrome: validation of the revised International Society for Cutaneous Lymphomas/European Organisation for Research and Treatment of Cancer staging proposal. *J Clin Oncol.* 2010;28(31):4730–4739.

Alberti-Violetti S, Torres-Cabala CA, Talpur R, et al. Clinicopathological and molecular study of primary cutaneous CD4+ small/medium-sized pleomorphic T-cell lymphoma. *J Cutan Pathol.* 2016;43:1121–1130.

Bekkenk MW, Vermeer MH, Jansen PM, et al. Peripheral T-cell lymphomas unspecified presenting in the skin: analysis of prognostic factors in a group of 82 patients. *Blood.* 2003;102(6):2213–2219.

Benoit BM, Jariwala N, O'Connor G, et al. CD164 identifies CD4+ T cells highly expressing genes associated with malignancy in Sézary syndrome: the Sézary signature genes, FCRL3, Tox, and miR-214. *Arch Dermatol Res.* 2017;309(1):11–19.

Brown DN, Wieser I, Wang C, et al. Leonine facies (LF) and mycosis fungoides (MF): A single-center study and systematic review of the literature. *J Am Acad Dermatol.* 2015;73(6):976–986.

Burg G, Kempf W, Dummer R. Cutaneous lymphoma, leukemia and related disorders. In: Schwartz RA, ed. *Skin Cancer: Recognition and Management.* 2nd ed. Oxford, UK: Blackwell; 2008:238–266.

Burg G, Kempf W. Therapy of cutaneous lymphomas. In: Burg G, Kempf W, eds. *Cutaneous Lymphomas.* London: Taylor & Francis; 2005:475–528.

Burg G. Systemic involvement in mycosis fungoides. *Clin Dermatol.* 2015;33:563–571.

Burg G, Kempf W, Cozzio A, et al. WHO/EORTC classification of cutaneous lymphomas 2005: histological and molecular aspects. *J Cutan Pathol.* 2005;32(10):647–674.

Chan JK, Sin VC, Wong KF, et al. Nonnasal lymphoma expressing the natural killer cell marker CD56: a clinicopathologic study of 49 cases of an uncommon aggressive neoplasm. *Blood.* 1997;89(12):4501–4513.

Clarijs M, Poot F, Laka A, et al. Granulomatous slack skin: treatment with extensive surgery and review of the literature. *Dermatology.* 2003;206(4):393–397.

Hodak E, Amitay-Laish I, Atzmony L, et al. New insights into folliculotropic mycosis fungoides (FMF): A single-center experience. *J Am Acad Dermatol.* 2016;75(2):347–355.

Jaffe ES, Krenacs L, Raffeld M. Classification of cytotoxic T-cell and natural killer cell lymphomas. *Semin Hematol.* 2003;40(3):175–184.

Jain S, Zain J, O'Connor O. Novel therapeutic agents for cutaneous T-cell lymphoma. *J Hematol Oncol.* 2012;5(1):24.

Jones GW, Hoppe RT, Glatstein E. Electron beam treatment for cutaneous T-cell lymphoma. *Hematol Oncol Clin North Am.* 1995;9(5):1057–1076.

Lambert WC, Schwartz RA. Dermatitic precursors of mycosis fungoides. In: Schwartz RA, ed. *Skin Cancer: Recognition and Management.* 2nd ed. Oxford, UK:Blackwell; 2008:227–237.

Larson K, Wick MR. Pagetoid reticulosis: report of two cases and review of the literature. *Dermatopathology (Basel).* 2016;3(1):8–12.

Mraz-Gernhard S, Natkunam Y, Hoppe RT, et al. Natural killer/natural killer-like T-cell lymphoma, CD56[+], presenting in the skin: an increasingly recognized entity with an aggressive course. *J Clin Oncol.* 2001;19(8):2179–2188.

Pimpinelli N, Olsen EA, Santucci M, et al. Defining early mycosis fungoides. *J Am Acad Dermatol.* 2005;53(6):1053–1063.

Pinter-Brown LC, Schwartz RA. Cutaneous T-cell lymphoma. *eMedicine Dematology 2016.* http://emedicine.medscape.com/article/1098342-overview

Ralfkiaer U, Hagedorn PH, Bangsgaard N, et al. Diagnostic microRNA profiling in cutaneous T-cell lymphoma (CTCL). *Blood.* 2011;118(22):5891–5900.

Sanz-Bueno J, Lora D, Monsálvez V, et al. The new Cutaneous Lymphoma International Prognostic index (CLIPi) for early mycosis fungoides failed to identify prognostic groups in a cohort of Spanish patients. *Br J Dermatol.* 2016;175:794–796.

Setoyama M, Katahira Y, Kanzaki T. Clinicopathologic analysis of 124 cases of adult T-cell leukemia/lymphoma with cutaneous manifestations: the smouldering type with skin manifestations has a poorer prognosis than previously thought. *J Dermatol.* 1999;26(12):785–790.

Smoller BR, Santucci M, Wood GS, et al. Histopathology and genetics of cutaneous T-cell lymphoma. *Hematol Oncol Clin North Am.* 2003;17(6):1277–1311.

van Santen S, Roach RE, van Doorn R, et al. Clinical staging and prognostic factors in folliculotropic mycosis fungoides. *JAMA Dermatol.* 2016;152:992–1000.

Vonderheid EC, Bernengo MG, Burg G, et al. Update on erythrodermic cutaneous T-cell lymphoma: report of the International Society for Cutaneous Lymphomas. *J Am Acad Dermatol.* 2002;46(1):95–106.

Wilcox RA. Cutaneous T-cell lymphoma: 2016 update on diagnosis, risk-stratification, and management. *Am J Hematol.* 2016; 91:151–165.

Willemze R, Jaffe ES, Burg G, et al. WHO–EORTC classification for cutaneous lymphomas. *Blood.* 2005;105(10):3768–3785.

Willemze R, Jansen PM, Cerroni, BE, et al. Subcutaneous panniculitis-like T-cell lymphoma: definition, classification, and prognostic factors: an EORTC Cutaneous Lymphoma Group Study of 83 cases. *Blood.* 2008;111:838–845.

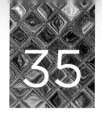

Diseases Affecting the Hair

Cheryl B. Bayart, MD, MPH and Wilma F. Bergfeld, MD

In most mammalian species, hair serves a variety of essential functions, including social and sexual communication, camouflage, proprioception, temperature regulation, and protection from the elements, insects, and parasites. Human hair plays a more limited functional role. Eyebrows and lashes protect the eyes from sweat and debris. Terminal hairs on the head and vellus hairs on the body provide a limited degree of warmth for the scalp and body, respectively. However, in many societies, hair plays an important role in personal appearance and sense of identity, including perceived masculinity and femininity. It is important to keep in mind that loss of hair on the scalp, an excessive amount of unwanted hair on other body parts, or abnormal appearance of hair may cause great distress. These psychosocial concerns may play a significant role in prompting a patient to seek care for a hair disorder.

The quantity and quality of an individual's hair are not only a reflection of age, sex, race, and hair care practices, but also provide insight into underlying physical and mental illness, and nutritional and endocrine status. A hair disorder may be a primary process or the presenting sign of systemic disease. The evaluating physician should perform a thorough history and physical examination, which in some cases may guide further laboratory studies, and/or referral to other specialists.

Hair disorders generally fall into three categories: disorders of excess hair (hirsutism and hypertrichosis), disorders of hair loss (alopecias), and hair shaft abnormalities (trichodystrophies).

HAIR ANATOMY AND PHYSIOLOGY

Knowledge of basic hair biology is helpful in understanding and classifying diseases of the hair. The hair fiber (or shaft) is composed of three layers: the central medulla, surrounding cortex, and outer cuticle. The medulla contains loosely connected cells which provide insulation in animals. The cortex contains keratins and associated proteins, and the cuticle maintains integrity of the hair fiber. The cells in these layers respond to signaling from the underlying dermal papilla to proliferate and differentiate. Surrounding the hair fiber below the surface of the skin is a supportive inner root sheath which undergoes enzymatic degradation, allowing the hair fiber to exit the skin alone. Together, these structures form the hair follicle. Associated with each follicle is a sebaceous (oil) gland and smooth muscle called the arrector pili, which contracts in response to various stimuli such as cold, stroking of the skin

and stress, causing hairs to stand on end. The hair follicle and its associated sebaceous gland and arrector pili muscle are collectively referred to as the pilosebaceous unit.

Human adults have two types of hair: terminal and vellus. Terminal hairs are medullated (have a medulla) and thicker in caliber than the inner root sheaths, which produce them (>0.06 mm diameter). They grow from large follicles rooted in the reticular (deep) dermis or subcutaneous fat. Terminal hairs grow from 1 to 50 cm in length, depending on the length of their anagen phase (discussed below). Hairs on the scalp and beard area of men are examples of terminal hairs. Vellus hairs are short (1 to 2 mm) and thin (<0.03 mm) and often unmedullated and unpigmented. They erupt from smaller follicles rooted in the superficial dermis and are seen on all body surfaces except the palms and soles. During puberty, the influence of androgens causes vellus hairs in sites such as the groin and axillae to enlarge and become terminal hairs. Miniaturization, or replacement of terminal with vellus hairs, is seen in androgenetic alopecia. Senescent thinning, in which hair follicles decrease slightly in density and caliber, may be observed after about 50 years.

Lanugo hairs are long, soft, downy, unmedullated hairs produced by fetal hair follicles in utero and shed at the end of gestation and during the first 3 to 4 months of life. Outside of infancy, the presence of lanugo hairs is considered pathologic and may be the presenting sign of malignancy (hypertrichosis lanuginosa acquisita). Lanugo hair may also be seen in the setting of malnutrition, anorexia nervosa, hyperthyroidism, acquired immune deficiency syndrome (AIDS), or use of certain medications.

Hair growth occurs in phases. In a healthy individual, an average of 80% to 90% of scalp hairs are in anagen (growth) phase, 1% are in catagen (involuting) phase, and 10% to 15% are in telogen (resting) phase. The length of the anagen phase determines the length of the hair. Scalp hair generally remains in anagen phase from 2 to 7 years, during which growth proceeds at approximately 1 cm/month. Patients with a rare condition called short anagen syndrome have a scalp anagen phase of 1 to 2 years and present as a patient who has never needed a haircut. Anagen phase is shorter for hairs on other areas of the body. Terminal hairs on mustache region, arms, and legs have anagen phases lasting 4 to 14 weeks, 6 to 12 weeks, and 19 to 26 weeks, respectively. Anagen phase for vellus hairs lasts only 6 to 12 weeks. Catagen phase lasts 2 to 3 weeks. Telogen phase is defined by the 2 to 4 months between the completion of follicular regression (catagen) and the onset of the next anagen phase. It is normal to lose approximately 100 to 200 (telogen) scalp hairs per day. Some authors describe a fourth phase of the hair cycle (exogen) in which hairs are actively shed.

The hair cycle is influenced by many factors, including seasonal changes, aging, and hormonal fluctuations. Seasonal changes in hair shedding are usually not noticeable but are important when conducting studies on treatment of hair loss. With aging and androgenetic (male or female pattern) hair loss, there is a shortening of the anagen phase and a lengthening of telogen phase. Increased estrogen levels during pregnancy increase the proportion of follicles in anagen, leading to increased hair growth. Postpartum hormonal shifts trigger many of these follicles to transition to telogen phase, resulting in marked shedding, or telogen effluvium, which is discussed in detail later in this chapter. Plucking the anagen hairs can advance the onset of the next anagen phase. Shaving hair does not affect the hair cycle. Hair cycle promoters such as minoxidil can help to lengthen short anagen cycles.

Graying or whitening of the hair (canities) is most commonly caused by an age-associated decrease or alteration in pigment-producing follicular melanocytes. Onset of graying generally occurs in the third-to-fourth decade of life and starts on the temples, spreading to the crown and occiput. By age 50, 50% of people are at least 50% gray. Graying prior to 20 years of age in whites and 30 years of age in blacks is considered premature. Premature graying has been associated with family history, obesity, smoking, osteopenia, and coronary artery disease. Other causes of pigment loss resulting in gray or white hair include autoimmune diseases such as alopecia areata and vitiligo, and a broad range of genetic disorders which affect melanin synthesis or distribution. Many people dye their hair to camouflage graying. Paraphenylenediamine (PPD) is a compound present in most hair dyes and is a common cause of allergic contact dermatitis.

DISORDERS OF EXCESS HAIR: HIRSUTISM AND HYPERTRICHOSIS

Excess hair growth is broadly categorized as hirsutism or hypertrichosis, and may be inherited, secondary to an underlying hormonal imbalance (namely hyperandrogenism), medical condition, or medication (Tables 35-1 and 35-2). Hypertrichosis is excessive hair growth on any part of the body. Hirsutism is a specific form of hypertrichosis defined by excessive growth of terminal hair in a male sexual pattern in a female. When assessing a patient with excess hair growth, it is important to consider the patient's ethnicity and elicit a thorough history regarding amount and pattern of hair growth in other family members. A complete medical history, including review of systems and use of medications and supplements, should be performed. Laboratory workup may be warranted.

Hirsutism

Hirsutism describes excess "male pattern" growth of terminal hairs in a woman, namely on the beard area, chest, shoulder,

abdomen, thighs, and buttocks (Fig. 35-1). The cause is usually hormonal: excess male hormone (androgen) production or increased sensitivity of hair follicles to these hormones. Androgen overproduction is generally adrenal or ovarian in origin. Regardless of origin, androgens are converted to dihydrotestosterone (DHT) by the 5-α-reductase enzyme in the hair follicles of the scalp, beard area, and chest. It is DHT that is implicated in the development of hirsutism and androgenetic alopecia. Importantly, when hirsutism is rapid in onset or progression, a neoplastic cause (hormone-producing adrenal or ovarian tumor) should be ruled out. This is particularly true if other signs of virilization are present: female pattern androgenetic alopecia (discussed later in this chapter), amenorrhea, clitoromegaly, increased muscle mass, or deepening of the voice (Table 35-3).

Adrenal hirsutism should be suspected in patients with central distribution of hair affecting the abdomen, central chest, neck, and chin. Coexisting androgenetic alopecia, signs of virilization, and thin body habitus are also suggestive. Adrenal

---

TABLE 35-1 • Causes of Hirsutism

Familial

Hyperandrogenism

    Androgen-producing tumor

    Adrenal hyperplasia

    Cushing syndrome

    PCOS
    Iatrogenic

TABLE 35-2 • Causes of Hypertrichosis

	Congenital	Acquired
Generalized	• Congenital hypertrichosis lanuginosa • Ambras syndrome	• Iatrogenic • Acquired hypertrichosis lanuginosa • Traumatic brain injury • Endocrinopathy • Malnutrition • Anorexia nervosa • HIV infection
Localized	• Neoplasm-associated • Familial • Spinal dysraphism • Porphyria • Genodermatoses	• Iatrogenic • Skin trauma • Porphyria • Juvenile dermatomyositis • Pretibial myxedema • Rosai-Dorfman disease • Reflex sympathetic dystrophy

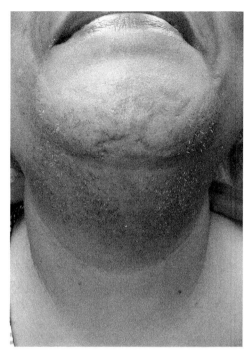

FIGURE 35-1: Hirsutism: a woman with extensive terminal hair growth of the beard area.

TABLE 35-3 • Adrenal Versus Ovarian Hyperandrogenism

Source of Excess Androgens	Adrenal	Ovarian
Elevated hormone	DHEA-S	Δ-4-androstenedione
Distribution of hair	Central	Lateral
Suggestive features	• Androgenetic alopecia • Virilization • Thin body habitus (+/−)	• Obesity • Menstrual abnormalities • Polycystic ovaries • Metabolic syndrome
Causative diseases	• Adrenal hyperplasia • Cushing syndrome • Adrenal tumors	• PCOS • Ovarian hyperthecosis • Ovarian tumors

polycystic ovarian syndrome (PCOS), ovarian hyperthecosis, and tumors (particularly in postmenopausal women). PCOS is the most common cause of hyperandrogenism, affecting 5% of women of reproductive age. Dermatologic manifestations are common. About 90% of PCOS patients have hirsutism, 70% have acne, and some who are obese develop acanthosis nigricans. Additional features include menstrual abnormalities including oligomenorrhea and amenorrhea (with or without associated infertility), obesity (in 50%), and polycystic ovaries. An associated "metabolic syndrome," including insulin resistance, dyslipidemia, and hypertension, is common. Elevated Δ-4-androstenedione and free testosterone levels indicate ovarian overproduction.

Hirsutism may be idiopathic. Inherited forms are common in certain ethnic groups, including women of the Mediterranean and South Asian ancestries. "SAHA syndrome" (seborrhea, acne, hirsutism, and alopecia) may be seen in association with PCOS, but also as isolated cutaneous findings. Anabolic steroids such as danazol and certain oral contraceptives can also cause hirsutism. Finally, hirsutism may be seen in association with other endocrinologic disorders including hyperprolactinemia, acromegaly, and thyroid dysfunction.

Workup of hirsutism includes thorough history and physical exam. If excess hair growth is moderate to severe or there are features suggestive of hyperandrogenism, laboratory workup may be warranted. Elevated free testosterone is the most sensitive marker of hyperandrogenism. DHEAS, prolactin, sex hormone binding globulin, Δ-4–androstenedione, and 3-α-androstanediol glucuronide (a metabolite of DHT) are also reasonable screening tests.

Treatment of hirsutism involves addressing the underlying cause, which may require the help of an endocrinologist. Anti-androgen therapies may be helpful in PCOS and idiopathic hirsutism. Oral spironolactone is a good first-line agent based on its availability and adverse effect profile. Other options include flutamide, finasteride, and cyproterone acetate. Spironolactone interferes with androgen biosynthesis, keeps androgens from acting on their receptors, and decreases 5-α-reductase levels in the follicle. An adequate trial consists of a 6-month trial at daily doses of 100 to 200 mg/day. Spironolactone should only be administered to women of childbearing age who are using reliable contraception, given its teratogenicity (pregnancy category D). The antihyperglycemic metformin reduces markers of insulin resistance in PCOS, and may help treat hirsutism. Hair loss was noted to be an adverse effect of eflornithine hydrochloride, a systemic treatment for African trypanosomiasis, and this property prompted its formulation as a cream (Vaniqa), which is FDA-approved for the treatment of facial hirsutism. Eflornithine hydrochloride cream is an irreversible inhibitor of ornithine decarboxylase, which slows hair growth and reduces hair fiber diameter and length (but does not remove hair). Maximal effect is seen by 8 to 24 weeks of use with marked improvement in 32% of users (compared to 8% marked improvement in the placebo group). Removal of hair as discussed under treatment of hypertrichosis may be a helpful adjunct.

causes of hirsutism include the adrenal hyperplasias (hirsutism is more common in congenital than late-onset forms), Cushing syndrome, and adrenal adenoma or carcinoma. The adrenal cortex characteristically produces DHEA-S, and elevated serum levels are a marker for adrenal hyperandrogenism.

Hirsutism in patients with ovarian androgen overproduction is more likely to be laterally distributed over the areolae and lateral face and neck. Ovarian causes of hyperandrogenism include

Hypertrichosis

Hypertrichosis is defined as excessive hair growth on any part of the body and can be classified as congenital or acquired and further subdivided into generalized and localized types. It may be characterized by a switch from vellus hairs to terminal hairs (which are pigmented) or lanugo hairs (which are fine and unpigmented).

Congenital Hypertrichosis

Congenital hypertrichosis lanuginosa is a rare, but striking, autosomal dominant disorder in which congenital lanugo hairs persist rather than being replaced by vellus hairs. Long, fine, unpigmented hairs cover nearly the entire body, growing up to 10 cm in length. Associated abnormalities have been reported, including abnormalities of teeth, ears, and eyes as well as pyloric stenosis and mental retardation.

Congenital generalized hypertrichosis (Ambras syndrome) is caused by a mutation in the trichorhinophalangeal syndrome I gene (*TRPS1*). In this disorder, anatomic patterning of hairs is disrupted, causing terminal hairs to grow at body sites where normally vellus hairs are seen. Associated abnormalities may include gingival hyperplasia, facial dysmorphism, skeletal defects, and mental retardation.

Congenital localized hypertrichosis may be seen overlying benign neoplasms such as congenital melanocytic nevi, neurofibromas, or Becker nevi (hamartomas). Congenital hypertrichosis of the midline spine raises suspicion for underlying spinal dysraphism: in these cases, magnetic resonance imaging (MRI) is warranted, as early identification and intervention may prevent permanent disability. Congenital localized hypertrichosis may also be seen as a feature of genetic disease. Hypertrichosis in sun-exposed areas is seen in porphyrias such as congenital erythropoietic porphyria. Low frontal hairline and synophrys (confluent brows) are seen in Cornelia de Lange syndrome. Congenital hypertrichosis of the ears may be seen in the babies of diabetic mothers or in babies with XYY syndrome. Hairy elbows may be present at birth or acquired, and may or may not be associated with other abnormalities.

Prepubertal hypertrichosis is benign and a common finding in children of Mediterranean and South Asian descent, the same groups in which familial hirsutism is seen (see above). Pigmented hairs involve the face (especially the forehead and brows, temples and preauricular areas), posterior hairline, extremities, and back. Mild elevation of serum free and total testosterone may be seen in some females with this condition.

Acquired Hypertrichosis

In *acquired hypertrichosis lanuginosa,* lanugo hairs appear over the body as in the congenital form of the disease, although with rapid onset, usually during adulthood. In some cases, only the face is affected. Acquired hypertrichosis lanuginosa is nearly always a paraneoplastic process, and has been associated with a broad spectrum of malignancies, most commonly of the lung, colon and breast. Patients without a known cancer diagnosis should undergo thorough evaluation and monitoring for malignancy.

TABLE 35-4 • Medications Which May Cause Excess Hair Growth	
Hirsutism	Androgens
	Danazol
	Progesterone
Hypertrichosis	Acetazolamide
	Corticosteroids
	Cyclosporine
	Diazoxide
	Interferon
	Latanoprost
	Minoxidil
	Penicillamine
	Phenytoin
	Psoralens
	Streptomycin

Apart from hypertrichosis lanuginosa, *acquired hypertrichosis* is characterized by the presence of terminal hairs in sites that usually bear vellus hairs. It may be generalized or localized. In generalized hypertrichosis, increased growth of terminal hairs is most commonly seen on the forehead, temples, flexural extremities, and trunk. It is most often caused by medications, but may also be associated with traumatic brain injury, endocrine disorders, malnutrition, and HIV infection (Table 35-4). Acquired localized hypertrichosis may be associated with local trauma, skin inflammation or systemic disease. Hypertrichosis can develop in areas of chronic friction, such as the skin underlying plaster cast. It has been reported transiently at the sites of vaccination, wart removal, laser epilation, and PUVA therapy. Hypertrichosis may also be seen as a manifestation of systemic disease, such as infrapatellar hypertrichosis in juvenile dermatomyositis, hypertrichosis of sun-exposed areas in porphyrias, and hypertrichosis in areas affected by pretibial myxedema, Rosai–Dorfman disease or reflex sympathetic dystrophy. Finally, iatrogenic hypertrichosis may occur at the site of application of potent topical corticosteroids, tacrolimus, mercury or iodine-containing creams. *Trichomegaly* refers to increased growth of eyelashes, which can be seen in association with genetic syndromes such as Cornelia de Lange syndrome and systemic diseases such as advanced HIV infection. Multiple medications can cause trichomegaly, including prostaglandin analogs (bimatoprost and latanoprost), epidermal growth factor receptor inhibitors, anticonvulsants (phenytoin and topiramate), antiretrovirals (zidovudine), immunosuppressants (cyclosporine and tacrolimus), and minoxidil. Many of these agents also cause hypertrichosis. Latanoprost has also been shown to cause hyperpigmentation of the lashes and is used for cosmetic purposes under the brand name Latisse.

Treatment of hypertrichosis may include shaving, topical depilatory creams, plucking, waxing (which results in simultaneous plucking of multiple hairs), laser, and electrolysis. Bleaching may lighten dark terminal hairs resulting in a cosmetically acceptable outcome. Shaving does not alter the hair cycle or amount of hair that regrows. Over-the-counter chemical depilatories and bleaching agents are effective, but may cause contact dermatitis. Patients should be instructed to test the product on a small area of the inner arm and wait for 72 hours prior to applying to the face or a large area of skin. Waxing and plucking have the advantage of removing the unwanted hair for longer periods without retreatment than does shaving or chemical removal. Shaving, waxing, and plucking may all result in ingrown hairs. Electrolysis and laser hair removal are the most permanent options, but are also the most costly and can result in scarring. As laser target melanin within the hair follicle, patients with fair skin and dark hair are ideal candidates. Patients with medium-to-dark skin tones risk dyspigmentation, and laser may be ineffective in those with light hair.

Pseudofolliculitis barbae is not a disorder of excess hair but is discussed here, as hair removal is an integral aspect of management. Pseudofolliculitis barbae typically presents as papulopustules, which lead to hyperpigmentation and scarring in the beard area of black men. Following close shaving, curly hairs may grow back into the skin surface resulting in the characteristically observed papulopustules. This can also occur following waxing or plucking of hairs in affected areas. The best treatment is to avoidance of close shaving. Standard and electric razors can be purchased for this purpose. For patients who prefer a clean-shaven look, such as may be required by an employer, topical depilatory agents or topical eflornithine hydrochloride may be helpful. Keratolytics such as topical tretinoin and benzoyl peroxide may help prevent ingrowing of hairs and decrease inflammation. A similar phenomenon can be seen when curly or kinky hair of the axillae, legs, and pubic areas is shaved. Treatment is similar. In patients who desire permanent removal of body hair in affected areas, laser removal is an option.

ALOPECIA (HAIR LOSS)

Loss of up to 50% of scalp hair may occur before the hair loss is clinically obvious. A thorough history and focused physical examination are of utmost importance in differentiating between the many potential causes of alopecia (Tables 35-5 and 35-6).

History should include:

- Nature of hair loss, namely thinning, shedding, or breakage. Breakage is more suggestive of mechanical causes of loss such as traction alopecia owing to hair care practices or underlying trichodystrophy.
- Pattern of loss: diffuse, patchy, or localized to certain areas
- Duration of the problem: when hair loss was first noted and if it has occurred in the past
- Associated symptoms: pain, itching, burning, or erythema, scale, pustules or rashes on the scalp
- Medical history, including underlying health conditions, use of medications and supplements, and potentially inciting illnesses, hospitalizations, or surgeries.

TABLE 35-5 • Causes of Alopecia

Nonscarring	Scarring (Cicatricial)
Androgenetic	Lymphocytic
Alopecia areata	Central centrifugal
Loose anagen syndrome	cicatricial alopecia
Hair cycle abnormality	(CCCA)
Telogen effluvium	Discoid lupus
Anagen effluvium	erythematosus
Trauma	Lichen planopilaris
Trichotillomania	Frontal fibrosing
Traction	alopecia
Pressure-induced	Neutrophilic
Infection	Folliculitis decalvans
Syphilis	Dissecting cellulitis
Tinea capitis	Mixed
Secondary	Acne keloidalis
Dermatitis (seborrheic,	Acne necrotica
atopic, psoriasis)	Erosive pustular
Systemic lupus	dermatosis
erythematosus	Secondary
	Neoplasia
	Sarcoidosis
	Scleroderma

TABLE 35-6 • Alopecia Evaluation: History and Physical Examination

History	Physical Examination
• Nature of problem	• General appearance
• Pattern of loss	• Scalp skin
• Duration	• Hair: scalp, eyebrows, eyelashes, body
• Associated symptoms	
• Medical history	
• Nutritional history	• Trichoscopy
• Hormonal and reproductive history	• Hair pull test +/− hair mount
• Psychosocial history	• Nails
• Hair care practices	• Thyroid
• Family history	

- Nutritional history, including avoidance of any foods or food groups and use of supplements
- Hormonal and reproductive history (women)
- Psychosocial history
- Hair care practices, past and current
- Family history

Physical examination should include:

- General appearance: May suggest an underlying medical condition, nutritional insufficiency, or psychosocial distress.
- Scalp: The extent and distribution of hair loss should be assessed, as well as hair color, texture, and length. The skin of the scalp should be assessed for erythema, scale, folliculitis, or dermatoses. Inflammatory conditions of the scalp, including seborrheic dermatitis, tinea capitis, and psoriasis may cause hair loss and breakage.

- Trichoscopy: A dermascope or dermatoscope is a specialized magnifying light designed for close examination of skin lesions. Examination of the scalp with a dermascope is referred to as trichoscopy. Trichoscopy is helpful in closely evaluating the scalp, including follicular ostia, and hair shafts.

- Hair pull test: A positive test is suggestive of telogen effluvium and is discussed later in this section.

- Eyebrows and lashes: Thinning may occur in multiple types of alopecia. Complete or patchy loss is most commonly seen in alopecia areata or trichotillomania.

- Body hair: Loss or excess should be noted. Causes of scalp alopecia such as anagen effluvium and alopecia areata can cause loss of hair anywhere on the body. Loss of the lateral third of the eyebrows may be seen in hypothyroidism. Complete loss of brows and lashes (madarosis) can be seen in infiltrative skin disorders such as cutaneous T-cell lymphoma and leprosy.

- Nails: Pitting may be noted in alopecia areata or psoriasis. Beau lines may be associated with telogen effluvium. Patients with nutritional deficiency may display nail fragility or koilonychia. Proximal pterygium is characteristic of lichen planus and can be observed in lichen planopilaris.

- Thyroid: Enlargement or nodularity warrants laboratory assessment and potentially endocrinology consult. Patients with undiagnosed or poorly controlled thyroid disease commonly present with telogen effluvium. Autoimmune thyroid conditions are associated with alopecia areata.

Laboratory workup should be guided by history and physical examination as above (Table 35-7). Some of the most common tests ordered include:

- Complete blood count: This is a screening to rule out and classify anemia, which is a common cause of telogen effluvium.

- Thyroid screening: Abnormal thyroid stimulating hormone (TSH) suggests underlying hypo- or hyperthyroidism, which may cause diffuse nonscarring alopecia. Microsomal or anti-thyroglobulin antibodies are seen in autoimmune thyroid disease, which is closely associated with alopecia areata.

- Nutritional screening: Deficiencies such as iron, zinc, vitamin C, vitamin D, and B vitamins may cause or contribute to hair loss.

- Hormonal screening: Elevated free or total testosterone or dehydroepiandrosterone-sulfate (DHEA-S) suggests female hyperandrogenism, which may be implicated in androgenetic alopecia.

Alopecias can be categorized as scarring or nonscarring. As a general rule, scarring alopecias entail permanent destruction of the regenerative stem cell region in the bulge of the hair follicle (Fig. 35-2). This is not seen in nonscarring alopecias, which are considered reversible.

TABLE 35-7 • Alopecia Evaluation: Laboratory Studies

Baseline
  Complete blood count
  Complete metabolic panel
  Thyroid stimulating hormone
  Ferritin
  Zinc
  1, 25 hydroxy-vitamin D
  Testosterone (free and total)[a]
  Dehydroepiandrosterone-sulfate[a]
  Microscopic examination of hair shaft
Additional studies
  T4, microsomal and thyroglobulin antibodies
  Vitamin C
  B vitamins
  Syphilis screen
  KOH prep
  Bacterial and fungal cultures
  Scalp biopsy

[a]In women.

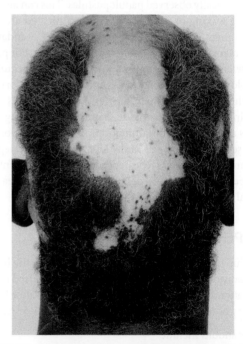

FIGURE 35-2: Discoid lupus erythematosus: note the scarring alopecia and dyspigmentation characteristic of this disorder.

Nonscarring Alopecias

The vast majority of alopecia patients have nonscarring disorders, including androgenetic (androgenetic, male pattern or female pattern), telogen effluvium, alopecia areata, trichotillomania, traction alopecia, and tinea capitis. As these entities are not associated with fibrosis leading to permanent hair follicle destruction, they are generally considered nonpermanent. However, androgenetic alopecia, alopecia areata and traction alopecia are considered biphasic: early disease is nonscarring, but in chronic forms, permanent follicular dropout may be seen.

Androgenetic alopecia (androgenetic alopecia, patterned hair loss, female pattern hair loss, male pattern hair loss, common baldness) is exceedingly common, affecting 50% of men by age 50 and 40% of women by age 70. In genetically-susceptible individuals, interplay between androgens and their receptors lead to gradual miniaturization of hairs. Androgen sensitivity varies depending scalp region. Follicles on the occipital scalp are androgen-independent and thus, spared. In men, thinning begins after puberty and initially occurs at the anterior hairline, both frontally and bi-temporally, and at the vertex. Advanced androgenetic alopecia is easily diagnosed in men and may progress to nearly complete baldness with sparing of a thin rim of occipital hair. Women present more commonly with a more diffuse pattern of hair loss, usually most pronounced on the vertex and mid-scalp. Bi-temporal thinning may also be seen (Fig. 35-3).

Androgenetic hair loss in men is likely autosomal dominantly inherited with variable penetrance and expression, a factor which should be elicited in the family history. Women with androgenetic alopecia represent a more heterogeneous group. Inheritance is likely polygenic, and hormonal factors play a role in some cases. Screening for hyperandrogenism should be considered, namely free and total testosterone and DHEAS, particularly if additional signs and symptoms such as acne or irregular menses are present. Androgenetic alopecia may also be seen in the setting of insulin resistance and PCOS, and appropriate metabolic screening should be performed in cases of clinical suspicion. However, most women with female pattern hair loss have normal hormone levels. In some women, telogen effluvium may "unmask" underlying androgenetic alopecia.

Topical minoxidil (Rogaine) is FDA-approved for treatment of androgenetic alopecia in men and women. 2% formulations are available, but 5% solution or foam is recommended, as this concentration is more effective. Efficacy of the solution and foam are comparable, but the foam does not contain propylene glycol and thus may be less irritating and less likely to cause contact dermatitis. Minoxidil's precise mechanism of action of is unknown, but vasodilatory, proliferative, anti-androgenic and anti-inflammatory effects are thought to be implicated in its efficacy. Potential adverse effects include irritant or allergic contact dermatitis and facial hypertrichosis in women. The latter may be prevented by avoiding contact with the facial area, limiting use along the frontal hairline and frequently changing pillow cases (at least every other day). Daily to twice-daily application is recommended, and continuous therapy is required to maintain hair growth.

Finasteride (Propecia), an oral 5-α-reductase inhibitor administered 1 mg/day, is an additional treatment option for men with androgenetic alopecia. Finasteride is given at a higher dose of 5 mg (Proscar) to treat benign prostatic hypertrophy (BPH). Finasteride blocks the action of enzyme 5-α-reductase, which normally catalyzes conversion of testosterone to the more potent dihydrotestosterone. Adverse effects in men are primarily sexual, and include decreased libido and erectile dysfunction. Like minoxidil, finasteride must be taken indefinitely to maintain hair growth.

Dutasteride (Avodart) is a more potent 5-α-reductase inhibitor than finasteride and is approved by the FDA for treatment of BPH. Studies have shown dutasteride to be superior to finasteride in the treatment of androgenetic alopecia in men. Drug interactions are a potential issue, as dutasteride is processed by CYP3A4 enzymes: it may affect the clearance of other potent CYP3A4 inhibitors such as ketoconazole, verapamil, diltiazem, cimetidine, and ciprofloxacin.

Although the only FDA-approved treatment for women with female pattern hair loss is minoxidil, other antiandrogens such as finasteride, dutasteride, spironolactone, cyproterone acetate, and flutamide may be helpful in treating the cutaneous signs of androgen excess in women, including acne, hirsutism and female pattern androgenetic alopecia. Of these, the safest and most readily available is finasteride. Finasteride 1 mg/day has been for treatment of androgen excess in females and has shown mixed results in the treatment of androgenetic alopecia in postmenopausal females. Greater efficacy has been seen with dutasteride. It is essential to bear in mind that all of these medications are teratogenic and should be avoided in pregnant or breast-feeding women, as well as those in childbearing age who are not using a reliable method of contraception. Women who are pregnant or lactating should not even handle finasteride or dutasteride pills, especially if crushed or broken.

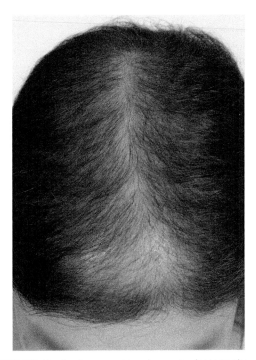

FIGURE 35-3: Androgenetic alopecia: hair is thinning over the crown and vertex with sparing of the frontal hairline.

SAUER'S NOTES

Empathy is important in all of medicine but no more important than in evaluation of women with hair loss. Friends, relatives, and well-meaning medical personnel may de-emphasize the importance of hair loss in women in our culture. To the patient it is important.

Telogen effluvium is another common cause of nonscarring alopecia. It is characterized by an abnormal increase in the number of scalp hairs in telogen (resting) phase compared with those in the anagen (growth phase), leading to the shedding of an abnormal number of hairs. Patients will generally note the loss of at least 25% of scalp hair and shedding of at least 150 to 200 scalp hairs per day (Figs. 35-4 and 35-5). Common triggers are summarized in Table 35-8 and include childbirth, major illness or hospitalization, underlying medical conditions such as hypothyroidism, surgical procedures, general anesthesia, high fever, medications (Table 35-9), rapid or marked weight loss, nutritional deficiency (most commonly anemia), and major psychosocial stressors such as the death of a child or spouse. However, any major physical or emotional stressor can induce an increase in the ratio of telogen to anagen hairs. As telogen phase lasts 2 to 4 months, an abnormally large shedding of hair is noted at this interval. If the inciting factor is removed, complete regrowth occurs in 4 to 6 months. However, acute telogen effluvium may rarely become chronic (last >6 months) if triggers are persistent.

A positive hair pull test with an excess of telogen hairs suggests a diagnosis of telogen effluvium. The hair pull test is performed by grasping 50 to 60 hairs between the thumb and second and third fingers and pulling firmly, but gently, perpendicular to the scalp. The test should be repeated in all four quadrants of the scalp. The goal of the hair pull test is to dislodge hairs in the telogen phase. Normally, 10% of scalp hairs are in telogen phase, which translates to 5 to 6 per quadrant. If more than 10 hairs are removed in a quadrant, this implies a positive test result and active shedding. It is important to keep in mind that shampooing on the day of the test or vigorous grooming may lead to a false-negative hair pull test result. A

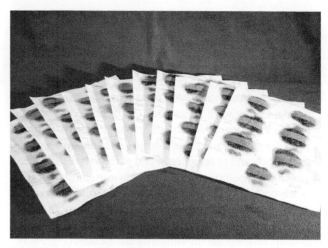

FIGURE 35-5: Hair collection: loss of >150 hairs can be demonstrated with daily hair collection.

TABLE 35-8 • Common Triggers of Telogen Effluvium
Medical illness
Acute
Chronic
Hormones
Thyroid dysfunction
Estrogen withdrawal
Postpartum
Nutritional deficiency
Iron
Zinc
Biotin
Vitamin D
Protein
Surgery/Anesthesia
Psychological stress or illness
Death of a family member
Divorce
Change in employment status or residence
Scalp inflammation
Psoriasis
Seborrheic dermatitis
Atopic dermatitis

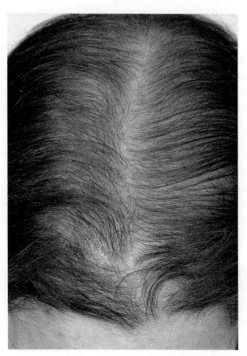

FIGURE 35-4: Telogen effluvium: diffuse, extensive thinning.

patient who has not shampooed or combed for several days (as may be done out of concern for shedding) may have a false-positive result. Hairs dislodged during the hair pull test should be examined microscopically at 2×. Telogen hairs can be identified by their lack of inner root sheath and lightly or nonpigmented "club shaped" bulbs. Marked hair shaft diameter variance is compatible with androgenetic hair loss. Anagen hairs, in contrasts, display pigmented bulbs with intact inner root sheaths. Numerous dystrophic anagen hairs are consistent with anagen effluvium owing to a cytotoxic medication, loose anagen syndrome, or alopecia areata, which are discussed below.

Beau lines are horizontal nail ridges, usually most prominent on the thumbs and great toenails, which represent transient

TABLE 35-9 • Selected Medications Which May Cause Alopecia

Psychotropics: most commonly lithium, valproic acid; also carbamazepine

SSRIs: most commonly fluoxetine; also sertraline, paroxetine

Tricyclic antidepressants: imipramine, desipramine

Low molecular weight heparins: enoxaparin, dalteparin, tinzaparin

Warfarin

β-blockers: metoprolol, propranolol

ACE-inhibitors (captopril, enalapril)

Amiodarone

Retinoids: isotretoin, acitretin, bexarotene

Isoniazid

Anti-retrovirals: most commonly indinavir, combination therapies

Antifungals: most commonly ketoconazole, fluconazole

Corticosteroids

Chemotherapeutics

Gout medications: allopurinol, colchicine

Leflunomide

---

thinning of the nail plate in response to an acute stressor (Fig. 35-6). They are analogous to telogen effluvium of the scalp hair. Nail findings which may suggest the cause of a telogen effluvium include koilonychia, or "spoon nails," which can be seen in anemia and nail thickening or onycholysis (detachment of the distal aspect of the nail plate), which are nonspecific, but can be observed in hypothyroidism. Given that telogen effluvium is triggered by specific inciting factor(s), identification and elimination of these factors is essential to treatment.

Loose anagen syndrome may occur sporadically or be inherited as an autosomal dominant trait. The prototypical patient is a young blond girl, but the disorder has been reported in adults, males and dark-haired patients. Patients will complain of diffuse or patchy hair loss and inability to grow hair long. As in telogen effluvium, a hair pull test (see above), will be positive. However, microscopic examination of the proximal ends of the hair in telogen effluvium reveals lightly or nonpigmented bulbs consistent with telogen hairs.

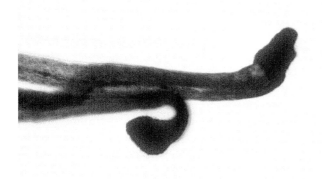

FIGURE 35-6: Dystrophic anagen hair.

Anagen hairs, in contrasts, display pigmented bulbs with intact inner root sheaths. In loose anagen syndrome, these anagen hairs are often dystrophic, with misshapen, irregular, shrunken roots that may have a "mousetail" or "loose-sock" appearance (Fig. 35-6).

Normal anagen hairs are not pulled out with a firm or gentle pull, but anagen hairs in this syndrome are easily and painlessly extracted. The underlying defect is thought to be faulty cornification of the inner root sheath, leading to poor adhesion with the hair shaft cuticle and anchoring of the hair. Loose anagen syndrome is usually an isolated finding, but may be associated with other entities such as alopecia areata, Noonan syndrome, and AIDS. Families may be reassured that loose anagen syndrome will likely improve with age.

Anagen effluvium, or diffuse shedding of anagen hairs, may be seen in the context of loose anagen syndrome, but is most commonly observed in patients receiving chemotherapeutic agents or radiation therapy which cause a sudden arrest in the mitotic activity of the matrix (regenerative) cells in the hair follicle (Table 35-9). In contrast to telogen effluvium, hair loss in anagen effluvium occurs in close proximity to the inciting event, usually within 1 to 2 weeks. History easily clinches the diagnosis. Approximately 90% of scalp hairs are shed, as this is the typical percentage found in anagen phase at a given moment.

Tinea capitis should be suspected in children with patchy hair loss on the scalp. The most common culprits in the United States and worldwide are *Trichophyton rubrum* and *Microsporum canis*, respectively. *T. tonsurans* infection classically presents with patches of "black dot alopecia" scattered throughout the scalp. Close examination reveals the "black dots" to be short, broken hair shafts. Surrounding nonadherent scale is often present. Posterior cervical lymphadenopathy is commonly present, and is a clue to diagnosis. Tinea capitis is uncommon in adults: when it is seen, there is often an identifiable exposure. Clinical diagnosis should ideally be performed with microscopic KOH examination or fungal culture of the hair. If cases of high clinical suspicion but negative confirmatory studies, empiric therapy should still be initiated. Topical treatments are insufficient, as dermatophytes track down the hair follicle below the surface of the skin. Adequate therapy entails prolonged (6 to 8 week) course of oral antifungals, typically griseofulvin or terbinafine (lamisil), administered at the upper range of the recommended weight-based daily dosing. Systemic absorption of griseofulvin is enhanced when it is taken with a high fat meal and can have an antabuse-like effect.

Alopecia areata causes nonscarring alopecia in an estimated 1% to 2% of the US population. Pathogenesis is incompletely understood, but is most likely an autoimmune process driven by T lymphocytes. Clinically, patients present with one or more round or oval areas of complete alopecia (Fig. 35-7). Close examination of the affected areas reveals patent follicular ostia, which may be plugged with yellow, keratinaceous material. Broken off "exclamation point" hairs with thicker proximal ends and tapered distal ends are characteristic. Very short "black dot" hairs may be observed as in tinea capitis. Patients may progress to or present with alopecia totalis (loss of all scalp

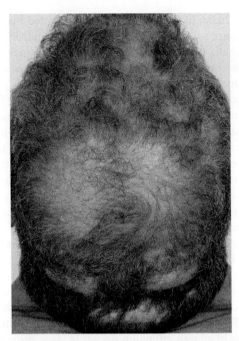

FIGURE 35-7: Alopecia areata: scattered round-to-oval areas of hair loss, with many areas of diffuse regrowth.

hair) or alopecia universalis (loss of all body, including scalp, hair). A diffuse pattern can be seen, but is the least common presentation. Diagnosis is usually clinical, but scalp biopsy demonstrating inflammatory cells (primarily lymphocytes, but also eosinophils) surrounding and infiltrating the bulbs of anagen hair follicles ("swarm of bees") can be helpful.

First presentation can occur at any age, but is most common between 15 and 30 years of age. Genetics are thought to be a predisposing factor, and 20% of patients with alopecia areata report a family history of the disease. Between 20% and 30% will develop an associated immune disorder. Autoimmune thyroiditis is the most common, but other conditions, including vitiligo, celiac disease, type I diabetes mellitus, inflammatory bowel disease, rheumatoid arthritis, and atopy have also been associated. Onset is usually abrupt, and particularly in adults, may be related to development or flaring of an underlying autoimmune condition. An inciting physical or psychosocial stressor may be noted. Alopecia areata typically follows a relapsing and remitting course. It is thought that pigment may be targeted by the immune system, and initial regrowth may be with fine, white colored hair. Factors portending a poor prognosis include young age of onset, associated immune disease and extensive early hair loss, namely alopecia totalis, universalis or ophiasis pattern loss, which occurs in a band-line distribution over the occipital and lateral aspects of the scalp.

Of patients with alopecia areata, 10% to 66% present with nail dystrophy, which precede, accompany or follow the hair disorder. Nail pitting (57.8%), onychorrhexis (11.6%), and onychomycosis (8.7%) are most common, but koilonychia, onycholysis, and onychomadesis have also been reported.

Treatment of alopecia areata is challenging, and no single treatment has been shown to induce lasting remission in a large percentage of patients. First-line treatment typically consists of mid to high-potency topical and/or intralesional corticosteroids. Systemic corticosteroids may be considered to abate an acute flare, but risks and benefits must be carefully weighed. Second line treatments fall into multiple categories. Contact sensitizers are applied to the scalp for short periods of time in an effort to alter the local inflammatory milieu and include anthralin, diphencyprone, and squaric acid. Systemic immunosuppressants and immunomodulators, including methotrexate, cyclosporine, azathioprine, and TNF-α inhibitors adalimumab, infliximab, and etanercept have been used with variable success. JAK kinase inhibitors tofacitinib and ruxolitinib also show promise. Research is underway to further understand the inflammatory mediators and mechanisms of alopecia areata, which will likely shed light on additional therapies. Adjunctive treatments may include phototherapy, topical minoxidil and nutritional supplements such as vitamin D and zinc. In patients with underlying atopy, daily antihistamine therapy may be helpful. The National Alopecia Areata Foundation (http://www.naaf.org) provides excellent patient information and support services.

Trichotillomania is a self-induced form of traumatic alopecia in which patients consciously or unconsciously pull or pluck out their own hair, resulting in notable hair loss. Most commonly, the scalp is affected, but patients may also remove hairs from other areas of the body, including the eyebrows and eyelashes.

The *DSM-5* criteria for trichotillomania are as follows:

- Recurrent pulling out of one's hair, resulting in hair loss
- Repeated attempts to decrease or stop the hair-pulling behavior
- The hair pulling causes clinically significant distress or impairment in social, occupational, or other important areas of functioning
- The hair pulling or hair loss cannot be attributed to another medical condition (e.g., a dermatologic condition)
- The hair pulling cannot be better explained by the symptoms of another mental disorder (e.g., attempts to improve a perceived defect or flaw in appearance, such as may be observed in body dysmorphic disorder)

Trichotillomania is most commonly seen in children, with peak presentation at school age. Adolescents and adults are less commonly affected and more likely to have a concomitant psychiatric disorder. Females are affected more often than males, with a larger gender discrepancy in older age groups. Etiology is unknown, but is likely multifactorial. Hair pulling has been hypothesized to develop as a repetitive habit, coping mechanism to deal with a stressor, form of disordered reward processing, or secondary to psychological factors or abnormalities of brain functioning. There appears to be a genetic component: trichotillomania and obsessive-compulsive disorder are frequently seen in the same families. Other associated disorders include anxiety disorder, attention-deficit disorder, depression, tic disorder, and body-focused repetitive behaviors such as thumb sucking, skin picking, or nail biting. It is important to be aware that associated trichophagia (swallowing) of plucked hairs is not an uncommon complication of trichotillomania. Patients should be asked about this, as well as vomiting, abdominal pain, constipation, or other gastrointestinal symptoms which could suggest the formation of a trichobezoar (mass of hair in the stomach or intestines).

The pattern of hair loss seen in trichotillomania is variable, but most often patchy and reminiscent of alopecia areata. As patients will often deny hair pulling, clinicians must have a high level of suspicion for the diagnosis. One clue on physical examination is the presence of hairs of different length within the alopecic patches, whose borders may not be as smooth and well defined as those seen in alopecia areata (Fig. 35-8). Trichoscopic examination may reveal broken hairs, which may have a corkscrew, wrinkled or wavy appearance. Scalp biopsy, when required to confirm the diagnosis, shows normal-appearing and damaged hairs within close proximity. Acute damage to the hair follicles results in characteristic "pigment casts" within follicles, as well as perifollicular and intra-follicular hemorrhage. An unusually large number of catagen follicles is also typical.

Trichotillomania often follows a relapsing–remitting course lasting for a year or more. Prognosis varies negatively with age. In children, hair pulling tends to be a time-limited behavior, and prognosis is excellent. Adolescents and adults are more likely to suffer severe disease and have associated psychiatric diagnosis. It is important to educate parents regarding the nature of this trichotillomania. Initial therapy involves parental interventions to address any inciting stressors, provide alternate outlets such as physical activity and provide behavioral guidance. It is invaluable to provide these patients with a warm, nonjudgmental environment. Professional cognitive behavioral therapy is the recommended second line therapy or treatment of choice in severe cases, or when parental interventions are unlikely to be successful. In patients with concurrent obsessive–compulsive disorder, oral selective serotonin reuptake inhibitors (SSRIs) may be helpful. There is also evidence as to the efficacy of N-acetylcysteine and olanzapine. The Trichotillomania Learning Center provides educational materials and support at http://www.trich.org.

Temporal triangular alopecia (congenital triangular alopecia, congenital temporal alopecia) typically presents as a singular triangular or oval-shaped alopecic patch on the frontotemporal scalp. Alopecia is usually noted at 2 to 6 years of age with the growth of surrounding hairs. Trichoscopy (and biopsy if performed) reveal vellus hairs in the area of involvement. Temporal triangular alopecia is benign and nonprogressive, but should be considered in the patient presenting with a nonscarring alopecia to avoid unnecessary workup. Patients may respond to topical minoxidil, as is used for androgenetic alopecia (see above).

Traction alopecia (traumatic hair loss) results from chemical or physical trauma to the hair caused by grooming procedures such as permanents, relaxers, dyes, hot combs, and pulling the hair into tight braids. This results in hair breakage and complete loss, usually accentuated at the frontal scalp (Fig. 35-9). Over time, widening of the part and scarring alopecia may occur. Patients should be instructed to minimize heat treatments such as blow-drying and straightening, chemical treatments such as permanents and relaxers, and physical agents such as extension, which may pull at the hair. For patients who wear their hair in tight braids or buns, alternative styling such as loose twists or braids and allowing hair to assume its "natural" texture should be encouraged.

Pressure-induced (postoperative) alopecia is most commonly seen following surgical procedures, during which one area of the patient's scalp is in prolonged contact with the operating table. It may also be seen following blunt trauma to the scalp.

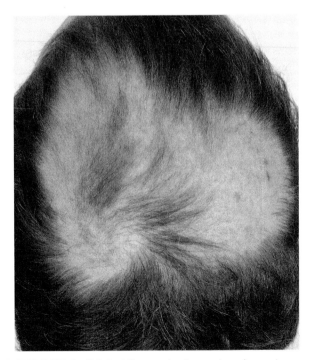

FIGURE 35-8: Trichotillomania: irregular alopecic patches with scattered regrowing hairs and excoriations.

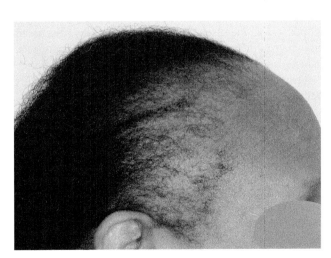

FIGURE 35-9: Traction alopecia.

Pathogenesis is similar to that of a pressure ulcer. Patients present with a solitary, ovoid, erythematous, indurated, alopecic plaque at the site of greatest pressure. Full regrowth usually occurs.

Secondary syphilis is becoming a less common cause of alopecia. However, syphilis should be ruled out in patients with known risk factors, including HIV infection. Characteristically, the alopecia is patchy or "moth-eaten" alopecia, but can be diffuse. Serologic testing can confirm the diagnosis. Alopecia may be scarring or nonscarring depending on the duration of infection.

Scarring (Cicatricial) Alopecias

Scarring alopecias are far less common than nonscarring forms of hair loss and can be broadly categorized as primary or secondary forms. In primary scarring alopecias, the hair follicle is directly targeted for destruction. In secondary scarring alopecias, the hair follicle is affected as an adjacent "bystander" to a nonfollicular process, such as sarcoidosis, systemic sclerosis, infection, or radiation dermatitis. This section will focus on the primary scarring alopecias, which can be subdivided into lymphocyte-associated, neutrophil-associated and mixed inflammatory primary scarring alopecias based on the composition of associated inflammatory cells.

On physical exam, scarring alopecias are characterized by a smooth, shiny appearance of the scalp. Trichoscopy fails to reveal patent follicular ostia. Patients with later stages of disease may display polytrichia or "tufted folliculitis" with the appearance of "doll's hair," in which numerous hair shafts exit from one follicular orifice, often in an area which is otherwise scarred and alopecic. While many of these entities can be diagnosed clinically, scalp biopsy is often useful in confirming the diagnosis and ruling out a secondary process. Biopsy is most useful during the active (inflammatory) stage of disease, as biopsy of quiescent disease may simply reveal scarring and fibrosis of the follicular tracts. Early and aggressive treatment is essential to halting disease progression. While regrowth of hair may be seen, patients must be counseled that this is not guaranteed, and that the goal of therapy is prevention of further scarring.

Causes of lymphocyte-associated primary scarring alopecias include discoid lupus erythematosus (discussed elsewhere in the text), central centrifugal cicatricial alopecia, lichen planopilarias and its variants, and alopecia mucinosa. Neutrophil-associated scarring alopecias include folliculitis decalvans and dissecting cellulitis. Cicatricial alopecias associated with a mixed inflammatory infiltrate include acne keloidalis, acne necrotica, and erosive pustular dermatosis.

Central centrifugal cicatricial alopecia (CCCA) is most commonly seen in black women (Fig. 35-10). As hair loss begins on the crown, early disease may resemble androgenetic alopecia. Alopecia is progressive and slowly spreads centrifugally. Trichoscopic exam reveals the surface of the scalp to be smooth with obliteration of the follicular ostia. Scalp biopsy is rarely necessary given the characteristic clinical presentation, but when performed reveals lymphocytic folliculitis with destruction of the pilosebaceous unit. Premature desquamation of

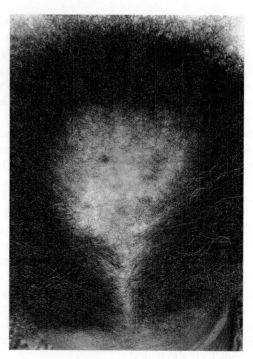

FIGURE 35-10: Central centrifugal alopecia (CCCA).

the inner root sheaths may also be seen. Etiology is unknown. Initially dubbed "hot comb alopecia," CCCA has traditionally been attributed to processing of the hair, namely the use of hot combs and caustic chemicals such as relaxers. However, CCCA is observed in patients without history of such procedures. It is thought some patients may be genetically predisposed to premature desquamation of the inner root sheaths, which renders hairs more fragile and susceptible to damage. Given that chemical and heat processing of the hair may be implicated, patients with CCCA should avoid such procedures. Treatment options include mid to high-potency topical steroids, oral antibiotics (namely minocycline and doxycycline), and daily use of 5% topical minoxidil.

Lichen planopilaris (LPP) and its variant *frontal fibrosing alopecia* (FFA) most commonly affect white women. Perifollicular erythema and hyperkeratotic papules are characteristic of active disease. Pruritus and tenderness are common. In LPP, patches of alopecia are scattered throughout the scalp (Fig. 35-11). Approximately half of LPP patients will develop additional cutaneous, mucous membrane, or nail changes consistent with lichen planus. Scalp biopsy reveals lichenoid dermatitis (affecting the epidermal–dermal junction) as seen in lichen planus, which involves the follicular epithelium. FFA is a similar process affecting the frontal hairline and frequently the eyebrows (Fig. 35-12). Progressive recession of the frontal hairline is characteristic. LPP and FFA are notoriously refractory to treatment. Therapeutic options include corticosteroids (topical, intralesional, and oral), oral antimalarials such as hydroxychloroquine, topical tacrolimus, oral tetracycline, and PPAR-agonist pioglitazone hydrochloride. Some success has also been reported with systemic immunosuppressants such as cyclosporine, mycophenolate mofetil, methotrexate and

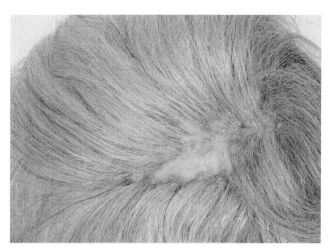

FIGURE 35-11: Lichen planopilaris (LPP).

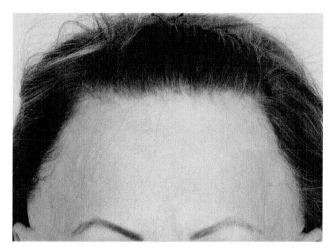

FIGURE 35-12: Frontal fibrosing alopecia (FFA).

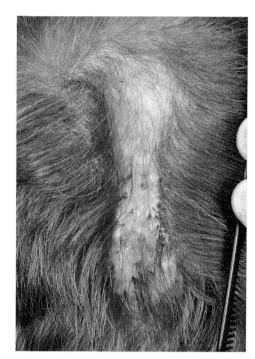

FIGURE 35-13: Folliculitis decalvans.

increased risk for hidradenitis suppurativa, acne conglobata, and pilonidal sinuses, which are collectively referred to as the follicular occlusion tetrad. Patients present with deep-seated, inflammatory nodules on the crown, vertex and occipital scalp, which progress to confluent, boggy, plaques (Fig. 35-14). As in hidradenitis suppurativa, disfiguring scars with overlying alopecia and underlying sinus tracts draining purulent material are often seen. Interestingly, discomfort may be minimal.

retinoids. Patients with LPP and FFA may enter remission, either spontaneously or secondary to treatment, but others have a prolonged and progressive course.

Folliculitis decalvans is a highly inflammatory scarring folliculitis. *Staphylococcus aureus* is frequently cultured and likely plays a role in pathogenesis. Patients present with round to irregular patches of alopecia with folliculocentric pustules at the advancing margin, which give way to atrophic scars (Fig. 35-13). If initiated early, aggressive antibacterial and anti-inflammatory therapy may abate the process. Anti-staphylococcal antibiotics are often administered according to culture results. Doxycycline 100 mg twice daily is often used as a first line therapy, with clindamycin and rifampin as second line treatment. Clarithromycin, dapsone, cephalexin, minocycline and tetracycline are also options. Some authors advocate isotretinoin as a more effective first line treatment. Adjuncts may include fusidic acid, oral zinc and topical, intralesional and systemic corticosteroids and photodynamic therapy. Advanced or extensive cases may require surgical intervention.

Dissecting cellulitis (perifolliculitis capitis abscedens et suffodiens) is a scarring form of suppurative folliculitis most commonly observed in young black men. Patients are at

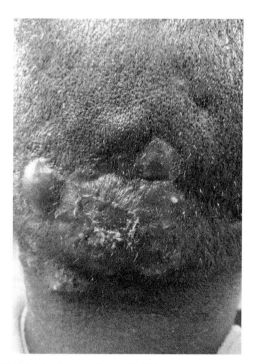

FIGURE 35-14: Dissecting cellulitis.

Treatment is often challenging. Oral antibiotics such as those used in folliculitis decalvans may be considered as a first-line therapy, but are often inadequate. Isotretinoin 0.5 to 1.5 mg/kg/day for 4 to 5 months has been shown to be effective. Some success has been reported with the off-label use of TNF-α inhibitors for dissecting cellulitis, which is unsurprising, given that adalimumab has been FDA-approved for the treatment of hidradenitis suppurativa. Intralesional corticosteroids can be injected into inflammatory nodules. Surgical interventions include excision with grafting and laser hair removal.

Acne keloidalis (acne keloidalis nuchae, folliculitis keloidalis) is a misnomer, as this entity is not related to acne and results in hypertrophic scars, rather than true keloids. Like dissecting cellulitis, this is most commonly seen in young black men. Patients develop smooth papules and pustules on the occipital scalp and posterior neck, which evolve into scarred alopecic plaques. Superinfection with suppurative drainage may occur. Oral antibiotics such as those used in folliculitis decalvans (see above) are helpful in suppurative cases. Perifollicular scars can be treated with intralesional corticosteroids injected every 4 to 6 weeks until they flatten. In advanced cases, surgical excision or laser of scarred areas may be warranted.

TRICHODYSTROPHIES

Trichodystrophies (hair shaft abnormalities) can be congenital or acquired. Patients may complain of a slow rate of hair growth, despite normal or near-normal hair density. Acquired trichodystrophies commonly occur secondary to exogenous factors, namely hair styling and processing. There are many genetic syndromes in which hair shaft abnormalities are a feature. Most of these are relatively rare, and only the most common and clinically relevant are discussed below. Trichodystrophies can be categorized as to whether or not they are associated with hair fragility and increased breakage. A hair mount or 1- to 2-in proximal sections of cut hairs is the optimal means of displaying a trichodystrophy. Most can be diagnosed with routine light microscopy. In some disorders, electron microscopy and amino acid analysis may be useful adjuncts (Table 35-10).

TABLE 35-10 • Trichodystrophies

Trichodystrophy	Characteristic Finding	Cause/Associated Disorders

Trichorrhexis nodosa[a]	Tiny white specks on the hair shaft on light microscopy resemble the bristles of two broom ends	Acquired (hair grooming)
		Genetic disease
		  Menkes disease
		  Urea cycle defects

Trichoptilosis[a]	"Split ends": longitudinal splitting of distal hair shaft	Trauma
		  Hair grooming
		  Trichotillomania

"Bubble hair"[a]	Area of abnormally stiff, straight, fragile, uneven hairs: irregularly shaped air bubbles on light microscopy	Heat drying and styling
Monilethrix[a]	Elliptical nodes and constrictions on light microscopy ("beaded hair")	Autosomal dominant inheritance
Trichorrhexis invaginata[a]	"Bamboo hair": "ball in socket" defect on light microscopy	Netherton syndrome Idiopathic

Pili torti[a]	Flat, twisted hair shaft on light microscopy	Genetic
		  Björnstad syndrome
		  Menkes disease
		  Urea cycle defects
		  Mitochondrial disorders
		  Ectodermal dysplasias
		Acquired
		  Anorexia nervosa
		  Oral retinoids

Trichothiodystrophy[a]	Light microscopy: transverse fractures (trichoschisis) and alternating "tiger's tail" light and dark bands under polarization. Amino acid analysis: sulfur-deficient hair shafts	Autosomal recessive inheritance +/− associated anomalies of the skin, nails, bones, neurologic and immune systems
Uncombable hair syndrome	"Spun glass" hair which appears unruly. Hair shafts with triangular cross-sections on light microscopy and longitudinal grooves on electron microscopy	Likely sporadic inheritance Improves with age, biotin treatment

TABLE 35-10 • Trichodystrophies (*continued*)

Trichodystrophy	Characteristic Finding	Cause/Associated Disorders
Acquired progressive kinking of the hair	Acquired curling of hair	Androgenetic alopecia
Pili annulati	"Ringed hair": bright and dark bands when light reflects off hairs. Air-filled clusters on light microscopy	Sporadic or autosomal recessive inheritance
Woolly hair	Tightly curled, kinky hair with variable microscopic findings	Woolly hair nevus (circumscribed) Associated with PPK

a Associated with increased hair fragility.

Trichodystrophies With Increased Hair Fragility

Trichorrhexis nodosa is the most common structural abnormality of the hair shaft and is usually acquired through damage from hair grooming procedures. It may also be associated with hypothyroidism and genetic syndromes such as Menkes disease, argininosuccinic aciduria, and citrullinemia. Clinically, it presents as tiny white specks on the hair shaft that may superficially look like nits from head lice. When viewed microscopically, these specks resemble the bristles of two broom ends interlocked and are the site of fractures (Fig. 35-15). Pathogenesis is thought to be cuticular damage.

Trichoptilosis (split ends) is the longitudinal splitting of the distal hair shaft. It is induced by trauma, styling of hair, use of cosmetic products, and grooming procedures. Trichoptilosis and trichorrhexis nodosa may both be seen in hair pulling (trichotillomania) and scratching.

"Bubble hair" typically presents in young women as a localized area of abnormally stiff, straight, fragile, uneven hairs. Light microscopy reveals irregularly shaped air bubbles, which expand to thin the hair cortex (Fig. 35-16). Fracture occurs at the site of larger bubbles. The cause is usually excessive heat from hair dryers.

Monilethrix (beaded hair) occurs secondary to autosomal dominantly inherited point mutations, usually in hair cortex-specific keratin genes *KRT86* and *KRT81*. Within the first few months of life, normal lanugo hairs are replaced by fragile, brittle hair. Light microscopy reveals uniform elliptical nodes and abnormal constrictions, where breakage can occur (Fig. 35-17). The scalp

is always involved. Involvement of the eyebrows, eyelashes, and nails is variable.

Trichorrhexis invaginata ("bamboo hair") is seen most commonly in association with Netherton syndrome, but can also occur in the absence of a genetic disorder. Netherton syndrome is caused by a mutation in the *SPINK5* gene. Affected individuals have short, sparse hair from infancy, as well as atopy and the characteristic skin finding of ichthyosis linearis circumflexa. Light microscopy reveals a "ball" in "socket" defect at breakage points (Fig. 35-18). Eyebrows and body hair are also affected. Scalp involvement tends to improve with time.

Pili torti is characterized by a flat, twisted hair shaft (Fig. 35-19). Scalp hair is brittle and fragile. Body hair is

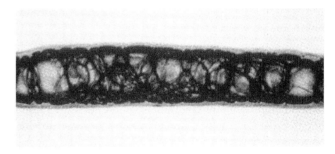

FIGURE 35-16: Bubble Hair.

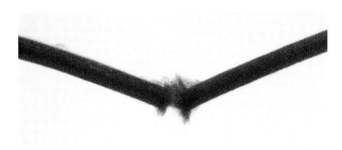

FIGURE 35-15: Trichorrhexis nodosum.

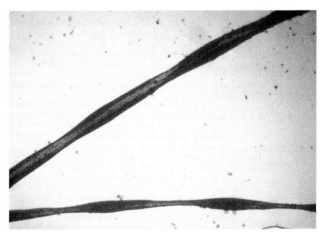

FIGURE 35-17: Monilethrix.

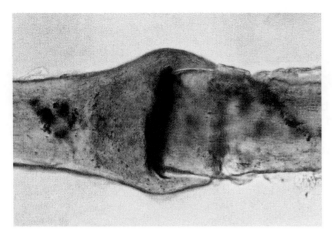

FIGURE 35-18: Trichorrhexis invaginata.

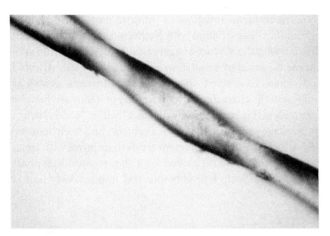

FIGURE 35-19: Pili torti.

absent or sparse. Pili torti is associated with multiple genetic disorders, including Björnstad syndrome, Menkes disease, Bazex–Dupré–Christol syndrome, hypotrichosis with juvenile macular dystrophy, Laron syndrome (primary growth hormone insensitivity), ectodermal dysplasias, mitochondrial disorders, and urea cycle defects, namely citrullinemia and argininosuccinic aciduria. As Björnstad syndrome is associated with sensorineural hearing loss, children presenting with pili torti should receive auditory screening. Acquired pili torti can be seen in the settings of anorexia nervosa and oral retinoid therapy. There is no treatment for pili torti, but it may improve at puberty.

Trichothiodystrophy is an autosomal recessive disorder characterized by brittle, hair which is sulfur-deficient on amino acid analysis. Microscopic examination of hair shafts reveals transverse fractures (trichoschisis), with alternating light and dark bands resembling a tiger's tail under polarization. Electron microscopy reveals severely damaged cuticles. Hair findings may occur in isolation or with a variety of other anomalies, including those of the skin (photosensitivity, ichthyosis,) neurologic system (mental retardation, spasticity, tremor, ataxia), bones (dental caries, bony defects, short stature), nail dystrophy, and immunodeficiency.

Trichodystrophies Not Associated With Hair Fragility

Uncombable hair syndrome (spun glass hair) is an interesting hair shaft abnormality in which the hair shafts in cross-section are triangular and on electron microscopy there are longitudinal grooves. The onset is usually around 3 years of age when the hair seems particularly wild and unruly. Typically, the hair is of a silver blond color and the problem may be generalized (usually) or localized (Fig. 35-20). Spontaneous improvement may occur in childhood. Oral biotin may prove helpful. This same triangular hair shaft abnormality has been described in loose anagen syndrome and after spironolactone therapy.

Acquired progressive kinking of the hair is refers to acquired curling of scalp hair, which may be localized or diffuse. Most commonly, this is seen in young men who develop frizzy hair at the androgen-dependent frontotemporal regions or vertex of the scalp. This is followed by progression to androgenetic alopecia in affected areas.

Pili annulati (ringed hair) may be sporadic or inherited in an autosomal dominant fashion. On microscopy, hair shafts reveal irregularly distributed air-filled clusters (Fig. 35-21).

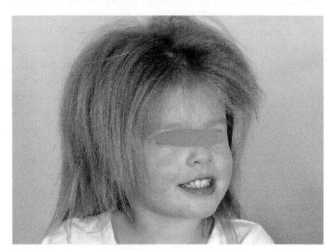

FIGURE 35-20: Uncombable hair syndrome.

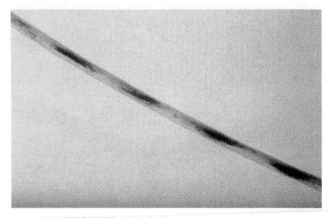

FIGURE 35-21: Pili annulati: microscopic view demonstrating regular placement of air bubbles.

Unlike "bubble hair," however, these clusters do not lead to increased breakage and fragility of hair. Bright and dark bands are seen when light reflects off affected hairs (Fig. 35-22).

Woolly hair presents diffusely or as a circumscribed patch (woolly hair nevus, Fig. 35-23). It is usually inherited and may be congenital. Microscopic examination of the hair shafts may reveal a variety of findings, including elliptical cross-sections, pili torti, and trichorrhexis nodosa. Woolly hair is associated with multiple genetic disorders, many of which also have palmoplantar keratoderma (PPK) as a feature.

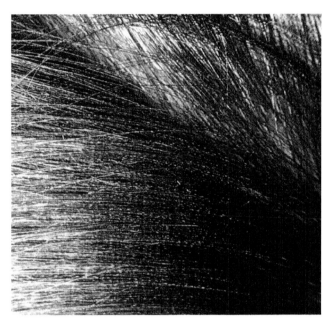

FIGURE 35-22: Pili annulati: alternating bright and dark bands on gross inspection.

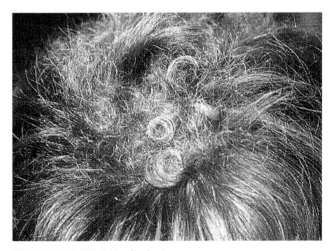

FIGURE 35-23: Woolly hair nevus.

Suggested Readings

Sperling LC, Sinclair RP, El-Shabrawi-Caelen L. Alopecias & hair shaft abnormalities. In Bolognia JL, Jorizzo JL, Schaffer JV, eds. *Dermatology.* Spain: Mosby (Elsevier Limited); 2012.

American Psychiatric Association. *Diagnostic and Statistical Manual of Mental Disorders.* 5th ed. Washington, DC: American Psychiatric Association; 2013:251–254.

Atanaskova Mesinkovska N, Bergfeld WF. Hair: what is new in diagnosis and management? Female pattern hair loss update: diagnosis and treatment. *Dermatol Clin.* 2013;31(1):119–127.

Bayart CB, Bergfeld WF. Telogen effluvium. In: McMichael A, Hordinsky M, eds. *Hair and Scalp Disorders.* 2nd ed. Boca Raton: CRC Press. 2016:chap 11.

de Berker D, Higgins CA, Jahoda C, et al. Biology of hair & nails. In Bolognia JL, Jorizzo JL, Schaffer JV, eds. *Dermatology.* 3rd ed. Spain: Mosby (Elsevier Limited); 2012.

Blazek C, Megahed M. Lichen planopilaris: successful treatment with tacrolimus. *Hautarzt.* 2008;59(11):874–877.

Bunagan MJ, Banka N, Shapiro J. Retrospective review of folliculitis decalvans in 23 patients with course and treatment analysis of long-standing cases. *J Cutan Med Surg.* 2015;19(1):45–49.

Camacho-Martinez FM. Hypertrichosis & hirsutism. In Bolognia JL, Jorizzo JL, Schaffer JV, eds. *Dermatology.* 3rd ed. Spain: Mosby (Elsevier Limited); 2012.

Delamere FM, Sladden MM, Dobbins HM, et al. Interventions for alopecia areata. *Cochrane Database Syst Rev.* 2008;(2). doi:10.1002/14651858.

Georgala S, Korfitis C. Dissecting cellulitis of the scalp treated with rifampicin and isotretinoin: case reports. *Cutis.* 2008;82:195–198.

Jackson J, Caro J, Caro J, et al. The effect of eflornithine 13.9% cream on the bother and discomfort due to hirsutism. *Int J Dermatol.* 2007;46:976–981.

Kaur S, Mahajan BB. Eyelash trichomegaly. *Indian J Dermatol.* 2015;60(4):378–380.

Koudoukpo C, Abdennader S, Cavelier-Balloy B, et al. Dissecting cellulitis of the scalp: a retrospective study of 7 cases confirming the efficacy of oral isotretinoin (Article in French). *Ann Dermatol Venereol.* 2014;141(8–9):500–506.

McDonough PH, Schwartz RA. Premature hair graying. *Cutis.* 2012;89(4):161–165.

Mubki T, Rudnicka L, Olszewska M, et al. Evaluation and diagnosis of the hair loss patient: part I. History and clinical examination. *J Am Acad Dermatol.* 2014;71(3):415.e1–415.e15.

Mubki T, Rudnicka L, Olszewska M, et al. Evaluation and diagnosis of the hair loss patient: part II. Trichoscopic and laboratory evaluations. *J Am Acad Dermatol.* 2014;71(3):431.e1–431.e11.

Palomba S, Santagni S, Falbo A, et al. Complications and challenges associated with polycystic ovary syndrome: current perspectives. *Int J Womens Health.* 2015;7:745–763.

Rothbart R, Stein DJ. Pharmacotherapy of trichotillomania (hair pulling disorder): an updated systematic review. *Expert Opin Pharmacother.* 2014;15(18):2709–2719.

Sand FL, Thomsen SF. Off-label use of TNF-alpha inhibitors in a dermatological university department: retrospective evaluation of 118 patients. *Dermatol Ther.* 2015;28(3):158–165.

Schmidt TH, Shinkai K. Evidence-based approach to cutaneous hyperandrogenism in women. *J Am Acad Dermatol.* 2015;73(4):672–690.

Shin H, Ryu HH, Yoon J, et al. Association of premature hair graying with family history, smoking, and obesity: a cross-sectional study. *J Am Acad Dermatol.* 2015;72(2):321–327.

Tietze JK, Heppt MV, von Preußen A, et al. Oral isotretinoin as the most effective treatment in folliculitis decalvans: a retrospective comparison of different treatment regimens in 28 patients. *J Eur Acad Dermatol Venereol.* 2015;29(9):1816–1821.

Vañó-Galván S, Molina-Ruiz AM, Fernández-Crehuet P, et al. Folliculitis decalvans: a multicentre review of 82 patients. *J Eur Acad Dermatol Venereol.* 2015;29(9):1750–1757.

Yin Li VC, Yesudian PD. Congenital triangular alopecia. *Int J Trichology.* 2015;7(2):48–53.

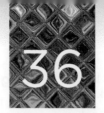

36

Diseases Affecting the Nail Unit

Richard K. Scher, MD, FACP, Bradley Merritt, MD, FACMS,
Alex Lombardi, MD, and Patrick Retterbush, MD

The nail unit is an essential component of the integumentary system and can be affected by primary disease, dermatologic disorders with nail involvement, and systemic illnesses that alter the appearance of the nails.

Primary nail disorders, as in the case of subungual melanoma and subungual squamous cell carcinoma, can be life threatening.

Secondary nail changes can be a sign of underlying life-threatening diseases such as advanced renal, hepatic, and cardiovascular disease.

The nail unit's most important functions are to protect the distal digit and to improve dexterity in manipulating small objects. By providing counterpressure, the nail plate enhances the transmission of delicate sensations. Perhaps more important from an evolutionary standpoint, the nail unit facilitates scratching and grooming. Disorders of the nail unit can be physically and psychologically distressing to patients, because nails often serve socially as a cosmetic enhancement. This chapter reviews common and serious nail disorders, including those caused by infectious, traumatic, neoplastic, congenital, and primary dermatologic disorders.

A complete history and physical examination should be included in any evaluation of a patient with a nail disorder. Medication history is important and systemic disease should be noted, as these factors often affect the appearance of the nail unit. Family history can give clues to hereditary nail abnormalities as can be found in nail-patella syndrome (osteo-onychodysplasia), ectodermal dysplasia, pachyonychia congenita, and Darier disease (keratosis follicularis). An occupational history can provide insight into possible allergic or irritant exposures. Treatments of the nail, including prior medical/surgical modalities, home remedies, and manicures/pedicures, are important to note because they can be factors contributing to persistent nail disease. All 20 nails should be examined. A magnifying glass can be used to enhance fine details. A dermatoscope can be helpful when evaluating the nail folds for signs of connective tissue disease and the nail plate for melanonychia striata. A complete skin examination, including the oral mucosa, is also important. Subtle lesions can give clues as to the cause of nail disorders. Laboratory tests useful in the evaluation of nail disease include biopsy of the nail plate, cuticle, bed, or matrix, fungal cultures, bacterial cultures, and potassium hydroxide preparations. Imaging modalities including plain film and magnetic resonance imaging (MRI) can be helpful in determining the extent of disease and evaluating possible involvement of bone underlying the nail apparatus.

ANATOMY OF THE NAIL UNIT

The nail unit is a specialized appendage of the skin, composed of unique structures not found elsewhere in the body. The nail unit consists of the nail plate, proximal and lateral nail folds, cuticle, nail matrix, nail bed, and the hyponychium (Fig. 36-1). What most people consider *the nail* refers to the nail plate, the clear, hard portion of the nail made of keratin. The nail plate is divided into two sections: the dorsal plate created by the proximal nail matrix, and the ventral plate created by the distal nail matrix, with some contribution from the nail bed. The nail matrix is composed of a group of germative cells located proximal to the nail plate. The nail matrix contains a layer of actively dividing keratinocytes that mature and, after death, contribute to the formation of the nail plate. The nail plate is bordered by the proximal nail fold and two lateral nail folds. The lunula is the most distal portion of the matrix, visible as a white, half-moon–shaped area under the nail plate bordered by the proximal nail fold. The nail plate rests on the highly vascular nail bed. The hyponychium is the section of the skin located under the free edge of the nail plate between the nail bed and the distal nail groove.

Fingernails grow constantly at a rate of 0.1 mm/day or 3 mm/month. At this rate, a fingernail can be totally replaced in 4 to 6 months. Toenails, however, grow at about half this rate and can take 8 to 12 months to be replaced. Certain disease states including psoriasis, minor trauma, pityriasis rubra pilaris, brittle nail syndrome, hyperpituitarism, and hyperthyroidism can cause nails to grow at a faster rate than normal. Slower nail growth has been noted in patients with malnutrition, acute infections, peripheral neuropathy, onychomycosis, and hypothyroidism, as well as in smokers. The rate of nail growth can also be affected by a variety of medications.

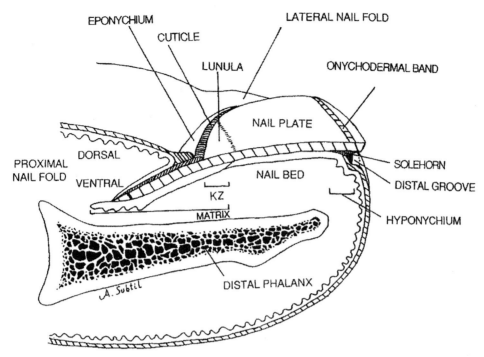

FIGURE 36-1: Anatomy of the nail unit. KZ, keratogenous zone. (Reprinted from Hordinsky MK, Sawaya ME, Scher ME. Histology of the normal nail unit. In: *Atlas of Hair and Nails*. 1st ed. Philadelphia: Churchill Livingstone; 2000:19. Copyright 2000, with permission from Elsevier.)

ONYCHOMYCOSIS

Onychomycosis, or fungal infection of the nail, is the most common nail disorder and accounts for up to half of all nail problems encountered in clinical practice. The prevalence of onychomycosis increases with age. Other risk factors for developing onychomycosis include smoking, peripheral arterial disease, recurrent trauma, diabetes mellitus, family history, and immunosuppression including HIV infection. Fungal infections of the nail may be caused by dermatophytes (tinea unguium), nondermatophyte molds, or yeast. More than 90% of cases of onychomycosis are caused by the dermatophytes *Trichophyton rubrum* and *Trichophyton mentagrophytes*. Onychomycosis has been classified into five major types:

- distal and lateral subungual onychomycosis (DLSO)
- superficial white onychomycosis (SO)
- proximal subungual onychomycosis (PSO)
- endonyx onychomycosis, and
- total dystrophic onychomycosis

Clinical signs of onychomycosis include

- thickening of the nail bed and nail plate
- subungual debris
- onycholysis (separation of the nail plate from the nail bed)
- nail discoloration (white/yellow or orange/brown patches or streaks)
- ridging of the nail
- nail pitting

Diagnosis

Before treating patients with clinical evidence of onychomycosis, the diagnosis can be confirmed by (1) direct microscopy (48% sensitivity) of nail debris using a preparation of potassium hydroxide (KOH) with or without dimethyl sulfoxide or chlorazol black, or (2) fungal culture (53% sensitivity), or (3) histologic examination of the nail plate with periodic acid–Schiff (PAS) stain (82% sensitivity). Collection of an appropriate specimen is crucial. In general, it is best to obtain a sample from the most proximal central area of involved nail. Direct microscopy allows for rapid diagnosis but does not provide speciation. Fungal culture, while less sensitive, can be important for identifying the causative organism, especially in treatment-resistant cases. Histologic examination with PAS is the most sensitive test for onychomycosis and has the highest negative predictive value. When combined with culture, the sensitivity is 96%. It is also the most expensive test at approximately $150, and should be reserved for cases when direct microscopy is unavailable or negative but clinical suspicion is high.

Presentation and Characteristics

Distal and lateral subungual onychomycosis (DLSO) is the most common form of onychomycosis (Fig. 36-2). The first sites of fungal invasion are the hyponychium or the lateral nail fold. Onycholysis occurs when subungual keratotic debris separates the nail plate from the nail bed. Paronychia can also occur. The nail bed is the ideal site for obtaining a specimen for microscopic examination. The most common organism associated with DLSO is the dermatophyte *T. rubrum*. Candida

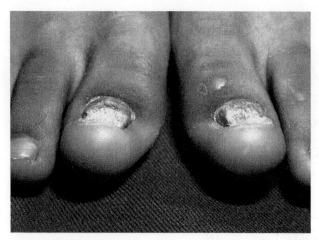

FIGURE 36-2: Distal and lateral subungual onychomycosis.

species are less frequently responsible, while the nondermatophyte molds, including *Scopulariopsis brevicaulis*, Aspergillus species, Acremonium species, and *Fusarium oxysporum*, are the least common causative organisms.

Superficial onychomycosis (SO) can be divided into white and black variants. White SO is the most common. The first, second, and third toenails are more likely to be affected, and the exposed dorsal surface of the nail plate is the site of fungal invasion. Clinically, white SO presents on the nail plate as white, opaque islands with distinct edges. Untreated lesions can develop a yellow color. Because of the superficial nature of the infection, organisms can often be scraped from the nail plate surface. White SO is most often caused by the dermatophyte *T. mentagrophytes var. interdigitale* but can also be caused by *T. rubrum* as well as by molds including Aspergillus, Acremonium, and *Fusarium spp*. White SO caused by *T. rubrum* often leads to more extensive nail involvement and is seen in otherwise healthy children and in patients infected with HIV. White SO secondary to molds can be clinically indistinguishable from disease caused by dermatophytes, but can also lead to deeper, more extensive involvement of the nail. Black SO presents with black, opaque plaques on the nails secondary to invading fungi that are pigmented. This variant occurs with *Scytalydium dimidiatum* and *T. rubrum*.

Endonyx onychomycosis is a fungal infection of the nail in which both the superficial and deep layers of the nail plate are affected without resulting in nail bed inflammatory changes. Tunnels formed by and filled with invading fungi may be present. Clinically, this appears as a milky-white discoloration of the nail plate that is not accompanied by subungual hyperkeratosis or onycholysis. There is lamellar splitting of the nail plate. Endonyx onychomycosis is caused by *Trichophyton soudanense* and *Trichophyton violaceum*.

Proximal subungual onychomycosis (PSO) is a relatively uncommon subtype that occurs secondary to fungal invasion at the proximal nail fold through the cuticle. PSO with rapid progression is a variant most often associated with immunocompromised conditions, especially HIV infection. *T. rubrum* is the most common pathogen. Because of the association with

HIV, clinicians should consider laboratory testing to investigate immune status when a diagnosis of PSO is made.

Clinically, PSO demonstrates a whitish discoloration of the proximal nail plate along with proximal subungual hyperkeratosis and onycholysis. The distal end of the nail plate appears normal in early infection. PSO can be seen with or without paronychia. In patients without paronychia, proximal subungual onychomycosis is usually caused by *T. rubrum*. In patients with paronychia, PSO is usually secondary to *C. albicans* but can also be caused by Aspergillus, Fusarium, and *Scopulariopsis spp*.

Total dystrophic onychomycosis can be primary or secondary. Secondary total dystrophic onychomycosis usually occurs because of extensive fungal infection involving the entire nail plate from distal and lateral subungual onychomycosis or proximal subungual onychomycosis. The entire nail plate is extensively thickened and can easily collapse. Primary total dystrophic onychomycosis is seen in patients with chronic mucocutaneous candidiasis and is caused by infection of all portions of the nail unit by Candida.

Differential Diagnosis

A variety of diseases of the nail can mimic onychomycosis and must be considered in the differential diagnosis. Only 40% to 50% of abnormal-appearing toenails are actually due to onychomycosis. Possible simulators of onychomycosis include psoriasis, chronic onycholysis, lichen planus, alopecia areata, chronic paronychia, hemorrhage/trauma, onychogryphosis, aging, median canaliform dystrophy, pincer nail deformity, yellow nail syndrome, subungual malignant melanoma, and subungual squamous cell carcinoma. Any of these disease states can coexist with onychomycosis, and proof of dermatophyte infection in the nail (Fig. 36-3) does not exclude a separate, concurrent disease of the nail unit.

Treatment

Therapy for onychomycosis depends on the pattern, pathogen, and degree of involvement. Treatments include oral and topical medications, as well as periodic clipping and filing of infected portions of the nail plate. White superficial onychomycosis involving less than the distal two-thirds of the nail plate and moderate distal and lateral subungual onychomycosis can be treated effectively with the topical fungicidal lacquers/solutions efinaconazole, tavaborole, ciclopirox, and amorolfine. These lacquers have a broad range of antifungal activity against dermatophytes, as well as *C. albicans*. Additionally, ciclopirox has antibacterial and anti-inflammatory action. Lacquers are less effective (7% to 18% complete cure rate with 48 weeks of treatment) than oral treatments, but can be useful in patients with onychomycosis who cannot tolerate oral antifungals because of liver or kidney disease, or those taking multiple systemic medications where drug interactions may be a concern.

The first-line treatment for onychomycosis is oral terbinafine, an allylamine fungicidal. A meta-analysis of randomized clinical trials found terbinafine to be superior to placebo, itraconazole, fluconazole, and griseofulvin in achieving mycologic cure in

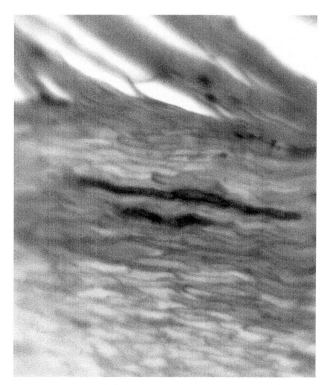

FIGURE 36-3: High-power microscopic view of a dermatophyte in the nail plate (PAS stain; original magnification 400×). (Courtesy of Dr. George W. Niedt.)

patients with onychomycosis. Terbinafine also demonstrates the lowest recurrence rates. Typical dosing for terbinafine is 250 mg daily for 12 weeks for toenails and 6 weeks for fingernails. While previously considered cost-prohibitive by many patients, the cost of treatment with terbinafine has been reduced significantly with the advent of $4 generic plans available at many pharmacies.

Other systemic medications used to treat onychomycosis include the azole antifungals itraconazole and fluconazole, as well as the newer agent posaconazole. Itraconazole can be given as 100 mg twice daily for 12 weeks for toenails or 6 weeks for fingernails. Alternatively, itraconazole can be pulsed at 200 mg twice daily for 1 week per month for 3 months for toenails and 2 months for fingernails, lowering the risk for hepatotoxicity. Various pulse therapies have also been advocated for oral terbinafine therapy but are generally less effective than continuous therapy. Fluconazole can be dosed from 150 to 300 mg once per week until the nails are clear, but has a low clearance rate. Posaconazole is dosed at 200 mg daily for 24 weeks, and has shown equivalency to terbinafine but at a significantly higher dose. Griseofulvin is a fungistatic medicine that must be taken until the entire nail is replaced. For this reason, as well as inferior efficacy compared to newer treatments and potential interactions with warfarin and oral contraceptives, griseofulvin is no longer used frequently for onychomycosis. Ketoconazole is also used infrequently for onychomycosis because of possible hepatotoxicity.

Hepatotoxicity has been reported with itraconazole, fluconazole, posaconazole, and terbinafine, in decreasing order of frequency. Baseline liver enzyme levels should be documented to confirm normal liver function, but monitoring of liver enzymes during continuous therapy is likely unnecessary. Systemic treatments for onychomycosis are well tolerated, with gastrointestinal side effects, skin changes, and headaches most common. Serious side effects with the first-line agent terbinafine are rare, occurring in 0.04% of patients. Combining oral and topical treatments may allow for shorter courses with higher cure rates.

Factors leading to a poor response to treatment with oral therapy include lateral nail disease, proximal nail disease, involvement of the entire nail unit, longitudinal streaks of fungal infection in the nail plate, presence of a dermatophytoma (mass of fungi between the nail plate and the nail bed), and extensive onycholysis. If a dermatophytoma is present, removing the portion of nail plate overlying it and removing the concentration of fungi can help to achieve a cure. Candida onychomycosis also can be more difficult to treat. Terbinafine is slightly less effective than itraconazole in curing onychomycosis secondary to *Candida spp.*

Onychomycosis is difficult to cure permanently. Many patients have recurrent infection. Factors associated with recurrence include persistent predisposing conditions such as peripheral vascular disease, diabetes mellitus, recurrent trauma, older age, as well as insufficient treatment from premature termination or inadequate dosing. Several measures have been suggested to avoid recurrence, include wearing footwear when walking in areas of high concentrations of dermatophytes (e.g., communal areas by pools, spas), avoiding shoes that may have dermatophytes present, drying feet and interdigital spaces after a bath or shower, using socks made of absorbent material (highly wicking socks), treating concurrent tinea pedis, using powder such as Zeasorb AF (very absorbent and contains the antifungal miconazole) to shake into shoes or socks, and prophylactic use of topical antifungal agents. In refractory cases, surgical removal of the entire nail can be performed with subsequent topical and systemic therapy until full nail regrowth.

SAUER'S NOTES

Remember that onychomycosis or candida often colonizes a damaged nail from any cause. So more than one culprit may be involved in the diseased nail that you see before you.

PARONYCHIA

Paronychia is defined as acute or chronic inflammation of the nail fold, typically with an associated infection. Acute paronychia is usually preceded by trauma that facilitates bacterial inoculation of the nail fold. It affects the digit with rapid development of erythema, tenderness, and in more advanced disease, purulent discharge. Untreated, acute paronychia can lead to a subungual abscess and nail dystrophy. The most commonly associated organism is *Staphylococcus aureus*, but *Streptococcus pyogenes, Pseudomonas pyocyanea, Proteus vulgaris,* and anaerobic bacteria have also been cultured from acute paronychia. Herpes simplex virus can cause recurrent acute paronychia in the form of herpetic whitlow. Pemphigus vulgaris is also associated with acute paronychia.

Chronic paronychia is defined as inflammation of the nail fold present for at least 6 weeks that develops from repeated exposure to moisture, irritants, and allergens. Patients present with erythema, swelling, and tenderness of the nail folds. Nail plate thickening, ridging, and discoloration can occur. Chronic paronychia most commonly affects patients with repeated exposure to a moist environment, including cooks, dishwashers, laundry workers, and nurses. Candida is often present, but its role in the pathogenesis is unclear. Chronic paronychia has been associated with isotretinoin (Accutane), protease inhibitors, and the epidermal growth factor inhibitors.

Diagnosis

Squamous cell carcinoma, subungual melanoma, and metastatic carcinoma can simulate paronychia and are important to exclude. In patients with acute paronychia that responds poorly to conventional treatment, cultures can be beneficial in identifying the causative organism. The prevalence of skin infections secondary to methicillin-resistant *S. aureus* is increasing, and culture may be necessary to rule out this pathogen. If vesicles are present, herpetic whitlow should be suspected and a Tzanck smear and/or HSV culture or less often PCR should be performed. Biopsy should be considered in treatment of refractory cases or if there is any suspicion of a neoplastic process.

Treatment

Mild acute paronychia responds well to warm compresses and topical antibacterial treatment. More severe and persistent disease often requires oral antibiotics or incision and drainage. Surgical drainage effectively treats acute paronychia and is indicated if an abscess has formed. Herpetic whitlow can be treated with acyclovir, valacyclovir, or famciclovir. Incision and drainage should be avoided if the presence of HSV is confirmed.

Chronic paronychia is best treated by avoidance of moisture and irritants. Patients should be advised to avoid manipulation of the cuticle, which is important in preventing entry of microorganisms. Topical antifungal treatment is also recommended because of the presence of Candida. Topical corticosteroids are the treatment of choice, however, especially if inflammation is prominent. A randomized trial found greater improvement of chronic paronychia treated with topical steroids compared to topical antifungal therapy.

NAIL PSORIASIS

Nail involvement in psoriasis is common, occurring in up to half of all patients with psoriasis. Psoriatic nail changes are especially common in patients with psoriatic arthritis. Most patients with nail involvement have classical skin lesions as well, but nail disease can occur in the absence of cutaneous psoriasis. Clinical features of nail psoriasis include:

- pitting
- discoloration
- onycholysis
- subungual hyperkeratosis
- nail plate crumbling and grooving and
- splinter hemorrhages

Nail changes in psoriasis are variable, ranging from a few pits to total nail dystrophy. Nail pits, while not specific for psoriasis, are the most common finding and are formed by small psoriatic lesions in the proximal nail matrix. Nail pitting in psoriasis is typically irregular and nongeometric as opposed to the regular nature of nail pitting seen in alopecia areata. Oil drop or salmon-colored spots are yellow-red discolorations of the nail bed caused by inclusion of neutrophilic exudates between the nail plate and the nail bed. While less frequent in nail psoriasis, they are pathognomonic when seen. Psoriasis can affect all of the components of the nail unit, and biopsy from affected areas including the proximal nail fold, nail plate, nail bed, and matrix may be appropriate to establish the diagnosis.

Pustular psoriasis of the nails (also known as acrodermatitis continua of Hallopeau) is a variant of nail psoriasis in which the characteristic clinical features include periungual or subungual pustules (Fig. 36-4). Pustular psoriasis of the nails can be difficult to distinguish from other nail disorders. In an evaluation of 38 patients with pustular psoriasis of the nails, all of whom had been evaluated by a prior physician, 35 (92%) had not been correctly diagnosed. The diagnosis of pustular psoriasis of the nails should be considered in patients with recurrent subungual and periungual pustules, recurrent painful onycholysis, and in patients with painful dystrophic and crusted nails. Nail bed biopsy can be useful in confirming the diagnosis of pustular psoriasis of the nails.

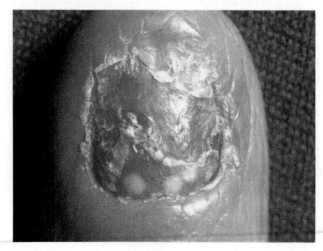

FIGURE 36-4: Pustular nail psoriasis.

Diagnosis

Nail psoriasis almost always occurs along with classical cutaneous lesions, in which case diagnosis is straightforward. In patients without skin involvement, the diagnosis can be difficult unless a characteristic cluster of nail changes is present. Nail pits can be seen as a normal variant as well as in diseases such as chronic eczema, alopecia areata, and lichen planus. The pits in nail psoriasis are typically deeper and less regular than in other nail conditions. Onycholysis is a nonspecific nail change that can also be seen in nail infections, chronic dermatitis, repetitive trauma, and as a side effect of medications. Onycholysis increases the risk for infection, which should be excluded. The majority of patients with psoriatic arthritis have nail changes, so concomitant arthritis can be a clue to the diagnosis. Biopsy of the nail plate, bed, or matrix may be necessary for confirmation of the diagnosis.

Treatment

Treatment of nail psoriasis requires counseling of basic nail care to avoid repetitive trauma that can exacerbate the disease (Koebner phenomenon), as well as patience, as correction of abnormal findings can require up to 6 months for fingernails and longer for toenails. About 30% of affected patients have concomitant onychomycosis that may also require treatment. The treatment of choice for nail psoriasis is individualized, based on the local severity, number of nails affected, and whether concurrent psoriatic arthritis and/or cutaneous psoriasis is present.

First-line therapies for isolated mild nail psoriasis (less than 1 to 2 nails without severe pain or functional loss) include high-potency topical corticosteroids, topical vitamin D analog, and/or combination topical corticosteroid and topical vitamin D analog. First-line therapies for isolated moderate-to-severe nail psoriasis or nail psoriasis with concurrent psoriatic arthritis and/or severe cutaneous psoriasis include biologic therapies (TNF-α inhibitors or ustekinumab), methotrexate, and/or intralesional corticosteroids. Intralesional steroids are generally preferred for disease with primarily nail matrix involvement. Injections with triamcinolone acetonide (2.5 to 10 mg/mL) are performed at multiple sites within the proximal nail fold at monthly intervals typically for up to 5 to 6 months with improvement noted usually within the first 3 months.

Treatment for acrodermatitis continua of Hallopeau (pustular psoriasis,) consists of topical therapies with superpotent topical corticosteroids, systemic therapies with local phototherapy (topical PUVA or NB-UVB therapy). Systemic retinoids (acetretin) may be required as this variant is typically more refractory to standard treatments. Other effective systemic therapies include cyclosporine, methotrexate, and biologics.

SUBUNGUAL HEMATOMA

Subungual hematoma is a common problem encountered by clinicians. A sudden, strong, external force or repeated minor trauma to the digit can cause bleeding of the nail bed, which is highly vascular. The collection of blood under the nail plate causes a bluish or violaceous discoloration (Fig. 36-5).

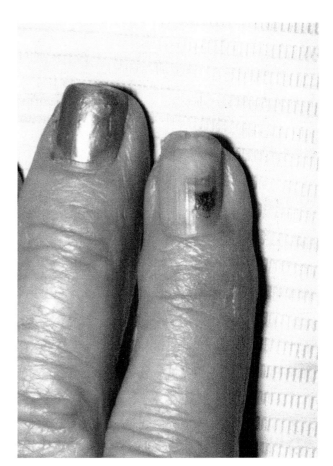

FIGURE 36-5: Subungual hematoma.

Repeated minor trauma often leads to subungual hematoma that can simulate melanonychia striata. Increased pressure in the space between the nail bed and the nail plate can cause intense pain, and larger hematomas can lead to shedding of the nail plate and permanent nail dystrophy.

Diagnosis

The most important distinction to make when evaluating discoloration under the nail plate is differentiating subungual hematoma from subungual melanoma. Information obtained by taking a history can clarify the diagnosis. A rapidly developing lesion that occurs after trauma is more likely to be a subungual hematoma, but patients with subungual melanoma also occasionally report a history of trauma, and bleeding can be the first sign of a subungual melanoma. Distinguishing pigment secondary to blood from pigment of melanocytic origin can sometimes be accomplished using dermoscopy, but only a biopsy can establish a definitive diagnosis.

Additional work-up includes physical exam to detect injury to the extensor tendon and plain films to exclude fracture of the distal phalanx. The PIP and MCP joints can be stabilized to isolate the extensor tendon to test for active range of motion. Pain and swelling over the DIP joint with the inability to extend the distal phalanx and a flexed DIP at rest (mallet finger deformity) are indicative of injury. These patients should be referred to a hand surgeon.

Treatment

Treatment for subungual hematoma consists of evacuation and decompression via nail trephination for uncomplicated hematomas (intact nail plate and nail fold) or nail plate removal for complicated hematomas. Trephination facilitates relief of pressure and immediate pain relief. For complicated hematomas, nail plate removal allows repair of nail bed or nail matrix lacerations.

In patients with larger hematomas involving >50% of the nail, there is a high probability of concurrent distal phalanx fracture, and thus plain films are recommended. Nondisplaced distal phalanx fractures should be splinted for 3 to 4 weeks. Complicated, displaced, or intra-articular distal phalanx fractures require referral to a hand surgeon.

Nail trephination can be performed without local anesthesia. A number of instruments have been used including a heated paper clip or 18-gauge needle, #11-blade scalpel, 2- to 4-mm punch biopsy tool, electrocautery device, and carbon dioxide laser. When performing trephination, care should be taken to avoid the lunula. A large-enough hole (3 to 4 mm) or multiple holes should be created to allow for adequate drainage. If the presentation is greater than 24 to 48 hours after injury, trephination is typically ineffective owing to clot maturation.

PINCER NAIL

The pincer nail deformity is a hereditary or acquired condition defined as a transverse overcurvature of the nail plate that leads to progressive pinching of the nail bed and compression of the underlying dermis. The lateral edges of the nail plate can break through the skin, resulting in the formation of granulation tissue and paronychia (Fig. 36-6). Any nail can be involved, but less often with fingernails, and with the great toenails being most commonly affected. Pincer nail is usually asymptomatic, but can lead to inflammation, pain, difficulty with footwear, and an undesirable cosmetic appearance. Although not frequently seen, pain, recurrent or chronic infections, or underlying osteomyelitis can complicate pincer nail. This condition may be an autosomal dominant inherited condition or may result from trauma. In the hereditary form, involvement is usually symmetric, whereas acquired pincer nail generally does not show symmetric involvement.

Pincer nail can be divided into three clinical types. The most common form is the trumpet nail deformity that occurs when the curvature increases from the proximal to distal portion. The second clinical type of pincer nail is the tile-shaped nail, which displays an even, transverse overcurvature with the lateral nail plate edges remaining parallel. The third form of pincer nail is the plicated nail, which shows a less drastic overcurvature with one or both lateral nail plate edges forming a vertical sheet pressing into the lateral nail groove.

Diagnosis

Pincer nail deformity is usually diagnosed easily by the characteristic clinical appearance. It is important to determine the underlying cause, however, as there are a variety of treatable causes of acquired pincer nail. The most common cause is deviation of the phalanges of the feet secondary to poorly fitting shoes. Diseases associated with acquired pincer nail deformity include renal disease, lupus erythematosus, Kawasaki disease, psoriasis, onychomycosis, subungual exostosis, epidermal cyst, or myxoid cyst. Pincer nails have also been reported in association with metastasis of colon carcinoma, placement of an arteriovenous fistula for hemodialysis, and the use of β blockers or pamidronate. Pincer nail deformity can also be seen in association with osteoarthritis. Imaging with plain film or MRI can help identify the presence of osteophytes or hyperostosis, which unless treated, can lead to recurrence.

Treatment

Pincer nail can be treated nonsurgically by placement of a brace on the nail plate that is fixed to the lateral edges. The brace is gradually adjusted, resulting in flattening of the nail plate. Recurrences are common with this method. Nail avulsion has also been shown to be an ineffective long-term treatment that can actually exacerbate the overcurvature of the nail plate. Several surgical treatments are effective in correcting pincer nail deformity. These include widening and flattening of the nail bed, tunneled dermal graft placement for flattening of the matrix, and selective destruction of the lateral matrix horns by phenol, electrocautery, or CO_2 laser. Urea ointment under occlusion has also been reported to be effective. Improvement is more likely to be permanent when bony defects that contribute to the nail deformity are removed. Destruction of the entire nail matrix by phenol or surgical ablation may be required in recurrent cases.

ONYCHOCRYPTOSIS (INGROWN NAILS)

Onychocryptosis occurs when the lateral edge of the nail plate grows into the nail fold, resulting in inflammation and soft tissue hypertrophy that can become secondarily infected.

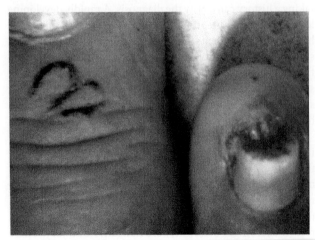

FIGURE 36-6: Pincer nail.

Pressure necrosis, edema, and granulation tissue may also be seen. The great toenail is most often affected (Fig. 36-7). This condition can be extremely painful and restrict mobility. Onychocryptosis has been classified based on the extent of disease. Stage I is typified by pain with mild nail fold erythema and swelling without drainage. Stage II is characterized by swelling, purulent drainage, and ulceration of the nail fold. Stage III is characterized by chronic inflammation with granulation tissue and extensive nail fold hypertrophy.

Diagnosis

Onychocryptosis is typically apparent clinically, but in patients presenting with this condition, it is important to explore all potential etiologies. Onychocryptosis is usually caused by poorly fitting shoes or improper trimming of the nail. Other causes include onychomycosis that results in a thickened and dystrophic nail, arthritis, hyperhidrosis, obesity, injury to the nail, and medications. Isotretinoin is one of the more commonly reported causative medications, while the epidermal growth factor inhibitors have recently been found to cause onychocryptosis. Radiologic studies may be needed in patients more prone to infection and/or with other complications, like diabetes mellitus or peripheral vascular disease. Osteomyelitis should be excluded owing to the need for anti-staphylococcal antibiotic and orthopedic referral for immediate treatment.

Treatment

Treatment of onychocryptosis depends on the extent of involvement. Early disease can be treated conservatively with warm soaks and local care, such as separating the nail plate from the nail fold using a piece of cotton, a wedge of fabric treated with antiseptic solution, or a plastic tube splint. These stay in place until the nail plate grows beyond the lateral nail fold. In more advanced disease, the portion of nail plate pressing on the nail fold should be removed via partial matricectomy and if secondary infection is suspected, drainage should be cultured and antibiotics should be prescribed. Chemical partial matricectomy can also be performed, and in an office setting. For stage III, despite high recurrence rate of onychocryptosis, avulsion of

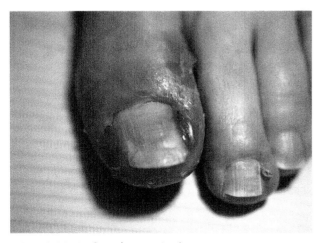

FIGURE 36-7: Onychocryptosis.

the lateral nail plate plus ablation of the corresponding lateral nail matrix using phenol, sodium hydroxide, or CO_2 laser is the preferred treatment. A Cochrane review found simple nail avulsion combined with the use of phenol for matrix ablation to be more effective at preventing symptomatic recurrence but more likely to be complicated by postoperative infection compared to surgical excision without phenol. In cases where the lateral nail fold is hypertrophied, excision of extra lateral nail fold tissue reduces pain and the risk of recurrence.

The technique of performing a partial nail avulsion combined with phenol chemical ablation is as follows: (Fig. 36-8)

1. Achieve digital block with local anesthetic. A wing block around the proximal fold may also alleviate pain. Epinephrine is safe on digits.
2. Tourniquet is applied for hemostasis for up to 15 minutes.
   a. Cut end of a rolled glove is an alternative
   b. Phenol must be applied in a bloodless field as it is inactivated by blood
3. Partial nail avulsion.
   a. Nail splitter or scissors used to cut nail, separating portion to be avulsed
   b. Nail freer (or careful use of a hemostat) used to separate the nail plate from the bed
   c. Hemostat used to pull plate away from the nail fold (prevent embedding of nail spicules)
4. Phenol application.
   a. Protective petroleum ointment applied to adjacent normal periungual tissue, preventing chemical cellulitis of normal tissue
   b. About 88% to 90% phenol applied with fine-tipped cotton applicator in a rotating fashion for 2 to 3 applications of 30 to 60 seconds (total duration 3 to 4-minutes); neutralize/rinse phenol via flushing with 70% isopropyl alcohol or saline

RACKET NAIL

Racket nail is a short, broad, flat nail named after its similarity in shape to a tennis racket. The nail shape usually results from an underlying, shortened distal phalanx of the thumb. Other digits may be involved as well. Women are more often affected. Racket nails may be inherited in an autosomal dominant manner. One or both hands can be involved. Racket nails can be a source of cosmetic concern to patients, but do not otherwise affect function of the digit. Most cases of racket nail are congenital, but an acquired case has been reported in association with tertiary hyperparathyroidism.

HABIT-TIC DEFORMITY

Habit-tic deformity presents as evenly spaced, parallel transverse grooves with a central depression of the nail plate (Fig. 36-9). The lunula is enlarged and the cuticle is often disrupted. The thumbnail is most commonly affected, but other nails can also be involved. This deformity is caused by

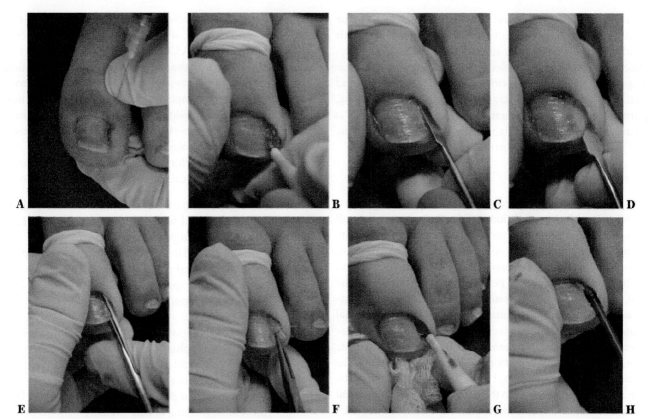

FIGURE 36-8: Partial nail avulsion. **A:** Distal bloc is performed. **B:** Granuloma tissue is removed with a curette. **C and D:** Nail plate is freed from nail groove and nail bed. **E and F:** Nail plate is cut and removed. **G:** Nail matrix, nail bed, and lateral nail fold are curetted. **H:** Phenol solution 88% is applied. (From Di Chiacchio N, Belda W, Gabriel FV, et al. Nail matrix phenolization for treatment of ingrowing nail: technique report and recurrence rate of 267 surgeries. *Dermatol Surg.* 2010;36:534–537.)

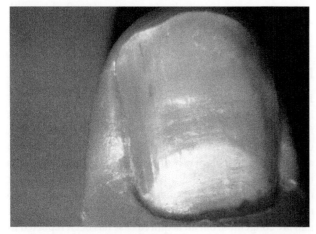

FIGURE 36-9: Habit-tic deformity.

repeated trauma to the nail matrix at the proximal nail fold secondary to picking from a conscious or unconscious habit. Body dysmorphic disorder, obsessive–compulsive disorder, and other psychiatric illnesses that involve a loss of impulse control can include ritualistic nail picking. Habit-tic deformity is responsive to outside trauma being ceased. Interventions shown to be effective include physical barriers to external

trauma such as tape or applying instant glue to the nail folds. A case of the habit-tic deformity has been reported to respond to treatment with fluoxetine (Prozac).

MEDIAN CANALIFORM DYSTROPHY

Median canaliform dystrophy, also known as dystrophia unguium mediana canaliformis, is a nail plate defect in which a median (central) ridge develops, with short transverse ridges running from both sides of the central split. This has been described as an "inverted fir tree configuration." The thumbnails are most commonly affected, and any affected digits frequently exhibit enlarged lunulae. Median canaliform dystrophy can be hereditary. In most cases, an inciting cause cannot be identified and the nails normalize over a period of months to years.

Diagnosis

Lichen planus and nail psoriasis should be included in the differential diagnosis for canaliform nail dystrophy, owing to the shared characteristic of longitudinal splitting of the nail between these conditions. Lichen planus is most likely suspected when pterygium unguius (winged nail) deformity is seen with a central elevated ridge ultimately causing nail deformity or destruction. Nails affected by habit-tic deformity also show multiple transverse ridges, but lack the longitudinal splitting seen in median canaliform dystrophy. This condition is also frequently incorrectly diagnosed as onychomycosis, making recognition of this deformity vital for avoiding unnecessary prescription of antimycotic agents.

Although the pathogenesis of this disorder is not known, it is speculated that localized dyskeratinization of the nail matrix may be responsible. Self-inflicted damage to the middle part of the posterior nail fold has also been hypothesized to be the cause of median canaliform dystrophy. Repeated pressure forced onto the nail bed is the most common identifiable cause of this condition. There are three case reports of patients who developed median canaliform dystrophy after treatment with isotretinoin for acne. All cases had nail changes revert to normal after discontinuation of the drug. The condition will also typically resolve with cessation of traumatic activity. Although not frequently done, treatment with topical ointments or injection of triamcinolone acetonide directly into the proximal nail fold has been shown to improve median canaliform dystrophy.

TRACHYONYCHIA

Trachyonychia or "rough nails" can be associated with a variety of dermatoses including

- lichen planus
- psoriasis
- alopecia areata
- atopic dermatitis
- ichthyosis vulgaris

Trachyonychia has also been associated with immunoglobulin A deficiency. Trachyonychia is described as having a sand-paper appearance, with a rough, lusterless nail plate (Fig. 36-10). The presence of numerous small, superficial pits in the nail plate in less severe cases can cause the nail to appear shiny. One or more nails can be affected. When all 20 nails are affected, the condition is often termed "twenty-nail dystrophy." The peak incidence is between 2 and 12 years of age. Identification of a specific cause may require nail matrix biopsy. Trachyonychia associated with lichen planus in children usually resolves over time without treatment.

Treatment

Local treatment of trachyonychia is best accomplished with intralesional triamcinolone acetonide into the proximal nail folds. A case report has demonstrated a beneficial effect of topical 5-fluorouracil cream in the treatment of psoriatic trachyonychia. Emollients or nail sticks with 50% urea may be beneficial.

BRITTLE NAILS

Brittle nail syndrome is characterized by dry, easily damaged nail plates with onychorrhexis (longitudinal ridging), onychoschizia (horizontal layering), and excessive cracking and/or splitting (Fig. 36-11). A grading system based on the degree of lamellar and longitudinal splitting has been proposed. Dehydration of the nail plate is believed to be the main cause of brittle nails, leading to loss of flexibility and inelasticity of the nail plate. This can occur in patients exposed to organic solvents, acetone, alkaline liquids, and frequent handwashing. Psoriasis, lichen planus, and alopecia areata can be associated with brittle nails. Several systemic diseases are associated with brittle nails, including:

- tuberculosis
- endocrinopathies
- iron deficiency anemia
- hemochromatosis
- osteoporosis
- glucagonoma
- vitamin deficiencies

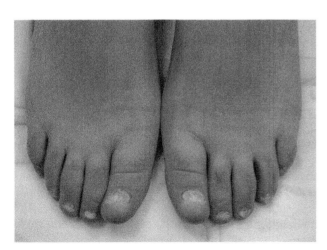

FIGURE 36-10: Trachyonychia.

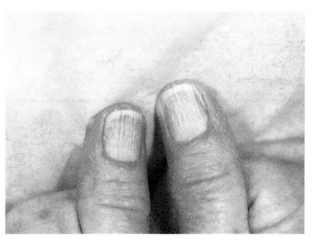

FIGURE 36-11: Brittle nails.

Treatment

Treatment of brittle nails should first address underlying dermatologic or systemic disease. Determining the moisture content of the nail plate can also dictate treatment. There appears to be an optimal humidity for nail strength, and brittle nails can be divided into cases in which the plate is hard and brittle and those in which the plate is soft and brittle. Hard and brittle nails result from dehydration that may be exacerbated by low-humidity environments. In these cases, the goal of treatment is nail plate rehydration, accomplished by the addition of daily emollients, a humidifier, and nighttime nail soaks in water followed by application of urea or lactic acid creams. After soaking, the nail plate can also be massaged with mineral oil to prevent drying. Soft and brittle nails result from excess moisture, a condition that may worsen in high humidity. Treatment in these cases should focus on minimizing exposure to moisture by the use of cotton gloves under vinyl gloves for wet work and avoidance of irritants.

Oral biotin, a B-complex vitamin, has proven effective in the treatment of brittle nails. The recommended dose is 2.5 mg/day, taken for 3 to 6 months. The average time before clinical improvement is 2 months. Silicon has also shown efficacy in improving brittle nails.

> **SAUER'S NOTES**
>
> A quick look at the nails may give you a quick insight into internal disease.

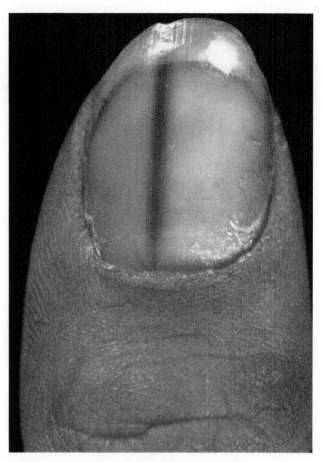

FIGURE 36-12: Longitudinal melanonychia.

LONGITUDINAL MELANONYCHIA (MELANONYCHIA STRIATA)

Longitudinal melanonychia refers to a tan, brown, or black longitudinal band or streak affecting a nail (Fig. 36-12). One or multiple nails can be involved. When multiple bands are present, the inciting cause is most likely nonneoplastic. Causes of multiple bands of longitudinal melanonychia include:

- racial variation (African American, Hispanic, Indian, Japanese)
- dermatologic disorders (Laugier–Hunziker syndrome, lichen planus, pustular psoriasis, lichen stratus, and localized bacterial and fungal infections)
- trauma (nail biting, frictional trauma from shoes, manicure)
- radiation and drugs (many chemotherapeutic agents, esp. hydroxyurea, zidovudine, psoralens, antimalarials, minocycline, ketoconazole, and more)
- endocrine abnormalities (Addison disease, Cushing syndrome after adrenalectomy, pregnancy, hyperthyroidism, and acromegaly)
- systemic diseases (Peutz–Jeghers syndrome, systemic lupus erythematous, scleroderma, HIV, hyperbilirubinemia, malnutrition, porphyria, and others).

Causes of isolated LM include:

- conditions that mimic longitudinal melanonychia (exogenous sources, subungual hematoma, onychomycosis, and bacterial infection)
- matrix melanocytic neoplasms (melanocytic activation, benign and atypical melanocytic hyperplasia, acquired and congenital melanocytic nevi, and subungual melanoma)
- nonmelanocytic nail tumors (Bowen disease, onychopapilloma, and onychomatricoma)
- overlap with causes of multiple bands (most often trauma)

Exogenous pigmentation can occur from tobacco dirt, tar, and nail lacquers. Exogenous pigment typically does not present as a longitudinal streak but follows the shape of the surrounding nail folds and can usually be scratched off the nail plate. Chronic subungual hematomas are caused by repeated, asymptomatic minor trauma usually from shoe friction. Fungal melanonychia most often results from *Scytalidium dimidiatum* and *Trichophyton rubrum var. nigricans*. Clinically, other signs of distal subungual onychomycosis are present in addition to a hyperpigmented streak usually wider distally than proximally. Nail plate infection with gram-negative bacteria such as *Klebsiella* and *Proteus spp.* can cause longitudinal melanonychia. When a greenish discoloration is present, infection with *Pseudomonas aeruginosa* is likely. Bacterial infection causing a pigmented streak usually presents at the junction of the lateral and proximal nail folds. The border of this streak is usually variable.

A variety of melanocytic lesions, including acquired and congenital melanocytic nevi, benign and atypical melanocytic hyperplasias, and melanoma, can cause longitudinal melanonychia. Nail unit melanoma should always be in the differential diagnosis of isolated longitudinal melanonychia and can only be confirmed or excluded by biopsy.

Diagnosis

The most important diagnosis to exclude in longitudinal melanonychia is subungual melanoma. When multiple bands are present, the inciting cause is most likely nonneoplastic, but biopsy is often the only definitive way to evaluate pigmented nail bands. Situations in which a biopsy is warranted to rule out subungual melanoma include LM that:

- begins in a single digit of an adult especially in the fourth-to-sixth decade
- develops abruptly in a previously normal nail plate
- develops a sudden change in shape, color, or width (>3 to 5 mm)
- has blurred, uneven borders
- occurs in an isolated nature or unique manner in dark-skinned patient
- includes pigmentation of proximal nail folds, lateral nail folds, cuticles, and/or hyponychium (i.e., Hutchinson sign)
- is accompanied by nail dystrophy
- other benign causes of isolated LM are unlikely (i.e., trauma and chronic subungual hematoma)

Dermoscopy can be used as a tool to aid in the decision to biopsy longitudinal melanonychia. Melanoma is more likely to be associated with irregular longitudinal lines varying in color, spacing, thickness, and parallelism. End-on nail plate dermoscopy can be used to determine the site of pigment origin in the matrix. Dorsal plate pigment corresponds to the proximal matrix and ventral plate pigment corresponds to the distal matrix.

When malignancy is suspected, biopsy of the site of origin in the matrix is critical for an accurate diagnosis. There are several different techniques to perform a biopsy of the nail matrix to determine the underlying cause. The method of choice depends on the width of the pigment band (<3 mm or >3 mm), band location (midline vs. lateral), and origin of pigment (proximal matrix vs. distal matrix).

To achieve nail matrix exposure for obtaining a biopsy, a partial proximal nail plate avulsion can be performed (Fig. 36-13). This is preferred to a complete nail plate avulsion because there is less risk for complications and nail dystrophy.

If the pigment band is located in the midline and <3 mm in width, a punch biopsy can be performed. If the midline band is larger/or in the distal matrix, an excisional biopsy can be

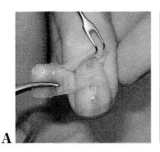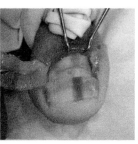

FIGURE 36-13: Partial proximal nail plate avulsion. Two examples **(A and B)** of partial proximal nail plate avulsion in setting of longitudinal melanonychia. Note broad exposure of entire matrix and proximal bed. In each case, pigmented band in nail plate points proximally to origin of pigmentation in matrix. (From Collins SC, Cordova K, Jellinek NJ. Alternatives to complete nail plate avulsion. *J Am Acad Dermatol.* 2008;59:619–626.)

performed. If a punch biopsy greater than 3 mm is performed, then the matrix should be re-approximated with a 6-0 absorbable suture. The nail matrix (proximal > distal matrix) is the site with highest risk of nail plate dystrophy/permanent scarring from procedures. Biopsies involving the proximal nail matrix can result in nail plate splitting. Thus, an elliptical biopsy in the distal nail matrix should be orientated in the horizontal/transverse direction rather than in a longitudinal fashion to minimize this risk. Additionally, the complication of dorsal pterygium can occur as a result of adherence and scar tissue formation between the ventral part of the proximal nail fold and healing proximal matrix. Suturing the nail plate between the nail matrix and ventral proximal nail fold can prevent adhesion and pterygium formation.

Shave biopsy is an alternative approach to excisional or punch biopsies. The advantage to this method is lower risk of nail dystrophy with healing by second intention but potentially offset by greater recurrence and inadequate sampling owing to lack of proper depth.

For longitudinally orientated pigmented bands, biopsy can be obtained by the technique of lateral longitudinal excisional biopsy. This removes the entire lateral nail unit en-bloc for pathologic examination but results in a narrower nail plate width with possible unique complications of nail spicules.

LM in children is evaluated on a case-by-case basis and biopsy should be performed only when appropriate. The majority of cases of childhood LM are benign even when occurring with concerning features such as a wide pigment band, Hutchinson sign, multiple colors, and history of change. Only 10 cases of childhood subungual melanoma in situ have been reported and, more importantly, no cases of invasive subungual melanoma have been reported. Thus, given the indolent clinical behavior of childhood LM, current recommendations are in favor of conservative management with clinical follow-up alone with digital photography and measurements. Biopsy can be reserved for those with very concerning clinical features given the risk of nail dystrophy. Nail unit excision should be avoided unless melanoma cannot be ruled-out after expert review.

Treatment

Treatment of longitudinal melanonychia depends on the underlying cause.

TUMORS OF THE NAIL UNIT

SAUER'S NOTES

If nail dystrophy and pigment act atypically, think biopsy. Malignant melanoma and squamous cell cancer are truly incognito in the nail unit.

Subungual Melanoma

The nail apparatus is an uncommon site for melanoma, making up between 0.7% and 3.5% of all cases. Timely diagnosis is critical, however, because the prognosis for melanoma involving the nail is significantly worse than cutaneous melanoma of the same thickness and stage. The prognosis may be worse because subungual melanoma is diagnosed later (mean Breslow depth of 4.7 mm), is felt to grow more aggressively than cutaneous melanoma, and has earlier metastasis. Patients most commonly present with subungual melanoma between the fifth and seventh decades. Amelanotic melanoma makes up a much higher percentage of melanomas affecting the nail compared to other sites, further complicating accurate diagnosis. The most important factors affecting prognosis are Breslow depth of invasion, presence of tumor mitotic rate, and presence of bone invasion.

Diagnosis

Subungual melanoma can be misdiagnosed as onychomycosis, pyogenic granuloma, subungual hematoma, benign nevus, and paronychia, causing delay in potentially lifesaving treatment. Two important signs of subungual melanoma are longitudinal melanonychia (discussed before) and Hutchinson sign (Fig. 36-14). Hutchinson sign refers to the spread of

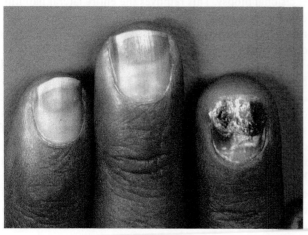

FIGURE 36-14: Subungual melanoma.

pigment from the nail bed, matrix, and nail plate onto the adjacent cuticle and proximal and/or lateral nail folds. Pseudo-Hutchinson sign refers to periungual pigmentation unrelated to melanoma that can be found in Laugier–Hunziker syndrome, as a side effect of certain medications, as a result of nail infection, as a normal variant, and with a variety of systemic diseases.

The ABCDEF acronym for clinical detection of subungual melanoma is a useful screening method:

- A stands for African Americans, Asians, and Native Americans, the races most commonly affected by subungual melanoma.
- B stands for the diagnostic sign of a brown- to black-pigmented nail band with blurred borders and a breadth of 3 mm or more.
- C stands for a recent, sudden, or rapid change in the size of the nail band or lack of change despite treatment.
- D stands for the digit most commonly affected by subungual melanoma, the thumb, followed by the hallux or index finger. A single digit affected by a pigmented band should raise the suspicion of subungual melanoma more than a situation where multiple digits are affected by pigmented bands.
- E stands for extension of pigment onto the proximal and/or lateral nail fold (Hutchinson sign).
- F stands for a family or personal history of the dysplastic nevus syndrome or previous melanoma, which would indicate an increased overall risk for subungual melanoma.

Final diagnosis of subungual melanoma requires a biopsy.

Treatment

Treatment of subungual melanoma depends on the extent of disease and the presence or absence of systemic metastases.

Wide local excision is the only treatment proven to reduce mortality. For invasive tumors, most authors advocate distal amputation, but some suggest that digit sparing may be possible for in situ lesions and thinner invasive lesions. Sentinel lymph node mapping provides information regarding prognosis but has not shown any survival benefit and lymph node dissection itself carries morbidity.

Subungual Squamous Cell Carcinoma

Subungual squamous cell carcinoma is rare. It is often associated with predisposing factors including prior radiation therapy (especially in physicians and dentists), infection with human papillomavirus, tar exposure, and trauma. The incidence of subungual squamous cell carcinoma is highest in men between 50 and 69 years of age. Most reported cases of subungual squamous cell carcinoma occur on the fingers, but cases have been described occurring on the toes as well. Usually one digit is affected, the most common site being the thumb (Fig. 36-15).

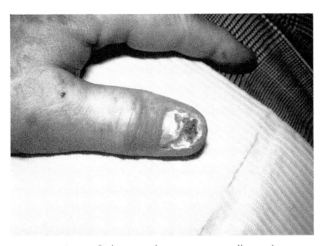

FIGURE 36-15: Subungual squamous cell carcinoma.

Diagnosis

Definitive diagnosis of subungual squamous cell carcinoma requires a biopsy. Delay in diagnosis is common as the tumor can be confused with onychomycosis, verruca vulgaris, or paronychia. Subungual squamous cell carcinoma involves the bone in 20% to 55% of cases. Squamous cell carcinoma of the nail unit is considered to have a good prognosis when compared with squamous cell carcinomas of other cutaneous sites. Lymph node and visceral metastasis are uncommon.

Treatment

Invasive tumors and in situ lesions are effectively treated with Mohs micrographic surgery. If there is bone involvement, amputation of the affected digit is recommended. Radiation therapy has been used successfully in the treatment of unresectable subungual squamous cell carcinoma.

Subungual Metastases

A comprehensive review of 133 patients diagnosed with subungual metastases shows that the three most common sites of primary malignancy are the lung (41% of cases), kidney (11% of cases), and breast (9% of cases). The appearance of these lesions takes a variety of forms, with some cases masquerading as pyogenic granuloma, acute paronychia, erysipelas, and herpes zoster. Subungual metastases are usually painful. Anatomic sites of presentation include both the hands and feet. One or multiple digits can be affected. An x-ray of the affected digit should be performed to evaluate bone involvement, which is a common complication of subungual metastases. A review of 39 patients with subungual metastases showed that in 44% of the cases the metastatic lesion was the initial presentation of an undiagnosed malignancy or appeared in the same month that the primary tumor was discovered.

Digital Myxoid Cyst

Digital myxoid cyst is also known as a digital mucoid cyst, digital mucous cyst, myxoid pseudocyst, and synovial cyst. The variety of terms for this disorder reflects the controversial origin of cyst development. It usually presents as an asymptomatic, single, soft-to-rubbery nodule on the dorsal surface of a finger, located between the proximal nail fold and distal interphalangeal joint, lateral to the midline. The material encased in the cyst has been described as viscous or gelatinous. The surface of the cyst is usually smooth, but verrucous variants have also been reported. Most cases occur in patients between the ages of 40 and 70 years. Women are more often affected than men. The most commonly affected anatomic sites are the middle and index fingers, but myxoid cysts are also sometimes found on the toes. Because of their location, cysts can exert pressure on the nail matrix, resulting in a linear nail plate dystrophy and a groove in the nail. Occasionally, these cysts can have a connection with the nearby distal interphalangeal joint.

Treatment

When surgically excised, care must be taken to remove any communicating tracts between the cyst and joint to prevent recurrence. Other treatment options include cryotherapy, carbon dioxide laser vaporization, and injection of sclerosing solutions. Treatment by aspiration of the cyst contents and injection of intralesional steroids can have high recurrence rates.

NAIL MANIFESTATIONS OF SYSTEMIC DISEASE

The nails can provide important clues in the diagnosis of systemic disease. Many morphologic changes can occur that point to an underlying renal, hepatic, pulmonary, and cardiac disease. Clubbing can suggest pulmonary infection, chronic pulmonary disease, and lung cancer. Koilonychia usually signifies underlying iron deficiency anemia. Transverse depressions in all nails are called Beau lines and indicate recent illness causing cessation of nail growth. Mees lines are transverse white bands that can be associated with arsenic poisoning, congestive heart failure (CHF), and Hodgkin disease. Muehrcke lines are pairs of white lines extending across the nail that disappear with pressure (Fig. 36-16). They are classically associated with hypoalbuminemia.

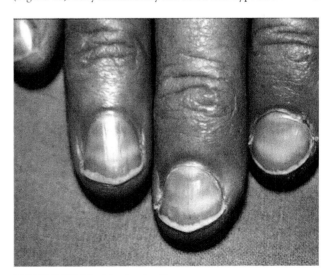

FIGURE 36-16: Muehrcke lines.

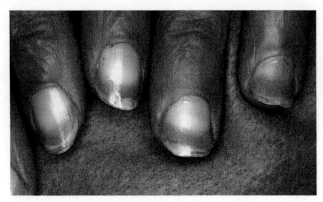

FIGURE 36-17: Half-and-half nails.

Terry nails are described as white nails with sparing of the tip of the nail plate. They are found most commonly in hepatic disease. Renal disease can be associated with nails with a half-white proximal portion and half-brown distal portion called half-and-half nails (Fig. 36-17). Yellow nail syndrome consists of thickened yellow nails with absent lunula, pleural effusions, and lymphedema. Increased nail fold capillaries are best seen by dermoscopy and are indicative of connective tissue disease like lupus erythematosus, dermatomyositis, rheumatoid arthritis, or scleroderma. Diffuse pigmentation of the nails suggests medication side effects. Changes in the color of the lunula can be seen in Wilson disease, CHF, connective tissue disease, and medication side effects.

Suggested Readings

Armstrong AW, Tuong W, Love TJ, et al. Treatments for nail psoriasis: a systematic review by the GRAPPA nail psoriasis work group. *J Rheumatol.* 2014;41(11):2306–2314.

Baran R, Dawber RPR. *Baran and Dawber's Diseases of the Nails and their Management.* 3rd ed. Malden, MA: Blackwell Science; 2001.

Baran R, Hay RJ, Tosti A, et al. A new classification of onychomycosis. *Br J Dermatol.* 1998;139:567–571.

Braun RP, Baran R, Le Gal FA, et al. Diagnosis and management of nail pigmentations. *J Am Acad Dermatol.* 2007;56:835–847.

Cohen PR, Metastatic tumors to the nail unit: subungual metastases. *Dermatol Surg.* 2001;27:280–293.

Collins SC, Cordova K, Jellinek NJ. Alternatives to complete nail plate avulsion. *J Am Acad Dermatol.* 2008;59(4):619–626.

Cooper C, Arva NC, Lee C, et al. A clinical, histopathologic, and outcome study of melanonychia striata in childhood. *J Am Acad Dermatol.* 2015;72(5):773–779.

de Berker D. Management of nail psoriasis. *Clin Exp Dermatol.* 2000;25:357–362.

Di Chiacchio N, Di Chiacchio NG. Best way to treat an ingrown toenail. *Dermatol Clin.* 2015;33(2):277–282.

Eekhof J, Van Wijk B, Knuistingh A, et al. Interventions for ingrowing toenails. *Cochrane Database Syst Rev.* 2012;4(4):1–83.

Faergemann J, Baran R. Epidemiology, clinical presentation and diagnosis of onychomycosis. *Br J Dermatol.* 2003;149(suppl 65):1–4.

Farber EM, Nall L. Nail psoriasis. *Cutis.* 1992;50:174–178.

Fawcett RS, Linford S, Stulberg DL. Nail abnormalities: clues to systemic disease. *Am Fam Physician.* 2004;69:1417–1424.

Finch JJ, Warshaw EM. Toenail onychomycosis: current and future treatment options. *Dermatol Ther.* 2007;20:31–46.

Fountain JA. Recognition of subungual hematoma as an imitator of subungual melanoma. *J Am Acad Dermatol.* 1990;23(4):773–774.

Gupta AK. Types of onychomycosis. *Cutis.* 2001;68(suppl 2):4–7.

Haneke E, Baran R. Longitudinal melanonychia. *Dermatol Surg.* 2001;27:580–584.

Hay R. Literature review. Onychomycosis. *J Eur Acad Dermatol Venereol.* 2005;19(suppl 1):1–7.

Hordinsky MK, Sawaya ME, Scher RK. *Atlas of Hair and Nails.* 1st ed. Philadelphia: Churchill Livingstone; 2000.

Jellinek NJ. Primary malignant tumors of the nail unit. *Adv Dermatol.* 2005;21:33–64.

Jellinek N. Nail matrix biopsy of longitudinal melanonychia: diagnostic algorithm including the matrix shave biopsy. *J Am Acad Dermatol.* 2007;56:803–810.

Jiaravuthisan MM, Sasseville D, Vender RB, et al. Psoriasis of the nail: anatomy, pathology, clinical presentation, and a review of the literature on therapy. *J Am Acad Dermatol.* 2007;57(1):1–27.

Peterson SR, Layton EG, Joseph AK. Squamous cell carcinoma of the nail unit with evidence of bony involvement: a multidisciplinary approach to resection and reconstruction. *Dermatol Surg.* 2004;30:218–221.

Piraccini BM, Dika E, Fanti PA. Tips for diagnosis and treatment of nail pigmentation with practical algorithm. *Dermatol Clin.* 2015;33(2):185–195.

Rich P. Nail biopsy: indications and methods. *Dermatologic Surg.* 2001;27(3):229–234.

Rich P, Scher RK. *An Atlas of Disease of the Nail.* 1st ed. New York: Parthenon Publishing Group; 2003.

Rigopoulos D, Larios G, Gregoriou S, et al. Acute and chronic paronychia. *Am Fam Physician.* 2008;77:339–346.

Rounding C, Bloomfield S. Surgical treatments for ingrowing toenails. *Cochrane Database Syst Rev.* 2005;2:CD001541.

Scher RK, Daniel CR III. *Nails: Therapy, Diagnosis, Surgery.* 3rd ed. Philadelphia: WB Saunders; 2005.

Scher RK, Tavakkol A, Sigurgeirsson B, et al. Onychomycosis: diagnosis and definition of cure. *J Am Acad Dermatol.* 2007;56:939–944.

Seaberg DC, Angelos WJ, Paris PM. Treatment of subungual hematomas with nail trephination: a prospective study. *Am J Emerg Med.* 1991;9(3):209–210.

Sonnex TS. Digital myxoid cysts: a review. *Cutis.* 1986;37:89–94.

Thai KE, Young R, Sinclair RD. Nail apparatus melanoma. *Australas J Dermatol.* 2001;42:71–81; quiz 2–3.

Usman A, Silvers DN, Scher RK. Longitudinal melanonychia in children. *J Am Acad Dermatol.* 2001;44:547–548.

Uyttendaele H, Geyer A, Scher RK. Brittle nails: pathogenesis and treatment. *J Drugs Dermatol.* 2003;2:48–49.

Diseases of the Mucous Membranes

John C. Hall, MD

The mucous membranes of the body adjoin the skin at the oral cavity, nose, conjunctiva, penis, vulva, and anus. Histologically, these membranes differ from the skin in that the horny layer and the hair follicles are absent. Disorders of the mucous membranes are usually associated with existing skin diseases or internal diseases. Only the most common diseases of the mucous membranes are discussed herein. At the end of the chapter is a listing of the uncommon conditions of these areas.

GEOGRAPHIC TONGUE

Geographic tongue is an extremely common condition of the tongue that usually occurs without symptoms. When these lesions are noticed for the first time by the individual, they may initiate fears of cancer.

Presentation and Characteristics

Clinical Appearance

Irregularly shaped (map-like or geographic) pale red patches are seen on the tongue (Fig. 37-1). Close examination reveals that the filiform papillae are flatter or denuded in these areas. The patches slowly migrate over the tongue surface and heal without scarring.

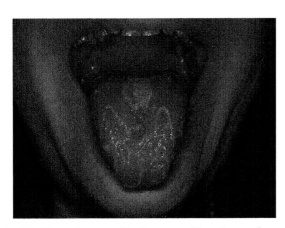

FIGURE 37-1: Geographic tongue. (Courtesy of Neutrogena Corp.)

Course

The disorder may come and go but may be constantly present in some persons.

Cause

The cause is unknown, but the lesions seem to be more extensive during a systemic illness. It has been suggested by some authors that geographic tongue is a form of psoriasis.

Subjective Symptoms

Some patients complain of burning and tenderness, especially when eating sour or salty foods.

Differential Diagnosis

- *Syphilis,* secondary mucous membrane lesions: similar clinically, but acute in onset; usually more inflammatory; other cutaneous signs of syphilis; dark field examination and serology positive (see Chapters 25 and 29); does not come and go as rapidly.

Treatment

1. Reassure patient that these are not cancerous lesions.
2. There is no effective or necessary therapy. However, if patient complains of burning and tenderness, prescribe triamcinolone (Kenalog) in Orabase 15.0
   Sig: Apply locally q.i.d. half hour p.c. and h.s.

GINGIVAL ENLARGEMENT

Excessive growth of periodontal tissue with raising and blunting of the gingival margins.

Presentation and Characteristics

Clinical Appearance

If inflammation is present, the gingiva appears shiny, red, smooth, soft, and friable, with easy bleeding. If noninflammatory, it is firm with loss of stippling and contains a reddish-purple hue.

Course

Improvement is common if the underlying cause is treated.

Cause

Systemic diseases include primary amyloidosis, sarcoidosis, acromegaly, Kaposi sarcoma, Wegener granulomatosis, leukemia, aplastic anemia, lymphomas, Crohn disease, scurvy, and neurofibromatosis.

Drug causes include phenytoin, calcium channel blockers, and cyclosporine. Less common drugs include lithium, tacrolimus, sertraline, birth control pills, ketoconazole, erythromycin, and other antiseizure medicines in addition to phenytoin. Poor dental hygiene with chronic gingivitis may be causative. It can be congenital, idiopathic, or physiologic in pregnancy or puberty.

Symptoms

Pain, tenderness, halitosis, poor speech, difficult mastication, and unsightly appearance are all reasons to initiate therapy.

Treatment

Therapy is focused on the treatment of the underlying cause as well as aggressive oral hygiene. Surgical reduction is the last approach to be considered.

APHTHOUS STOMATITIS

Canker sores are extremely common, painful, superficial ulcerations of the mucous membranes of the mouth (Fig. 37-2).

Presentation and Characteristics

Course

One or more lesions develop at the same time and heal without scarring in 5 to 10 days. They can recur at irregular intervals. It is the most common oral inflammatory disease (affects 20% of population). It usually begins in adolescence and peaks in incidence in the third-to-fourth decade, after which the disease becomes less severe and less frequent.

Clinical Appearance

Lesions are usually located on nonkeratinized mucosa (buccal, labial sulci, lateral and ventral tongue, soft palate, oropharynx).

There are three subtypes: (1) minor lesions (80%) are less than 5 mm to 1 cm, especially buccal and labial, and heal spontaneously in 7 to 10 days without a scar, (2) major (10%) are 5 to 10 mm deep, heal in weeks to months and often scar; other names are Sutton ulcers or periadenitis mucosa necrotica recurrens, and (3) herpetiform (10%) occur on dorsal tongue, palate, or other keratinized mucosa, are small (1 to 3 mm) and grouped on coalescent ulcers, and heal in 1 to 4 weeks.

Cause

The cause is unknown, but certain foods, especially chocolate, nuts, and fruits, can precipitate the lesions or may even

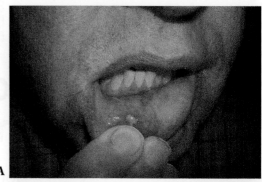

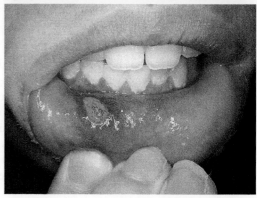

FIGURE 37-2: A: Atrophic ulcer of lower lip covered with a white pseudomembrane. Patient had accidently bitten his lip illustrating pathergy of an aphthous ulcer. **B:** Aphthous ulcer in a patient with cyclic neutropenia. (Courtesy of Neutrogena Corp.)

be causative. Trauma from biting or dental procedures can initiate lesions (pathergy). Some cases in women recur in relation to menstruation. A viral cause has not been proved. A pleomorphic, transitional L-form of an α-hemolytic *Streptococcus* sp (*Streptococcus sanguis*) has also been implicated as causative. Stress, nutritional deficiency, smoking cessation, and allergy may be triggers. Numerous underlying illnesses include Behçet disease, human immunodeficiency virus (HIV), inflammatory bowel disease, cyclic neutropenia, FAPA (fever, aphthous stomatitis, pharyngitis, adenitis), and MAGIC (mouth and genital ulcers with inflamed cartilage and gluten-sensitive enteropathy). The disease can also be a sign of deficiencies of iron, zinc, folate, and B vitamins 1, 2, 6, and 12.

Differential Diagnosis

- *Syphilis,* secondary lesions: clinically similar; less painful; other signs of syphilis; dark field examination and serology positive (see Chapters 25 and 29)
- *Herpes simplex virus:* usually a single lesion of grouped vesicles that erode. The first episode can be much more severe and widespread. Recurrence is usually at or near the original site and seldom intraoral. Can culture virus or see viral effect on biopsy (see Chapter 26)

Treatment

Most persons who get these lesions learn that very little can be done for them and that the ulcers heal in a few days.

1. Toothpaste swish therapy: Brush the teeth and swish the toothpaste around in the mouth after each meal and at bedtime. If done soon after the onset of ulcers, extension of the lesions can be prevented and early healing can be helpful in many cases.
2. Triamcinolone in Orabase (prescription needed) applied locally after meals relieves some of the pain.
3. Tetracycline therapy: An oral suspension in a dosage of 250 mg per teaspoonful (or the powdery contents of a 250-mg capsule in a teaspoon of water) kept in the mouth for 2 minutes and then swallowed, four times a day, is beneficial. This mixture can be applied with a piece of cotton soaked in this solution.
4. Systemic corticosteroids may occasionally be used for severe ulcers.
5. A few reports in the literature have suggested limited benefit from the helicobacter elimination antibiotic regimen.

SAUER'S NOTES

1. I wish to emphasize the value of the toothpaste swish therapy for aphthous stomatitis. It is especially valuable if begun soon after lesions appear.
2. The toothpaste swish also aids healing of self-inflicted tongue-bite sores.

BEHÇET DISEASE

Behçet disease is a triad of ulcers of oral and genital mucous membranes and uveitis. The "silk route disease" is so named because of its increased prevalence in the Middle East, Asia, and the Mediterranean (especially Turkey).

Presentation and Characteristics

O'Duffy Criteria for Behçet Disease

Aphthous stomatitis
Genital ulcers
Uveitis
Cutaneous pustular vasculitis
Synovitis
Meningoencephalitis
At least three criteria, one being recurrent aphthous ulcers.
Incomplete form
At least two criteria, one being recurrent aphthous ulcers.
Must exclude inflammatory bowel disease, systemic lupus erythematosus, Reiter disease, and herpes simplex virus infection.

International 1990 Study Group for Diagnosis of Behçet Syndrome: Oral aphthae at least three times a year, plus two of the following:

Recurrent genital ulcers
Uveitis or retinal vasculitis
Papulopustular vasculitis or erythema nodosum
Pathergy—oblique insertion of 20-gauge needle showing perivascular neutrophils
Leukocytoclastic vasculitis at 24 to 48 hours

Course

Behçet disease can affect people of all ages, with no symptoms for weeks, months, or years and cycles of disease lasting days, weeks, or months. Oral aphthae can be the only sign of the disease for years (6 to 7 years on average). Blindness can occur in the 50% to 90% of Behçet patients with eye disease. The disease affects the gastrointestinal tract (ulcers throughout the gastrointestinal tract), the neurologic system (vasculitis), the cardiopulmonary system (vasculitis), and the renal system. The oral and genital ulcers can be very debilitating.

Cause

The cause is unknown, but it is hypothesized that exogenous trigger factors induce vasculitis in genetically predisposed individuals. Infectious triggers that may play a role are herpes simplex virus or streptococci. There may be an immunologic or cytokine imbalance.

Treatment

1. Topical and systemic corticosteroids are the mainstay of therapy
2. Nonsteroidal anti-inflammatory drugs, colchicines, and dapsone
3. Immunosuppressives and cytotoxic agents
4. Other therapies tried include tacrolimus, thalidomide, interferon-γ, etanercept, and infliximab

HERPES SIMPLEX

Herpes simplex virus infection can occur as a group of umbilicated vesicles on the mucous membranes of the lips, the conjunctiva, the penis, and the labia. Frequently recurring episodes of this disease can be quite disabling (see Chapter 26). Recurrent intraoral herpes simplex is uncommon, but the primary outbreak can have extensive intraoral mucous membrane involvement.

FORDYCE DISEASE

This is a physiologic variant of oral sebaceous glands in which more than the normal number exists. When they are suddenly noticed, the person becomes concerned as to the diagnosis. The lesions are asymptomatic and yellowish orange, and there are 1- to 2-mm papules on the lips and labia minora. No treatment is necessary; they are benign.

OTHER MUCOSAL LESIONS AND CONDITIONS

Mucosal lesions can also be caused by the following:

- *Physical causes:* Sucking of lips, pressure sores, burns, actinic or sunlight cheilitis, factitial disorders, tobacco, and other chemicals. Contact dermatitis almost never occurs owing to constant bathing of the mucous membranes with saliva.

- *Infectious diseases* (from viruses, bacteria, spirochetes, fungi, and animal parasites): Gangrenous bacterial infections are called *noma. Ludwig angina* is an acute cellulitis of the floor of the mouth caused by bacteria, abscesses, and sinuses and may be owing to dental infection. *Trench mouth,* or *Plaut–Vincent disease,* is an acute ulcerative infection of the mucous membranes caused by a combination of a spirochete and a fusiform bacillus.

- *Systemic diseases:* These include lesions seen with hematologic diseases (e.g., leukemia, agranulocytosis from drugs or other causes, thrombocytopenia, pernicious anemia, cyclic or periodic neutropenia), immunocompromised conditions (such as the acquired immunodeficiency syndrome, organ transplants, lymphomas), collagen diseases (such as lupus erythematosus, scleroderma), pigmentary diseases (e.g., Addison disease, Peutz–Jeghers syndrome), and autoimmune diseases, which cross over in several categories but include pemphigus and benign mucosal pemphigoid.

- *Drugs:* Phenytoin sodium causes a hyperplastic gingivitis; bismuth orally and intramuscularly causes a bluish-black line at the edge of the dental gum (see Fig. 8-12B); certain drugs cause hemorrhage and secondary infection of the mucous membranes.

- *Metabolic diseases:* Mucosal lesions are seen in primary systemic amyloidosis, lipoidosis, reticuloendothelioses, diabetes, and other disorders.

- *Tumors, local or systemic:* These include leukoplakia, squamous cell carcinoma, epulis, and cysts.

RARER CONDITIONS OF ORAL MUCOUS MEMBRANES

- *Halitosis:* Halitosis, or fetor oris, is a disagreeable odor of the breath.

- *Periadenitis mucosa necrotica recurrens* (Fig. 37-3): Also known as Sutton disease, this is a painful, recurrent, ulcerating disease of the mucous membranes of the oral cavity. The single or multiple deep ulcers exceed 10 mm and heal with scarring. Systemic corticosteroids may be indicated. It is considered by some to be a very severe type of aphthous ulcer.

- *Hand–foot–mouth disease:* This is a common vesicular eruption of the hands, feet, and mouth. Usually

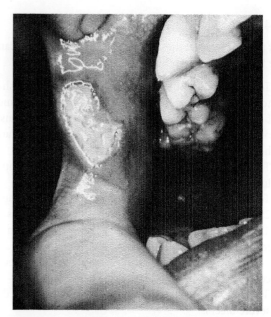

FIGURE 37-3: Periadenitis mucosa necrotica recurrens.

affecting children, it lasts up to 2 weeks. Most cases are caused by Coxsackievirus A16 or Enterovirus 71. A more severe form has been associated with Coxsackie A6 virus with fever, joint pains, and widespread painful eruptions sometimes requiring hospitalization.

- *Koplik spots:* Bright red, pinpoint-sized lesions on the mucous membranes of the cheek are seen in patients before the appearance of the rash of measles.

- *Erythema multiforme* (Fig. 37-4): This causes "bull's eye" lesions on the skin and erosions of the mucous membranes that may be severe. The commonest causes are herpes simplex and drug allergies.

- *Burning tongue* (glossodynia): This rather common complaint, particularly among middle-aged women, is usually accompanied by no visible pathology. The cause is unknown, and therapy is of little value, but the many diseases and local factors that cause painful tongue must be ruled out from a diagnostic viewpoint. The entire mouth can also burn. Tricyclic antidepressants have been used with some success.

- *Black tongue* (hairy tongue, lingua nigra); (Fig. 37-5): Overgrowth of the papillae of the tongue, apparently caused by an imbalance of bacterial flora, is owing to the use of antibiotics and other agents. Black tongue without papillae hypertrophy can be seen with tobacco abuse, crack cocaine smoking, lansoprazole, chewing bismuth, methyldopa, minocycline, and hydroxychloroquine.

- *Hairy leukoplakia of the tongue:* This is a slightly raised, poorly demarcated lesion with a corrugated or "hairy" surface that appears on the sides of the tongue. It is seen mainly in immunosuppressed homosexual men infected with HIV. Human papillomavirus and

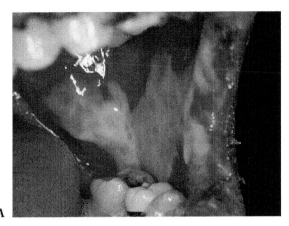
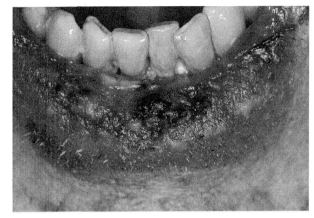

A   **B**

FIGURE 37-4: Erythema multiforme of the left buccal mucosa **(A)** and on the lower lip **(B)**.

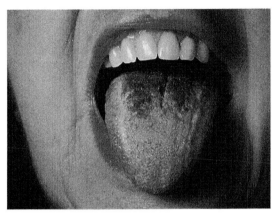

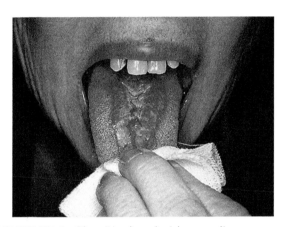

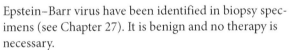

FIGURE 37-5: Black tongue. (Courtesy of Neutrogena Corp.)

FIGURE 37-6: Glossitis rhomboidea mediana. (Courtesy of Neutrogena Corp.)

Epstein–Barr virus have been identified in biopsy specimens (see Chapter 27). It is benign and no therapy is necessary.

- *Moeller glossitis:* This painful, persistent, red eruption on the sides and the tip of the tongue persists for weeks or months, subsides, and then recurs. The cause is unknown.

- *Furrowed tongue* (grooved tongue, scrotal tongue): The tongue is usually larger than normal, containing deep longitudinal and lateral grooves of congenital origin owing to syphilis or as part of Melkersson–Rosenthal syndrome (see Dictionary–Index).

- *Glossitis rhomboidea mediana* (median rhomboid glossitis) (Fig. 37-6): This rare disorder, characterized by a smooth reddish lesion, usually occurs in the center of the tongue. This term is poor because there is no inflammation and the reddish plaque may not always be in the center.

- *Sjögren syndrome:* This rare entity is characterized by dryness of all of the mucous membranes and of the skin in middle-aged women. *Keratoconjunctivitis sicca* is used to describe the severe dryness of the eyes seen in this syndrome. The primary form of this syndrome is in many cases associated with a cutaneous

vasculitis. The secondary type of Sjögren syndrome is associated with rheumatic and collagen diseases. Evoxac is an oral medication that may help with the dry mouth. Sucking on hard lemon candy and artificial saliva can be tried.

- *Cheilitis glandularis:* This chronic disorder of the lips is manifested by swelling and secondary inflammation caused by hypertrophy of the mucous glands and their ducts. There is up to a 35% risk of deterioration to squamous cell carcinoma. Surgical intervention has usually been the mainstay of therapy. Topical calcineurin inhibitors such as tacrolimus (Protopic) have been used with some success.

RARER CONDITIONS OF GENITAL MUCOUS MEMBRANES

- *Fusospirochetal balanitis:* This uncommon infection of the penis is characterized by superficial erosions. It must be differentiated from syphilis by a dark field examination and blood serology.

- *Balanitis xerotica obliterans* (see *Atrophies of the Skin* in the Dictionary–Index): This whitish atrophic lesion on the penis is to be differentiated from leukoplakia. The female counterpart is lichen sclerosus et atrophicus.

- *Lichen sclerosus et atrophicus:* This is a rare atrophy of the skin, usually of the genital and perirectal mucous membranes. In children (Fig. 37-7), it is the most common chronic genital dermatitis. The prognosis is better in younger patients. In older patients, there is a slight increase in the incidence of squamous cell cancer (approximately 5%). (See *Atrophies of the Skin* in the Dictionary–Index.)

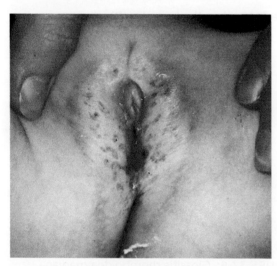

FIGURE 37-7: Peripheral erythema and central atrophic white plaque that has scattered over the surface.

LIPSCHÜTZ ULCER

Nonsexually related acute genital ulcers: Formerly called ulcus vulvae acutum, they are considered a variant of complex aphthosis, and are often preceded by an acute systemic illness or fever. They are in the vulvae and are seen most in otherwise healthy adolescent patients. They are very painful and appear as well-demarcated shallow erosions with a clean fibrinous base and sometimes with ensuing necrosis. They may be recurrent, multiple, and be accompanied by oral involvement.

Suggested Readings

Axell T. The oral mucosa as a mirror of general health or disease. *Scand J Dent Res.* 1992;100:9–16.

Chi CC, Baldo M, Lewis F, et al. Systematic review and meta-analysis of randomized controlled trials on topical interventions for genital lichen sclerosus. *J Am Acad Dermatol.* 2012;67(2):305–312.

Daley TD. Common acanthotic and keratotic lesions of the oral mucosa: a review. *J Can Dent Assoc.* 1990;56:407–409.

Eisen D. The clinical features, malignant potential, and systemic associations of oral lichen planus: a study of 723 patients. *J Am Acad Dermatol.* 2002;46(2):207–214. D, Lynch DP. *The Mouth: Diagnosis and Treatment.* St. Louis: Mosby; 1998.

Eisen D, Lynch DP. *The Mouth: Diagnosis and Treatment.* St. Louis: Mosby; 1998.

Eversole LR. Immunopathology of oral mucosal ulcerative, desquamative and bullous disease: selected review of the literature. *Oral Surg Oral Med Oral Pathol.* 1994;77:555–571.

Kavala M, Topaloglu Demir F, Zindanci I, et al. Genital involvement in pemphigus vulgaris(PV): correlation with clinical and cervicovaginal Pap smear findings. *J Am Acad Dermatol.* 2015;73(4):655–659.

Novick NL. Diseases of the mucous membrane. *Clin Dermatol.* 1987;5:123–136.

Sami N. Approach to the patient with autoimmune mucocutaneous blistering disease. *Dermatol Ther.* 2011;24:173–186.

van der Waal I. *Diseases of the Salivary Glands: Including Dry Mouth and Sjögren's Syndrome Diagnosis and Treatment.* New York: Springer; 1997.

Skin Diseases in Ethnic Skin

Cheryl M. Burgess, MD, and Beverly A. Johnson, MD

LEARNING OBJECTIVES/GOALS

- Recognize diversity among skin types.
- Describe the changing demographics among ethnic populations in the United States.
- Recognize the market growth of ethnic consumers of dermatologic services.
- Recognize differences between white skin and ethnic skin.
- Identify skin types using established classification systems.
- Assess therapeutic considerations and identify potential for adverse effects in ethnic skin.
- Select treatment plans with respect to the potential for tissue response in ethnic skin.
- Identify the most common cosmetic concerns in ethnic skin.

CHAPTER OVERVIEW

Doctors must take adequate steps for maintaining the necessary knowledge and instruction to provide all patients with thorough and comprehensive services. Therefore, additional knowledge and training must be considered to deliver the greatest efficacy with the lowest risk of adverse events when using state-of-the-art products and procedures in ethnic skin. This is especially true in light of daily advances in dermatologic services and growing diversity of skin types in the ethnic patient population. Clinicians must be fully prepared to recognize common problems in ethnic skin, identify appropriate treatments, and take steps to limit risk for any adverse events within this patient population.

TERMINOLOGY

Throughout the burgeoning research on ethnic skin, it has been difficult to provide consistent terminology in the medical literature that conveys appropriate categorization and accurate description of skin types. To address this challenge, the following conventions are used throughout this chapter: The term "white skin" refers to skin having a Fitzpatrick classification of I, II, or III. The term "Caucasian" is avoided because this term refers to a larger group of skin types, beyond people with white skin. The term "ethnic skin" refers to skin that has a Fitzpatrick classification of IV, V, and VI, which applies to skin types in people of Black, Latino, and Asian ethnic groups. The term "Blacks" is used in place of "African Americans" because the latter term refers to only a subgroup of a much larger category of people with pigmented skin. These conventions have been selected to provide consistency, accuracy, and clarity in the following discussion. These conventions should not be substituted for careful clinical descriptions.

INTRODUCTION AND BACKGROUND

Demographic Trends and the Growth of Dermatologic Services in Ethnic Consumers

Diversity of Skin Types

The buzz phrase, "Skin of Color," has often been thought to refer primarily to black skin. However, in the United States, individuals with pigmented skin come from a variety of racial and ethnic groups. These groups are summarized in Table 38-1. The diversity of ethnic and racial groups yields a broad spectrum of pigmented skin types that is continuously changing. For example, the 1990 US Census Bureau listed 6 races with 23 racial subtypes. Only 10 years later, the same 6 race categories included at least 67 subtypes. The largest ethnic populations—Black, Hispanic, and Asian—are expected to make up almost half of the total US population by the year 2050; the predictions are 25% Hispanic, 14% Black, 8% Asian, and 1% other. Trends in the growth of diversity must drive the practice of dermatology to new levels of knowledge and awareness, so that clinicians are prepared to meet the challenges of today's patient populations and provide the highest level of care to the largest possible number of patients.

Categorizing Pigmented Skin Types

Fitzpatrick Skin Phototype Classification System

In the United States, individuals with pigmented skin come from a large collection of racial and ethnic groups. The diversity of racial and ethnic groups yields a broad spectrum of pigmented skin types that defy easy categorization. Throughout the years, the fields of dermatology and cosmetics have

---

TABLE 38-1 • Racial and Ethnic Groups in the United States

- African-American Black persons (including Caribbean-American Black persons)
- Asian and Pacific Islanders (including those of Filipino, Chinese, Japanese, Korean, Vietnamese, Thai, Malaysian, Laotian, Hmong)
- Latino or Hispanic (including those of Mexican, Cuban, Puerto Rican, Central American, Spanish descent)
- People traditionally categorized as Caucasoid (including a majority of Indians, Pakistanis, and those of Middle Eastern origin)
- Native Americans
- Alaskans
- Aleuts

---

struggled to characterize pigmented skin types adequately. After its development in the 1970s, the Fitzpatrick Skin Phototype classification became a surrogate classification system for this purpose.

The Fitzpatrick Skin Phototype classification system was originally developed to categorize the skin's response to UV radiation. Over time, doctors became accustomed to using the system to classify both UV sensitivity and skin color. However, the system has limited utility for accurately communicating patient information for either research or clinical purposes and is of almost no value for helping clinicians treat ethnic skin effectively and safely. Patients with ethnic skin would benefit more from a classification system based on the propensity of the skin to scar and/or become hyperpigmented—a unique characteristic of pigmented skin. Several classification systems have been developed or proposed to meet these obvious needs. However, none have risen to an industry standard.

Roberts Skin Type Classification System

The recently introduced Roberts Skin Type classification system may provide the most comprehensive information to meet the needs of clinicians. This system uses a four-part serial profile to characterize the skin's likely response to insult, injury, and inflammation through a quantitative and qualitative assessment that includes a review of ancestral and clinical history, visual examination, test site reactions, and physical examination of the patient's skin. Skin is categorized using a numeric descriptor that provides information on the phototype, hyperpigmentation, photoaging, and scarring characteristics. The Roberts classification system can provide a means to help facilitate study designs and communicate data in the medical literature.

Distinguishing Characteristics of Black Skin

Structure and Function

There are several distinguishing characteristics of black skin (Table 38-2). For example, in the skin of Blacks, the stratum corneum layer counts are significantly higher and more compact, with thicker collagen bundles present in the dermis. The most evident difference between ethnic skin and white skin is epidermal melanin content. While no differences exist in the number of melanocytes, variations do exist in the number, size, packaging, and distribution of melanosomes. In the skin of Blacks, melanosomes are larger and more dispersed. Moreover, the epidermal melanin unit in ethnic skin contains more melanin overall and may undergo slower degradation. These differences in melanin and melanosomes provide superior UV protection in ethnic skin. In fact, the minimal erythema dose in black skin is 30-fold greater than that of white skin. In addition, black skin has increased apocrine and sebaceous glands that are associated with increased follicular responses. Transdermal water loss is also increased in the skin of Blacks.

> **SAUER'S NOTES**
>
> Inflammatory skin conditions (such as atopic dermatitis) are more apt to be papular in black skin.

Because of these differences in skin structure and function, ethnic people suffer less photodamage than Whites do. In fact, one study of adults living in Tucson, Arizona, found that the epidermis of Black participants was largely spared the gross photodamage observed in White participants. Most of the

---

TABLE 38-2 • Characteristics of Darker Complexions

- Black skin has larger, more dispersed melanosomes
- The minimal erythema dose of black skin is 30-fold greater than that of white skin
- The skin becomes darker in response to injury
- Thicker, more compact stratum corneum
- Thicker collagen bundles in the dermis
- Blacks have increased apocrine and sebaceous glands associated with increased follicular responses
- Increased transepidermal water loss

Source: Stephens TJ, Oresajo C. Ethnic sensitive skin: a review. *Cosmet Toiletries.* 1994;109:75–80; Draelos ZD. Is all skin alike? *Cosmet Dermatol.* 2002;15(9):81–83.

TABLE 38-3 • Most Common Dermatologic Concerns in Ethnic Skin

- Pseudofolliculitis barbae and acne keloidalis nuchae
- Acne vulgaris and acne rosacea
- Seborrheic dermatitis
- Scarring alopecia
- Scalp folliculitis

White women, aged 45 to 50 years, had wrinkles in the area of the lateral epicanthus (this is also known as crow's feet) and on the corners of the mouth, while none of the Black women of comparable age had obvious crow's feet wrinkles or perioral rhytides. The skin of Blacks was also felt firmer, and the histology of the dermal elastic fibers in black skin was similar to the appearance of these fibers in sun-protected white skin.

COMMON DERMATOLOGIC CONCERNS IN ETHNIC SKIN

Pseudofolliculitis Barbae and Acne Keloidalis Nuchae

These chronic inflammatory disorders are among the most common dermatologic concerns in ethnic skin (Table 38-3). It is observed primarily in individuals with tightly curled hair, and found most commonly in Black men, followed by Hispanic men. It is also found in women of all races due to shaving in the bikini region where natural folds of the crural area in friction from underwear promote epidermal reentry of even straight hair (Fig. 38-1).

All treatments should target elimination or reduction of the foreign body reaction surrounding an ingrown hair. Cessation of shaving is the first choice of treatment but is typically insufficient to break the cycle of ingrown hairs because many men must have a clean-shaven face, and discontinuation of shaving can continue to cause problems in approximately 10% to 20% of affected individuals. Shaving with single-blade razors can result in the extrafollicular reentry of the hair follicle. New or multiple blade systems can lead to transfollicular penetration. Plucking hairs can also lead to transfollicular penetration. An inflammatory response associated with these processes can lead to papules and pustules, which has the propensity to leave hyperpigmented macules and keloids.

Treatment

To minimize pseudofolliculitis barbae, it is necessary to discontinue close shaves. This can be achieved by the use of a correct shaving tool with proper training of the patient. Single-bladed razors or The Bump Fighter Razor is an effective shaving tool for this purpose. Treatment can also be accomplished with fairly good success by the AM/PM alternation of a topical steroid and a topical retinoid. Treatment may also consist of depilatories, adjunctive topicals, electrolysis, chemical peels, and laser hair removal therapy. Ingrown hair follicles may be prevented by the use of retinoids, glycolic acid or salicylic acid preparations, topical anti-inflammatory agents, or the use of a soft toothbrush to lift the hair follicles above the skin.

Seborrheic Dermatitis

Seborrheic dermatitis occurs in all types of skin and is commonly found in areas of the scalp and along the hairline; in and behind the ears; along the side of the nostrils, eyebrows,

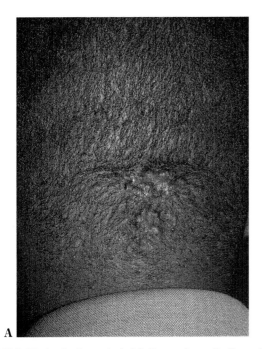
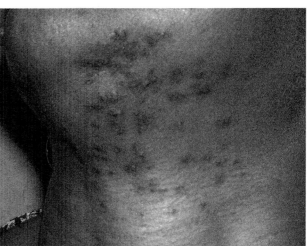

A   **B**

FIGURE 38-1: **A:** Acne keloidalis nuchae. **B:** Pseudofolliculitis barbae.

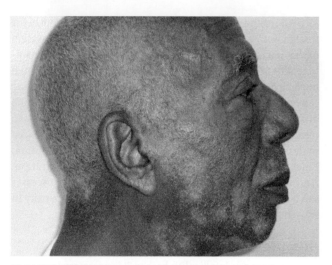

FIGURE 38-2: Seborrheic dermatitis.

or T-zone of the face; midchest; and in the beard and mustache of men. Contrary to what the references have said regarding black skin, applying pomades and oils and lotions to these areas only exacerbates the condition. Seborrheic dermatitis may cause hypo- or hyperpigmented changes in skin color in affected areas of black skin (Fig. 38-2).

Treatment

Treatment for seborrheic dermatitis includes topical medications and dandruff shampoos containing selenium sulfide, coal tar, sulfur, salicylic acid, pyrithione, zinc, ketoconazole, and mild steroids. When dandruff shampoos are recommended, patients must routinely shampoo their scalp for a minimum of 5 minutes once or twice a week.

SAUER'S NOTES

All tightly curled hair must be oiled in Black patients to prevent breakage. To keep this oil from causing seborrhea, which is a condition of oily skin, 5% to 10% sulfur can be added to any oil used. A product with less smell is to add 3% to 5% salicylic acid or 1% hydrocortisone to the hair oil of choice. A midstrength corticosteroid such as triamcinolone ointment can be mixed with equal parts of a hair oil as another option.

Frequent shampooing can lead to dry brittle hair and subsequent breakage; therefore, dandruff shampoos are not commonly used or recommended. Topical preparations with active ingredients containing ketoconazole or corticosteroids can be used as an alternative to the daily use of dandruff shampoos. Topical preparations are applied directly to the scalp several times a week until the condition is brought under control. The use of topical preparations limits the need to shampoo the scalp on a daily basis. With proper treatment, skin discoloration typically returns to normal.

Scarring Alopecia

General Information

Scarring alopecia is a condition that commonly occurs in Black women and some Hispanic women and is typically the result of some unique biologic attribute. For men and women of all ages, hair loss can be devastating and can cause serious psychologic and financial consequences. The spectrum of hair loss is broad. Causes of hair loss vary from controllable to uncontrollable circumstances such as genetic predisposition to disease for unknown reasons. In addition, it is important to acknowledge and accommodate cultural differences that can serve as a barrier to the patient's acceptance of a recommended treatment protocol. Accurate diagnosis requires taking a comprehensive history of the patient, including influences from social and economic influences. For example, take into consideration weekly or twice-monthly hair shampooing, the use of braids or twists, as well as home remedies. Black patients may also have a presumed preference for oily vehicles and medications to treat dermatitis of the scalp (Fig. 38-3).

Common causes of alopecia may be due to (1) scarring alopecia (traction alopecia, discoid lupus erythematosus [DLE], chronic tinea capitis, central centrifugal cicatricial alopecia [CCCA]); (2) nonscarring alopecia (alopecia areata, tinea capitis); or (3) grooming alopecia.

Traction Alopecia

Traction alopecia is a common cause of hair loss due to pulling forces exerted on the scalp hair. This excessive tension leads to breakage in the outermost hairs. The two types of traction alopecia are marginal and nonmarginal. Traction alopecia is unintentionally induced by various hairstyling practices (use of braids, hair rollers, weaves, twists, locks, or cornrows). When tensile forces are chronically present, an irritant type of folliculitis develops. Follicular scarring and permanent alopecia may result. Hair loss is reversible in the initial stages, but with prolonged traction, alopecia can be permanent. Therefore, the key is early prevention (Figs. 38-4 and 38-5).

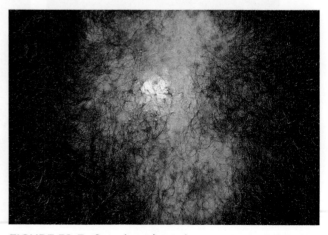

FIGURE 38-3: Scarring alopecia.

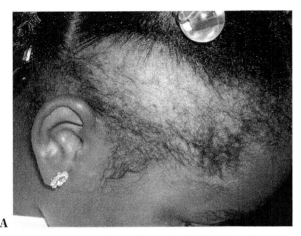
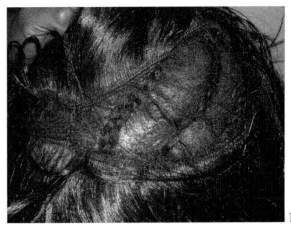

A   **B**

FIGURE 38-4: **A:** Traction alopecia. **B:** Hair tracks.

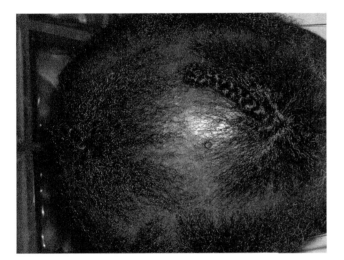

FIGURE 38-5: Traction alopecia due to braids.

Discoid Lupus Erythematosus

DLE is a chronic skin disease that produces atrophic lesions of sores with inflammation and scarring on the face, ears, and scalp, and to a lesser degree, on other areas of the body. When lesions occur in hairy areas such as the beard or scalp, permanent scarring and hair loss can occur. The exact cause of DLE is unknown, but the condition is thought to be an autoimmune disease. This condition tends to run in families and occurs about three times more often in females. In some patients with DLE, sunlight and cigarette smoking may trigger the lesions (Fig. 38-6).

Treatment: Treating DLE lesions with topical corticosteroids often reduces the severity of the involved areas and slows their progression. A cortisone injection into the lesions is typically more effective than the topical form of cortisone. Alternatively, calcineurin inhibitors such as pimecrolimus cream or tacrolimus ointment may be used. Additionally, imiquimod has been identified as a successful treatment. Patients whose condition is sensitive to sunlight should use a UVA/UVB blocking sunscreen daily and wear a hat while outdoors. Follow-up with the doctor is important and necessary every 6 to 12 months to check for internal organ involvement and to minimize scarring.

Grooming Alopecia

Hair breakage can occur in natural hairstyles because of friction that develops from dry hair grooming through narrow combs or brushes. Hair breakage can also be caused by chronic use of chemical treatments. Hair processing solutions that contain sodium hydroxide (lye) or potassium hydroxide (non-lye) contribute to hair breakage by breaking disulfide bonds. Non-lye hair relaxers were developed for safe use at home by novices. However, contrary to popular belief, lye- and non-lye relaxers are equally damaging to hair. Therefore, most doctors and hair stylists prefer the use of lye relaxers. This is because the shorter processing time reduces the chemical contact exposure to the hair, which limits the degree of breakage.

Ammonium thioglycolate, ammonium sulfate, and ammonium bisulfate are known as perm salts that weaken the internal structures of the bonds, but stop short of breaking up disulfide bonds. Although these solutions are milder, they remove natural oils and moisture. Furthermore, after using ammonium thioglycolate, a mild alkaline solution is necessary to fix the perm.

Other products and practices that can contribute to hair breakage include hot comb and pomade use combined with blow-drying, the use of hot iron curling, hair rollers, hair dyes, and the use of various hairstyles, such as ponytails, extensions, and microbraids.

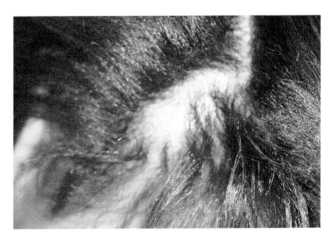

FIGURE 38-6: Scarring alopecia from discoid lupus erythematosus.

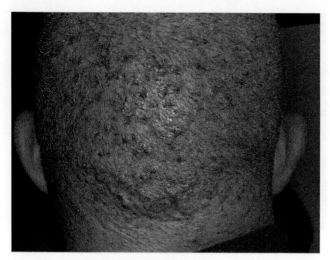

FIGURE 38-7: Scalp folliculitis.

Scalp Folliculitis

Individuals with scalp folliculitis often develop uncomfortable and embarrassing symptoms such as intense itching, tenderness, persistent bumps, sores, pus discharge, and even bleeding of the scalp. In some cases, these symptoms subside and the scalp returns to its normal condition. However, these symptoms often progress, leading to the loss of individual hair follicles, with permanent hair loss and scarring in later stages. Early intervention is crucial to successful treatment and can lead to the slowing or reversal of hair loss in many individuals (Figs. 38-7 and 38-8).

The etiology of scalp folliculitis is unclear. However, clinical observations suggest that variants of scalp folliculitis develop most often in Black men and women. It is believed that the condition refers to folliculitis occurs more often in women than in men, although the apparent prevalence of this condition in women may only be a reflection of women's tendency to seek medical attention more often than men, in the case of hair loss. Doctors have speculated that the condition is associated with hair care products and grooming practices used by Blacks. Pressing of the hair, pomades, chemical relaxers, permanent wave agents, braiding, and other physically aggressive combing techniques are examples of possible causes suggested by this theory. However, doctors remain puzzled about the specific role of hair care products and grooming practices. For example, women and men with no prior use of these products or hair grooming practices develop scalp folliculitis. Other causes have also been proposed. For example, a family trait or genetic cause has been suggested by some experts, and a weakened immune system or hormonal change has also been suggested. Like many other skin conditions, a single cause may not be responsible for developing the condition; it may be multifactorial.

Throughout the years, doctors have explored a variety of treatments for scalp folliculitis with little or no success. Treatments have included the use of such medications as antibiotics, steroids, and oral retinoids. The prognosis (outcome) based on these treatments is not good. Either the condition persists through the treatment, or the condition briefly dissipates, only to stubbornly resurface shortly after halting the treatment. **Treatment:** It had been reported in the literature that a combination of rifampicin 300 mg and cephalexin 500 mg given twice daily for 2 weeks led to nearly 100% improvement of symptoms in a majority of patients. Moreover, hair regrowth occurred in almost half of the patients treated. However, if the patient has experienced a long-standing, chronic condition, treatment may be less successful, because permanent damage to the hair follicle prevents regrowth of hair in the affected areas.

Central Centrifugal Cicatricial Alopecia

CCCA can be divided into two categories: primary and secondary. Primary cicatricial alopecias are caused by an intrinsic process that specifically targets the hair follicle, leading to its destruction and replacement by fibrous tissue. Primary cicatricial alopecias are further classified as lymphocytic or neutrophilic according to the type of predominant inflammatory infiltrate. CCCA is a lymphocytic primary cicatricial alopecia.

CCCA begins with a patch of hair loss on the vertex of the scalp that expands centrifugally over the course of months to years. Affected areas of the scalp have a shiny appearance

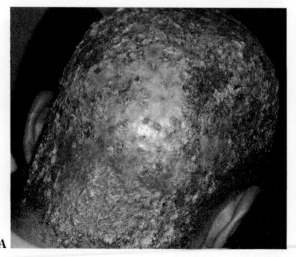

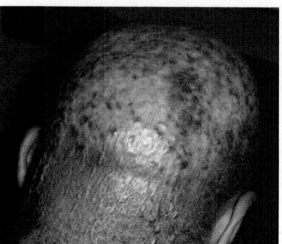

FIGURE 38-8: **A:** Dissecting cellulitis and folliculitis. **B:** After oral antibiotic treatment.

and can develop into large affected areas in late stages, while tenderness, pruritus, burning, and a "pins and needles" sensation are common associated symptoms. Histopathologically, CCCA is characterized by perifollicular lymphocytic inflammation and premature desquamation of the inner root sheath. Lamellar fibroplasia and follicular fibrosis are also seen. Biopsies taken of end-stage lesional scalp reveal diffuse scarring with a marked reduction or absence of hair follicles. Although the prevalence has not been studied, CCCA is one of the leading causes of hair loss in Black women.

The cause of CCCA is poorly understood. Although thermal and chemical straightening of the hair has been implicated, conclusive evidence for this association is lacking. In particular, the term CCCA encompasses the previously described entity, hot comb alopecia, which refers to a scarring alopecia that is associated with the long-term use of heat and oil ("hot combing") to straighten the hair. However, CCCA has also been rarely reported in men who do not straighten the hair. Therefore, the etiology of CCCA is likely a combination of genetic and environmental factors.

COMMON DERMATOLOGIC DISEASES IN ETHNIC SKIN

Pityriasis Alba

Pityriasis Alba is a variation of atopic eczema that occurs in ethnic children. The round, light patches are covered with fine scale, but are otherwise asymptomatic. The condition can occur on any part of the body, but is usually first noticed on the face and upper arms, and can also involve the trunk. It is more noticeable in the summer months when the normal skin darkens and the affected skin looks paler by contrast. The loss of color is temporary and is not related to vitiligo. Treatment with topical immunomodulators is preferable to topical corticosteroids (which can further depigment the skin). Patients should be educated on sun protection and reassurance that the condition will not evolve into vitiligo. If the disease is widespread, topical PUVA is effective (Fig. 38-9).

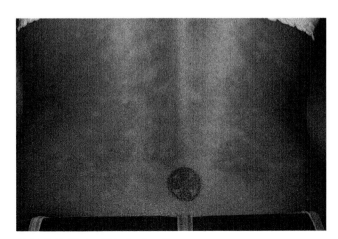

FIGURE 38-9: Pityriasis alba.

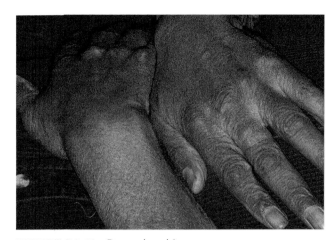

FIGURE 38-10: Dry ashy skin.

Dry or "Ashy" Skin

When dry or "ashy" skin develops in individuals with darker skin tones, the skin takes on a noticeable grayish or ashen hue that is easily observed. When dry skin occurs on the scalp, the ashiness may be mistaken for seborrhea. Treatment should include the use of moisturizers and avoidance of long hot baths or showers, or bath gels containing alcohol. To improve the condition of the scalp, patients should avoid the use of some of the antiseborrheic shampoos that can increase the dryness of the scalp and exacerbate the situation. Patients with dry ashy skin suffer more during cold weather seasons when dry air causes dry skin to worsen. Treatment can include humidifiers, and moisturizers applied immediately after showering while the skin is still damp. Moisturizing twice daily may be necessary for extremely dry skin (Fig. 38-10).

Acne Vulgaris and Acne Rosacea

The morphology of acne lesions is the same in pigmented and white skin. However, there are several differences in the occurrence of acne between Black and White individuals. Acne in Blacks is often due to cultural preferences. For example, products such as pomades are typically applied to the hair for controlling hair and treating dryness, but can also cause comedonal acne on the forehead, hairline, and temples. The most significant difference in the acne of Blacks is dramatic inflammation and subsequent development of postinflammatory hyperpigmentation (Fig. 38-11).

Treatment

When treating ethnic patients, it is important to recognize that many topical products are poorly tolerated by Black and Hispanic patients, especially women. In addition, clinicians should be careful to avoid hyperpigmentation or hypopigmentation that can be caused by the acne treatment, such as benzoyl peroxide, azelaic acid, and retinoids. The use of test spots with dermabrasion and chemical peeling treatments is strongly recommended before attempting dermal grafting, punch grafting, and punch elevation.

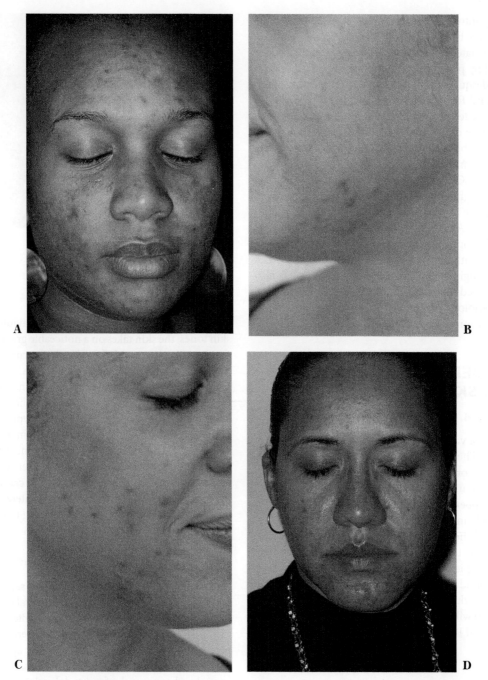

FIGURE 38-11: A–C: Acne. **D:** Rosacea.

Occasionally, doctors will want to use acne treatments that hypopigment the skin when dark macules are present. In such cases, it is important to blend the complexion. In addition, reports have suggested that among Blacks, the incidence of "sensitive skin" and rosacea is more common than previously thought. Blacks have reported skin sensitivities as high as 50% in undocumented observations. Even though the prevalence of sensitivity might not be as high as reported by ethnic patients, doctors should have an increased awareness of potential irritation from acne products.

<table>
<tr><td>

TABLE 38-4 • Unusual Variants of Diseases in Ethnic Skin

- Inverse pityriasis rosea
- Pitted keratolysis
- Hypopigmented cutaneous T-cell lymphoma
- Ichthyosiform sarcoidosis

</td></tr>
</table>

Unusual Variants of Disease in Ethnic Skin

With few exceptions, skin disease incidence is the same in all people, regardless of skin color. However, doctors should be aware of certain diseases with a higher incidence in ethnic skin (Table 38-4). For black skin, these diseases include inverse pityriasis rosea, hypopigmented cutaneous T-cell lymphoma (CTCL), pitted keratolysis, and ichthyosiform sarcoidosis.

Inverse Pityriasis Rosea

Inverse pityriasis rosea is a papulosquamous eruption that occurs on ethnic skin. More frequently, the eruption is mostly papular with prominent scales and occurs in distal regions such as on the legs, feet, arms, wrists, and neck, sparing the trunk. Prolonged dyspigmentation can cause suffering in ethnic patients with this disease (Fig. 38-12).

Hypopigmented Cutaneous T-cell Lymphoma

Hypopigmented CTCL has a high prevalence in Black patients. In a retrospective study at Howard University Hospital, 12.1% of skin cancers in Black patients were due to CTCL. The disease is aggressive in Black patients, and late-stage disease at the time of diagnosis contributes to a poor prognosis. These patients have a history of generalized eczematoid or psoriasiform dermatitis,

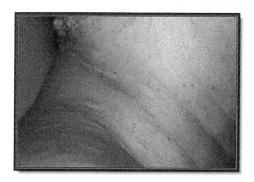

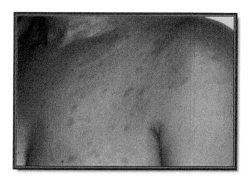

FIGURE 38-12: Inverse pityriasis rosea.

which does not respond to routine therapy for those conditions. The hypopigmented variant can also be mistaken for pityriasis alba or postinflammatory hypopigmentation. Skin biopsy should include immunophenotyping studies for definitive diagnosis. Repeated histologic evaluation is usually necessary when patients with "eczema" are not improving with therapy. The hypopigmented form is more common in ethnic patients and is often seen in adolescents and children with CTCL (Fig. 38-13).

Ichthyosiform Sarcoidosis

Black patients with cutaneous sarcoidosis are the only patients who seem to express ichthyosiform sarcoidosis. The skin lesions are clinically identical to those found in acquired ichthyosis or ichthyosis vulgaris and must be biopsied to determine the correct diagnosis. Noncaseating granulomas are observed even when the skin lesions precede the systemic disease. The skin findings are usually on the distal extremities and may precede the development of systemic disease.

COMMON COSMETIC CONCERNS IN ETHNIC SKIN

Keloid/Hypertrophic Scars

Growth of Cosmetic Products and Procedures in Ethnic Populations

Growing diversity of skin types and shifting trends in US demographics are driving the increased growth of the ethnic patient population. However, products and procedures that target the ethnic market are also bringing more ethnic patients into the clinic. According to recent surveys, 11.7 million cosmetic procedures were performed in 2007, an overall increase of 8% in surgical procedures. As the total number of cosmetic procedures continues to increase, doctors can expect greater numbers of healthcare consumers from specialized ethnic populations. For example, of the total 11.7 million cosmetic procedures performed in 2007, 2.48 million (22%) procedures were performed in ethnic groups. Hispanics accounted for 9%; Blacks accounted for 6%; Asians, 5%; and other non-Caucasians, 2%. This represents an increase of more than 65% in ethnic groups since 2004. Therefore, it is especially important for the doctor or primary care physician to incorporate safe and effective, ethnic-specific treatment procedures.

Keloids in Ethnic Populations

Keloids are among the most common cosmetic concerns in ethnic skin (Table 38-5). These scars are benign, sometimes painful and/or pruritic, proliferative growths of dermal collagen that typically occur in ethnic skin because of excessive tissue response to trauma. These growths typically occur 3 to 18 times more often in ethnic skin than in white skin. Patients with a Fitzgerald Phototype of IV–VI are at greater risk for keloid formation and keloid recurrence after treatment. A higher incidence occurs in younger females due to ear piercing. Keloids have also developed from tattoos. People aged 65 years or older seldom experience keloids; however, the incidence is increasing as more individuals experience

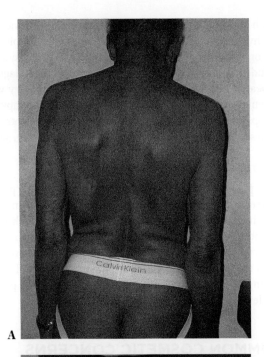

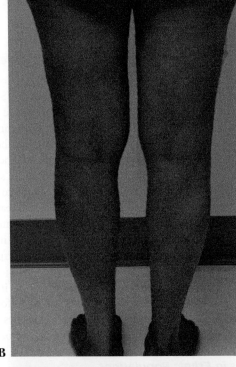

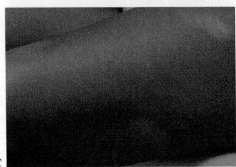

TABLE 38-5 • Common Cosmetic Concerns in Ethnic Skin

- Dyschromia (postinflammatory hyperpigmentation/hypopigmentation, melasma, vitiligo)
- Scarring (hypertrophic scars, keloid scars) (surgical vs. nonsurgical) and discoloration
- Dermatosis papulosa nigra
- Seborrheic keratosis and acrochordons
- Striae distensae
- Accentuated facial lines of expression (especially glabellar frown lines)
- Lipoatrophy (deep nasolabial folds, skin laxity, and cheek festooning)

coronary artery bypass surgery and midchest operations. Treatment success is variable and the first rule of keloid therapy is prevention. Success rates are low and the rate of recurrence is high—for example, 50% to 80% of lesions recur after excision therapy. Patients should be aware of familial keloid history, especially in Blacks. Therapy is more complex for large, nonpedunculated earlobe keloids, or keloids with wide bases (Figs. 38-14 to 38-17).

Treatment: For many years, injection with triamcinolone acetonide (10 to 40 mg/mL) was the standard of care for treating keloids. Patients should be told in advance that injected areas might become hypopigmented for 6 to 12 months. Pain can be minimized by using topical anesthetic preparations prior to injection. With the exception of treating midsternal keloids, the current gold standard of treatment is primary excision followed by adjuvant therapy. Excision can be followed up

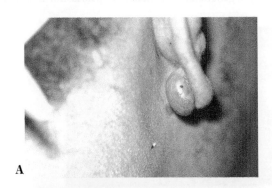

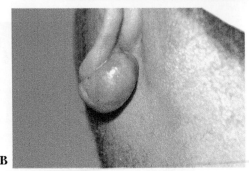

FIGURE 38-13: **A–C:** Hypopigmented cutaneous T-cell lymphoma.

FIGURE 38-14: **A:** Keloid that was not excised. **B:** Keloid after surgical intervention.

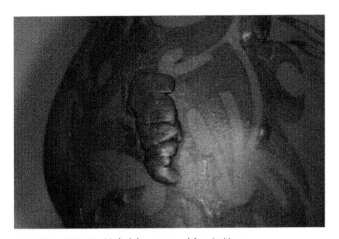

FIGURE 38-15: Keloids caused by tattoos.

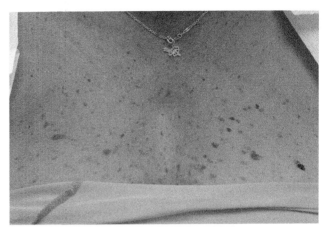

FIGURE 38-17: Seborrheic keratosis.

with corticosteroid injection, radiation therapy, and pressure gradient garments. Other primary therapies include lasers and silicone gel-sheeting.

Dermatosis Papulosa Nigra

Dermatosis papulosa nigra (DPN) presents as small (1 to 3 mm in diameter), discrete, rounded, brownish-black skin growths on the face, and develops most often, on a person's cheeks, neck, upper chest, and back. Lesions begin to appear in the mid-20s as flesh-colored to black papules and/or plaques on the face, neck, and upper torso. The condition is chronic, with new lesions continually developing as the person ages. The exact reason for the growth of these lesions remains unknown. However, researchers are confident that the appearance of DPNs has a hereditary tendency, which leads to DPNs observed on the skin of family members and relatives. DPN occurs more often in females, and overall, affects one in three Blacks. Although most doctors believe that these growths are unique to black skin, some doctors think these same growths occur on the skin of Asians.

Treatment

Treatment of Dermatosis Papulosa Nigra/Seborrheic Keratoses/Acrochordons: Some patients choose to treat DPNs

for cosmetic reasons or as a medical necessity. For example, medical reasons for removing these lesions might include chronic irritations about the neck, caused by chains or collars rubbing on the lesions, or interference with the line of vision, caused by lesions that occur on the eyelids (Fig. 38-18). More commonly, however, these lesions are removed for cosmetic reasons, as the DPNs are histologically and biologically benign. Effective cosmetic therapy is available to treat DPN/seborrheic keratoses/acrochordons. Treatment of these "skin tags" can effectively reduce the appearance of age by 10 years. Low-voltage electrodesiccation is an effective treatment for more common smaller, flat macules. Electrodesiccation causes very little pain, since the procedure is normally done under local anesthesia using a topical anesthetic cream. In about a week's time, the individual lesions begin to drop off the skin, leaving a normal skin appearance. Advise the patient not to pick the treated areas. Pedunculated lesions respond well to scissor excision of papules; use local anesthesia to alleviate pain. If a person has hundreds of DPNs, several treatment sessions may be required to completely remove all of the lesions. Although cryosurgery is commonly used to destroy DPNs/seborrheic keratoses, the method has a high incidence of causing hyperpigmentation and hypopigmentation, and therefore, should be considered the last treatment option. Cryosurgery requires significant caution; risks should be minimized by using only short bursts

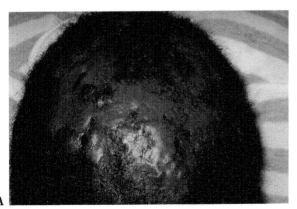

A

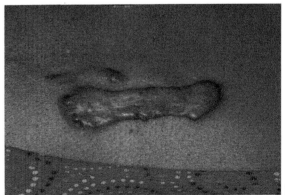

B

FIGURE 38-16: **A and B:** Spontaneous keloids.

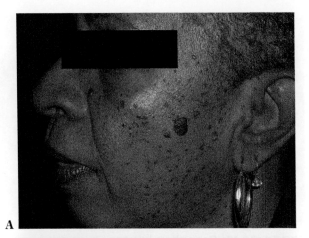

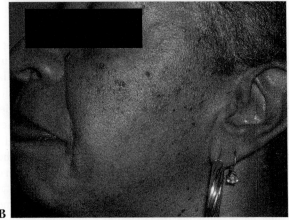

FIGURE 38-18: Dermatosis papulosa nigra. **A:** Before treatment. **B:** After electrodesiccation treatment.

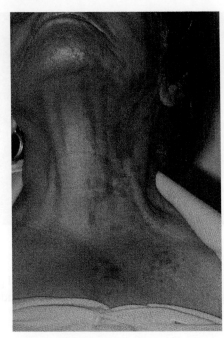

FIGURE 38-19: Postinflammatory hyperpigmentation.

of nitrogen since the risk for discoloration increases with the length of freezing. Trichloroacetic acid (50%) can be used for large seborrheic keratotic plaques.

Dyschromia

Oftentimes, Black patients will indicate that they want to be treated for a scar. However, in many cases, the purported scars are in fact postinflammatory hyperpigmentation (Fig. 38-19).

It is important to discuss the significant differences between true scarring and postinflammatory hyperpigmentation since there are differences in the specific therapies and relative difficulty between treating true scarring and postinflammatory hyperpigmentation. In addition, problems involving misdiagnosis may occur with pityriasis alba, tinea versicolor, seborrheic dermatitis, and trichrome vitiligo (Figs. 38-20 to 38-22).

Pigmentary disorders are especially prevalent and distressing for Blacks, Latinos, Asians, and Middle Easterners. Postinflammatory hyperpigmentation is caused by various inflammatory skin disorders, such as eczema, allergic contact or irritant contact dermatitis, acne, or other causes. In fact, ethnic patients are commonly more distressed by the resulting dark areas than the initial culprit–the acute acne lesion. Dermal incontinence of pigment also occurs in melasma and hereditary dyschromias. Postinflammatory hypopigmentation

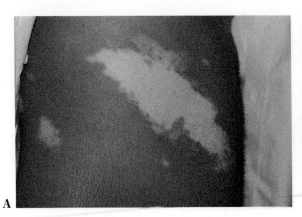

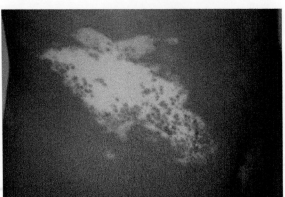

FIGURE 38-20: A: Vitiligo. **B:** Stimulation of pigment with psoralen + UVA light treatment.

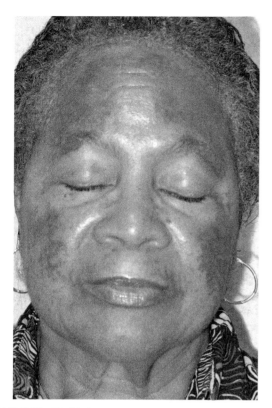

FIGURE 38-21: Melasma.

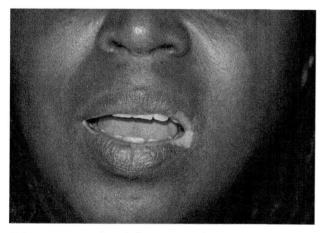

FIGURE 38-22: Postinflammatory hypopigmentation caused by laser hair removal device.

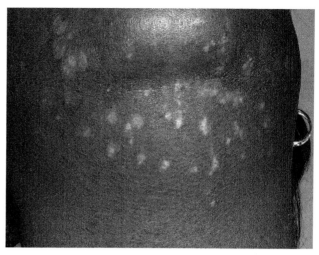

FIGURE 38-23: Hypopigmentation.

Treatment

Hyperpigmentation can be evaluated to provide a general idea of the prognosis and length of treatment. The evaluation can consist of both qualitative diagnosis and quantitative analysis (Table 38-6). A positive Wood lamp examination reveals superficial (epidermal) incontinence of pigment, whereas a negative Wood lamp examination reveals a deep (dermal) incontinence of pigment. Although not commonly used, quantitative analysis can be performed with a colorimeter.

Although disorders of hyperpigmentation may be difficult to treat, several therapeutic agents have been used over the years and others are in development (see Table 38-6). Epidermal incontinence of pigment can be seen in postinflammatory hyperpigmentation. Product ingredients of lightening agents containing hydroquinone 4% to 6%, mequinol, kojic acid, azelaic acid, licorice (glabridin), citric acid, retinol, soy, arbutin,

can develop from laser hair removal (Figs. 38-22 and 38-23). Unprotected sun exposure is also a significant source of additional skin discoloration because it prolongs melanin production in active melanocytes in various inflammatory conditions. Sun protection is typically required during procedures to blend skin discoloration. Chemical (organic) sun protection includes Parsol 1789 (avobenzone), ecamsule (Mexoryl), oxybenzone, and octinoxate. These are preferred because physical (inorganic) sun protection such as titanium dioxide, zinc oxide, and mineral makeup can leave a chalky or ashy residue on brown skin. Other options for sun protection include clothing, hats, and umbrellas.

TABLE 38-6 • Some Drugs That Can Cause Alopecia

Qualitative Diagnosis

- +Wood lamp examination
  Superficial (epidermal) incontinence of pigment
- −Wood lamp examination
  Deep (dermal) incontinence of pigment

Quantitative Analysis
Colorimeter
- Delta L, a and b
- L (98.4) white-black
- a (0.2) red-green
- b (1.2) yellow-blue

Source: Wolff K, Goldsmith LA, Katz SI, et al. *Fitzpatrick's Dermatology in General Medicine.* 7th ed. New York: McGraw-Hill Publishing; 2008; Shriver MD, Parra EJ. Comparison of narrow-band reflectance spectroscopy and tristimulus colorimetry for measurements of skin and hair color in persons of different biological ancestry. *Am J Phys Anthropol.* 2000;112(1):17-27.

N-acetylglucosamine, nicotinamide, and mulberry are used once to twice daily.

Topical agents are generally classified as phenolic or non-phenolic compounds. The goal of these therapeutic agents is to inhibit key regulatory steps of hyperactive melanocytes by regulating (1) melanin synthesis via transcription inhibition of tyrosinase or TRP-1, (2) the uptake and distribution of melanosomes in keratinocytes, and (3) melanosome degradation and cell turnover. Hydroquinone has been the standard for many years but has occasionally been mired in controversy pertaining to safety. Lightening agents are also used for pretreatment of areas that will undergo cosmetic procedures. The agents are typically applied in advance as a cautionary measure to minimize any hyperpigmentation that may result from procedures.

Hydroquinone: The most commonly used ingredient in bleaching preparations to treat hyperpigmentation is hydroquinone. The concentration of hydroquinone can range from 2% (over-the-counter) to 4% to 8% prescription formulations. Currently, the Food and Drug Administration (FDA) is monitoring the use of hydroquinone products in the United States since they have been outlawed in several countries in Africa and Asia. The FDA is concerned about ochronosis or persistent darkening of the skin with chronic use of hydroquinone-containing products, in addition to the potential of hydroquinone to cause cancer in lab mice. Although the concern is noteworthy, the countries where hydroquinone has been outlawed have routinely overused large quantities of hydroquinone-containing products to lighten the entire body. Those who use the ingredient in excess are at risk for systemic absorption. There is little concern among doctors in the United States partly due to the standard use of smaller quantities or application to dark spots only and because it is not being routinely used to lighten the entire body. Therefore, in the United States, there is not significant systemic absorption from topical hydroquinone bleaching, and if systemic levels are detected, it is primarily from natural sources of hydroquinone as seen with consumption of coffee, tea, red wine, wheat germ, pears, and berries and/or exposure to cigarette and wood smoke. The American Academy of Dermatology reports no incidences of cancers associated with hydroquinone in the United States and supports the need for further clinical science information on the safety of hydroquinone.

SUMMARY

Although differences in the structure of ethnic skin can be beneficial, some of these differences can have the opposite effect. For example, the photoprotection afforded by differences in melanosome and melanin characteristics also causes frequent hyperpigmentation in ethnic skin and may be responsible for divergent responses observed in burn injuries. Indeed, individuals with darker skin experience more frequent post-inflammatory hyperpigmentation compared to patients with lighter complexions. Moreover, surveys found that uneven skin tone was a chief complaint in more than one-third of Black women, while pigment disorders were rated the third most commonly treated dermatoses. In a survey of 100 ethnic women, complaints about dark spots reached 86%, while 49% of women complained of sensitive or very sensitive skin.

SAUER'S NOTES

Members of ethnic groups will soon comprise a majority of the international and domestic population. As the importance of ethnic markets continues to increase, doctors and cosmetic surgeons will require more expertise in the treatment of ethnic skin. Ethnic consumers are increasingly seeking out products and procedures to provide dermatologic and cosmetic solutions in these patients. However, when treating ethnic patients, issues specific to ethnic skin such as skin sensitivity, hyperpigmentation, and keloid scarring require special consideration by clinicians. As with patients of all skin colors, a comprehensive approach to assessment and treatment is absolutely necessary. With proper training and technique, clinicians can provide successful outcomes with little risk of adverse events to patients with pigmented skin.

Suggested Readings

Callender VD, McMichael AJ, Cohen GF. Medical and surgical therapies for alopecias in black women. *Dermatol Ther.* 2004;17(2):164–176.

Kelly AP. Pseudofolliculitis barbae and acne keloidalis nuchae. *Dermatol Clin.* 2003;21(4):645–653.

Kelly AP. Medical and surgical therapies for keloids. *Dermatol Ther.* 2004;17(2):212–218.

Olsen EA, Bergfeld WF, Cotsarelis G, et al. Summary of North American Hair Research Society (NAHRS)-sponsored Workshop on Cicatricial Alopecia, Duke University Medical Center, February 10 and 11, 2001. *J Am Acad Dermatol.* 2003;48(1):103–110.

Olsen EA, Callender V, Sperling L, et al. Central scalp alopecia photographic scale in African American women. *Dermatol Ther.* 2008;21(4):264–267.

Ross EK, Tan E, Shapiro J. Update on primary cicatricial alopecias. *J Am Acad Dermatol.* 2005;53(1):1–37; quiz 38–40.

Sperling LC. Scarring alopecia and the dermatopathologist. *J Cutan Pathol.* 2001;28(7):333–342.

Tan E, Martinka M, Ball N, et al. Primary cicatricial alopecias: clinicopathology of 112 cases. *J Am Acad Dermatol.* 2004;50(1):25–32.

Taylor SC, Burgess CM, Callender VD, et al. Postinflammatory hyperpigmentation: evolving combination treatment strategies. *Cutis.* 2006;78(2 suppl 2):6–19.

39

Military Dermatology

Tracy V. Love, MD and Jon H. Meyerle, MD

Military dermatology is overall very similar to civilian dermatology. As in civilian practice, its primary mission includes delivery of health care to its beneficiary population, research, and graduate medical education. However, owing to the nature of military operations, there are several unique aspects of military dermatology. The military medical organization and dermatologic disease and nonbattle injury will be reviewed, followed by a discussion of several military-relevant dermatologic topics. These include telemedicine, scar management, and amputations.

ORGANIZATION OF MILITARY MEDICINE

Delivery of military medicine is organized into levels of care to facilitate the triage, treatment, and evacuation of service members. At the lowest level, it begins with self-care at the point of injury; at the highest level, it ends in the military's largest medical centers in the continental United States. Each service branch differs slightly in this organization, so for simplicity of instruction, Army doctrine will be used as the example.

There are five levels of care in the Army. Levels are defined by their capabilities and personnel, and each level can provide and expand upon the care delivered by lower levels.

Level 1 is characterized by immediate first aid delivered by one's self, "battle buddy," or combat medic. A physician or physician assistant also provides care at the level 1 treatment facility, which is known as a battalion aid station (BAS). The purpose of the BAS is to quickly triage, treat, and stabilize patients for evacuation. It is usually not a fixed building or structure, and it does not have facilities for surgery or prolonged observation of patients.

Level 2 provides additional services in primary care, optometry, and mental and dental health. It is further supported by basic laboratory and plain radiograph services. Limited inpatient beds are available, but the facility is completely mobile, similar to level 1. Unless augmented by a Forward Surgical Team (FST), level 2 does not have surgical capabilities. If an FST is attached, 20-person teams can perform resuscitative surgeries and basic general, orthopedic, and neurosurgical procedures.

Level 3 provides the highest level of care available within combat zones. It is also known as a Combat Support Hospital (CSH) and has expanded surgical services, including urologic and oral maxillofacial surgery, and multiple intensive care wards.

The CSH is designed to be modular and can be customized to the needs of a commander.

Level 4 consists of a Field or General Hospital outside of the combat zone but near or within the theater of operations. This hospital can provide definitive medical and surgical care and is where patients requiring more intensive rehabilitation or convalescence are evacuated. These types of hospitals were located in Europe during the Iraq and Afghanistan wars.

Level 5 is the highest level of care and is most closely recognizable to civilian hospitals. These facilities are located within the continental United States and ultimately retain the most medical, surgical, and rehabilitative capabilities within the military medical system. On a case-by-case basis, predetermined civilian hospitals can provide additional facilities.

DERMATOLOGIC DISEASE AND NONBATTLE INJURY

Medical diagnoses that are not attributable to combat wounds are classified as disease and nonbattle injuries. Their distinction is important not only for data collection and disease surveillance, but also because they are responsible for the majority of clinical encounters in the deployed setting and can contribute to significant combat ineffectiveness. Dermatology complaints account for many of these visits (Table 39-1).

TABLE 39-1 • Dermatologic Disease and Nonbattle Injury in the Deployed Setting

Cold injury
Heat injury
Photodermatitis
Immersion foot syndromes
Cutaneous reactions to nuclear, biologic, and chemical warfare
Contact dermatitis
Cutaneous trauma
Arthropod infestations
Arthropod and other animal bites
Rickettsial disease
Parasitic infections
Bacterial skin disease
Atypical mycobacterial infections
Fungal infections
Sexually transmitted diseases

Approximate numbers obtained during World War II estimate that skin disorders were responsible for 15% to 25% of outpatient visits in temperate climates and 60% to 75% of visits in tropical climates. By the end of the war, from late 1944 into early 1945, dermatologic disease even became a more frequent cause for evacuation than battlefield injury.

This data trend continued into the Vietnam War. During the entire conflict, skin conditions were the number one reason for all outpatient visits and the third highest cause for hospital admission. Within a 1-year period (1968 to 1969), skin disease was responsible for 47% of all man-days lost within the Ninth Infantry Division. For some infantry battalions within this division, this number increased to more than 80%.

TELEMEDICINE

Telemedicine is the delivery of health care to a geographically separate location through the use of technology and communication systems. It can be used by health care providers of varying expertise including physicians and health care extenders such as physician assistants, nurses, and medical technicians. These providers collect clinical information at the point of care, then upload it to a server, and transmit the information to a consulting provider (Fig. 39-1).

This technology is beneficial given the environments in which the military operates. The US military executes combat operations, training exercises, and humanitarian missions worldwide. Frequently, these locations are austere with minimal health care resources. Military telemedicine allows access to specialized health care in these remote locations.

Patients often receive more expedited care through telemedicine than they would if they were seen by a military or civilian dermatologist in the continental United States. Between 2004 and 2012, the U.S. Army Medical Department's telemedicine program recorded more than 4,000 dermatology teleconsultations. Of these, the average reply time was 5 hours and 14 minutes, with 98% of all consultations answered within 24 hours.

Telemedicine also assists with disposition and identification of patients requiring evacuation. During the aforementioned time frame, 46 evacuations were avoided, while 41 cases were recommended for evacuation. Diagnoses warranting evacuation included suspicion for melanoma, guttate psoriasis, mastocytosis, and methicillin-resistant *Staphylococcus aureus* (MRSA) infection.

Forestalling unnecessary evacuations frees up medical and logistic resources for more critical patients. In addition to the inherent risks associated with the civilian emergency response system, military evacuations face added challenges. These challenges include hostile enemy fire, hazardous environmental conditions, logistic coordination with aircraft, extra personnel for ground security, and the need to hold and stabilize patients during transport. Moreover, evacuation of a service-member from the battlefield entails the broader impact of possibly requiring troop replacements.

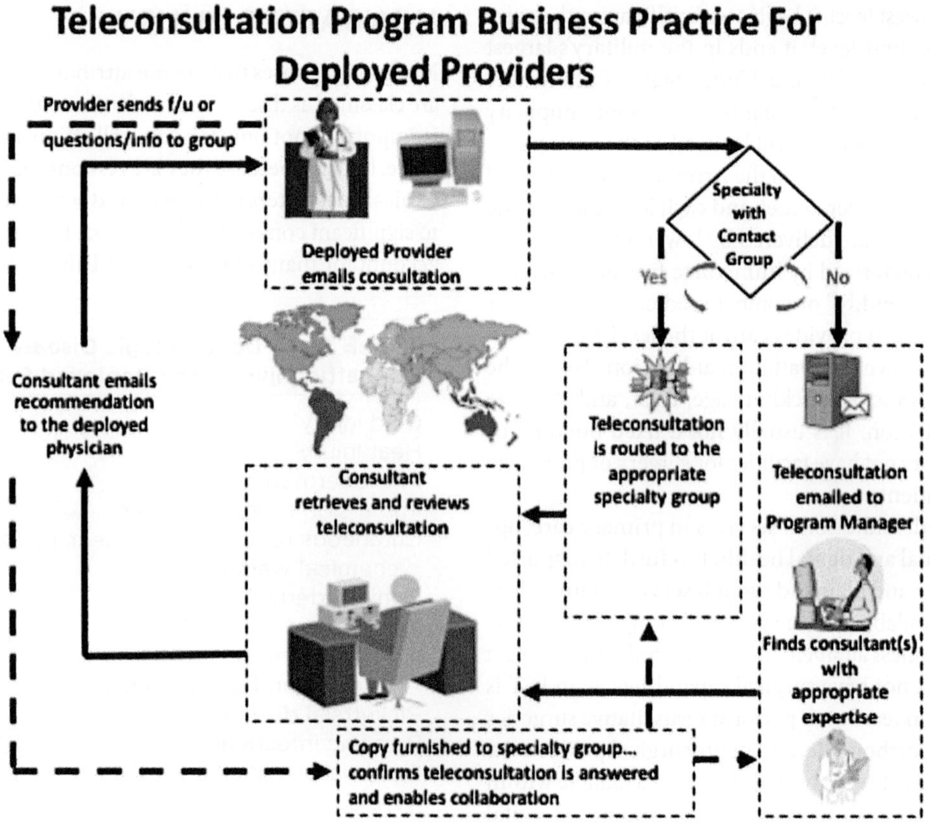

Teleconsultation Program Business Practice For Deployed Providers

FIGURE 39-1: Telemedicine workflow. Diagram courtesy of LTC Jon H. Meyerle, MD, Department of Dermatology, Walter Reed National Military Medical Center.

SCAR MANAGEMENT

More than 50,000 US service members have been wounded in the wars in Iraq and Afghanistan. Consequently, scar revision and care is a significant area of research among military physicians and scientists.

Lasers have been identified as especially useful in improving the appearance of scars. The fractionated carbon dioxide laser and pulsed-dye laser are used to treat hypertrophic and hyperemic scars in order to improve collagen architecture and decrease scar thickness, pruritus, and pain (Fig. 39-2). Tattoo lasers are now used to remove gun powder and materials that have been traumatically embedded by improvised explosive devices. Hair removal lasers are used to treat hairs that have regrown through scars and become niduses for chronic infection.

Another important aspect of scar management is restoring skin's function. After scarring, adnexal glands can become nonfunctional. This impairs the body's normal thermoregulatory mechanisms and can predispose an individual to heat injury. For a burn patient with scarring over most of his body, this can be occupationally limiting. However, in one case series of patients treated with the fractionated carbon dioxide laser, one patient demonstrated restored sweat function.

Conversely, sweating may also be undesirable after trauma and subsequent injury. The residual limbs of amputees can sweat profusely when wearing a prosthetic, causing a socket to lose function and the prosthetic to fall off. By adapting the use of onabotulinum toxin for hyperhidrosis on residual limbs, amputees are now better able to obtain proper prosthetic fits.

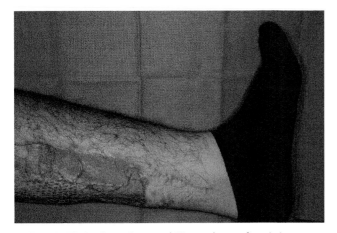

FIGURE 39-2: Scarring and tissue loss after injury from an improvised explosive device and subsequent reconstruction with split-thickness skin graft. This patient reported stiffness and decreased range of motion at the site of the graft. Ablative fractional laser resurfacing may be used to improve patient mobility and comfort. Photo courtesy of CAPT Peter R. Shumaker, MD, Department of Dermatology, Naval Medical Center San Diego.

AMPUTATIONS

More than 1,600 veterans from the Iraq and Afghanistan wars have at least one amputated limb. In contrast to amputees in the civilian sector who frequently have a history of peripheral vascular disease, diabetes, or malignancy, amputees as a result of trauma frequently do not suffer from poor blood perfusion or neuropathy issues prior to amputation.

Residual skin at an amputation site is different from normal skin. The vasculature, nerve bundles, and lymphatic structures have all been altered as a result of the amputation. This alteration disrupts neuromediator signaling and transport of immunologic cells, and leads to a localized immunocompromised state. In addition, the skin of the residual limb is not well suited for the occlusive environment of a prosthetic. Within a socket, the skin is exposed to high compressive and shear forces, increased temperature, and increased humidity. All of these factors make the skin more susceptible to problems including opportunistic infections, tumors, and malignancies.

Two types of amputations are of particular dermatologic relevance. Transtibial amputations are the most common type of amputation; so it is more likely for the doctor to encounter these amputees. Meanwhile, transfemoral amputations have the greatest risk of skin disease owing to the large surface area of skin on the residual limb. Common to both these amputation types is that the distal limb bares most of the pressure in a prosthetic and corresponds with the area of the most skin problems.

Skin diseases common among the general population are common among amputees as well. Several of these diseases include eczema, psoriasis, folliculitis, ulcers, and both irritant and allergic contact dermatitis. Other skin diseases more specific to amputees include hyperemia, acroangiodermatitis, and choke syndrome.

Hyperemia is the accumulation of hemosiderin at the distal end of a residual limb, which can occur when an amputee first begins to wear a prosthetic. Clinically, the amputee presents with a well-defined area of erythema that directly corresponds to an area of negative pressure within the socket. It results from vascular and lymphatic insufficiency within the limb, and although transient, may be prevented by postoperative wear of compression bandages. Poor prosthetic fit and weight fluctuations can further exacerbate this condition.

Acroangiodermatitis is the proliferation of preexisting vasculature within an amputee's residual limb and manifests as painful and erythematous papules, plaques, and nodules. It results from poor circulation and hypoxia, and in the case of amputees is often secondary to poor suction of a prosthetic. Although modification of the prosthetic often leads to improvement, medications or surgical intervention may be required in more advanced cases.

In choke syndrome, loss of contact between the residual limb and the socket leads to impairment of venous return and verrucous hyperplasia (Fig. 39-3). This is because the socket fits too tight proximally and too loose distally. Progressive erythema and edema develops over the residual limb, followed by vesicles, and eventually lichenification and induration. Improvement

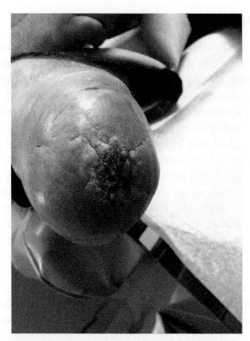

FIGURE 39-3: Verrucous hyperplasia at site of residual limb. Photo courtesy of LTC Jon H. Meyerle, MD, Department of Dermatology, Walter Reed National Military Medical Center.

can be obtained through prosthetic adjustment such as evening the distribution of pressure across the residual limb.

Amputees continue to endure site-specific skin conditions decades after amputation. In a 2012 study of Vietnam veteran amputees, almost half of the respondents reported skin breakdown or a rash within the previous year. Of these, many attributed their skin problems to the prosthetic, more than half reported having to temporarily discontinue use of the prosthetic, and almost half eventually modified or replaced their prosthetic.

Proper care of the residual limb by the amputee can help prevent skin irritation and infection. The prosthetic socket and liners should be removed and cleaned every day, and the residual limb should be washed nightly. The patient should also inspect the residual limb for evidence of redness, swelling, or skin breakdown. If skin breakdown occurs, the patient may need to stop wearing the prosthesis to allow the skin to heal.

SAUER'S NOTES

1. Dermatologic disease and nonbattle injury are responsible for a significant proportion of troop morbidity and combat ineffectiveness.
2. Telemedicine facilitates health care delivery in the world's most remote locations.
3. Laser therapies can help improve the appearance and function of scars.
4. After amputation, residual limbs are more prone to a variety of skin conditions including dermatitis, infections, and tumors.

Suggested Readings

Buikema KE, Meyerle JH. Amputation stump: privileged harbor for infections, tumors, and immune disorders. *Clin Dermatol.* 2014;32:670–677.

Fischer H. A Guide to U.S. Military Casualty Statistics: Operation Freedom's Sentinel, Operation Inherent Resolve, Operation New Dawn, Operation Iraqi Freedom, and Operation Enduring Freedom. http://www.fas .org/sgp/crs/natsec/RS22452.pdf. Updated August 7, 2015. Accessed March 1, 2016.

Hwang JS, Lappan CM, Sperling LC, et al. Utilization of telemedicine in the U.S. military in a deployed setting. *Mil Med.* 2014;179:1347–1353.

James, WD. *Military Dermatology.* Falls Church, VA: Office of the Surgeon General, US Department of the Army; 1994.

Shumaker PR. Laser treatment of traumatic scars: a military perspective. *Semin Cutan Med Surg.* 2015;34:17–23.

Yang NB, Garza LA, Foote CE, et al. High prevalence of stump dermatoses 38 years or more after amputation. *Arch Dermatol.* 2012;148:1283–1286.

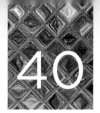

Pigmentary Dermatoses

John C. Hall, MD

There are two types of pigmentation of the skin: hyperpigmentation and hypopigmentation. The predominant skin pigment discussed in this chapter is melanin, but other pigments can also be present in the skin. A complete classification of pigmentary disorders appears at the end of this chapter.

The melanin-forming cells and their relationship to the tyrosine–tyrosinase enzyme system are discussed in Chapter 1. The common clinical example of abnormal hyperpigmentation is *chloasma*, but secondary melanoderma can result from many causes. The most common form of hypopigmentation is *vitiligo*, but secondary leukoderma does occur.

CHLOASMA (MELASMA)

Presentation and Characteristics

Clinical Lesions

An irregular hyperpigmentation of the skin that varies in shades of brown is seen. It is well demarcated and located most often on the face in sun-exposed areas (Fig. 40-1).

Distribution

The lesions usually occur on the sides of the face, forehead, and sides of the neck.

Course

The disorder is slowly progressive, but remissions do occur. It is more obvious in the summer.

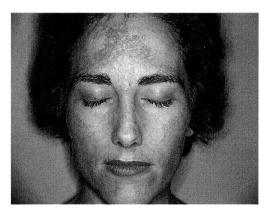

FIGURE 40-1: Chloasma of the face. (Neutrogena Skin Care Institute.)

Cause

The cause is unknown, but some cases appear during pregnancy (called "mask of pregnancy") or with chronic illness. There is an increased incidence of chloasma in women taking contraceptives, postmenopausal hormone replacement, or fertility hormones. The melanocyte-stimulating hormone of the pituitary may be excessive and affect the tyrosine–tyrosinase enzyme system.

> ### SAUER'S NOTES
>
> 1. Skin pigmentation is the most socially significant skin marker, and care must be taken not to underestimate its importance to the patient even if it is not harmful to the patient's medical well-being.
> 2. Change in skin pigmentation can be an important marker for underlying illness.
> 3. The safest and most beneficial therapy may be camouflage, that is, Lydea O'Leary Covermark or Dermablend.

Differential Diagnosis

The causes of *secondary melanoderma* should be ruled out (see end of this chapter).

Treatment

1. The patient should not be promised great therapeutic results. Most cases associated with pregnancy slowly fade or disappear completely after delivery. The pigmentation may be prolonged if the patient elects to breastfeed.
2. For a mild case in an unconcerned patient, cosmetic coverage can be adequate. Dermablend or Lydia O'Leary Covermark are two useful products.
3. Sunlight intensifies the pigmentation, so a sunscreen should be added to the routine each morning all year round.
4. Hydroquinone preparations (any of the following):
   Comment: Tri-Luma contains a retinoid, a class VI corticosteroid, and hydroquinone. This product should show a response within 8 weeks, and some authors restrict its use to this time period and then have a rest period because it contains a

corticosteroid. They then switch to a sunscreen and hydroquinone combination. There are many variants of these topicals, all with hydroquinone and some with sunscreens, glycolic acid, and retinoids. They all tend to be expensive with the exception of over-the-counter hydroquinone. Insurance considers these products cosmetic and seldom defrays the cost.

Sig: Apply locally b.i.d. Stop if irritation develops.

Comment: The treatment with any of these hydroquinone preparations should be continued for at least 2 to 3 months. Response to therapy is slow. When they are stopped, the disease tends to recur. Prolonged use over many months to years can cause increased pigmentation owing to an acquired ochronosis. This resolves on discontinuing the hydroquinone.

Melanex solution 3%

Lustra cream 4%

Eldopaque Forte cream (tinted)

Solaquin Forte cream (nontinted)

Eldoquin Forte

Lustra AF (sunscreen)

Lustra-Ultra (sunscreen, retinol) 4% hydroquinone cream is an inexpensive generic preparation.

Tri-Luma (fluocinolone, tretinoin)

EpiQuin (microsponge)

Glyquin (glycolic acid)

5. Retinoic acid (Retin-A cream [0.025%, 0.05%, 0.1%] or gel, Renova [0.02%]) applied at night can slowly decrease the pigmentation, if tolerated.

6. Kojic acid is advocated by some authors.

7. Surgical procedures used by experienced physicians include microdermabrasion, laser, and chemical peels. Beware of the danger of hypopigmentation.

VITILIGO

Presentation and Characteristics

Clinical Lesions

Irregular areas of depigmented skin are seen with a hyperpigmented border (Fig. 40-2). There is a segmental variety that has pigment loss in a dermatomal (especially trigeminal) distribution. Segmental vitiligo is not usually associated with thyroid abnormalities, does not have hyperpigmented rims surrounding the patches of vitiligo, has less Koebner phenomenon, and has less frequent progression of disease.

Distribution

It is estimated to affect 1% to 2% of the population. It is a more severe cosmetic problem in darker-skinned patients. Most commonly, the lesions occur on the face and the dorsum of hands and feet, but they can occur on all body areas.

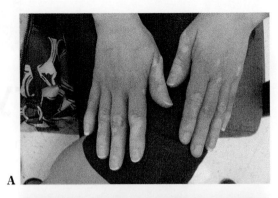
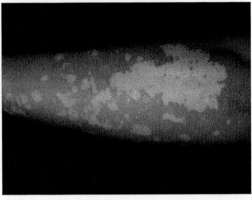

FIGURE 40-2: A: Sharply demarcated, macular areas of depigmentation over the dorsal hands in a patient with vitiligo and hypoparathyroidism. **B:** Vitiligo of the forearm in a black patient. (Neutrogena Skin Care Institute.)

Course

The disease is slowly progressive, but remissions and changes are frequent. It is more obvious during the summer because of the tanning of adjacent normal skin.

Cause

The cause is unknown but believed by some to be an autoimmune disease. Heredity is a factor in some cases. Autoimmune diseases, especially thyroiditis and pernicious anemia, can be associated with vitiligo.

Differential Diagnosis

Causes of *secondary hypopigmentation* need to be ruled out (see end of this chapter and Fig. 40-3).

Treatment

Case Example: A young woman with large depigmented patches on her face and dorsum of hands asks if something can be done for her "white spots." Her sister has a few lesions.

■ *Cosmetics:* The use of the following covering or staining preparations is recommended: pancake-type cosmetics, such as Covermark, by Lydia O'Leary; Vitadye (Elder); dihydroxyacetone-containing self-tanning creams, gels, and foams; walnut juice stain; or potassium

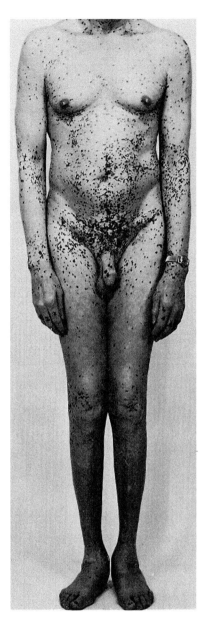

FIGURE 40-3: Secondary hypopigmentation. A marked example of loss of pigment that occurred in an African American man following healing of an exfoliative dermatitis. Corticosteroids were used in the therapy.

permanganate solution in appropriate dilution. Many patients with vitiligo become quite proficient in the application of these agents. A sunscreen used on the surrounding skin makes the contrast of light and dark skin less apparent.

- *Corticosteroid cream therapy:* This is effective for early mild cases of vitiligo, especially when one is mainly concerned with face and hand lesions. Betamethasone valerate (Valisone) cream 0.1% can be prescribed for use on the hands for 4 months or so and for use on the face for only 3 months. It should not be used on the eyelids or as full-body therapy. Class I topical corticosteroids can also be used for a while if appropriate precautions are observed.

- *Protopic 0.1% ointment* used twice a day avoids topical corticosteroid side effects and may be quite beneficial. Concern over induction of cutaneous lymphoma has been hypothesized but not proven and discredited by many.

- *Sun avoidance:* Sun tanning should be avoided because this accentuates the normal pigmentation and makes the nonpigmented vitiligo more noticeable. The white areas of vitiligo are more susceptible to sunburn. If the patient desires a more specific treatment, the following can be suggested with certain reservations.

- *Psoralen derivatives:* For many years, Egyptians along the Nile River chewed certain plants to cause the disappearance of the white spots of vitiligo. Extraction of the chemicals from these plants revealed the psoralen derivatives to be the active agents, and one of these, 8-methoxypsoralen, was found to be the most effective. This chemical is available as Oxsoralen in 10-mg capsules and also as a topical liquid form. The oral form is to be ingested 2 hours before exposure to measured sun radiation. The package insert should be consulted. Our results with this long-term therapy have been disappointing.

- Trisoralen is a synthetic psoralen in 5-mg tablets. The recommended dosage is two tablets taken 2 hours before measured sun exposure for a long-term course. Detailed instructions accompany the package. Some dermatologists believe this therapy to be more effective than Oxsoralen.

- A short 2-week course of Oxsoralen capsules (20 mg/day) has been advocated for the purpose of acquiring a better and quicker suntan. The value of such a course has been questioned. The sun exposure must be gradual. Oral psoralens plus self-administered UVA or UVB in "tanning booths" can produce severe burns, which may be fatal.

- *Psoralens and ultraviolet light (PUVA) therapy:* The combination of topical or oral psoralen therapy with UVA radiation has been somewhat successful in re-pigmenting vitiligo. The psoralen can be given orally, topically, or as a bath. Precautions concerning photoaging and skin cancer apply. Narrowband UVB has less short-term side effects with no photoprotective goggles needed, less cost, less phototoxicity, less skin cancer, and less photoaging than PUVA or broadband UVB.

- *Depigmentation therapy:* In the hands of experts, mono-benzyl ether of hydroquinone (Benoquin) can be used to remove skin pigment to even out the patient's skin color. Beware of this therapy because pigment loss is permanent. The author has never attempted this therapy.

- *Skin grafting:* Autologous minigrafting and other similar surgical procedures have been used with success by some.

- *Surgical therapy:* Various grafting procedures are valuable in recalcitrant disease. Epidermal or full-thickness autographs have been advocated by some authors.

- Narrowband UVB therapy has been advocated and may be safer than PUVA or broadband UVB. Afamelanotide has been used in combination with light therapy with good results.
- Intralesional Triamcinolone 3 mg/mL has been used with benefit in some patients.

CLASSIFICATION OF PIGMENTARY DISORDERS

Melanin Hyperpigmentation or Melanoderma

1. Chloasma (melasma) (see Fig. 40-1)
2. Incontinentia pigmenti
3. Secondary to skin diseases
   a. Chronic discoid lupus erythematosus
   b. Tinea versicolor
   c. Stasis dermatitis
   d. Lichen planus
   e. Fixed drug eruption
   f. Many cases of dermatitis in African Americans and other dark-skinned individuals (Fig. 36-3)
   g. Scleroderma
   h. Porphyria cutanea tarda (Fig. 40-4)
   i. Dermatitis herpetiformis
4. Secondary to external agents
   a. X-radiation
   b. Ultraviolet light
   c. Sunlight
   d. Tars
   e. Photosensitizing chemicals, as in cosmetics, causing development of clinical entities labeled as Riehl melanosis, poikiloderma of Civatte on the sides of the neck resulting from chronic sun exposure, berloque dermatitis resulting from application of certain colognes or perfumes to the skin (Fig. 40-5), and others
5. Secondary to internal disorders
   a. Addison disease (Fig. 40-6)
   b. Chronic liver disease

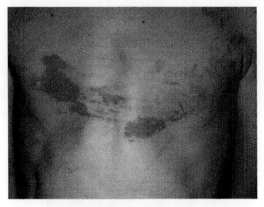

FIGURE 40-5: Berloque dermatitis: photosensitivity reaction from mother's perfume, age 7 years. (Neutrogena Skin Care Institute.)

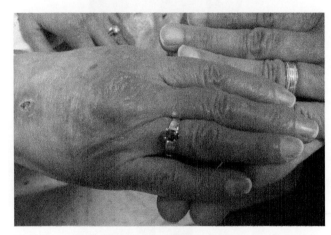

FIGURE 40-6: Blue-gray discoloration over the back of a hand owing to 20 years of daily usage of nose drops that contained silver.

   c. Pregnancy
   d. Hyperthyroidism
   e. Internal carcinoma causing a malignant form of acanthosis nigricans
   f. Hormonal influence on benign acanthosis nigricans
   g. Intestinal polyposis causing mucous membrane pigmentation (Peutz–Jeghers syndrome)
   h. Albright syndrome
   i. Schilder disease
   j. Fanconi syndrome (in HIV-positive patients)
6. Secondary to drugs such as adrenocorticotropic hormone, estrogens, progesterone, melanocyte-stimulating hormone, minocycline, nonsteroidal anti-inflammatory drugs, amiodarone, psychotropic drugs, antimalarials, tetracyclines, heavy metals, zidovudine, retigabine, porokeratosis, ptychotropica (see porokeratosis), and fluoroquinolones
7. Vitamin B_{12} Deficiency

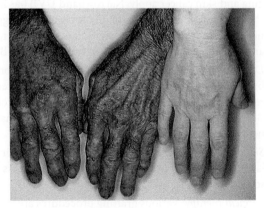

FIGURE 40-4: Porphyria cutanea tarda hyperpigmentation. (Neutrogena Skin Care Institute.)

Nonmelanin Pigmentations

1. Argyria (Fig. 40-6) owing to silver salt deposits
2. Arsenic pigmentation caused by ingestion of inorganic arsenic, as in Fowler solution and Asiatic pills
3. Pigmentation from heavy metals such as bismuth, gold, and mercury
4. Tattoos
5. Black dermographism, the common bluish black or green stain seen under watches and rings in some persons because of the deposit of the metallic particles reacting with chemicals already on the skin or the granules in talc (Fig. 40-7)
6. Hemosiderin granules in hemochromatosis, stasis dermatitis, or pigmented purpuric eruptions (see Chapter 13)
7. Bile pigments from jaundice
8. Yellow pigments following atabrine and chlorpromazine ingestion
9. Carotene coloring in carotenemia and lycopene coloring in lycopenia
10. Homogentisic acid polymer deposit in ochronosis
11. Minocycline hyperpigmentation (characteristic histopathology) diffuse and also localized at scar sites (and rarely teeth)
12. Hyperpigmentation of Ito or Ota

Hypopigmentation

1. Albinism
2. Vitiligo
3. Nevus achromicus (nevus depigmentosus) (Fig. 40-8)
4. Vogt–Koyanagi–Harada syndrome
5. Whitaker syndrome
6. Chediak–Higashi syndrome
7. Hypomelanosis of Ito
8. Leukoderma or acquired hypopigmentation (Fig. 40-9)
   a. Secondary to skin diseases such as tinea versicolor, chronic discoid lupus erythematosus, localized scleroderma (may show perifollicular pigment retention), psoriasis, secondary syphilis, or pinta (Fig. 40-3)

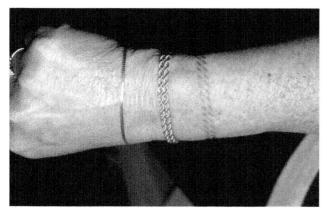

FIGURE 40-7: Black dermographism on the wrist owing to metal particles reacting to chemicals on the skin or talc.

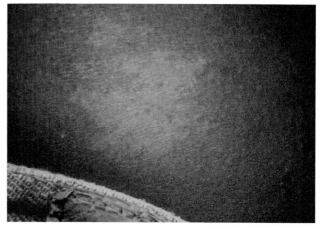

FIGURE 40-8: Nevu achromicus (nevus depigmentosus) on the buttock of a person of color. Since this is in an adult without underling sequelae, an ash leaf macule is unlikely. Vilitigo is unlikely since this is a single lesion and has been stable for years. Macular, well-demarcated loss of pigment, which is characteristic, can be seen on any site in any ethnic group.

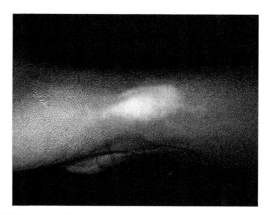

FIGURE 40-9: Leukoderma on the wrist from intralesional corticosteroid injections in a black patient. (Neutrogena Skin Care Institute.)

   b. Secondary to chemicals such as mercury compounds, monobenzyl ether of hydroquinone, and cortisone-type drugs given intralesionally, especially in people of color (Fig. 40-6)
   c. Secondary to internal diseases, such as hormonal diseases, and in Vogt–Koyanagi syndrome
   d. Associated with pigmented nevi (halo nevus or leukoderma acquisitum centrifugum)
   e. Hypopigmented patch-stage mycosis fungoides
   f. Indeterminate leprosy with anesthesia
   g. Pinta
   h. Imatinib treatment for chronic myelogenous leukemia
   i. Idiopathic guttate hypomelanosis
9. Waardenburg syndrome
10. Ash-leaf macule of tuberous sclerosis
11. Idiopathic guttate hyponelanosis (acquired depimented macular spots) (Fig. 40-10)
12. Nevus anemicus (Fig. 40-11)

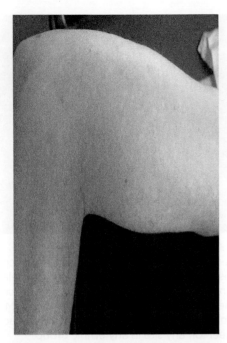

FIGURE 40-10: Idiopathic guttate hypomelanosis on the extensor arm. Well-demarcated 3-mm macule are seen that will become more easily seen when the patient gets a tan. Treatment is unsatisfactory and the cause is idiopathic. Also common on extensor legs.

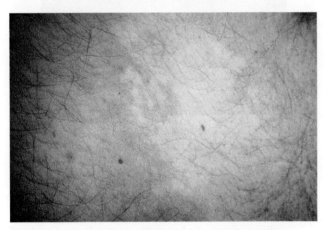

FIGURE 40-11: Nevus anemicus on the back. The well-demarcated area disappears on pressure with a clear glass slide (diascopy). There is no known treatment, and it is not a sign of underlying disease.

Suggested Readings

Boersma BR, Westerhof W, Bos JD. Repigmentation in vitiligo vulgaris by autologous minigrafting: results in nineteen patients. *J Am Acad Dermatol*. 1995;33(6):990–995.

Drake LA, Dinehart SM, Farmer ER, et al. Guidelines of care for vitiligo. American Academy of Dermatology. *J Am Acad Dermatol*. 1996;35:620–626.

Fulk CS. Primary disorders of hyperpigmentation. *J Am Acad Dermatol*. 1984;10:1–16.

Grimes PE. New insights and new therapies in vitiligo. *JAMA*. 2005;293:730–735.

Kovacs SO. Vitiligo. *J Am Acad Dermatol*. 1998;38(5, pt 1):647–666.

Levine N. *Pigmentation and Pigmentary Disorders*. Boca Raton, FL: CRC Press; 1994.

Lio PA. Little white spots: an approach to hypopigmented macules. *Arch Dis Child Educ Pract Ed*. 2008;93:98–102.

Nordlund JJ, Boissy R, Hearing VJ, et al. *The Pigmentary System: Physiology and Pathophysiology*. New York: Oxford University Press; 1998.

Sheth VM, Pandya AG. Melasma: a comprehensive update: part I and II. *J Am Acad Dermatol*. 2011;65(4):689–716.

Taieb A, Picardo M. Clinical practice. Vitiligo. *N Engl J Med*. 2009;360(2):160–169.

Victor FC, Gelber J, Rao B. Melasma: a review. *J Cutan Med Surg*. 2004;8:97–102.

Autoimmune Connective Tissue Diseases

Robin S. Lewallen, MD, Lindsay C. Strowd, MD, and Joseph L. Jorizzo, MD

Autoimmune connective tissue diseases are a group of autoimmune disorders that include lupus erythematosus (LE), scleroderma, dermatomyositis (DM), rheumatoid arthritis, Sjögren syndrome, and mixed connective tissue disease. LE, scleroderma, and DM are discussed in detail in this chapter. There is a great deal of overlap in the cutaneous and laboratory findings among these disorders. These diseases are characterized by circulating autoantibodies (aAbs), cutaneous as well as internal manifestations. Cutaneous findings, such as cuticular dystrophy or poikiloderma, may be the presenting or dominant feature of autoimmune connective tissue disease. Nevertheless, systemic multiorgan disease needs to be excluded in each case.

A thorough laboratory evaluation is required in all patients with autoimmune connective tissue disease. Much has been written about antinuclear antibody (ANA) testing. This assay identifies aAbs present in serum to autoantigens present in nuclei of mammalian cells. ANA testing is reported as a titer, and most commercial kits report ANA titers of 1:40 or 1:80 as abnormal. Having a low titer, of 1:40 or 1:80, usually is not pathologic and is the result of DNA recycling during normal cell turnover. Approximately 5% of otherwise healthy young individuals have an ANA titer of 1:160 or higher. The prevalence of this false-positive ANA increases with age and is more common in females. Therefore, it is important not to label patients with LE or another autoimmune disease simply based on a single laboratory test. In addition, ANA positivity is seen in multiple other autoimmune diseases and is not specific for LE. There are many subtypes of ANA such as anti-Ro, anti-La, anti-smith, anti-topoisomerase/Scl-70, anti-dsDNA, antihistone, and anticentromere. Additional subtype testing after obtaining a positive ANA may aid in the diagnosis. For example, anti-smith antibodies are the most specific autoantibodies for LE, whereas antihistone antibodies are commonly found in drug-induced LE.

After securing a diagnosis, much important work remains. A thorough medical history, including medicinal and social history, should be obtained. Paraneoplastic phenomena should also be considered, especially in the setting of DM, and patients should be questioned about family history of malignancy as well as the status of their age-appropriate cancer screening including, but not limited to, colonoscopy, mammograms, and PSA levels. Finally, understanding the systemic effects of each disease is crucial for initial screening tests as well as appropriate referral.

LUPUS ERYTHEMATOSUS

Chronic cutaneous lupus erythematosus (CCLE) (Fig. 41-1), subacute cutaneous lupus erythematosus (SCLE) (Fig. 41-2), acute cutaneous lupus erythematosus (ACLE), and systemic lupus erythematosus (SLE) are the four types of LE.

It has been estimated that cutaneous variants of LE are two to three times more common than systemic disease. LE is much more common in women than in men; the female-to-male ratio is at least 6:1. Young, fertile women are most commonly affected, and pregnancy issues should be addressed. LE is more common in African Americans or black Africans than in Caucasians, and Africans have a higher frequency of systemic disease. Diagnosis of LE and its subtypes depends on a constellation of findings that include history, physical examination, histopathologic correlation, and laboratory evaluation that focuses on published American College of Rheumatology criteria (Table 41-1).

There are three major specific forms of LE: CCLE, SCLE, and ACLE (Table 41-2). CCLE includes discoid LE, tumid lupus,

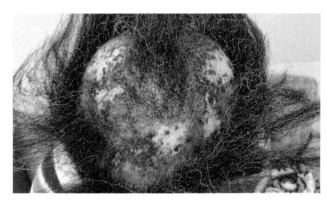

FIGURE 41-1: CCLE with discoid lesions–erythematous, hyper- and hypopigmented plaques with scarring characteristic of CCLE with discoid lesions.

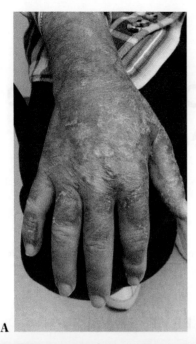

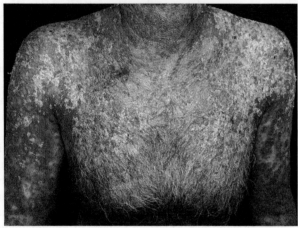

FIGURE 41-2: SCLE. **A:** Erythematous papules and plaques on dorsal hands; typical distribution spares the knuckles. **B:** Erythematous papules and plaques in a typical sun-exposed distribution of the chest and arms, with sparing photoprotected aspect of the neck.

lupus panniculitis, and chilblain lupus. The localized form of discoid LE is the most common cutaneous manifestation; if confined to the head and neck, there is ≤5% risk of SLE. Patients with widespread disease (skin involvement outside of the head and neck) have an increased risk of progression to SLE of up to 20%. SCLE is characterized by annular and/ or papulosquamous plaques and is often photodistributed. Approximately 70% of SCLE patients have anti-Ro/SSA aAbs, and there is a 10% to 15% risk of SLE. Neonatal LE (NLE) is a special form of SCLE and is discussed separately in the following paragraph, but it is also associated with positive anti-Ro/ SSA aAbs. Finally, ACLE is the form most closely associated with SLE, and anyone with ACLE should be evaluated for SLE.

NLE is seen in newborns whose mothers have anti-Ro/SSA aAbs. Nearly 100% of patients with NLE also have anti-Ro aAbs. SCLE-like lesions are usually seen on the face of newborns. Congenital heart block is an important complication, is usually present at birth, and is the leading cause of this condition. Therefore, screening for heart disease should be performed in all patients with NLE. Children with this complication have a 20% mortality rate, and two-thirds require pacemakers. Other associated systemic findings include elevated hepatic manifestations including elevated liver function testing and hepatosplenomegaly as well as hematologic manifestations including anemia, neutropenia, and thrombocytopenia.

Drug-induced lupus is separated into three categories: drug-induced CCLE, drug-induced SCLE, and drug-induced SLE. The most common medications implicated in the subacute form include hydrochlorothiazide, terbinafine, calcium channel blockers, angiotensin-converting enzyme inhibitors (captopril), TNF-α inhibitors, and proton pump inhibitors . The cutaneous findings are identical to SCLE with photodistributed annular and papulosquamous lesions usually in the absence of systemic symptoms. Drug-induced SCLE is associated with positive anti-Ro/SSA aAbs. Drug-induced SLE is most commonly associated with procainamide and hydralazine; other associated medications include isoniazid, quinidine, minocycline, and TNF-α inhibitors. Antihistone aAb is a serologic marker that occurs in patients with drug-induced LE; however, Anti-dsDNA aAbs are seen in patients with drug-induced LE to TNF-α inhibitors.

TABLE 41-1 • 1997 Update of the 1982 American College of Rheumatology Revised Criteria for Classification of Systemic Lupus Erythematosus (4 of 11 Needed for Diagnosis of Systemic Disease)

1. Malar Rash (butterfly rash)
2. Discoid Rash
3. Photosensitivity
4. Oral or Nasopharyngeal Ulcers (usually painless)
5. Nonerosive Arthritis (involving two or more peripheral joints)
6. Pleuritis or Pericarditis
7. Renal Disorder (persistent proteinuria or cellular casts)
8. Neurologic Disorder (seizures or psychosis)
9. Hematologic Disorder (hemolytic anemia, leukopenia, lymphopenia, or thrombocytopenia)
10. Immunologic Disorder (Anti-DNA, Anti-smith, or antiphospholipid autoantibodies)
11. Positive Antinuclear Antibody

TABLE 41-2 • Comparison of Three Most Common Types of LE Encountered by Doctors

LE Subtype	CCLE	SCLE	ACLE
Distribution	Face, scalp, ears, extensor arms	V of the neck, upper back, shoulders, extensor arms, and, less commonly, face	"Butterfly" malar distribution on face, V of the neck, arms, hands (sparing knuckles)
Clinical features	*Early lesions:* sharply demarcated erythematous papules and plaques with prominent scale, follicular plugging, and early scarring; *late lesions:* atrophic plaques with central scarring, telangiectasia, and hypopigmentation; photosensitivity	Erythematous papules and scaly, hyperkeratotic, annular/polycyclic plaques; photosensitivity; nonscarring	Poorly marginated erythematous macules, fine scaling, poikiloderma, edema; photosensitivity; nonscarring
Course	Chronic with disease progression without treatment; 5%–10% eventually meet ACR criteria for SLE	50% meet ACR criteria for SLE	Acute onset, usually with systemic signs and symptoms
Histopathology	Vacuolar change; dyskeratotic keratinocytes; follicular plugging; basement membrane thickening; superficial and deep perivascular and perifollicular lymphohistiocytic infiltrate; increased dermal mucin	Vacuolar change; dyskeratotic keratinocytes, epidermal atrophy; superficial and mid perivascular lymphohistiocytic infiltrate; increased dermal mucin	Vacuolar change; dyskeratotic keratinocytes; superficial perivascular lymphohistiocytic infiltrate; dermal edema
Laboratory findings	Positive ANA (5%)	Positive ANA, anti-Ro aAb (>90%)	Positive ANA (99%); double-stranded DNA (60%); anemia (normocytic); leukopenia; thrombocytopenia; elevated ESR; proteinuria; cellular casts
Differential diagnosis	Polymorphous light eruption; psoriasis; sarcoidosis; lichen planus; granuloma faciale	Annular erythemas; atopic dermatitis; psoriasis; dermatophyte infection; secondary syphilis	Sunburn; rosacea; DM; phototoxic drug eruption; seborrheic dermatitis

Abbreviations: ACLE, acute cutaneous lupus erythematosus; ACR, American College of Radiology; ANA, antinuclear antibody; CCLE, chronic cutaneous lupus erythematosus; DM, dermatomyositis; ESR, erythrocyte sedimentation rate; LE, lupus erythematosus; SCLE, subacute cutaneous lupus erythematosus; SLE, systemic lupus erythematosus.

See Table 41-2 for a comparison of CCLE, SCLE, and ACLE. The treatment approach is outlined in Table 41-3.

SCLERODERMA

Localized scleroderma (morphea), systemic (diffuse) sclerosis, and limited scleroderma (CREST syndrome, calcinosis cutis, Raynaud phenomenon, esophageal dysfunction, sclerodactyly, and telangiectasias) are variants included under the general heading of scleroderma (Fig. 41-3).

Systemic sclerosis (SSc) is a systemic disease that affects the skin, lungs, heart, gastrointestinal tract, and other organ systems. It is up to 15 times more common in women,

and the age of onset is between 30 and 50 years. Ten-year survival of patients with SSc is less than 70%. Pathogenesis of SSc is unknown, but endothelial cell damage as well as activation of T lymphocytes is suspected as the key pathogenic abnormality.

aAbs are often detected in nonlocalized forms of sclerosis. ANA may be used as a screen, while additional subtype testing with antitopoisomerase/Scl-70 antibodies differentiate SSc from the anticentromere antibody-associated limited scleroderma (CREST syndrome). Cutaneous and systemic findings of SSc and other variants of scleroderma are summarized in Table 41-4. Treatment options are often directed toward the symptoms and are summarized in Table 41-4.

TABLE 41-3 • Therapeutic Options for LE

Mild local disease	Sunscreens (high SPF with UVA blocker) Topical or intralesional corticosteroids Topical immunomodulators (e.g., tacrolimus) Hydroxychloroquine (may add quinacrine)
Extensive cutaneous disease	Oral retinoids Dapsone/sulfapyridine Clofazimine Methotrexate Thalidomide Azathioprine
Systemic disease	Prednisone Azathioprine Mycophenolate mofetil Cyclophosphamide Cyclosporine Interferon IVIG Newer biologic therapies Extracorporeal immunomodulation Androgen therapy Stem cell transplantation

Abbreviations: IVIG, intravenous immunoglobulin; SPF, sun protective factor; UVA, ultraviolet A.

DERMATOMYOSITIS

DM is an autoimmune proximal extensor inflammatory myopathy with specific cutaneous manifestations (Fig. 41-4). Polymyositis is an inflammatory myopathy without any skin involvement. DM sine myositis presents with the characteristic skin eruption of DM without muscle involvement.

Cutaneous disease is characteristic (Table 41-5) and can either precede or follow muscle disease. Adult and juvenile variants exist. Differential diagnosis of skin disease includes SLE, psoriasis, allergic contact dermatitis, phototoxic drug eruption, cutaneous T-cell lymphoma, atopic dermatitis, flat warts, and scleroderma. Overlap with other autoimmune diseases such as Sjögren syndrome, SLE, scleroderma, or vasculitis is not uncommon.

The pathogenesis of DM is unclear, but it is believed to be an autoimmune disease triggered by outside factors in genetically predisposed individuals. Ultraviolet radiation plays an important trigger role in cutaneous DM. Average age of onset of adult disease is 52 years and of juvenile disease is 8 years. Adult DM is more common in women; the male-to-female ratio is 1:6. Juvenile DM is slightly more common in boys. Drug-induced DM has been reported secondary to hydroxyurea, statins, penicillamine, quinidine, and phenylbutazone.

The inflammatory myopathy affects proximal muscle groups, especially the triceps and quadriceps. Patients present with proximal muscle weakness, muscle tenderness, and fatigue. Muscle workup should include creatine phosphokinase and aldolase levels, as well as magnetic resonance imaging, electromyography, and/or a triceps muscle biopsy. Pulmonary fibrosis can be seen in 15% to 30% of patients and is more common in patients with anti–transfer-RNA syndrome (which may include Jo-1 aAbs).

Internal malignancy is estimated to occur in 10% to 50% of patients with adult DM and has been associated with anti-p155 aAbs. Ovarian, breast, lung, and gastric cancers have been described. The risk of malignancy may return to normal after 2 years. Juvenile DM is not associated with increased malignancy risk.

Histopathology reveals vacuolar change, sparse lymphocytic infiltrate, epidermal atrophy, and basement membrane degeneration. aAbs to Jo-1 and Mi-2 are found in 30% of patients with polymyositis and 10% of patients with DM, respectively.

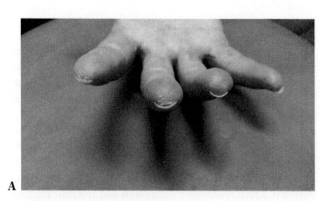

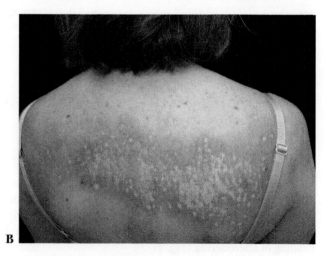

A

B

FIGURE 41-3: Scleroderma. **A:** Distal fingertip ulceration and keratosis consistent with "rat-bite" necrosis in a patient with limited scleroderma. **B:** Salt-and-pepper pigmentation of the upper back in a patient with systemic sclerosis.

TABLE 41-4 • Clinical Features of Scleroderma Variants

Scleroderma Subtype	Systemic Sclerosis	Limited Scleroderma (CREST syndrome)	Morphea
Cutaneous findings	Sclerodactyly (induration of fingers, waxy, shiny, hardened, bound down skin, loss of wrinkling), Raynaud phenomenon (coldness, triphasic color changes, i.e., pallor, cyanosis, rubor), diffuse and salt-and-pepper hyperpigmentation, cutaneous ulcers ("rat-bite necrosis"), trunk involvement	Telangiectasias, Raynaud phenomenon, calcinosis cutis (especially over bony prominences), cutaneous ulcers ("rat-bite" necrosis), sclerodactyly	*Plaque type:* erythematous, edematous plaque that becomes sclerotic and scarlike with hypopigmentation and hyperpigmentation; *deep (profunda) morphea:* deep tissue sclerosis; *en coupe de saber:* linear morphea affecting the forehead and scalp; *Parry–Romberg syndrome:* hyperpigmentation and soft tissue atrophy affecting the entire distribution of the trigeminal nerve leading to facial asymmetry
Systemic findings	*Esophagus:* reflux disease, dysmotility, dysphagia; *GI tract:* decreased peristalsis leading to constipation, diarrhea, bloating, malabsorption; *heart:* constrictive pericarditis, conduction abnormalities; *lungs:* diffuse pulmonary fibrosis; *kidneys:* uremia, renal hypertension	*Esophagus:* reflux disease, dysmotility, dysphagia; *GI tract:* telangiectasias	None
Histopathology	Diffuse dermal sclerosis, mild vacuolar change, excessive collagen deposition, decreased adnexal structures, mild perivascular infiltrate with plasma cells	Same (For sclerodactyly)	Same
Laboratory findings	Positive ANA (90%–95%), anti–Scl 70 aAb (DNA topoisomerase I; 60%)	Positive ANA, anti-centromere aAb (80%)	Possibly a positive ANA (especially linear morphea), anti–fibrillin-1 aAb
Differential diagnosis	Eosinophilic fasciitis, scleromyxedema, scleredema, ʟ-tryptophan syndrome, nephrogenic fibrosing dermopathy, toxic oil syndrome, graft-versus-host disease, drug reaction (bleomycin)	Pathognomonic if all features are present	Toxic oil syndrome, drug reaction (bleomycin), silicosis, chemical exposure (vinyl chloride, organic solvents, pesticides, and epoxy resin), graft-versus-host disease
Treatment	*Skin sclerosis:* physical therapy, prednisone (controversial), methotrexate, ᴅ-penicillamine; *Raynaud phenomenon:* calcium channel blockers, Viagra; *calcinosis cutis:* excision; *renal disease:* ACE inhibitors; *esophageal disease:* proton pump inhibitors; *pulmonary disease:* cyclophosphamide	*Calcinosis cutis:* excision; *Raynaud phenomenon:* calcium channel blockers, Viagra; *esophageal disease:* proton pump inhibitors; *skin sclerosis:* physical therapy, methotrexate, ᴅ-penicillamine	*Mild disease:* topical/intralesional corticosteroids, topical immunomodulators (e.g., tacrolimus), with keratolytics; *severe disease:* hydroxychloroquine, methotrexate, ᴅ-penicillamine, cyclosporine, phototherapy, physical therapy

Abbreviations: ANA, antinuclear antibody; ACE, angiotensin-converting enzyme; GI, gastrointestinal.

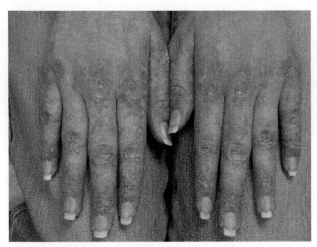

FIGURE 41-4: Gottron papules on the dorsal hands of a patient with juvenile DM.

TABLE 41-5 • Cutaneous Manifestations of Dermatomyositis

Gottron papules (see Fig. 41-4)	Violaceous papules overlying dorsal interphalangeal and metacarpophalangeal joints
Gottron sign	Confluent violaceous erythema overlying dorsal interphalangeal and metacarpophalangeal joints
Periorbital heliotrope rash	Confluent violaceous erythema and edema of the eyelids and periorbital tissue
Poikiloderma	Violaceous erythema with hypopigmentation, hyperpigmentation, and atrophy in sun-exposed distribution and over extensor surfaces

The presence of these aAbs is associated with a decreased risk of internal malignancy. ANA positivity is seen in 60% to 80% of patients. Treatment is outlined in Table 41-6.

TABLE 41-6 • Therapeutic Options for Treatment of Dermatomyositis

Cutaneous lesions	Sunscreens (high SPF with UVA blocker) Topical corticosteroids Topical immunomodulators (e.g., tacrolimus) Hydroxychloroquine Methotrexate Mycophenolate mofetil Retinoids
Systemic disease	Oral prednisone Methotrexate Mycophenolate mofetil Cyclosporine Cyclophosphamide Chlorambucil Rituximab IVIG

Abbreviations: IVIG, intravenous immunoglobulin; SPF, sun protective factor; UVA, ultraviolet A.

Suggested Readings

Connolly MK. Systemic sclerosis (scleroderma) and related disorders. In: Bolognia JL, Jorizzo JL, Rapini RP, eds. *Dermatology*. 3rd ed. St. Louis: Elsevier; 2012:643–655.

Chung L, Lin J, Furst DE, et al. Systemic and localized scleroderma. *Clin Dermatol*. 2006;24:374–392.

Hochberg MC, Boyd RE, Ahearn JM, et al. Systemic lupus erythematosus: a review of clinico-laboratory features and immunogenetic markers in 150 patients with emphasis on demographic subsets. *Medicine*. 1985;64:285–295.

Jacobe HT, Sontheimer RD, Saxton-Daniels S. Autoantibodies encountered in patients with autoimmune connective tissue diseases. In: Bolognia JL, Jorizzo JL, Rapini RP, eds. *Dermatology*. 3rd ed. St. Louis: Elsevier; 2012:603–614.

Jorizzo JL, Vleugels RA. Dermatomyositis. In: Bolognia JL, Jorizzo JL, Rapini RP, eds. *Dermatology*. 3rd ed. St. Louis: Elsevier; 2012:631–641.

Petri M, Orbai AM, Alarcon GS, et al. Derivation and validation of the Systemic Lupus International Collaborating Clinics classification criteria for systemic lupus erythematosus. *Arthritis Rheum*. 2012;64(8):2677–2686.

Simard JF, Costenbader KH. What can epidemiology tell us about systemic lupus erythematosus? *Int J Clin Pract*. 2007;61(7):1170–1180.

Sontheimer RD. Skin manifestations of systemic autoimmune connective tissue disease: diagnostics and therapeutics. *Best Pract Res Clin Rheumatol*. 2004;18:429–462.

Strowd LC, Jorizzo JL. Review of dermatomyositis: establishing the diagnosis and treatment algorithm. *J Dermatolog Treat*. 2013;24(6):418–421.

Sugai DY, Gustafson CJ, De Luca JF, et al. Trends in the outpatient medication management of lupus erythematosus in the United States. *J Drugs Dermatol*. 2014;13(5):545–552.

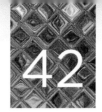

42

The Skin and Internal Disease

Tracy T. Hung, BS, Maryam Liaqat, MD, and Warren R. Heymann, MD

A practicing doctor must be cognizant of the potential cutaneous manifestations of systemic diseases. Although certain skin findings are pathognomonic for particular maladies, more often than not, cutaneous eruptions must be interpreted in the context of the complete clinical picture. It is the interplay between the skin and internal medicine that underscores the importance of a cutaneous evaluation as a routine part of a complete physical examination.

Cutaneous findings can be classified as specific and nonspecific. *Specific changes* demonstrate the same pathologic process as internal disease and can therefore be diagnostic of the disease. *Nonspecific changes* do not demonstrate the primary disease process (Figs. 42-1 and 42-2). These changes can be helpful in establishing the diagnosis only if interpreted within the context of the clinical data. The following cases are a few selected examples of the many systemic diseases with skin involvement. Table 42-1 lists some internal diseases and their dermatologic manifestations.

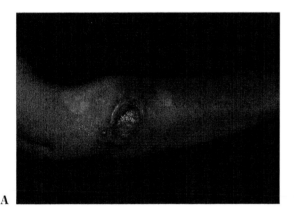
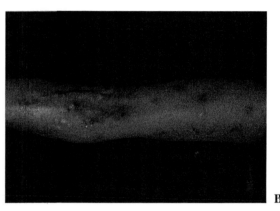

FIGURE 42-1: Nonspecific skin changes indicating an underlying psychological disease state. **A:** Delusional excoriation on the arm ("have to get the hairs out"). **B:** Neurotic excoriations on the arm.

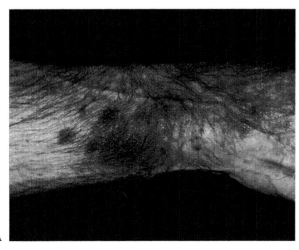
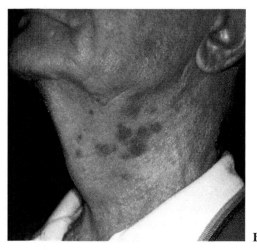

FIGURE 42-2: Nonspecific skin changes resulting from an internal disease. Purpura of the arm **(A)** and folliculitis of the neck **(B)** in a patient with myelogenous leukemia. (Courtesy of Syntext Laboratories, Inc.)

TABLE 42-1 • Internal Malignancies With Cutaneous Manifestations

Disorder	Cutaneous Findings	Associated Malignancies
Acanthosis nigricans	Velvety hyperpigmentation of flexures and, less commonly, mucosal surfaces and palms (tripe palms)	Adenocarcinoma of genitourinary or gastrointestinal tract. Most commonly associated with adenocarcinoma of the stomach (55.5%)[a]
Acquired ichthyosis	Adult onset hyperkeratosis indistinguishable from ichthyosis vulgaris	Hodgkin lymphoma, mycosis fungoides, multiple myeloma, leiomyosarcoma
Acrokeratosis paraneoplastica (Bazex syndrome)	Acral psoriasiform plaques with nail dystrophy	Carcinomas of upper digestive and respiratory tracts. Also described in association with transitional cell bladder carcinoma[b]
Carcinoid syndrome	Deeply erythematous or violaceous flushing of upper body associated with pruritus, diaphoresis, lacrimation, and facial edema	Foregut, midgut, and bronchial neuroendocrine tumors
Cushing syndrome	Generalized hyperpigmentation, including areolae, palmar creases, and scars; hirsutism; central obesity; moon facies, striae	Ectopic ACTH production by small cell lung cancer, bronchial carcinoid tumors and cancers of the thyroid, pancreas, and adrenals
Dermatomyositis	Heliotrope dermatitis, proximal nail fold telangiectasias, Gottron papules, cutaneous necrosis	Ovarian, gastrointestinal, and nasopharyngeal carcinomas; adenocarcinomas of the lung and prostate; hematologic malignancies
Erythema gyratum repens	Migratory figurate erythema with "wood grain" pattern	Malignancies of the lung, breast, female reproductive tract, gastrointestinal tract, and prostate
Hypertrichosis lanuginosa acquisita	Excessive growth of vellus hairs on neck and face, but can involve any body surface	Most commonly observed with colorectal, breast, and lung cancers
Necrolytic migratory erythema	Acral and intertriginous papulosquamous dermatitis with occasional vesiculation	Pancreatic α-cell tumor presents with glucagonoma syndrome
Paget disease	(1) Unilateral eczematous nipple plaque (2) Eczematous plaque of the anorectal, genital, and axillary regions (extramammary Paget disease)	(1) Associated with ductal adenocarcinoma (2) Regional associations are (a) anorectal—adenocarcinoma of the anus and colorectum, (b) vulvar—epithelial, eccrine, and apocrine neoplasms, and (c) male genitourinary reproductive tract malignancies
Paraneoplastic pemphigus	Diffuse mucocutaneous involvement with blisters, erosions, lichenoid, and erythema multiforme–like lesions. Head and neck skin is usually spared. Extensive oral erosions are notable	Hematologic malignancies
Porphyria cutanea tarda	Vesicles and bullae with subsequent scarring, skin fragility on the dorsal hands, milia formation, and hypertrichosis on sun-exposed surfaces	Hepatocellular carcinoma, hematologic malignancies, myelodysplastic syndromes
Sweet syndrome—atypical bullous pyoderma gangrenosum overlap	Indurated erythematous to violaceous plaques with or without bulla formation and ulceration	Hematologic malignancies, myeloproliferative disorders
Sign of Leser–Trélat	Eruptive multiple seborrheic keratoses	Adenocarcinomas of the lung and gastrointestinal tract

Abbreviations: ACTH, Adrenocorticotropic hormone.

[a] From Rigel DS, Jacobs MI. Malignant acanthosis nigricans: a review. *J Dermatol Surg Oncol.* 1980;6(11):923–927.

[b] From Arregui MA, Raton JA, Landa N, et al. Bazex's syndrome (acrokeratosis paraneoplastica)—first case report of association with a bladder carcinoma. *Clin Exp Dermatol.* 1993;18(5):445–448.

CARDIOLOGY

Kawasaki Syndrome

Kawasaki syndrome, also known as *mucocutaneous lymph node syndrome*, is a self-limited acute vasculitis of childhood. It has a propensity for coronary artery involvement with aneurysms, angina pectoris, or myocardial infarction in up to 18% to 23% of untreated cases. With proper treatment, the percentage of coronary artery aneurysms decreases to 4% to 8%. It is most commonly seen in children under age 5, with a slight female preponderance. The criteria for diagnosing Kawasaki syndrome includes fever lasting at least 5 days, nonsuppurative cervical adenopathy, bilateral nonpurulent conjunctival injection, reddening and fissuring of the lips, "strawberry tongue," and several cutaneous findings.

The skin changes begin with erythema of the palms and soles that may spread to the trunk. Then the syndrome progresses with the presence of an indurative edema and desquamation starting on the tips of the fingers and toes and around the nails. A polymorphous rash that can vary from morbilliform to scarlatiniform may also be present. Although many forms of treatments have been proposed, aspirin and intravenous immunoglobulins (IVIG) are used as standard therapies.

LEOPARD Syndrome

Multiple lentigines syndrome is an autosomal dominant disorder with abnormalities of various clinical expressions. LEOPARD is an acronym for the following abnormalities that may be present in an individual patient with this syndrome:

- *Lentigines:* Multiple lentigines are present at birth and may cover the entire body, including the palms and soles but sparing the lips and oral mucosa. The pigment can be seen in the iris and retina as well
- *Electrocardiogram conduction defects*
- *Ocular hypertelorism*
- *Pulmonary stenosis*
- *Abnormalities of the genitalia*
- *Retardation of growth*
- *Deafness (sensorineural)*

As much as 85% of the affected patients are found to have a missense mutation in PTPN11. More recently, missense mutations in RAF1 were detected in patients who are PTPN11-negative.

Pseudoxanthoma Elasticum

Pseudoxanthoma elasticum is a genetic connective tissue disease characterized by progressive mineralization of elastic fibers with cutaneous, cardiovascular, and ophthalmologic complications. Several loss-of-function mutations in the *ABCC6* gene are largely responsible for the pathomechanisms of this disease. The disease manifests as angioid streaks of the retina, retinal and gastrointestinal hemorrhages, hypertension, and occlusive vascular disease secondary to progressive calcification and fragmentation of the elastic fibers in the eye and blood vessels. Characteristic yellowish papules that appear like a "plucked chicken" are seen in the flexural areas of the neck, periumbilical areas, as well as the oral, vaginal, and rectal mucosa. Currently, no effective treatment is available for the connective tissue mineralization, although therapies, such as low calcium diet, phosphate binders, and surgery for cosmetic improvement of the skin manifestations, have been documented.

ENDOCRINOLOGY

Diabetes Mellitus

Cutaneous manifestations associated with diabetes mellitus may correlate with metabolic derangements or may present as chronic degenerative changes with no apparent correlation with the degree of hyperglycemia. Metabolic changes in patients with poorly controlled diabetes tend to lead to a higher risk for the development of cutaneous infections by bacterial, fungal, and yeast pathogens. Diabetic dermopathy (atrophic, circumscribed, brownish plaques on the pretibial surfaces; Fig. 42-3) or bullous diabeticorum (spontaneous development of bullae on the extremities) can be seen as a result of chronic degenerative changes. Peripheral neuropathy, further compounded by vascular compromise, may eventuate in neuropathic foot ulcers (Fig. 42-4).

Necrobiosis lipoidica (NL) is seen in less than 1% of diabetics, but the majority of patients with NL have diabetes mellitus (Fig. 42-5). One-third of patients will have diabetes when NL is diagnosed, and one-third will develop diabetes. Gestational and corticosteroid diabetes are also more common if NL is present. When diabetes is diagnosed, the term NLD (necrobiosis lipoidica diabeticorum) is used. NL begins as sharply circumscribed, dusky-red nodules or papules located most commonly on the anterior and lateral surfaces of the lower extremities. The lesions expand to form atrophic, waxy, yellowish, telangiectatic plaques with active brawny borders. The plaques occasionally ulcerate, and squamous cell carcinoma has been reported to arise in the area of NL as a nonhealing ulcer.

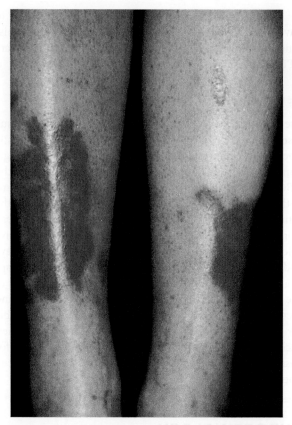

FIGURE 42-3: Diabetic dermopathy with atrophic areas seen on right leg just above the NLD and a little higher up on the left leg. (Courtesy of Smith Kline & French Laboratories.)

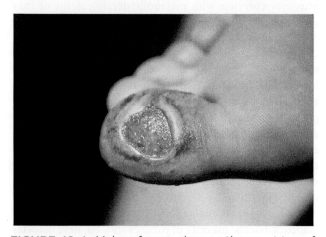

FIGURE 42-4: Mal perforans ulcer on the great toe of a diabetic man.

DISORDERS OF THE HYPOTHALAMIC-PITUITARY-ADRENAL AXIS

Cushing syndrome of glucocorticoid excess is caused by either endogenous overproduction of corticosteroids by the adrenal glands or by iatrogenically administered steroids, whereas Cushing disease is caused by an adrenocorticotropic hormone–secreting anterior pituitary or nonpituitary neoplasm. The most profound cutaneous manifestations of

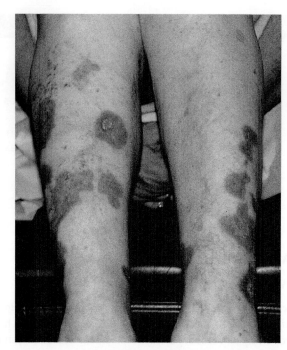

FIGURE 42-5: Necrobiosis lipoidica.

Cushing syndrome (and disease) include epidermal atrophy, striae, plethoric moon facies, buffalo hump, supraclavicular fat pads, and central obesity. There is a marked susceptibility to cutaneous fungal infections. The following findings may be observed in Cushing syndrome:

- Addisonian hyperpigmentation
- Precocious puberty
- Virilization
- Pattern alopecia in females

Patients with Addison disease, or primary adrenocortical insufficiency, suffer from a deficiency of glucocorticoids as well as mineralocorticoids. There is a hyperpigmentation of sun-exposed surfaces, flexural areas, pressure points, scars, and palmar creases (Fig. 42-6). Women may experience loss of axillary and pubic hair.

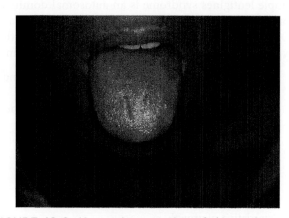

FIGURE 42-6: Hyperpigmentation of skin and tongue in a white woman with Addison disease.

Multiple Mucosal Neuroma Syndrome

Multiple mucosal neuroma syndrome is also known as *multiple endocrine neoplasia IIB* (MEN IIB). In this autosomal dominant disorder, medullary thyroid carcinoma (MTC) and pheochromocytoma are associated with oral, nasal, upper gastrointestinal tract, and conjunctival neuromas. A mutation in the germline activating RET proto-oncogene is responsible for MEN IIB in the majority of patients, although other RET mutations also cause MEN IIA. Screening for this mutation can detect disease predisposition in patients during the preclinical stage. The skin lesions typically range from soft to firm intradermal nodules that can precede or, occasionally, follow the MTC. Additional skin findings include "blubbery" lips, lentigines, café-au-lait macules, and localized intense unilateral pruritus on the back (notalgia paresthetica).

Thyroid Disease

The activity of the thyroid gland is intimately reflected by changes in the skin and its appendages. In hyperthyroidism, the skin is thin, warm, moist, and flushed secondary to vasodilation of the dermal vasculature. Erythema and hyperhidrosis of the palms and soles may be present. Adnexal changes include rapidly growing, fine, soft hair with attendant nonscarring alopecia and soft nails with distal onycholysis. Graves disease is associated with ophthalmopathy (proptosis, exophthalmos, and lid lag), thyroid dermopathy (pretibial myxedema), and acropachy.

In hypothyroidism, the skin is cold, dry, and pale secondary to vasoconstriction of the cutaneous vessels (Fig. 42-7). There is a generalized thinning and hyperkeratosis of the epidermis. Fine wrinkling and a yellow discoloration of the skin are also sometimes present. The hair is coarse, dry, brittle, and slow growing. Patchy or diffuse alopecia may be seen. Loss of the outer third of the eyebrow (madarosis) is a characteristic finding. Madarosis, however, can also be seen in other diseases including leprosy. Myxedema may be generalized in its distribution. Hypothyroid facies is typically expressionless, with thickening of the lips, broadening of the nose, drooping of the upper eyelids, and overall puffiness.

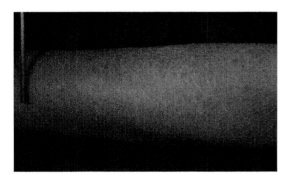

FIGURE 42-7: Year-round dry skin associated with hypothyroidism. (Courtesy of Reed and Carnick.)

GASTROENTEROLOGY

Dermatitis Herpetiformis

Also known as Duhring disease, dermatitis herpetiformis manifests as grouped (herpetiform) vesicles on the buttocks, elbows, and knees. Dermatitis herpetiformis is associated with celiac sprue (gluten-sensitive enteropathy), which can be confirmed by jejunal biopsy. Dermatitis herpetiformis should be suspected in children presenting with recalcitrant eczema or individuals with recalcitrant pruritus and ill-defined dermatoses. A gluten-free diet is the only documented treatment that can lead to complete resolution, although dapsone, an antibacterial agent, can provide symptomatic relief if tolerated by patients. Dapsone should be given with cimetidine to prevent anemia.

Inflammatory Bowel Disease

Ulcerative colitis is most commonly associated with pyoderma gangrenosum, a destructive neutrophilic dermatosis (Fig. 42-8). In pyoderma gangrenosum, a painful violaceous nodule or pustule breaks down to form an enlarging ulcer with a raised, undetermined border and a boggy, necrotic base. Pyoderma gangrenosum has also been observed with Crohn disease as well as hematologic malignancies, monoclonal gammopathies (notably IgA), and various arthritides.

Peutz–Jeghers Syndrome

Peutz–Jeghers syndrome (PJS) is an autosomal dominant disorder characterized by hamartomatous gastrointestinal polyposis and mucocutaneous pigmentation. Up to 145 mutations in the serine threonine kinase (STK11) that lead to a truncated protein and subsequent clinical manifestations have been documented in patients with PJS. Patients may present with abdominal pain, rectal bleeding, rectal prolapse, or intussusception. There is an increased risk of gastrointestinal tumors, ovarian and breast malignancies in females, and Sertoli cell tumors in males. Lentigines may be present at birth or develop in early childhood, with the palmar and plantar areas being the most common sites. Discrete brown, blue, or blue-brown macules are almost always located on the lips and oral mucosa, especially on buccal surfaces. Lentigines may also appear on the nail beds, hands, and feet, especially on palmar and plantar areas. With age, the cutaneous lesions may fade and even disappear, but the buccal mucosal lesions tend to persist into adulthood.

HEMATOLOGY-ONCOLOGY

Although cutaneous manifestations of systemic neoplastic disorders are diverse and often nonspecific, a practitioner must be vigilant for warning signs that warrant further investigation. For example, a patient presenting to a doctor with generalized pruritus may trigger a workup for underlying malignancy. Criteria of association pioneered by Curth and later expanded by Hill (Table 42-2) are applied to determine whether any given malignancy and dermatologic condition are correlated.

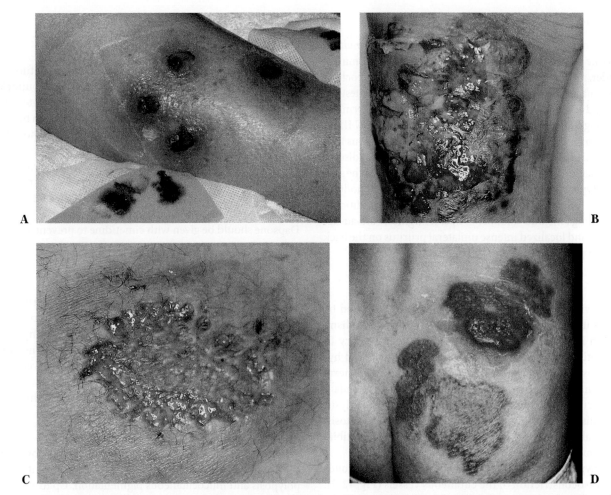

FIGURE 42-8: Pyoderma gangrenosum associated with ulcerative colitis. (Part D courtesy of Schering Corp.)

TABLE 42-2 • Criteria for Establishing Relationship Between Dermatosis and Internal Malignancy. (Curth's Criteria With Modifications Noted.)

- Both conditions develop at about the same time.
- Both conditions follow a parallel course.
- In certain syndromes, the course and onset of the dermatosis do not depend on the course and onset of the malignancy (and vice versa) because the two conditions are part of a genetic syndrome and they are coordinated with one another. Modified: Now classified as genodermatoses with malignant potential.
- A specific tumor occurs in connection with a certain dermatosis.[a]
- The dermatosis is usually uncommon.[a]
- The two conditions are strongly associated.[a]

Note: Curth's Criteria with modifications noted.
[a]These criteria are not essential for a mucocutaneous condition to be considered a paraneoplastic syndrome.
Source: From Cohen PR. Cutaneous paraneoplastic syndromes. *Am Fam Physician.* 1994;50(6):1273–1282.

Examples of these associations include the following: Acquired ichthyosis (Fig. 42-9), which clinically appears as severely dry skin, is most often associated with lymphoproliferative disorders and other malignancies, including

- Hodgkin disease
- Mycosis fungoides
- Multiple myeloma
- Kaposi sarcoma
- Leiomyosarcomas
- Breast, cervical, and lung cancers

Erythroderma is a diffuse erythema of the skin, usually accompanied by induration and scaling. When scaling is diffuse, the condition is diagnosed as an exfoliative erythroderma. Erythrodermas are seen more commonly with hematologic malignancies, especially leukemia, lymphoma, and Sézary syndrome.

Acanthosis nigricans (AN) presents as hyperpigmented, velvety skin in flexural areas (Fig. 42-10). "Benign" forms are generally seen in obese patients or associated with endocrinopathies such as hyperandrogenism and insulin resistance as well as diabetes mellitus and the polycystic ovarian syndrome. AN

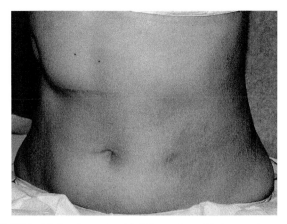

FIGURE 42-9: Acquired ichthyosis, which can be a sign of lymphoproliferative disorders.

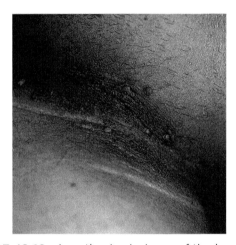

FIGURE 42-10: Acanthosis nigricans of the base of the neck.

is also observed in a number of genetic disorders. Occasionally, AN is induced by systemically administered corticosteroids, somatotropin, nicotinic acid, and insulin. AN in metabolic disturbances appears to be related to insulin and insulinlike growth factor (IGF) and their interaction with corresponding keratinocytic receptors (IGFR-1), and it is likely to be a reflection of insulin resistance.

"Malignant" AN is suspected in thin, older individuals with extensive involvement of the mucocutaneous integument. These gray-brown, symmetric, velvety, papillomatous plaques involve the axillae, neck, groin, antecubital fossae, vermilion border of the lip, and eyelids. Mucosal AN presents with verrucous pigmented plaques on the oral mucosa and conjunctivae, and is especially suggestive of a neoplastic process. Association with rugated, velvety plaques of palmar surfaces (tripe palms) is observed. This variant of AN is most often associated with lung, ovarian, breast, gastric, bladder, and endometrial carcinomas.

Necrolytic migratory erythema (NME) is an integral part of a paraneoplastic syndrome observed in the context of glucagonoma (a neuroendocrine pancreatic tumor). Although no longer considered pathognomonic of glucagonoma, NME

accompanied by the new onset of diabetes, weight loss, glossitis, and angular cheilitis may be observed in a majority of patients with a glucagonoma. NME frequently presents as an annular psoriasiform eruption in an acral distribution affecting the central face, extremities, and groin. The lesions tend to have a waxing and waning course, healing without scarring. The NME course does not reflect the activity of the underlying tumor.

The classical paraneoplastic rheumatologic syndrome is dermatomyositis. Although malignancy-associated and nonparaneoplastic rheumatologic disturbances can present similarly, there are certain laboratory and clinical findings that may suggest malignancy in otherwise typical cases. Rapid onset, cutaneous necrosis, extensive vasculitis, and a history of malignancy are all likely predictors of a concurrent neoplasm. Rheumatic symptoms and primary tumors may follow parallel clinical courses. Dermatologic manifestations of some lymphoproliferative disorders are shown in Fig. 42-11.

INFECTIOUS DISEASES

> ### SAUER'S NOTES
>
> Hepatitis C behaves as an autoimmune disease as well as an infection. Evidence of this is pruritus, cryoglobulinemia, necrolytic acral erythema, porphyria cutanea tarda, cryoglobulinemia (purpura, arthralgias, and weakness), urticaria, sicca syndrome, paresthesias, and vasculitis. Positive serologies include anti-nuclear antibody (ANA) and positive smooth muscle antibodies. Recent treatments have given us a cure in almost all cases.

Hepatitis C

Skin conditions can often be the first indication of the patient's underlying hepatitis C infection. The more common manifestations include generalized pruritus, mixed cryoglobulinemia, necrolytic acral erythema, porphyria cutanea tarda (PCT), and lichen planus.

Generalized pruritus is a presenting symptom that raises flags for many underlying diseases. It is seen in about 20% of patients with hepatitis C and can be associated with nonspecific lesions such as prurigo nodules or excoriations.

Mixed cryoglobulinemia (types II and III) is a disorder of monoclonal or polyclonal immunoglobulins that reversibly precipitate at low temperatures. Hepatitis C infection is thought to cause an immune dysregulation that leads to the development of cryoglobulinemia. The classic presentation is a triad of purpura, arthralgias, and weakness. Palpable purpura appears in crops on the lower extremities, lasting 3 to 10 days, and is thought to be secondary to deposition of immune complexes in the vessels. Livedo reticularis, a netlike pattern of reddish-blue discoloration with central pallor, ischemic ulcers, acrocyanosis, and hemorrhagic bullae are also seen with mixed cryoglobulinemia.

Although rare, necrolytic acral erythema is a pathognomonic complication of hepatitis C infection. Well-circumscribed, annular, hyperkeratotic, violaceous plaques with raised scaly

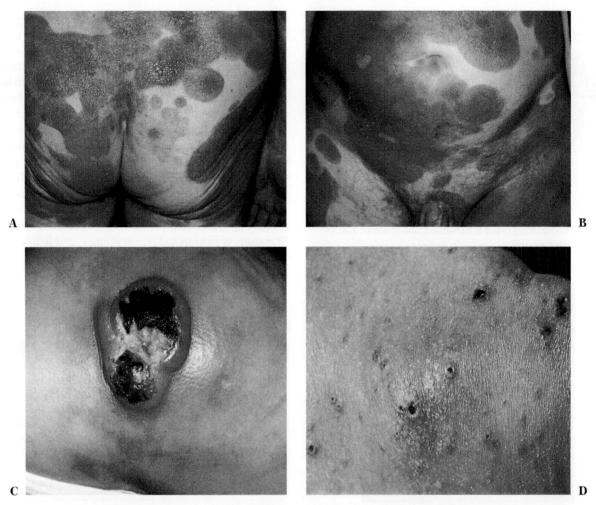

FIGURE 42-11: Dermatoses associated with lymphomas. Mycosis fungoides in plaque stage of the buttocks **(A)** and abdomen **(B)** of a 79-year-old man. **C:** Mycosis fungoides in tumor stage on the thigh. **D:** Nonspecific pyoderma with lymphocytic leukemia.

borders or vesiculobullous lesions appear on acral surfaces. Patients report burning and pruritus associated with the lesions.

Lichen planus may also be seen in association with hepatitis C, especially in patients from southern Europe and Japan. Oral and genital mucosal lesions begin as white, lacy papules; they may become erosive and are more commonly associated with hepatitis C than the cutaneous form. Cutaneous lichen planus is characterized by pruritic, purple, polygonal papules with an overlying reticulate pattern of white lines called Wickham striae. These lesions are typically distributed over the flexor surfaces of the wrists and forearms, dorsal hands, the anterior aspect of the lower legs, the presacral area, and the neck.

Human Immunodeficiency Virus

Untreated human immunodeficiency virus (HIV) infection may be associated with a host of dermatologic disorders and an increased risk of malignancies. With the advent of increased routine HIV screening and the institution of antiretroviral therapy, the incidence of dermatologic diseases associated with terminal HIV infection has decreased significantly. A full discussion of cutaneous diseases associated with HIV is presented in Chapter 27.

Lyme Disease (See more information in bacteria chapter)

Lyme borreliosis is a spirochetal, multisystem illness borne by *Ixodes* spp. (ticks). It is prevalent in the Northeastern, North Central, and Pacific coastal regions in the United States. *Borrelia burgdorferi* is the most commonly isolated causative organism in the United States, whereas in European countries, *B. afzelii* and *B. garinii* predominate. Erythema chronicum migrans (ECM) is pathognomonic for new-onset Lyme disease (Fig. 42-12). Early lesions display homogeneous erythema at the site of the tick bite that subsequently spreads centrifugally. In North America, this lesion is less likely to show central clearing. However, in Europe, the center of the lesion may fade or clear completely, leaving an annular, expanding erythema. ECM usually presents with a single lesion. Although ECM is by far the most common Lyme-associated dermatosis in the United States and Europe, other cutaneous disorders such as borrelial lymphocytoma (BL) and acrodermatitis chronica atrophicans (ACA) are observed more frequently in Europe. BL, also known as *lymphadenosis benigna cutis,* is usually noted at or near the tick bite site. Typically, BL presents as a solitary

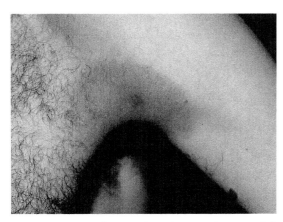

FIGURE 42-12: Erythema chronicum migrans of the axilla.

bluish-red nodule with regional lymphadenopathy commonly on the earlobe, nipple and areola, scrotum, and nose. Patients with BL may present with or without preceding or concomitant ECM. Late Lyme disease may be associated with ACA, a chronic acral dermatitis that develops 6 months to 10 years after the initial arthropod assault. ACA has been found to be caused exclusively by *B. afzelii*. The onset is insidious, with waxing and waning edema and a reddish-blue discoloration of distal extremities, reminiscent of venous insufficiency. With time, the epidermis and dermis become atrophic and translucent. Late findings include fibrotic bands and nodule formation.

Of note, a Lyme disease mimic known as southern tick–associated rash illness (STARI) is an emerging entity in the United States. Although the etiology is still under investigation, physicians need to be aware of this clinical presentation when diagnosing and testing suspected cases, especially in areas that are not endemic for Lyme disease.

Syphilis

> **SAUER'S NOTES**
>
> Syphilis remains the great mimic, and worldwide incidence is once again on the increase.

With its incidence on the rise and its increasing prevalence coincident with HIV infection, syphilis has reemerged as an important treponemal disease. Syphilis (lues) is caused by the spirochete *Treponema pallidum*. The mode of acquisition (sexual vs. vertical) and stage determine cutaneous and systemic manifestations. Cutaneous manifestations of syphilis are addressed in detail in Chapter 25. Briefly, lesions of primary syphilis present as a syphilitic chancre—a firm, painless, eroded plaque at the site of treponemal entry. Often, syphilitic chancres are unrecognized as such because of their perianal, anal, intravaginal, or oral locations. They heal spontaneously without treatments. If the chancre is coinfected with other sexually transmitted agents, the presentation may be atypical.

Approximately one-third of patients with untreated primary syphilis progress to secondary syphilis. More than 80%

of these patients develop generalized cutaneous eruptions—syphilids that vary widely in their presentations including macular, maculopapular, papular, annular, and, less frequently, nodular and pustular lesions (Fig. 42-13). Condyloma lata are pathognomonic, patchy alopecia is rare, and mucous membrane lesions may be seen. Mucous patches are especially common on the tongue and lips. These lesions are highly infectious.

Nearly one-third of untreated patients develop tertiary syphilis, which also presents with polymorphous lesions. Gummas are painless, pink to dusky-red nodules that can ulcerate and cause local tissue destruction. They are often seen in the skin and can also involve visceral organs and skeletal structures. Neurosyphilis and cardiovascular syphilis each affect 25% of patients with tertiary syphilis.

Presenting signs and symptoms of cerebrovascular syphilis range from the Argyll Robertson pupil that accommodates and converges but does not react to light, blindness, deafness, and dementia. Tabes dorsalis is the degeneration of the posterior columns of the spinal cord leading to lancinating pain, ataxia, urinary incontinence, and loss of proprioception with resultant joint deterioration (Charcot joints). Cardiovascular syphilis leads to a spectrum of manifestations: uncomplicated aortitis, aortic aneurysm (usually affecting the ascending aorta), aortic valvulitis with aortic insufficiency, coronary artery ostial stenosis, and myocarditis. Interestingly, early atherosclerosis in individuals with no known risk factors has been associated with tertiary syphilis.

Congenital syphilis tends to present soon after birth. However, a delay in presentation of up to 2 years may occur. Early manifestations are remarkably similar to syphilids in adults. In neonates, pemphigus syphiliticus with vesiculobullous lesions of the palms and soles, as well as other areas, has been described. Classically, syphilitic rhinitis (snuffles) is one of the more frequent specific signs of congenital syphilis. Mucosanguineous discharge with attendant nasal obstruction

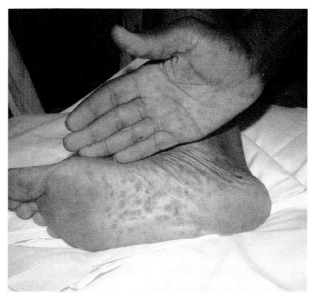

FIGURE 42-13: Ham-colored, scaly papules of the palm and sole in secondary syphilis.

is present early in the disease; saddle nose deformity with septal perforation and perioral rhagades are stigmata of late congenital syphilis. Hutchinson triad of congenital syphilis consists of Hutchinson teeth (notched incisors), interstitial keratitis, and sensorineural deafness. Other important signs include bone lesions (saddle nose deformity, epiphysitis with resultant pain on motion—Parrot pseudoparalysis), Higoumenakis sign (unilateral clavicular thickening lateral to the patient's dexterity), neurosyphilis (seizures, hydrocephalus, cranial nerve palsies, tabes dorsalis), lymphadenopathy, and hepatosplenomegaly.

NEPHROLOGY

Acquired Perforating Disease

Acquired perforating disease (APD) of end-stage renal disease presents as a clinical aggregate of three primary perforating disorders:

- Kyrle disease
- Reactive perforating collagenosis
- Perforating folliculitis

APD has also been associated with patients on dialysis. As with primary perforating disorders, an alteration in connective tissue (collagen or elastin) and transepithelial elimination have been implicated in the pathophysiology of APD. The lesions appear clinically as dome-shaped papules with keratotic plugs on the trunk and extensor extremities. Severe pruritus may accompany cutaneous eruption of APD. Koebnerization is frequently observed.

Calcinosis Cutis and Calciphylaxis

Abnormal calcium and phosphate metabolism with subsequent secondary hyperparathyroidism predisposes patients with renal disease to metastatic calcifications. Calcinosis cutis frequently affects periarticular soft tissues. Discrete, mobile, skin-colored subcutaneous nodules are tender when present on the digits, and may be productive of pasty or chalky contents. Calciphylaxis is a systemic vascular disease with mural calcification of small- and medium-sized arteries and is associated with a high mortality rate. Typical lesions are exquisitely tender, poorly defined, deep subcutaneous nodules and plaques with overlying livedoid purpura of proximal thighs and buttocks. Stellate ulcerations may be accompanied by marked cutaneous necrosis. The medical treatments focus mainly on normalizing hypercalcemia and hyperphosphatemia. Of these treatments, cinacalcet acts as a calcimimetic for secondary hyperparathyroidism, and sodium thiosulfate serves as a chelating agent in tissue calcifications.

Chronic Renal Failure and Dialysis

Several cutaneous changes are particularly prevalent in patients on dialysis. Generalized pruritus without a primary cutaneous eruption could be a sign of various underlying disorders, including uremia or chronic renal failure. Dialysis seems to be an important trigger of pruritus. Although rare, uremic frost can be seen as white, crystalline precipitation on the skin. Pallor of the proximal nail bed, known as Lindsay nail (half-and-half nail), may be observed in azotemic patients.

Henoch–Schönlein Purpura

Henoch–Schönlein purpura is an immunoglobulin (Ig) A–mediated systemic leukocytoclastic vasculitis of small vessels that typically affects the skin, joints, gastrointestinal tract, and kidneys (see Chapter 13). Clinically, pediatric patients present with the classic tetrad of abdominal pain, polyarthritis, nephritis, and a purpuric eruption. Palpable purpura, typically of the lower legs and buttocks, occurs in almost every case and is the presenting sign in more than 50% of cases. Petechiae and ecchymoses may also be present. Urticarial and erythematous maculopapular lesions preceding the purpura have been described. A characteristic finding in children is painful edema of the face, scalp, ears, periorbital region, extremities, and genitalia. Scrotal edema and bruising are observed in up to one-third of male patients. Rare cases of penile edema and purpura involving the glans penis have been reported.

Fabry Disease (also called Anderson-Fabry Disease)

Fabry disease is an X-linked recessive defect in the activity of a lysosomal enzyme, α-galactosidase A, causing accumulation of glycosphingolipids in tissues. The glycosphingolipid deposits primarily affect the vascular endothelium, which leads to cardiovascular, cerebral, and renal manifestations. Cutaneous findings give rise to vascular lesions known as angiokeratoma corporis diffusum universale, which appears in childhood and may be one of the earliest signs of the disease. These are nonblanchable, punctate, red to blue-black keratotic papules with slight hyperkeratosis in the larger lesions. Angiokeratomas, with time, increase in size and number. Lesions are mostly located between the umbilicus and the knees and are usually symmetrically distributed. Acroparesthesias and hypohidrosis with resultant heat intolerance have been described. Enzyme replacement therapy is the standard of treatment and has been shown to decrease both organ dysfunction and cutaneous manifestations.

Nephrogenic Systemic Fibrosis

Owing to the identification of gadolinium as a presumptive cause, the incidence of nephrogenic systemic fibrosis (NSF), formerly nephrogenic sclerosing (fibrosing) dermopathy, has significantly declined in patients with renal insufficiency. NSF occurs equally in males and females without ethnic predilection. Clinically, patients initially present with erythematous papules as well as a peau d'orange appearance of distal extremities. These primary lesions coalesce into woody, sclerodermoid, red-brawny plaques with an edge that advances proximally. Dependent areas are more severely involved. There is accompanying pruritus, burning, and lancinating pain. A marked decrease in the affected joints' range of motion may progress to joint contractures, thereby incapacitating patients. Systemic involvement with extensive calcifications and fibrosis of vital structures has been reported. The disease course closely parallels that of renal function. Patients may or may not require hemodialysis.

Porphyria Cutanea Tarda

PCT is a photosensitivity disorder and can be familial. It can be associated with renal disease as well as with hepatitis C and hemochromatosis. The renal disease variant is most often of the sporadic type. Clinical and laboratory findings are analogous to those of the inherited form of PCT, with photodistributed tense bullae that tend to rupture and heal with scars and milia. Hypertrichosis and hyperpigmentation are common. Pseudoporphyria, a bullous dermatosis clinically similar to PCT, has been described in patients on chronic hemodialysis or those taking one of several medications that have been reported to cause the condition. Patients with pseudoporphyria lack abnormal porphyrin levels and do not exhibit either hypertrichosis or sclerodermoid changes.

PULMONARY

Atopic Dermatitis

Asthma, penicillin allergy, urticaria, marked reaction to insect bites, multiple food allergies, allergic rhinitis, and conjunctivitis have all been associated with atopic dermatitis (see Chapter 11). These disorders may occur concomitantly or independently, and most patients develop only one or two components of an atopic diathesis. Several genetically inherited cutaneous disorders include atopic dermatitis as an integral part of the syndrome. Netherton syndrome is an autosomal recessive genodermatosis characterized by pathognomonic erythematous patches with a double-edged scale termed *ichthyosis linearis circumflexa,* a "ball-and-socket" hair deformity (trichorrhexis invaginata), and atopic dermatitis. Other diseases associated with atopic dermatitis include ichthyosis vulgaris and the Wiskott–Aldrich syndrome. Phenylketonuria has also been associated with a type of skin disease similar to atopic dermatitis. The association between atopic dermatitis and CD30$^+$ cutaneous lymphoma has been documented, although the causal relationship remains uncertain.

Adequate skin care and the use of moisturizer are strongly recommended, and pharmacologic therapies are suggested if conservative measures fail. Topical corticosteroid is the mainstay anti-inflammatory, as well as maintenance, treatment. Other topical treatments include calcineurin inhibitors (tacrolimus and pimecrolimus). A novel human monoclonal antibody (dupilumab) has been shown to be effective in treating atopic dermatitis. Another monoclonal antibody (omalizumab) can also be used effectively (anecdotal experience of editor JH).

Sarcoidosis

Sarcoidosis is a granulomatous process affecting various organ systems (see Chapter 18). The most characteristic cutaneous

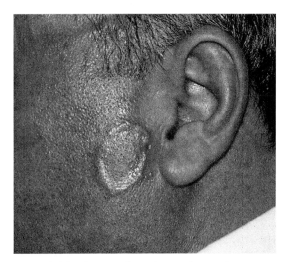

FIGURE 42-14: A granulomatous plaque in a man with sarcoidosis.

sarcoidal lesion is lupus pernio. Lesions of lupus pernio consist of chronic, reddish-brown to violaceous, indurated papules and plaques with a predilection for the nose, ears, and lips (Fig. 42-14). They can also present on the limbs, back, and buttocks. These plaques may have central atrophy or a hypopigmented appearance. Erythema nodosum is the most common nonspecific cutaneous manifestation of sarcoidosis. It is a hypersensitivity reaction to various agents, appearing clinically as tender, erythematous, subcutaneous nodules predominantly on the anterior shins. Löfgren syndrome presents with erythema nodosum, fever, hilar adenopathy, and polyarthralgia. Lupus pernio is more frequent in African American patients; erythema nodosum is commonly found in European and Latin American patients. Heerfordt syndrome is a manifestation of acute sarcoidosis and presents with fever, uveitis, parotitis, and Bell's palsy. Although rare in the general population, this syndrome has been most often reported in young Japanese female patients. Koebnerization of sarcoidal lesions is observed. Uncommon manifestations such as leonine facies, psoriasiform or lichenoid plaques, and pyoderma gangrenosum have been reported. Other nonspecific skin findings include scarring and nonscarring alopecia, hypopigmented patches, erythroderma, erythema multiforme, acquired ichthyosis, and dystrophic calcifications.

NEUROLOGY

Neurofibromatosis

Neurofibromatosis (NF) is an autosomal dominant genodermatosis (see Chapter 44). There are two subtypes of NF: Recklinghausen disease (NF-1) and bilateral acoustic neurofibromatosis (NF-2). NF-1 is caused by a mutation in the *NF1* gene on chromosome 17, whereas NF-2 is caused by a mutation in the *NF2* gene on chromosome 22. Both types involve congenital and acquired hamartomatous tumors of the central nervous system (CNS), skin, bone, endocrine glands, and eyes. Café-au-lait macules develop shortly after birth and may be found anywhere on the body. These hyperpigmented lesions can be found in normal individuals, but the presence of six or more macules 1.5 cm or greater in adults (≥0.5 cm in children) is highly suggestive of NF. Intertriginous freckling (Crowe sign) and pigmented hamartomas of the iris (Lisch nodules) are virtually diagnostic of NF. The principal dermatologic manifestations of this disease are cutaneous, subcutaneous, or plexiform neurofibromas (Fig. 42-15). Less common features include total or partial limb enlargement (elephantiasis neuromatosa), multiple lipomas, or a cutaneous sclerosing perineurioma. Recent reports suggest an association with nevus anemicus. Segmental involvement with either NF subtype may represent a postzygotic mutation.

Sturge–Weber Syndrome

Recent studies have shown that the capillary malformation (port-wine stain, or nevus flammeus) in this neurocutaneous syndrome appears to follow the pattern of embryonic vasculature, instead of the distribution of the ophthalmic division of the trigeminal nerve. A somatic mutation in the *GNAQ* gene is consistently detected in affected individuals. Typically, the cutaneous involvement precedes the cerebral involvement, which appears later in childhood as a contralateral spastic

hemiparesis, unilateral seizures, hemisensory defects, mental retardation, glaucoma, and homonymous hemianopia. Although plain skull x-rays reveal the classic "tram-track" calcifications, these do not appear until later in life. Therefore, either MRI/MRA (magnetic resonance imaging/angiography) or PET (positron emission tomography) scans are better modalities to screen for leptomeningeal angiomatosis and brain involvement.

Tuberous Sclerosis

Tuberous sclerosis is a highly penetrant, genetically heterogeneous, autosomal dominant genodermatosis characterized by the triad of multiple hamartomas, seizures, and developmental difficulties. Hamartomas can involve any organ system, especially the skin, CNS, renal system, and cardiovascular system. Facial angiofibromas (adenoma sebaceum) (Fig. 42-16), Koenen tumors (Fig. 42-17), and fibrous plaques are the major cutaneous findings.

Angiofibromas are pink to red papules appearing after 4 years of age and localizing to the nasolabial folds, cheeks, and chin. Fibrous forehead plaques may present as early as the first weeks of life. The Koenen tumor is an ungual angiofibroma. A later finding appearing during childhood or adolescence is the shagreen patch, a connective tissue hamartoma. It is

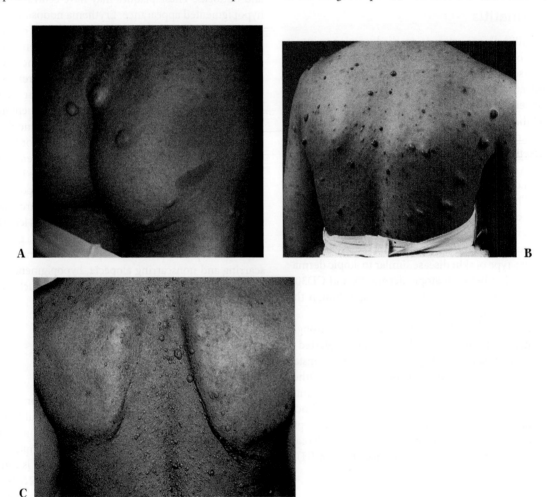

FIGURE 42-15: Neurofibromatosis of the buttocks **(A)**, with café-au-lait lesions on the back **(B and C)**. (Part B courtesy of KUMC; Reed and Carnick.)

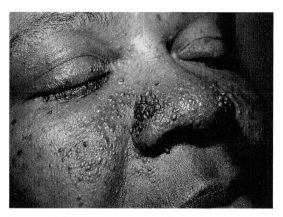

FIGURE 42-16: Angiofibromas (adenoma sebaceum) on the face of a patient with tuberous sclerosis.

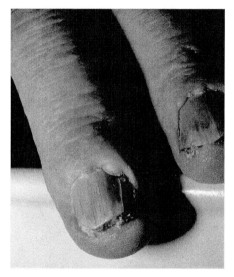

FIGURE 42-17: Periungual fibromas (Koenen tumor) associated with tuberous sclerosis.

characteristically found in the lumbosacral region and appears as a skin-colored, slightly elevated plaque with the texture and appearance of an orange peel. Hypomelanotic macules have been found in up to 90% of patients with tuberous sclerosis. These lesions, typically located on the trunk and limbs, appear before any other skin findings. Their configurations vary from guttate leukodermatous "confetti" macules to lance ovate ash-leaf macules. One or two hypopigmented macules may be seen in normal individuals; when three or more are present, the diagnosis of tuberous sclerosis must be considered. Although the most common renal lesion in tuberous sclerosis is the angiomyolipoma, tuberous sclerosis is associated with an increased risk of renal cancer, specifically clear cell carcinoma. Patients must be radiologically monitored because these tumors are likely to be multifocal, bilateral, and present at a younger age than the general population (30 vs. 60 years of age). Until recently, surgery remained the only effective treatment. However, a growing understanding of the dysregulation of the mTOR pathway has allowed rapamycin, an mTOR inhibitor, to be a potential treatment for these patients.

RHEUMATOLOGY (SEE CHAPTER 41)

Dermatomyositis

Dermatomyositis is a complex autoimmune disease of adults and children that causes progressive muscular inflammation and weakness. Myositis preferentially involves the shoulder and hip girdles, manifesting as difficulty with such activities as combing hair or getting up from a chair. Interstitial lung disease may be a presenting sign of dermatomyositis, with 65% of newly diagnosed patients affected by it. In approximately 15% of patients, dermatomyositis may be complicated by associated malignancies, including cancers of the lung, ovary, and hematopoietic systems.

The cutaneous manifestations are pathognomonic. The most specific skin finding is Gottron papules, which are erythematous papules of distant interphalangeal joints, elbows, and knees. The heliotrope rash, a subtle, erythematous or violaceous blush on the eyelids and periorbital region, is seen in approximately 60% of cases. Erythema may develop on sun-exposed areas, and chronic changes may include poikilodermatous lesions on the trunk and proximal extremities. Periungual telangiectasias and cuticular thromboses may also be observed. Of note, myositis and cutaneous manifestations often have divergent courses in terms of onset, progress, and severity. "Amyopathic" dermatomyositis displays classic cutaneous findings without an associated myopathy. These patients may also be at risk for associated malignancies.

Lupus Erythematosus

Systemic lupus erythematosus (SLE) is an autoimmune connective tissue disease characterized by multiorgan involvement and the presence of autoantibodies to nuclear antigens (see Chapter 41). The stringent diagnostic criteria for SLE were originally set forth by the American College of Rheumatology in 1982 and revised in 1997. The butterfly rash is the sine qua non of an acute SLE eruption (Fig. 42-18), which presents as erythematous to violaceous edematous plaques over the malar

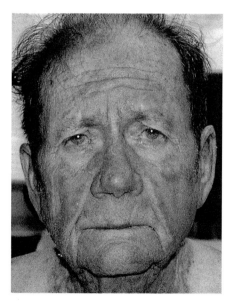

FIGURE 42-18: Butterfly appearance in a patient with SCLE.

cheeks and dorsal nose. The nasolabial folds are typically spared (compared to dermatomyositis, where they are usually involved). As with all SLE cutaneous manifestations, the malar rash typically appears after sun exposure. Other sites of predilection are the V of the chest, extensor extremities, mid-upper back, and shoulders (Fig. 42-19). On rare occasions, the atrophic, hyperpigmented scarring lesions of chronic cutaneous lupus erythematosus (discoid lupus erythematosus) may develop; the annular or papulosquamous lesions of subacute cutaneous lupus erythematosus have a more frequent association with systemic disease than discoid lupus erythematosus. Subacute cutaneous lupus can mimic psoriasis or erythema annulare centrifugum.

The palatal and buccal mucosa may also be affected. The former is involved with honeycombed plaques, hyperemia, and punched-out ulcerations, whereas lichen planus–like lesions appear on the latter. Discoid lesions may be observed on both areas. Panniculitis (lupus profundus), alopecia, livedo reticularis, and periungual telangiectasias are other cutaneous features that may be seen in SLE.

Scleroderma

Systemic scleroderma is a chronic disease of unknown origin that affects the connective tissue and the vasculature. The disease is characterized by fibrosis and obliteration of the vessels in the skin, lungs, heart, gastrointestinal tract, and kidneys (Fig. 42-20). Patients with systemic scleroderma have been shown to be at a higher risk of developing malignancies, particularly lung cancer and hematologic neoplasms. Morphea (localized scleroderma) is only rarely associated with systemic disease (when such lesions are multiple and diffuse).

There are two forms of systemic scleroderma: progressive and limited. Limited systemic scleroderma or CREST syndrome (*c*alcinosis, *R*aynaud phenomenon, *e*sophageal dysmotility, *s*clerodactyly, *t*elangiectasias) predominantly affects the hands and may start as Raynaud phenomenon or nonpitting edema of the hands and fingers (Fig. 42-21). Flexion contractures and sclerodactyly may eventually supervene. Progressive systemic scleroderma may

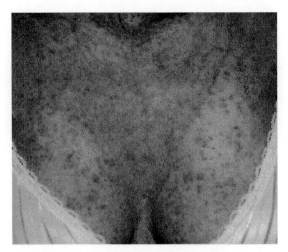
FIGURE 42-20: Hypopigmentation with perifollicular pigment retention and skin tightening of scleroderma.

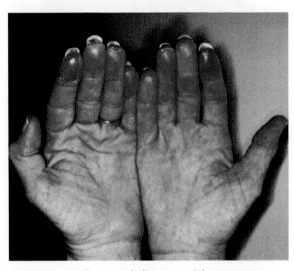
FIGURE 42-21: Raynaud disease with gangrene.

also present with Raynaud phenomenon and, as the name implies, evolve to affect viscera and the skin. The disease slowly extends to involve upper extremities, face, trunk, and possibly the lower extremities. It begins as a painless edema that leads to tightening of the skin. In the final or atrophic stage, the skin becomes taut, smooth, and discolored, being tightly bound to underlying bony structures, with a resultant decrease in range of motion. The face takes on a masklike quality with microstomia, radial furrowing around the mouth, a beaked nose, and an unnaturally youthful countenance. Matlike telangiectasias of the face, palms, and upper trunk, alopecia, and anhidrosis are also seen.

Suggested Readings

Abdelmalek NF, Gerber TL, Menter A. Cardiocutaneous syndromes and associations. *J Am Acad Dermatol.* 2002;46:161–183.
Beck LA, Thaçi D, Hamilton JD, et al. Dupilumab treatment in adults with moderate-to-severe atopic dermatitis. *N Engl J Med.* 2014;371(2):130–139.

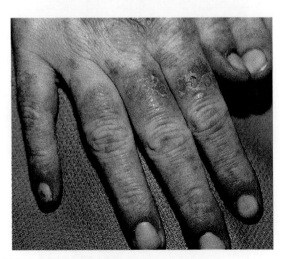
FIGURE 42-19: Sparing of the knuckles in systemic lupus erythematosus (the opposite of dermatomyositis).

Bonifazi M, Tramacere I, Pomponio G, et al. Systemic sclerosis (scleroderma) and cancer risk: systematic review and meta-analysis of observational studies. *Rheumatology (Oxford)*. 2013;52(1):143–154.

Borkowska J, Schwartz RA, Kotulska K, et al. Tuberous sclerosis complex: tumors and tumorigenesis. *Int J Dermatol*. 2011;50(1):13–20.

Bratton RL, Whiteside JW, Hovan MJ, et al. Diagnosis and treatment of Lyme disease. *Mayo Clin Proc*. 2008;83(5):566–571.

Brewster UC. Dermatological disease in patients with CKD. *Am J Kidney Dis*. 2008;51(2):331–344.

Cahill J, Sinclair R. Cutaneous manifestations of systemic disease. *Aust Fam Physician*. 2005;34(5):335–340.

Callen J. *Dermatological Signs of Internal Disease*. 3rd ed. Philadelphia: WB Saunders; 2003.

Centers for Disease Control and Prevention. Lyme disease-United States, 2003–2005. *MMWR Morb Mortal Wkly Rep*. 2007;56(23):573–576.

Dutkiewicz AS, Ezzedine K, Mazereeuw-Hautier J, et al. A prospective study of risk for Sturge-Weber syndrome in children with upper facial port-wine stain. *J Am Acad Dermatol*. 2015;72(3):473–480.

Eichenfield LF, Tom WL, Berger TG, et al. Guidelines of care for the management of atopic dermatitis: section 2. Management and treatment of atopic dermatitis with topical therapies. *J Am Acad Dermatol*. 2014;71(1):116–132.

Greco A, De Virgilio A, Rizzo MI, et al. Kawasaki disease: an evolving paradigm. *Autoimmun Rev*. 2015;14(8):703–709.

Gudi VS, Campbell S, Gould DJ, et al. Squamous cell carcinoma in an area of necrobiosis lipoidica diabeticorum: a case report. *Clin Exp Dermatol*. 2000;25(8):597–599.

Heymann WR, Ellis DL. Borrelia burgdorferi infections in the United States. *J Clin Aesthet Dermatol*. 2012;5(8):18–28.

Hoa M, Slattery WH. Neurofibromatosis 2. *Otolaryngol Clin North Am*. 2012;45(2):315–332, viii.

Holman JD, Dyer JA. Genodermatoses with malignant potential. *Curr Opin Pediatr*. 2007;19(4):446–454.

Ianuzzi MC, Rybicki BA, Teirstein AS. Sarcoidosis. *N Engl J Med*. 2007;357(21):2153–2165.

Kent ME, Romanelli F. Reexamining syphilis: an update on epidemiology, clinical manifestations, and management. *Ann Pharmacother*. 2008;42(2):226–236.

Kirsner RS, Federman DG. Cutaneous clues to systemic disease. *Postgrad Med*. 1997;101:137, 144–147.

Kleyn CE, Lai-Cheong JE, Bell HK. Cutaneous manifestations of internal malignancy: diagnosis and management. *Am J Clin Dermatol*. 2006;7(2):71–84.

Launonen V. Mutations in the human LKB1/STK11 gene. *Hum Mutat*. 2005;26(4):291–297.

Li Q, Jiang Q, Pfendner E, et al. Pseudoxanthoma elasticum: clinical phenotypes, molecular genetics and putative pathomechanisms. *Exp Dermatol*. 2009;18(1):1–11.

Marconi B, Bobyr I, Campanati A, et al. Pseudoxanthoma elasticum and skin: clinical manifestations, histopathology, pathomechanism, perspectives of treatment. *Intractable Rare Dis Res*. 2015;4(3):113–122.

Martucciello G, Lerone M, Bricco L, et al. Multiple endocrine neoplasias type 2B and RET proto-oncogene. *Ital J Pediatr*. 2012;38:9.

Mendes FB, Hissa-Elian A, Abreu MA, et al. Review: dermatitis herpetiformis. *An Bras Dermatol*. 2013;88(4):594–599.

Nakashima M, Miyajima M, Sugano H, et al. The somatic GNAQ mutation c.548G>A (p.R183Q) is consistently found in Sturge-Weber syndrome. *J Hum Genet*. 2014;59(12):691–693.

Ostezan LB, Callen JP. Cutaneous manifestations of selected rheumatologic diseases. *Am Fam Physician*. 1996;53:1625–1633.

Pipkin CA, Lio PA. Cutaneous manifestations of internal malignancies: an overview. *Dermatol Clin*. 2008;26(1):1–15, vii.

Sarkozy A, Digilio MC, Dallapiccola B. Leopard syndrome. *Orphanet J Rare Dis*. 2008;3:13.

Tabor CA, Parlette EC. Cutaneous manifestations of diabetes. Signs of poor glycemic control or new-onset disease. *Postgrad Med*. 2006;119(3):38–44.

Varela CU, Prieto-Rayo JC. Causal relationship between the use of gadolinium based contrast media and nephrogenic systemic fibrosis [in Spanish]. *Rev Med Chil*. 2014;142(12):1565–1574.

Wohlrab J, Wohlrab D, Meiss F. Skin diseases in diabetes mellitus. *J Dtsch Dermatol Ges*. 2007;5(1):37–53.

Wollina U. Update on cutaneous calciphylaxis. *Indian J Dermatol*. 2013;58(2): '87–92.

Yell JA, Mbuagbaw J, Burge SM. Cutaneous manifestations of systemic lupus erythematosus. *Br J Dermatol*. 1996;135(3):355–362.

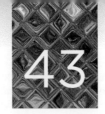

Dermatologic Reactions to Ultraviolet, Visible Light, and Infrared Radiation

Laurie L. Kohen, MD, James L. Griffith, MD, and Henry W. Lim, MD

SOLAR RADIATION

Although the sun emits nearly all of the electromagnetic spectrum, transmission of sunlight to the earth's surface is primarily limited to ultraviolet (UV), visible light (VL), and infrared radiation (IR). In recent years, each of these spectral bands has been found to induce clinically-relevant photobiologic effects, such as development of erythema, photoaging, malignancy, pigmentation, and photodermatoses. Molecularly, these photobiologic effects vary from direct or indirect alteration of chemical bonds to thermal and/or mechanical destruction based on the wavelength's energy, depth of penetration, and molecular target. Thus, in order to prevent or mitigate these photo-induced effects, it is important to be aware of the photobiologic properties of solar spectrums and the photodermatoses associated with each of these bands.

Ultraviolet Radiation

By convention, UV radiation is divided into the photobiologic spectral bands of UVA (320 to 400 nm), UVB (290 to 320 nm), and UVC (200 to 290 nm). Each UV spectral band differs from the other by its photobiologic properties and transmission capabilities. For example, UVC poses the greatest risk to genomic DNA being the only ionizing UV radiation. However, its inability to penetrate the earth's atmosphere negates the relevance of this photobiologic effect of sunlight. UVB, on the other hand, is a nonionizing radiation whose transmission is mitigated by the ozone and blocked by glass. Between 10:00 AM and 2:00 PM, while 65% of UV radiation emitted by the sun reaches the earth's surface, UV radiation at noon consists of 95% UVA, 5% UVB, and 0% UVC. Twenty to thirty percent of this UVA radiation will then penetrate to the deep dermis, whereas only 10% of UVB reaches the superficial dermis. Thus, broad-spectrum sunscreens with good UVA and UVB filters are recommended, especially for those with UVA- or UVB-induced photodermatoses.

Visible Light and Infrared Radiation

VL is another band of nonionizing radiation which spans the entire color spectrum, from blue to red (400 to 700 nm). VL spectrum is used therapeutically in photodynamic therapy, and it is the spectrum range of most lasers used in dermatology. VL in sunlight historically has been considered photobiologically "inert." However, recent studies have shown that compared to UVA1 (340 to 400 nm), VL induced more prolonged pigmentary darkening that lasts up to 3 months, and blue light was more efficient that red light in inducing these changes. As importantly, these changes were observed only in individuals with darker skin, but not in fair skinned subjects. These results suggest that VL may play a role in pigmentary alterations such as melasma and postinflammatory hyperpigmentation that are seen predominantly darker skinned individuals. VL wavelengths also can induce reactive oxygen species, pro-inflammatory cytokines, and matrix metalloproteinase.

IR, another nonionizing radiation, is responsible for a warm sensation. It is classified into three IR bands: IRA (750 to 1,440 nm), IRB (1,440 to 3,000 nm) and IRC (3,000 nm to 1 mm). Dermatologically, IRA appears to be the primary IR band of clinical significance, as it comprises 65% of the rays penetrating into the dermis and 30% of IR overall. Photobiologically, this deep penetration induces dermal heating and matrix metalloproteinase 1 expression, resulting in wrinkles. Chronic exposure contributes to photoaging and the clinical and histopathologic findings of erythema ab igne: epidermal atrophy, pigment incontinence, collagen degradation, dermal elastosis, and distension of vessels with subsequent hemosiderin deposition. Aside from photoaging and erythema ab igne, no other definitive conditions have been associated with IR exposure in human.

SUNBURN AND TANNING: ACUTE EFFECTS OF SOLAR RADIATION

Skin phototype plays an important role in the clinical outcome of sun exposure. Fitzpatrick classification of skin types (FST) is widely used for this purpose (Table 43-1). However, sensitivity to UV is best assessed by the determination of minimal erythema dose (MED), which is defined as the smallest dose of radiation causing perceptible erythema covering the entire

TABLE 43-1 • Fitzpatrick Skin Types

Skin Type	Characteristics
I	Never tan, always burn
II	Occasionally tan, usually burn
III	Usually tan, occasionally burn
IV	Easily tan, rarely burn
V	Brown skin
VI	Black skin

irradiated area. For individuals with skin type I, the MED of broadband UVB (MED-B) is between 20 and 40 mJ/cm^2 and then 1,000 fold higher for broadband UVA (MED-A) (20 to 40 J/cm^2).

Presentation and Characteristics

UVA-induced erythema is typically apparent by the end of the irradiation period and fades gradually over the next 24 to 72 hours. UVA induces significantly more pigmentary alteration than erythema. Exposure to UVA radiation results in three types of pigmentation changes: immediate pigment darkening (IPD), persistent pigment darkening (PPD), and delayed tanning. IPD occurs immediately after exposure and fades within 10 to 20 minutes; it presents as a bluish-gray discoloration of the skin. The mechanism of IPD is oxidation of preexisting melanin in the epidermis; there is no neo-melanogenesis. PPD occurs by the same mechanism and follows IPD if the UVA dose is sufficiently high. It lasts from 2 to 24 hours. Delayed tanning is due to the formation of new melanin in the epidermis. This pigmentation lasts for several days and may blend with IPD and PPD.

UVB-induced erythema consists of an immediate and a delayed phase; the former starts within the first 2 to 6 hours before peaking in 24 to 36 hours. There is no apparent IPD/PPD seen with UVB, just a delayed tanning reaction that is always preceded by erythema. UVB-induced delayed tanning peaks at 72 hours and fades rapidly. Similar to UVA-induced delayed tanning, neo-melanogenesis also takes place.

VL-induced erythema can be observed immediately after exposure in dark-skinned individuals, and fades within 30 minutes. Delayed tanning is significantly more intense and prolonged than UVA, but only present in individuals with FST III–VI. VL-delayed tanning also persists notably longer (up to 3 months) than UVA-induced delayed tanning.

SAUER'S NOTES

1. UVB is the most efficient at inducing a sunburn, while UVA is the primary driver of delayed tanning.
2. VL has now been shown to induced prolonged delayed tanning (up to 3 months), seen only individuals with FST III–VI.

3. Photoprotection includes seeking shade between 10 AM and 2 PM and using photoprotective clothing, long sleeves and pant legs, socks, photoprotective fabric (UPF of 50 or greater), wide-brimmed hats with neck protector, sun protective glasses, and broad-spectrum sunscreen with SPF of 30 or above.
4. Sunscreen should be applied generously 20 minutes before outdoor activities and then reapplied every 2 hours.
5. Using "water-resistant" sunscreens provides additional benefit when perspiring or performing water-sports.

Sunburn reactions present as erythema, edema, vesiculation, and pain, followed by scaling, desquamation, and hyperpigmentation. Acute reactions, when severe, may be accompanied by weakness, fatigue, and pruritus.

Treatment

■ *Photoprotection*: Photoprotection consists of minimizing sun exposure between 10 AM and 2 PM, the use of photoprotective clothing, wide-brimmed hats, sunglasses, and the application of "broad-spectrum" sunscreens. Sunscreens with a sun protection factor (SPF) of 30 or greater should be applied 20 minutes before sun exposure and then reapplied every 2 hours, especially if sweating or swimming. "Water-resistant" sunscreens are labeled either 40 or 80 minutes to denote the duration of water immersion of the subjects during testing. Sunscreens should be applied generously: 1 oz (30 mL) is needed to cover the entire body surface. Broad-spectrum sunscreens, which protect against both UVB and UVA radiation, are recommended. The United States Food and Drug Administration (USFDA)-approved sunscreen ingredients are listed in Table 43-2.

TABLE 43-2 • FDA-Approved Sunscreen Ingredients in the United States

UVB Filters	UVA Filters
Cinoxate	Avobenzone (Parsol 1789)
Ensulizole	Dioxybenzone Ecamsule*
Homosalate	Meradimate
Octinoxate	Oxybenzone
Octisalate	Sulisobenzone
Octocrylene PABA	Titanium dioxide
Para-aminobenzoic acid	Zinc oxide
Padimate O	
Trolamine salicylate	

*Ecamsule is currently approved through the New Drug Application for use in four specific, branded formulations: Anthelios SX, Capital Soleil, Anthelios 20, and Anthelios 40.

■ *Nonsteroidal anti-inflammatory agents and corticosteroids:* These should be taken within 4 to 6 hours after sun exposure. Topical corticosteroids and cool compresses are helpful in reducing the inflammation. Oral prednisone (1 mg/kg) may be used for 5 to 7 days in severe cases.

SAUER'S NOTES

Sunscreens work best when broad-spectrum UVA and UVB are applied thick enough, applied 20 minutes before sun exposure, reapplied after sweating or water exposure, and reapplied every 1 to 2 hours. For all these reasons, editor opinion is that they are not a substitute for protective clothing or shade in many instances.

PHOTOAGING: CHRONIC EFFECTS OF UV RADIATION

Presentation and Characteristics

Photoaging accounts for 90% of age-associated cosmetic problems. The effects of photoaging can be broken down into the following categories:

■ Pigmentation changes
■ Texture changes
■ Vascular changes
■ Papillary changes

Pigmentary changes result from UV damage to the epidermis; the other changes result from dermal pathology. UVA, UVB, and IR radiation contribute to the process of photoaging.

The prototypical pigmentary change seen in older adults is a solar lentigo. Solar lentigines, or "age spots," appear in chronically sun-exposed areas, usually starting at around 40 years of age. They are macules with well-demarcated borders that vary in color from yellowish-brown to dark brown. The mechanism of occurrence is thought to be an increase in melanin content within the keratinocytes and possibly reactive hyperplasia of melanocytes. Areas near the lentigines may be hypopigmented, creating an overall mottled appearance of the skin.

The leathery texture and deep wrinkling of the skin from photoaging is called *solar elastosis*. This is very characteristic of severe chronic sun damage, and typically occurs on the face and neck. It gives the skin a yellowish hue. The pathologic hallmark for this condition is deposition of amorphous elastotic material in the papillary dermis that does not form functional elastic fibers. This altered connective tissue does not demonstrate the resilient properties of normal elastic tissue. There is also epidermal acanthosis seen on histology. Furthermore, collagen destruction, induced by downstream effects of oxidative and direct DNA damage from UV radiation and thermal destruction from IR, plays a role in the loss of the skin's tensile strength.

Photoaging also damages blood vessels as well. With cumulative photoaging the vessel wall thickness, perivascular connective tissue, and even the number of vessels diminish. Thus, these fragile vessels develop ecchymoses (senile purpura) after minimal trauma and even become visible as telangiectasias in chronically sun-exposed regions.

A common example of a papillary change seen in photoaging is a seborrheic keratosis. This "wisdom spot" results from disrupted keratinocyte maturation imposed by accumulated UV radiation. Seborrheic keratoses appear "stuck on" the skin, and arise more frequently on sun-exposed areas like the face, trunk, and extremities. They are completely benign growths and pose no risk of malignant transformation. Inheritance plays a more important role in occurrence (editor's opinion).

Treatment

■ *Topical retinoids:* These can cause slight reversal of photoaged skin. They increase collagen levels, which effaces wrinkles. Retinoids also stimulate epidermal hyperplasia, which manifests clinically as smoother skin with fewer fine lines. Deeper wrinkles from chronologic aging persist. Retinoids also lighten pigmentary changes associated with photodamage. Side effects include peeling, erythema, and dryness. Tolerance often occurs over weeks of use.

■ *Photorejuvenation:* This entails stimulation of dermal collagen synthesis by exposure to laser, intense pulse (visible) light, radiofrequency, or photodynamic therapy. This is a rapidly evolving area with numerous methods and equipment on the market. More studies are needed for many of the methods used.

■ *Resurfacing:* This can occur at a superficial, medium, or deep level. Techniques employed include microdermabrasion, chemical peels, and, less commonly, laser resurfacing. Efficacy depends on the depth of wound infliction. The mechanism of wrinkle reduction is stimulation of wound healing with new collagen formation. Re-epithelialization occurs from stem cells located in adnexal appendages. Side effects of resurfacing include permanent pigmentary changes and scarring.

■ *Microneedling:* Various depths of tissue injury can be obtained based upon needle length. Improvement in wrinkle appearance occurs through wound healing with new collagen formation similar to fractionated photorejuvenation. Tram-track scarring from microneedling has been reported in the literature.

SAUER'S NOTES

1. Photoaging changes include the formation of solar lentigines, solar elastosis, telangiectasias, and inelastic skin.
2. Treatments include topical retinoids, photorejuvenation, resurfacing, and microneedling.

PHOTOCARCINOGENESIS

Actinic Keratoses

Presentation and Characteristics

Actinic keratoses (AKs) (Fig. 43-1) are premalignant lesions that predominately arise on chronically sun-exposed areas of skin types I and II (see Table 43-1) patients, but may occasionally appear in type III and type IV individuals as well. Clinically, they present as discrete, rough, hyperkeratotic, and often sensitive to touch areas with a scale. They may be brown, yellowish-brown, flesh-colored, or red. When the lower lip is involved, the term *actinic cheilitis* is used. Texture is the key to diagnosis. Histologically, an AK is an abnormal proliferation of cells confined to the epidermis with some evidence of cellular atypia. It has been estimated that over 10 years, 10.2% of AKs would evolve into invasive squamous cell carcinoma, thus necessitating the treatment of lesions that do not spontaneously remit. AKs are considered to be precursors of squamous cell carcinoma; hence, they should be treated appropriately. Preventative measures of photoprotection and nicotinamide supplementation reduce the rate of AK formation by limiting DNA damage.

Treatment

- *Cryotherapy:* This is the treatment of choice for most superficial lesions. For AK lesions that appear indurated, painful, or with a thick crust, surgical removal may be required and a specimen should be sent for pathologic examination to rule out squamous cell carcinoma.

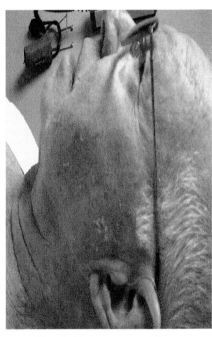

FIGURE 43-1: Keratotic tumors arizing on an ill-defined erythematous face over the side of the face in a fair-skinned man with dramatic solar skin damage.

- *Topical agents:* 5-Fluorouracil, imiquimod cream, ingenol mebutate, and diclofenac sodium gel are useful for patients with multiple or recurrent lesions.
- *Photodynamic therapy:* This modality utilizes 5-aminolevulinic acid (which gets converted into protoporphyrin) and blue light, or methyl aminolevulinate and red light. It has been shown to successfully eliminate AKs.
- *Cosmetic resurfacing:* Medium-to-deep chemical peels, ablative resurfacing, and dermabrasion are another set of treatment options if the entire epidermis is removed. This technique depends upon the experience and expertise of the practitioner, and is often not covered by insurance.

Nonmelanoma Skin Cancer

Basal cell carcinomas (BCCs) comprise 80% of nonmelanoma skin cancers (NMSCs) diagnosed; squamous cell carcinomas (SCCs) comprise 20%. SCCs demonstrate a more linear correlation to the amount of UV exposure than do BCCs. Among Caucasians, the incidence of NMSCs and melanomas has been increasing annually for several decades. It has now been shown that consistent use of sunscreens reduces the formation of NMSCs and melanoma.

Squamous Cell Carcinoma

Presentation and Characteristics: The in-situ form of SCC is known as Bowen disease. Clinically, it appears as a well-demarcated, red, scaly patch, usually in sun-exposed areas. It is more likely to be found on the lower extremity of women and the scalp and ears of men. Treatment options include electrodessication and curettage, cryosurgery, and surgical excision.

Risk factors for development of SCCs include fair skin, light-colored iris, intermittent burns during childhood, ionizing radiation, immunosuppression, chronic inflammation, environmental carcinogens, certain genodermatoses, proximity to the equator, and cumulative exposure to UV radiation—specifically UVB radiation. UVB damages DNA and mutates tumor suppressor genes, such as *p53*. UVA also damages DNA and is thought to enhance the carcinogenic potential of UVB radiation.

SCCs are typically distributed on the scalp, dorsal hands, and pinna and have greater risk for metastasis than BCCs. Their risk of metastasis depends on a multitude of factors including location of the primary lesion, immune status, tumor size, degree of differentiation on histopathologic examination, immune state of the patient, and depth of invasion. A 12.5-year study done in Australia has shown that the use of broad-spectrum sunscreens could significantly decrease the development of SCCs. Systemic nicotinamide also has shown promise for reducing new SCC formation in a recent phase III trial.

Treatment: Treatment entails electrodessication and curettage, surgical excision, radiation, or Mohs micrographic surgery. Thin, early SCCs can be treated with PDT, laser destruction, or chemotherapy creams, such as 5-fluorouracil.

Basal Cell Carcinoma

Presentation and Characteristics: BCCs are the most common human malignancies and occur typically after the age of 40 years. Although sun exposure is an important cause of BCCs, other factors, such as ethnicity and skin type, play a role in its etiology. Cumulative, rather than intermittent, sun exposure is more indicative for the development of BCCs. BCCs can appear in areas protected from the sun, such as behind the ear. Approximately 25% to 30% of BCCs occur on the nose.

Clinically, BCCs appear as pink or white pearly papules with areas of telangiectasia. As lesions progress, they may develop central ulceration and look as if they have been gnawed upon (i.e., the classical "rat bite" description). There are five histologic patterns of BCCs: nodular, superficial, micronodular, infiltrative, and morpheaform. Microscopically, BCCs are nests of basophilic cells originating from basal keratinocytes and hair follicles. Peripheral palisading is a hallmark histologic feature.

Risk factors include poor ability to tan, fair skin, immunosuppression, old age, and exposure to UV radiation. There are also genodermatoses associated with the development of BCCs, such as Gorlin syndrome. Just as with SCCs, UVB radiation is thought to be more effective than UVA in photocarcinogenesis. DNA mutations involving the Sonic hedgehog pathway are thought to play a role.

BCCs grow by direct extension; therefore, the incidence of metastasis is low. Diagnosis is made only from biopsy.

Treatment: Treatment options include electrodessication and curettage, surgical excision, Mohs micrographic surgery, or radiation therapy for elderly patients who cannot tolerate surgical procedures. Photodynamic therapy, imiquimod, and 5-fluorouracil have been used successfully for superficial tumors. In the rare cases of BCC metastasis or advanced tumors that cannot be excised or treated by radiation, vismodegib should be considered.

Melanoma

Presentation and Characteristics: Melanoma demonstrates a less clear-cut relationship with sun exposure. Multiple studies have shown increased risk of melanoma with indoor tanning bed use. A meta-analysis of 7 studies revealed a 1.75 relative risk of melanoma if tanning bed use started before the age of 35 years; another study noted a 16% increased risk in those with >10 tanning bed sessions. DNA mutations associated with UV radiation also were identified in a genomic study of melanoma. However, unlike BCCs, melanoma does not localize to skin receiving the most cumulative UV radiation. In fact, although the incidence of melanoma is low in people of color, when it occurs, the palms, soles, and proximal nail matrix of the thumb and great toe are common sites. Furthermore, melanoma has a peak incidence in younger patients, who have acquired less lifetime sun exposure than their elderly counterparts. Melanoma occurs more frequently in people who work indoors, as opposed to outdoors. One proposed explanation for why indoor workers have a higher incidence of melanoma is that melanoma may be related to intense, intermittent sun exposure of untanned skin. This also supports the distribution pattern of melanoma seen on the trunk in men and lower extremities in women.

A helpful guideline to distinguish melanomas from benign nevi (moles) is the ABCDE rule. Melanoma tends to be asymmetrical, with border irregularity, color variegation, and a diameter >6 mm. Lesions that are evolving must also be evaluated. Moles that look different (outliers or ugly ducklings) from the other moles on the patient are another clinical clue that should be considered. However, dermoscopy has evolved into a well-researched and effective tool for such requirement with a higher specificity and sensitivity when performed by trained practitioners compared to nondermoscopic examinations.

There are four major clinical histopathologic subtypes:

- Superficial spreading
- Lentigo maligna
- Nodular
- Acral lentiginous

They differ with respect to the pattern of sun exposure and location. A more detailed discussion of these subtypes is beyond the scope of this chapter. Other risk factors for melanoma include the following:

- A first-degree relative with melanoma
- The presence of atypical, dysplastic, or giant congenital (>20 cm) nevi
- Fair skin and light eyes
- A history of severe childhood sunburns
- A history of NMSC
- Immunosuppression

Multiple genes have been linked to melanoma in certain families. These include tumor suppressor genes, such as *CDKN2A*, *PTEN*, *p53*, and *BAP-1*, encoding protein products for cell cycle arrest and DNA repair mutations, such as BRCA, that allow DNA damage to continue unrepaired, leading to oncogenesis.

Diagnosis: The diagnosis of melanoma is only made by biopsy. Under the microscope, melanomas appear as clusters of large and atypical melanocytes with visible mitotic figures proliferating above in the epidermis. The pathology report includes the Breslow depth (full tumor thickness), mitoses (>1 per high-power field), and the presence or absence of ulceration. The depth of the lesion is the strongest histologic factor influencing prognosis. Thus, superficial shave biopsies are not appropriate in cases of suspected melanoma because they have the potential to obscure an accurate report of tumor depth. Wide local excision is the only acceptable treatment, and surgical margins are determined by Breslow depth and the diameter of the lesion. α-Interferon is considered for adjuvant therapy in certain cases. Additional treatment options for metastatic melanoma include BRAF/V500E wild-type inhibitors, PD-1, and immune checkpoint inhibitors CTLA-4, C-KIT, and IL-2. Lastly, an oncolytic immunotherapeutic vaccine, talimogene laherparepvec, has recently been approved for the treatment of metastatic melanoma. Melanomas, especially the deeper ones, are frequently lethal. They are responsible for 75% of skin cancer deaths.

SAUER'S NOTES

1. Chronic sun exposure, or repeated sunburn, is associated with the development of AKs, BCCs, and SCCs. The association of melanomas and sun exposure is less clear.

2. Treatment
   a. *Actinic keratoses:* cryotherapy, topical 5-fluorouracil, imiquimod cream, diclofenac sodium gel, photodynamic therapy. Nicotinamide and sunscreen for prevention.
   b. *BCCs, SCCs:* electrodessication and curettage, surgical excision, Mohs micrographic surgery, radiation, photodynamic therapy and topical chemo/immunotherapy (for early lesions only). Vismodegib for rare cases of metastatic or nonoperable BCC. Oral nicotinamide for prevention of SCC.
   c. *Melanomas:* wide local excision, α-interferon, IL-2, CTLA-4, C-KIT, oncolytic immunotherapeutic vaccine, and various inhibitors of immune checkpoint, BRAF, and PD-1.

PHOTODERMATOSES

Although the aforementioned acute and chronic effects of UV radiation occur in exposed skin of all individuals, there are some abnormal reactions to sunlight that only manifest in the predisposed. These reactions are known as *photodermatoses*. The more commonly encountered ones (Table 43-3) are discussed below. Photoprotection is an integral part of the management of all photodermatoses.

Immunologically Mediated Dermatoses

Polymorphous Light Eruption

Presentation and Characteristics: Polymorphous light eruption (PMLE) is the most common photodermatosis in humans. It affects patients of all backgrounds and races and occurs more often in women than in men. Its peak onset is during the third and fourth decades of life. In temperate climates, it flares during the spring and summer, after exposure to a certain threshold of UV radiation. Association with lupus erythematous and thyroid disease has been reported.

Patients are usually susceptible to broadband UVA and UVB radiation, with either able to elicit the symptoms. In most patients, however, the minimal dose of UV needed to induce redness in the skin is normal. There is evidence to indicate

TABLE 43-3 • Commonly Encountered Photodermatoses
Immunologically Mediated Photodermatoses
Polymorphous light eruption
Chronic actinic dermatitis
Solar urticaria
Endogenous Photodermatoses
Porphyria cutanea tarda
Erythropoietic protoporphyria
Exogenous Photodermatoses
Phototoxicity
Photoallergy
Photoaggravated Dermatoses
Lupus erythematosus
Dermatomyositis
Atopic dermatitis
Seborrheic dermatitis
Some Patients with Psoriasis

that patients with PMLE are less susceptible to UV-induced immunosuppression. Therefore, PMLE is considered a delayed type of hypersensitivity response to a photo-induced antigen.

Clinically, PMLE presents minutes to hours after exposure to UV radiation and can persist from 1 day to weeks. Initial symptoms include mild burning and pruritus. Grouped erythematous papules appear in a symmetrical distribution on sun-exposed skin—notably, the forehead, upper chest, dorsum of hands, and forearms (Fig. 43-2). There are several different clinical manifestations, such as papules, plaques, nodules, and, rarely, vesicles. In individuals with skin of color, pinhead-sized papules are the most common presentation. General malaise,

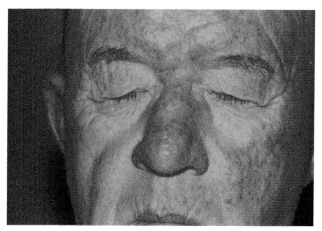

FIGURE 43-2: Polymorphous light eruptions with coalescing inflammatory papules photodistributed over the face.

headache, fever, and nausea may infrequently accompany the cutaneous findings.

Histologically, PMLE appears as a nonspecific, dermal, lymphocytic, perivascular infiltrate. Diagnosis is made by history and clinical findings in the context of a negative rheumatologic (lupus erythematosus, dermatomyositis) serology workup. Biopsy is not typically helpful, and phototesting is often unnecessary.

Treatment

- *Desensitization:* This is attained by narrowband UVB phototherapy, two to three times per week for 15 treatments, usually done in the spring.
- *Antimalarials:* They have been shown to provide moderate protection during the spring and summer. Most commonly, hydroxychloroquine, 200 mg twice a day, is used.
- *Oral antioxidants: Polypodium leucotomos* extract has been reported to result in downregulation of UVB- and PUVA-induced changes on the skin. Lycopene, *β*-carotene, and *Lactobacillus johnsonii* in combination have been found to diminish symptoms in a 12-week randomized, placebo-controlled, double-blinded study.

Once the outbreak has occurred, the symptoms are best treated with topical or oral corticosteroids.

Chronic Actinic Dermatitis

Description: Chronic actinic dermatitis is a chronic photodermatosis that occurs more commonly among older men. It is most severe during the summer months. Clinically, it presents with lichenified papules or plaques on sun-exposed areas (Fig. 43-3). The lesions are usually pruritic. Histologically, there is mild epidermal spongiosis, perivascular lymphocytic infiltrate, and not infrequently, there are atypical mononuclear cells in the dermis and epidermis. Therefore, histologic changes of chronic actinic dermatitis may resemble those of cutaneous T-cell lymphoma. Diagnosis is confirmed by phototesting; there is an abnormal response to UVB and/or UVA and/or visible radiation.

Treatment

- *Corticosteroids and tacrolimus:* Symptom relief is accomplished with the use of topical and oral corticosteroids. Topical tacrolimus has been used with success in some patients.
- *Others:* Management of refractory cases includes low-dose PUVA, mycophenolate mofetil, cyclosporine, and azathioprine.

Solar Urticaria

Presentation and Characteristics: Solar urticaria occurs slightly more often in females and is associated with atopic dermatitis in 21% to 48% of patients. Patients typically present in their 20s and 30s. The pathogenic mechanism is thought to involve mast cell degranulation in response to a yet-unidentified photosensitized allergen.

Patients present with urticaria minutes after exposure to the instigating wavelength (Fig. 43-4). Like all urticarias, lesions disappear within hours. The wheals may be pruritic and occasionally burn. In rare instances, patients may also experience a systemic anaphylactic reaction. Biopsy of the lesion shows mild dermal edema with a perivascular infiltrate consisting of neutrophils and eosinophils. Upon phototesting with the activating wavelengths, urticaria is induced within a few minutes after the exposure.

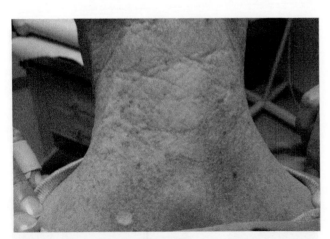

FIGURE 43-3: Actinic dermatitis (persistent light reactor), as sometimes seen, in an AIDS patient. Photodistributed lichenified dermatitis over the back of the neck.

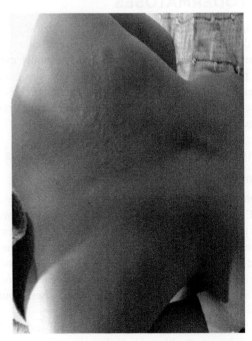

FIGURE 43-4: Solar urticaria with raised white papules and plaques of the upper central back in a patient who had been in a sunbed.

Treatment

- *Antihistamines*
- *Desensitization:* This is done with incrementally increasing doses of UVA or PUVA.

Endogenous Photodermatoses: The Cutaneous Porphyrias

The porphyrias are a group of disorders caused by congenital defects of enzymes in the heme biosynthesis pathway. Plasma porphyrin determination is an excellent screening test, since it is elevated in all types of cutaneous porphyrias. This section discusses the two most common porphyrias that exhibit skin involvement most prominently.

Porphyria Cutanea Tarda

Presentation and Characteristics: Porphyria cutanea tarda (PCT) is the most common cutaneous porphyria. There are two forms: an inherited autosomal dominant form (20% of patients) and an acquired form (80% of patients). Men present with PCT slightly more commonly than women. Men with PCT are more likely to use alcohol and women are more likely to be exposed to estrogen replacement. Most patients present after their 40s, although childhood onset has been infrequently reported. There is a strong association of PCT with hepatitis C as well as with hemochromatosis. Association of PCT with human immunodeficiency virus (HIV) infection has been well reported. Therefore, HIV testing should be offered to all newly diagnosed patients with acquired PCT.

PCT is caused by a defect in hepatic uroporphyrinogen decarboxylase activity, which results in an excess of uroporphyrinogen, 7-, 6-, 5-, and 4-carboxyl porphyrinogens. All porphyrinogens are spontaneously oxidized to the corresponding porphyrins. These porphyrins are phototoxic when exposed to VL (Soret band, 400 to 410 nm).

Clinically, PCT manifests with skin fragility, blisters, erosions, crusting, and milia on sun-exposed areas (Fig. 43-5). Mottled hyper- and hypopigmentation and hypertrichosis on

the periorbital areas are frequently observed. Scarring alopecia and sclerodermoid lesions are uncommon presentations. The latter can occur in both sun-exposed and sun-protected areas.

Histologically, a subepidermal blister with cell-poor dermal infiltrate is seen. Diagnosis is confirmed by the characteristic porphyrin profile. There are elevated levels of uroporphyrin, 7-, 6-, 5-, and 4-carboxyl porphyrins in urine and plasma and elevated isocoproporphyrin in the stool.

Treatment

- *Photoprotection:* Because the action spectrum is in the VL range, photoprotection with physical agents (non-micronized titanium dioxide or zinc oxide, clothing, etc.) is required.
- *Iron load reduction:* Phlebotomy or chelation therapy can be performed to decrease the iron load. Phlebotomy is the most effective treatment for patients. One unit of blood is usually removed weekly for 10 to 15 treatments. Erythropoietin alfa can help stimulate the division and differentiation of progenitor cells to accelerate iron consumption. Alcohol, other hepatic toxins, and iron should be avoided. Interferon-α or ledipasvir may be beneficial in the treatment of PCT in those patients with concomitant hepatitis C virus infection.
- *Antimalarials:* Low-dose (weekly or twice a week) chloroquine or hydroxychloroquine also produces a therapeutic response. Its mechanism of action is to form a porphyrin—antimalarial complex that can be excreted renally.

Erythropoietic Protoporphyria

Presentation and Characteristics: Unlike PCT, erythropoietic protoporphyria (EPP) presents in children, usually by 2 years of age. It is inherited in an autosomal dominant fashion with variable penetrance. The enzyme deficient in EPP is ferrochelatase, which converts protoporphyrin into heme by insertion of iron. Elevated levels of phototoxic protoporphyrin in erythrocytes, plasma, and stool are seen in EPP. Because protoporphyrin is lipophilic, urine porphyrin level is normal in EPP (Fig. 43-6).

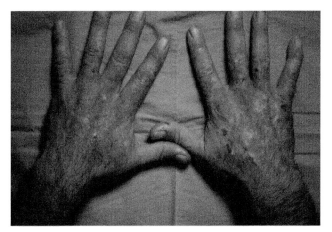

FIGURE 43-5: A man with porphyria cutanea trade. Note the bullae on the left dorsal hand in the center. The stellate tears are also characteristic. These are due to easy skin fragility. The patient benefitted greatly from decreased alcohol abuse.

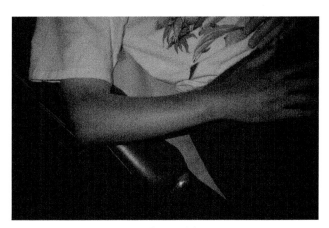

FIGURE 43-6: Teenage boy with severe photodermatitis over extensive upper extremities with porphyrin studies indicating EPP.

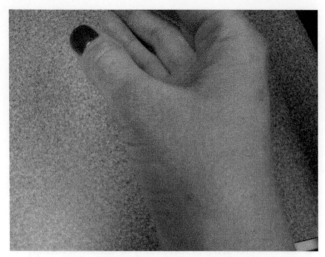

FIGURE 43-7: Contact photo dermatitis from a nail lacquer seen over dorsal hand and thumb. Redness occurs after repeated use of the nail-care product.

TABLE 43-4 • Common Exogenous Photosensitizers

Common Phototoxic Agents	Common Photoallergic Agents
Antiarrhythmics	Sunscreen filters
Diuretics	Fragrances
NSAIDs	Antibacterials
Phenothiazines	
Psoralens	
Quinolones	
Tetracyclines	
Thiazides	
Sulfonamides	
Sulfonylureas	

Abbreviation: NSAIDs, nonsteroidal anti-inflammatory drugs.

Clinically, children with EPP usually cry or scream in pain minutes after exposure to sunlight. Sometimes this is misdiagnosed as psychoneurosis. The burning sensation lasts for hours and is followed by erythema, induration, and purpura. Vesicles are rarely seen. With repeated attacks, shallow erosions on the forehead and nasal bridge and waxy thickening of the skin of knuckles may be apparent. In rare instances, hepatic failure may occur. Histologically, thickening of the dermal–epidermal junction and blood vessel walls of superficial capillaries is observed.

Treatment

- *Photoprotection:* Same as PCT, see previous section.
- *PUVA or narrowband UVB:* These are utilized to induce tolerance.
- *Afamelanotide:* Provides a significant improvement in quality of life and pain-free time compared to placebo group. Currently approved by the European Medicine Agency.

Exogenous Photodermatoses

Phototoxicity and Photoallergy

Presentation and Characteristics: Exogenous agents can be categorized by whether they cause a phototoxic or photoallergic cutaneous reaction. *Phototoxic responses* occur when UV radiation activates a drug or chemical that subsequently produces tissue injury. It occurs in 100% of individuals provided they are exposed to sufficient doses of a phototoxic agent and the radiation (Fig. 43-7). *Photoallergy* is a delayed-type hypersensitivity reaction, consisting of a sensitization phase on first exposure. Subsequent exposures precipitate a photoallergic response. Commonly encountered photosensitizers are listed in Table 43-4.

Clinically, phototoxic eruptions consist of erythema, edema, stinging, and burning in sun-exposed areas (Fig. 43-8). Relatively sun-protected areas such as the submental,

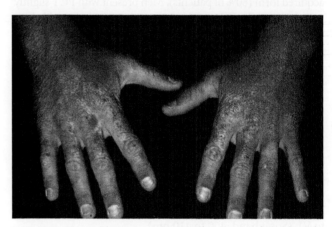

FIGURE 43-8: Phototoxicity on the back of the hands from tetracycline. Note it is the dorsal hands, and the left hand has sparing under the fourth finger where the patient wore his ring.

retroauricular areas and eyelids are usually spared. Occasionally, vesicles, bullae, and onycholysis may be observed. Symptoms resolve with hyperpigmentation over the course of days to weeks. Histologically, phototoxic reactions present with lymphocytic and neutrophilic dermal infiltrates and occasional necrotic keratinocytes.

UVA is the most common action spectrum for systemic, drug-induced phototoxicity. Exposure to furanocoumarin-producing plants causes a topical phototoxic reaction called *phytophotodermatitis* (Fig. 43-9). Common plants evoking this condition include celery, parsnip, lime, and parsley.

Photoallergic reactions present with pruritus and eczematous dermatitis. Bullae and vesicles are rarely seen. The histologic changes are similar to those of contact dermatitis, namely, lymphohistiocytic dermal infiltrates and spongiosis. Currently, the most common cause of photoallergic reactions is sunscreen filters. However, it should be noted that considering the large number of individuals exposed

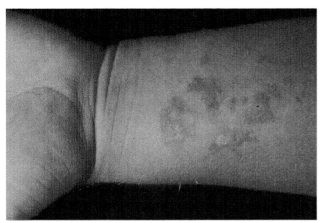

FIGURE 43-9: Bizarre angulated red dermatitis on flexor wrist of phytophotodermatitis in a boy pulling weeds. Areas should be expected to leave dramatic hyperpigmentation.

to sunscreens, the incidence of photoallergy to sunscreen agents is very low.

Taking a careful history and paying special attention to both medication and recent chemical exposures is crucial for diagnosis. Photoallergy can be confirmed by photopatch testing.

Treatment: Treatment includes avoidance of the offending agents along with appropriate photoprotection; symptomatic treatment, including topical or systemic corticosteroids, may be necessary in severe cases.

PHOTOAGGRAVATED DERMATOSES

Exacerbation of cutaneous lesions in lupus erythematosus following sun exposure is frequently seen, especially in subacute lupus erythematosus and in tumid lupus erythematosus. Patients with dermatomyositis also frequently complain of photosensitivity. Photoexacerbation of atopic dermatitis and, less commonly, psoriasis and seborrheic dermatitis have been well reported.

Treatment

In addition to treatment of the primary disease, photoprotection is the appropriate management for these conditions.

Suggested Readings

Baron ED, Suggs AK. Introduction to photobiology. *Dermatol Clin.* 2014;32(3):255–266.

Chen AC, Martin AJ, Choy B, et al. A phase 3 randomized trial of nicotinamide for skin-cancer chemoprevention. *N Engl J Med.* 2015;373(17):1618–1626.

Frank J, Poblete-Gutierrez P. Porphyria. In: Bolognia JL, Jorizzo JL, Schaffer, JV, eds. *Dermatology.* London: Mosby; 2012:717–727.

Green AC, Williams GM, Logan V, et al. Reduced melanoma after regular sunscreen use: a randomized trial follow-up. *J Clin Oncol.* 2011;29(3):257–263.

Langendonk JG, Balwani M, Anderson KE, et al. Afamelanotide for erythropoietic protoporphyria. *N Engl J Med.* 2015;373:48–59.

Lim HW, Paek SY, eds. Photodermatology. *Dermatol Clin.* 2014;32(3):xiii.

Mahmoud BH, Ruvolo EC, Hexsel CL, et al. Impact of long wavelength ultraviolet A and visible light on melanocompetent skin. *J Invest Dermatol.* 2010;130(8):2092–2097.

SAUER'S NOTES

1. Photoprotection is essential in the management of photodermatoses.
2. Treatment
   a. *PMLE:* narrowband UVB, and antimalarials. Preliminary results show that *Polypodium leucotomos* extract, and combination vitamin: Lycopene, *β*-carotene, and *Lactobacillus johnsonii* might also be helpful.
   b. *Chronic actinic dermatitis:* topical and oral corticosteroids, topical tacrolimus, low-dose PUVA, mycophenolate mofetil, cyclosporine, azathioprine.
   c. *Solar urticaria:* antihistamines, low-dose UVA or PUVA.
   d. *PCT:* phlebotomy, chelation, erythropoietin alfa, avoidance of hepatotoxins and iron, low-dose antimalarials.
   e. *EPP:* Afamelanotide, narrowband UVB, PUVA.
   f. *Phototoxicity and photoallergy:* avoidance of precipitating agent.

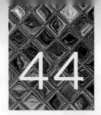

44

Genodermatoses

Margaret L. McKinnon, MD, BSc and Deepti Gupta, MD

The inherited skin disorders are individually rare, but together comprise a significant proportion of dermatologic practice. Some are of minimal medical significance; others are life threatening, life shortening, or debilitating. For some, treatment is available. For others, there is no management beyond diagnosis. For a growing number of conditions, both the causal mutations and the specific perturbations in cellular function are known.

Genetic skin disorders are unique in that the diagnosis automatically invokes the issues of recurrent risk to relatives and potential for prenatal diagnosis. Identification of a genodermatosis may require referral for medical genetics evaluation and counseling. The availability and applicability of molecular (DNA) testing change daily. Medical genetics centers are most likely to be aware of these resources. Online resources include:

- Gene Tests

  https://www.genetests.org/

  GeneTests is a medical genetics information resource developed for physicians, genetic counselors, other healthcare providers, and researchers that includes a listing of laboratories offering molecular testing for research and/or clinical purposes.

- Gene Reviews

  http://www.ncbi.nlm.nih.gov/books/NBK1116/

  GeneReviews are published online, expert-authored, peer-reviewed disease descriptions that are authored by experts in the field presented in standardized "chapter-based" formats. Each topic focuses on clinically relevant information regarding diagnosis, management, links to support groups and genetic counseling for patients and families with specific inherited conditions. Chapters are updated by the author(s) in a formal comprehensive process every 2 to 3 years and revised whenever significant changes in clinical information occur.

- OMIM

  http://www.ncbi.nlm.nih.gov/omim/

  A comprehensive catalog of human genes and related phenotypes, the online "Mendelian Disorders In Man" is updated daily with references, clinical synopses, and hyperlinks to other databases.

Many common skin disorders also have a significant genetic component. The risk for psoriasis, atopic dermatitis, vitiligo, alopecia areata, or systemic lupus erythematosus is much higher among close relatives of affected individuals than for the general population. Even acne and onychomycosis enjoy genetic contribution. These disorders are discussed in Chapters 15 and 36, respectively, and will not be further addressed here. This chapter will deal with only a handful of the many inherited skin disorders.

DISORDERS OF KERATINIZATION

Ichthyoses

The term ichthyosis or disorders of cornification refers to an inherited group of conditions where there are molecular defects causing that keep the epidermis from forming properly. (Table 44-1; Figs. 44-1 to 44-4) Clinically, they share common features of a thickened stratum corneum, which results in scaly skin. The distribution and severity of scaling, the presence of erythroderma, the mode of inheritance, and associated abnormalities differ among them. The degree to which life is impaired ranges from minimal to lethal. The genetic alterations responsible for some of these conditions are known. Treatment remains general and nonspecific. A mainstay of treatment includes hydration of skin through the use of bland

TABLE 44-1 • Ichthyoses

Disorder	Inheritance	Basic Defect	Major Dermatologic Findings	Associated Features	Miscellaneous
Ichthyosis vulgaris	Autosomal Semi-dominant	Mutations in Profilaggrin (FLG)	Fine white scale that can be generalized and can involve the face. Larger scale can be present especially on the legs. Relative sparing of the flexures. Hyperlinear palms.	Increased risk of atopic dermatitis and keratosis pilaris	Improves with age and warm weather
X-linked ichthyosis (sterol sulfatase deficiency)	XLR	Deletion of arylsulfatase C (ARSC1) steroid sulfatase gene	White-brown large scale with accentuation of the neck and behind the ears. Relative sparing of the flexures and face	Corneal opacities Possible increased risk of testicular malignancy	Pregnancies with affected males have low to absent estriol levels; failure of spontaneous initiation of labor is common
Bullous congenital ichthyosiform erythroderma (epidermolytic hyperkeratosis)	AD	Mutations in K1 or K10 (suprabasal keratins)	Red skin with blisters and scale evident at birth Marked hyperkeratosis Face usually least affected Inter- and intrafamilial variability	Secondary skin infection, bacterial and fungal common	Skin is tender; skin fragility improves with age
Lamellar ichthyosis/ nonbullous congenital ichthyosiform erythroderma/ congenital autosomal recessive ichthyosis	AR	Heterogenous. Some caused by mutations in transglutaminase 1 (*TGM1*), 12-R lipoxygenase (ALOX12B), lipoxygenase-3 (*ALOXE3*), ATP-binding cassette transporter 2 (*ABCA2*)	LI: mild erythroderma; brown, adherent plate-like scale NCIE: Erythroderma; fine, white scale Many cases with overlap in phenotype	Secondary tinea infection common	Collodion membrane common at birth Ectropion/ ecla-bium common
Harlequin fetus	AR	Unknown; probably heterogenous	Severe, armor plate-like hyperkeratosis In survivors, phenotype becomes similar to BCIE	Among survivors, mental retardation has been noted in a few	Rare spontaneous survival; handful of survivors treated with oral retinoids
Conradi Hunermann	XLD AR	XLD: mutation in gene encoding delta(8)-delta(7) sterol isomerase emopamilbinding protein AR: mutations in *PEX7* gene	Feathery scale on erythrodermic base Follicular atrophoderma	Seizures; MR Chondrodysplasia punctata Cataracts	Asymmetry typical in XLD form

TABLE 44-1 • Ichthyoses (*continued*)

Disorder	Inheritance	Basic Defect	Major Dermatologic Findings	Associated Features	Miscellaneous
Sjögren–Larsson syndrome	AR	Fatty aldehyde dehydrogenase deficiency	Mild-to-moderate fine, adherent scale Pruritus	Progressive spastic paraparesis Mild retardation Glistening white dots on retina	
Netherton syndrome	AR	Mutations in *SPINK5* gene	Variable erythroderma and scale Classical pattern of ichthyosis linearis circumflexa	Trichorrhexis invaginata (bamboo hair)	Failure to thrive Food allergies
Collodion baby	AR if isolated Otherwise, depends on underlying disorder	Heterogenous	Plastic wrap-like membrane peels within few weeks after birth, revealing underlying skin, which may range from minimally xerotic to lamellar ichthyosis	This is a feature of many disorders including lamellar ichthyosis, hypohidrotic ectodermal dysplasia, Gaucher disease and lamellar exfoliation of the newborn	

Abbreviations: AD, autosomal dominant; AR, autosomal recessive; BCIE, bullous congenital ichthyosiform erythroderma; K, keratin; MR, mental retardation; XLR, X-linked recessive.

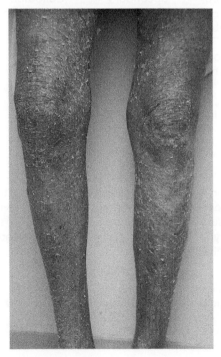

FIGURE 44-1: X-linked ichthyosis. (Reprinted from Sybert VP. *Genetic Skin Disorders*. New York: Oxford University Press; 1997.)

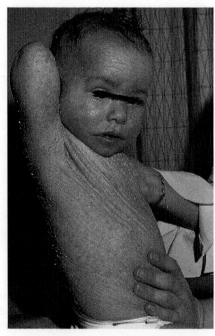

FIGURE 44-2: A young girl with nonbullous congenital ichthyosiform erythroderma. (Reprinted from Sybert VP. *Genetic Skin Disorders*. New York: Oxford University Press; 1997.)

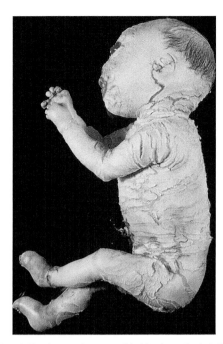

FIGURE 44-3: A newborn with Harlequin ichthyosis. (Reprinted from Sybert VP. *Genetic Skin Disorders*. New York: Oxford University Press; 1997.)

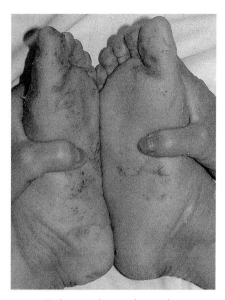

FIGURE 44-5: Palmar–plantar hyperkeratosis. The hands and soles are thickened, with erythroderma evident at the margins. A young girl shares the same condition as her father. (Reprinted from Sybert VP. *Genetic Skin Disorders*. New York: Oxford University Press; 1997.)

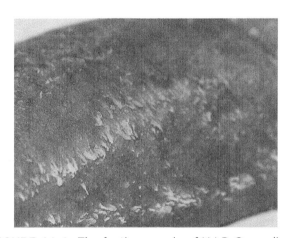

FIGURE 44-4: The feathery scale of X-LD Conradi Hunermann disease. (Reprinted from Sybert VP. *Genetic Skin Disorders*. New York: Oxford University Press; 1997.)

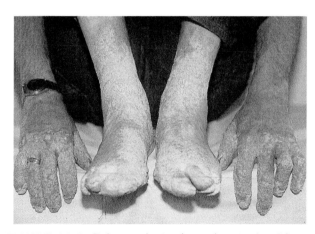

FIGURE 44-6: Palmar–plantar hyperkeratosis with severe palm/sole involvement and extension onto the wrists and shins. Some of these patients have involvement of the elbows, knees, and gluteal cleft. (Reprinted from Sybert VP. *Genetic Skin Disorders*. New York: Oxford University Press; 1997.)

emollients. Use of keratolytics (α-hydroxy acids such as lactic acid, glycolic acid, and urea-based emollients) can be helpful. Oral retinoids are effective and should be considered in the more severe forms of ichthyoses. Their long-term use is limited by significant side effects including dryness of the mucous membranes, alterations in serum lipids, musculoskeletal pain, bony alterations, and teratogenicity.

Palmar–Plantar Keratodermas

Palmar–plantar keratodermas (PPK) (Figs. 44-5 and 44-6) are conditions in which thickening of the stratum corneum and scaling, with or without erythroderma, are limited primarily to the palms and soles. They are distinguished, as are

the more generalized ichthyoses, by mode of inheritance and associated findings. One autosomal dominant form (caused by mutations in the *RHBDF2* gene) is associated with esophageal carcinoma. Papillon–Lefèvre syndrome is an autosomal recessive PPK caused by mutations in the cathepsin C gene (*CTSC*) that is associated with gingivitis and premature tooth loss. Nonepidermolytic hyperkeratosis (formally referred to as "Unna-Thost" disease) results primarily from heterozygous mutations in *KRT1*, with rare diffuse forms caused by mutations in the *AQP5* gene and the *SERPINB7* gene and other focal forms caused by mutations in *KRT16* and *TRPV3*. PPK with epidermolytic hyperkeratosis (formally known as

Vörner disease) is also caused by heterozygous mutations in *KRT1* and in *KRT9*.

DISORDERS OF ADHESION

The epidermolysis bullosa (EB) syndromes (Table 44-2; Figs. 44-7 to 44-9) are mechanobullous disorders that share in common fragility of the skin. They are distinguished, one from the next, by the degree of involvement, mode of inheritance, associated cutaneous features and categorized according to the histologic level of blister formation via a sequential "onion skin" approach. Although many new genes and rare subtypes are now described, the four major types remain and were retained in the most recent consensus classification scheme: EB simplex (EBS), junctional EB (JEB), dystrophic EB (DEB), and Kindler. Most forms present at birth or soon thereafter. Scarring is primarily limited to the dystrophic forms, where the separation of the skin occurs below the basement membrane of the dermis. Extensive involvement in the newborn period can

TABLE 44-2 • Epidermolysis Bullosa

Disorder	Mode of Inheritance	Basic Defect Mutations In	Major Dermatologic Findings	Associated Features	Level of Skin Cleavage and Immunohistochemistry Findings
Epidermolysis Bullosa -Simplex (EBS) -localized (formerly Weber–Cockayne-type)	AD	Basal keratins *KRT 5* *KRT 14*	Blisters primarily limited to hands and feet. Onset can be at birth but usually thereafter. Occasionally delayed until adolescence. Palmar–plantar hyperkeratosis may occur	None	Level of split within basal keratinocytes
Epidermolysis bullosa simplex (EBS)-generalized (formerly Koebner-type)	AD	Basal keratins *KRT 5* *KRT 14*	Blisters soon after birth, generalized. May have oral involvement/nail involvement	None	Level of split within basal keratinocytes
Epidermolysis bullosa simplex (EBS)-generalized severe (formerly Dowling Meara or EBS-herpetiformis)	AD	Basal keratins *KRT 5* *KRT 14*	Marked blistering at birth. With time clustering of small blisters in rosettes may occur. Oral involvement common. Nails often dystrophic. Progressive palmar–plantar hyperkeratosis common. Dyspigmentation common	Can result in neonatal/infant death. Blistering tends to diminish with age	Clumping of tonofilaments within basal cells with cytolysis
EBS with muscular dystrophy	AR	Plectin *PLEC1*	Relatively severe simplex disease, may be mistaken for junctional EB +/− nail dystrophy	Muscular dystrophy of various types has been described	Split at basal epidermis within hemidesmosomal attachment plate
EBS with mottled hyperpigmentation	AD	Basal keratin *KRT 5*	Blisters similar to EBS-K. Development of hyper/hypopigmented spots +/− nail dystrophy	None	Level of split within basal keratinocyte

TABLE 44-2 • Epidermolysis Bullosa (*continued*)

Disorder	Mode of Inheritance	Basic Defect Mutations In	Major Dermatologic Findings	Associated Features	Level of Skin Cleavage and Immunohistochemistry Findings
Junctional epidermolysis bullosa (JEB)—generalized severe (formerly JEB-Herlitz)	AR	Various components of laminin *LAMA3* *LAMC2* *LAMB3*	Widespread severe. GI, respiratory, and GU mucosa often involved. Usually lethal.		Level of split within lamina lucida, expect decreased laminin 332 staining
JEB, generalized intermediate	AR	*COL17A* *ITGB4* *LAMA3* *LAMC2* *LAMB3*	More mild, gradual atopic appearance of healed skin	None	Level of split within lamina lucida; expect decreased level of relevant protein (i.e., collagen XVII staining).
JEB with pyloric atresia (JEB-PA)	AR	Integrins *ITGB4* *ITGB6*	Severe, skin and mucosal involvement, usually lethal	Pyloric atresia, intestinal malabsorption	Level of split within lamina lucida, absent or reduced staining for Integrin $\alpha6\beta4$.
Dominant dystrophic epidermolysis bullosa (DDEB)—generalized (formerly DDEB-Cockayne-Touraine)	AD	Type 7 collagen *COL7A1*	Blistering and scarring limited and localized to areas of greatest trauma. Mild oral involvement. Milia	None	Dermal split (sublamina densa) May see decrease or normal Collagen VII staining
Recessive dystrophic epidermolysis bullosa (RDEB)—generalized severe (formerly (Hallopeau-Siemens)	AR	Type 7 collagen *COL7A1*	Widespread, severe blistering, progressive scarring. Pseudo-amputation of digits. Development of cutaneous malignancy common in adult life. Oral mucosa involved. Milia	Failure to thrive. Anemia, GI involvement is progressive	Dermal split (sublamina densa) Absence or marked reduction in Collagen VII staining

occur in EBS-generalized severe, recessive dystrophic epidermolysis bullosa (RDEB), and in junctional epidermolysis bullosa (JEB). Neonatal or infant death owing to sepsis or intestinal protein loss is common in the most severe forms. Respiratory mucosa is often involved in the generalized severe form of JEB. Accurate diagnosis requires examination of a skin biopsy by transmission electron microscopy (TEM), immunofluorescent antibody/antigen mapping, or molecular genetic testing (via targeted sequencing, or via multi-gene panel analysis). Treatment consists of protection of skin surfaces and avoidance of trauma, lancing of small blisters to prevent lateral spread by the pressure of blister fluid, topical antibiotics, and nonadherent dressings. More severe forms require a team approach to management of complications.

DISORDERS OF PIGMENTATION

There are many molecules that contribute to skin color. This discussion is limited to alterations in melanin, the major contributor to color in the skin. Perturbations in pigment production can be as a result of alterations or defects anywhere along the pathway from the differentiation and migration of neural crest derivatives, through the enzymatic production of melanin, to the packaging and transport of melanosomes.

Hypopigmentation

Waardenburg syndromes I through III and piebaldism (Fig. 44-10) share in common white patches of skin, a white forelock, premature graying of the hair, and autosomal

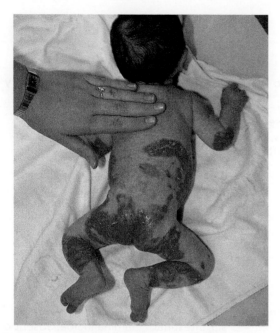

FIGURE 44-7: A newborn with junctional epidermolysis bullosa-generalized severe.

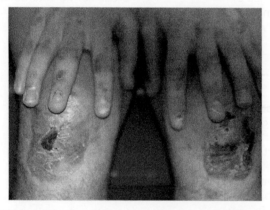

FIGURE 44-8: Scarring in a patient with DEBD.

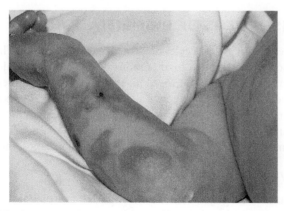

FIGURE 44-9: Extensive superficial blistering in a patient with EBS-generalized severe.

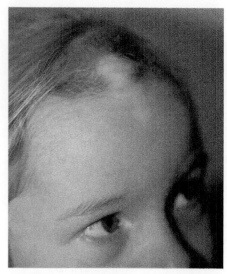

FIGURE 44-10: A white forelock and patch of unpigmented skin in young girl with piebaldism.

dominant inheritance. All are due to a failure of migration and invasion of melanocytes into the epidermis, resulting in lack of melanocytes in the depigmented areas. Individuals with Waardenburg syndrome may also have deafness and heterochromia irides. Those with Waardenburg syndromes I, III, and rarely IV, have dystopia canthorum. Waardenburg III is associated with limb abnormalities. Hirschsprung disease occurs in Waardenburg syndrome type IV and rarely in piebaldism. Waardenburg I and III are owing to mutations in *PAX3*. Mutations in *MITF*, *SNAI2*, or *SOX 10* have been found in some cases of Waardenburg II, while mutations in *EDNRB*, *EDN3*, or *SOX10* have been identified in Waardenburg IV, confirming genetic heterogeneity within this group. Piebaldism, which is caused by mutations in the c-kit proto-oncogene, is usually characterized only by skin changes, although deafness has been reported in some patients.

The oculocutaneous albinisms (OCAs) are a group of autosomal recessive disorders that are distinguished from each other by the degree of pigment production. Affected individuals have pink skin, transillumination of the irises, white to light-yellow hair, and often visual disturbances, foveal hypoplasia, and nystagmus. Many mutations in the tyrosinase gene have been identified in both OCA1A (the most severe form classically known as "tyrosinase-negative" with complete lack of tyrosinase activity) and OCA1B (with partial tyrosinase activity) forms of OCA, and many affected individuals are compound heterozygotes for mutations at this locus. In addition, mutations in other genes account for milder forms of OCA: *OCA2* on chromosome 15 in OCA2; *TYRP1* on chromosome 9 in OCA3; and *SLC45A2* gene on chromosome 5 in OCA4.

Tuberous sclerosis complex (TSC) is an autosomal dominant disorder that results from mutations in genes at one of at least two loci: one on chromosome 9 (*TSC1*-hamartin) and the other on chromosome 16 (*TSC2*-tuberin). It is characterized by a number of cutaneous changes including angiofibromas, connective tissue nevi (shagreen patches), periungual fibromas, and hypopigmented macules (ash-leaf spots) (Fig. 44-11).

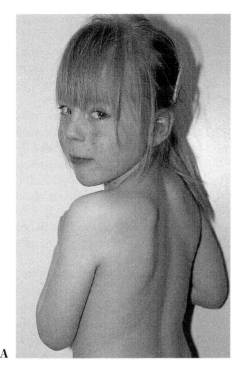

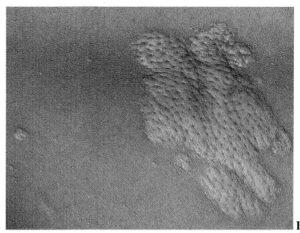

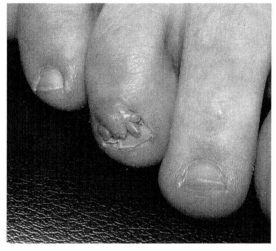

FIGURE 44-11: **A:** A young girl with tuberous sclerosis; hypopigmented macules; angiofibromas on the cheeks. **B:** Shagreen patches (collagenoma). (B, reprinted from Burkhart C, Morrell D, Goldsmith LA, et al. *VisualDx: Essential Pediatric Dermatology*. Philadelphia: Lippincott Williams and Wilkins; 2010.) **C:** Periungual fibroma. (C, reprinted from Sybert VP. *Genetic Skin Disorders*. New York: Oxford University Press; 1997.)

Melanocytes and keratinocytes in these lightly-colored areas contain "effete" or poorly melanized small melanosomes. Mental retardation, seizures, and renal and pulmonary involvement are the other major features of this condition that has very variable expression.

Hypomelanosis of Ito is the term given to the presence of hypopigmentation (or hyperpigmentation) distributed along the lines of Blaschko (Fig. 44-12). Individuals with these skin changes often have additional structural malformations and mental retardation, with almost two-thirds of such patients showing detectable mosaicism for chromosomal aneuploidy. Mosaicism for X-chromosome alterations, tetrasomy 12p, triploidy, trisomy 18, and chimerism are the more common abnormalities reported. It appears that it is the presence of two

chromosomally distinct lines, rather than specific cytogenetic alterations, that confers this striking pigment anomaly.

Individuals with hypopigmentation owing to any cause need to be protected from excessive sun exposure.

Hyperpigmentation

Neurofibromatosis type I (Fig. 44-13) is a relatively common (1/3,000) autosomal dominant disorder caused by mutations in the *NF1* (neurofibromin) gene that resides on chromosome 17.

It is a disorder of neural crest cells, including the melanocyte. Affected individuals manifest pigment abnormalities including café-au-lait spots (brown macules and patches), usually numbering more than five (>5 mm in children and

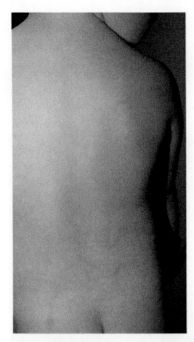

FIGURE 44-12: Streaky pigment variegation, along the lines of Blaschko in a patient with mosaicism for 46, XX/47, XX + rea (12).

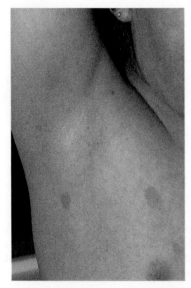

FIGURE 44-13: Café-au-lait spots and axillary freckling in neurofibromatosis. (Reprinted from Sybert VP. *Genetic Skin Disorders*. New York: Oxford University Press; 1997.)

>1.5 cm in adults); axillary, inguinal, and inframammary freckling (Crowe sign) and a general increase in skin color (hypermelanosis). Pigment in these areas is packaged in giant melanosomes—a feature also common in café-au-lait spots not associated with neurofibromatosis. Over time, affected persons develop benign tumors, neurofibromas, which arise from Schwann cells and can occur along any myelinated nerve. These may be few or may number in the hundreds. Severe complications include: plexiform neurofibromas—which

are large disfiguring growths, pseudoarthrosis, intellectual disability (5% to 10%), specific learning issues (40% to 60%), sarcomatous degeneration of benign growths (malignant peripheral nerve sheath tumors), optic glioma, and leukemia (<1%). This is a condition which is extremely variable in its expression both within and among families.

The clinical features of McCune Albright syndrome (Fig. 44-14) are giant café-au-lait spots, polyostotic fibrous dysplasia, and endocrine abnormalities, primarily precocious puberty. It results from a postzygotic mutation in the *GNAS* gene. Affected individuals are mosaic for this otherwise lethal dominant mutation. The severity and location of clinical features depends upon the proportion of normal to abnormal cells that are present. Affected individuals who reproduce have no risk for affecting offspring, as embryos with the abnormal gene present in all cells cannot develop.

Incontinentia pigmenti (IP) (Fig. 44-15) is an X-linked dominant condition caused by mutations in the *IKBKG* gene (coding for the NEMO protein) that affects females almost exclusively. It is usually lethal prenatally in affected males. Newborns present with blistering distributed along the lines of Blaschko (see Dictionary/Index). Over weeks to months, these areas become hyperkeratotic and warty in appearance. This gradually subsides and hyperpigmentation develops, also along the lines of Blaschko, but not necessarily in or limited to the areas of blistering. This hyperpigmentation persists throughout childhood, but may fade to hypopigmented hairless skin in adult life. The severity of associated problems varies. These include central nervous system (CNS) abnormalities including seizures and mental retardation, retinal vascular dysplasia and visual defects, alopecia, hypodontia and peg-shaped teeth, nail dysplasia, and skeletal abnormalities. Surviving males with IP are usually mosaic owing to a postzygotic mutation in *IKBKG* or have Klinefelter syndrome (47, XXY) so that the presence

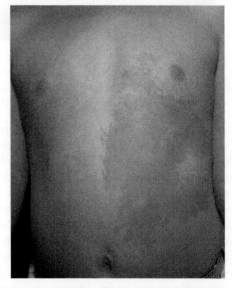

FIGURE 44-14: Giant café-au-lait in a patient with McCune–Albright syndrome. (Reprinted from Sybert VP. *Genetic Skin Disorders*. New York: Oxford University Press; 1997.)

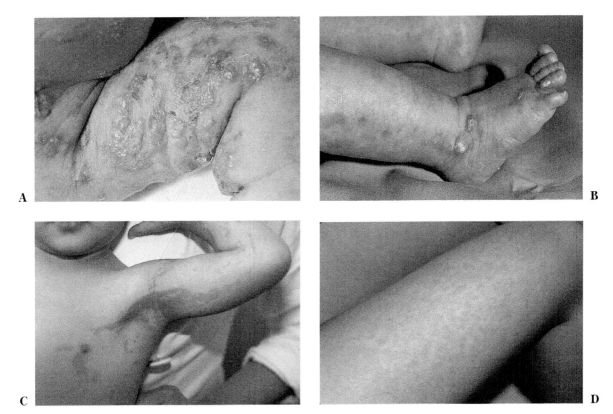

FIGURE 44-15: **A–D:** Stages I to IV of incontinentia pigmenti. (Reprinted from Sybert VP. *Genetic Skin Disorders*. New York: Oxford University Press; 1997.)

of the additional X chromosome with a normal *IKBKG* gene "rescues" them from the usual lethality in males. Mutations in a different region of the *IKBKG* gene give rise to an X-linked recessive condition in which affected males have a phenotype similar to hypohidrotic ectodermal dysplasia, along with additional immune defects.

DISORDERS OF ELASTICITY

Ehlers–Danlos syndrome (EDS) is the eponym given to a group of conditions, some of which share little in common. Recently, efforts have been made to limit application of this eponym to those conditions in which fragility, thinness, and/ or hyperelasticity of the skin is a primary finding.

The classical type of EDS is characterized by soft, velvety hyperextensible skin that is fragile, tears easily, and heals poorly with thin cigarette paper scars. There is easy bruising. Over time, elastosis perforans serpiginosa can become a significant management problem. Patients have marked ligament laxity. In some families, mutations in type 5 collagen (*COL5A1* or *COL5A2*) or type 1 collagen (*COL1A1*) have been identified. Individuals with the hypermobility type of EDS have minimally affected skin, but marked hyperextensibility of large and small joints. Electron microscopy of the skin shows abnormal collagen bundles in these conditions. The vascular type of EDS is autosomal dominant, as are the classical and hypermobility types. The skin in the vascular type of EDS is

thin and taut, rather than velvety and soft. This is a disorder of type III collagen (*COL3A1*) that is distributed in the lining of vessels and viscera. Rupture of these is the major medical complication and death is common before age 50.

Cutis laxa is a heterogeneous group of autosomal recessive and X-linked recessive conditions, which share laxity, not elasticity, of the skin. The skin is soft and progressively loses tone. Affected individuals have a prematurely aged "hound dog" appearance to the face. X-linked cutis laxa, now known as occipital horn syndrome (OHS), is caused by a defect in the *ATP7A* gene, whose product transports copper. Causative mutations result in secondary deficiency of copper-dependent enzymes. Internal involvement includes progressive hydronephrosis and bladder diverticula, emphysema and pulmonary blebs, and hernias. Intellect ranges from mild mental retardation to normal. Allelic mutations in *ATP7A* also cause Menkes syndrome, which is a much more severe disorder. In Menkes, the skin of affected males is thin, pale, with a prominent venous pattern. The hairs are fine, sparse, and fragile and demonstrate pili torti (twisting). Neurologic involvement is usually severe and progressive. Prenatal diagnosis is available for both OHS and Menkes syndrome. Daily use of a dietary copper histamine supplementation when instituted shortly after birth may have some benefit in slowing the progression of neurologic symptoms.

In pseudoxanthoma elasticum (PXE), there is progressive deterioration of elastic fibers in the dermis, choroid of the eye, and blood vessels. The changes in PXE are progressive. The skin becomes progressively involved by cobblestoned, yellowish plaques, especially at the nape and in the folds. These are clinically similar to solar elastosis. Progressive atherosclerotic disease, presumably owing to calcified plaques developing on abnormal vessel walls, results in claudication, gastrointestinal (GI) bleeding, and stroke. Breaks in Bruch membrane of the eye are seen as angioid streaks upon eye examination. This is a feature typical of the disorder. Making the diagnosis is unusual in childhood unless there is a positive family history and a high index of suspicion. Homozygosity or compound heterozygosity for mutations in the *ABCC6* gene underlies this autosomal recessive condition. Pedigrees with apparent autosomal dominant inheritance of PXE appear to be the result of pseudodominance.

DISORDERS OF APPENDAGES

Hair

Inherited defects in hair can affect the development of follicles, hair growth, and hair structure. Congenital alopecias are rare. They may be isolated or associated with other organ involvement. Most are autosomal recessive. A disorder of hair growth in early childhood is the loose anagen syndrome—a condition in which the anagen roots are structurally abnormal, the hairs are poorly anchored and easily plucked, and the growth period is reduced. Affected children have thin, short hair which "never needs to be cut." It tends to improve with time and by adult life hair may appear normal although still relatively loosely anchored. Inheritance is uncertain. Structural hair shaft abnormalities are listed in Table 44-3.

Nails

Isolated inherited disorders of nails are rare and most abnormalities are usually part of syndromes. Pachyonychia congenita (PC) (Fig. 44-16A) is a term used for the autosomal dominant genodermatosis with the main clinical features of hypertrophic nail dystrophy, painful and highly debilitating plantar keratoderma, oral leukokeratosis, follicular keratosis at the elbows and knees with or without other features such as epidermal cysts

TABLE 44-3 • Hair Disorders

Name	Inheritance	Basic Defect	Microscopic Features	Associated Abnormalities
Monilethrix	AD	Mutations in type II hair keratins: *hHb6 hHb1*	Beaded hairs; regular or irregular narrowing and widening of hair shaft	None
Pili annulati	AD	Unknown. Bands are owing to air-filled cavities in cortex	Ringed hair; alternating bands of light and dark	None
Pili torti	XLR AD	Mutations in *MNK1* (*ATP7A*) Unknown	Twisting along longitudinal axis of hair shaft	Menkes syndrome None
Pili trianguli et canaliculi (uncombable; spangled hair)	AD	Unknown	Grooved, triangular hair	None
Trichorrhexis invaginata	AR	Unknown	Nodal swelling of hair shaft; similar to bamboo	Netherton syndrome
Trichorrhexis nodosa	AD	Unknown	Fraying of medulla owing to abnormal cuticle. Appearance of opposing broom heads	Argininosuccinic aciduria
	AR Acquired	Unknown Argininosuccinate lyase deficiency		Trauma can be seen in any fragile hair
Trichothiodystrophy	AR	Decrease in disulfide bonds. Decrease in cysteine in hair	Thin fragile hairs with birefringent regions in polarized microscopy	Heterogeneous; may be associated with any of the four major types of EB simplex: Ichthyosis
		Mutations in *ERCC2/XPD* and *ERCC3/XPB* in some with *PIBIDS*		Mental retardation Failure to thrive Short stature Infertility or maybe isolated

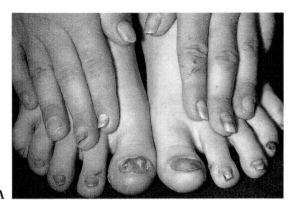
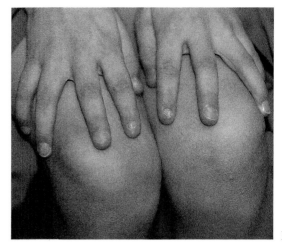

FIGURE 44-16: A: Nails in pachyonychia congenita. **B:** Nails in nail-patella syndrome. (Reprinted from Sybert VP. *Genetic Skin Disorders*. New York: Oxford University Press; 1997.)

and steatocystoma multiplex. In all PC types, the nail plates are thickened or may be small or absent. Nail changes may appear within the first few years of life or not until later. Not all nails are necessarily involved. Originally the condition was divided into two conditions: type 1–Jadassohn–Lewandowsky (PC1) and type 2—Jackson–Lawler (PC2). Palmar–plantar hyperkeratosis and leukokeratosis of the oral mucosa were more common in PC1, and. epidermal cysts, steatocystoma multiplex, and natal teeth are more typical of PC2. With molecular characterization, and as patients are found to have a mixed characterization of features, PC is now divided according to genotype, with mutations described in associated keratins, *KRT16* (PC1), *KRT17* (PC2), *KRT6A* (PC3), and *KRT6B* (PC4).

Nail-patella syndrome (see Fig. 44-16B) is an autosomal dominant disorder marked by variable nail dystrophy with usually symmetric involvement. Skeletal abnormalities are also a feature and include hypoplasia to absence of the patellae, malformations of the elbows and scapulae, and iliac horns. Renal involvement ranges from glomerulonephritis to severe renal failure and occurs in up to a third of affected individuals. The causal gene, *LMX1B* (LIM-homeodomain protein), is linked to the ABO blood group on the long arm of chromosome 9.

ECTODERMAL DYSPLASIAS

There are over 100 genetic conditions whose major findings involve alterations in two or more of the primary ectodermal derivatives—hair, teeth, sweat glands, and nails. Historically, the ectodermal dysplasias have been divided into those with relatively normal sweating—hidrotic and those with heat intolerance, hypohidrotic, or anhidrotic. The most common of the ectodermal dysplasias is X-linked recessive hypohidrotic ectodermal dysplasia (Christ–Siemens–Touraine syndrome), which is caused by mutation in the gene encoding ectodysplasin A (*ED1*) (Fig. 44-17). Affected males may present with a collodion membrane at birth, have heat intolerance because of inability to sweat, hypodontia and peg-shaped teeth, and

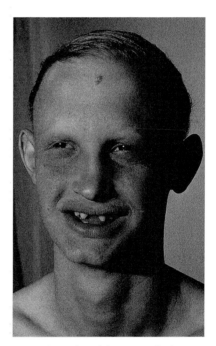

FIGURE 44-17: A male with sparse hair; peg-shaped teeth, hypodontia, and the typical facies of hypohidrotic ectodermal dysplasia. (Reprinted from Sybert VP. *Genetic Skin Disorders*. New York: Oxford University Press; 1997.)

sparse hair. Female carriers may have patchy hair loss, patchy distribution of sweat glands, with minimal to significant tooth involvement.

HAMARTOMAS/MALIGNANCIES

A number of genetic skin conditions are marked by development of cutaneous and extracutaneous malignancy. Table 44-4 lists some of these.

TABLE 44-4 • Disorders Associated With Malignancy

Disorder	Mode of Inheritance	Gene	Major Dermatologic Findings	Associated Features	Typical Malignancy
Ataxia telangiectasia	AR	*ATM*	Progressive telangiectases on skin conjunctiva. Premature graying of the hair	Ataxia CNS degeneration Immunodeficiency	Leukemia Lymphoma Others (ovarian, breast, gastric, sarcoma)
Basal cell nevus syndrome	AD	PTCH SUFU (5%)	Basal cell nevi Palmar–plantar pits Epidermal cysts	Many, including odontogenic keratocysts and skeletal abnormalities	Basal cell carcinoma Medulloblastoma Cardiac and ovarian fibromas
Bloom syndrome	AR	*BLM*	Malar telangiectases Photosensitivity	Immunodeficiency Growth failure Infertility in males	Myelodysplasia Many subtypes of common cancers: Hematologic Adenocarcinomas
Cowden syndrome	AD	*PTEN*	Tricholemmomas Acral keratoses Palmar–plantar keratoses Oral papillomas Lipomas Vascular malformations	Macrocephaly Thyroid abnormalities Fibrocystic breast disease GI polyps Intellectual disability	Breast Ovarian Thyroid (follicular) Uterine Renal
Dyskeratosis congenita	XLR AD AD + AR Other AD and AR	DKC1 TERC TERT Other genes	Progressive reticular hyperpigmentation Nail dystrophy Oral leukoplakia Premature graying	Bone marrow failure Pulmonary fibrosis	Squamous cell cancer Leukemia risk
Fanconi anemia syndrome	AR	Mutations in multiple complementation groups including: *FANCA FANCB FANCC FANCD2*	Café-au-lait spots Patchy hyperpigmentation Sweet syndrome	Bone marrow failure Radial ray defects Short stature Microcephaly Renal anomalies	Hematopoietic (AML and Myelodysplastic) Squamous cell Hepatocellular
Gardner syndrome (Familial Adenomatous Polyposis [FAP])	AD	*APC*	Epidermal inclusion cysts Fibromas Desmoid tumors	Intestinal polyps Mandibular osteomas Congenital hypertrophy of retinal pigment epithelium (CHRPE)	GI malignancies (Colon, Gastric) Other (thyroid, hepatic, medulloblastoma)
MEN 2A/2B	AD	*RET*	Mucosal neuromas	Marfanoid habitus Ganglioneuromas of GI tract	Pheochromocytoma Medullary thyroid carcinoma Parathyroid adenoma

TABLE 44-4 • Disorders Associated With Malignancy (*continued*)

Disorder	Mode of Inheritance	Gene	Major Dermatologic Findings	Associated Features	Typical Malignancy
Peutz-Jeghers	AD	*STK11*	Lentigines (hyperpigmented macules) on lips, mucosa palms, soles, fingertips	GI (colorectal and gastric) hamartomatous polyposis	Gastrointestinal carcinoma Breast Thyroid Lung Pancreatic Uterine Sertoli cell testicular Ovarian sex cord
Rothmund-Thomson syndrome	AR	*RECQL4* in some cases	Facial telangiectases Poikiloderma Alopecia	Short stature Radial ray defects Hypogonadism Cataracts	Squamous cell cancer Osteogenic sarcoma
Xeroderma pigmentosa	AR	*Mutations in multiple complementation groups including: ERCC2 ERCC3 ERCC5 XPC XPA*	Progressive dyspigmentation Telangiectases Atrophy Progressive actinic changes	Neurologic involvement in XPA, XPC, XPD	Susceptibility to skin cancer: Squamous cell cancer Basal cell cancer Malignant melanoma

ACKNOWLEDGMENT

The authors wish to acknowledge Amy Y. Jan, MD, PhD and Virginia P. Sybert, MD for their work on the previous version of this chapter.

Suggested Readings

Beighton P, De Paepe A, Steinmann B, et al. Ehlers–Danlos syndromes: revised nosology, Villefranche, 1997. Ehlers-Danlos National Foundation (USA) and Ehlers-Danlos Support Group (UK). *Am J Med Genet*. 1998;77:31–37.

Byers PH. Disorders of collagen biosynthesis and structure. In: Scriver CR, Beaudet al, Sly WS, et al, eds. *The Metabolic and Molecular Bases of Inherited Disease*. 8th ed. New York: McGraw-Hill; 2001:chap 205.

Callewaert B, Malfait F, Loeys B, et al. Ehlers–Danlos syndromes and Marfan syndrome. *Best Pract Res Clin Rheumatol*. 2008;22(1):165–189.

Chassaing N, Martin L, Calvas P, et al. Pseudoxanthoma elasticum: a clinical, pathophysiological and genetic update including 11 novel ABCC6 mutations. *J Med Genet*. 2005;42(12):881–192.

Ehrenreich M, Tarlow MM, Godlewska-Janusz E, et al. Incontinentia pigmenti (Bloch-Sulzberger syndrome): a systemic disorder. *Cutis*. 2007;79(5):355–362.

Fine JD, Bruckner-Tuderman L, Eady RA, et al. Inherited epidermolysis bullosa: updated recommendations on diagnosis and classification. *J Am Acad Dermatol*. 2014;70:1103–1126.

Freire-Maia N, Pinheiro M. *Ectodermal Dysplasias: A Clinical and Genetic Study*. New York: Alan R. Liss; 1984.

Gronskov K, Ek J, Brondum-Nielsen K. Oculocutaneous albinism. *Orphanet J Rare Dis*. 2007;2:43. http://www.OJRD.com/content/2/1/43

Hu X, Plomp AS, van Soest S, et al. Pseudoxanthoma elasticum: a clinical, histopathological, and molecular update. *Surv Ophthalmol*. 2003;48:424–438.

Juhlin L, Baran R. Hereditary and congenital nail disorders. In: Baran R, Dawber RPR, de Berker DAR, et al, eds. *Diseases of the Nails and their Management*. 3rd ed. Oxford: Blackwell; 2001.

King RA, Hearing VJ, Creel DJ, et al. Albinism. In: Scriver CR, Beaudet al, Valle ED, et al, eds. *The Metabolic and Molecular Bases of Inherited Disease*. 8th ed. New York:McGraw-Hill; 2001:chap 220.

Lamartine J. Towards a new classification of ectodermal dysplasias. *Clin Exp Dermatol*. 2003;28(4):351–355.

Neldner KH. Pseudoxanthoma elasticum. *Clin Dermatol*. 1988;6:1–159.

Oji V, Traupe H. Ichthyoses: differential diagnosis and molecular genetics. *Eur J Dermatol*. 2006;16(4):349–359.

Passeron T, Mantoux F, Ortonne J-P. Genetic disorders of pigmentation. *Clin Dermatol*. 2005;23(1):56–67.

Somoano B, Tsao H. Genodermatoses with cutaneous tumors and internal malignancies. *Dermatol Clin*. 2008;26(1):69–87, viii.

Sprecher E. Genetic hair and nail disorders. *Clin Dermatol*. 2005;23(1):47–55.

Steinmann B, Royce PM, Superti-Furga A. The Ehlers-Danlos syndrome. In: Royce PM, Steinmann B, eds. *Connective Tissue and its Heritable Disorders*. New York: Wiley-Liss; 1992:351–407.

Stratigos AJ, Baden HP. Unraveling the molecular mechanisms of hair and nail genodermatoses. *Arch Dermatol*. 2001;137(11):1465–1471.

Sybert VP. Hypomelanosis of Ito: a description, not a diagnosis. *J Invest Dermatol*. 1994;103:141S–143S.

Sybert VP. *Genetic Skin Disorders*. New York: Oxford University Press; 1997.

Uitto J, Richard G. Progress in epidermolysis bullosa: from eponyms to molecular genetic classification. *Clin Dermatol*. 2005;23(1):33–40.

Pediatric Dermatology

Kimberly A. Horii, MD, and Rachel L. Laarman, MD

Skin disorders in infants and younger children may be different from the same diseases in older children or adults (Figs. 45-1 and 45-2). Certain skin conditions such as diaper dermatitis are typically seen only in infants; other conditions such as atopic dermatitis may appear different in children when compared with adults. Pediatric dermatology can be divided into neonatal dermatoses and dermatoses of infants and children. It is useful to describe a lesion by its morphology to develop a differential diagnosis of what the disorder might be.

NEONATAL DERMATOSES (BIRTH TO 1 MONTH)

A few lesions may be noted at birth or shortly thereafter (Table 45-1). In the newborn period, an infectious etiology for a skin eruption needs to be ruled out because some neonatal infections can be life threatening.

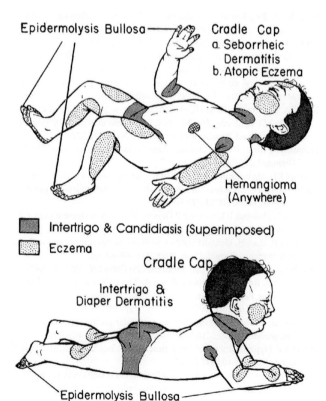

FIGURE 45-1: Pediatric dermograms (infancy).

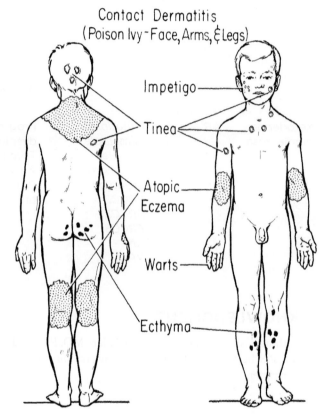

FIGURE 45-2: Pediatric dermograms (childhood).

Blistering (Vesiculobullous) Lesions

Blistering lesions can be mechanically induced or caused by infections.

- *Sucking blisters:* Usually seen as oval bullae on the hand or forearm and thought to be caused by sucking in utero. They resolve rapidly.
- *Epidermolysis bullosa* (Fig. 45-3): A group of inherited disorders with fragile skin and bullous lesions that develop spontaneously or as a result of trauma.
- *Infections* (Fig. 45-4): Herpes simplex, congenital varicella, candidiasis, and congenital syphilis can present as blisters in the newborn. Herpes simplex is important to recognize and refer for treatment because neonatal herpes infection can be fatal.

TABLE 45-1 • Neonatal Dermatoses (Birth to 1 Month)

Blistering (Vesiculobullous Lesions)
Mechanical
   Sucking blisters
   Epidermolysis bullosa
   Bullous ichthyosiform erythroderma
     (ichthyosis)

Infectious
   Herpes simplex
   Congenital varicella
   Candidiasis
   Congenital syphilis

Pustular Lesions
Candidiasis
Erythema toxicum
Transient neonatal pustular melanosis
Neonatal acne
Milia

Birthmarks
White
   Albinism
   Piebaldism
   Ash leaf macules
   Nevus anemicus
   Nevus depigmentosus

Brown
   Café-au-lait spots
   Congenital melanocytic nevus
   Dermal melanosis
   Epidermal nevus

Vascular
   Nevus simplex (Salmon patch)
   Capillary malformation (port-wine stain)
   Hemangioma of infancy

Yellow
   Nevus sebaceous

Papulosquamous Lesions
Ichthyosis
Neonatal lupus erythematosus

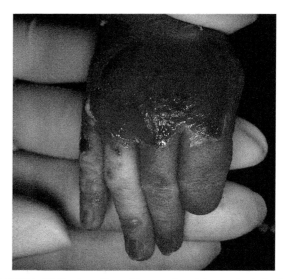

FIGURE 45-3: Junctional type of epidermolysis bulls with sloughing of epidermis on the dorsal hand and blisters over the dorsal fingers.

Pustular Lesions

Some pustular dermatoses are self-limited and require no treatment; others may be a result of an infection requiring therapy.

- *Candidiasis* (see Fig. 45-4): Apart from blisters, candidiasis may also present with erythematous papules and pustules.
- *Erythema toxicum:* A common, benign, and self-limited condition of the newborn, usually noted during the first few days of life. Erythematous macules, papules, and sterile pustules may occur anywhere on the body.
- *Transient neonatal pustular melanosis* (Fig. 45-5): A benign, self-limited disorder characterized by sterile pustules that rupture and evolve into hyperpigmented macules.
- *Neonatal acne:* Papules and pustules develop at 2 to 4 weeks of age. It is self-limited and usually does not scar. Topical erythromycin or benzoyl peroxide may be helpful. Neonatal cephalic pustulosis is considered synonymous by some authors, and response to topical ketoconazole has been reported. The role of yeast is yet to be determined.
- *Milia:* Occurs commonly on the cheeks, nose, chin, and forehead. It presents as 1- to 2-mm white or yellow papules, which are frequently grouped. The lesions resolve without therapy.

Birthmarks

Newborns may have many different types of birthmarks that can be categorized by color.

White

- *Albinism:* An uncommon inherited disorder with lack of pigment in the skin, hair, and eyes. A partial lack of pigmentation is termed *piebaldism* or *partial albinism*.
- *Ash leaf macules:* Lance-shaped hypopigmented macules on the trunk, arms, or legs, usually associated with tuberous sclerosis.

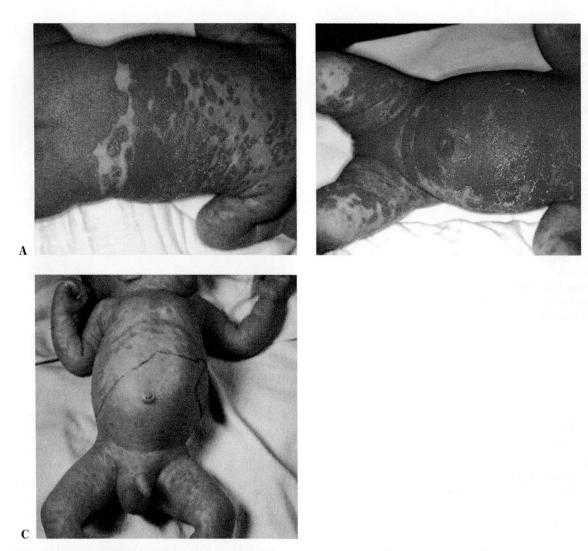

FIGURE 45-4: Candidiasis and syphilis. **A and B:** Extensive candida albicans with confluent bright erythema and satellite papules. **C:** Congenital syphilis with hepatomegaly and splenomegaly.

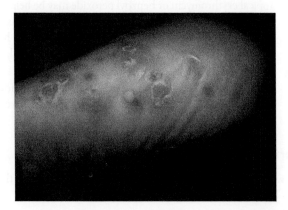

FIGURE 45-5: Transient neonatal pustular melanosis. Pustules and vesicles. Some have ruptures and are developing hyperpigmentation.

- *Nevus anemicus:* A solitary hypopigmented macule resulting from a localized vascular reaction. The surrounding borders classically blanch with pressure.
- *Nevus depigmentosus:* A unilateral hypopigmented patch with poorly defined borders.

Brown

- *Café-au-lait spots* (Fig. 45-6): Light brown, round or oval macules. These can be normal findings but may be seen in association with neurofibromatosis type I. This condition should be suspected if six or more café-au-lait spots greater than 0.5 cm in diameter are present in association with other clinical findings.
- *Congenital melanocytic nevus* (Fig. 45-7): A tan to dark brown, well-circumscribed papule or plaque. Nevi vary in size from small to large, and often have associated hypertrichosis. Congenital nevi have the rare potential of developing into a melanoma depending on their size (more so for large nevi >20 cm), location, border (irregular), color (especially black and multicolored), and texture (nodules).
- *Dermal melanosis* (Mongolian spots) (Fig. 45-8): Deep brown, slate gray, or blue-black macules found mostly over the lumbosacral area and buttocks in darker-pigmented infants. These are benign and self-limited.

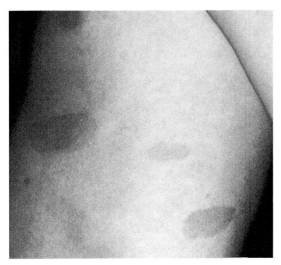

FIGURE 45-6: Café-au-lait lesions. Macules and patches of oval evenly colored and evenly edged brown areas.

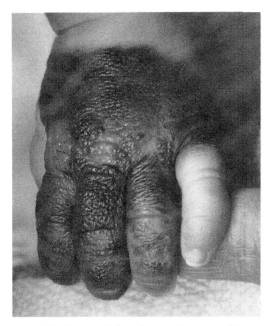

FIGURE 45-7: Congenital melanocytic nevus. Verrucous brown and black plaque over dorsal hand and fingers.

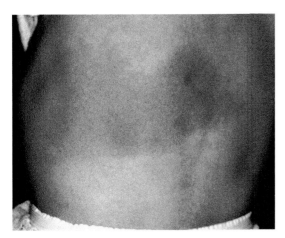

FIGURE 45-8: Dermal melanosis (mongolian spots) on the back. Bruise-like patch of brown-black pigment over lower back.

- *Epidermal nevus* (Fig. 45-9): Tan to brown verrucous linear lesions often noted at birth. They may rarely have other associated neurologic or skeletal abnormalities.

Vascular

- *Nevus simplex (Salmon patch)* (Fig. 45-10): Dull pink macules on the glabella, upper eyelids, (also referred to as angel kisses), or nape of the neck (also referred to as a *stork bite*). Angel kisses usually fade when present on the face, but stork bites do not.
- *Port-wine stain (capillary malformation)* (Fig. 45-11): A congenital vascular malformation composed of dilated capillaries. These are reddish purple macules or patches that do not involute. Laser therapy is a treatment option. Neurologic and ophthalmologic abnormalities (Sturge–Weber syndrome) may accompany a port-wine stain located on the face above the palpebral fissure.
- *Infantile hemangioma* (Fig. 45-12): Benign tumors of infancy composed of proliferating vascular endothelium.

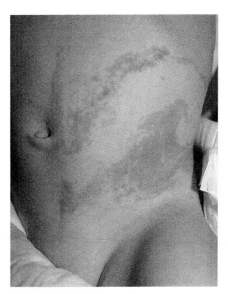

FIGURE 45-9: Epidermal nevus. Linear unilateral whorls of pink, slightly verrucous plaques over the abdomen.

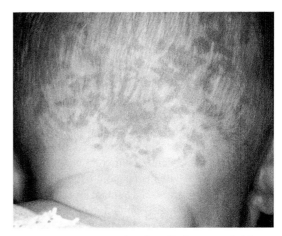

FIGURE 45-10: Nevus simplex (Salmon patch). Mottled pink plaque over back of scalp and nape of neck. Called the "devil's bite." It is usually permanent.

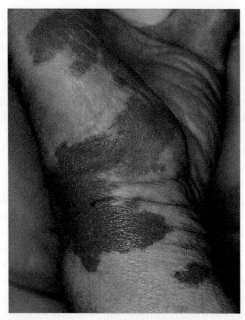

FIGURE 45-11: Capillary malformation (port-wine stain). Deep-red slightly elevated plaques over wrist and hand.

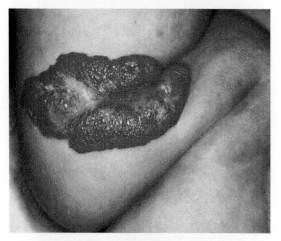

FIGURE 45-12: Infantile hemangioma-superficial. Bright-red "strawberry" tumor of the groin.

They grow rapidly in infancy, stabilize, and involute in childhood, many resolving by 10 years of age. They may be superficial, deep, or mixed. A newer classification system separates hemangiomas based upon their configuration. Localized hemangiomas are symmetric and confined to a limited space. Segmental hemangiomas are large and appear to follow a geographic territory of the body (Fig. 45-13). Segmental hemangiomas can be associated with underlying anomalies and have been associated with more complications and may require treatment more frequently. Numerous cutaneous lesions may be associated with hemangiomas in the viscera, such as the liver. Large facial hemangiomas may be associated with neurologic, ophthalmologic, and cardiac abnormalities (PHACE syndrome). Management may consist of observation alone, oral prednisolone, oral propranolol, topical timolol, laser treatment, or surgery.

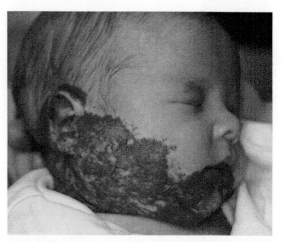

FIGURE 45-13: A large segmental hemangioma on the face may be a sign of an underlying anomaly. Bright-red tumor in a beard-like distribution in an infant.

Yellow

- *Nevus sebaceous:* Noted at birth as a yellow-orange, oval or linear area of alopecia on the scalp. At puberty, they become raised and warty. Basal cell carcinomas can rarely develop within the nevus later in life. A benign warty tumor called *syringocystadenoma papilliferum* may occur in conjunction with a nevus sebaceous.

Papulosquamous Lesions

- *Ichthyosis* (Fig. 45-14): Associated with dry, fishlike adherent scales. The rarer and more severe forms of autosomal recessive congenital ichthyosis usually present at birth with a shiny, tight layer of skin called a *collodion membrane.* Ichthyosis vulgaris is the commonest form, and X-linked ichthyosis is usually not present at birth.
- *Neonatal lupus erythematosus* (Fig. 45-15): Characterized by annular papulosquamous skin lesions on the forehead and cheeks. The skin lesions usually fade by 6 to 7 months of age. Other systemic symptoms can include congenital heart block, hepatic transaminitis, leukopenia, and thrombocytopenia. Because this is maternally transmitted, the mother also needs to be evaluated for lupus or another underlying collagen vascular disorder. Anti-Ro or Sjogren syndrome type A (SSA) and anti-La or Sjogren syndrome type B (SSB) antibodies may be present in the mother and/or newborn.

DERMATOSES OF INFANTS AND CHILDREN

See Table 45-2 for a summary of these dermatoses.

Blistering Lesions (Vesiculobullous)

- *Impetigo* (Fig. 45-16): Typically presents as small pustules that may develop into large, flaccid bullae (bullous impetigo). The pustules eventually rupture leaving

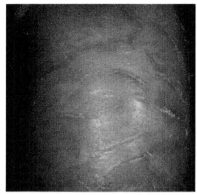
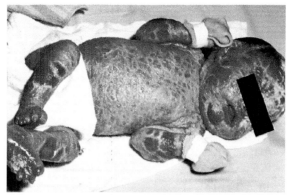

FIGURE 45-14: Ichthyosis. **A:** Lamellar ichthyosis with large laminated plaques divided into plates by linear fissures. **B:** Harlequin fetus covered with sheets of reddish-brown plates. As is often the case, this was fatal in this newborn.

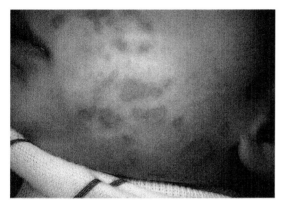

FIGURE 45-15: Neonatal lupus erythematosus.

erosions covered by a honey-colored crust. Impetigo is usually caused by *Staphylococcus aureus* and less commonly by *Streptococcus pyogenes*. Staphylococcal scalded skin syndrome is a desquamating disorder caused by an exfoliative toxin that results in perioral crusting, erythema, and superficial desquamation most prominent in the intertriginous and flexural regions. In the newborn, it is known as Ritter disease.

- *Viral blisters* (Fig. 45-17): Herpes simplex, varicella (chicken pox), and Coxsackie (hand–foot–mouth disease) can present with vesicles on an erythematous base.

- *Bullous disease of childhood (linear IgA dermatoses):* Sausage-shaped bullae in a "string of pearls" configuration most commonly noted on the buttocks, groin, and lower extremities. It is usually a self-limited disease. Rarely, when treatment is needed, it responds well to dapsone. Direct immunofluorescence is positive for IgA at the dermal–epidermal junction.

- *Dermatitis herpetiformis:* Recurrent crops of severely pruritic grouped vesicles or bullae on the extensor surfaces of the extremities, shoulders, and buttocks. The eruption is often associated with celiac disease and may improve with a gluten-free diet.

- *Incontinentia pigmenti* (Fig. 45-18): An inherited disorder presenting with vesicles and pustules in a linear distribution following lines of Blaschko during the first

TABLE 45-2 • Dermatoses of Infants and Children

Blistering Lesions
Impetigo
Viral blisters
Bullous disease of childhood
Dermatitis herpetiformis
Incontinentia pigmenti

Pustular Lesions
Acropustulosis of infancy
Impetigo
Candidiasis

Papules/Nodules
Skin color
 Warts
 Molluscum contagiosum
 Keratosis pilaris
 Granuloma annulare
 Angiofibroma

Brown
 Melanocytic nevi
 Urticaria pigmentosa

Yellow papules
 Juvenile xanthogranuloma
 Nevus sebaceous

Red papules
 Papular acrodermatitis
 Papular urticaria
 Urticaria
 Erythema multiforme
 Pyogenic granuloma
 Viral exanthems
 Drug eruption

Vascular Lesions
Blanching
 Spider angioma

Nonblanching
 Idiopathic thrombocytopenic purpura
 Henoch–Schönlein purpura
 Meningococcemia
 Vasculitis

TABLE 45-2 • Dermatoses of Infants and Children (*continued*)

Papulosquamous
Psoriasis
Pityriasis rosea
Tinea versicolor

Eczematous Lesions
Atopic dermatitis
Seborrheic dermatitis
Immunodeficiency
Allergic contact dermatitis
Diaper dermatitis

Diseases Affecting the Hair
Congenital/hereditary hair defects
Alopecia areata
Tinea capitis
Trichotillomania

Diseases Affecting the Nails
Congenital nail defects
Twenty-nail dystrophy
Psoriasis/atopic dermatitis
Warts
Paronychia

Dermatoses Owing to Physical Agents and Photosensitivity Dermatoses
Sunburn
Thermal burn
Child abuse
Polymorphous light eruption
Phytophotodermatitis

few months of life. The vesicles are replaced by a warty stage followed by a pigmented stage. There may be associated ophthalmologic and dental abnormalities.

Pustular Lesions

- *Acropustulosis of infancy:* Noted between birth and 2 years of age. Recurrent crops of pruritic papulopustules or vesiculopustular lesions develop on the palms, soles, dorsum of hands, and feet. It is self-limited and often misdiagnosed as scabies.
- *Impetigo:* (See earlier) may also be pustular.
- *Candidiasis* (Fig. 45-19): Can present with pustules and erythematous papules in the diaper and intertriginous regions.

Papules/Nodules

Skin Color

- *Warts:* Verrucous papules caused by the human papillomavirus and transmitted by skin contact. They may resolve without therapy. In children, they are common on the face, hands, and feet. When they are noted in the genitalia, sexual abuse should be considered.
- *Molluscum contagiosum:* Viral disease caused by a member of the pox virus group. They present as single or multiple dome-shaped and often umbilicated papules found anywhere on the body. There may be an associated dermatitis near the molluscum lesions. Spread is by skin contact or autoinoculation. Molluscum is also more common in individuals with atopic dermatitis. They may dissipate without therapy.
- *Keratosis pilaris:* An autosomal dominant disorder characterized by minute follicular papules on the outer aspects of the arms, thighs, and cheeks. It is often seen in association with atopy and dry skin. Topical keratolytic creams may be helpful.
- *Granuloma annulare* (Fig. 45-20): Asymptomatic skin-colored or dull red papules that spread peripherally, forming a ring with a normal appearing center. These are usually found on the dorsum of the hands and feet. The cause is unknown, and spontaneous resolution without treatment occurs in months to years.
- *Angiofibroma:* Firm pink to skin-colored papules. They may be associated with tuberous sclerosis when seen in a symmetric distribution on the face.

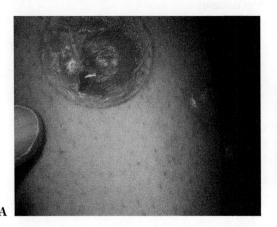

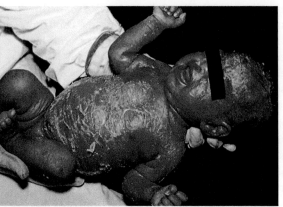

A **B**

FIGURE 45-16: **A:** Flaccid bullae on the leg of a child with methicillin-sensitive staphylococcal aureus grown on culture. **B:** Ritter disease or staphylococcal-scalded skin syndrome in a neonate. Generalized exfoliative dermatitis with thick adherent scale.

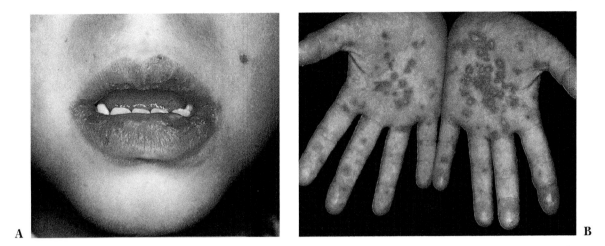

FIGURE 45-17: Viral exanthem. **A:** Erosions of the lips. **B:** Blisters on the palms.

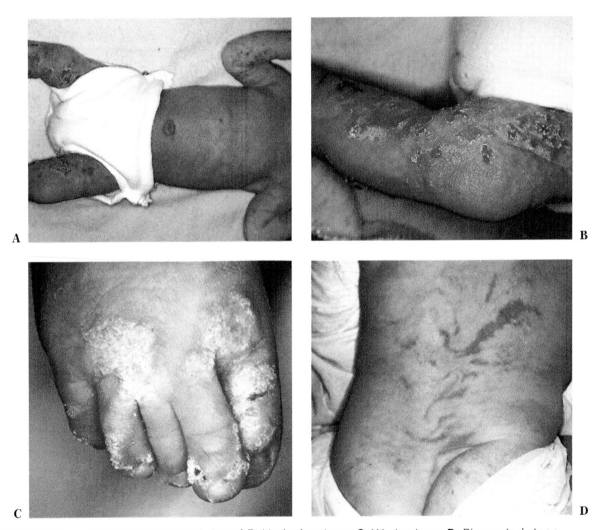

FIGURE 45-18: Incontinentia pigmenti. **A and B:** Vesicular stage. **C:** Warty stage. **D:** Pigmented stage.

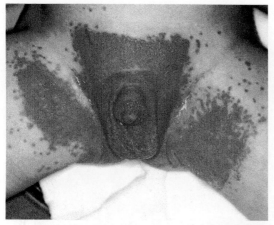

FIGURE 45-19: Candidal rash. Bright-red dermatitis worse in the folds of the skin with distinctive satellite papules.

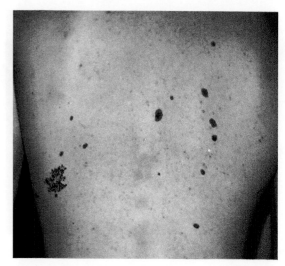

FIGURE 45-21: Melanocytic nevi. Junctional nevi on the back and speckled lentiginous nevus far left midback.

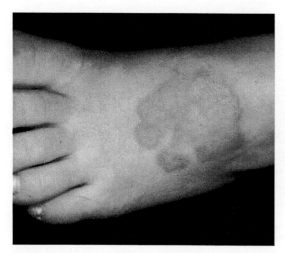

FIGURE 45-20: Granuloma annulare. On the dorsum of the foot.

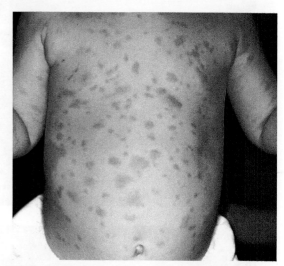

FIGURE 45-22: Urticaria pigmentosa. Urticaria pigmentosa in a 2-year-old patient (note the red, urticating lesion below the left nipple indicating a positive Darier sign).

Brown

- *Melanocytic nevi* (Fig. 45-21): Depending on the location of the nevus cells, these may be called junctional (at the border of the dermal–epidermal junction, usually flat and brown in color), intradermal (within the dermis, usually flesh colored and elevated), or compound nevi (both at the dermal–epidermal junction and in the dermis, usually elevated and brown). They occur anywhere on the body and may be flat, elevated, verrucous, or papillomatous. If they are black, multicolored, large (>6 mm), or have an irregular border, or are noted to change quickly, an excisional biopsy should be considered.

- *Urticaria pigmentosa* (Fig. 45-22): Tan to brown macules and papules that urticate when stroked (Darier sign). It usually has an excellent prognosis if there is no systemic involvement. Lesions eventually resolve without therapy. Signs of systemic involvement could include chronic diarrhea and flushing.

Yellow

- *Juvenile xanthogranuloma:* Usually develops in the first year of life and disappears around 5 years of age. They present as either solitary or multiple small yellow papules on the scalp or body. There may be associated ocular involvement if multiple lesions are present.

- *Nevus sebaceous:* See earlier.

Red

- *Papular acrodermatitis (Gianotti–Crosti syndrome):* Nonpruritic, flat-topped papules on acral surfaces, especially elbows and knees. It was originally associated with the hepatitis B virus, but recently other viruses have been implicated. Usually, it is benign and self-limited but can last for several weeks.

- *Papular urticaria:* A delayed hypersensitivity reaction to a variety of arthropod bites. It presents as pruritic erythematous papules with a surrounding wheal on exposed skin such as arms and legs. Recurrent crops occur in the summer.
- *Urticaria:* Commonly seen in infants and children, associated with an underlying infection or a reaction to a medication or food. It presents as pruritic, erythematous, and edematous wheals that migrate over a 24-hour period.
- *Erythema multiforme (EM):* Acute hypersensitivity syndrome presenting with macular, urticarial, or vesiculobullous lesions commonly on the palms and soles. Target or "bull's eye" lesions are the hallmark of this condition with a central dusky hue and surrounding concentric erythema. It is commonly divided into EM minor, which is a benign, recurrent, and self-limited condition also involving one mucous membrane surface. EM minor is often associated with a recurrent herpes simplex virus infection. EM major presents with the involvement of at least two mucous membrane surfaces, widespread bullous lesions, and more systemic symptoms. EM major is frequently associated with *mycoplasma pneumoniae* infection or drugs.
- *Pyogenic granuloma:* Bright red, rapidly growing papule that bleeds easily. It may arise spontaneously or at sites of trauma. Excision is usually required.
- *Viral exanthems:* Roseola, rubeola, rubella, adenovirus, erythema infectiosum, and enterovirus infections may present with erythematous macules and papules. Fever may also accompany the cutaneous manifestations.
- *Drug eruption:* Multiple medications may cause a diffuse cutaneous eruption. Typically, morbilliform drug eruptions present with blanchable erythematous macules and papules.

Vascular Lesions

Blanching

- *Spider angioma:* Small telangiectatic lesion on the cheeks, nose, dorsum of hands, or sun-exposed areas. Lesions are benign and often resolve spontaneously.

Nonblanching (Petechiae and Purpura)

- *Idiopathic thrombocytopenic purpura:* Low platelet disorder presenting with nonblanching petechiae and purpura especially on areas of trauma. Intravenous immunoglobulin is the treatment of choice.
- *Henoch–Schönlein purpura* (Fig. 45-23): Form of a leukocytoclastic vasculitis presenting with petechiae followed by palpable purpura on the buttocks and lower extremities. Abdominal pain, joint swelling, and renal involvement may occur.
- *Meningococcemia:* Presents with nonblanching petechiae and purpura along with fever and signs of

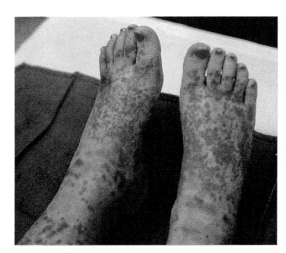

FIGURE 45-23: Showers of vasculitic papules becoming confluent reddish-brown plaques over the feet in Henoch–Schoenlein purpura.

meningitis. Early diagnosis and treatment can be lifesaving.

- *Vasculitis:* Nonblanching palpable petechiae and purpura commonly found on the extremities. Associated causes can include underlying medication, infection, and rarely a collagen vascular disease.

Papulosquamous

- *Psoriasis* (Fig. 45-24): Seen fairly frequently in children, especially "guttate psoriasis," which is often associated with an underlying streptococcal infection. See Chapter 16 for more details.
- *Pityriasis rosea:* See Chapter 17.
- *Tinea versicolor:* See Chapter 17.

Eczematous Lesions

- *Atopic dermatitis* (Fig. 45-25): Hereditary disorder usually beginning around 1 to 4 months of age. In infants, the involvement is usually of the face, scalp, trunk, and extensor extremities. Toddlers have involvement of flexural skin surfaces, and adolescents have more

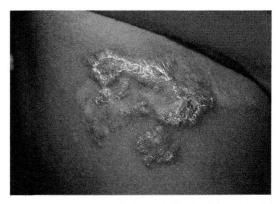

FIGURE 45-24: Psoriasis in an infant with typical silvery-white scale.

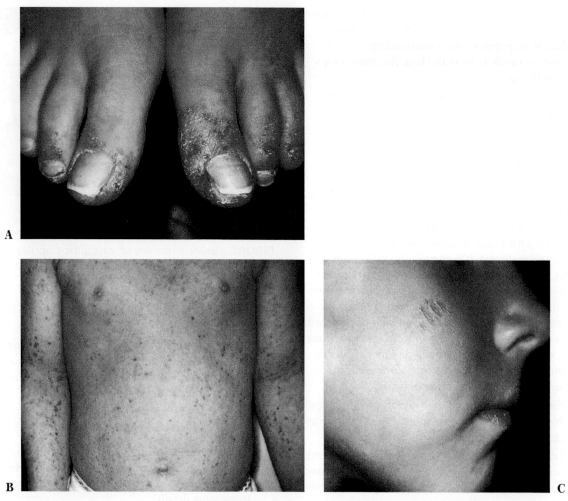

FIGURE 45-25: Atopic dermatitis. **A:** Atopic dermatitis of the toes. **B:** Atopic dermatitis of the chest and antecubital fossae in a 9-year-old child. **C:** Hypopigmented patches on the cheeks (pityriasis alba).

severe involvement of the hands and feet. Individuals with atopic dermatitis may also have hypopigmented scaly patches on the cheeks and extensor arms referred to as *pityriasis alba*. First-line therapy remains to be emollients and topical steroids. The topical calcineurin inhibitors are considered second-line therapeutic options for the treatment of children 2 years of age and older.

■ *Seborrheic dermatitis* (Fig. 45-26): Scaly, erythematous eruption in the "seborrheic areas," which include the scalp, face, postauricular, groin, and intertriginous areas.

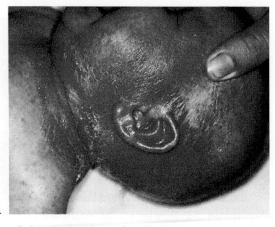
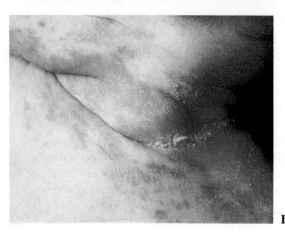

FIGURE 45-26: **A:** Bright-red well-demarcated erythema covering an infant's head and neck. **B:** Salmon-pink erythema over an infant's neck with yellow, greasy scale in a skin fold.

It appears in infancy and usually clears spontaneously. It is also seen in adolescents. Langerhans cell histiocytosis may be misdiagnosed as seborrheic dermatitis.

- *Immunodeficiency:* Severe combined immunodeficiency, Omenn syndrome (familial reticuloendotheliosis with eosinophilia), HIV infection, and Wiskott–Aldrich syndrome can present with a widespread erythematous scaly eruption in early infancy.
- *Allergic contact dermatitis* (Fig. 45-27): The distribution and shape of these pruritic lesions are helpful in making the diagnosis. The lesions can range from vesicles to erythematous papules and eczematous plaques. Generalized reactions to poison ivy/oak are common in children. An eczematoid rash in the infraumbilical area may be seen in association with a "nickel" contact dermatitis to belt buckles and/or metal snaps on pants. Generalized "ID" reactions can occur.
- *Diaper dermatitis* (Fig. 45-28): Irritant (secondary to stool or urine) or contact dermatitis is usually confined to the buttocks and perineal areas, and typically spares the creases. Pustular eruptions are often seen secondary

to *Candida albicans* or staphylococcal infections. "Punched out" erosions can be seen in a severe form of irritant diaper dermatitis (Jacquet dermatitis). Atopic dermatitis usually spares the diaper region.

Disease Affecting the Hair

- *Congenital/hereditary hair defects* (Fig. 45-29): Congenital hair shaft defects can present with broken-off hairs, twisted, or spun-glass appearing hair. There is no satisfactory treatment for these conditions. Abnormal hair findings may be suggestive of other underlying disorders.
- *Alopecia areata* (Fig. 45-30): Common disorder presenting with the sudden appearance of patches of smooth, sharply defined alopecia. Short, tapered, "exclamation point" hairs tend to narrow as they enter the scalp. It is considered to be an autoimmune process involving the hair follicle and has been associated with thyroiditis. The prognosis depends on the extent of the hair loss (the less the better), the area involved, and chronicity. There may be associated nail pitting. The most commonly prescribed therapy for children remains to be topical or intralesional corticosteroids.

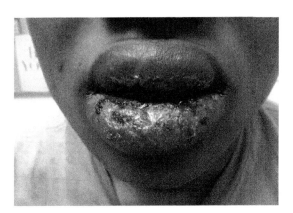

FIGURE 45-27: Oozing, crusting, blister, and erosions, as well as well-demarcated lesion are all characteristic of a contact dermatitis. This time on the lips due to eating mangoes.

> ### SAUER'S NOTES
>
> Pediatric patients have a larger surface area/body mass ratio.
>
>   This necessitates more careful consideration for absorption of topical medications.
> - *Tinea capitis* (Fig. 45-31): Common organisms are *Trichophyton tonsurans* (the most common cause of tinea capitis in the United States) and *Microsporum canis*. "Black dot" tinea, caused by *T. tonsurans*, often presents with broken-off hairs and minimal inflammation. Tinea capitis may be asymptomatic or can present with scale, pruritus,

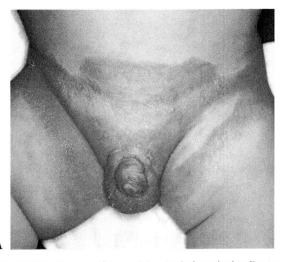
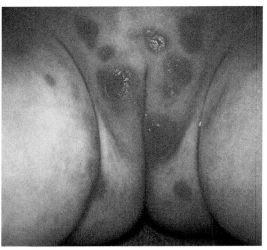

FIGURE 45-28: Diaper dermatitis. **A:** Seborrheic diaper dermatitis. Salmon-pink well-demarcated intertrigo without satellite papules. **B:** Jacquet diaper dermatitis. Genital area with redness and large circular erosions.

alopecia, or pustules. A kerion, which is an inflammatory, pus-filled, boggy mass with associated hair loss, can be seen in more severe cases. Occipital lymphadenopathy is commonly noted in patients with tinea capitis. Fungal culture and potassium hydroxide mount can be diagnostic. Treatment is with oral griseofulvin for at least 2 months or oral terbinafine for 4 to 6 weeks.

• *Trichotillomania* (Fig. 45-32): Commonly seen between 4 and 10 years of age in both genders. Patients pluck, twirl, or rub hair-bearing areas either consciously or subconsciously as a result of a habit. It usually affects the scalp, but may also involve eyebrows and eyelashes. It is usually self-limited.

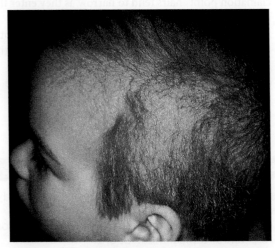

FIGURE 45-29: Diffuse alopecia with ectodermal defect in a 3-year-old child. Oval red-brown circinate smooth plaque with no scale.

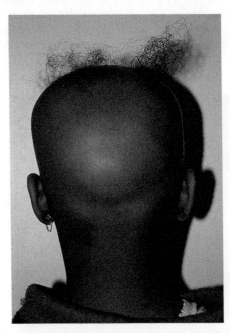

FIGURE 45-30: Alopecia areata. Note completely smooth bald area.

Disease Affecting the Nails

■ *Congenital nail defects:* Absent or poorly developed nails are associated with many syndromes, usually representing nail matrix disorders. Ectodermal dysplasias (Fig. 45-33) are syndromes associated with abnormal nails, skin, hair, and teeth.

■ *Twenty-nail dystrophy:* Presents as thickened nails with exaggerated longitudinal ridges, noted in all nails of the hand (ten-nail dystrophy) (Fig. 45-34) or hands and feet (twenty-nail dystrophy). This dystrophy is self-limited and may resolve over time.

■ *Psoriasis:* Nails may be thickened, shiny, and contain ridges or pitting with these conditions.

■ *Warts:* Children frequently develop warts around (periungual) and under the nail (subungual). These warts can pose a therapeutic challenge.

■ *Paronychia:* Usually presents as a red, painful, inflamed lesion around the nail fold, which may drain pus. It can be acute or chronic. *S. aureus* is the most common organism causing acute infection. The chronic form is often seen in thumb suckers, nail biters, and nail pickers and is commonly associated with *C. albicans.*

Dermatoses Owing to Physical Agents, and Photosensitivity Dermatoses

■ *Sunburn:* On the first sunny days, parents tend to underestimate the effects of the sun rays and overexpose their children. Parents should be taught the ABCs of sun exposure. *Always stay out of the sun between 10 AM and 4 PM. Block the sun with sunscreens that protect against both UVA and UVB rays with a sun protection factor (SPF) of at least 30. Clothes, especially a hat and shirt, should be worn when outside. Adolescents should also be cautioned to avoid tanning salons.*

> **SAUER'S NOTES**
>
> Sun exposure prior to 15 years of age is crucial to the development of skin cancer and is a true public health issue.

■ *Thermal burn:* Severe pain. May be partial thickness with erythema and blisters, or full thickness with loss of skin and subsequent scar formation.

■ *Child abuse:* Well-demarcated atypical appearing purpura, erosions, or scars should raise the suspicion of possible child abuse.

■ *Polymorphous light eruption (PMLE):* Idiopathic sensitivity to UV rays characterized by pruritic, eczematous, papulovesicular, or plaque-like lesions on sun-exposed areas such as the cheeks, ears, nose, neck, or dorsum of the hands. If no additional sunlight exposure occurs, lesions will involute spontaneously in 1 to 2 weeks.

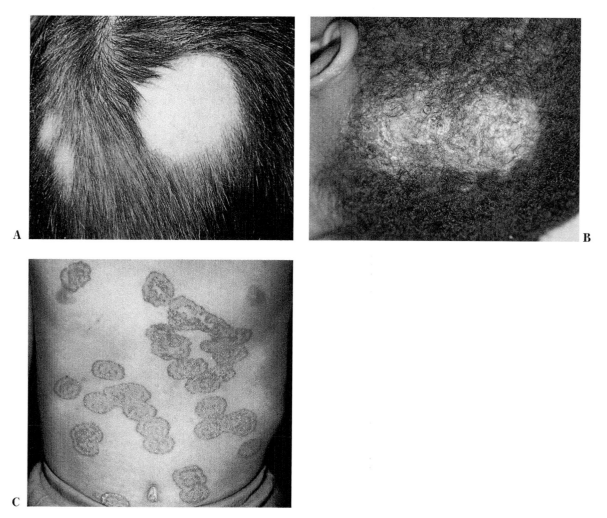

FIGURE 45-31: Tinea. **A:** Tinea of the scalp due to *Microsporum audouinii*. **B:** Erythematous crusted plaque with hair loss—kerion on scalp. **C:** Tinea of the body due to *Microsporum canis*.

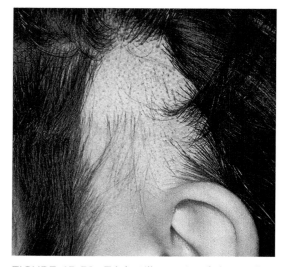

FIGURE 45-32: Trichotillomania of the scalp. Note that there is no complete baldness, and hairs are of varying lengths.

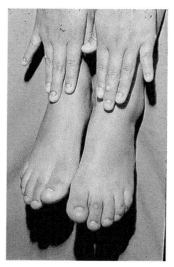

FIGURE 45-33: Ectodermal defect with hypoplasia of the fingernail and toenails.

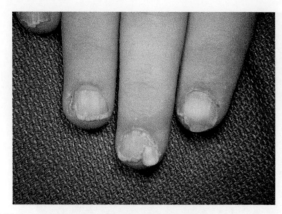

FIGURE 45-34: Twenty-nail dystrophy (trachyonychia) with roughness, longitudinal striations, linear ridges, and splitting.

Broad-spectrum sunscreens providing protection against UVB and UVA are helpful.

■ *Phytophotodermatitis:* Well-demarcated erythema (often linear) with residual hyperpigmentation on sun-exposed skin. This dermatitis is more common in the spring and summer in children who have been exposed to a plant that contains furocoumarin psoralen, a photosensitizing agent. The hyperpigmentation can last for several months.

Suggested Readings

Alikhan A, Ibrahimi OA, Eisen DB. Congenital melanocytic nevi: where are we now? Part I. Clinical presentation, epidemiology, pathogenesis, histology, malignant transformation, and neurocutaneous melanosis. *J Am Acad Dermatol.* 2012;67(4):495.e1–495.e17.

Bolognia JL, Jorizzo JL, Schaffer JV, eds. *Dermatology.* 3rd ed. Philadelphia: Saunders; 2012.

Castelo-Soccio L. Diagnosis and management of alopecia in children. *Pediatr Clin North Am.* 2014;61(2):427–442.

Chen X, Anstey AV, Bugert JJ. Molluscum contagiosum virus infection. *Lancet Infect Dis.* 2013;10:877–888.

Coughlin CC, Eichenfeld LF, Frieden IJ. Diaper dermatitis: clinical characteristics and differential diagnosis. *Pediatr Dermatol.* 2014;31(suppl 1):19–24.

Council on Environmental Health, Section on Dermatology, Balk SJ. Ultraviolet radiation: a hazard to children and adolescents. *Pediatrics.* 2011;127(3):588–597.

Darrow DH, Greene AK, Mancini AJ, et al. Diagnosis and management of infantile hemangioma: executive summary. *Pediatrics.* 2015;136(4):786–791.

Dyer JA. Childhood viral exanthems. *Pediatr Ann.* 2007;36(1):21–29.

Eichenfeld LF, Boguniewicz M, Simpson EL, et al. Translating atopic dermatitis guidelines into practice for primary care providers. *Pediatrics.* 2015;136:554–565.

Eichenfeld LF, Frieden IJ, eds. *Neonatal and Infant Dermatology.* 3rd ed. Philadelphia: Saunders; 2015.

Eichenfeld LF, Krakowski AC, Piggott C, et al. Evidence-based recommendations for the diagnosis and treatment of pediatric acne. *Pediatrics.* 2013;131(suppl 3):S163–S186.

Eichenfield LF, Tom WL, Chamlin SL, et al. Guidelines of care for the management of atopic dermatitis: section 1. Diagnosis and assessment of atopic dermatitis. *J Am Acad Dermatol.* 2014;70(2):338–351.

Farvolden D, Sweeney SM, Wiss K. Lumps and bumps in neonates and infants. *Dermatol Ther.* 2005;18:104–116.

Ibrahim OA, Alikhan A, Eisen DB. Congenital melanocytic nevi: where are we now? Part II. Treatment options and approach to treatment. *J Am Acad Dermatol.* 2012;67(4):515e1–515e13.

Kelly BP. Superficial fungal infections. *Pediatr Rev.* 2012;33(4):e22–e37.

Paller AS, Mancini AJ. *Hurwitz Clinical Pediatric Dermatology.* 4th ed. Philadelphia: Elsevier; 2011.

Püttgen KB. Diagnosis and management of infantile hemangiomas. *Pediatr Clin North Am.* 2014;61(2):383–402.

Schachner LA, Hansen, RC eds. *Pediatric Dermatology.* 4th ed. Philadelphia: Mosby; 2011.

Song JE, Sidbury R. An update on pediatric cutaneous drug eruptions. *Clin Dermatol.* 2014;32(4):516–523.

Swerdlin A, Berkowitz C, Craft N. Cutaneous signs of child abuse. *J Am Acad Dermatol.* 2007;57:371–392.

Wassef M, Blei F, Adams D, et al. Vascular anomalies classification: recommendations from the International Society for the Study of Vascular Anomalies. *Pediatrics.* 2015;136(1):e203–e214.

Weston WL, Lane AT, Morelli JG, eds. *Color Textbook of Pediatric Dermatology.* 4th ed. Philadelphia: Mosby; 2007.

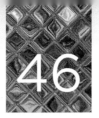

46

General Principles of Skin Aging

Rachel T. Pflederer, MD, Tiffany J. Herd, MD, Anand Rajpara, MD, and Daniel Aires, MD, JD

The approach to the older patient is similar to the approach to any other patient. Some disorders increase in prevalence with increasing age, which creates differences in management strategies. These disorders range from potentially life-threatening skin cancers to harmless benign neoplasms such as seborrheic keratoses.

Common skin conditions in elderly patients are shown in Figure 46-1.

INCIDENCE OF GERIATRIC SKIN DISEASES

According to one study by Gip and Molin (see Suggested Readings), the 10 most prevalent dermatologic disorders in a large group of elderly Swedish patients are as follows (the numbers in parentheses refer to the total number of dermatologic disorders found in the 286 patients examined):

- Pigmented nevus (143)
- Discoloration of the toenails (133)
- Seborrheic keratosis (84)
- Plantar hyperkeratosis (36)
- Stasis dermatitis of the legs (31)
- Seborrheic dermatitis (27)
- Dermatitis of the legs (unspecified) (23)
- Marked atrophy of the skin (19)
- Xanthelasma (12) (Fig. 46-2)
- Capillary hemangiomas (10)

These investigators studied 286 patients over 60 years of age who were hospitalized in a Swedish geriatric clinic. Each patient underwent a full-body skin exam. Histopathologic, bacteriologic, or mycologic examinations were undertaken in some cases. In the 107 men, there were 231 skin diagnoses (2.2 per person), and in the 179 women, 372 skin diagnoses were made (2.1 per person). The number of skin diagnoses per person ranged from 1 to 5. No skin diagnoses were registered

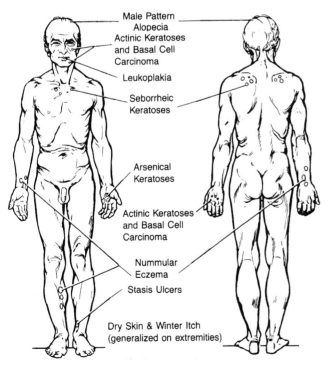

FIGURE 46-1: Geriatric dermagrams.

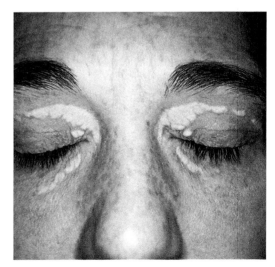

FIGURE 46-2: Xanthelasma.

in 22 cases (8% of patients, 5 men and 17 women). A similar study conducted in a Taiwanese population in 2001 by Liao and Chen showed general dermatitis to be the most prevalent skin condition in the elderly.

SAUER'S NOTES

1. Aging is part of living.
2. There will be a never-ending attempt to be forever young, and the doctor will not be neglected in this pursuit.
3. The need to be helpful to our patients should not lead to unrealistic recommendations for fighting the inevitable changes of time.
4. We are physicians first and businessmen/businesswomen a distant second.

Based on common and concerning skin conditions in the elderly, we provide some general advice (Table 46-1). Understanding the most common dermatologic problems that are seen in elderly patients requires an appreciation of the mechanisms of aging in the skin. Thus, the next part of this chapter addresses the clinical and histologic features and prevention and treatment of intrinsic aging and photoaging.

Intrinsic Versus Extrinsic Skin Aging

Although much remains to be known, a brief overview of the science of aging skin can provide a basis for understanding clinical changes. Aging skin results from two forces: (1) intrinsic chronologic factors, and (2) extrinsic factors such as lifestyle and sun damage.

TABLE 46-1 • General Skin Advice for Elderly Patients

- Monthly self skin exams for new or changing lesions, especially if there is a history of previous skin cancers. May require assistance from family members or caregivers.
- Vitamin D_3 800–1,000 IU supplement with meal unless there is a history of kidney stone; this pertains to elderly skin because elderly people generally get less sun exposure.
- When cleansing, limit soap to strategic areas (groin, axillae, feet); avoid scrubbing and excessive handwashing/bathing.
- Moisturize liberally with petrolatum or lactic acid and urea, especially in winter and/or dry climates.
- Clip toenails with squared-off ends to avoid ingrown toenails. Choose properly fitting shoes. Apply Vicks VapoRub daily to toenails for incipient onychomycosis.
- Wear support hose for early signs of stasis dermatitis.

Intrinsic Aging

Intrinsic factors cause the clinical, histologic, and physiologic changes observed in sun-protected aged skin. These changes include reductions in epidermal regeneration rate, collagen production, rete ridge depth, dermal thickness, thermoregulatory ability, immune defense, wound healing, mechanical defense, sensory perception, sweat and sebum production, and vitamin D synthesis.

Clinical signs of intrinsic skin aging result mainly from thinning, fragility, and loss of elasticity. In the dermis, both intrinsic and extrinsic aging begin with fragmentation of the dermal collagen matrix. Collagen is the principle structural component of the dermis, offering strength and support to the skin. In aging skin, collagen synthesis decreases, creating a shift in the balance between synthesis and degradation. Collagen fragmentation is a normal process resulting from the actions of matrix metalloproteinases (MMPs). Fibroblasts typically keep the activity level of these collagen-degrading enzymes in balance with new collagen production. It is now known that a decrease in fibroblasts occurs with age. This, combined with a loss of function of the fibroblasts relative to the collagen fragmentation leads to a self-perpetuating cycle of decreased fibroblast attachment to intact collagen, decreased collagen production, increased MMP activity, and ultimately increased collagen fragmentation.

Other underlying mechanisms of intrinsic aging include progressive telomere shortening, exacerbated by low-grade oxidative damage to telomeres and other cellular components.

Regarding hair, chest, axillary, and pubic hair all decrease in density with age. In men, there is often increased hair growth in other body sites like eyebrows, and nostrils, and decrease of hair growth on the scalp. In elderly women, there is a similar conversion of vellus to coarse terminal hairs on the chin and moustache areas. Hair graying seems to be a consequence of an overall depletion of hair bulb melanocytes. Specific genes like *PAX3* and *MITF* change the balance between melanocyte stem cell maintenance and differentiation and lead to the gradual loss of melanocyte stem cells, resulting in gray hair.

Extrinsic Aging/Photoaging

Most of what we see as aging is in fact extrinsic aging, due mainly to cumulative exposure to sunlight and certain lifestyle habits like smoking. Clinical signs of photoaging include: lentigines, keratosis, rhytides, purpura, loss of elasticity, and telangiectasias. Photoaging is characterized by a chronic inflammatory response to UV light.

UV irradiation upregulates MMPs, which decrease collagen production, and generates deleterious reactive oxygen species, which then start the cycle of chronic inflammation. Smoking contributes greatly to this increased inflammation, further exacerbating oxidative stress, and causing expression pathways within the skin cells that contribute to the aging processes.

UV irradiation decreases collagen production. Wrinkling is caused by a loss of collagen fibers, as well as the deposition of abnormal degenerative elastotic material within the dermis. The resultant product is called solar elastosis.

Fisher et al. showed that solar UV irradiation reversibly reduces collagen production by approximately 80% within 24 hours after a single short exposure. In aged skin, it has been shown that decreased fibroblasts and elevated levels of partially degraded collagen act to reduce collagen synthetic activity.

Immune regulatory function is also impaired by effects of UV irradiation and smoking. Aging skin is unable to produce certain cytokines, like interleukin-2, while the production of other proinflammatory cytokines seems to be increased (e.g., epidermal growth factor, interleukin-1β, interleukin-4,6,8, intercellular adhesion molecule-1, and tumor necrosis factor-α). This results in a decreased ability of the skin to perform its normal immune regulatory functions, and makes the skin more prone to infections.

On a cellular level, photoaging changes the structure and function of both the dermis and the epidermis. Photoaged epidermis, for example, can become either hyperplastic or atrophic. Histologic examination of severely photodamaged skin reveals atypical keratinocytes and loss of epidermal polarity, both of which can signify premalignant or malignant changes. In photoaged dermis, degraded and/or irregularly thickened collagen and elastic fibers can present clinically as wrinkling and yellow-brown discoloration. In addition, irregular dilation and increased fragility of dermal blood vessels can result in telangiectasias and senile purpura.

Kadunce showed that cigarette smoking is an independent risk factor in the development of wrinkles regardless of sun exposure. Heavy cigarette smokers (>50 packs per year) were five times more likely to be wrinkled than nonsmokers. Premature wrinkling occurred most commonly in combined cigarette smoking and excessive sun exposure.

In brief, sun damage and lifestyle choices like smoking cause the majority of age-related cosmetic and clinical problems on facial skin, including skin cancers, irregular pigmentation, rhytides, and increased skin fragility and coarseness.

Histologic Changes

Histologically, the epidermis of aged skin demonstrates decreased numbers of all major cell types in the skin—keratinocytes, melanocytes, Langerhans cells, and fibroblasts. Accordingly, the function of these cell types is decreased. Keratinocytes, which form the basic barrier that confers the primary mechanical and immunologic defense to our skin, exhibit decreased proliferation, cell signaling, and response to growth factors with aging. These changes result in a reduction of the barrier function leading to increased skin fragility. The decrease in melanocytes, which results in decreased melanin synthesis for UV protection, is evident in the decreased number of nevi present as we age. Conversely, an increase in production of melanin of certain remaining melanocytes may cause solar lentigos, which to many is a marker for aging. Langerhans cells are antigen presenting cells that play an important role in fighting skin infections and malignancy, and a decrease in these cells contribute to a weakened immune system of the skin.

The dermoepidermal junction of aged skin becomes flatter, which results in a lower threshold for separation and blister formation. Likewise, reductions in fibroblasts result in a thinned dermis with less collagen and mucopolysaccharide, especially hyaluronic acid. Capillary loops also shrink, resulting in decreased cutaneous blood flow and nutrient supply. Appendages such as hair follicles, eccrine and apocrine glands, and Pacinian and Meissner corpuscles are similarly decreased, resulting in drier, less hairy, less sensitive skin.

Prevention and Treatment

Primary photoprotection (reviewed in Chapter 7) is the most effective way to prevent photoaging. Daily liberal use of a high sunprotection factor (SPF), broad-spectrum sunscreen that shields both UVA and UVB radiation, reduces photodamage and prevents skin cancer.

That being said, diligent sunscreen use carries a risk of vitamin D deficiency, which is already common among elderly patients. Vitamin D is naturally produced in the skin after sun exposure, and is necessary for important functions in the body including bone health, immune system, and gut health. Emerging data indicate that it probably plays important roles in prevention of cancer, including skin cancer, and in prevention of autoimmune disease, such as multiple sclerosis. For those who practice diligent sun protection, we recommend oral supplementation of vitamin D. The recommended dose is 800 to 1,000 IU/day for persons over the age of 71 years. The American Academy of Dermatology recommends "smart sun" precautions such as applying sunscreen every day, wearing sun-protective clothing including hats and gloves when doing outdoor activities like gardening and fishing, and also trying to stay out of the sun between 10:00 AM and 4:00 PM. These precautions can help prevent sunburns and reduce the risk for skin cancer.

Retinoids

Topical retinoids are a popular choice to treat photodamage. Tretinoin (all *trans*-retinoic acid) has well documented rejuvenating effects on both chronologically aged and photodamaged skin. Work by Fisher has shown that through complex molecular pathways, retinoid compounds can cause deposition of new, nonfragmented collagen in photoaged human skin, thereby markedly improving skin texture and appearance. Tretinoin has been proven to block UV induction of nuclear transcription factors *AP-1* and NF-κB, along with three collagen damaging MMPs. Fisher's study also showed an increase in interstitial collagenases and gelatinases in irradiated skin samples that were pretreated 48 hours prior to exposure. The restorative effects of tretinoin have also been demonstrated histologically in non–sun exposed, chronologically aged skin. Daily application of 0.025% tretinoin cream for 9 months in women aged 68 to 79 years resulted in thickened epidermal layers with corresponding increased height in the dermoepidermal junction, increased uniformity in keratinocyte density, and decreased melanocyte vacuolization. Dermal morphology showed new microvasculature and increased numbers and sizes of fibroblasts, collagen, elastin, microfibrils, and anchoring fibrils. These dramatic results make topical retinoids a wonderful option for treating aging skin.

α-Hydroxy Acids

Studies show that α-hydroxy acids (AHAs), which include the compounds listed in Table 46-2, are known to increase epidermal thickness. Papillary dermal changes include increased acid mucopolysaccharides, increased thickness, and increased density of collage. Application of AHAs in higher concentrations can be useful in treating actinic keratosis, warts, and seborrheic keratoses.

Polyphenols

Polyphenols are reviewed in Chapter 7 and therefore will be discussed here only briefly. A well-balanced diet rich in fruits and vegetables is a good source for polyphenols. Coffee, chocolate, and red wine are also excellent sources. In regard to oral supplements, there has been some debate regarding the efficacy and even safety of oral vitamin supplements. One study even suggested that high doses of Vitamins E and C could potentially reduce life expectancy. Additional studies are needed to clarify such results.

Several other less controversial supplements are available, and have shown some benefit to reduce signs of aging. Oral supplements containing ingredients such as L-proline, L-lysine, manganese, copper, zinc, quercetin, grape seed extract, and N-acetyl-D-glucosamine sulfate have been touted as potential wrinkle reducers.

Topical vitamin C prevents erythema following UV exposure. Studies have shown that vitamin C can upregulate collagen and tissue inhibitor of metalloproteinases (TIMP) synthesis as well as decrease wrinkles. Topical CoQ_{10} has been shown to reduce wrinkles through its antioxidant properties. α-Lipoic acid may have a role in the treatment of photoaging by reducing transcription factors, such as NF-κB, that affect the production of cytokines.

Chen et al. published a study in the *New England Journal of medicine* in 2015 showing supplementation with Niacinamide (vitamin B_3) 500 mg twice a day can result in a significant reduction of nonmelanoma skin cancers (squamous cell, basal cell, actinic keratosis). This may be especially beneficial in patients who are at a higher risk for skin cancers, like the immunosuppressed.

Interventional Treatments

More details on interventional treatments are discussed elsewhere, but a brief overview is included here.

Botulinum toxin A inhibits neuromuscular transmission by blocking acetylcholine release. Cosmetically, botulinum (Botox) relaxes the underlying musculature of the face, lessening the appearance of wrinkles. Understanding underlying anatomy is important for optimal outcome.

Soft tissue augmentation, or "fillers," can partially offset age-associated subcutaneous atrophy. Maintenance is required every 6 to 12 months, depending on location, depth, and choice of filler. Immunogenicity can present a major drawback. Acellular dermal grafts from human cadavers show less immunogenicity than bovine collagen but have fallen out of favor since the development of newer lab-generated fillers. Both hyaluronic acid and calcium hydroxyapatite derivatives are less immunogenic, and calcium hydroxyapatite is also potentially more durable.

A variety of resurfacing techniques have been used to improve the appearance of aged skin. Microdermabrasion exfoliates the superficial epidermis, and microablation uses low-frequency radiofrequency via an electrode. The goal of therapy is to injure the superficial epidermis enough to activate cytokines, MMPs, and type I procollagen mRNA to trigger a healing cascade. Other radiofrequency devices aim to improve cheek and neck laxity via heat generation. Adverse effects range from burning and erythema to subcutaneous atrophy.

Laser systems treat multiple age-associated changes such as mottled pigmentation, wrinkling, and dermal atrophy. Fractionated-delivery laser systems have fewer side effects. Care must be taken to avoid ablating the surface of a potentially malignant pigmented lesion, thus allowing a deeper component to proliferate undetected.

Tumorigenesis

Cumulative UV exposure rises with age, and the link between UV radiation exposure and the development of skin cancer is well established (Fig. 46-3). Furthermore, there is a lag between exposure and tumor development. The combination of these factors leads to a dramatically increased incidence of many skin tumors in the elderly. Basal cell carcinomas (BCCs) and squamous cell carcinomas (SCCs), the two most common skin cancers, tend to occur on sun-exposed skin in older people with skin types 1 and 2. Sunlight consists mostly of infrared (52% to 55%), visible (44%), and UV light (3%). The vast majority of the sun's UV rays are blocked by the atmosphere, and the remaining UV rays that reach the planet's surface consist of >95% UVA (400 to 315 nm) and 5% UVB (315 to 280 nm). UVA rays penetrate deep into the skin's dermis and connective tissue, causing an increased risk in skin cancer. UVB rays only penetrate as deep as the epidermis where they can cause sunburn, tanning, inflammation, as well as skin cancer

---

TABLE 46-2 • α-Hydroxy Acids

- Glycolic acid
- Lactic acid
- Glycolic acid + ammonium glycolate
- α-Hydroxyethanoic acid + ammonium α-hydroxyethanoate
- α-Hydroxyoctanoic acid
- α-Hydroxycaprylic acid
- Hydroxycaprylic acid
- Mixed fruit acid
- Triple fruit acid
- Tri-α-hydroxy fruit acids
- Sugarcane extract
- α-Hydroxy and botanical complex
- L-α-Hydroxy acid
- Glycomer in cross-linked fatty acids alpha nutrium

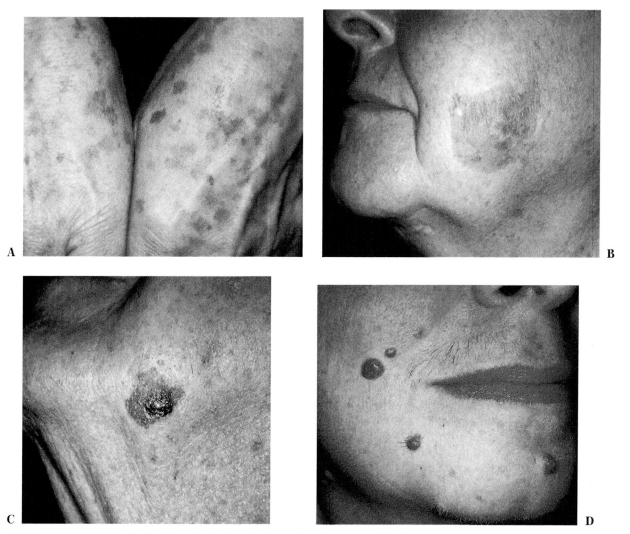

FIGURE 46-3: A: Senile freckles (solar lentigo) on the dorsum of the hands. **B:** Lentigo on the cheek. **C:** Malignant melanoma in a lentigo, on the jaw area. **D:** Compound nevi on the face. (Syntex Laboratories, Inc.)

formation. UVA rays may have a greater role in photoaging, as it affects the epidermis and dermis, where the collagen lies. UVA and UVB both induce genetic alterations in DNA that are associated with BCCs and SCCs. Superficial spreading and nodular melanomas are associated with intermittent and intense UV exposure, and lentigo maligna melanoma and SCC/BCC are related to cumulative sun exposure. Tanning beds, which emit predominantly UVA, are associated with melanoma, SCC, and BCC.

Premalignant Lesions

Clinically, actinic keratoses (AKs) are flat or slightly elevated, pink, tan, or brownish, rough, poorly demarcated, scaly, adherent papules. Though generally under 1 cm in size, AKs may become larger and even become confluent. As previously mentioned, these papules occur mainly on sun-exposed skin such as the face, ears, neck, and dorsum of the hands, especially in fair-skinned people. Cutaneous horns can arise as a proliferative variant of AK. If left untreated, up to 10% of these lesions may

progress to SCC. Lesions with palpable induration, marked inflammation, or recurrence after treatment may merit further evaluation by biopsy. Shave biopsies are adequate as long as enough tissue is obtained to examine whether dermal invasion has occurred. Cryotherapy works well for single or scattered lesions. Treatment options for multiple and confluent lesions that cover a large surface area include topical 5-fluorouracil, imiquimod, diclofenac gel as well as photodynamic therapy with aminolevulinic acid and an activating light source.

Leukoplakia is clinically a white patch on the oral mucosa that cannot be easily removed with simple rubbing and may be premalignant. If a biopsy reveals the lesion to be premalignant, there is a 20% to 30% progression rate to SCC and the lesion should be managed aggressively, as SCC of the mucous membranes has a metastatic rate of 40% to 50% compared to 4% to 5% in the skin. Actinic cheilitis is the lip counterpart of AKs and is defined as involvement of the cutaneous aspect of the upper or lower lip. Metastatic SCC has a poor prognosis as discussed in the following text.

Malignant Lesions

BCC is the most common malignant skin cancer, and incidence increases with age. Although the risk of metastasis is very low, untreated tumors can become very locally destructive over time.

SCC is the second most common skin malignancy in the elderly, and the incidence of it too increases with age. The rate of metastasis is higher than that of BCC, though lower than that of malignant melanoma. Although metastases are fairly uncommon, once the SCC becomes invasive to the lymph node, survival rates decline dramatically. Some types of SCC appear to be more aggressive than others. SCCs from chronic injuries, burns, or scars (termed Marjolin ulcers) tend to be more aggressive, as do mucous membrane SCCs.

Common treatment options include surgical excision and electrodessication and curettage with or without subsequent adjuvant topical 5-fluorouracil, diclofenac, or imiquimod treatment. Radiation therapy is generally reserved for elderly patients not able to tolerate surgery. Some studies show that elderly patients with superficial SCCs or nodular or superficial BCCs who cannot tolerate surgery or elect not to undergo surgical excision may benefit from curettage followed by the application of imiquimod 5% cream five to seven times weekly for 6 weeks (BCCs) or a maximum of 16 weeks (SCCs). Patients should wait 2 weeks after curettage before starting imiquimod to allow partial re-epithelialization. Recent studies have demonstrated clearance rates of 96% to 100% in the treatment of BCCs at 12 to 36 months' follow-up; 80% to 100% clearance in the treatment of superficial SCCs at a mean of 31 months' follow-up; and 71.4% clearance in the treatment of invasive SCCs at a mean of 31 months' follow-up—all with relatively good cosmetic outcomes and tolerance.

Merkel cells carcinomas (MCCs) are rare aggressive skin tumors that account for less than 1% of cutaneous malignancies and are seen more common in the elderly. A study published by Agelli in 2003 described 76% of MCCs occurring in patients over 65 years old, and more commonly in White males. These tumors usually present as shiny, solitary, dome-shaped, red or violaceous nodules or firm plaques on the head or neck. Risk factors for MCC include chronic immunosuppression, organ transplantation, B-cell lymphoma, erythema ab igne, and congenital ectodermal dysplasia. Once an MCC is diagnosed, wide local excision, if clinically feasible, and a referral to a surgical and medical oncologist as well as a radiation therapist are indicated.

Melanoma is the most common aggressive skin malignancy. The incidence of melanoma actually peaks before old age, but it, too, often presents in elderly patients. Any new mole in an older person should be carefully assessed, since new moles do not generally arise after age 40. The link between UV radiation exposure and melanoma is an area of active research. Lentigo maligna melanomas occur overwhelmingly in areas that have received the greatest cumulative exposure to sunlight. Other types of melanoma like superficial spreading type and nodular type melanomas appear to be related to intense episodic exposure rather than total lifetime sun exposure.

Common Benign Lesions

Actinic lentigines (i.e., solar lentigo, liver spots, age spots) are hyperpigmented macules, typically arising on sun-exposed skin such as the face or dorsal hands, and result from an increase in melanocyte number. These benign pigmented lesions are seen in middle to late age and, to the chagrin of many patients, do not fade with time.

In severely photodamaged skin of the neck and chest, a mottled, reddish-brown discoloration known as poikiloderma of Civatte (Fig. 46-4) may be seen. Large, open comedones in the periorbicular area are also often seen in severely photodamaged patients. This is known as Favre–Racouchot syndrome.

Seborrheic keratoses (known as "seborrheic warts" in Europe) (Fig. 46-5) typically appear as waxy, warty, stuck-on, flesh-colored, tan, brown, or black papules on the head, neck, trunk, and extremities. These lesions are common in the elderly and are often the most worrisome to the patient owing to their appearance. However, they are completely benign and are generally asymptomatic, so no treatment is required. If a lesion does become inflamed or if a patient desires cosmetic destruction, cryotherapy generally works well. Cryotherapy for these lesions is best performed at a lateral angle rather than head-on in order to minimize damage to surrounding tissue and decrease the potential for scarring. Although seborrheic keratoses usually have a characteristic appearance, they can sometimes be difficult to distinguish from other skin cancers, especially when they become inflamed. A biopsy should be performed if any doubt exists.

Dermatosis papulosa nigra (DPN) affects up to 35% of the African-American population in the United States and can also be seen in Asians. Histologically, this condition appears the same as a seborrheic keratosis. Females are more frequently affected than males, and the incidence as well as the number and size of lesions increases with age, beginning

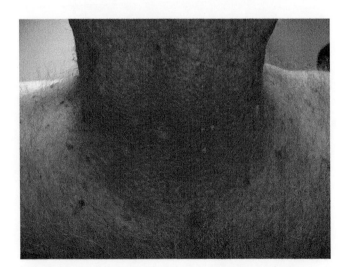

FIGURE 46-4: Poikilodermatous changes on the sides of the neck with sparing of the anterior neck where there was shading by the chin. This is typical of poikiloderma of Civatte and is a good way to gauge amount of sun exposure.

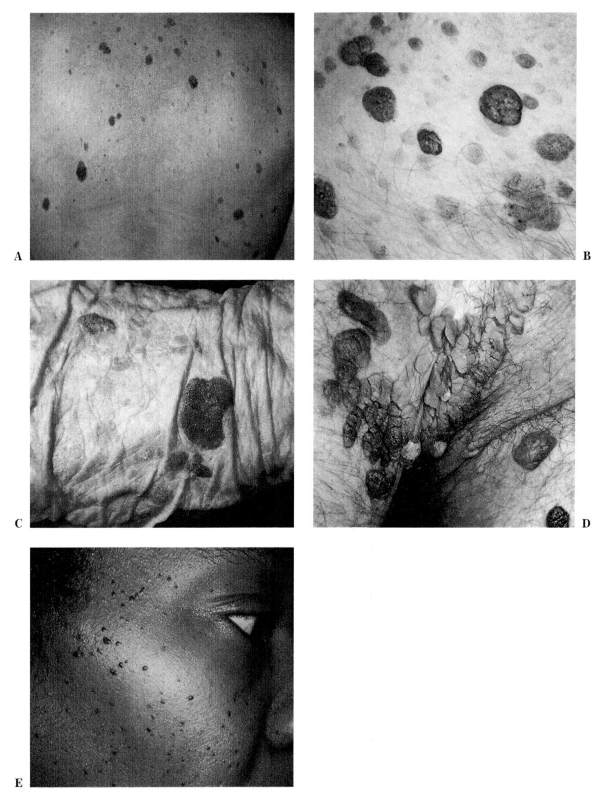

FIGURE 46-5: A: Seborrheic keratoses over the back of a 71-year-old man. **B:** Seborrheic keratoses, close-up. **C:** Large seborrheic keratosis on the hand in an 84-year-old woman. **D:** Multiple seborrheic keratoses of the crural area. **E:** Seborrheic keratoses or dermatosis papulosa nigra on the face.

in adolescence. Lesions may be removed for cosmetic reasons, but the risk of keloid formation or hypopigmentation may outweigh the benefit.

Pedunculated fibromas (also known as acrochordons or skin tags) are extremely common on the neck and axilla. They

are usually not a cause for concern and require no treatment unless they are inflamed or bothersome to the patient. Treatment options include cryotherapy or excision.

Benign vascular neoplasms, most notably cherry angiomas and venous lakes, occur in a significant proportion of elderly patients (see Chapter 30) and are typically found on the trunk, lips, and ears, respectively. Laser treatments can help if lesions are cosmetically troublesome.

Sebaceous gland hyperplasia on the face is common. It is a benign condition that appears as small yellowish papules with a central dell on the cheeks, nose, and forehead.

Xerosis and Contact Dermatitis

Xerosis (Fig. 46-6), or dry skin, is characteristic of chronologically aged skin and can be attributed to intrinsic and extrinsic changes discussed earlier in this chapter. Dry skin can be asymptomatic or can present as irritation or pruritus, most commonly on the lower extremities and in winter (winter itch). Patients may also complain of drier mucous membranes. Should pruritus persist after xerosis is treated, it is important to consider an underlying systemic process, such as cutaneous T-cell lymphoma (CTCL) or a paraneoplastic syndrome. Generalized pruritus is discussed in more detail in Chapter 12.

Treatment of xerosis (see Table 46-1) should include minimizing time spent immersed in hot water and avoidance of excess washing. In addition, we recommend using synthetic unscented surfactant soaps, which are less drying, and limiting the application of soap to the hands, feet, face, groin, and axillae. Baths should be lukewarm, and harsh scrubbing should be discouraged. Fragrance-free and dye-free moisturizers should be applied immediately after bathing in order to minimize transepidermal water loss. Plain petroleum jelly ointment is effective if tolerated by the patient. Humectants containing ammonium lactate or urea are useful, especially in hyperkeratotic areas, but may sting if the area being treated is fissured or raw. Oral antihistamines to relieve pruritus should be utilized with caution, owing to their sedative effects and possible association with Alzheimer disease.

In elderly individuals, ACD (allergic contact dermatitis) is less common owing to both decreased sensitization to new allergens and diminishing responses in previously sensitized patients. However, although the development of ACD may be delayed, the dermatitis may be more persistent once developed.

Impaired Circulation and Ulcers

Stasis Dermatitis

Stasis dermatitis (Fig. 46-7) is a common inflammatory skin condition of the calves and shins of middle-aged and elderly patients with chronic venous insufficiency and venous hypertension. It usually occurs after the fifth decade of life. If a patient presents with stasis dermatitis before the fifth decade of life, the clinician should consider venous insufficiency secondary to trauma, surgery, or thrombosis. The prevalence of stasis dermatitis is 6% to 7% in patients over 50, and the risk steadily increases with age. In adults over 70, the prevalence of stasis dermatitis may be greater than 20%.

Patients with stasis dermatitis typically have a history of dependent leg edema resulting from comorbidities such as congestive heart failure or long-standing hypertension with diastolic dysfunction. A slight female prevalence has been reported.

Early stasis dermatitis typically presents as a gradual onset of pruritus or xerosis affecting one or both lower extremities, sometimes accompanied by reddish-brown skin discoloration. Petechiae may be seen overlying the brawny discoloration. In time, these early changes can progress to erythematous, swollen, scaling plaques. An acute erysipelas-like eruption has been described. The medial ankle is most frequently involved because of its relatively poor blood flow. Secondary bacterial or candidal infection can cause crusting. Lichenification, hyperpigmentation, edema, varicosities, atrophy, and induration can result from chronic scratching and rubbing. Severe chronic inflammation and thickening can lead to lipodermatosclerosis with its characteristic inverted champagne bottle appearance. The patient should be advised that these chronic changes generally persist despite treatment. The goal is generally to prevent progression.

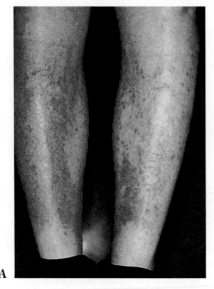
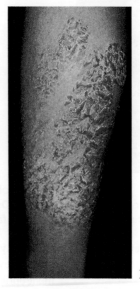
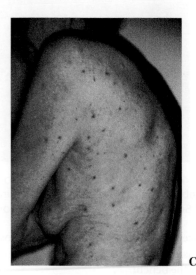

FIGURE 46-6: Xerosis. **A:** Redness of winter itch on the legs. **B:** Xerosis with secondary infection on the legs. **C:** Senile pruritus in 74-year-old woman. (Courtesy of Johnson & Johnson.)

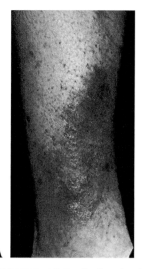 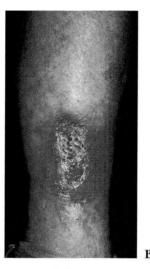

A   B

FIGURE 46-7: **A:** Stasis dermatitis of the leg aggravated by contact allergy to neomycin. **B:** Stasis ulcer of the leg with varicose veins.

Treatment for stasis dermatitis focuses mainly on mitigating venous insufficiency. This involves leg elevation, properly fitted compression stockings, elastic wraps, Unna boots, and/or end-diastolic compression boots. The patient's peripheral arterial circulation must be assessed before starting compression therapy as compression therapy is contraindicated if arterial circulation is compromised.

In early stages, low-potency topical steroids and topical calcineurin inhibitors (tacrolimus, pimecrolimus) can be helpful for reducing inflammation and pruritus in acute flares. However, high-potency topical corticosteroids carry risks of systemic absorption and steroid-induced atrophy.

Stasis can look like cellulitis, but stasis is generally bilateral, while cellulitis is usually unilateral. Suspected cellulitis should always be treated with oral or intravenous antibiotics. Superficial bacterial infections should be cultured and may be treated empirically with topical mupirocin or an appropriate systemic antibiotic with activity against *Staphylococcus* and *Streptococcus* species. Mild superficial bacterial superinfections can be treated with wet-to-damp gauze dressings soaked with water or with a drying agent such as aluminum acetate, Domeboro, or a 1:1 water:white vinegar mix. Complications of chronic stasis dermatitis include increased incidences of allergic contact dermatitis, nonhealing lower extremity ulceration(s), cellulitis, lipodermatosclerosis, and id reactions on other parts of the body.

Allergic contact dermatitis commonly results from use of topical antibiotics such as neomycin and bacitracin. In addition, patients may become sensitized to rubber products found in some wraps and stockings. Topical corticosteroid allergy, while uncommon, should be considered when stasis dermatitis worsens despite seemingly appropriate prescription therapy. To minimize risk of allergies, patients with chronic but stable stasis dermatitis can be treated with bland topical emollients such as plain white petrolatum with elimination of other potential allergens.

Arterial Insufficiency

Manifestations of arterial insufficiency include erythema, local hair loss, ulcers, stellate scars, and atrophie blanche. Associated pain and gangrene are more common with arterial insufficiency than with venous insufficiency. Ulcers due to arterial insufficiency typically appear on the dorsal feet, toes, and lateral legs as punched-out lesions with intense pain. Patients with diabetes are at an increased risk of complications. The treatment of ulcers owing to arterial insufficiency should include consultation by a vascular surgeon and is beyond the scope of this chapter.

Ulcers

As life expectancies have increased over the past several decades, the incidence of chronic venous leg ulcers, pressure ulcers, and diabetic ulcers in patients over 65 has steadily risen as well. Multifactorial age-related declines in skin repair and sensation can cause skin breakdown, which is then exacerbated by excessive inflammatory responses, with associated proteolysis, vascular compromise, fibroblast dysfunction, and bacterial infection.

Diabetic foot ulcers are seen in 15% to 25% of diabetic patients and remain the most common cause of lower limb amputation. Peripheral neuropathy is the most significant risk factor related to diabetic foot ulcers. Sensory, autonomic and motor neuropathy may lead to the development of diabetic ulcers while vascular occlusion and inflammation perpetuate the cycle. Diabetic foot ulcers typically present overlying pressure-bearing sites with a thick hyperkeratotic callus. Treatment includes prevention such as protective footwear, callus removal, non–weight bearing, and immobilization.

Pressure ulcers result from chronic immobilization and occur most frequently in the pelvic girdle region and lower limbs. One and a half to three million Americans suffer from bedsores at an annual estimated cost of 5 billion dollars. Risk factors include poor circulation, decreased nerve sensation, skin atrophy, and the lack of strength, immobility, and mental capacity to turn oneself to redistribute pressure. Prophylactic measures are paramount. A bed-bound patient should be turned at least every 2 hours, and the bed needs to be kept clean and dry. Special cushion supporters and mattresses that can redistribute pressure are indicated. Surgical dressings such as Opsite, Duoderm, Tegaderm, Mepilex, and PolyMem may be applied to incipient wounds. Vinegar soaks may be helpful in controlling potential bacterial infections, especially pseudomonas.

Ulcer Colonization

Bacterial colonization of ulcers is common and does not necessarily impair wound healing or require treatment. For recalcitrant or exudative ulcers bacterial superinfection should be considered. A surface swab culture may be obtained after the wound is cleansed. Clinically apparent infections may be seen with a bacterial bioburden of $>1 \times 10^6$ or any wound with Group A β Hemolytic Streptococcal infection. *S. aureus* is the most common cause of wound infection although chronic wounds tend to be polymicrobial. Treatment should include empiric antibiotics for *S. aureus* for 2 to 4 weeks. Antibiotic therapy should be tailored based on culture results.

Skin Infections

Candidiasis

Although fungal infections are discussed in detail in Chapter 28, a brief summary is in order here. Candidiasis is the most common mycologic infection in the elderly, especially those who are obese, diabetic, debilitated, and/or chronic users of antibiotics. Debilitation can lead to increased bed rest and decreased cleansing, which greatly increases the risk. Cutaneous candidiasis may present in the groin, inframammary folds, axillae, or inguinal areas. Treat with topical antifungal agents or with oral fluconazole if severe. Urinary and fecal incontinence can contribute to candidiasis, along with primary skin irritation and corrosion. Corrosion of skin owing to urinary incontinence may require temporary use of an indwelling catheter.

Onychomycosis

Onychomycosis is as significant and treatable change in the nails of the elderly. Onychomycosis increases with age, reaching 20% at 60 years with the great toenail, which is most commonly affected. Other risk factors include male gender, diabetes, smoking, family history, psoriasis, concurrent intake of immunosuppressive drugs, human immunodeficiency virus (HIV) infection, and peripheral vascular disease.

Dermatophytes are by far the most common cause of onychomycosis. Nondermatophyte molds can also be seen in the elderly (*Scopulariopsis brevicaulis, Hendersonula toruloidea, Scytalidium hyalinum*). *Scopulariopsis* tends to be found in conjunction with paronychia. This is of particular concern in immunocompromised patients, owing to an associated increased risk of cellulitis.

Onychomycosis is difficult to treat permanently, especially in the elderly. Oral antifungals are notorious for having multiple drug interactions, and older individuals are more likely to be on multiple medications. Also, the metabolic capabilities in the elderly liver decline, making the medications less tolerable even without drug interactions.

Topical treatments are a safer alternative in the elderly and can work well even though onychomycosis is usually thought to be less easily treated than other superficial fungal infections. One safe and cheap method is application of Vicks VapoRub daily to the affected nails, including the base. Forty percent urea cream can be used as an adjunct, owing to its keratolytic properties. Compliance may be a disadvantage of this method, as complete clearance of an infection may take up to 16 months. However, a clear band of healthy nail has been seen in as little time as 2 months. Another topical treatment option is ciclopirox lacquer (Penlac). Ciclopirox has a broad range of antifungal activity as well as antibacterial and anti-inflammatory actions. Kerydin and Jublia are also used.

A simple but often overlooked issue in elderly patients, especially men, is foot hygiene. Many elderly patients have worn the same pair of occlusive shoes for literally decades. These shoes should be discarded.

Other common nail changes in the elderly include increased ridging (onychorrhexis) and discoloration of the nail plate. Some patients with thinning nails may benefit from oral biotin supplementation.

Scabies

Sarcoptes scabiei infection classically presents with excoriated papules on the flexor surfaces of wrists, interdigital webs, axillae, ankles, lower abdomen and back, pubic area, and perineum. Scabies transmission results mainly from close contact but can also occur via fomites. In chronic care facilities, vulnerability is usually limited to those with skin-to-skin contact such as healthcare workers. Although elderly persons who live independently can contract scabies, those in large care facilities are at a much higher risk. Scabies is often missed when itching is incorrectly attributed to dry skin or senile pruritus, especially in confused patients. In a 1-year Canadian study, 25% of surveyed institutions reported cases, with 11% reporting one or more infested healthcare workers. Mean number of infestations per outbreak was 18. All affected persons should be treated at the same time. Because of the large number of people involved, this can present a major management problem.

Elderly and immunocompromised patients are more likely to develop atypical presentations such as crusted scabies, also known as Norwegian scabies. This form can go unrecognized owing to lack of itching and can spread. Norwegian scabies is associated with a much higher mite count: 2 million versus the more typical 10 to 15 mites per patient. Laboratory studies and treatments are the same as in normal adults and are discussed in detail in Chapter 20. Treatment with oral ivermectin is recommended if crusted scabies is suspected. This has a psoriasiform look and can be mistaken for psoriasis.

Varicella-Zoster Virus

Viral skin infections are discussed in detail in Chapter 26. Varicella-Zoster virus (Fig. 46-8) is mentioned here owing to its elevated incidence of recurrence as herpes zoster (HZ) in the elderly. HZ has a lifetime prevalence of 10% to 20% and

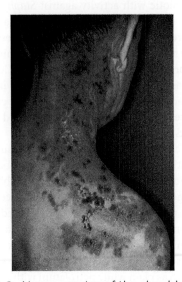

FIGURE 46-8: Herpes zoster of the shoulder and neck.

increases with age. Vaccination can help decrease morbidity and mortality of HZ. The Advisory Committee on Immunization Practices of the CDC (Centers for Disease Control and Prevention) recommends vaccination with the live attenuated virus (Zostavax) in adults over 60 years. Infections may be treated with a 7- to 10-day course of acyclovir, valacyclovir, and famciclovir. Treatment should start as soon as symptoms occur, preferably within 72 hours of onset. All three medications shorten the duration of acute pain, rash, viral shedding, and acute- and late-onset anterior horn complications.

Of adults over age 60, 20% to 40% develop neuropathic pain following HZ. This is termed "postherpetic neuralgia" or PHN. PHN can be severely debilitating and can last several months or years. Valacyclovir and famciclovir decrease the incidence and severity of PHN, but they do not prevent it.

If PHN does occur, pain control is very important. One option is tricyclic antidepressants (TCAs). Nortriptyline and desipramine are relatively newer TCAs and are better choices for elderly patients than amitriptyline. The dose is generally 25 to 50 mg at bedtime, which is approximately half the dosage needed for antidepressant activity. Antiseizure medications have also been effective. These include gabapentin 600 mg two to six times daily and pregabalin 300 to 600 mg daily. These medications reduce the need for opioids and are synergistic with TCAs. Topical analgesics (5% lidocaine, lidocaine/prilocaine, capsaicin) can be added to any of the above treatments. In severe cases, opioids may be needed.

Postherpetic itch can be treated with antihistamines, but caution is advised when prescribing oral antihistamines to elderly patients as they are more likely to experience adverse reactions such as sedation, orthostatic hypotension, and urinary retention.

Several subtypes of HZ deserve special attention. Ophthalmic HZ involves the first division of the trigeminal nerve (CN V1). This branch is involved 20 times more often than CN V2 or V3. Ophthalmic HZ may lead to corneal scarring and secondary panophthalmitis with loss of vision. Characteristic signs include lesions on the tip of the nose (innervated by CN V1) and sensations of a foreign body in the eye. A second important subtype involves the facial nerve (CN VII), leading to Ramsay–Hunt syndrome, which can result in deafness. It can present with lesions in the external auditory meatus, pinna of the ear, and soft palate. This type is also associated with unilateral facial paralysis, aka Bell palsy. A third important subtype of HZ is the disseminated form. Disseminated HZ involves more than three dermatomes or more than 20 lesions outside of a single dermatome. It is more common in patients with lymphoproliferative disorders or advanced HIV. HZ can disseminate to internal organs leading to hepatitis, pneumonitis, meningoencephalitis, myelitis, or motor radiculopathy. All three of these important subtypes should be treated with IV acyclovir.

Systemic Diseases With Cutaneous Manifestations

Cutaneous manifestations of systemic diseases, including malignancies, are discussed in Chapter 30. Some of these have aspects that are more common in elderly people.

Metastatic Cancer

Cutaneous metastases are seen in 1% to 10% of patients with metastatic disease. In women, breast carcinoma and melanoma are the most common causes of cutaneous metastasis; while for men, melanoma and head/neck carcinoma are the most commonly seen. Breast carcinoma is the most likely malignancy to metastasize to the skin. Cutaneous malignancy may present with alopecia (alopecia neoplastica). Renal carcinoma metastases are classically found on the scalp. In addition, metastases to the upper abdominal wall are usually from gastrointestinal (GI) tumors. The Sister Mary Joseph nodule is a carcinoma metastasis to the umbilicus, most commonly from adenocarcinoma of the stomach. Lower abdominal wall metastases are more likely to be genitourinary (GU) tumors.

Cutaneous metastases are usually hard, fixed, subcutaneous or dermal nodules that may be of any color. Rarely, tumor cells may appear to have a zoster-like distribution owing to perineural invasion. Ulceration is rare. The nodules may be solitary or multiple. A general rule is that any nodule with dermal or subcutaneous involvement of unknown origin should undergo biopsy.

Paget Disease

Paget disease of the breast presents as a unilateral, pruritic, eczematous eruption of the nipple and areola indicative of underlying invasive ductal carcinoma or ductal carcinoma in situ.

Signs of Internal Cancers

Internal cancers can present with cutaneous symptoms. These include paraneoplastic syndromes as well as other nonspecific lesions. Bazex syndrome (acrokeratosis paraneoplastica) is a well-known paraneoplastic syndrome presenting as psoriasiform lesions involving acral sites, ears, and nails. Primary squamous cell carcinoma of the pharynx, larynx, or esophagus is the most common etiology.

Acanthosis Nigricans

Acanthosis nigricans (AN) is discussed in Chapter 42. It is characterized by pigmented velvety plaques on intertriginous areas and on the sides and nape of the neck. Acrochordons often arise within acanthotic plaques. AN can be caused by obesity, insulin resistance, or, less commonly, internal malignancy. Extensive AN has been linked with adenocarcinomas, particularly GI cancers. Severe AN may become verrucous and can be associated with papillomatous changes in the oral cavity.

The mechanism underlying AN is not yet known. An association with tumor-produced insulin-like growth factors in the skin has been proposed. Another possible explanation is that elevated systemic transforming growth factor alpha (TGF-α) induces epidermal growth factors, leading to acrochordons and AN. A similar explanation has been proposed for the sudden appearance of multiple rapidly growing seborrheic keratoses in the setting of an internal malignancy, also known as the sign of Leser–Trélat. The sign of Leser–Trélat is frequently seen along with malignancy-associated AN. However, both seborrheic keratoses and cancer are common in elderly people, so assessing the significance of Leser–Trélat is difficult.

Clubbing

Fingertip clubbing may be associated with internal malignancy. Clubbing can be seen in 10% of patients with primary or metastatic lung cancer. This can also be seen in other pulmonary diseases. Clubbing is caused by subperiosteal bone formation of the phalangeal shaft. Associated symptoms such as joint swelling, synovitis, hyperhidrosis, and palmar erythema can mimic early rheumatoid arthritis.

Dermatomyositis

Up to 25% of patients with adult-onset dermatomyositis have an internal malignancy. Dermatomyositis is most commonly associated with ovarian, breast, lung, and GI malignancy. Cutaneous findings include heliotrope dermatitis, proximal nail fold telangiectasias, Gottron papules, and cutaneous necrosis. All patients with adult-onset dermatomyositis should undergo age-appropriate cancer screening with emphasis on the above malignancies. After 2 to 5 years of disease, the risk of associated malignancy is mitigated.

Conditions Secondary to Cancer Treatment

In addition to skin conditions from active cancers, there are also changes that can occur as a result of prior cancer treatments. As cancer treatments become more effective and survivors live longer, the skin changes associated with these treatments are becoming increasingly common.

Radiodermatitis typically includes poikiloderma, telangiectasia, and atrophy. A more concerning symptom is nonhealing ulceration. The increased risk of SCC in irradiated skin makes regular skin examination important for these patients.

Radiation-induced morphea has been reported in breast cancer survivors. It is important to rule out recurrence of cancer with a biopsy. Morphea can be treated with local steroid injections, psoralens and ultraviolet A (PUVA), or UVA-1. Efficacy, however, is variable. The mechanism of action underlying PUVA may involve a reduction in cytokine activity, including TGF-β, which is a stimulator of fibroblast activity. If these less invasive therapies do not offer improvement, reconstructive plastic surgery can help reduce morphea-associated pain and disfiguration. Chapter 41 gives a more detailed description of morphea.

OTHER NOTEWORTHY SKIN ISSUES IN THE ELDERLY

Other notable diseases that present more commonly in the elderly include pemphigus vulgaris (Fig. 46-9) and bullous pemphigoid (Fig. 46-10). These are discussed further in Chapter 21.

It is important to remember that elderly patients are often on many medications which may alter the pharmacokinetics and dosing of medications. As alterations in adiposity and muscle mass occur over time, the volume of distribution may be altered. In addition, some of these have cutaneous side effects (Fig. 46-11). Medications that increase photosensitivity are reviewed in Chapter 43. Photosensitizers especially relevant to

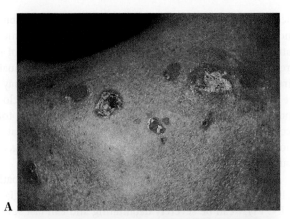

A

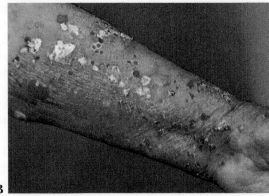

B

FIGURE 46-9: **A:** Pemphigus vulgaris of the upper back area. **B:** Pemphigus vulgaris of the forearm.

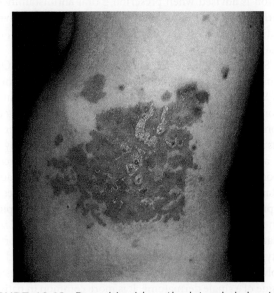

FIGURE 46-10: Pemphigoid on the lateral abdominal area.

the elderly include diuretics, nonsteroidal anti-inflammatory drugs (NSAIDS), phenothiazines, and antiarrhythmics. It is important to ask about blood thinners, as these can affect procedures performed in the office as well as contribute to easy bruising. Blood thinners, particularly warfarin, also have a number of drug interactions.

Changes in hair occur throughout life. Hair is discussed in detail in Chapter 35. Elderly people experience a change

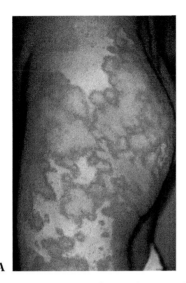 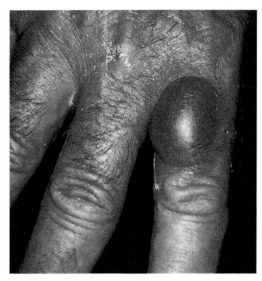

FIGURE 46-11: A: Drug eruption from phenacetin. **B:** Fixed bullous drug eruption owing to tetracycline. (Courtesy of Johnson & Johnson.)

in hair color, with eventual transition to gray or pure white. Male pattern alopecia can begin as early as late adolescence and tends to be progressive. Elderly patients who have not suffered typical male pattern alopecia often show a youthful hairline with diffuse thinning of scalp hair. This so-called senile alopecia can occur in both men and women. Diffuse hair loss also occurs in the axilla and pubic area. Excess facial hair is common in elderly women and can require treatment. Shaving facial hair blunts the otherwise tapered visible tip of the hair, but does not cause increased hair density or thickness.

Some conditions are seen less frequently in the elderly. These include atopic dermatitis, acne, pityriasis rosea, impetigo, syphilis, herpes simplex, warts, exanthemas, chloasma, and sunburns. If acne is present, the patient should be asked about testosterone intake and corticosteroid drugs. Seborrheic dermatitis can become less bothersome with age but can worsen following a stroke or in the presence of Parkinson disease.

Elder mistreatment and abuse is a special consideration in this population. In those over the age of 60 years, 1% to 10% are suspected of suffering from abuse. A 2003 survey revealed that 44% of nursing home residents may have been physically abused. Risk factors include, increasing age, female gender, and functional or cognitive impairment. Cutaneous findings that are suspicious for abuse include a patterned distribution suggesting an external source, lesions in multiple stages of healing, symmetric injuries from restraints, and irregular hair patches of hair loss from traumatic pulling.

ACKNOWLEDGMENT

We would like to acknowledge Deede Liu, MD, Emily Stevens, MD, and Daniel West, MD, for their contributions to previous versions of this chapter.

Suggested Readings

Agelli M, Clegg LX. Epidemiology of primary Merkel cell carcinoma in the United States. *J Am Acad Dermatol.* 2003;49:832–841.

Brennan M, Bhatti H, Nerusu KC, et al. Matrix metalloproteinase-1 is the major collagenolytic enzyme responsible for collagen damage in UV-irradiated human skin. *Photochem Photobiol.* 2003;78(1):43–48.

Chang AL, Wong JW, Endo JO, et al. Geriatric dermatology: part II risk factors and cutaneous signs of elder mistreatment for the dermatologist. *J Am Acad Dermatol.* 2012;68(4):533.e1–533.e10.

Chen AC, Martin AJ, Choy B, et al. A phase 3 randomized trial of nicotinamide for skin-cancer chemoprevention. *N Engl J Med.* 2015;373:1618–1626.

Dancey AL, Waters RA. Morphea of the breast. Two case reports and discussion of the literature. *J Plast Reconstr Aesthet Surg.* 2006;59:1114–1117.

El-Mofty M, Mostafa W, Esmat S, et al. Suggested mechanisms of action of UVA phototherapy in morphea: a molecular study. *Photodermatol Photoimmunol Photomed.* 2004;20:93–100.

Feldser DM, Greider CW. Short telomeres limit tumor progression in vivo by inducing senescence. *Cancer Cell.* 2007;11:461–469.

Fisher G, Kang S, Varani J, et al. Mechanisms of photoaging and chronological skin aging. *Arch Dermatol.* 2002;138:1462–1470.

Geller AM, Zenick H. Aging and the environment: a research framework. *Environ Health Perspect.* 2005;113:1257–1262.

Gonsalves WC, Chi AC, Neville BW. Common oral lesions: part I. Superficial mucosal lesions. *Am Fam Physician.* 2007;75:501–507.

Hall G, Phillips TJ. Estrogen and skin: the effects of estrogen, menopause, and hormone replacement therapy on the skin. *J Am Acad Dermatol.* 2005;53(4):555–568.

Harpaz R, Ortega-Sanchez IR, Seward JF. Prevention of herpes zoster. Recommendations of the Advisory Committee on Immunization Practices. *MMWR Recomm Rep.* 2008;57:1–30.

Hocker T, Tsao H. Ultraviolet radiation and melanoma: a systematic review and analysis of reported sequence variants. *Hum Mutat.* 2007;28(6):578–588.

Jones KR, Fennie K, Lenihan A. Evidence-based management of chronic wounds. *Adv Skin Wound Care.* 2007;20:591–600.

Jucgla A, Sais G, Berlanga J, et al. Hyperpigmentation of the flexures and pancytopenia during treatment with folate antagonists. *Acta Derm Venereol.* 1997;77(2):165–166.

Kaufman SC. Anterior segment complications of herpes zoster opthalmicus. *Opthalmology.* 2008;115:S24–S32.

Kwangsukstith C, Maibach HI. Effect of age and sex on the induction and elicitation of allergic contact dermatitis. *Contact Dermatitis*. 1995;33(5):289–298.

Lambert EM, Dziura J, Kauls L, et al. Yellow nail syndrome in three siblings: a randomized double-blind trial of topical vitamin E. *Pediatr Dermatol*. 2006;23(4):390–395.

Liao YH, Chen KH, Tseng MP, et al. Pattern of skin diseases in a geriatric patient group in Taiwan: a 7-year survey from the outpatient clinic of a university medical center. *Dermatology*. 2001;203:308–313.

Lowe NJ, Meyers DP, Wieder JM, et al. Low doses of repetitive ultraviolet A induce morphologic changes in human skin. *J Invest Dermatol*. 1995;105(6):739–743.

Maldonado F, Tazelaar HD, Wang CW, et al. Yellow nail syndrome: analysis of 41 consecutive patients. *Chest*. 2008;134(2):375–381.

Mori K, Ando I, Kukita A. Generalized hyperpigmentation of the skin due to vitamin B12 deficiency. *J Dermatol*. 2001;28(5):282–285.

Nishimura EK, Granter SR, Fisher DE. Mechanisms of hair graying: incomplete melanocyte stem cell maintenance in the niche. *Science*. 2005;307(5710):720–724.

O'Donnell JA, Hofmann MT. Skin and soft tissues: management of four common infections in nursing home patients. *Geriatrics*. 2001;56:33–38.

Pavan-Langston D. Herpes zoster antivirals and pain management. *Opthalmology*. 2008;115:S13–S20.

Penn I, First MR. Merkel's cell carcinoma in organ recipients: report of 41 cases. *Transplantation*. 1999;68(11):1717–1721.

Perrem K, Lynch A, Conneely M, et al. The higher incidence of squamous cell carcinoma in renal transplant recipients is associated with increased telomere lengths. *Hum Pathol*. 2007;38(2):351–358.

Ramsewak RS, Nair MG, Stommel M, et al. In vitro antagonistic activity of monoterpenes and their mixtures against [toe nail fungus] pathogens. *Phytother Res*. 2003;17(4):376–379.

Rostan EF. Laser treatment of photodamaged skin. *Facial Plast Surg*. 2005;21(2):99–109.

Sato S. Iron deficiency: structural and microchemical changes in hair, nails, and skin. *Semin Dermatol*. 1991;10(4):313–319.

Scheinfeld N. Infections in the elderly. *Dermatol Online J*. 2005;11:8.

Sinclair R. There is no clear association between low serum ferritin and chronic diffuse telogen hair loss. *Br J Dermatol*. 2002;147(5): 982–984.

Singh G, Haneef NS, Uday A. Nail changes and disorders among the elderly. *Indian J Dermatol Venereol Leprol*. 2005;71(6):386–392.

Stone SP, Buescher LS. Life-threatening paraneoplastic cutaneous syndromes. *Clin Dermatol*. 2005;23:301–306.

Tanaka K, Hasegawa J, Asamitsu K, et al. Prevention of the ultraviolet B-mediated skin photoaging by a nuclear factor kappaB inhibitor, parthenolide. *J Pharmacol Exp Ther*. 2005;315(2):624–630.

Theirs BH. Dermatologic manifestations of internal cancer. *CA Cancer J Clin*. 1986;36:130–148.

Tobin DJ. Introduction to skin aging. *J Tissue Viability*. 2016. http://dx.doi .org/10.1016/j.jtv.2016.03.002

Vaziri H, Benchimol S. From telomere loss to p53 induction and activation of a DNA-damage pathway at senescence: the telomere loss/DNAdamage model of cell aging. *Exp Gerontol*. 1996;31:295–301.

Vorou R, Remoudaki HD, Maltezou HC. Nosocomial scabies. *J Hosp Infect*. 2007;65:9–14.

Wenk J, Schüller J, Hinrichs C, et al. Overexpression of phospholipidhydroperoxide glutathione peroxidase in human dermal fibroblasts abrogates UVA irradiation-induced expression of interstitial collagenase/matrix metalloproteinase-1 by suppression of phosphatidylcholine hydroperoxide-mediated NFkappaB activation and interleukin-6 release. *J Biol Chem*. 2004;279(44):45634–45642.

Wolpowitz D, Gilchrest, BA. The vitamin D questions: how much do you need and how should you get it? *J Am Acad Dermatology*. 2006;54(2): 301–317.

Obesity and Dermatology

David J. Rosenfeld, MD, BS and Nora K. Shumway, MD

OBESITY AND DERMATOLOGY

Obesity is a growing epidemic in the United States affecting more than one-third (34.9% or 78.6 million) of U.S. adults. As the number of patients with obesity has increased, so has the importance of physician awareness of its many associated dermatologic complications. The physician's role in treatment must include targeted therapy to address these specific complications as well as encouragement of the patient to improve their overall health through diet and exercise. While all physicians have the responsibility to encourage weight loss in obese patients, doctors have the unique role of recognizing and treating many of its most deforming and easily observable complications. Obesity is defined as a body mass index greater than 30, and patients affected by this condition may experience direct skin changes (owing to an increased body size) as well as skin changes secondary to systemic complications. These changes will be reviewed here.

Direct Skin Changes

Due to the change in body size, there are direct skin changes that can be seen.

Plantar Hyperkeratosis

Plantar hyperkeratosis is the thickening of the skin on the plantar surface of the feet. This is presumed to be secondary to increased pressure from the increased weight the feet are bearing. In the setting of diabetes, this can be a source of ulceration development, and therefore, appropriate management is key. Surgical removal of this hyperkeratosis, often with the assistance of podiatry, can be helpful. Other early treatments include urea cream and salicylic acid, which help to soften the hyperkeratosis. Both of these serve as keratolytic agents within the stratum corneum. Salicylic acid works through corneocyte disaggregation to promote shedding of scales, whereas urea promotes protein denaturation through increased water uptake.

Acanthosis Nigricans

Acanthosis nigricans (Fig. 47-1) presents as brown velvety plaques that develop in intertriginous areas; most commonly on the neck. However, it can also develop in the axilla and along the inframammary fold. Acanthosis nigricans in both children and adults can be associated with insulin resistance prior to the diagnosis of diabetes. When acute in onset and in locations

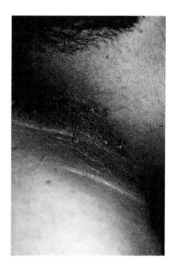

FIGURE 47-1: Acanthosis nigricans and skin tags on the side of the neck.

other than intertriginous areas, such as palms and mucosa, malignancy should be considered. Adenocarcinomas are the most commonly associated malignancy; however, many solid tumors have been reported. While the exact mechanism behind acanthosis nigricans is not entirely determined, particularly when malignancy related, it appears that insulin and insulin growth factor-1 act on keratinocytes and fibroblasts to result in hyperplasia. Treatment should focus on weight loss and improvement of insulin resistance. Additionally, a trial of ammonium lactate, topical retinoids, or keratolytic creams (salicylic acid or urea containing) could be considered. Due to risk of irritation, however, these treatments should be used with caution.

Acrochordons (Skin Tags)

Acrochordons are common in patients who are obese. They present as soft hyperpigmented or flesh-colored papules, which are often pedunculated. Acrochordons usually develop in areas of friction such as the neck and axilla. Although they are benign growths, they are a frequent source of discomfort particularly when irritated from frictional forces. These can be treated with either cryotherapy or excisional removal.

Striae

Due to the expansive growth associated with obesity and the resulting tension placed on the skin, striae or stretch marks commonly develop. While many patients who are obese have striae, not all patients who have striae are obese. Pregnancy and the growth spurt of adolescence can result in striae as well. The striae of obesity arise along cleavage lines perpendicular to the direction of greatest tension in areas with the most adipose tissue—the breasts, buttocks, lateral abdomen, and thighs. Striae are characterized by linear smooth bands of atrophic-appearing skin that are sometimes initially erythematous, then purple, and finally, white and depressed. Current hypotheses suggest that striae are a type of dermal scarring with an aberrant healing response and replacement of collagen. While there is currently no treatment to completely remove striae, the use of a pulse dye laser may improve their appearance particularly during the erythematous phase.

Cellulite

Cellulite is a dimpling of the skin that occurs most commonly on the thighs and buttocks. This occurs most commonly in women who often have no health concerns and are not obese. It is rarely, if ever, noted in men. While the pathophysiology is not completely understood, its increased prevalence in women indicates a possible anatomic predisposition. The appearance of cellulite is caused by herniations of fat, and it is characterized by the presence of focally enlarged fibrosclerotic strands that partition the subcutis. The mainstay of cellulite treatment is weight loss.

Secondary Skin Changes

Obesity has many systemic complications ranging from decreased ability for venous return in lower extremities to increased risk of diabetes and vascular disease. Associated with these systemic complications come dermatologic manifestations.

Venous Stasis

Central obesity causes increased abdominal pressure resulting in venous stasis and lymphedema that leads to swelling in the lower extremities and associated skin changes. Early on, this manifests as soft pitting edema. Over time, this progresses to woody induration which is prone to breakdown and slow healing ulcers. Eventually, the skin can take on a pebbly and then verrucous appearance termed *elephantiasis nostra verrucosa*. For these patients, the most important treatment and prevention strategy is to limit swelling with compression stockings and weight loss.

Stasis Dermatitis

Stasis dermatitis (Fig. 47-2) is the epidermal change associated with lymphedema and results in brown-red scaly patches and plaques, most commonly on the shins. It is thought to occur owing to the decreases in microcirculation resulting from obesity, peripheral vascular disease, diabetes, coronary artery disease, and hyperlipidemia. Key treatment strategies include compression, topical emollient, and steroid use when actively inflamed. If possible, it is important to avoid the use of topical antibiotics owing to an increased risk of developing allergic contact dermatitis.

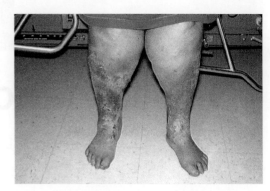

FIGURE 47-2: Stasis dermatitis with hyperpigmentation, oozing and crusting on the pretibial area in an obese patient. Also with lipodermatosclerosis with an "inverted champagne bottle" deformity.

Lipodermatosclerosis

Lipodermatosclerosis is one of the results of venous stasis. It has two phases. In the acute phase, it presents as erythema, pain, and warmth, which is often mistaken for cellulitis. This diagnosis should be considered for any patient with "recurrent" or "treatment-resistant" cellulitis. The persistence of lesions despite antibiotic therapy in the setting of other changes of venous stasis is often a clue. The chronic stage of this disease results in woody induration of the distal leg that results in an "inverted champagne bottle" appearance. First-line therapy includes compression, elevation, and use of topical or intralesional corticosteroids. Pentoxifylline is thought to be helpful by some authors.

Leg Ulcerations

Leg ulcerations are the feared and long-term complications of persistent venous stasis. They are often slow healing and result in significant morbidity in affected patients. These chronic wounds result in an increased risk of bacterial penetration leading to an increased risk of cellulitis. Ulcers are best prevented with early intervention of venous stasis as mentioned above. While leg ulcerations can also develop in peripheral arterial disease, this will not be discussed in this chapter. To also help prevent cellulitis in patients with venous stasis, it is also important to evaluate and treat tinea pedis as resulting fissures can also serve as portal of entry.

Obesity Impairs the Integrity of the Skin

Due to the friction, neural changes, tension, and pressure-related changes seen in the enlarged skin folds in obese patients, the skin is more prone to breakdown, infection, and dermatoses. Infections that are related to changes in epidermal integrity include cutaneous candidiasis (including erosio interdigitalis blastomycetica, candidal folliculitis, and tinea cruris). The vascular disease and diabetes mellitus often seen in the setting of obesity also play a role in the development of these infections owing to direct immune impairment.

Intertrigo

Intertrigo is a common complication of obesity secondary to the increased depth and amount of body folds. Intertrigo frequently develops in the area below the abdominal pannus, inguinal folds, gluteal cleft, axilla, and inframammary folds. Factors that predispose obese patients to intertrigo include friction, maceration, moisture, warmth, and occlusion. Colonization of the skin and intertriginous areas with bacteria, yeast, and dermatophytes may exacerbate the intertrigo. Candidal colonization and infection is the most common pathogenic factor. Patients often complain of pruritus, irritation, and burning. Treatment includes reducing moisture collection by ensuring adequate drying after bathing, moisture wicking materials placed directly in folds, using anti-candida/bacterial agents when needed and encouraging weight loss to reduce skin folds.

Hyperhidrosis

Hyperhidrosis, or excessive sweating, can be seen in the setting of obesity. This increased sweating can be distressing to patients. While encouraging weight loss is essential, other interventions include topical agents such as aluminum chloride 20%, oral therapies such as anticholinergics (i.e., glycopyrrolate), and/or the targeted use of Botox.

Other Dermatologic Diseases Associated With Obesity

Hypothyroidism

Hypothyroidism is the result of decreased circulating thyroid hormone or rarely, peripheral resistance to hormonal action. Dermatologic manifestations include dry skin, obesity, macroglossia, swollen lips, cold hands and feet, brittle nails, alopecia, and a mucinosis of the skin called myxedema. There can also be a reduction of the basal metabolic rate. Hypothyroidism can respond well to treatment with thyroid hormone, often with complete resolution of the cutaneous findings.

Psoriasis

Patients with psoriasis have been shown to have an increased risk of developing obesity. While there is no demonstrable causation between the two, these conditions do share a common link of chronic low-grade inflammation. Obesity is not only associated with higher incidences of psoriasis, but also with greater severity of the disease. Therefore, when managing psoriasis in obese patients, it is equally important to address the skin manifestations of their disease as well as their underlying obesity.

> **SAUER'S NOTES**
>
> Psoriasis is now considered a cutaneous marker of the metabolic syndrome. The importance of this association is essential for attempted management of psoriasis and the overall health of the patients.

Hidradenitis Suppurativa

Similar to psoriasis, obesity (as well as smoking) is a significant risk factor for hidradenitis and can also increase its severity. The treatment of hidradenitis involves addressing the associated obesity and encouraging weight loss.

Polycystic Ovarian Syndrome

Dermatologic manifestations of PCOS include acne, androgenic alopecia, and increased terminal hair growth. While PCOS has many other systemic complications, insulin resistance and obesity are commonly seen. The adipocyte is highly metabolic and has significant consequences on steroid metabolism. In obese women (including those with PCOS), a positive correlation has been shown between BMI and serum androgen levels. Excess androgen production is responsible for many of the manifestations of PCOS, including those that affect the skin and hair. As with many of the dermatologic diseases associated with obesity, weight loss should be encouraged in the management of PCOS. In fact, in many obese women with PCOS, even minor weight loss (up to 5%) has been shown to improve many of its symptoms.

Suggested Readings

Schwarzenberger K, Callen JP. Dermatologic manifestations in patients with systemic disease. In: Bolognia JL, Jorizzo JL, Schaffer JV, eds. *Dermatology.* 3rd ed. Philadelphia, PA: Elsevier Limited; 2012:761–781.

Shipman AR, Millington GWM. Obesity and the skin. *Br J Dermatol.* 2011;165(4):743–750.

Yosipovitch G, DeVore A, Dawn A. Obesity and the skin: skin physiology and skin manifestations of obesity. *J Am Acad Dermatol.* 2007;56(6):901–916.

Skin Disease in Transplant Patients

Edit B. Olasz, MD, PhD and Marcy Neuburg, MD

Since the first successful cadaver kidney transplant in 1962, the field of solid organ transplantation has undergone a remarkable journey, resulting in an ever-growing number of transplantations and increased transplant and recipient survival. The success of transplant survival is built on the advances in our understanding of physiology, immunology, improved surgical techniques, more efficient immunosuppressive treatments, and the multidisciplinary care of solid organ transplant recipients (OTRs). Longer recipient survival has led to an increased understanding of the consequences of long-term immunosuppression. Potent immunosuppressive drugs allow for long-term organ and patient survival. However, these drugs have numerous side effects, many of which manifest in the skin. These include direct effects from the individual drugs, immune-mediated effects from the grafted organ, and indirect effects of acute and chronic immunosuppression such as opportunistic infections and an increased incidence of skin cancers. The recognition of the accelerated and accentuated cutaneous carcinogenesis and the increased risk for cutaneous infections in OTRs opened the field of transplant dermatology. In 2001 the International Transplant Skin-Cancer Collaborative (ITSCC) was formed, joined by its European counterpart Skin Cancer in Organ Transplant Patients, Europe (SCOPE), in an effort to educate and care for the growing number of OTRs. The following sections outline the broad scope of skin diseases observed in OTRs.

SAUER'S NOTES

1. Transplant patients will continue to increase in the foreseeable future and dermatologists need to help meet the challenge of their complex care.
2. Infections of the skin tend to be associated with less common organisms, to be more aggressive, and to be more recalcitrant to therapy.
3. Malignancies of the skin tend to be more common, more aggressive, and more apt to recur.
4. The skin is the window to other organ systems of the body. In this challenging group of patients, "this window" needs to be used to detect systemic infections and malignancies.

EPIDEMIOLOGY

According to the United Network for Organ Sharing, over 28,000 solid organ transplants are performed in the United States each year and 74,000 worldwide. Approximately 250,000 solid OTRs are alive in the United States today, while over 90,000 people await transplantation. The overall five-year survival rate has steadily increased in the past 10 years, reaching 80% to 90% in kidney, 72% to 86% in liver, 70% in cardiac, and 42% in lung transplant recipients.

CUTANEOUS EFFECTS OF IMMUNOSUPPRESSIVE MEDICATIONS

The cutaneous adverse effects of commonly used immunosuppressive agents are detailed in the following text and summarized in Table 48-1.

Corticosteroids

Cushing Syndrome

Cushing syndrome is caused by the administration of excess glucocorticoids as part of an OTR patient's immunosuppressive regimen. The patient may have any of the following typical physical stigmata: moon facies, facial plethora, supraclavicular fat pads, buffalo hump, truncal obesity, and purple striae. Individuals often complain of proximal muscle weakness, easy bruising, weight gain, hirsutism, and impaired wound healing. Reduction or discontinuation of glucocorticoid therapy should be managed by, or in conjunction with the transplant physician due to the risks of (1) steroid withdrawal syndrome, (2) organ rejection, and (3) possible suppression of HPA axis with secondary adrenal insufficiency.

Steroid Acne

Steroid acne presents with monomorphous, erythematous papules and pustules that appear relatively abruptly on the upper trunk, often sparing the face. The monomorphous nature and abrupt appearance distinguish steroid acne from acne vulgaris, which typically has a slower onset and is composed of acneiform lesions in different stages of development, usually involving the face. Cysts and comedones are common in acne vulgaris.

TABLE 48-1 • Cutaneous Adverse Effects of Commonly Used Immunosuppressive Agents

Drug	Common Cutaneous Side Effects
Corticosteroids	Cushing syndrome
	Acne
	Striae
	Fragile skin
Cyclosporine	Hirsutism
	Sebaceous hyperplasia
	Gingival hyperplasia
	Gynecomastia
Tacrolimus	Alopecia
Azathioprine	Hypersensitivity reaction
Mycophenolate Mofetil	Nonspecific eruptions
	Acne
Sirolimus	Impaired wound healing
	Acne/folliculitis
	Edema

Source: Modified from Otley CC, Stasko T. *Skin Disease in Organ Transplantation.* New York: Cambridge University Press; 2008.

Treatment: Topical retinoids is the treatment of choice in steroid acne. Lowering systemic steroid dosage is curative.

Striae

Striae rubra distensae are linear bands of atrophic, cigarette paper-like skin, which are originally red and indurated, later becoming hypopigmented and atrophic. These may be widely distributed, especially over the abdomen, lower back, buttocks, and thighs.

Treatment: In the early erythematous stage, pulsed-dye laser has been shown to be somewhat helpful. After striae reach the late atrophic stage, treatment is very difficult. Topical retinoids, cryotherapy, and ablative laser resurfacing have been used with inconsistent results.

Cutaneous Fragility and Ecchymosis

The skin may become thin and fragile. Spontaneous tearing may occur with trivial trauma. Purpura and ecchymoses are most commonly located on the dorsal forearms and dorsal hands. Avoidance of shearing trauma on the dorsal hands and forearms may help prevent the ecchymoses. Adhesive bandages should be removed with extreme care as skin may tear.

Cyclosporine

Hypertrichosis

Hypertrichosis is a cosmetically undesirable dose-dependent side effect of cyclosporine therapy, characterized by excessive hair growth not localized to the androgen-dependent areas of the body. It appears months after initiation of cyclosporine therapy in about 75% of patients. The cessation of cyclosporine therapy results in a progressive resolution of hypertrichosis. Laser-assisted hair removal or switching to tacrolimus may improve the hypertrichosis.

Sebaceous Hyperplasia

Sebaceous hyperplasia is a well-known side effect of cyclosporine therapy, presenting within several years after starting treatment. About 10% to 15% of patients taking cyclosporine develop multiple small, yellowish umbilicated papules measuring 2 to 6 mm located usually on the central face. However, ectopic sites such as the oral mucosa may be affected as well. These lesions are benign but can be cosmetically bothersome to patients. Electrosurgery, laser treatment, shave excision, and photodynamic therapy (PDT) have been employed to treat sebaceous hyperplasia.

Gingival Hyperplasia

Gingival overgrowth affects 30% to 50% of patients. It is first observed approximately 3 months following the initiation of cyclosporine therapy. Topical or systemic azithromycin may induce marked improvement. In some cases, periodontal surgery may be necessary. In addition, changing cyclosporine to tacrolimus has been reported to improve this condition.

Tacrolimus

Alopecia

Tacrolimus-induced hair loss presents in about 29% of patients as widespread hair thinning, occurring at a mean of 30 to 422 days after initiating tacrolimus. Rapid reversal of alopecia has been reported with the use of minoxidil. Reducing the dose of tacrolimus or switching to cyclosporine is helpful.

Azathioprine

Azathioprine (AZA) has been reported to cause cutaneous hypersensitivity reactions including urticarial, maculopapular, and vasculitic eruptions. Less commonly reported side effects are mucositis, photosensitivity, and increased susceptibility to verrucae, herpes zoster, and Norwegian scabies. In addition, AZA has been shown in laboratory models to have direct carcinogenic effects.

Mycophenolate Mofetil

Nonspecific cutaneous eruptions have been reported in 8% to 22% of patients on mycophenolate mofetil (MMF). Acne and peripheral edema, as well as exacerbation of dyshidrotic eczema, have been linked to MMF therapy.

Sirolimus

Infections and Pilosebaceous Eruptions

Infections and acne-like eruptions are common cutaneous side effects of sirolimus. More specifically, 34% of patients developed viral infections, 4% developed bacterial, and 16% of patients developed fungal infections. With predominance in men, inflammatory eruptions resembling acne were noted in 46% of renal transplant patients on sirolimus. Scalp folliculitis and hidradenitis suppurativa, as well as other skin eruptions resembling seborrheic dermatitis involving almost every body part, have also been reported. Topical and systemic antibiotics, benzoyl peroxide, and topical or systemic retinoids are recommended.

Edema

Chronic edema, mainly affecting the lower legs (98%) was noted in more than half of OTRs (65%) treated with sirolimus. In some patients, upper extremity edema or angioedema involving the face and oral cavity was observed. The exact mechanism of sirolimus-induced edema is unknown, but it is thought to be due to vasculitis, lymphatic obstruction, or capillary obstruction. Sirolimus-induced edema is often resistant to diuretics; therefore, dietary restrictions, blood pressure control, and compression therapy are advised. Discontinuation of the inciting drug is often necessary. Depending on the severity of angioedema, airway support, antihistamines, glucocorticoids, and epinephrine may be required.

Impaired Wound Healing

Sirolimus has been found to cause delayed wound healing, wound dehiscence, and superficial and deep wound fluid collections. The mechanism of impaired wound healing has been shown to be due to the inhibitory effect of sirolimus on fibroblast and endothelial cells through the blockade of growth factors, leading to anti-angiogenesis. Appropriate medical or surgical wound care, drainage of seromas, and in severe cases discontinuation of the drug are necessary. Temporary use of alternate immunosuppressive agents in anticipation of elective surgery is advised.

CUTANEOUS EFFECTS OF THE TRANSPLANTED ORGAN

Graft Versus Host Disease (GVHD)

Although GVHD is most frequently associated with bone marrow or stem cell transplantation, it is also a rare but severe complication of solid organ transplantation. Transplanted solid organs contain a variable amount of lymphoid tissue, enabling the allografts to function as a mini bone marrow transplant and initiate an immunologically mediated and injurious set of reactions by cells genetically disparate to their host. In OTRs, GVHD is seen most frequently after liver transplantation, but the incidence of GVHD is highest after small bowel transplantation (about 5%), possibly owing to a large number of donor lymphocytes present in the gut. Risk factors for developing GVHD in liver transplant recipients include age greater than 65, closely matched HLA recipients, and a donor more than 40 years younger than the recipient.

The diagnosis of acute GVHD is established by clinical judgment, imaging studies, laboratory workup, and biopsy results. Skin involvement often precedes hepatic (except in liver transplant patients), hematologic, or gastrointestinal symptoms and presents from 2 days to 6 weeks posttransplant with an erythematous maculopapular eruption. The eruption has a predilection for the palms and soles and in severe cases can progress to generalized erythema with bullae

and desquamation, often making it difficult to distinguish it from a severe drug eruption. Skin biopsy and the presence of other systemic symptoms including diarrhea, pancytopenia, and fever aid in confirming the diagnosis. When evaluating a maculopapular eruption in an OTR, in addition to GVHD, drug eruption, chemotherapy toxicity, and viral eruption should be considered in the differential diagnosis. The mortality rate of GVHD in OTRs is high (75% to 90%), with death usually resulting from overwhelming sepsis, gastrointestinal bleeding, pneumonia, or renal failure. Management of acute GVHD after solid organ transplantation requires a multidisciplinary approach. Current therapies include antilymphocyte regimens and various approaches resulting in either increased or decreased immunosuppression. New biologics including basiliximab, a chimeric mouse–human monoclonal antibody to the IL-2Rα receptor (CD25) of T cells, have been successfully used in some cases.

INFECTIOUS DISEASES OF THE SKIN IN OTR PATIENTS

Due to their suppressed host immune defense mechanism, OTRs are more susceptible to bacterial, fungal, and viral infections. Most infections during the first month are related to surgical complications. Opportunistic infections typically occur from the second to the sixth month post-transplant. During the late post-transplant period (beyond 6 months), OTRs suffer from the same infections seen in the general community. Opportunistic bacterial infections seen in transplant recipients include those caused by *Legionella spp.*, *Nocardia spp.*, *Salmonella spp.*, and *Listeria monocytogenes*. Cytomegalovirus (CMV) is the most common cause of viral infections. Herpes simplex virus (HSV), varicella-zoster virus (VZV), Epstein–Barr virus (EBV), human papillomavirus (HPV), and others are also significant pathogens. Fungal infections caused by both yeasts and mycelial fungi are associated with the highest mortality rates. Mycobacteria, pneumocystis, and parasitic diseases may also occur. Due to the heightened risk of infection, the clinician should maintain an increased index of suspicion. More aggressive and earlier diagnostic approaches including skin biopsy with special stains, superficial and tissue culture, and diagnostic imaging modalities may be warranted. Many systemic antimicrobials require dose adjustments in the setting of renal insufficiency. Use of these drugs in renal transplant recipients should include co-management by transplant nephrologists.

Bacterial Infections

Staphylococcal Infections

Staphylococcus aureus is a common pathogen and causes the majority of pyodermas and soft tissue infections seen in solid OTRs. It often colonizes the anterior nares as well as superficial skin breaks and skin disruptions in these patients. Treatment of *S. aureus* colonization with topical mupirocin ointment has been shown to decrease the occurrence of *S. aureus* pyodermas including folliculitis, furuncles, carbuncles, impetigo, bullous impetigo, and ecthyma in certain non-immunosuppressed patients. However, the same results in OTRs have not been proven. Topical treatment with clindamycin, mupirocin, retapamulin, or oral antibiotics according to sensitivities is recommended. Methicillin-resistant *S. aureus* is an increasing concern in OTRs (Fig. 48-1). Use of Vancomycin or treatment with Linezolid 600 mg b.i.d. may be employed if sensitivities are determined and infection is of significant concern.

Streptococcus Infections

Group A *β*-hemolytic streptococci can cause superficial pyodermas presenting as impetiginized skin and soft tissue infections. Necrotizing fasciitis is a severe form of soft tissue infection extending into the subcutaneous fat and deep fascia caused by *β*-hemolytic streptococcus or a combination of non-group A streptococci and anaerobe bacilli. Pain out of proportion to clinical signs should raise the clinical suspicion of necrotizing fasciitis. Treatment includes clindamycin and gamma globulin in addition to extensive, emergency surgical debridement and intensive care monitoring.

Gram-negative bacteria, such as *Klebsiella pneumoniae*, *Escherichia coli*, *Pseudomonas aeruginosa*, *Proteus mirabilis*, and *Enterobacter*, may cause cellulitis in OTR patients, presenting with varying morphology including bullae, ulcers, or cutaneous necrosis with vascular involvement. Initial empiric coverage with gentamicin is helpful until tissue and blood cultures return.

Nocardiosis

Nocardial infections have been reported primarily in renal and heart transplant patients, fewer than 4% of whom develop this type of infection. Nocardial infection is most commonly caused by *Nocardia asteroides*, a gram-positive, weakly acid fast bacterium. It can be directly introduced to the skin or more commonly spread by the hematogenous route from the lung. Primary cutaneous infection can present as abscesses, ulcers, granulomas, soft tissue infection, mycetoma, or lymphocutaneous infection. Sulfonamides, either alone or in combination with trimethroprim, are the treatment of choice

for nocardiosis. Antimicrobial therapy should be continued for a prolonged period after cure because there is a tendency to relapse and the optimal duration of therapy is not known.

Bartonella Infection

Infection by *Bartonella henselae*, a gram-negative bacillus, has been reported in kidney, liver, and heart transplant recipients as early as 11 months and as late as 14 years after transplantation. The clinical manifestation of Bartonella infection in OTRs can vary greatly. Patients may present with the typical features of cat-scratch disease with regional lymphadenopathy and fever, but this will usually progress to a more severe, systemic illness if not treated promptly. Transplant recipients have also been reported to develop bacillary angiomatosis, the form of Bartonella infection caused by *B. henselae* and *B. quintana*, commonly seen in individuals with HIV infection. Patients with bacillary angiomatosis present with red-to-violaceous, dome-shaped friable papules and nodules, ranging in size from a few millimeters up to 2 to 3 cm in diameter. Culture of the organism from the skin or a lymph node may be difficult to obtain and requires an incubation period of as long as 30 days. For this reason, polymerase chain reaction of the tissue specimen may be preferable. The antibiotics of choice are erythromycin 250 to 500 mg PO four times daily or doxycycline 100 mg two times daily, continued for 3 months.

Vibrio Vulnificus

Vibrio vulnificus, a gram-negative rod, may contaminate shellfish and oysters. Infection occurs either through ingestion or direct inoculation through open wounds from seawater mainly along the Atlantic seacoast. Skin lesions begin within 24 to 48 hours after exposure as erythematous plaques and rapidly progress to hemorrhagic bullae, subsequently becoming necrotic ulcers. Aggressive early surgical debridement is mandatory. Mortality is not insignificant. It is important to remember that infection with *V. vulnificus* can lead to sepsis in immunocompromised hosts and these patients should be cautioned about eating uncooked shellfish. Treatment with Doxycycline 100 mg twice daily is recommended.

Fungal Skin Infections

Fungal skin infections in OTR patients include classical dermatomycosis, opportunistic fungal infections, and infections with rare fungal pathogens. Fungal infections in solid OTRs continue to be a significant cause of morbidity and mortality. *Candida spp.* and *Aspergillus spp.* account for most invasive fungal infections. The incidence of fungal infection varies with the type of solid organ transplant. Liver transplant recipients have the highest reported incidence of Candida infections while lung transplant recipients have the highest rate of Aspergillus infections.

The classic superficial fungal infections, such as tinea cruris, corporis, and pedis, are seen in up to 50% of OTR patients and are most commonly caused by *Trichophyton rubrum*. Onychomycosis is also a frequent finding. Onychomycosis more commonly involves multiple toe- or fingernails in OTRs,

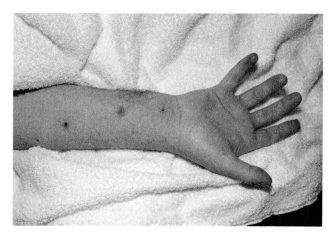

FIGURE 48-1: Heart transplant patient with 24-hour history of impetigo and swollen forearm, wrist, and hand. Culture was positive for CA-MRSA.

and more importantly it is frequently caused by molds, such as *Scopulariopsis spp.* In an immunosuppressed host this fungus may cause subcutaneous infection or fatal systemic infection. Proximal white subungual onychomycosis is a pathognomonic sign of immunosuppression, involves the nail plate adjacent to the proximal nail fold, and is produced by *T. rubrum* and *T. megnini.* In addition to topical antifungal medications, treatment with terbinafine for extensive superficial fungal infections is a good option because the potential for drug interactions with immunosuppressants is minimal.

Opportunistic Infections

Opportunistic fungal infections in OTRs may be caused by fungi normally occurring in our environment that do not typically cause infection in a normal host, such as *Candida, Aspergillus, Cryptococcus, Zygomycetes,* and *Scedosporium spp.* In a severely immunocompromised host these saprophytes can cause serious infections. *Candida spp.* are found in the human gastrointestinal tract, from the oropharynx to the anus, in the female gynecologic tract, and on the skin. Small numbers of yeast colonies are normally present, increasing in number when the normal microbial flora is altered by antibiotics or when there is a defect in immune competence. Thrush (candidiasis of the oral mucosa) is the most common fungal infection in transplant patients, affecting up to 64% of patients. Treatment with oral fluconazole 200 mg on the first day, then 100 mg once daily for at least 2 weeks to decrease the likelihood of relapse, is recommended. Candida infection may also involve the skin folds and nails and can cause chronic paronychia. Additionally, it can present as Candida folliculitis or appear granulomatous, as seen in mucocutaneous candidiasis. Disseminated candidiasis is one of the most common serious opportunistic mycoses in severely immunocompromised patients.

Invasive aspergillosis remains among the most significant opportunistic infections in OTRs. The incidence of invasive aspergillosis varies from relatively low rates in renal transplant recipients to approaching 15% in lung transplant recipients. Mortality rates in transplant recipients with Aspergillus infections have ranged from 68% to 92%. An estimated 9.3% to 16.9% of deaths in the first post-transplant year have been considered to be attributable to invasive aspergillosis. Primary cutaneous aspergillosis is rare and most cases occur at the site of intravenous cannulas. Infection presents with erythematous nodules, and hemorrhagic bullae or ulcers. Pulmonary involvement is usually present in invasive Aspergillus infection, with associated cutaneous involvement in only 10% of cases. Biopsy of the skin lesion may establish the diagnosis, and tissue culture will provide definitive diagnosis. Lipid formulation of Amphotericin B is the drug of choice for treatment of aspergillosis. Voriconazole and the new echinocandins have also proven to be useful.

Cutaneous *Cryptococcus spp.* (Fig. 48-2) infection occurs secondarily in up to 15% of patients with disseminated disease as described in renal, liver, and lung transplant patients. Skin infection occurs most commonly on the head and neck, presenting with variable morphology, such as molluscum-like lesions, ulcers, papules, pustules, nodules, acneiform eruptions,

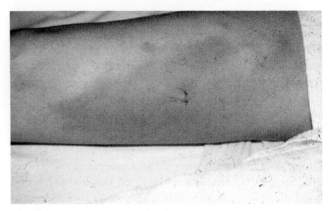

FIGURE 48-2: Cryptococcal cellulitis in a renal transplant that was diagnosed by culture and viewing fungal organisms in tissue.

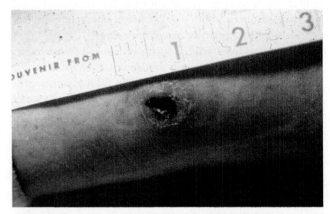

FIGURE 48-3: Ulcer on the inner calf of a heart transplant patient that showed mucormycosis on tissue stains from a skin biopsy at the ulcer's edge.

and cellulitis. Initial intravenous Amphotericin B followed by oral fluconazole is the standard treatment.

Infection with other opportunistic fungi, including *Mucorales spp.* (Fig. 48-3) dematiaceous and nondematiaceous fungi also pose a real threat to immunosuppressed patients. In addition, these patients are at increased risk to develop infection by rare or endemic fungi, including *Sporothrix schenckii, Histoplasma capsulatum,* and *Coccidioides immitis,* and *Blastomyces* and *Penicillium spp.* Geographic location and travel history of the patient can be crucial when taking a complete medical history from these patients.

Viral Diseases

Viral infections cause a wide variety of complications in solid OTRs, some of them are life threatening. Approximately 10% of patients have chronic or progressive infection with HBV, HCV, CMV, EBV, or papillomavirus. Such viral infections may cause injury to the infected organ (the liver in the case of the hepatitis viruses and the retina in the case of CMV) or contribute to the development of cancer (e.g., hepatocellular carcinoma following HBV or HCV infection, lymphoma due to EBV, and squamous cell cancer due to papillomavirus).

Herpes Simplex Virus-1 and -2

The majority of HSV infections in OTRs are reactivation of latent infections, typically occurring in the first 3 months posttransplantation. The lesions commonly present with typical grouped vesicles in a localized distribution in the perioral, anogenital, or digital area. However, with increasing immunosuppression, chronic large ulcers, widespread vesicular eruption, eczema herpeticum, or disseminated visceral infection (hepatitis, pneumonitis, encephalitis) may occur. Infection can be diagnosed by isolation of the virus from lesional smears. Treatment with valacyclovir, famciclovir, or acyclovir is recommended. Intravenous acyclovir should be considered in severe infections.

Varicella-Zoster Virus

Primary infection with VZV via the airborne route causes varicella (chickenpox). Reactivation of VZV in the dorsal root ganglia, and subsequent replication in the epithelial cells produces the characteristic vesicular eruption of herpes zoster. Unlike HSV infections that usually occur in the immediate post-transplant period, VZV reactivation usually occurs after day 100 in OTRs. Herpes zoster in transplant recipients can follow one of three clinical patterns. In most instances, the patients develop a dermatomal skin eruption similar to what is seen in immunocompetent patients; however, the risk of dissemination is higher (40%). Less commonly, OTR patients develop varicella-like eruption with no obvious primary dermatomal eruption, a syndrome that is termed "atypical generalized zoster." Finally, some patients may develop subclinical reactivation of latent VZV, with no evidence of cutaneous lesions. Cutaneous complications in immunocompromised children include bullous or hemorrhagic varicella lesions, necrotizing fasciitis, purpura fulminans, and bacterial superinfections. Complications related to herpes zoster may include postherpetic neuralgia, cutaneous scarring, and bacterial superinfections. Hematogenous dissemination of VZV to the eye can cause acute retinal necrosis and blindness. Fewer than 5% of transplant patients experience a second episode of herpes zoster. A positive Tzanck test confirms diagnosis of either VZV or HSV. Detection of viral antigen on a smear from the base of a vesicle is diagnostic. Treatment is with the same drugs as approved for HSV but with higher doses. Varicella vaccination is currently recommended prior to transplantation in children and adolescents. The vaccination has been used post–renal transplantation with no adverse affects to the vaccine and a 66% rate of seroconversion.

Epstein–Barr Virus

Primary cutaneous EBV-associated post-transplant lymphoproliferative disease (PTLD) is the most common cutaneous manifestation of EBV infection in OTRs. Disease localized to the skin is rare and presents with polymorphic lesions characterized by maculopapular eruption, single or multiple erythematous nodules or ulcers.

Cytomegalovirus

The most important pathogen affecting transplant recipients is CMV, with infection occurring mainly after the first month post-transplant. CMV can present as primary infection, reinfection, or reactivation of latent disease. Classically, CMV presents with fever, constitutional symptoms, visceral disease including colitis, esophagitis, hepatitis, laboratory evidence of bone marrow suppression, and rarely pneumonitis. Cutaneous manifestations are variable and rare, often with delayed diagnosis. Multiple skin morphologies have been reported, including maculopapular eruption, petechiae, vesiculobullous lesions, indurated hyperpigmented nodules, and plaques. Ulceration, particularly involving the genital, perineal, and perianal areas, as well as necrosis of mucosal membranes, can occur in more severe cases. However, none of these appearances is pathognomonic for CMV. Despite the morphologic cutaneous variances, all exhibit uniform histologic appearance, including typical vascular endothelial cytopathic changes with intracytoplasmic and intranuclear inclusions affecting skin capillaries. Definitive diagnosis relies on histopathologic examination. Treatment of clinical CMV disease usually requires administration of intravenous ganciclovir for 2 to 4 weeks; clearance of viremia should be documented before intravenous therapy is discontinued.

Human Herpesvirus-8

Human herpesvirus (HHV8), a gamma herpesvirus, is associated with Kaposi sarcoma (KS), Castleman disease, and primary effusion lymphoma. KS, by far the most common HHV8-associated disease (Fig. 48-4), has been observed most frequently in patients suffering from acquired immunodeficiency syndrome (AIDS). Solid organ recipients show an increasing incidence of KS. According to the Cincinnati Transplant Tumor Registry up to 6% of all de novo cancers following solid organ transplantation are KS. The risk of developing this type of malignancy for renal recipients is approximately 500 times more than that seen in the nontransplant population. The clinical presentation of Kaposi sarcoma in transplant recipients is often limited to the skin, although visceral Kaposi sarcoma has been described. The lesions present as red to purple, infiltrated macules, plaques,

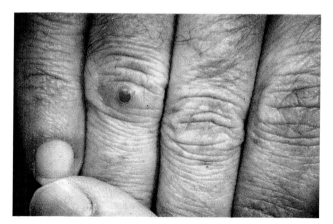

FIGURE 48-4: Purple papule on the dorsal finger in a renal transplant patient was proven Kaposi sarcoma by biopsy. This tumor and similar other ones dissipated when immunosuppression was decreased. Kaposi sarcoma is by far the most common HHV-8 disease in solid transplant recipients.

and nodules that vary in number and size depending on the level of immunosuppression. In most transplant patients KS is located predominantly on the lower legs, similarly to the classical form of KS, and often associated with lymphedema. Mucosal lesions show a predilection for the nasal mucosa and hard palate.

A diagnosis of KS should be established by skin biopsy, which should be taken from the center of the most infiltrated plaque. The main approach to managing transplant-associated Kaposi sarcoma is to reduce or even discontinue immunosuppressive therapy. The addition of rapamycin in place of other immunosuppressant medication, in particular cyclosporine, has been associated with regression of KS. Isolated KS lesions can be treated with surgical excision or cryotherapy. Radiotherapy should be avoided due to the risk of additional cutaneous malignancies. Systemic immunotherapy or chemotherapy can be considered for indolent, disseminated KS.

Molluscum Contagiosum Virus

In contrast to the general population, molluscum contagiosum virus (MCV) infection is commonly found in the adult OTR patients in addition to the pediatric transplant recipients, where the incidence has been reported to be 6.9%. Molluscum lesions present as 1 to 3 mm pink papules with a characteristic central umbilicated keratinous plug. In addition, giant molluscum lesions larger than 1 cm may occur in OTRs as well. Diagnosis is easily made based on the characteristic appearance. Treatment of cosmetically disturbing lesions with cryotherapy is recommended. Reduction of immunosuppression is the most efficacious treatment but is rarely required.

Human Papillomavirus

There is a wide diversity of high levels of HPV, in particular, the epidermodysplasia verruciformis (EDV)–type HPV (HPV 5 and 8) detected in cutaneous warts, dysplastic keratoses, and squamous cell carcinomas (SCCs) in solid organ recipients. The epidemiologic data and the high prevalence of HPV DNA in premalignant and neoplastic skin lesions in OTRs may suggest an etiologic role of HPV in NMSC oncogenesis even though the exact mechanism is still unknown. Common warts present as skin colored or pink verrucous (verruca vulgaris) or flat topped (verruca plana) papules, which upon close examination characteristically disrupt the normal dermatoglyphics. As opposed to the general population, common warts appear predominantly on sun-exposed sites, tend to be more numerous or grouped, and display fewer tendencies for spontaneous regression in OTRs. More importantly, in immunocompromised patients, HPV-induced lesions have the potential for malignant transformation, particularly on sun-exposed areas (Fig. 48-5). Therefore, rapidly enlarging hyperkeratotic verrucae should be biopsied to rule out malignant transformation. HPV-induced anogenital in situ and invasive SCC is 10 times more common in transplant recipients. Screening of the anus and cervix with Pap test and lesional biopsy is warranted.

Treatment of viral warts is similar to that in general population and includes conventional ablative therapies, such as cryotherapy, topical application of 40% salicylic acid and

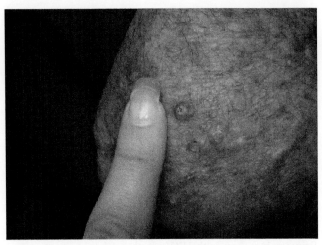

FIGURE 48-5: Multiple squamous cell carcinomas on the elbow of a renal transplant patient.

pulsed-dye laser treatment. In certain cases, intralesional injection of bleomycin may be attempted. Patients with extensive warts should be managed by reduction of sun exposure, sunscreen use, reduction of immunosuppression, and close follow-up to detect the development of malignant lesions. Therapy for condyloma acuminatum includes topical podophyllotoxin applied twice daily on 3 consecutive days per week for 4 to 5 weeks. Use of imiquimod 5% cream, a topical immune modulator, in OTR patients is still controversial. Small studies with the use of imiquimod cream in OTRs showed moderate efficacy for condyloma without deleterious effects on the transplanted organ. For genital warts, it is recommended once daily three times a week for 16 weeks. Surgical removal of the genital wart may be a first option if there are a few small warts or a large number of warts over a large area. Several other modalities are available, including local excision, laser therapy, cryotherapy, and electrosurgical excision. Recurrence is frequent and close follow-up is recommended.

Mycobacterial Diseases

Solid OTRs are at risk for mycobacterial infections because of their depressed cell-mediated immunity and the effects of chronic corticosteroid administration. *M. tuberculosis* infection occurs in approximately 1% of solid OTRs in North America and Europe. Solid OTRs are at increased risk for both primary and reactivation infection. Disseminated disease is also more common in this population than in nonimmunocompromised populations. There is a 30% mortality rate associated with *M. tuberculosis* infection in transplant recipients. *M. tuberculosis* is acquired primarily by inhalation of aerosolized droplets containing the organism. This leads to infection of the respiratory tract and occasional subsequent dissemination via the lymphatic system or bloodstream. Atypical mycobacteria comprise slow-growing organisms including *M. marinum, M. kansasii, M. avium*–intracellulare complex, and *M. ulcerans* and rapid-growing organisms including *M. fortuitum, M. chelonae,* and *M. abscessus.* The spectrum of cutaneous manifestations of *M. tuberculosis* and atypical mycobacteria is diverse and range from indurated plaques, to nodules, to ulcers, at times with purulent drainage. Similarly to the general population, infection with *M. marinum* usually occurs following exposure to fish tank water and presents with nodules on the hands and arms often with a sporotrichoid spread. Solid organ transplantation recipients should be warned of the hazards of infection from home fish tanks. Failure to respond to standard antimicrobial therapy should raise the question of infection with an unusual organism such as a nontuberculous mycobacterium. Aspiration or biopsy of lesions for histopathologic testing, staining for mycobacteria, and mycobacterial culture are essential for diagnosis. Tissue culture may be delayed up to 6 weeks due to the slow-growing nature of most mycobacterial species. Importantly, the tuberculin skin test is positive in only one quarter to one third of solid organ transplantation recipients with tuberculosis; therefore, serologic testing using the interferon-γ assay specific to *M. tuberculosis* may prove to be a better option. Treatment of mycobacterial infections is complex and depends on the infecting organism and the severity of the infection. For tuberculosis, therapeutic guidelines are similar to the general population. However, special consideration should be made regarding drug interactions between certain antimycobacterial agents, such as rifampicin and rifabutin and immunosuppressive medications that are also metabolized via cytochrome P-450 enzymes, such as cyclosporine, sirolimus, and tacrolimus. In most cases of atypical mycobacterium infections, a course of antibiotics is necessary. These include rifampicin, ethambutol, isoniazid, minocycline, ciprofloxacin, clarithromycin, azithromycin, and co-trimoxazole. Usually treatment consists of a combination of drugs. *M. marinum* species are often resistant to isoniazid. Treatment with other antibiotics should be for at least 2 months. *M. kansasii* should be treated for at least 18 months. *M. chelonae* is best treated by clarithromycin in combination with another agent. Sometimes surgical excision is the best approach.

Benign Tumors Occurring in Increased Frequency in OTRs

Verrucal keratoses present in large numbers in transplant patients as gray-white flat or hyperkeratotic papules mainly on sun-exposed sites. Consistent use of moisturizers, topical urea products, or topical retinoids may improve appearance and texture, but these lesions are often resistant to topical therapy. Liquid nitrogen may be used to treat individual bothersome lesions.

Skin Cancer in Organ Transplant Recipients

Skin cancer encompasses 42% of all post-transplant malignancies. Population-based standard incidence ratios for SCCs are increased 65- to 250-fold and for basal cell carcinomas (BCCs) 10- to 16-fold in OTRs compared with nontransplanted patients (Table 48-2). Within 20 years of transplantation, approximately 40% to 50% of white patients in most western countries and 70% to 80% of white Australians will have developed at least one nonmelanoma skin cancer (NMSC). An increased incidence of melanoma in transplant patients has been reported, but recent studies have failed to confirm these findings. Kaposi sarcoma has been reported in excess among OTRs, especially from patient

TABLE 48-2 • Population-Based Standard Incidence Ratios of Skin Cancer in Transplant Patients Compared to the General Populations

Skin Cancer	Incidence Ratio in Transplant Patients Compared to the General Population
SCC	65–250
SCC of lip	20
BCC	10–16
Melanoma	1.6–3.4
Kaposi sarcoma	84

populations in which the disease is endemic, such as patients of Mediterranean, black African, or Caribbean origin. In addition, Merkel cell carcinoma (MCC) appears to be more common in OTRs and has a high mortality rate. Lymphomas affect up to 5% of all OTRs, but purely cutaneous lymphomas are rare.

Incidence of Skin Cancer by Allograft Type

Cardiac OTRs are reported to have a higher incidence of NMSC in comparison to other OTRs, which is attributed to the significantly higher doses of immunosuppressant medications used to prevent allograft rejection in this subset of OTR patients. It has been postulated that another possible factor is that heart OTRs are generally 15 years older at transplantation than renal OTRs, and therefore are at a higher risk for skin cancer. The time interval between transplantation and development of skin cancer was found to be much shorter in heart OTRs (3.9 years) compared to the renal OTRs (8.6 years). There are few studies concerning skin cancer in liver, pancreas, or lung OTRs, but it has been suggested that the incidence of NMSC in liver OTRs is less than in heart or kidney OTRs because the level of immunosuppression is lower and the drug regimens differ from those employed for other solid OTRs.

Incidence of Skin Cancer by Age

Although older transplant patients develop more skin cancer, probably due to higher cumulative sun exposure before transplantation, younger transplant recipients have a higher risk relative to others of their same age. The reversal of SCC/BCC ratio compared to the general population was found to be even more pronounced in children than in adult OTRs (2.8:1 vs. 1.7:1).

Evaluation of OTR Patients for Risk Factors

When evaluating an OTR patient, careful history taking about risk factors for transplant-associated dermatologic problems is crucial. There are multiple well-defined risk factors for ultraviolet-induced skin cancer in the general population that are accentuated in transplant patients, including increasing age, skin type, history of extensive ultraviolet exposure, and a history of previous NMSC (Table 48-3). Additional risk factors include blue or gray eyes, a Celtic background, infection with HPV, and a low CD4 count. Cancer risk appears to be higher for heart transplant recipients who are maintained on high

TABLE 48-3 • Risk Factors for NMSC in Solid Organ Transplant Patients

	General Population	Transplant Population
Increasing age	++	++++
Fair skin, light hair, light eyes	++	++++
Sun exposure	++	++++
History of previous skin cancer	50% risk of second cancer	>70% risk of second skin cancer
Intensity and length of immunosuppression	N/A	Positive correlation

levels of immunosuppression and lower for kidney and liver transplant patients who require less immunosuppression. The duration and intensity of immunosuppression positively correlates with the risk for skin cancer and cutaneous infections. Exposure to chronic immunosuppression severely depresses specific components of host immunity including both antitumor immune surveillance and antimicrobial host defense. The link between immunosuppression and cancer formation is further evidenced by observed decrease in skin cancer formation with reduction or cessation of immunosuppressive therapy. This has prompted an expert consensus panel to recommend reductions in immunosuppressive medication for those patients with numerous or life-threatening skin cancers. Additionally, there has been recent evidence that some immunosuppressive agents, most notably azathioprine, have direct procarcinogenic effects, whereas others may have anticarcinogenic properties, as shown with sirolimus. Nevertheless, determining the relative contribution of the individual immunosuppressive drug to the development of skin cancer has been difficult to quantify.

Actinic Keratosis

Actinic keratosis (AK) (Fig. 48-6) is a partial thickness proliferation of atypical keratinocytes confined to the epidermis, with the potential to progress to invasive SCC. AKs present as pink, rough, scaly papules on sun-exposed sites, with a predilection for the bald scalp, face, ears, dorsal hands, and forearms. Diffuse AKs of the lower vermillion lip is called actinic cheilitis and presents with diffuse scaling as well as erythematous, keratotic, or non-healing erosions. Within the first 5 years of immunosuppression, about 40% of OTRs may develop AKs. Similar to the general population, fair skin and extensive sun exposure predisposes to the development of AKs. However, in transplant patients, AKs not only appear with increased frequency, but also appear earlier, in greater numbers, and progress more rapidly to invasive SCC. Because of the increased risk for malignant transformation, early and aggressive treatment of lesions is recommended.

Treatment: There are a wide variety of treatment options that need to be tailored to the patient risk factors for skin cancer, the number, and anatomic location of these lesions. For low-risk patients with a limited number of AKs, the recommended treatment is cryotherapy of the individual AKs. For best results, cryotherapy should be applied for 15 to 20 seconds with two freeze–thaw cycles. Curettage, electrosurgery, carbon dioxide laser, and surgical excision are less common treatment options. For areas with diffuse, severe actinic damage and a large number of AKs, the best approach is to perform "field therapy" with topical 5-fluorouracil (5-FU), topical diclofenac, PDT, imiquimod cream, or topical ingenol mebutate. Other modalities, including topical retinoids, ablative lasers, chemical peels, and dermabrasion, have been used to treat AKs. Most importantly, regular use of high SPF sunscreen should be recommended, as it has been shown to reduce the development of AKs and increase the rate of remission of existing AKs in transplant patients.

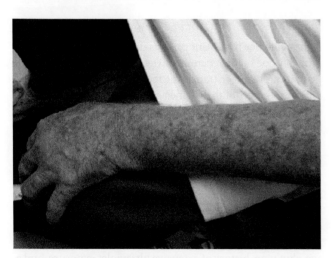

FIGURE 48-6: Multiple hyperkeratotic tumors over the extensor forearm in a renal transplant patient. Frequent observation, aggressive therapy, and biopsy when necessary are needed to control these premalignant tumors.

Basal Cell Carcinoma

BCCs are most common in the heart transplant population where they develop 15 years earlier compared to the general population. In the general population the incidence of SCC is less than that of BCC, with an SCC/BCC ratio of about 1:4. It is well recognized that the SCC/BCC ratio is reversed in transplant recipients. BCCs have a predilection for sunexposed areas and appear as erythematous, slightly scaly plaques (superficial type), pearly translucent telangiectatic papules which may ulcerate (nodular and infiltrative type), or shiny scar like plaques (morpheaform type). Most importantly, BCCs in transplant patients do not seem to display increased "aggressive" behavior. Metastasis is extremely rare. Treatment is similar to nonimmunosuppressed patients and listed in Table 48-4.

TABLE 48-4 • Treatment Options for AK, BCC, and SCC in Transplant Patients

Treatment	Actinic Keratosis	Basal Cell Carcinoma	Squamous Cell Carcinoma	Comments
Destructive				
Cryosurgery	First line of individual lesions	Only for superficial BCC	Only for in situ SCC	Lack of margin control Scarring
Electrodesiccation and curettage	Not indicated	For low-risk BCC	For low-risk SCC	Lack of margin control Scarring
Topical				
5-Fluorouracil	Individual or field treatment	For superficial BCC	Not FDA approved	Rare contact hypersensitivity Application site reaction
Imiquimod	Individual or field treatment	For superficial BCC	Not FDA approved	Potential risk of immune activation Local inflammation and irritation
Diclofenac	Individual or field treatment	Not FDA approved	Not FDA approved	Potential risk to effect renal function
Ingenol Mebutate	Field treatment	Not FDA approved	Not FDA approved	Local inflammation and irritation
Retinoids	Field treatment	Not indicated	Not indicated	Chronic irritation
Photodynamic therapy	Field treatment	For superficial BCC	Not indicated	Provider controlled
Chemical peel	Field treatment	Not indicated	Not indicated	Medium-to-deep peels needed
Excisional				
Excision with postoperative margin evaluation	Not indicated	For low-risk lesions	For low-risk lesions	4-mm margin re-excision
Mohs micrographic surgery	Not indicated	For high-risk lesion	For high-risk lesions	Needs specialized provider Removal of skin cancer with maximal tissue preservation
Systemic				
Oral retinoids	Field treatment	Chemoprevention	Chemoprevention	Retinoid side effect (Rebound)
Vismodegib	Not indicated	For metastatic or locally advanced disease	Not indicated	Has not been rigorously studied in a transplant population
Systemic chemotherapy	Not indicated	Adjuvant	Adjuvant	Significant adverse effects
Reduction of immunosuppression	Adjuvant	Adjuvant	Adjuvant	
Radiotherapy	Not indicated	Poor surgical candidates in-transit metastasis	Poor surgical candidates in-transit metastasis	Radiation dermatitis Recurrence

Vismodegib, a smoothened receptor inhibitor and Hedgehog signaling pathway targeting agent, has been approved by the FDA for the use in metastatic and locally invasive BCC; however, this drug has not been studied in the immunosuppressed population such as transplant patients. One case report of its use in a heart transplant patient on cyclosporine has been published, but only a subjective improvement in tumor burden was observed. More rigorous clinical trials should be performed to validate its efficacy and safety in OTRs.

Squamous Cell Carcinoma

SCC is the most common skin cancer in the organ transplant population and may have a somewhat different presentation and clinical course compared to the general population. SCCs tend to occur in a younger age, typically first appearing 3 to 8 years after transplantation. They may develop in large numbers and follow an aggressive clinical course, resulting in significant morbidity and mortality. Approximately 6% to 9% of SCCs metastasize, most often during the 2 years after excision, with a 50% 3-year disease-specific survival in those patients with metastasis. SCCs in OTRs most frequently occur in chronically sun-damaged areas and often present as red, pink scaly, hyperkeratotic papules and plaques within a field of diffuse keratotic lesions that may include verrucae, verrucal keratoses, porokeratoses, and AKs, making it difficult to distinguish clinical borders. The most common locations for SCC in OTRs include the scalp, face, ears, neck, dorsal forearms, and hands. The history of a chronic, nonhealing lesion, which may be painful or bleeding, aids the diagnosis. Physical examination should include careful examination of the surrounding skin, assessment of the fixed nature of the lesion, facial nerve examination (for facial lesions), and palpation of regional lymph nodes to evaluate for invasive tumor and metastasis. It is important to identify clinical features of high-risk tumors (Table 48-5) because these lesions have an aggressive clinical course and may require a cooperative management by dermatologists and transplant physicians, as well as surgical, medical, and radiation oncologists. In situ SCC and low-risk SCC are managed similarly to that in general population, while high-risk SCCs need excision with intraoperative margin evaluation by Mohs micrographic surgery with or without reduction of immunosuppression and chemoprevention with oral retinoids (see Table 48-4). If a tumor shows high-grade atypia or a pattern of perineural invasion, postoperative adjuvant radiation therapy may be indicated. Sentinel lymph node biopsy may provide some aid in evaluation and management, but there are no studies demonstrating survival benefit. Patients with high-risk tumors are usually subjected to preoperative staging examination with PET/CT. Chemoprevention with oral retinoids (acitretin and isotretinoin); nicotinamide and capecitabine have been shown to reduce the incidence of precancerous and SCC lesions while on therapy.

Malignant Melanoma

Malignant melanoma (MM) is the most aggressive skin tumor and commonly presents as an atypical pigmented lesion. The incidence of MM in transplant patients compared to the general population is debated. Prior studies have shown variable rates ranging from no increase to an eightfold increase in incidence. Risk factors for development of MM are similar to the general population and include those with fair skin, red or blonde hair, blue eyes, history of sunburns, atypical nevi, numerous nevi, and a personal or family history of MM. MM in transplant patients appears most commonly on the trunk, followed by the upper arms. Transplant recipients with a history of MM before transplantation may have a high incidence of recurrence after transplantation. In addition, MM is one of the most common donor-transmitted cancers in OTRs. Current treatment recommendations are based on the guidelines established for the general population; in addition, a decrease in the level of immunosuppression should be attempted in collaboration with the transplant team.

Other Malignant Skin Tumors in OTRs

Merkel Cell Carcinoma

MCC is a rare neuroendocrine tumor with very high mortality rate and greater than 10-fold increased incidence rate in organ transplant patients. Clinically, these lesions appear as rapidly growing, firm, red-to-violaceous nodules with a shiny surface and overlying telangiectasia. Distribution is similar among OTRs and the general population and includes the head and neck, followed by the upper extremities and the trunk. Five-year disease-specific survival in transplant patients is reported to be 46%. Management is similar to that of general population and includes excision, with or without sentinel node mapping, followed by radiotherapy or chemotherapy if needed.

Other rare cutaneous neoplasms reported in OTRs include atypical fibroxanthoma, malignant fibrous histiocytoma, leiomyosarcoma, sebaceous carcinoma, microcystic adnexal carcinoma, angiosarcoma, and dermatofibrosarcoma protuberans. None of these have been reported to occur with significantly increased frequency in OTRs.

Chemoprophylaxis

The prevention of NMSCs in OTRs has been described with previously approved medications. Oral retinoids (acitretin and isotretinoin) have been shown to decrease the number

---

TABLE 48-5 • Characteristics of High-Risk SCCs

- Rapid growth or recurrence
- Ulceration
- Location: forehead, temple, ear, nose, lip, mid face, genitalia
- Large size
  - >1.0 cm cheeks, forehead, neck, and scalp
  - >0.6 cm other areas of face
  - >2.0 cm trunk and extremities
- Poor differentiation
- Deep invasion (fat, muscle, cartilage, bone)
- Perineural/neural invasion

of new NMSCs in several small studies; however, these medications are associated with serious adverse effects including hepatotoxicity, teratogenicity, and hyperlipidemia and are not always well tolerated due to excessive dry skin. Capecitabine, a precursor to 5-FU, is used for the treatment of metastatic breast and colon cancer. Reductions in NMSCs have been reported sparingly but consistently with the use of low-dose capecitabine (500 to 1,500 mg/m^2 twice daily on days 1 to 14 in a 21-day cycle). While prevention numbers look attractive, with nearly a 70% reduction in SCCs per month in those receiving treatment up to 1 year, many patients experience significant adverse events, including: fatigue, gout, palmar-plantar erythrodysesthesia, gastrointestinal distress and reduced renal function. Another molecule shown to have protective effects against NMSCs in OTRs is nicotinamide (vitamin B$_3$). A phase 3, double-blind, randomized, controlled trial reported the use of 500 mg twice daily nicotinamide significantly decreased the development of new NMSCs by 23% compared to placebo. Of note this difference was largely attributed to new SCCs (30% lower rate), and as expected the number of AKs were also reduced (20% lower at 9 months). For high-risk patients such as OTRs these agents are a strategy for the prevention of NMSCs even though the chemoprevention is not sustained after they are discontinued.

Education and Management of OTRs

It is imperative to repetitively educate patients about the importance of sun protection, which should include the use of sunscreen with SPF greater than 30, avoidance of direct sun exposure in the midday, and sun protective clothing. The goal of education and preventive treatments is to decrease future skin cancer formation. Early recognition and treatment of skin cancers is important in this population. The patients should be risk stratified and undergo regular surveillance with a frequency based on their skin cancer risk (Table 48-6). Furthermore, adjustment of a patient's immunosuppressive regimen may be considered in certain cases. It has been shown that renal transplant patients placed on sirolimus develop significantly fewer NMSCs (in addition to reduced overall malignancies) as compared to other standard immunosuppressive regimens. Conversion to an mTOR inhibitor may be in the best interest of a patient who develops numerous skin cancers, but can be limited by impaired graft function or other systemic complications. A multidisciplinary approach involving the transplant team and oncologist in caring for patients with life-threatening skin cancers is highly recommended.

TABLE 48-6 • Recommended Follow-Up Intervals for Organ Transplant Patients

Clinical Exam and History	Follow-Up Intervals (Months)
No history of skin cancer, no risk factors	12–24
No history of skin cancer, positive risk factors	6–12
Actinic keratosis or viral warts	3–6
One BCC or SCC	3–6
Multiple NMSC	3
High-risk SCC	3
Metastatic SCC	1–3

Suggested Readings

Ablashi DV, Chatlynne LG, Whitman JE Jr, et al. Spectrum of Kaposi's sarcoma-associated herpesvirus, or human herpesvirus 8, diseases. *Clin Microbiol Rev.* 2002;15:439–464.

Berg D, Otley CC. Skin cancer in organ transplant recipients: epidemiology, pathogenesis, and management. *J Am Acad Dermatol.* 2002;47(1):1–17; quiz 18–20.

Dantal J, Soulillou JP. Immunosuppressive drugs and the risk of cancer after organ transplantation. *N Engl J Med.* 2005;352(13):1371–1373.

Euvrard S, Kanitakis J, Claudy A. Skin cancers after organ transplantation. *N Engl J Med.* 2003;348(17):1681–1691.

Fishman JA. Infection in solid-organ transplant recipients. *N Engl J Med.* 2007;357(25):2601–2614.

Harwood CA, McGregor JM, Swale VJ, et al. High frequency and diversity of cutaneous appendageal tumors in organ transplant recipients. *J Am Acad Dermatol.* 2003;48(3):401–408.

Harwood CA, Proby CM. McGregor JM, et al. Clinicopathologic features of skin cancer in organ transplant recipients: a retrospective case-control series. *J Am Acad Dermatol.* 2006;54(2):290–300.

Nindl I, Gottschling M, Stockfleth E. Human papillomaviruses and non-melanoma skin cancer: basic virology and clinical manifestations. *Dis Markers.* 2007;23(4):247–259.

Neuburg M. Transplant-associated skin cancer: role of reducing immunosuppression. *J Natl Compr Canc Netw.* 2007;5(5):541–549.

Otley CC, Berg D, Ulrich C, et al. Reduction of immunosuppression for transplant-associated skin cancer: expert consensus survey. *Br J Dermatol.* 2006;154(3):395–400.

Otley CC, Stasko T. *Skin Disease in Organ Transplantation.* New York: Cambridge University Press; 2008.

Snydman DR. Infection in solid organ transplantation. *Transpl Infect Dis.* 1999;1(1):21–28.

Stasko T, Brown MD, Carucci JA, et al. Guidelines for the management of squamous cell carcinoma in organ transplant recipients. *Dermatol Surg.* 2004;30(4, pt 2):642–650.

Stockfleth E, Ulrich C, Meyer T, et al. Epithelial malignancies in organ transplant patients: clinical presentation and new methods of treatment. *Recent Results Cancer Res.* 2002;160:251–258.

49

Cutaneous Manifestations of Child Abuse

Lawrence A. Schachner, MD, Kate E. Oberlin, MD,
Andrew M. Margileth, MD, and Walter F. Lambert, MD

The pediatric patient may pose a unique challenge in the dermatologic arena given the lack of ability to personally describe the temporal nature of their lesions and the exacerbating or ameliorating factors associated with their lesions. Observation and history-taking skills from the family are crucial in examining the skin lesions of young children. Inconsistencies in stories of presentation or a description that places the child performing an act above their expected motor or cognitive function should be alarming red flags for physicians. Recognition of particular patterns of abuse is necessary for both the primary physician and dermatologist given that the majority of child abuse occurs in toddler-aged children, too young to report details. Even in older pediatric patients, fear and anxiety may make a history very challenging, and visual cues for foul play are imperative not to miss. Child abuse can be classified into the following divisions for ease of diagnosis and management:

- Physical abuse
- Burn injuries
- Chemical injuries
- Sexual abuse

This chapter will explore each division, as well as various disease mimickers of each presentation, so that a valid and timely diagnosis can be constructed.

PHYSICAL ABUSE

> ### SAUER'S NOTES
>
> Physical abuse of the pediatric patient presents in a vast array of manifestations. One must be cognizant of certain distribution patterns, history inconsistencies, and systemic signs that can point to the vital diagnosis of child abuse.

Presentation and Characteristics

Primary Lesions

The cutaneous lesions of physical abuse due to brute force can manifest in unique presentations. Peculiar bruises in different stages of evolution, linear or circumferential lacerations secondary to exogenous tools, bite marks with spacing of the teeth analogous to an adult's anatomy, and hematomas can be highly specific and suggestive of child abuse (Fig. 49-1). Unusual or geometric morphology of lesions not otherwise explained by a common pediatric dermatological diagnosis should raise suspicion for abuse. The specific color of the lesions may help delineate the timeline of the act and lead to an incongruous historical presentation. Characteristic thumb and fingerprint impressions, particularly around the ears, buttocks, and outer thighs, are highly indicative of aggressive or foul play. In comparison, normal bruising in a pediatric patient typically presents on the forehead, chin, and distal anterior lower extremities as toddlers are first learning to walk.

Secondary Lesions

Erosions and crusting can ensue from repetitive trauma due to physical forces and the specific objects inflicting trauma.

Course

Care must be undertaken for a thorough evaluation of a pediatric patient suspected of residing in an abusive environment. A meticulous physical examination with detailed photography should be documented. A complete dermatological evaluation of the entire body, including mucous membrane and genital skin, should be performed. Weight should be recorded to investigate concomitant indications of neglect. If there are signs of possible head injury or impaired consciousness, an ophthalmologic examination should be pursued to evaluate for retinal hemorrhages, which are highly suggestive of abusive head trauma and subdural hematomas. Social work and Child Protective Services must be notified in a timely manner to ensure patient safety.

Causes

Physical abuse includes any form of contact between the adult and child in a forceful, inappropriate, and harmful manner. Belts, shoes, ropes, and other accessory objects may be involved in inflicting harm to the child.

Laboratory Findings

Systemic investigation may be warranted to rule other visceral organ involvement. Retinal hemorrhage, rib fractures, and ruptured internal viscera can ensue from aggressive force.

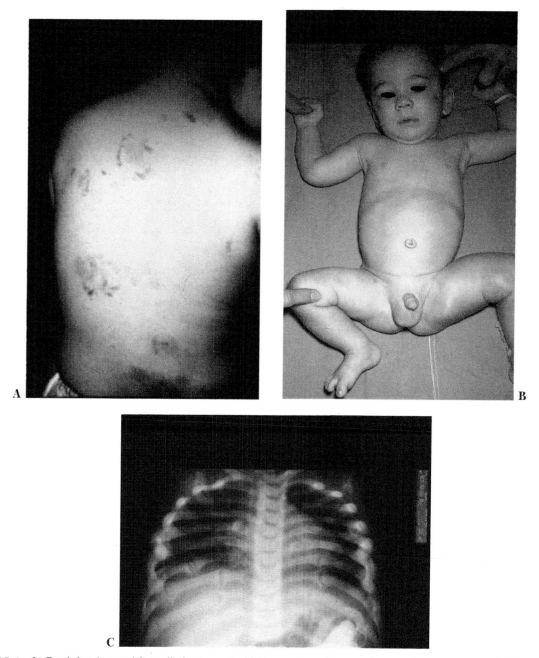

FIGURE 49-1: **A:** Back bruises with well-demarcated bite marks with spacing analogous to an adult bite. **B:** An irritable 5-month-old presenting with a vague history for scattered ecchymoses and abrasions resulting from nonaccidental trauma. **C:** CXR from the 5-month-old patient demonstrating 14 rib fractures.

A head CT, CXR, abdominal ultrasound, or KUB may be necessary based on the location of the bruises or cutaneous lesions. The physical examination should provide clues to the mechanism of injury and help guide the necessary imaging.

Differential Diagnosis

- *Cultural therapies*: A number of cultural therapies can additionally mimic signs of physical abuse and, likewise, will display unique geometric configurations. A listing of the more commonly recognized cultural therapies are displayed in Table 49-1 (also see Fig. 49-2).

- *Mongolian spots*: Dermal melanosis that can mimic bruises; more common in darker-skinned patients.

- *Bleeding disorder*: Hemophilia can lead to spontaneous hemarthroses or increased susceptibility to bruising with minor trauma; associated with a positive family history of a bleeding diathesis.

- *Vasculitis*: Henoch–Schönlein purpura involves inflammation of the small blood vessels, which can be confused with widespread bruising of the buttocks and lower extremities. The kidney and gastrointestinal tract may additionally be involved.

TABLE 49-1 • Cultural Therapies Mimicking Physical Child Abuse	
Coining or "Cao gio" (Fig. 49-4)	More common in SE Asia; thought to rid the body of maladies by bringing blood to the surface. A coin is vigorously rubbed in a downward, linear fashion against the back until bruising is elicited. Resulting linear postinflammatory hyperpigmentation ensues across the affected areas.
Spooning	Chinese and Vietnamese cultures; analogous to cupping; however, a spoon is used and repeated pressurized strokes against the back are performed.
Cupping	More common in Asian cultures; utilized to reduce ailments. A cup is coated with alcohol, placed upside down, and suction is created via open flame or a lit match. The cup is then placed against the skin creating a vacuum.
Moxibustion	Chinese culture; used to alleviate pain. Moxa herbs are either rolled and burned directly onto the skin or burned in conjunction with an acupuncture needle, which is placed onto the skin.

- *Erythema multiforme:* Widespread erythematous macules can be confused as diffuse bruising and foul play; secondary to drugs or infection.
- *Acute hemorrhagic edema of infancy:* Purpuric macules or edematous plaques involving the face and extremities that can be misdiagnosed as bruises; self-limiting cutaneous vasculitis.

Treatment

Documentation is imperative. If a human bite is involved in physical abuse, the patient may need antibiotic therapy. Wound care is necessary to prevent scarring of deep lacerations. Child psychiatry may be warranted for older children to avoid and minimize long-term mental incapacities from such trauma. Child Protective Services and social workers will help guide the necessary exit strategy for the patient.

BURN INJURIES

Burn injuries can be due to a vast number of exogenous sources. Most commonly, burns are secondary to immersion injuries into scalding water, cigarette burns, or burns from electrical or radiation sources.

Presentation and Characteristics

Primary Lesions

Abuse due to burns must be carefully examined because both accidental and nonaccidental injuries can lead to acute vesicles and bullae with surrounding edema on the face and extremities. Immersion lesions are normally symmetric and well demarcated with a sharp cutoff line between involved and uninvolved adjacent skin (Fig. 49-3). Cigarette burns will display a typical punched out, circular red to purple configuration. A geometric configuration will be displayed with the characteristic shape of a heated metal object or appliance.

Secondary Lesions

The lesions may develop secondary erosions or ulceration; yellow–brown crust may be present over actively healing lesions.

Course

Documentation with a body diagram outlining the cutaneous involvement is again, imperative. A detailed history will help to clarify the difference between an accidental and intentional injury. Depending on the depth of cutaneous involvement, ulcerations may heal with postinflammatory hyperpigmentation and scarring.

Causes

The pattern of blistering can help decipher the nature of the injury. Suspected immersion injuries into a bathtub will characteristically display a lack of distant skin involvement

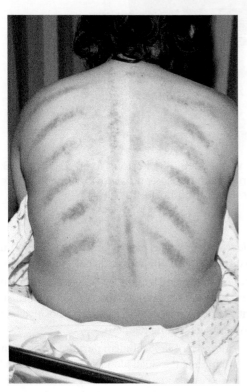

FIGURE 49-2: Coin rubbing (Cao gio) in a patient with pneumonia.

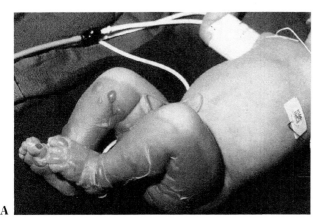

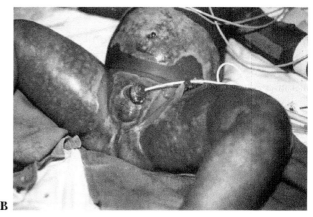

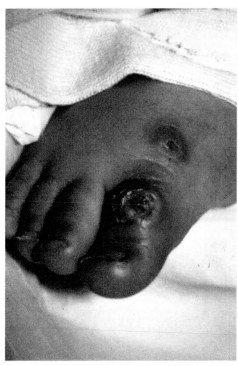

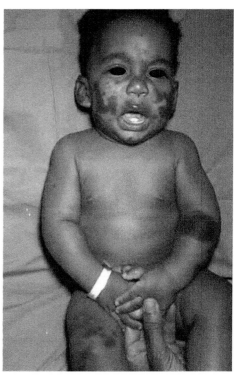

FIGURE 49-3: **A:** Forced immersion burn in an infant involving the bilateral lower extremities with a well-demarcated line of uninvolved adjacent skin. **B:** Forced immersion highlighting the crescents of normal skin on lower abdomen where the infants' thighs are drawn up to protect the skin from hot water. **C:** Infant with new and old (healed) cigarette burns resulting in scars on the foot. **D:** Presentation of acute hemorrhagic edema of infancy, which can mimic purpuric lesions of child abuse.

related to the absence of splash marks; distant involvement would otherwise suggest the child had the ability to recoil from the painful stimulus and was not being forcefully submerged. Additional manifestations of child abuse including purpuric ecchymoses secondary to physical abuse may coexist and help elucidate the diagnosis.

Laboratory Findings

No specific laboratory investigation is necessary in the scenario of most limited burn injuries. However, if a vast area of body surface is involved, the child may need fluids and should be monitored for electrolyte abnormalities as well as a predisposition to acquiring a secondary infection. Vitals should be documented with the physical examination to assess for stability.

Differential Diagnosis

- *Chronic bullous disease of childhood:* Blistering neutrophilic disorder presenting with annular and grouped bullae over the extensor surfaces and groin. A punch biopsy will help confirm the diagnosis showing subepidermal bullae with neutrophils.
- *Bullous impetigo:* Contagious skin infection common in children resulting in flaccid bullae or characteristic golden crust; common in periorificial regions.
- *Epidermolysis bullosa simplex:* Hereditary bullous disease with varied presentations involving both limited and widespread bullae with and without scarring. At sites easily traumatized such as hands, feet, and extensor extremities.

Treatment

In addition to removing the child from the abusive home and reporting the incident, local wound care is mandatory to facilitate proper healing, prevent infection, and minimize disfiguring scars. Admission may be necessary to stabilize the pediatric patient.

CHEMICAL INJURIES

Presentation and Characteristics

Primary Lesions

Caustic injuries due to chemicals can be categorized into acidic and alkaline sources. The lesions consist of well-demarcated linear or geometric superficial erosions, vesicles, or bullae. In comparison to intentional injury, an accidental chemical injury can display adjacent linear or grouped bullae as the hot fluid has fallen off the extremities (Fig. 49-4).

Secondary Lesions

Erosions and fissures can coexist with primary lesions based on the extent and depth of involvement.

Course

Once the chemical has been thoroughly removed with irrigation as applicable, the lesions will have the opportunity to heal with possible ensuing scarring.

Causes

Common causes of household acidic substances include acetic acid found in vinegar, sulfuric acid found in cleaning products and car batteries, and sulfurous acid from bleach products. Alkaline etiologies can include ammonia or lye from cleaning products. Overall, acidic substances are usually less harmful; however, if abuse is suspected, no injury should be overlooked.

Laboratory Findings

For limited cutaneous involvement, laboratory evaluation may be unnecessary. However, it is imperative to examine the mucosa of the pediatric patient to rule out accidental or nonaccidental ingestion as well as conjunctival involvement if a fluid source is suspected. If confirmed, an upper gastrointestinal scope or ophthalmology examination, respectively, may be warranted to assess involvement.

Differential Diagnosis

- *Phytophotodermatitis:* Cutaneous reaction provoked by contact with certain plants and fruits containing psoralens followed by sun exposure.
- *Contact dermatitis:* Allergic or irritant dermatitis caused shortly after contact with the inciting material; usually in a linear or geometric presentation that outlines the site of contact.
- *Herpes virus infection:* Common viral infection that can similarly manifest with grouped vesicles.

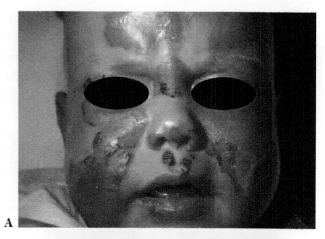

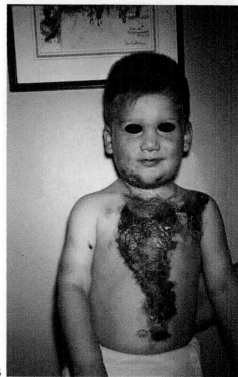

FIGURE 49-4: **A:** Traumatic nonaccidental chemical burn with resulting edema and erosions of the face. **B:** Accidental coffee burn in a linear distribution on the chest of a pediatric patient.

- *Incontinentia pigmenti:* Rare genodermatosis characterized by stages of linear vesicular and verrucous lesions with resulting dyspigmentation.

Treatment

Poison control is an accommodating resource for providing supplementary information and treatment guidelines based on the specific chemical involved. The timing of the incident as well as a history of whether or not irrigation was utilized is a critical point to discuss. Minimizing permanent long-term disabling side effects from the injury is the mainstay of therapy.

SEXUAL ABUSE

Presentation and Characteristics

Primary Lesions

The cutaneous manifestations of sexual abuse are numerous and can be due to physical forces alone or due to concomitant transmission of sexually transmitted diseases. Ecchymoses, lacerations, and erythematous macules in the genital or anal area are indicative of physical trauma and may be accompanied by distant cutaneous involvement as well. Grouped erythematous vesicles are characteristic of transmission of herpes simplex virus (Fig. 49-5A). Skin-colored papules can be a manifestation of genital warts, or condyloma acuminatum from the human papilloma virus. Primary syphilis can present with a painless ulcer, whereas secondary syphilis can present with palmoplantar macules and papules in addition to skin-colored wartlike papules of condyloma lata (Fig. 49-5B).

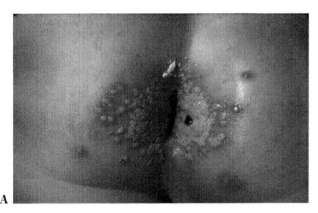

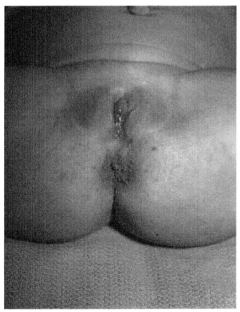

FIGURE 49-5: **A:** Perianal pink to skin-colored vesicles indicative of HSV. **B:** Characteristic skin-colored papules of condyloma acuminatum in the genital area.

Secondary Lesions

Lesions may be in various stages of evolution with scarring, fissuring, and erosions owing to repetitive trauma.

Course

> **SAUER'S NOTES**
>
> Trained personnel are necessary to identify the cutaneous manifestations and to remove the child from the perpetrator. Child psychiatry and/or psychology is a valuable resource for both younger and older pediatric patients to help cope with the incident and necessary environmental changes.

Causes

Lesions may result from physical trauma or sexually transmitted diseases. The most commonly transmitted diseases include herpes simplex virus, warts owing to human papilloma virus, bacterial infection owing to chlamydia or gonorrhea, syphilis, and HIV.

Laboratory Findings

A thorough workup is mandatory to rule out disease transmission and investigate the probability of suspected abuse. Specialized teams for this precise evaluation are becoming universal in emergency department settings. Urinary analysis with polymerase chain reaction testing for gonorrhea and chlamydia should be performed, including serologic testing for HSV, HIV, and syphilis.

Differential Diagnosis

- *Lichen sclerosus:* Autoimmune disorder affecting the genitals; presents as pruritic white to pink plaques in the vulvar and perianal area.
- *Crohn disease:* Can manifest as erythematous plaques of the buttocks or with labial or scrotal swelling and erythema in children.
- *Genital lichen planus:* May present on glans penis or as vulvar erosions that coexist with oral lesions.
- *Morphea:* Autoimmune disorder with ivory alopecic patches with a lilac-colored edge; more common in females.
- *Vulvar eczema:* Inflammatory skin condition causing dry or itchy skin that can be associated with underlying atopic dermatitis.
- *Perianal strep:* Perianal, painful erythema that is well demarcated.

Treatment

After a documented thorough examination and workup, treatment of sexually transmitted disease with the appropriate antibiotic or HAART therapy for prophylaxis, if indicated, is implemented.

Suggested Readings

Carlsen, K, Weismann, K. Phytophotodermatitis in 19 children admitted to hospital and their differential diagnoses: child abuse and herpes simplex virus infection. *J Am Acad Dermatol*. 2007;57:S88–S91.

Ciarallo L, Paller AS. Two cases of incontinentia pigmenti simulating child abuse. *Pediatrics*. 1997:100:e6.

Ellerstein NS. The cutaneous manifestations of child abuse and neglect. *Am J Dis Child*. 1979;133:906–909.

Findlay, J, Mudd S. The cutaneous manifestations and common mimickers of physical child abuse. *J Pediatr Health Care*. 2004;18:123–129.

Kos L, Shwayder T. Cutaneous manifestations of child abuse. *Ped Derm*. 2006;23:311–320.

Ravanfar P, Dinulos JG. Cultural practices affecting the skin of children. *Curr Opin Pediatr*. 2010;22:423–431.

Saulsbury FT, Hayden GF. Skin conditions simulating child abuse. *Pediatr Emerg Care*. 1985;1:147–150.

Tsokos M. Diagnostic criteria for cutaneous injuries in child abuse: classification, findings and interpretiation. *Forensic Sci Med Pathol*. 2015;11:235–242.

50

Tropical Diseases of the Skin

Francisco G. Bravo, MD and Salim Mohanna, MD

A chapter on tropical diseases is essential in this era of globalization. By tropical diseases, one may think of diseases limited to the tropical and subtropical areas of the world. The term actually implies the study of infectious diseases endemic to specific areas of the world, not always located in the tropics (i.e., human T-cell lymphotropic virus [HTLV]-1 in Japan). Previously a domain of European doctors traveling to colonies in the 19th century, tropical disease now has implications for every specialty in medicine, including, of course, dermatology. Traveling, either for tourist, business, or military purposes or just as immigrants in search of a better future for their families, has expanded the limits of places that the diseases discussed in this chapter can be seen. Let us keep an open mind and not forget to ask where the patient was born and where he or she is coming from.

VIRAL DISEASES

HTLV-1

The HTLV-1 is a retrovirus of the subfamily Oncovirinae, with the ability to infect CD4 cells and induce different degrees of immunosuppression. An estimated 10 to 20 million people are infected with the virus worldwide. There are multiple endemic areas in the world, in Africa (Gabon, Zaire, Ivory Coast), Asia (Japan, Iran), and Australia (the aborigines group). In the American continent, its presence is well established in Caribbean countries such as Jamaica, Trinidad, Barbados, and Haiti. In South America, countries affected include Brazil, Colombia, and Peru. In the United States, Canada, and Europe, the incidence of seroprevalence is low, but when one looks at specific migratory populations, the number can increase exponentially.

The infection propagated to the Americas from three different sources: early migration of Mongoloid population to the American continent in ancient times, the trade of African slaves in the 19th century, and migration of the Japanese as a labor force in the 19th and 20th centuries.

Presentation and Characteristics

The most common routes of transmission are breastfeeding, sexual contact, and blood transfusions. As opposed to HIV infection (the other well-known retrovirus), most HTLV-1–infected patients will remain asymptomatic for the rest of their lives, and no more than 10% will develop some clinical manifestations, either inflammatory or neoplastic.

HTLV-1 infection can induce disease due to an altered immune system (infective dermatitis, crusted scabies, and disseminated dermatophyte infections), autoimmunity (tropical spastic paraparesis, uveitis), and neoplasia (adult T-cell leukemia/lymphoma or ATLL). Most dermatologists may have heard of HTLV-1-related cutaneous T-cell lymphomas, but, in fact, cutaneous disease due to immune dysfunction may be more common in endemic areas of the world.

- Infective dermatitis was first described in Jamaican children in 1966. Louis La Grenade described its relation to HTLV-1 infection in 1990. The clinical picture is that of a chronic, eczematous dermatitis affecting the scalp and intertriginous areas, such as the neck folds, axillae, and groin (Fig. 50-1). On the face, it may follow a seborrheic dermatitis–like distribution. The main affected population are children, although the disease also occurs in adults. An important component is the constant degree of superinfection by *Staphylococcus aureus* and *β*-hemolytic *Streptococcus*. This condition can be described as an "oozing, honey-crusted seborrheic dermatitis or intertrigo," as an "always impetiginized scalp psoriasis," or as "atopic dermatitis with predominant scalp involvement." This is, in fact, a viral-induced dermatitis that, in many ways, resembles atopic dermatitis. Most patients with infective dermatitis clear temporarily when they receive antibiotic

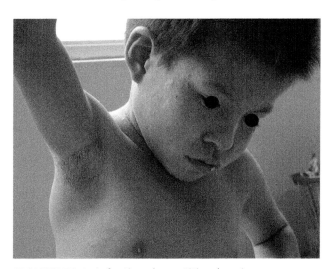

FIGURE 50-1: Infective dermatitis, showing an eczematous rash involving the face and axillae.

therapy, but the disease promptly recurs when the treatment is discontinued, adopting a chronic, recurrent course. Many affected children will go into remission when reaching puberty, in a way similar to atopic patients; adult patients have a more persistent disease. Some authors consider infective dermatitis a marker for a higher risk of developing ATLL.

■ Crusted scabies have been described in populations that are known to be endemic for HTLV-1, such as Australian aborigines. Also, in places with high prevalence, like in the Peruvian population, most cases are related to the retrovirus infection, even more commonly than immunosuppression secondary to HIV infection or chronic steroid therapy.

■ Pruritus, xerosis, and ichthyosis are considered by some researchers as the most common HTLV-1 manifestations, although they are not very specific.

■ ATLL was described and linked to HTLV-1 in the Japanese population in 1977 and is actually seen in all endemic areas. Between 25% and 40% of cases will have some sort of cutaneous involvement. Four subtypes have now been recognized including acute leukemia, chronic leukemia, lymphoma, and a smoldering subtype; a purely cutaneous tumoral form, with a worse prognosis than the smoldering type has been proposed by some authors. The skin lesions may vary: A number of cases will be indistinguishable from mycosis fungoides, whereas others will present with a more varied morphology including papules, nodules, tumors, and even erythroderma and ichthyosiform eruptions.

Dengue

Presentation and Characteristics

Dengue, or breakbone fever, is one of the most prevalent viral diseases in the world, causing a systemic illness expressed as an acute febrile disease with arthropathy, hemorrhagic fever, and neurologic involvement. The etiologic agent is an RNA flavivirus, with four described serotypes. It is present around the world (100 million cases per year), in tropical and subtropical areas of Africa and Asia, and it is also becoming an increasing public health problem for some countries in South and Central America.

The disease is transmitted by the bite of mosquitoes belonging to the genus *Aedes*, mainly *A. aegypti*, which is also a carrier of yellow fever, and Zika virus. Dengue is present most commonly in urban areas with poor sanitary systems. The mosquitoes thrive whenever they find open water reservoirs. *Aedes* is also the main living reservoir for the virus.

The disease may adopt various clinical forms, from mild to classic to a more severe and dangerous hemorrhagic form, the so-called dengue hemorrhagic fever (DHF). Although the classical form is more common in new arrivals to endemic areas, the more severe DHF is more likely to affect children, residents of endemic areas, and those who have already had dengue in the past.

Clinical Appearance

The classical form starts as a sudden fever, lasting 2 to 5 days, and is associated with headache, intense myalgias and arthralgia, and retro-orbital pain. Cutaneous involvement varies, from facial flushing to a more diffuse macular or maculopapular morbilliform eruption. The erythematous areas become confluent, leaving small spared areas of normal skin, similar in a way to that seen in pityriasis rubra pilaris, although lacking its roughness; this image is described as "white islands on a red sea" (Fig. 50-2). The main area of involvement is the trunk, with the eruption spreading centrifugally toward the extremities. Petechial eruptions affecting the lower extremities may also be seen. Pruritus may be present, and a later state of desquamation may follow.

DHF presents with a more severe course, including vomiting, facial flushing, perioral cyanosis, and weakness with cool and clammy extremities. Hemorrhagic complications, such as gastrointestinal (GI) and genital bleeding, appear, and the patient may go into a dengue shock syndrome. This state may have a mortality rate as high as 10% if not given the appropriate support. A very similar eruption is seen in Zika virus infections.

Hemorrhagic Fevers

These febrile diseases result from infection by viruses from various viral families: Arenaviridae, Bunyaviridae, Filoviridae, and Flaviviridae. Not all viruses in these families cause hemorrhagic fever. These viruses have a higher occurrence in tropical areas, such as South America, Africa, and the Pacific Islands. Clinical manifestations of hemorrhagic fever include capillary permeability, leukopenia, and thrombocytopenia. Hemorrhagic fever manifest clinically as a sudden onset of fever, headache, generalized myalgia, backache, petechiae, conjunctivitis, and severe prostration. Intensive supportive care is necessary when dealing with most hemorrhagic fevers.

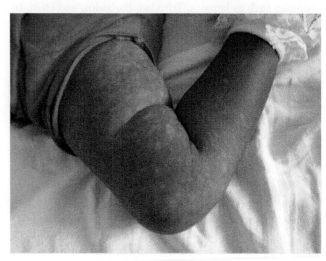

FIGURE 50-2: Dengue rash in a baby: "white islands in a red sea."

BACTERIAL INFECTIONS

Anthrax

Anthrax is an infection caused by *Bacillus anthracis*, an encapsulated gram-positive bacterium capable of surviving up to 20 years in dry grass. The disease is more common in people working or having contact with cattle. The infection is acquired either by contact through the skin or by inhalation of spores while slaughtering sick animals. The cutaneous lesion, called "malignant pustule," is usually located in exposed areas of the skin, especially the face, neck, arms, or hands and is usually solitary. A papule grows 1 to 5 days after the inoculation. A blister then forms on an edematous base that eventually breaks, leaving a hemorrhagic crust. Redness and edema may be very marked (Fig. 50-3). General symptoms appear on the third or fourth day; the condition may result in severe toxicity and even lead to death. When the spores are inhaled, the clinical presentation will be of an acute pneumonia that carries a high mortality rate.

Treatment

Treatment options include penicillin, doxycycline, and quinolones.

Diseases Caused by Bartonellas

Carrion Disease

Until the AIDS era, bartonellosis was one of those exotic diseases only studied for board examinations. The first description of *Carrion disease* can be dated back to the late 19th century; the disease was reported in very specific areas of the Peruvian Andes; the causal agent was identified as *Bartonella bacilliformis*. The bacterium, a gram-negative rod, is transmitted from the natural reservoirs to humans by the bite of mosquitoes belonging to the genus *Lutzomyia* (the same vector of leishmaniasis).

Presentation and Characteristics: The disease has two characteristic phases, one systemic and another purely cutaneous. The first phase, known as **Oroya fever**, produces an impressive bacteremia and parasitism of the reticuloendothelial system, in which microorganisms may be seen inside red blood cells on peripheral smears. The clinical picture is a systemic disease with fever, malaise, profound paleness, and a high susceptibility to other infections, such as salmonellosis or toxoplasmosis.

The most distinct and relevant phase for the dermatologist is the eruptive phase, known as **verruga peruana**. It may follow the bacteremia, or it may present de novo. Characteristically, an eruption of multiple papules, nodules, and tumors appears over a period of weeks. The more superficial lesions have an angiomatous appearance, resembling pyogenic granulomas (Fig. 50-4). The natural course of the disease is toward spontaneous involution, although antibiotic treatment may induce a more prompt remission.

Treatment: Oroya fever can be treated with ciprofloxacin or chloramphenicol. The chronic eruptive phase, that is, the true verruga peruana, can be effectively treated with rifampicin or azithromycin.

Bacillary Angiomatosis

At the beginning of the 1980s, some patients with AIDS presented with a clinical picture very similar to the eruptive phase of **verruga peruana**. This new disease was then named *bacillary angiomatosis* (BA). The histologic descriptions of the eruptive lesions of BA were identical to those described in verruga peruana, which was the only bartonellosis known at the time. The initial thought was to associate this new entity with cat-scratch disease. At a later time, isolation of

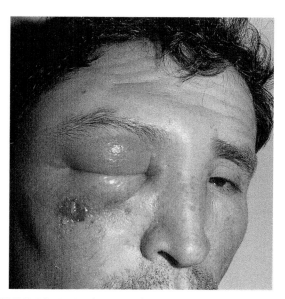

FIGURE 50-3: Anthrax, 48 hours after infection.

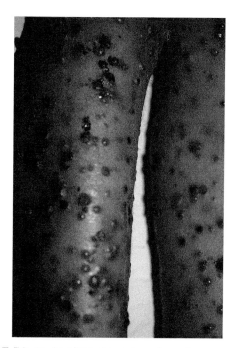

FIGURE 50-4: Angiomatous papules of verruga peruana.

a gram-negative rod from the lesions led to classifying it under a new genus of bacteria called *Rochalimaea*. Genetic studies demonstrated a close relation between Rochalimaeas and Bartonellas, resulting in a new grouping under the term *Bartonella*. The new species include *B. henselae*, *B. quintana* (both cause BA), and *B. elizabethae*, which causes septicemia and endocarditis in alcoholics. *B. henselae* is also the main cause of cat-scratch fever. *B. quintana* is now recognized as the cause of trench fever.

BA is currently recognized as a disease characteristic of immunosuppressed patients of all kinds, although it has been reported in immunocompetent patients. The most likely natural reservoir of bartonellas worldwide are domestic animals such as cats. BA is a cosmopolitan disease, as opposed to verruga peruana, which is still endemic and restricted to specific Andean areas of Peru and Ecuador.

The disease clinically is characterized by the appearance of one to several papules, nodules, and tumors that look vascular in nature; the lesions can extend to soft tissues. *B. henselae* is also capable of inducing the formation of large vascular spaces in the liver parenchyma, a change known as peliosis.

Treatment: BA is easily treated with erythromycin 500 mg, four times a day or doxycycline 100 mg, twice a day for 3 months. The truth is that BA, as a disease of HIV patients, has disappeared from practice because of prophylactic antibiotic therapy as well as the advances in retroviral therapy.

Rhinoscleroma

Presentation and Characteristics

Rhinoscleroma, also known as scleroma, is a chronic disease of very slow progression that can be incapacitating (due to the induced scarring) and potentially fatal. The etiologic agent is *Klebsiella pneumonia subsp. rhinoscleromatis* (Frish bacillus). Three stages are recognized as follows:

- The initial stage is that of rhinitis. The first symptoms are generally nasopharyngeal; the lesions grow slowly, and often the patient does not seek medical attention for years. This is an exudative stage, with symptoms similar to those of a common cold, including headache and difficulty in breathing. There is a very purulent, fetid secretion with crusts and occasional epistaxis.

- The second stage is proliferative, characterized by obstruction and infiltration of nasal tissues by a friable granulomatous tissue. By extending into the pharynx and the larynx, it may cause hoarseness. Later, during a nodular period, the nose increases in size, adopting a "tapir" shape, also named nose of Hebra. Respiration becomes difficult, and it may be necessary to do a tracheotomy.

- The third stage is fibrotic sclerosis (Fig. 50-5), and although associated with partial improvement and occasionally a spontaneous cure, it usually results in a marked distortion of the anatomic structures. Invasion of the bone and nasal sinuses, with eventual destruction of bone tissue, may occur. The diagnosis is based

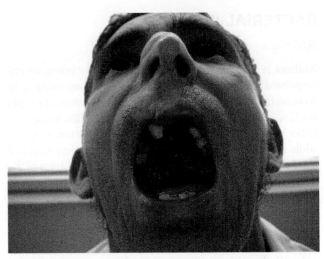

FIGURE 50-5: Rhinoscleroma, showing deformity of the nose and ulceration of the palate.

on the clinical and histologic picture and the presence of the Frish bacillus either on smear or tissue or its isolation in culture media.

Treatment

Treatment includes antibiotics such as tetracycline, azithromycin, cephalosporins, and trimethoprim. It does not respond to sulfa or penicillin. When using tetracycline, 2 g/day should be given for a period of 6 months.

Nonvenereal Treponematoses

Different species of the spirochete *Treponema* cause different infections in humans. *T. pallidum* causes venereal syphilis. *T. carateum* and *T. pertenue* cause pinta and yaws, respectively. Endemic syphilis or bejel is caused by *T. pallidum endemicum*.

Pinta has been restricted to lowland tropical areas of Central and South America. The last known descriptions have been made in autochthonous tribes of the Brazilian and Venezuelan Amazon. Transmission occurs during childhood by direct contact with lesions from infected individuals, but it is not transmitted by sexual contact. Patients go through three different stages, with early, secondary, and late lesions. The primary lesion is an erythematous papule that becomes scaly, psoriasiform, and even lichenified. It is usually located on lower extremities and becomes dyschromic with time. Secondary lesions appear about 2 months after the primary lesion. They are multiple and similar to the primary lesion, although smaller. The most prominent change is again the dyschromia, with hyper/hypopigmentation mixed in single lesions. The late lesions consist of extensive areas of hypopigmentation and achromia, resembling vitiligo (Fig. 50-6). Pinta should be suspected in patients from endemic areas with extensive dyschromias. Treatment is based on penicillin therapy. The changes in color do not reverse with antibiotic therapy.

Yaws, also called "pian" or "frambesia," is a contagious, nonvenereal disease that mainly occurs in children younger than 15 years. It is endemic to all tropical areas around the world,

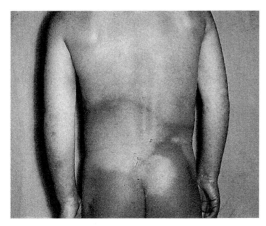

FIGURE 50-6: Pinta, showing hyper- and hypopigmented lesions.

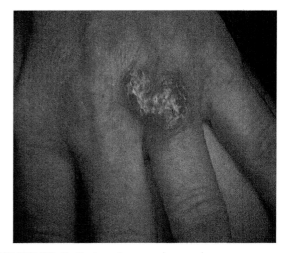

FIGURE 50-7: Swimming pool granuloma.

from Central and South America, to Africa, Asia, Australia, and the Pacific Islands. From 88 countries that were considered endemic in the 1950s, only 13 are still considered by the WHO to be affected by the disease. The clinical manifestations go through the three classical stages of early, secondary, and late lesions. The primary lesion is chancroid in appearance, whereas the secondary lesions are papillomatous verrucous, similar to condylomas. In skin, they resemble raspberries, giving origin to the French name, "frambesia." Bone involvement can be rather destructive, ending in severe deformities and mutilations. Tertiary lesions can be gumma-like and achromic, as in pinta, and can produce palmoplantar hyperkeratosis. Treatment is based on the use of penicillin.

Bejel is still reported in the Middle East, the African Sahara, and some areas of the tropical belt. Like yaws, it is a disease of infants and children. The clinical manifestations are similar to the mucosal lesions of secondary syphilis, with a condylomatous appearance. Tertiary lesions are similar to yaws.

Mycobacterial Infections Other than Tuberculosis and Leprosy

Tuberculosis and leprosy are diseases caused by mycobacteria. They are discussed in Chapter 24.

Mycobacterium marinum Infection (Swimming Pool Granulomas)

Mycobacterium marinum (formerly called *Mycobacteria balnei*) infection is characterized by the presence of an indolent verrucous papule that later evolves into a plaque or a nodule with central scarring that may eventually ulcerate.

Presentation and Characteristics: It is commonly located on the extremities, especially at points of trauma (hands, elbows) that are in contact with fresh water, salt water, or marine animals such as fish or turtles. The incubation period ranges from 2 to 6 weeks. Patients may present with a papule or nodule that subsequently ulcerates (Fig. 50-7). The lesion is usually solitary, and there is no systemic reaction. Satellite lesions may appear and may simulate a localized granuloma or

sporotrichoid lymphangitis. Both visualization of the bacteria on skin tissue and its isolation by culture are difficult.

Treatment: Although there is no comparative trial to establish the treatment of choice, most authors recommend simultaneous use of at least two drugs, such as clarithromycin and ethambutol until 2 months of complete resolution of symptoms or a minimum of 6 months. If deeper structures are affected, rifampin can be added to the regimen. Superficial cases can be treated with monotherapy with either doxycycline or minocycline.

Mycobacterium Ulcerans Infection (Buruli Ulcer)

This mycobacterial infection was first described in southern Australia as Bairnsdale ulcer and later in Africa (in the Buruli valley in Uganda, therefore its name) with additional cases reported in South America and Papua New Guinea. This is, in fact, the third most common worldwide mycobacterium infection in immunocompetent patients, after only tuberculosis and leprosy. It is considered a public health problem in many developing countries, especially in central Africa. Buruli ulcer affects mainly populations living in poverty, many of whom are children.

Presentation and Characteristics: The bacterium lives in the environment and is acquired by humans through contamination of mild traumatic wounds. The classical clinical presentation is an ulcer, located most commonly on extremities. The cavity extends laterally, undermining the edges of the lesion; so the defect is always larger than what is seen at first glance. The ulceration will continue to enlarge and produce marked destruction and mutilation of the affected areas. The morbidity of the disease is directly related to the skin lesion, with no systemic disease.

On histology, the pattern is of massive necrosis of fatty tissue. With stains such as Ziehl–Neelsen, a huge amount of bacteria is seen in the necrotic areas, in quantities only comparable to lepromatous leprosy. The necrosis is a direct effect of a bacterial toxin, mycolactone, which is a soluble polyketide.

Diagnosis: The diagnosis is made on the basis of the clinical and histologic findings. The bacteria are difficult to isolate, although it can be done on special mycobacterial media. More sophisticated diagnostic techniques such as polymerase chain reaction (PCR) allow early diagnosis in smaller lesions. Until recently, surgical excision of the completely necrotic area was considered the treatment of choice. However, in the recent years, the WHO has switched its recommendation to a therapeutic regimen based on the administration of oral rifampicin and intramuscular streptomycin for 8 weeks. The last drug can be replaced with either a quinolone or clarithromycin.

Rapidly Growing Mycobacteria (Mycobacterium Fortuitum group) Infections

This group includes a series of microorganisms causing chronic infections after traumatic surgical, cosmetic, or therapeutic inoculation. A growing number of cases are reported in South America and around the world as late complications of cosmetic procedures, such as liposuction or mesotherapy. Mycobacterium species implicated include *M. fortuitum*, *M. abscessus*, and *M. chelonae*.

Presentation and Characteristics: Patients present with cold abscesses at the site of trauma, injection, or surgery, weeks to months after the precipitating event (Fig. 50-8). Upon draining, a purulent fluid may be obtained. Direct examination shows the presence of acid-fast staining bacilli. Unless treated, the lesion becomes chronic, with fistula formation and progressive infiltration of surrounding tissues. Although these bacteria grow rapidly in culture, their isolation requires special media and low temperatures. *M. abscessus* is able to grow for more than a year in distilled water; contamination of surgical material

or injectable substances is considered a potential source of infection when dealing with epidemic outbreaks.

Treatment: Treatments of choice include clarithromycin and quinolones. Amikacin can be used in deep-seated infections. Surgical drainage is of great importance to speed up the resolution of the process.

FUNGI

Subcutaneous Mycosis

Chromoblastomycosis

Chromoblastomycosis is a chronic mycosis that affects the skin and subcutaneous tissues. It is characterized by a distinct clinical presentation as a verrucous plaque and the presence of the so-called sclerotic bodies on tissue cuts. A great variety of fungi are able to cause the disease, including *Fonsecaea pedrosoi*, *Fonsecaea compacta*, *Fonsecaea monophora*, *Phialophora verrucosa*, *Cladophialophora carrionii* (formerly *Cladosporium carrionii*), and *Rhinocladiella aquaspersa*. The disease has been reported worldwide, with most cases coming from the tropical and subtropical areas of South America and Africa. Some fungi have a preference for certain climates. *F. pedrosoi* is most common in wet and humid areas within the torrid zones, whereas *C. carrionii* prefers the dry and semidesert regions of the tropical–intertropical zones.

Presentation and Characteristics: The most commonly affected areas are the lower extremities, although in some geographic locations, like the arid plains of Venezuela, the upper girdle (shoulder, arm, or back) is the prevalent site of infection.

The primary process occurs at the site of inoculation, most probably through traumatized skin. The fungus is acquired from the environment, where it lives as a saprophyte of wood, vegetable debris, or soil. The disease is not transmitted from person to person. The primary lesion is exophytic, presenting as a papule, a nodule, or a tumor. The lesions multiply and tend to coalesce, forming plaques with a verrucous surface (Fig. 50-9). Ulceration may develop, but there is no fistula formation, as seen in mycetoma. Verrucous areas may alternate with extensive scarring. As a rule, both bone and muscle are spared. The affected limb may end up in elephantiasis.

Diagnosis: The diagnosis is easily made by direct examination of scrapings from the lesion with potassium hydroxide (KOH). The morphology adopted by the fungus is a cluster of oblong, round, pigmented cells with thick walls and flattened abutting surfaces, dividing by septation in more than one plane. They are known as *sclerotic bodies* or *muriform cells*. The histopathology shows pseudocarcinomatous hyperplasia with a granulomatous suppurative reaction in the dermis. On histology, the sclerotic bodies have a brown color and are easily identified because their size (4 to 12 mm) makes them appear similar to "copper pennies." Species identification is only possible after culture isolation on Sabouraud media, after 4 to 6 weeks.

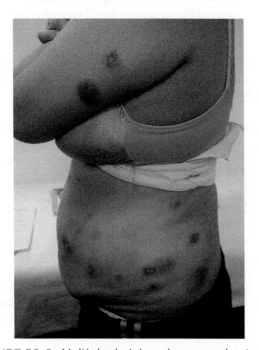

FIGURE 50-8: Multiple draining abscesses due to *Mycobacterium chelonae*, after mesotherapy.

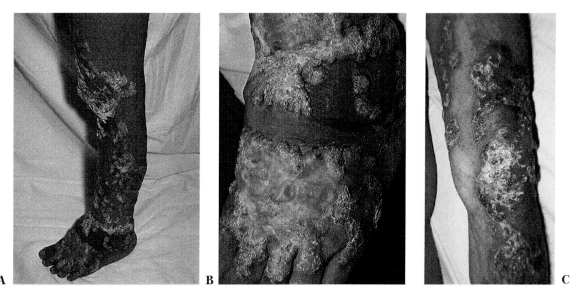

A   **B**   **C**

FIGURE 50-9: Chromoblastomycosis: cauliflower-like leg lesion **(A)**, with a closeup of the foot **(B)**. **C:** Another case of Chromoblastomycosis with verrucous surface and ulcerations.

Treatment: Treatment options include surgical excision when the lesion is small. Pharmacologic agents, reported to be useful but probably not curative by themselves, include 5-flucytosine, itraconazole, and newer drugs such as voriconazole or posaconazole. Cryotherapy is used in conjunction with antimycotics.

Mycetoma or Maduromycosis

Also known as Madura foot, mycetoma is a chronic subcutaneous infection with a distinct clinical picture of edema, fistula formation, and draining of grains. The disease is caused by at least 20 different species of fungi (eumycetoma) and actinomycetes (actinomycetoma). Among the true fungi, four are responsible for more than 90% of cases: *Madurella mycetomatis, Madurella grisea, Pseudallescheria boydii,* and *Leptosphaeria senegalensis.* Actinomycetomas are commonly caused by *Nocardia brasiliensis, Nocardia asteroides, Actinomadura madurae,* and *Streptomyces somaliensis.* The disease has a worldwide distribution. Originally described in India, with a high incidence in the region of Madura, it is typically seen in dry, tropical areas. Countries with the highest incidence include Sudan, Venezuela, Mexico, and India. Although eumycetomas predominate in Sudan (70% of cases), actinomycetomas represent 97% of all mycetomas seen in Mexico.

Presentation and Characteristics: The organisms gain entry into the body owing to trauma, and the disease is most common in adult males who work outdoors barefoot or who expose large areas of the skin, as stevedores do. The clinical picture manifests over a period of months or years as a nodule that later evolves into edematous areas with marked fibrosis, followed by the formation of a fistula that drains or expels "grains" (Fig. 50-10). Lesions are commonly located on the feet and legs; shoulder is a common location for actinomycetomas in Mexico. Bone involvement is characterized by periosteal

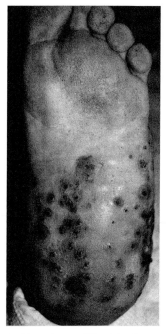

FIGURE 50-10: Mycetoma. The black granules are more indicative of a fungal rather than an actinomycotic etiology.

erosion and proliferation as well as the development of lytic lesions; otherwise, there is no systemic involvement.

Diagnosis: The presence of grains in the context of the clinical picture of edema and fistula formation favors mycetoma. However, grains can also be seen in the bacterial counterpart of mycetoma, a condition known as botryomycosis. Morphology of the grains may give an idea of the specific etiologic agent, but precise identification will require culture isolation. Dark grains are usually due to fungi; white to yellow grains can be either due to actinomyces or fungi.

Treatment: Treatment depends on the organism isolated. For cases where actinomycetes are isolated, sulfamethoxazole/trimethoprim and amikacin individually or a combination of them have been reported as successful; in fact, the combination has achieved cure rates of about 90%. Eumycetoma is more difficult to treat, with some response to oral imidazoles reported, including ketoconazole, itraconazole, voriconazole, and posaconazole. Surgery should be considered for more advanced eumycetomas, while is seldom required in actinomycetomas.

Sporotrichosis

Sporotrichosis is a mycotic infection produced by species of the environmental fungus *Sporothrix spp.* Medically relevant species include *S. schenkii (sensu stricto), S. brasiliensis, S. globose, S. mexicana, and S. luriei.* It has a worldwide distribution, although hyperendemic areas do exist, for example, in specific regions of the Peruvian Andes. More recently, a large number of cases has been reported in Rio de Janeiro, Brazil, occurring simultaneously to an epidemic in cats and dogs. In cosmopolitan cases around the world, it is commonly associated with trauma from a rose thorn or exposure to sphagnum moss and is considered an occupational hazard for florists and gardeners.

Presentation and Characteristics: The classical picture (about 70% of cases) is the so-called lymphocutaneous or sporotrichoid pattern characterized by a primary lesion, mostly an ulcerated plaque, followed by several satellite lesions, either papular, nodular, or crusted, in a linear distribution, following the lymphatic drainage (Fig. 50-11). It is commonly located on an extremity and, in children of endemic areas, on the face. There is a second type of presentation with only one isolated lesion, either a plaque, a nodule, or an ulcer (Fig. 50-12). This is known as the fixed cutaneous form of sporotrichosis. Rarely, the infection can disseminate to involve multiple sites and organs, usually associated with some form of immunosuppression, such as alcoholism, diabetes, or HIV infection. The most common extracutaneous sites of involvement are the joints.

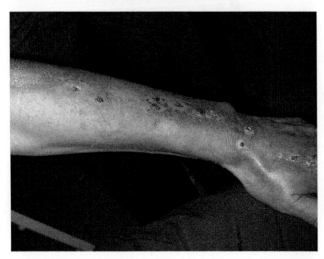

FIGURE 50-11: Sporotrichosis, classical sporotrichoid pattern.

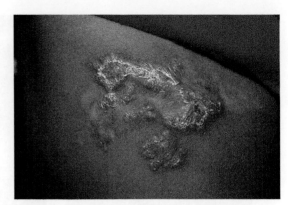

FIGURE 50-12: Sporotrichosis, fixed lesion.

Diagnosis: The fungus is rarely seen on direct examination or on tissue cuts, even with special stains. When visible, it has a levaduriform, cigar-shaped morphology. On histology, when it is seen, it is identified at the center of an asteroid body. However, the fungus easily grows on Sabouraud media, which is the easiest and most reliable method for diagnosis. Nested PCR can also be used in clinical samples to detect the microorganism.

Treatment: Treatment options include the use of potassium iodide solution and itraconazole; while the first option is cheap, the imidazole alternative is considered the treatment of choice because of good tolerance and fewer side effects. Therapy should be prolonged for up to 3 to 6 months, or 2 weeks after achieving total clinical remission.

Lobomycosis

This chronic skin infection is produced by *Lacazia loboi* (formerly *Loboa loboi*), a large fungus with a levaduriform morphology. The disease is endemic in tropical areas of South America.

Presentation and Characteristics: The disease is acquired by primary inoculation from the environment through traumatized skin. The clinical lesions take years to develop. The classical clinical manifestation is the formation of nodules with a keloid appearance (thus the name keloidal blastomycosis), usually located on the extremities, ears, face, and neck, with sparing of the scalp in most cases. Other primary lesions include infiltrated plaques, gummas, ulcers, and verrucoid nodules (Fig. 50-13). The histology consists of a massive histiocytic infiltrate, without the pseudocarcinomatous hyperplasia commonly seen in chromoblastomycosis. This is the reason that the nodules in lobomycosis tend to have a smooth surface, as opposed to the verrucous surface of chromoblastomycosis. The morphology of the fungus is quite distinctive, as globose, lemon-shaped buds, 9 to 10 mm in diameter, organized in short and long chains of uniform beads. The organism is readily seen in KOH preparations and tissue biopsies from lesions. The fungus has never been isolated in culture media.

Treatment: The only effective treatment is surgical excision. Recurrence is very common. Recent reports suggest that the

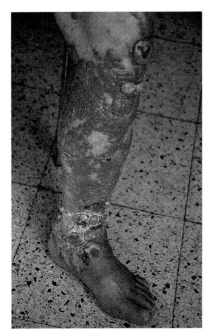

FIGURE 50-13: Lobomycosis: Compare the smooth surface with what is seen in chromoblastomycosis.

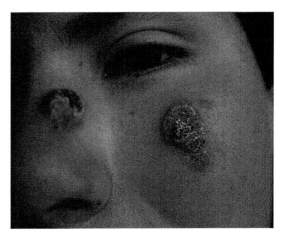

FIGURE 50-14: Ulceration due to histoplasmosis.

combination of itraconazole and clofazimine, or posaconazole alone may be of some benefit.

Systemic Mycosis

Histoplasmosis

This disease is caused by *Histoplasma capsulatum*. Found throughout the world in temperate areas, *H. capsulatum* is a saprophytic fungus that grows in the soil, prevalently in the soil of caves inhabited by bats. The disease is transmitted by the inadvertent inhalation of the spores. Epidemics have occurred while exploring infested caves or cleaning sites where bat excrement (guano) may be present.

Presentation and Characteristics: A benign clinical form mimicking a common cold may leave a calcified nodule in the lung similar to that of tuberculosis. In its most severe form, the disease can disseminate, involving the reticuloendothelial system. Nowadays, most cutaneous cases are seen in patients with AIDS. In such patients, the disease is seen in its most severe form. Lesions can be papules, plaques, ulcerations (Fig. 50-14), umbilicated lesions mimicking molluscum contagiosum, and deep-seated nodules, mimicking cellulitis or panniculitis. Primary cutaneous histoplasmosis is caused by direct inoculation. It is a nodular or indurated chancroid ulcer with accompanying lymphadenopathy. Occasionally, an allergic response has been seen appearing as urticaria or as erythema annulare centrifugum.

Diagnosis: The diagnosis is made by demonstrating the presence of small, intracellular *H. capsulatum* in sputum, bone marrow, or skin biopsy specimens. Serology can be helpful.

Treatment: Treatment in cases of disseminated disease consist of amphotericin B followed by prolonged administration of itraconazole.

Coccidioidomycosis or San Joaquin Valley Fever

This disease is caused by *Coccidioides immitis*, a soil inhabitant. Infection in both humans and animals is acquired by the inhalation of fungus-laden dust particles or, rarely, through a primary infection of the skin.

Presentation and Characteristics: The severity of coccidioidomycosis can range from very mild, simulating a common cold, to an acute disseminated fatal disease, especially in patients with AIDS. The classical skin manifestations include papules, pustules, plaques, abscesses, and draining sinuses, most commonly on the face and trunk. Other lesions include ulcerations, toxic erythema, and allergic reactions such as erythema multiforme or erythema nodosum. The basic symptoms of malaise and fever may suggest coccidioidomycosis if the patient has traveled through an endemic area. HIV patients may also develop molluscum-like lesions.

Diagnosis: Diagnosis is made by KOH mounts of sputum or isolation of the fungus in culture. Colonies of *Coccidioides immitis* in the fast-growing phase are dangerous to handle, and the greatest care should be taken when manipulating cultures.

Treatment: Treatment includes amphotericin B, ketoconazole, and itraconazole.

Paracoccidioidomycosis

Paracoccidioidomycosis is a systemic disease with hematogenous spreading from a primary pulmonary focus. The infection has a specific geographic distribution through Central and South America. The agent, *Paracoccidioides brasiliensis*, is a dimorphic fungus with special preference for tropical and subtropical forest with mild temperature and high humidity.

Presentation and Characteristics: The infection is acquired by inhalation, resulting in a primary lesion located in the lung.

From there on, it may take one of two forms: a subacute or juvenile form, seen commonly in young males, with marked involvement of the reticuloendothelial system (lymph nodes, liver, and spleen) and many skin lesions, or a chronic form, mostly affecting oral, nasal, or anal mucosae. Both forms are associated with chronic pulmonary disease. The typical patient is a male agricultural worker. The patients may present to the dermatologist with involvement of either the mucosae or the skin. Mucosal lesions are commonly located on the lips, buccal mucosae, gums, palate, and pharynx, and consist of infiltrating, ulcerated plaques and nodules (moriform stomatitis), with subsequent destruction and scarring deformities, such as severe limitation in opening the mouth (Fig. 50-15).

On the skin, the lesions vary widely. They may begin as small acneiform pustules 2 to 3 mm in size that later ulcerate, or they can adopt an ulcerated pattern related to the affected lymph nodes. A cold abscess may develop. In some instances, multiple symmetric papules, either with verrucous or umbilicated surfaces, may be present. On soles, they could be easily misinterpreted as warts (Fig. 50-16), whereas on the face, they may look like molluscum contagiosum.

Diagnosis: The size of the fungus and its characteristic morphology allow easy identification on sputum preparations and scrapings from the mucosal and cutaneous lesions. It is easy to recognize the blastospores with multiple budding giving the "pilot wheel" appearance (Fig. 50-17). Identical structures are seen on histologic examination of the affected tissues. The reaction pattern seen on biopsy is a granulomatous reaction with multiple giant cells, some of them engulfing the budding elements. The fungus grows on Sabouraud medium in 4 or more weeks, as a mold at 20° to 26°C and as a yeast at 34° to 37°C.

Treatment: Treatment choices have evolved, from sulfonamides to ketoconazole up to the new triazoles (itraconazole and fluconazole). At present, itraconazole is considered the drug of choice because of the lower doses required, shorter period of treatment, and fewer side effects.

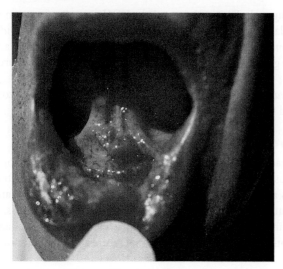

FIGURE 50-15: An infiltrative, deforming lesion of paracoccidioidomycosis.

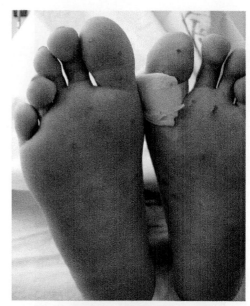

FIGURE 50-16: Wartlike lesions of paracoccidioidomycosis on the soles.

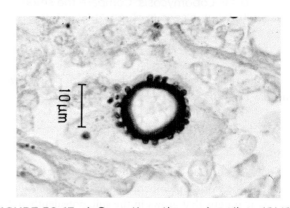

FIGURE 50-17: A Grocott methenamine silver (GMS) stain in tissue demonstrating the blastospore with the characteristic "pilot wheel" appearance. (Courtesy of Dr. James Fishback, University of Kansas Medical Center.)

PARASITIC DISEASES

Protozoal Dermatosis

Leishmaniasis

Leishmaniasis is an infectious process caused by intracellular parasites of the *Leishmania* genus. The disease is transmitted from natural reservoirs to humans through the bite of infected female sandflies belonging to the genuses *Phlebotomus* and *Lutzomyia*.

Presentation and Characteristics: The different forms of cutaneous disease are produced by species of *Leishmania* specific for certain regions of the world, like those seen in the Middle East (*L. tropica*), the Mediterranean region (*L. major*), Central America (*L. mexicana*), and South America (*L. peruviana* and *L. braziliensis*). Different local names are given to the disease depending on the geographical location:

Oriental sore in Asia, chiclero ulcer in Mexico, Uta in the Andes, and Espundia in the Amazon basin.

The classical cutaneous lesion consists of a round, isolated ulceration, with slightly elevated and indurated borders (Fig. 50-18). However, the clinical spectrum includes other types of lesions such as plaque-like, sporotrichoid, pustular, impetigo-like, eczematoid, sarcoidosis-like, lupoid, erysipeloid, papulotuberous, verrucous, disseminated, and diffuse cutaneous leishmaniasis. Common locations are areas of the body not covered by clothing and therefore exposed to the mosquito bite such as the face, neck, and extremities. The lesion itself is painless and commonly tends to regress spontaneously.

The variety known as mucocutaneous leishmaniasis, which is caused by *L. braziliensis*, is characterized by its ability to produce, after a dormant period, an ulceration on the mucosae of the nasal septum. This can progress externally, mutilating the whole nose and nasolabial area (Fig. 50-19). When the progression is on the mucosal side, it may destroy the palate, producing a granulomatous infiltration of the pharynx, the larynx, and even the upper respiratory airway. Disseminated cutaneous leishmaniasis refers to a clinical presentation consisting of a primary classical ulcerated lesion and multiple secondary lesions with similar morphology to the primary lesion but occurring at distant sites. Diffuse cutaneous leishmaniasis, also known as anergic leishmaniasis, is a quite distinct form, where the lesions have a completely different morphology, consisting of nodules and tumors, almost keloidal in aspect, which, on histology, translate into a massive infiltration of histiocytes loaded with amastigotes, in a manner quite similar to that seen in lepromatous leprosy.

The tissue destruction seen in leishmaniasis is in fact a result of the great inflammatory reaction induced by the parasite, rather than the virulent effect of the microorganism itself. In an early lesion, a heavy infiltration of histiocytes, many of them engulfing the *Leishmania* organisms, is mixed with lymphocytes and plasma cells. The more organized the granulomas, the less likely *Leishmania* will be seen on the biopsy specimens.

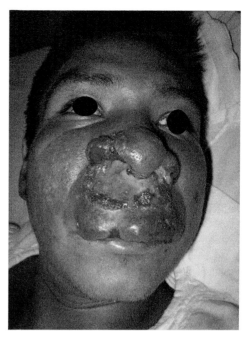

FIGURE 50-19: Nasal ulceration and upper lip infiltration and destruction typical of mucocutaneous leishmaniasis

Diagnosis: There is no single method of diagnosis that will have high sensitivity and specificity; rather, the diagnosis is based on the simultaneous utilization of several methods, including direct examination of smear and aspirate from the lesions, culture in specific media, skin biopsy, and PCR techniques. The Leishmanin response or Montenegro test, an intradermal reaction to fragments of the parasite, is useful when working up a diagnosis in someone who is just an occasional visitor to endemic areas. The high sensitivity of the test makes it very useful to rule out rather than to confirm the diagnosis.

Treatment: Treatment, when indicated, is based on the use of antimonial preparations and, in difficult cases, of amphotericin B. Always consider leishmaniasis in the differential diagnosis of chronic cutaneous ulcerations, especially when there is a history of living in or traveling to endemic areas, especially those that are very popular among the adventurous tourist. Reports have occurred in military personnel returning from the Middle East.

African/American Trypanosomiasis

African trypanosomiasis or "sleeping sickness" is transmitted to humans by bites of infected tsetse flies. A painful and indurated trypanosomal chancre appears in some patients 5 to 15 days after the inoculation of the parasite and resolves spontaneously over several weeks. Transient edema is common and can occur on the face, hands, feet, and other periarticular areas. Enlargement of the lymph nodes of the posterior cervical triangle, referred to as Winterbottom sign, is a classic finding in the West African form. Pruritus is frequent, and an irregular maculopapular rash is often present. This rash is located on the trunk, shoulders, buttocks, and thighs and consists of annular,

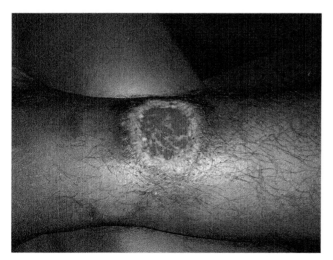

FIGURE 50-18: Round ulceration with slightly elevated borders typical of cutaneous leishmaniasis.

blotchy, erythematous areas with clear centers, called trypanids. Eventually, the parasitic invasion reaches the central nervous system (CNS), causing behavioral and neurologic changes, resulting in what is known as sleeping sickness.

American trypanosomiasis or Chagas disease is transmitted by the reduviid *Triatoma infestans* (kissing bug). Infections occur when the bug bites near the skin, mucous membranes, or conjunctivae. The resulting wound then becomes contaminated with bug feces containing infective parasites. When the organisms enter the skin, an indurated area of erythema and swelling (chagoma) will develop, accompanied by local lymphadenopathy. The Romaña sign, which consists of unilateral, painless edema of the palpebrae and periocular tissues, occurs in cases of entry through the conjunctiva. The initial local signs may be followed by malaise, fever, anorexia, and edema of the face and lower extremities. Some patients may also develop a rash that clears in several days. Cardiac involvement is the most frequent and serious defined manifestation of chronic Chagas disease. Treatment is unsatisfactory, with only two drugs (nifurtimox and benznidazole) available for this purpose.

Amebiasis, Including Free-Living Amebas and Entamoeba Histolytica

Free-living amebas are usually associated with disease of the CNS. The infection is acquired by swimming in ponds and streams with slow-moving or stagnant water. There are two types of meningoencephalitis produced by these organisms. The *Naegleria* species cause an acute form, with no skin manifestations. The subacute, granulomatous form is produced by two genera, *Acanthamoeba* and *Balamuthia*. *Acanthamoeba* infection is known to induce chronic ulcerative lesions in AIDS patients and, rarely, isolated, centrofacial plaques in immunocompetent hosts. In the 1990s, a new variety, named *Balamuthia mandrillaris*, was recognized as the causative agent of many cases of free-living ameba granulomatous meningoencephalitis around the world, especially in South America, the United States, and Australia. The cases reported in the United States concentrate in the states of California, Texas, and the Southwestern states.

The classical presentation will include a primary skin lesion, in the form of a central face plaque, of granulomatous appearance, usually located on the nose but also in extremities, especially around the knee. In the months following the cutaneous involvement, most patients will develop focal CNS symptoms, marking the beginning of a necrotizing encephalitis. Except for a few cases reported in the last few years, the outcome is always fatal. However, the early recognition of the skin lesion as a marker of the infection may allow early treatment with a combination of antiparasitic and antifungal drugs, with subsequent improvement of the survival rates.

Entamoeba histolytica can produce cutaneous lesions, most commonly in the anal margin and genital region (Fig. 50-20) but also beyond those areas, such as in the abdominal wall. The lesions are large cutaneous ulcerations, vegetative lesions, and even abscesses. They are, characteristically, extremely painful.

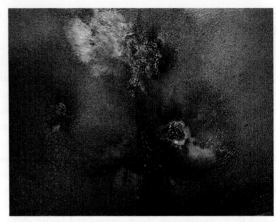

FIGURE 50-20: Cutaneous amebiasis with deep ulcers on the buttocks, due to *Entamoeba histolytica*. (Courtesy of Dr. A. Gonzalez-Orchoa.)

Helminthic Dermatosis (Roundworm)

Cutaneous Larva Migrans

Presentation and Characteristics: This is a disease caused by hookworms, usually parasites of dogs and cats. The ova are excreted through the feces, and they evolve into a larvarial state in sandy, moist ground. The larva penetrates the skin of bathers or people who walk on the contaminated ground. Usually, the "culprits" are *Ancylostoma braziliense, A. caninum, Uncinaria stenocephala,* and *Bunostomum phlebotomum*. Clinically, the parasite causes a serpentine, erythematous, papular, pruritic eruption in the skin (Fig. 50-21). The parasite is usually ahead of the tract. Vesicles, excoriations, and crusts are present.

Treatment: Treatment includes topical thiabendazole or oral albendazole, 200 mg twice a day for 3 days.

Larva Currens due to Strongyloidiasis

As opposed to cutaneous larva migrans, in which lesions migrate over a period of days, in the cutaneous form of strongyloidiasis, the movement occurs over a period of hours, thus the reason for the "currens" denomination. This infection, produced by *Strongyloides stercoralis,* is more common in immunosuppressed patients, in whom multiple tracts are seen. Lesions are commonly located in the abdominal wall, especially around the umbilicus, adopting the clinical appearance of "thumb-printing" purpura. Ivermectin is the treatment of choice, 200 μg/kg; in immunosuppressed patients, an early intervention will actually be lifesaving.

Gnathostomiasis

Gnathostomiasis is the infection produced by the third-stage larvae of nematodes of the genus Gnathostoma. It was described initially as a parasite of large felines by Owen in 1886, whereas the first human case was described in Thailand in 1889 as cited by Herman. Nowadays, it is a disease seen in endemic countries with a high consumption of raw fish or in travelers to such countries.

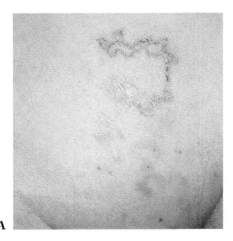
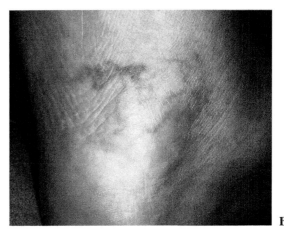

A   **B**

FIGURE 50-21: **A:** Larva migrans. **B:** Creeping eruption of larva migrans on the sole.

Presentation and Characteristics: Several species of *Gnathostoma* are capable of causing the disease, most commonly *G. spinigerum* and *G. binucleatum*. Clinically, it produces a nodular, migratory, eosinophilic panniculitis. The adult parasite normally inhabits the stomachs of domestic animals such as dogs and cats. The eggs are excreted in the stools of these animals. When the eggs reach the rivers, they hatch in the water, reach the first larvarial stage, and then, they are ingested by crustaceans of the *Cyclops* species, where they develop into a second larval stage. Fish later ingest the *Cyclops*, developing a third larval stage in their muscular tissue. Humans, who are not the definitive host, could acquire the disease by eating contaminated raw fish, in the form of ceviche or sushi. The parasite migrates through the tissues, most commonly to the skin, but it may go to any of the internal organs; in the worst scenario, it may go into the eye or the CNS. Clinically, after a variable incubation period of 4 weeks to 3 years, patients develop the classical symptom of a pruritic, migratory, edematous panniculitis, or a more superficial form, which can be identical to that seen in cutaneous larva migrans (Fig. 50-22). Exceptionally, either spontaneously or after administration of an antiparasitic drug, the larvae get very close or even emerge through the epidermis, and give rise to what is called the furuncular form. The clinical picture will be accompanied by either peripheral or tissue eosinophilia, therefore the name "migratory eosinophilic panniculitis."

Treatment: Treatment alternatives include albendazole 400 to 800 mg for 2 to 3 weeks or ivermectin 200 µg/kg in a single dose given every 2 weeks.

Filariasis

Three species of filarial parasites are known to cause human filariasis: *Wuchereria bancrofti*, *Brugia malayi*, and *Brugia timori*. Although *W. bancrofti* is a cause of filariasis worldwide, those caused by *B. malayi* and *B. timori* are seen only in South and East Asia. Mosquitoes belonging to the Culex family are the main vectors for the disease.

Presentation and Characteristics: The major symptoms of filariasis relate to damaged lymphatics. Acute lymphangitis and

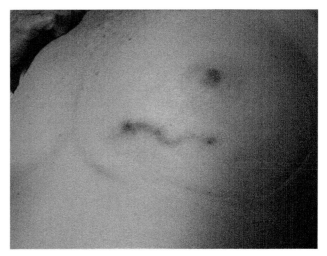

FIGURE 50-22: Gnathostomiasis showing superficial and deep patterns of migration.

lymphadenitis may affect limbs, breasts, and genitalia. Urticaria may be part of the clinical presentation. Late changes are due to obstruction of lymphatics, giving rise to different forms of elephantiasis with massive edema. Some patients with elephantiasis develop a crusty, verrucous skin change, referred to as elephantiasis nostras verrucosa. The chronic changes of elephantiasis in filariasis affect mostly the lower extremities and genitalia.

Diagnosis: Diagnosis is accomplished by detecting the presence of microfilaria in blood smears and by serologic testing.

Treatment: Treatment with diethylcarbamazine (6 mg/ kg daily for 12 days) remains the treatment of choice for the individual with active lymphatic filariasis. In efforts to eradicate the disease in endemic countries, single doses of the drug are given massively to specific populations. Additional therapy includes the use of doxycycline, aiming to eradicate an endosymbiotic bacteria of the *Wolbachia* family, helping to eliminate the microfilaria and adult worms. The treatment of the altered lymphatic circulation is of pivotal importance in chronic cases with elephantiasis.

Onchocerciasis

Onchocerciasis is a chronic infestation of the skin by *Onchocerca volvulus*. This is a microfilarial nematode whose natural hosts are humans and flies from the genus *Simulium*.

The disease was first described in Africa and later in Central America. It has been reported occasionally in the northern countries of South America. As in 2013, eradication has been almost completed in several central and South American countries.

Presentation and Characteristics: The transmission occurs when flies become infected by biting infected people. After a short period of maturation, the microfilaria moves to the buccal apparatus of the insect and enters the skin of a noninfected human with the next blood meal. The microfilaria become adults in an year inside cutaneous nodules called onchocercomas, where they start to produce new microfilariae; these new microfilariae are mainly responsible for the damage seen clinically. The nodules are firm, often flattened or bean-shaped, usually movable, and nontender. They can be up to several centimeters in diameter. Other clinical presentations include acute and chronic papular forms, facial erythema, facial livedoid discoloration, facial aging, and a prurigo-like eruption on the buttocks and extremities. Later signs are extensive lichenification and dyschromia similar to vitiligo. Ocular involvement is due to the direct invasion of eye structures by the microfilaria, causing uveitis, conjunctivitis, keratitis, optical nerve atrophy, and glaucoma. It may evolve into complete and permanent loss of vision, thus the reason for naming the disease "river blindness."

Diagnosis: Diagnosis is easy to confirm, either by direct scraping or histologic analysis of skin lesions in which adult forms and microfilariae are identified.

Treatment: Ivermectin is extremely effective, even as a single-dose therapy. Its massive administration to entire populations has allowed for complete eradication in several countries.

Trematodes Dermatosis (Flukes)

Cercarial Dermatitis

Cercarial dermatitis or swimmer's itch is caused by the penetration of the skin by schistosoma of birds or mammals. The cercaria is found in bodies of fresh water. It can penetrate the skin of a mammal and, if the host is receptive, reach the bloodstream and spread to other organs. In humans, who are not the definitive host, the cercariae are unsuccessful in reaching the blood. They are retained at the epidermal level and finally destroyed, resulting clinically in a form of dermatitis. Clinically, pruritic macules, papules, hemorrhages, and excoriations develop in the exposed areas. This resulting dermatitis is a product of the sensitization to the cercarial proteins. In massive or repeated infestations, the signs and symptoms are consequently more severe.

Cercarial dermatitis should be distinguished from *seabather's eruption*. The latter is an eruption that generally occurs in the area under swimwear after bathing in the ocean. Occasionally, it may affect other areas such axilla, neck, and flexures

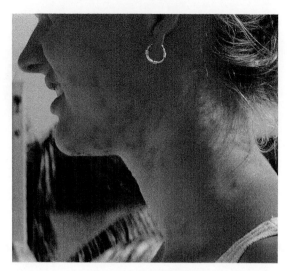

FIGURE 50-23: Seabather's eruption, caused by thimble jellyfish off the coast of Belize. (Courtesy of Dr. Kate Schafer.)

(Fig. 50-23). It is characterized by a papular pruritic eruption that will develop within hours of leaving affected waters. Occasionally, systemic symptoms may appear, including fatigue, malaise, fever, chills, nausea, and GI complaints. These episodes appear to be more severe after repeated attacks. The causative agent is the cnidarian larvae of *Linuche unguiculata* (thimble jellyfish). This larva has been found in water samples of tropical and subtropical beaches; in affected patients, high immunoglobulin G (IgG) levels specific to *L. unguiculata* have been demonstrated. Symptomatic treatment is accomplished with antihistamines, topical corticosteroids, and even oral steroid therapy. It is a self-limiting condition, lasting up to 12 days.

Schistosomiasis and Bilharziasis

Schistosomiasis and bilharziasis occur when humans come into contact with water infested by the flukes belonging to the genus *Schistosoma*. The disease manifests itself by the immune response to invading and migrating larvae. Cercarial dermatitis refers to the clinical picture elucidated by the penetration of cercaria into the skin. The clinical findings are those of an acute pruritic, papular rash at the site of the cercarial penetration, accompanied by a prickling sensation. Other manifestations include Katayama fever, a late nonspecific dermatitis, perigenital granulomas, and extragenital infiltrative lesions. Treatment of cercarial dermatitis and acute schistosomiasis should be directed toward treating the symptoms. Chronic schistosomiasis can be effectively treated with a single-day dose of praziquantel.

DERMATOSIS CAUSED BY ARTHROPODS

Human Scabies

Presentation and Characteristics

This disease is transmitted through prolonged personal contact and less often by clothing and bed linens. The mite's location

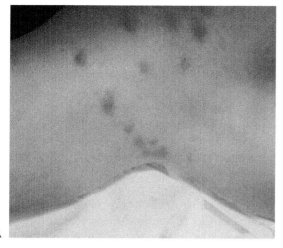

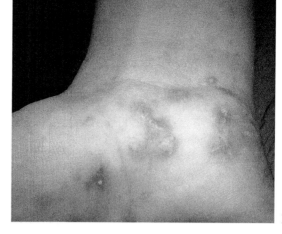

FIGURE 50-24: **A and B:** Scabies.

is in a "burrow" in the stratum corneum where it deposits its eggs. An allergic sensitization to the mite and/or its products causes the clinical picture. Itching appears 2 to 4 weeks after the infestation and is classically more severe at night. As a clinical finding, the burrow is pathognomonic and diagnostic. The remaining lesions are secondary to scratching, secondary infection, and allergic reaction. The burrow is a skin-colored, tortuous, elevated line of 1 to 1.5 cm in length. It is usually found in the finger webs, flexor surfaces of the wrists, nipples, axillae, and elbows (Fig. 50-24). In children, the lesions can be vesicular and located on the face, palms, and soles.

Diagnosis

The diagnosis is confirmed by a scraping preparation of the skin and identification of the parasite.

Treatment

One 8-hour application at night of permethrin, 5% solution or cream, is considered the standard treatment nowadays. The gamma isomer of hexachlorobenzene (lindane), 1% in a vanishing cream, was used for years, but it is used less commonly nowadays because of its toxicity; it should not be used in pregnant women or infants. With both medications, a second application is recommended after 1 week. Note that this application should cover the entire body very thoroughly. Areas not to be missed include the umbilicus, genital area, and the area under the nails. Ivermectin, 200 μg/kg, in a single dose has been found to be very effective. A 6% sulfur precipitate in petroleum jelly for 3 consecutive days is employed in infants and pregnant women. The nails should be cut short and scrubbed vigorously. Clothing and bed linen should be washed thoroughly.

Clinical Varieties of Scabies

Crusted scabies, also known as Norwegian scabies, is a form of scabies seen mostly in immunosuppressed individuals. HTLV-1 infection is a particular condition that predisposes the affected individual to develop crusted scabies. Typically, the lesions are extensive, crusted hyperkeratotic plaques where itching may not be a prominent feature. The direct examination of scrapings shows a massive amount of mites, and the patient is much more contagious.

Nodular scabies consists of brown or red firm nodules on the penis, scrotum, or buttocks. Such lesions may persist for months despite specific scabicidal treatment. Their prolonged course is the result of a delayed allergic reaction that does not require a viable mite to be present.

Animal Scabies

In this disease, very similar to papular urticaria, the mites invade the surface human skin, but they do not become established in it. There are varieties from dogs, sheep, birds, and others. Excoriated, crusted papules can be seen, and pruritus can be very severe, especially in the evening.

Arachnidism

Latrodectism

Latrodectus mactans are small, dark spiders called "black widows." They have a black or brown underside with a red, orange, or white hourglass marking on the back. They are commonly found near protected places such as the undersides of stones and logs, in the angles of doors, windows and shutters, and in outhouses. Their venom is neurotoxic; they usually bite on the genitalia or buttocks. Pain develops within about an hour, with accompanying reddening and swelling. Systemic symptoms include muscle cramping, rigidity, and later weakness, sweating, bradycardia, hypothermia, and hypotension. The mortality rate is about 5% in children.

Treatment: Treatment includes intravenous 10% calcium gluconate and corticosteroids. However, the most effective therapy is systemic antivenom.

Loxoscelism

The *Loxosceles* spiders are light brown to chocolate in color, with nocturnal habits, and are commonly found seeking warmth in discarded clothing. *Loxosceles reclusus* is mostly seen in the United States, and *Loxosceles laeta* is seen in Central and South America.

Presentation and Characteristics: Usually, affected areas include the arm and thigh of adults or the face in children. Pain develops 2 to 8 hours after the bite. The lesion becomes indurated and red, with a central blister and subsequent necrosis that can be quite large; the combination of erythema, cyanosis, and paleness can give rise to what is known as the marble plaque (Fig. 50-25). The necrotic area eventually becomes mummified. Around the 14th day, the eschar may slough off.

Rarely, general symptoms include fever, chills, vomiting, petechiae on the skin, as well as thrombocytopenia and hemolytic anemia, especially in children. Treatment is with antivenom, corticosteroids, and dapsone, which has been described as effective in limiting the size and extension of the necrosis.

Diseases Caused by Chiggers

These mites, also known as *harvest mites*, are the cause of the infestation known as trombiculiasis. It is seen worldwide, although most frequently in tropical areas. The disease is acquired while walking through low vegetation, and the affected area is usually exposed skin depending on the type of clothing worn. The offending chigger is the larval stage of the mite, 0.25 to 0.4 mm in diameter, orange to red in color, and with three pairs of legs. It gets fixed to the skin by its buccal apparatus and starts a process of liquefying and sucking the skin elements. As a consequence, it produces a type of papular urticaria and multiple red itchy papules that are extremely pruritic and sometimes purpuric (Fig. 50-26).

Treatment: Topical treatment is with steroids and antipruritic lotions. Occasionally, this condition requires systemic antibiotic therapy as well as systemic steroids.

Diseases Caused by Nigua

Tungiasis is a human infestation produced by *Tunga penetrans*, a sand flea that thrives on moist, sandy ground near pigsties and cowsheds. It is widely distributed in tropical and subtropical areas of South America and Africa. It is known by various names (*pique, nigua, bicho dos pes*). It is commonly acquired when walking barefoot in contaminated areas, including residential gardens recently fertilized with cattle manure.

Presentation and Characteristics: The infection is produced by the female flea, which burrows into the skin between the toes and near the nail. The flea inserts her body full of eggs, to die at a later time. The initial clinical manifestation is a black dot representing the burrow full of eggs that can later be seen on top of a papule or vesicle (Fig. 50-27). The walls of the burrow are horny tissue from the epidermis itself. The flea tissue produces a foreign body reaction that terminates in suppuration and opening of the cavity. Coalescing lesions may form a honeycomb plaque. This may serve as a port of entry for a more severe bacterial infection and even gangrene.

Treatment: The best treatment is the extraction of all insect parts. The best prevention is to wear closed shoes in high-risk areas.

Paederus Dermatitis

Blister beetle dermatitis, or *paederus dermatitis*, is caused by contact of human skin with the body fluids of *Paederus spp.*, a member of the order Coleoptera, family Staphylinidae. These blister beetles are closely related to the Spanish fly, the producer of cantharidin. An increased incidence has been seen in Peru and Ecuador during years of presentation of the El Niño phenomenon. The same disease, following an identical cycle during El Niño years, is seen in other continents like Africa. In Kenya, different species of *Paederus*, mainly *P. crebinpunctatis*, and *P. sabaeus*, are responsible for the disease (*Nairobi fly*). Clinically, an initial burning is felt followed by erythema and, later, the appearance of a blister, usually in a linear fashion ("latigazo" or whiplash) in exposed parts of the body (Fig. 50-28). The vesication

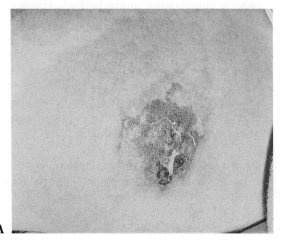
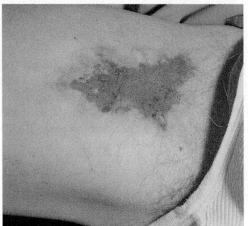

FIGURE 50-25: A: Spider bite (*Loxosceles laeta*), with erythema, central necrosis, and blister formation. **B:** Spider bite (*L. laeta*), with vertical extension of necrosis due to gravity.

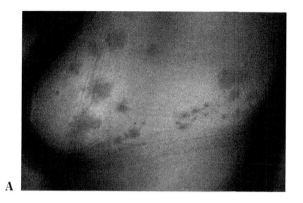

A

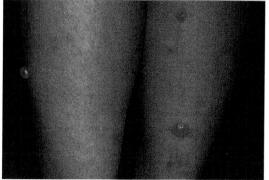

B

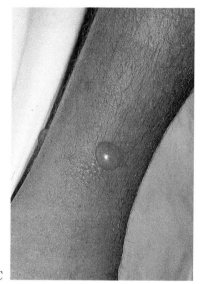

C

FIGURE 50-26: **A:** Chigger bites collected under the bra. **B:** Bullous chigger bites on the legs. **C:** Chigger bite blister formation.

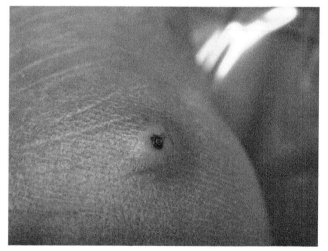

FIGURE 50-27: *Tunga penetrans* on the heel: classic morphology of a black dot at the center of a pustule.

is produced by *paederin*, a protein from the exoskeleton of the insect.

Treatment

Treatment includes compresses, topical corticosteroids, and in some serious cases, oral prednisone and antibiotics.

Papular Urticaria

Papular urticaria defines an exuberant reaction to arthropod bites. Initially, the bite results in a wheal formation, and, later, an intensely pruritic papule develops at the site. Lesions may evolve into hemorrhage, a vesicle, or even a blister, especially in children. A linear array of the lesions, known as breakfast–lunch–supper pattern, is a common characteristic (Fig. 50-29). The number and localization of the lesions depends on the type of exposure and feeding habits of the arthropod. New bites may exacerbate quiescent old bites. Because of scratching, lesions can become infected and crusted. Localization of the affected areas helps reveal the causative arthropod. Involvement of clothing-covered areas and sparing of underwear areas suggests fleas, involvement of the waist and thighs suggests chiggers, involvement of the abdomen and arms suggests sarcoptic mange of dogs, and a generalized eruption suggests bird mites. Flying insects, such as mosquitoes and sandflies, will bite on the face and arms.

Treatment

Treatment consists of oral antihistaminics, topical corticosteroids, and fumigation of the dwelling.

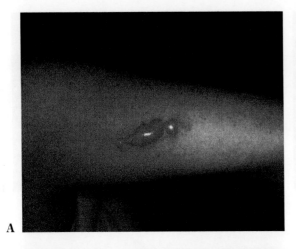

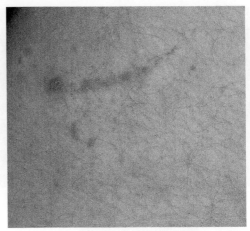

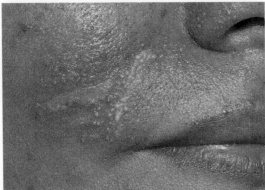

FIGURE 50-28. A: Blister beetle bullous reaction on the arm. **B and C:** Beetle dermatitis, whiplash effect (latigazo).

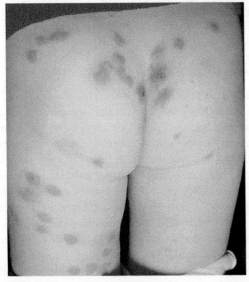

FIGURE 50-29: Papular urticaria: Note how lesions group in a linear array, three or four in a row.

NONINFECTIOUS MISCELLANEOUS DERMATOSES

Pityriasis Alba

This is a very common condition in children. It consists of hypopigmented, poorly defined, scaly macules and plaques found on the face and arms. It is believed to be a mild form of atopic eczema. Lesions accentuate during the summer, and the surrounding sun-affected skin becomes tan.

Treatment

Treatment consists of topical 1% hydrocortisone cream at night and sunscreens during the day. Topical tacrolimus is considered an alternative treatment.

Miliaria

Also known as *prickly heat, sudamina,* or *lichen tropicus,* this condition results from the obstruction of the sweat ducts caused by a combination of extreme heat and humidity. Depending on the level of obstruction, different clinical pictures can be seen. In the so-called *miliaria crystallina,* obstruction is very superficial, resulting in tiny vesicles. In *miliaria rubra,* the obstruction is deeper and clinically more pruritic. The lesions have an erythematous base and consist of tiny, red papules. In *miliaria profunda,* there can be associated anhydrosis, compensatory hyperhydrosis, and so-called *tropical asthenia.* Secondary infections are common. Treatment consists of a cooler environment, loose clothing, fluids by mouth, and antibiotics where indicated for secondary infection.

Pemphigus Foliaceus (Fogo Selvagem)

Fogo selvagem is an endemic type of pemphigus foliaceus, described in the Amazon regions of Brazil and to a lesser extent in other countries in South America. It is clinically identical to the common type of pemphigus foliaceus, except for the young age of the population affected and its common presentation in families. Genetic as well as environmental factors have been implicated in the pathogenesis. Field studies have demonstrated that healthy populations from endemic areas have circulating antibodies against desmoglein 1. The areas of prevalence are regions of wild jungle that have become colonized, for the purpose of farming. The disease may take a self-limited course or, most likely, progress to a generalized form that otherwise is identical to the cosmopolitan forms of pemphigus. The patient may become erythrodermic. The disease follows a chronic course; treatment is based on high-dose corticosteroid therapy as well as other forms of immunosuppressive therapy.

A FINAL WORD

The globalization of present times has made the word "exotic" useless. The patient that one might see in a clinic in a Midwestern city may have just returned from a trip to the Amazon—in less than a 23-hour flight—and the little ulceration he has on his right arm may not be just a simple impetigo but a cutaneous form of leishmaniasis or another heretofore remote condition. A global world means global patients and, thus, requires global thinking. A sufficient history for the dermatology patient should include questions about the faraway places to which he or she may have traveled and the surroundings to which he or she may have been exposed to. In jet age dermatology, just looking and not asking where the patient has been may no longer be enough.

SAUER'S NOTES

1. Ignore the plethora of diseases related to tropical climates in this globalized world, and you will run the risk of missed diagnoses.

2. Where your body has been may have a lot to do with where your health is going.

3. Once again, the skin is at the forefront of early signs of disease, when it is at its most treatable stage.

ACKNOWLEDGMENTS

We are grateful to Dr. Beatriz Bustamante, Dr. Carlos Seas, and the Leishmania Group of the Instituto de Medicina Tropical Alexander von Humboldt of the Universidad Peruana Cayetano Heredia for allowing us to use some of their clinical photos.

Suggested Readings

Bravo F, Sanchez MR. New and re-emerging cutaneous infectious diseases in Latin America and other geographic areas. *Dermatol Clin.* 2003;21(4):655–668.

Elmahallawy EK, Sampedro Martinez A, Rodriguez-Granger J, et al. Diagnosis of leishmaniasis. *J Infect Dev Ctries.* 2014;8(8):961–972.

Fisher AA. *Atlas of Aquatic Dermatology.* Orlando, FL: Grune & Stratton; 1978.

Herman JS, Chiodini PL. Gnathostomiasis, another emerging imported disease. *Clin Microbiol Rev.* 2009;22(3):484–492.

High WA, Bravo FG. Emerging diseases in tropical dermatology. *Adv Dermatol.* 2007;23:335–350.

Kamal SM, Rashid AK, Bakar MA, et al. Anthrax: an update. *Asian Pac J Trop Biomed.* 2011;1(6):496–501.

Koff AB, Rosen T. Nonvenereal treponematoses: yaws, endemic syphilis, and pinta. *J Am Acad Dermatol.* 1993;29(4):519–535; quiz 536–538.

Lotti T, Hautmann G. Atypical mycobacterial infections: a difficult and emerging group of infectious dermatosis. *Int J Dermatol.* 1993;321:499–501.

Lucchina LC, Wilson ME, Drake LA. Dermatology and the recently returned traveler: infectious diseases with dermatologic manifestations. *Int J Dermatol.* 1997;36:167–181.

Lupi O, Tyring SK. Tropical dermatology: viral tropical diseases. *J Am Acad Dermatol.* 2003;49(6):979–1000.

Merritt RW, Walker ED, Small PL, et al. Ecology and transmission of Buruli ulcer disease: a systematic review. *PLoS Negl Trop Dis.* 2010;4(12):e911.

Monge-Maillo B, López-Vélez R. Therapeutic options for old world cutaneous leishmaniasis and new world cutaneous and mucocutaneous leishmaniasis. *Drugs.* 2013;73(17):1889–1920.

Munayco CV, Grijalva CG, Culqui DR, et al. Outbreak of persistent cutaneous abscesses due to *Mycobacterium chelonae* after mesotherapy sessions, Lima, Peru. *Rev Saude Publica.* 2008;42(1):145–149.

Negroni R. Paracoccidioidomycosis. *Int J Dermatol.* 1993;32:847–859.

Owen R. *Gnathostoma spinigerum* n. sp. *Proc. Zool. Soc. (London).* 1836;4:123–126.

Steen CJ, Carbonaro PA, Schwartz RA. Arthropods in dermatology. *J Am Acad Dermatol.* 2004;50(6):819–842; quiz 842–844.

Tyring S, Lupi O, Hengge U. *Tropical Dermatology.* Philadelphia: Elsevier; 2006.

Vetter RS, Visscher PK. Bites and stings of medically important venomous arthropods. *Int J Dermatol.* 1998;37:481–496.

Werner AH, Werner BE. Sporotrichosis in man and animal. *Int J Dermatol.* 1994;33:692–700.

Sports Medicine Dermatology

Rodney S.W. Basler, MD

Parallel to the burgeoning interest of the general population in establishing personal fitness programs, sports-related conditions of the skin resulting from injury, infection, and exacerbation of preexisting dermatosis are presenting with increasing frequency in the offices of dermatologists across the country. In addition, athletes at all levels of competition from junior high school through professional sports are in need of the services of dermatologic practitioners who are well informed in this subset of cutaneous problems. By classifying the various categories of dermatologic issues related to sports medicine into these groupings, a problem-oriented approach to dermatology and sports medicine emerges that will enable the clinician to evaluate these problems in a direct, organized manner (Table 51-1).

ATHLETIC INJURIES

The integument, positioned at the interface between the athlete and the sporting environment, experiences disruption both from acute and long-term application of sports-related external forces. Preventing these injuries, or treating them aggressively to bring about an immediate resolution, greatly enhances a participant's ability to quickly return to workouts and competition.

Friction Injuries

Abrasions

Presentation and Characteristics: Abrasions occur when the granular and keratinized cells of the outer layers of the skin are abruptly removed from the underlying dermis or "true skin." This trauma exposes the lower papillary and reticular dermis, causing punctate bleeding from the severed arterials of the dermal papilla. These pinpoint areas of bleeding within a larger patch of tissue exudate produce the appearance of a lesion referred to in the vernacular as a "raspberry" or "strawberry."

Treatment: The treatment of acute abrasions, as with all other forms of injury, is determined by its severity. Minor abrasions can be treated by gentle cleansing with a mild detergent or a soapless cleanser such as Cetaphil antibacterial bar. A trick used by many trainers is to have a can of mentholated shaving gel in their treatment kit, which also works well for cleansing minor lesions and precludes the need for having clean water on the

TABLE 51-1 • Classification of Dermatologic Issues Related to Sports Medicine
Injury
Friction
Abrasions
Acute traumatic
Turf burn
Chronic
Calluses
Blisters
Chafing
Jogger's nipples
Pressure
Tennis toe
Acne mechanica
Talon noir
Ultraviolet damage
Infections
Bacterial
Impetigo
Occlusive folliculitis
Bikini bottom
Pitted keratolysis
Fungal
Tinea cruris
Tinea pedis
Viral
Plantar warts
Herpes gladiatorum
Molluscum contagiosum
Preexisting Dermatosis
Physical urticaria
Eczema

sideline, although the latter is usually present for preventing dehydration. Bacitracin ointment and a dry dressing can then be applied. This provides a moist environment promoting healing with a minimum of scarring. Larger abrasions, especially those that have been contaminated by the environment, require more aggressive immediate care. Treatments must minimize additional trauma, and aggressive scrubbing, especially with cleansers such as hydrogen peroxide or povidone iodine (which may be cytotoxic), should be avoided. A large "pistol-type" or plunger syringe should be used to irrigate the lesion. Nontoxic surfactant cleansers are the wash of choice.

Proper cleansing is followed by the application of a hydrocolloid or semiocclusive hydrogel dressing that provides a moist healing environment allowing for epithelial migration and prevents the formation of crust or eschar (Fig. 51-1). These artificial barriers can remain in place for 5 to 7 days, and may be covered with padding and tape to allow for continued participation in practice or competition.

Prevention: Preventing abrasions requires little more than a common sense approach to protecting skin potentially exposed to acute trauma. Areas at risk should be covered with protective equipment such as sliding pads, long-sleeved shirts, long socks, "biker" shorts, or a self-adhesive bandage such as Coban.

Turf Burn

Presentation and Characteristics: Turf burn is a related injury that develops when an athlete, most commonly a football or soccer player, has an exposed area of skin slide across artificial turf. Interestingly, the injury is also seen, with some frequency in an ancillary group of athletes, particularly at a collegiate or professional level, namely cheerleaders. As the name implies, the injury results as much from the generation of heat in the skin as from friction, producing an injury that is part abrasion and part burn; artificial turf has a lower coefficient of friction than natural grass, especially when wet.

Treatment: Because the injury is not as deep as that seen with most acute traumatic abrasions, treatment can be less aggressive with cleansing of the area and the application of an antibiotic ointment such as mupirocin or silver sulfadiazine (Silvadene), or an epithelium-stimulating emulsion (Biafine).

Prevention: As with other forms of abrasion, turf burns are best prevented by having specialized equipment, athletic tape, or Coban applied to areas of potential injury.

Chronic Friction Injury

Calluses

Presentation and Characteristics: Calluses present as thick hypertrophied stratum corneum without the characteristic puncta noted with clavi or "hard corns." They represent a compensatory protective response that forms a keratin shield between the outer layers of the skin and an article of equipment, by far the most common being athletic shoes. There is often a history or recently appearing clinical evidence of an anatomic defect underlying the callus. Significant calluses also may be observed on the palmar surface of the hands of boxers, golfers, oarsmen, tennis players (Fig. 51-2), and gymnasts. The latter usually consider calluses to be a competitive advantage, and for that reason, generally do not treat them.

Treatment: Because calluses often represent a protective mechanism of the skin, treatment is usually not necessary. The main reason to approach the lesions is to prevent the formation of painful blisters near the edges of the calluses. Careful paring, usually after soaking, followed by smoothing with a pumice stone or file, usually eliminates the calluses.

Prevention: To a certain extent, calluses are not preventable, and there is no particular reason for concern, unless they interfere with athletic performance or blister formation is a problem. Modification of footwear and the addition of gloves for tennis players and weightlifters are sometimes helpful.

Blisters

Presentation and Characteristics: The appearance of a tender vesicle or bullae, sometimes tinged with blood, over the site

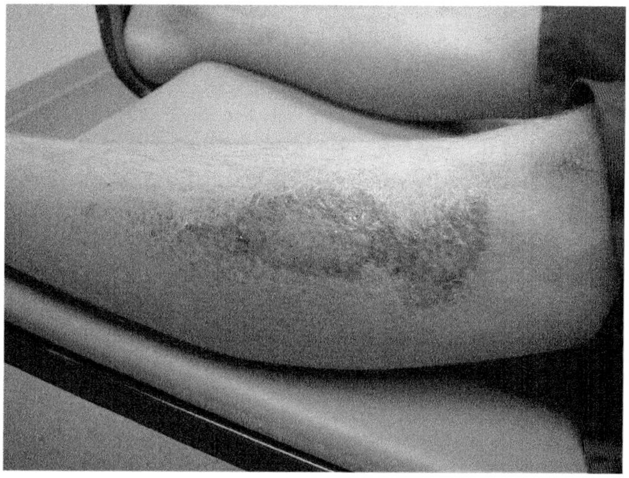

FIGURE 51-1: A resolving deep abrasion treated with hydrocolloid dressing.

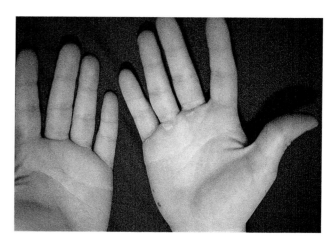

FIGURE 51-2: Calluses on the hand of a high-school tennis player.

of the application of applied force does not usually represent a diagnostic quandary (Fig. 51-3). Unfortunately, especially when unroofed, these lesions cause significant pain and tenderness to the athlete, and may seriously curtail the length or level of competitive activity. During a recent play of the US Open tennis tournament, it was noted that more participants visited the first-aid tent for skin-related problems rather than for all other injuries combined, and the great majority of the problems were blisters.

Treatment: As with most injuries, treatment depends on the size and location of the blister. Small blisters are usually self-limiting and respond to conservative management. It has been shown that the optimal approach to the epidermal "roof" is to leave it intact when possible. The blister should be drained three times at 12-hour intervals for the first 24 hours by using a flamed needle or scalpel. The blister is then covered with a hydrocolloid membrane or tape, either of which can be left in place for 5 to 7 days, allowing for repair of the epithelium.

> ### SAUER'S NOTES
> Leave small blisters intact. Drain large blisters, but leave the roof intact.

Prevention: In general, to help prevent blisters, athletes should increase the length and intensity of exercise workouts gradually, especially when breaking in new shoes or rackets. Early studies in the military proved, unequivocally, that moisture is a major contributory factor and needs to be minimized, especially over the feet. Newer acrylic-composition socks are designed to wick perspiration from the skin at the same time

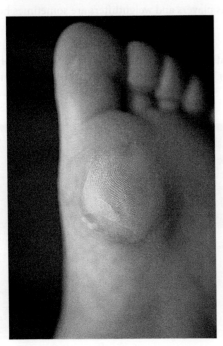

FIGURE 51-3: A large blister on the foot of a high-school tennis player.

that they diminish friction and should be changed every 30 to 60 minutes if they become drenched in sweat. Some athletes also find the application of petroleum jelly or Aquaphor over pressure points to be of considerable benefit.

Chafing

Presentation and Characteristics: Chafing is produced by the mechanical friction between the skin covering two apposing body parts or between the skin and an article of clothing. It is a common problem, familiar to participants of nearly all sports, and presents as bright red, inflamed, abraded patches that are sensitive to the touch. In extreme cases, bleeding may be noted from the area of involvement. Although it is annoying and distracting, the condition usually does not lead to cessation of play. The upper inner thighs and axillae represent the most common distribution, and excess muscle or fat may contribute to the problem.

Treatment: The application of both a lubricating ointment such as triple antibiotic and Aquaphor relieves the symptoms and helps prevent further friction injury.

Prevention: Merely changing the athletic clothing to a fabric that generates less friction may bring about very significant improvement. Any adjustment in the area of involvement that eliminates or diminishes the friction applied to the skin surface ameliorates chafing. As already mentioned, the application of petrolatum or Aquaphor may be very helpful. To decrease moisture, which may play a causative role, some athletes favor absorbent powders.

Jogger's Nipples

Presentation and Characteristics: A painful problem caused by long-term friction applied to a specific body part is the erosions that occur over the areolae and nipples of certain athletes. In extreme cases, the resulting injury may even cause hemorrhage into the clothing or uniform covering the area of involvement. Because the condition is particularly common in long-distance runners, it is usually referred to as *jogger's nipples*. Because most women athletes wear some type of soft protective sports bra, the problem is more common among men than women.

Treatment: Treatment is essentially the same as for all forms of superficial abrasion. The application of an antibiotic ointment covered by a simple dressing such as a Band-Aid is usually sufficient.

Prevention: The most obvious preventative action, of course, is to simply have athletes who are prone to this condition run without a shirt. However, for obvious reasons, this may not be practical. Changing to a softer fabric of running shirt, especially one that does not have a logo, may be beneficial. Friction-reducing ointments may also be helpful, but often are rubbed off over time. Affixing a piece of tape cut exactly to the size and shape of the areola is probably the best preventative measure.

Pressure Injuries

Subungual Hemorrhage

Presentation and Characteristics
The appearance of pooled blood under the plate of the great toenail (Fig. 51-4) is a manifestation of acute bleeding resulting from the repeated forceful contact of the anterior nail plate with the front part of the athletic shoe. Although the injury can be caused by shoes that are too short, it usually results from too small of a toe box. Although tennis players are more commonly affected than participants in other sports (giving rise to the epithet *tennis toe*), the injury is also noted in other sports with the associated terms *jogger's toe* and *skier's toe*. Although acute cases may cause some pain and tenderness, symptoms are usually minimal, and it is not necessary to shorten an exercise or competition schedule.

Treatment: In the acute phase, blood may be drained from beneath the nail with the time-honored flamed paperclip, or with a Geiger cautery if one is available. Soaking in warm water brings about some palliative benefit, as well, and tends to be more popular with affected athletes.

Prevention: Trimming the great toenail, in a straight tangential plane to the shortest point that it does not cause discomfort, is of major benefit. Careful attention to properly fitting shoes, especially ones with a generous toe box, is also recommended. Unfortunately, some athletes who are particularly prone to this condition notice some degree of involvement regardless of attempts to eliminate the problem.

Acne Mechanica

Presentation and Characteristics: Acne mechanica is a papulopustular eruption in the areas beneath heavy padding of certain contact sports, especially football and hockey. It varies in clinical presentation from acne vulgaris in that there is more inflammation, particularly around the papules, and the pustules appear to be more deep-seated. As first described by Mills and Klugman, the condition is produced by the combined factors of pressure, occlusion, friction, and heat. As would be expected, skin changes are most dramatic during the season when the equipment is worn and tend to spontaneously resolve after the season concludes.

Treatment: Acne mechanica responds to a certain, although lesser, extent to entities used to treat acne vulgaris. Rigorous cleansing with a moderately abrasive cleanser, and the use of a back brush, is recommended after each practice session or game. The application of an astringent or keratolytic agent, such as adapalene or retinol, may also be of considerable benefit. Because physical factors play an important role in pathogenesis, systemic antibiotics seem to be of considerably less help in treating the condition than in treating acne vulgaris, but may still be used.

Prevention: The simplest form of prevention of acne mechanica is the wearing of a clean, absorbent, cotton T-shirt under the equipment causing the problem, especially the shoulder pad in football players. The procedures and medications recommended for treatment might also be considered as part of prevention.

Talon Noir

Presentation and Characteristics: The skin change referred to as *talon noir* or *black heel* involves the skin over the calcaneal portion of the foot, and demonstrates asymptomatic color change owing to blue to black punctate petechiae, especially on the posterolateral aspect of the heel. In uncommon cases, the condition may also be seen on the palms of weight lifters, golfers, or tennis players, where it is referred to as *tache noir* or *black palm*. For reasons that are not entirely clear, talon noir is seen almost exclusively in older teenagers and young adults.

Treatment: No treatment is actually warranted, although paring of the overlying keratin will clinically improve or eliminate this essentially cosmetic condition. It usually comes to the attention of caregivers only because of the concern of the patient or their family about the possibility of it representing a malignant melanoma.

Prevention: Although there is probably little that can be done to prevent black heel, properly fitting shoes may contribute to fewer problems.

Ultraviolet Damage

Presentation and Characteristics: Photoinjury to the skin is characterized by the all too familiar, painful, erythematous to deep red, to violaceous changes that occur in exposed skin secondary to overexposure to the ultraviolet rays from the sun. In extreme cases, vesicles, bullae, and even systemic symptoms may accompany this reaction. Participants in nearly all of the outdoor sports are at risk, especially protracted activities, such as fishing, general water sports, and golfing. Long-term ultraviolet damage includes premature aging, premalignant keratosis, and cutaneous malignancy, all of which are among the most preventable diseases to afflict the integument.

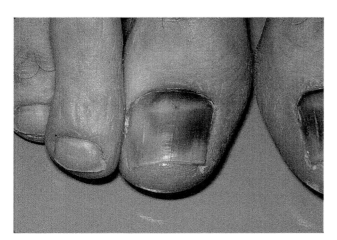

FIGURE 51-4: A subungual hematoma in a high-school tennis player.

Treatment: Although treatment definitely takes a backseat to prevention when dealing with solar injury, nearly all people who participate in any form of outdoor sports and lack deep natural melanotic pigmentation have experienced some level of sunburn. For the milder cases, topical application of an emollient moisturizing agent, with or without minimum potency corticosteroids, usually suffices to bring about significant palliation of symptoms. Systemic over-the-counter anti-inflammatories such as aspirin and ibuprofen are also of value, as are the more potent anti-inflammatories such as prescription nonsteroidal anti-inflammatories and corticosteroids for more severe photoinjury. Many practitioners and patients prefer spray steroids to cover the involved areas because they preclude further irritation and discomfort from an application. Usually a short course, generally 5 to 7 days, of treatment is adequate.

Prevention: The prevention of actinic damage of the skin in the general population is one of the most important and rigorously pursued challenges to face dermatologists. The basic recommendations of limiting outdoor athletic exposure to the hours before 10:00 AM and after 4:00 PM are sometimes impractical. Covering all exposed areas as much as possible with opaque clothing is important, but it might be also be not possible sometimes. Headcovering with a wide brim rather than a cap is advised, but represents protection no greater than a sun protective factor (SPF) of 2 unless a headcovering specifically for sunprotection is used. Ultraviolet Protection Factor or UPF should be 50 or higher. It means one-fiftieth of the ultraviolet rays penetrate the clothing. Sunscreen remains our most valuable line of defense and should optimally be applied 20 to 30 minutes before sun exposure and every 2 to 4 hours during sun exposure, according to the amount of water or perspiration that is diluting the product. An SPF of at least 15 is required, and a product with combined UVB and UVA protection is recommended. Of course, sunscreen must be applied even on cloudy days because the damaging rays can penetrate even through the cloud cover.

INFECTIONS

Bacterial Infections

Impetigo

Presentation and Characteristics: Superficial bacterial infection such as pyoderma or impetigo is a hazard of all contact sports. If community-acquired methicillin-resistant *Staphylococcus aureus* (CA-MRSA) is suspected, a sulfa-based systemic antibiotic should be empirically started, or clindamycin should be given if there is a sulfa allergy. Incision and drainage has been shown to be the procedure of greatest value in all types of bacterial abscesses. As with many sports-related infections, wrestling probably puts its participants at greatest risk, and bacterial skin infections may reach epidemic proportions among wrestling teams and at large wrestling meets. Any thin-roofed vesicle or bullae with purulent fluid or honey-crusted plaque on exposed areas of skin, particularly those extending from a mucous membrane, are suspects for this type of infection.

These may progress rapidly to sharply marginated erosions, sometimes with points of bleeding. Large furuncles or abscesses may rapidly appear with CA-MRSA infections.

Treatment: Treatment should be aggressive, straightforward, and immediate with systemic antibiotics being the main line of defense. The application of a compress made of warm water and antibacterial cleanser eliminates much of the surface bacteria, and the application of an antibacterial cream usually hastens healing as well.

Prevention: Any athlete suspected of carrying bacterial infection must be prohibited from competition. In wrestling, careful and regular sterilization of the mats with an appropriate disinfectant is also a necessity. Showering with an antibacterial soap immediately after competition often prevents infection in athletes as well.

Occlusive Folliculitis

Presentation and Characteristics: Occlusive folliculitis is seen under heavy, protective padding in sports such as football and hockey, much in the same way as is acne mechanica. The deep infection of the follicles with furuncle production and the lack of more superficial inflammatory papules (Fig. 51-5) differentiate these entities. In addition, the area of involvement is more limited and coincides exactly with overlying equipment.

Treatment: As with other bacterial infections, aggressive systemic antibiotic therapy is warranted in occlusive folliculitis, although it may need to be prolonged over several weeks or months during which the causative equipment is in contact with the skin. The topical application of antibiotics used to treat

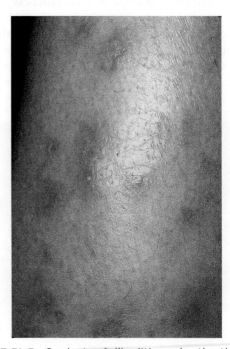

FIGURE 51-5: Occlusive folliculitis under the thigh pad of a collegiate football player.

acne, such as clindamycin or erythromycin, with or without benzoyl peroxide, is also of considerable benefit. If the follicular infection does not respond to these aggressive antibacterial measures, pityrosporum or yeast folliculitis must be considered. In these cases, systemic and topical ketoconazole therapy is usually warranted, sometimes over a protracted course.

Prevention: The application of an absorbent powder over the areas of involvement may be of considerable value. The causative equipment or padding should be removed as quickly as possible after a workout, and any clothing or equipment that comes into direct contact with the skin should be kept as clean as possible, even disinfected if necessary.

Pitted Keratolysis

Presentation and Characteristics: Pitted keratolysis is a superficial infection of the stratum corneum accompanied by the hallmark pungent odor, which has contributed to its alternative designation of *toxic SOCK syndrome*. Examination of the bottom of the foot shows macerated skin, often with a faintly erythematous border and characteristic "punched out" areas. It is only mildly symptomatic to the athlete.

Treatment: The application of over-the-counter acne gels, such as 10% benzoyl peroxide, may be curative for this condition. If this is not adequate treatment, prescription acne medicines such as benzoyl peroxide–clindamycin and benzoyl peroxide–erythromycin products are particularly beneficial.

Prevention: Careful washing of the feet with an antibacterial soap, followed by towel drying and air-drying, is a commonsense approach to the problem. Absorbent powders inside the stocking and the regular application of a 20% aluminum chloride solution also help prevent the condition.

Fungal Infections

Tinea Pedis

Presentation and Characteristics: *Athlete's foot* and *jock itch* indicate the close association of fungal infections with sports. The macerating effect of perspiration in nearly every athletic environment reduces the natural barrier of the epidermis, allowing invasion of fungal elements. Toe webs are usually the first, and generally the most common, site of infection, with spread to the keratin over the soles and lateral aspects of the feet. Marginated erythema and scaling, often with vesicle formation, are noted in areas of involvement. Unilateral distribution is also helpful in differentiating this entity from dyshidrotic eczema. Dystrophic onychomycosis may represent a reservoir of organisms that later spread over the skin.

Treatment: Topical antifungal creams, such as terbinafine and clotrimazole, may be effective in some early superficial cases, but systemic antifungals, such as griseofulvin, fluconazole, itraconazole, or terbinafine, are often required for treatment. When topical medications are used in the toe webs, solutions, sprays, and gels seem to work better than creams or ointments.

If there is a deep commensal infection of the toe web where the infection seems to be potentiated with bacterial overgrowth, broad-spectrum antibiotics such as ciprofloxacin may be indicated.

Prevention: Any procedure that helps keep the stratum corneum dry, thereby maintaining the natural physical barrier to fungal invasion, is beneficial in preventing this infection. The application of a foot powder such as Zeasorb AF or aluminum chloride in patients who show significant maceration is definitely helpful, and the use of shower thongs in the locker room may help those prone to chronic recurrent infections. The long-term administration of a systemic antifungal, such as fluconazole or itraconazole with a dosage as low as 200 mg/month, may be highly effective for prophylaxis.

Tinea Cruris

Presentation and Characteristics: Another time-honored epithet that underscores the association of fungal infection with athletes is *jock itch*. Although this infection presents in the groin, the source of infection is usually an indolent infection of the feet or toenails. When the causative organism is a dermatophyte, the involved area shows erythema and scaling, with a sharp margination, and rarely progresses to the genitals because of the fungistatic effect of sebum in this area. Fungal infections also lack the deep red coloration and satellite lesions seen when yeast is involved. Individual lesions may look particularly innocuous and imitate nummular eczema in wrestlers.

Treatment: Early localized infections may respond to prescription, or even over-the-counter, topical antifungals, such as miconazole, clotrimazole, or terbinafine. Some clinicians favor the older iodochlorhydroxyquin HC preparation. Systemic antifungals may be required in stubborn, persistent cases, and high-dose (250 mg b.i.d.) terbinafine may be required in particularly virulent infections in wrestlers, especially in the hair.

Prevention: Immediate showering after any exercise session with careful attention to removing soap and towel drying of intertriginous regions is strongly recommended. The daily change of sports briefs and attention to choosing those made of an absorbent fabric is also helpful. Absorbent powders in the groin as well as axillae may also prevent infection in these areas, particularly in susceptible wrestlers. Fluconazole at a dosage of 200 to 400 mg/week throughout the entire season may preclude missing important meets because of active fungal lesions.

Viral Infections

Plantar Warts

Presentation and Characteristics: Cutaneous invasion by the human papillomavirus, particularly of the skin of the feet, is relatively common among athletes. The macerating effect of perspiration is a contributing factor as with other forms of infection. In addition, the moist environment of the locker room, especially the showers, provides for a most hospitable environment for causative viruses to live and reproduce. Any area of the plantar portion of the foot may be involved with a very tender hyperkeratotic papule present, often revealing small black dots when the superficial portion is removed. Confluence of individual papules may result in relatively large mosaic warts, and lesions over the weight-bearing portions of the foot may cause considerable morbidity, especially in long-distance runners.

Treatment: In treating these localized viral infections, a conservative approach to therapy is recommended, particularly one that allows for continued practice and competition during therapy. If maceration appears to be a major contributory factor, the application of a 20% aluminum chloride solution or even stronger mixtures containing 10% to 25% formalin often bring about complete resolution with no morbidity. Some physicians and trainers favor the topical application of 50% trichloroacetic acid solution under a 40% salicylic acid plaster, applied once or twice weekly, and followed by vigorous paring. Aggressive ablative therapy, such as excision, electrodesiccation, or laser treatment, holds no curative advantage, and carries a significant risk of short-term disability and even permanent scarring.

Prevention: Wearing shower foot thongs in the locker room decreases the likelihood of coming into contact with the causative virus, whereas foot powders diminish maceration. The regular application of a 20% aluminum chloride solution may also be of considerable preventative value.

Herpes Gladiatorum

Presentation and Characteristics: As implied by its name, this superficial viral infection of the skin is noted almost exclusively in wrestlers, although it may sometimes be seen in other forms of contact and noncontact sports, including basketball. The head, neck, and upper extremities, which are exposed during periods of contact, are usually those noted, with the appearance of grouped vesicles on an erythematous to violaceous base (Fig. 51-6). Dermal edema is usually present, and burning and tenderness are experienced by the athlete.

Treatment: Systemic antivirals are, of course, the primary entity in the arsenal for treating this infection, and should be started immediately when symptoms occur, even before actual skin lesions are noted. Local improvement can be accelerated by unroofing the vesicles and applying benzoin topically, then injecting localized lesions intralesionally with a dilute triamcinolone solution.

Prevention: Athletes with a history of recurrent herpes lesions may greatly benefit from the prophylactic use of acyclovir or valacyclovir. Adequate dosage usually is 400 mg/day of acyclovir or 500 mg/day of valacyclovir. These medications should be started before the training season begins and continued through the course of the competitive schedule. Any athlete with active herpes must be prohibited from competition during the stage of intact or draining vesicles, usually requiring a quarantine period of 4 to 6 days, until all lesions are dry.

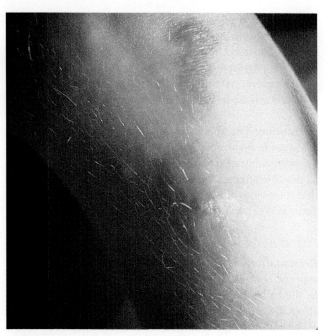

FIGURE 51-6: Herpes gladiatorum in a collegiate wrestler.

Molluscum Contagiosum

Presentation and Characteristics: Again, the venues of competitive wrestling seem to offer the primary athletic source of infection with the large pox virus that causes molluscum contagiosum. Less commonly, these lesions may also be seen in swimmers, and it has been speculated that the solutions used to sterilize pool water are not adequate to completely eliminate the virus. In addition, many athletes may be infected in nonsports arenas, such as "coed wrestling." Small, grouped, waxy papules are usually seen on exposed areas of skin, with individual papules showing a central umbilication in some cases. A linear distribution of lesions referred to as *pseudo-koebnerization* may also be noted, especially in wrestlers.

Treatment: Lesions are easily removed by curettage, even though this leads to superficial abrasions that may preclude contact for a short period of time. Curettage may be easily carried out following the application of a topical anesthetic gel. Liquid nitrogen and tape striping with a highly adhesive tape may also be effective.

Prevention: The prohibition of competition by infected participants is a necessity, and removal of localized individual lesions at their first appearance also helps prevent self-inoculation.

SAUER'S NOTES

Wrestlers are especially prone to staph, herpes simplex, and molluscum infections. These must be treated before competition can be resumed.

PREEXISTING DERMATOSES

Physical Urticarias

Presentation and Characteristics

The physical urticarias, particularly cholinergic urticaria, are most commonly diagnosed through history, although they have a distinctive form of papular erythema with a more punctate dermal edema than that seen with acute allergic urticaria. The erythematous papules are smaller and more distinct, and wheal formation is much less pronounced. The inner aspects of the arms and legs as well as the lateral flanks are common areas of involvement. By history, factors that induce physical urticaria are those indigenous to athletic endeavor, such as rapid temperature changes, especially cold to hot, physical exertion, and emotional stress. Cold urticaria and aquagenic urticaria also fall into this category and can be disabling to swimmers. Pressure urticaria usually appears under articles of athletic equipment.

Treatment

Because of its antiserotonin effect, cyproheptadine is particularly helpful in the physical urticarias. A dosage of 4 mg at bedtime may, in fact, be essentially curative in milder cases. Unfortunately, this antihistamine is quite sedating, and taking the drug the night before a morning competition may leave the athlete in less than prime condition in terms of competitive alertness. Combination therapy with H_1-H_2-inhibiting antihistamines usually works better than a single-drug regimen. In especially difficult cases, corticosteroids, sometimes on a long-term alternate-day schedule, may be required to eliminate the problem. Athletes being administered this course of treatment must be aware of the fact that the older, less specific means of steroid screening may reveal this use of corticosteroids causing them to test positive.

Prevention

The use of prophylactic antihistamines, especially cyproheptadine, as noted, is probably the best precaution to take for athletes who are prone to developing physical urticaria. Otherwise, elimination of the problem may be particularly difficult, short of complete cessation of athletic activity. If the reaction is seen secondary to changes in the temperature, gradual warming or cooling the body may diminish the severity to a certain extent.

Atopic Eczema

Presentation and Characteristics

Most atopes have a lifelong history of skin sensitivity with the characteristic flexural (Fig. 51-7) and facial involvement, and are usually well aware of their problem. Poorly marginated erythema and scaling in the commonly involved areas associated with persistent itching and evidence of excoriation are the hallmark of this condition. Unfortunately, increased body heat and perspiration, which are found in nearly all forms of athletic endeavor, generally exacerbate the condition.

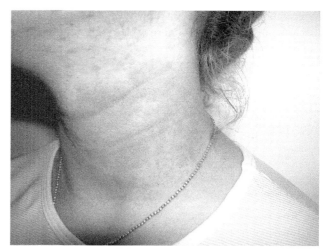

FIGURE 51-7: Eczema of the neck flaring mid-season in an atopic collegiate tennis player.

Treatment

The treatment of sports-induced eczema is essentially the same as that for any patient with atopic eczema, although there may be a need for more aggressive treatment in athletes during their competitive seasons. Topical corticosteroids in emollient creams or ointment bases are the traditional first line of defense, with the newer immunomodulators, tacrolimus and pimecrolimus, more beneficial in patients who have a long-standing history of atopic eczema. Tacrolimus and pimecrolimus may have a significant drawback, however, in that they usually impart a sensation of heat in the skin during periods of exercise, which the athlete may find annoying or distracting. Systemic corticosteroids over varying lengths of time may ultimately be required to bring the condition under control to a point that it does not interfere with athletic performance.

Prevention

Short, tepid showers, using an oil- or cream-based soap immediately following exercise periods to remove sweat are recommended, and should be followed with lubrication with an emollient cream or lotion, or a bath oil. Any of the medications used for treatment may also be considered to be preventative, including the use of antihistamines throughout the course of the season. It is particularly important for patients suffering from eczema to have the condition under the best possible control in the off season so as to preclude the need for aggressive therapy once conditioning becomes more intense.

CONCLUSION

Well-informed, up-to-date medical practitioners who deal with problems of the integument need to have a basic understanding of the care and prevention of cutaneous injuries that pertain to recreational and competitive athletes. Most skin problems that arise in the course of training or general fitness regimens can be treated aggressively and directly and can be prevented through thoughtful planning and preparation. When treated in an immediate and knowledgeable manner, very few of the skin conditions that arise as a result of sports participation need not interfere with an active lifestyle or the pursuit of lofty competitive goals.

SAUER'S NOTES

1. The science of sports medicine has advanced as the importance of exercise has become more apparent.
2. Dermatologists and general practitioners alike need to keep up with this explosion of information in order to keep the athlete off the couch and in the game.

Suggested Readings

Basler RS, Basler DL, Basler GC, et al. Cutaneous injuries in women athletes. *Dermatol Nurs*. 1998;10:9–18.

Basler RS, Basler GC, Palmer AH, et al. Special skin symptoms seen in swimmers. *J Am Acad Dermatol*. 2000;43:299–305.

Basler RS, Garcia MA, Gooding KS. Immediate steps for treating abrasions. *Phys Sportsmed*. 2001;29:69–70.

Basler RS, Garcia MA. Acing common skin problems in tennis players. *Phys Sportsmed*. 1998;25:37–44.

Basler RS. Acne mechanica in athletes. *Cutis*. 1992;50:125–128.

Basler RS. Managing skin problems in athletes. In: Mellion MB, Walsh W, Shelton GL, eds. *Team Physician's Handbook*. 3rd ed. Philadelphia: Hanley & Belfus; 2002:311–325.

Basler RS. Skin injuries in sports medicine. *J Am Acad Dermatol*. 1989;21:1257–1262.

Basler RSW. Sports related injuries in dermatology. In: Callen JP, ed. *Advances in Dermatology*. St Louis: Mosby; 1988:4, 29–50.

Bergfeld WF. Dermatologic problems in athletes. *Clin Sports Med*. 1982;1:419–430.

Eiland G, Ridley D. Dermatological problems in the athlete. *J Orthop Sports Phys Ther*. 1996;23:388–402.

Emer J, Sivek R, Marciniak B. Sports dermatology: traumatic or mechanical injuries, inflammatory conditions, and exacerbation of pre-existing conditions. *J Clin Aesthet Dermatol*. 2015 8(4):31–43.

Levine N. Dermatologic aspects of sportsmedicine. *Dermatol Nurs*. 1994;6:179–186.

Cutaneous Signs of Bioterrorism

Kevin C. Kin, DO, Dane Hill, MD, and Steven R. Feldman, MD, PhD

We are more than a decade out from 9/11, a devastating attack on the United States. There remains, however, significant upheaval and unrest throughout the world, and biologic warfare is an ever-present weapon that threatens people's safety. Physicians should know some fundamentals of recognizing and diagnosing an outbreak associated with biologic agents. Dermatologists have a particularly important role, because most illnesses that arise from biologic agents can have a cutaneous component.

> **SAUER'S NOTES**
>
> The skin is a valuable marker for the diagnosis of diseases associated with bioterrorism.

The Centers for Disease Control and Prevention (CDC) has identified six biologic agents as Category A agents, which pose the greatest risk for use in terrorism (Table 52-1). The assessment of risk is based on the ease of production, ease of dissemination, rate of subsequent person-to-person transmission, lethality, and psychosocial effects (how terrified the community will be). These six agents are smallpox, anthrax, botulism, tularemia, plague, and viral hemorrhagic fevers.

> **SAUER'S NOTES**
>
> Contact your health department or CDC if you have any question regarding a bioterrorism attack. If you are overcautious, then no one is harmed; if you are undercautious, then you have made a potentially grave error.

In smallpox, skin involvement is the most dramatic feature of the disease. For anthrax, cutaneous manifestations are not a central feature, but it is likely that the diagnosis of the index case will be made from cutaneous findings. The other four agents will be briefly discussed highlighting their cutaneous findings.

Category B and C agents, second- and third-highest priority, respectively, are presented in Tables 52-2 and 52-3.

SMALLPOX

> "The patient with smallpox presents a terrible picture. A picture that fully justifies the horror and fright with which smallpox is associated in the public mind."
>
> William Osler from *The Principles and Practice of Medicine*

Historical Aspects

The World Health Organization (WHO) regards smallpox, also called *variola,* as humankind's deadliest disease. Indeed, smallpox has caused perhaps 10% of all human deaths and, even during its waning years in the 20th century, smallpox killed half a billion people. One-third of its victims die. Survivors are usually maimed for life with pocked scars or blindness. Because of the mortality and morbidity associated with smallpox, people long sought ways to prevent, ameliorate, or cure the disease. Fortunately for humankind, smallpox had several characteristics that made it amenable to eradication: There is no subclinical carrier state in humans, the disease is not transmitted by food or water, and there are no animal reservoirs or vectors. The disease occurs only in humans and, during the smallpox era, it was readily diagnosed on a clinical basis alone. A person who survived a bout of smallpox achieved lifelong immunity, and most importantly, smallpox was preventable through vaccination.

The cowpox vaccine, which Edward Jenner used in 1796, and the vaccine that replaced it (one derived from the closely related vaccinia virus) confer near-complete immunity against smallpox. A concerted global vaccination program, led by the health organizations and governments around the world, used the vaccine to quell this disease. The last naturally occurring case was in Somalia in 1977, and in 1980 the WHO proclaimed the eradication of smallpox. Shortly afterward, all laboratory stocks of variola virus were destroyed except for two facilities designated by the WHO: the CDC in Atlanta, Georgia and the State Research Center of Virology and Biotechnology in Novosibirsk, Russia, that maintained small amounts of the virus, putatively for research purposes. There is speculation, however, that stocks of virus are in unmonitored hands. In addition, the ability to synthesize viral genomes in vitro brings these concerns to a new level as the altered or engineered viral strains could have virulence-enhancing properties. Consequently, there is a risk, at least theoretically, that smallpox might recur.

TABLE 52-1 • CDC Category A Agents: Biologic Agents Most Likely to Be Used in Terrorism or Warfare

Disease	Pathogen	Likely Presentation When Used as a Bioweapon	Cutaneous Manifestations	% of Patients in a Bioterrorism Setting Who Have Cutaneous Manifestations
Smallpox	*Variola*, an orthopoxvirus	Classic illness described in chapter	Exanthem followed by classic vesiculopustular eruption predominantly on acral surfaces; "pearls of pus"	100%
Anthrax	*Bacillus anthracis*, an aerobic encapsulated spore-forming gram-positive rod	Inhalational disease starts with flulike presentation and progresses	Edematous papule or plaque evolving into an ulcer surmounted by a black eschar	Roughly 50%
Plague	*Yersinia pestis*, an aerobic gram-negative rod with safety-pin bipolar staining	Fever, weakness, and rapidly developing pneumonia with dyspnea, chest pain, and bloody cough, leading to respiratory failure, shock, and rapid death	Bubonic form from fleabites produces painful tender enlarged lymph nodes (buboes); pneumonic plague may cause DIC with purpura	Not known
Tularemia	*Francisella tularensis*, an aerobic pleomorphic gram-negative coccobacillus	Hemorrhagic bronchopneumonia with fever	If acquired transcutaneously, then an ulceroglandular or lymphocutaneous presentation	Not known
Botulism	Toxin produced by the anaerobic gram-positive rod, *Clostridium botulinum*	Rapid onset of symmetric descending flaccid, paralysis starting in bulbar muscles; afebrile, normal mental status, and no sensory deficits	Facial nerve paralysis, dilated pupils, dry oral mucosa	Presumably most
Viral hemorrhagic fevers	Examples include arenaviruses (e.g., Lassa), filoviruses (Marburg and Ebola)	Flulike illness with fever, myalgia, and extreme fatigue; severe cases have uncontrolled internal and orofacial bleeding	Petechiae, purpura, and hemorrhage	Presumably most

Note: Biologic warfare is defined as the intentional use of microorganisms or toxins to produce death or disease in humans, animals, or plants.
Abbreviation: DIC, disseminated intravascular coagulation.

Presentation and Characteristics

Virology

Smallpox is caused by the variola virus, a member of the *Orthopoxvirus* genus within the poxvirus family. This genus also includes cowpox, vaccinia, monkeypox, and a few other viruses that cause mostly nonhuman disease. The poxvirus family has two other genera, one with the familiar molluscum contagiosum, and the other with the zoonotic disorders of orf and milker's nodules. All members in the poxvirus family are DNA viruses that replicate within the host cell's cytoplasm, unlike many other viruses that replicate inside the nuclei.

Clinical Disease

Smallpox is transmitted primarily in a respiratory manner by droplets from close contact with infected individuals. Fomite transmission, for example from skin crusts, can occur but is rare. It is feared that weaponized smallpox, on the other hand, will be spread long distances through aerosolization of the virus.

Smallpox has three clinical stages. The first, the incubation phase, starts when a person is initially infected with the virus. Incubation lasts approximately 12 to 14 days (range: 7 to 17 days), and during this time, individuals are unaware that they are infected. They feel well, have no clinical manifestations,

TABLE 52-2 • Category B Agents: Second-Highest Priority Biologic Agents to Be Used in Terrorism or Warfare

Agents/Diseases	Pathogen	Likely Presentation When Used as a Bioweapon	Cutaneous Manifestations
Brucellosis (undulant fever)	*Brucella* species	Flulike symptoms (fever, sweats, headache, back pain, and physical weakness)	May cause wound infection
Epsilon toxin	*Clostridium perfringens*	Pulmonary edema leading to renal failure and cardiovascular collapse[a]	None
Food safety threats	*Salmonella* species *Escherichia coli* 0157:H7 *Shigella*	GI symptoms	"Rose spots" in typhoid fever (*Salmonella typhi*)
Glanders	*Burkholderia mallei*	Pulmonary: malaise, headache, pleurisy	Inoculation nodule and lymphadenitis, ulcerated nodule, mucous membrane ulceration with granulomatous reaction
Melioidosis	*Burkholderia pseudomallei*	*Pulmonary*: symptoms of mild bronchitis to severe pneumonia, but normal sputum *Bloodstream*: Usually affects immunosuppressed patients and leads to septic shock *Chronic Suppurative*: Organ abscesses throughout the body	Inoculation through breaks in the skin may form nodules, pustules or subcutaneous abscesses (10%–20%); in children, suppurative parotitis
Psittacosis	*Chlamydia psittaci*	Fever, chills, headache, muscle aches, dry cough, pneumonia	Horder spots (pink macules similar to typhoid rose spots), acrocyanosis, superficial venous thrombosis, splinter hemorrhages, erythema multiforme, erythema nodosum
Q fever	*Coxiella burnetii*	Pneumonia with nonproductive cough due to aerosolization and inhalation of organism; high fever, vomiting, diarrhea	Occasionally can cause erythema nodosum and erythema annulare centrifugum
Ricin toxin	From *Ricinus communis* (castor beans)	*Inhalation*: Sudden onset congestion, respiratory distress (possibly leading to respiratory failure), flulike symptoms (fever, nausea, muscle pain) *Ingestion*: mucosal ulceration and hemorrhage leading to severe GI distress; splenic, hepatic, and renal bleeding[a,b]	Allergic reaction: Erythema, vesication, irritation, and pain may occur
Staphylococcal enterotoxin B	From specific strains of *Staphylococcus aureus*	*Inhalation*: Flulike symptoms, respiratory distress, chest pain, cough *Ingestion*: food poisoning symptoms (nausea, vomiting, abdominal cramping, diarrhea)[a,b]	None
Typhus fever	*Rickettsia prowazekii*	Malaise, myalgia, headache, fever, chills; neurologic symptoms such as meningismus and coma may develop	Centrifugally spreading eruption that spares the palms and soles; begins as erythematous, nonconfluent, blanching macules that become maculopapular and petechial

TABLE 52-2 • Category B Agents: Second-Highest Priority Biologic Agents to Be Used in Terrorism or Warfare (*continued*)

Agents/Diseases	Pathogen	Likely Presentation When Used as a Bioweapon	Cutaneous Manifestations
Viral encephalitis	Alphaviruses (Eastern equine encephalitis, Venezuelan equine encephalitis, and Western equine encephalitis)[c] Flaviviridae (Japanese encephalitis, St. Louis encephalitis, West Nile Virus) Bunyaviridae, Arenaviridae, Paramyxoviridae[d]	Decreased consciousness, seizures, focal neurologic signs, encephalitis,[c] fever, headache, flulike symptoms, nausea, vomiting, diarrhea[d]	Facial/periorbital edema, jaundice, flushing, lymphadenopathy, alopecia, palatal vesicular or petechial-eruption, cutaneous morbilliform or petechial eruption may be present[d]
Water safety threats	*Vibrio cholerae* (cholera) *Cryptosporidium parvum* (cryptosporidiosis)	Nausea, vomiting, headache, diarrhea (described as rice-water stool in cholera)	Skin infection through open wound and hemorrhagic bullous lesions have occurred with *Vibrio*, but are very rare

[a]Marks JD. Medical aspects of biologic toxins. *Anesthesiol Clin North America.* 2004;22:509–532, vii; Lupi O, Madkan V, Tyring SK. Tropical dermatology: bacterial tropical diseases. *J Am Acad Dermatol.* 2006;54:559–578.
[b]Henghold WB. Other biologic toxin bioweapons: ricin, staphylococcal enterotoxin B, and trichothecene mycotoxins. *Dermatol Clin.* 2004;22:257–262, v.
[c]Donaghy M. Neurologists and the threat of bioterrorism. *J Neurol Sci.* 2006;249:55–62.
[d]Bossi P, Tegnell A, Baka A, et al. Bichat guidelines for the clinical management of viral encephalitis and bioterrorism-related viral encephalitis. *Euro Surveill.* 2004;9:E21–E22.
Source: From the CDC website unless otherwise indicated.

TABLE 52-3 • Category C Agents: Third-Highest Priority Biologic Agents to Be Used in Terrorism or Warfare

Pathogen	Used as a Bioweapon	Likely Presentation When Cutaneous Manifestations	Disease
Nipah encephalitis	Nipah virus	Fever, headache, mental distortion (drowsiness, giddiness, confusion), possible respiratory illness, neurologic deficits	None
Hantavirus pulmonary syndrome	Hantavirus	Fatigue, fever, myalgia, headache, dizziness, vomiting, diarrhea, shortness of breath	Rash is uncommon

Source: From the CDC website unless otherwise indicated.

and cannot transmit the virus to others. The second stage, the prodrome, begins with a sudden high fever (typically 102° to 105°F) accompanied by severe headache, backache, and malaise. The patient is viremic, appears toxic, is often prostrate with pain, and may be delirious. After 2 to 4 days, the prodrome ends with a slight defervescence and the appearance of an oropharyngeal enanthem. This marks the beginning of the eruptive stage during which the patient is infectious. The classic exanthem has several distinctive features (Fig. 52-1). Individual lesions evolve gradually through several morphologic forms over 14 to 18 days. Lesions progress from macules to papules to vesicles to umbilicated vesicles to pustules to crusted scabs, with each form lasting 1 to 2 days. The smallpox patient is infectious from the onset of the enanthem until all scabs have

separated, roughly 20 to 25 days later. In people who received vaccinations less than 10 years before exposure to smallpox, historical case fatality rates were 1% to 3%.

An important diagnostic feature of smallpox is that at any one time, all lesions are in the same morphologic stage of development in the region of the body. In contrast, chickenpox lesions progress rapidly and asynchronously; thus, all morphologic forms (e.g., papules, vesicles, pustules, and crusts) are typically present at any moment in the same region of the body. Classic smallpox lesions are most abundant on acral surfaces (face, palms, and soles), whereas in chickenpox, lesions are most abundant centrally (on the trunk). Furthermore, the delicate lesions of classic chickenpox are described as "dewdrops on a rose petal," but firm smallpox lesions can

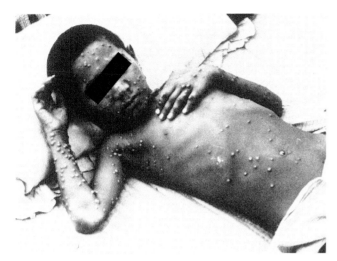

FIGURE 52-1: The classic exanthem of smallpox (variola major) shows pustules with uniform morphology, more prominent on acral surfaces. In the past, one-third of unvaccinated individuals who acquired smallpox died of the disease. The survivors were usually marked with pitted scars called *pocks*, and many were blinded by smallpox as well. (Courtesy of the James H. Graham, MD, and Gloria F. Graham, MD Dermatopathology Library.)

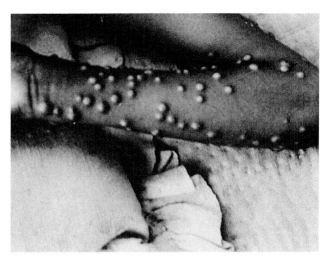

FIGURE 52-2: Smallpox lesions can be described as "pearls of pus"—they are firm, deep-seated, globose, opalescent papules, and pustules. (Courtesy of the James H. Graham, MD, and Gloria F. Graham, MD Dermatopathology Library.)

be described as "pearls of pus"—they are deep-seated, globose, opalescent papules and pustules (Fig. 52-2).

Types of Smallpox

About 90% of patients with smallpox present with ordinary type (see Fig. 52-1) in which individual pustules are either discrete (surrounded by normal-appearing skin) or coalesce with one or two neighboring pustules. Two variants of small-pox, the hemorrhagic type and the malignant (or flat) type, have especially poor prognoses. *Hemorrhagic smallpox* is characterized by disseminated intravascular coagulation (DIC) and purpura. It seems to occur more frequently in pregnant women. *Malignant smallpox* is characterized by innumerable flat lesions that cover the entire skin, producing an edematous appearance that resembles anasarca. This form produces neither classic pustules nor scabs. Both hemorrhagic and malignant smallpox have mortality rates of more than 95%.

Diagnosis

Naturally occurring disease has not existed since 1977, and there is no absolute confirmation that stocks of smallpox virus are in the hands of anyone who would use them. Therefore, practitioners confronted by a patient with fever and pustules should remind themselves to look for alternative explanations. The CDC has an algorithm for the evaluation of suspected smallpox and offers a differential (Table 52-4). The algorithm *Evaluating patients for smallpox: acute, generalized vesicular or pustular rash illness protocol* is available on the CDC's website (https://www.emergency.cdc.gov/agent/smallpox/diagnosis/). According to the CDC algorithm, if smallpox cannot be ruled

TABLE 52-4 • Differential Diagnosis for Febrile Patient With Vesicles and Pustules

Chickenpox

Disseminated herpes zoster

Disseminated herpes simplex

Impetigo

Pustular drug eruptions

Erythema multiforme

Enteroviral infections (especially hand, foot, and mouth disease)

Infected arthropod bites

Contact dermatitis

Monkeypox

Molluscum contagiosum (in immunocompromised patients)

out, then infectious disease and/or dermatology have to be consulted immediately consult and local and state public health authorities should be alerted.

A thousand years ago and today, the disease that most closely resembles smallpox is chickenpox. A typical presentation of chickenpox will not resemble smallpox, but as a variant presentation, one perhaps with a few more acral lesions and a higher temperature may resemble smallpox. If faced with a patient in whom smallpox is in the differential diagnosis, the physician should institute the same infection control precautions used for chickenpox or other respiratory diseases, then review the key clinical differences between the two diseases (Table 52-5), consult the CDC algorithm, and attempt to establish the diagnosis of another disease (see Table 52-4). In other words, by ruling in chickenpox or another disease, one can rule out smallpox. Disseminated herpes simplex and disseminated herpes zoster

TABLE 52-5 • Clinical Presentations of Classic Chickenpox and Smallpox

Chickenpox	Smallpox
Mild or no prodrome	Febrile prodrome
Superficial vesicles	Deep pustules
"Dew drops on a rose petal"	"Pearls of pus"
Individual lesions evolve rapidly	Individual lesions evolve gradually
Lesions with different morphologies	Lesions with same morphology
Central predominance	Acral predominance
Spares palms and soles	Involves palms and soles
Patient is rarely toxic	Patient is usually toxic or moribund

may also resemble smallpox. There are ongoing, scattered, small outbreaks of zoonotic monkeypox in equatorial Africa; this is a poxvirus infection that also resembles smallpox.

Although clinical judgment is important, laboratory confirmation of the cause of a patient's febrile, vesicopustular eruption is critical. In the past, electron microscopic examination was used to look for the classic brick- or dumbbell-shaped cytoplasmic virions of poxviruses. Viral culture was an effective but slow diagnostic technique. Today, polymerase chain reaction (PCR), direct flourescent antibody (DFA), immunohistochemical techniques, and in situ hybridization offer alternative—and more rapid—means to differentiate between poxviruses and herpesviruses.

Vaccination

The smallpox vaccine is the most successful immunization ever devised. Once the WHO declared smallpox's demise, there was no further need to continue to vaccinate populations with live vaccinia virus. In the United States and most other developed nations, compulsory vaccination against smallpox ceased in the early 1970s. Shortly after the attacks of September 11, 2001 and the 2001 anthrax attack, however, smallpox vaccination has been made available once again for certain emergency response personnel, law enforcement officials, medical staff, and the military. In 2003, the CDC recommended vaccination for persons who might be first-responders after a smallpox outbreak. Each state and territory was advised to maintain a smallpox response team that includes vaccinated individuals. Some of these teams would undoubtedly consist of dermatologists for their expertise in skin biopsies and diagnosis.

Unvaccinated health care workers who are exposed to a patient with smallpox can take reassurance in the rapid efficacy of the smallpox vaccine. It works so quickly that postexposure vaccination, even up to 4 to 5 days after exposure, prevents the disease from progressing through the 12-day asymptomatic incubation stage into the symptomatic or infectious stages of the disease. Furthermore, recent studies show that remote vaccination (i.e., smallpox vaccination several decades earlier) seems to confer longer-lasting immunity than originally believed.

Because there are many relative contraindications to vaccination, it is usually not necessary to vaccinate unless there has been a history of recent exposure. Because the vaccine contains a live virus, it should not be administered to persons who are pregnant or immunocompromised. Voluntary vaccination is not recommended for individuals with a history of heart disease or multiple risk factors for heart disease as there is risk for developing myopericarditis. Use of steroid eye drops, nonemergency vaccination of patients below 18 years of age, and emergency vaccination of patients below age 1 year are also contraindications.

Patients with atopic dermatitis—active or quiescent—or those who have a remote history of atopic dermatitis should not be vaccinated because of the risk of eczema vaccinatum (Fig. 52-3A). In this condition, the immunologic defects associated with atopic dermatitis render these individuals vulnerable to unchecked replication of the live vaccinia virus over the entire skin. Eczema vaccinatum can be fatal. Another possibly lethal complication is progressive vaccinia, which occurs in immunocompromised patients vaccinated by or inadvertently infected with vaccinia (Fig. 52-3B and C). The inoculation site lesion expands and becomes centrally necrotic. Vaccinia infection can spread inexorably through the compromised person's skin and organs. Other complications of smallpox vaccination include allergic reactions, vaccinia keratitis, generalized vaccinia, myopericarditis, postvaccinial encephalitis, and superinfection. Vaccinia immune globulin may be used to manage complications.

Institutions that administer the smallpox vaccine should maintain a vigilant monitoring program to examine the postvaccination response. The desired, normal response to vaccination is a "Jennerian pustule," an exuberant, umbilicated pustule at the vaccination site. Vaccination programs should instruct patients on hygiene practices to prevent autoinoculation and contact infection. If there is a laboratory-confirmed case of smallpox, vaccination guidelines would be modified to emphasize widespread protection of the potentially exposed population.

Treatment

CDC recommendations include supportive therapy and antibiotics for any secondary bacterial infections. Postexposure vaccination (with greatest efficacy if given within 1 to 3 days after exposure) can prevent disease or decrease disease severity. No antiviral has been approved for the treatment of smallpox, although cidofovir may be used in the event of an outbreak. Brincidofovir, a cidofovir prodrug, currently shows some promise. Research evaluating new treatments for both smallpox and adverse vaccination reactions is ongoing.

SAUER'S NOTES

Chickenpox and smallpox can be a difficult clinical differential. Questions about exposure from a lab that might harbor the smallpox is wise counsel.

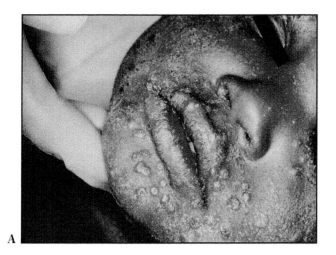

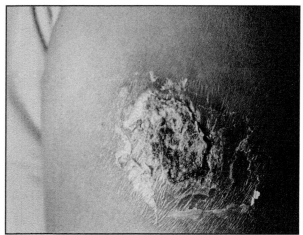

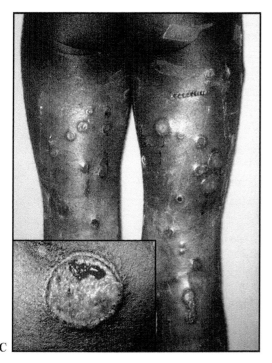

FIGURE 52-3: Smallpox vaccine reactions. **A:** Eczema vaccinatum. **B:** Necrotizing vaccinia. **C:** Progressive Vaccinia in AIDS. (Courtesy of the James H. Graham, MD, and Gloria F. Graham, MD, Dermatopathology Library.)

ANTHRAX

Anthrax is one of the oldest diseases known to humankind. It is a naturally occurring bacterial disease caused by the aerobic gram-positive rod, *Bacillus anthracis*. Typically, anthrax occurs in rural areas where it is associated with domesticated ruminants (sheep, cattle, and goats). Its historical importance includes several "firsts." It was the first bacterium seen under the microscope, the first organism to satisfy Koch's postulates, the first bacterial disease to have an effective vaccine, and the first bioterrorism agent of the 21st century.

When exposed to harsh environmental conditions, the rods of *B. anthracis* transform into spores that can remain dormant in soil for decades, impervious to heat, cold, desiccation, and solar radiation. These hardy spores are 1 to 2 μm in diameter and can be easily aerosolized and inhaled. *Woolsorter disease* is the name for the occupational illness caused by the inhalation of anthrax spores aerosolized during the handling

of unprocessed wool and animal hides. The mortality rate of untreated inhalational anthrax exceeds 90%. Thus, easy weaponization of this highly lethal agent makes it one of the most feared biologic weapons. During the Cold War, several nations produced massive quantities of weaponized anthrax, evidence of which became well known after a mishap at a Soviet bioweapons facility in 1979. A cloud of anthrax spores was accidentally released, and more than a hundred people downwind in the town of Sverdlosk died from inhalational anthrax.

Perhaps 95% of naturally occurring anthrax manifests as cutaneous disease, usually in agrarian settings. The Sverdlosk disaster, however, led to the notion that weaponized anthrax caused only inhalational illness. The letter-borne anthrax incidents of late 2001 in the United States, however, showed otherwise: Only 11 of the 22 victims had inhalational disease. The other 11 had cutaneous anthrax. Between 2009 and 2013, multiple outbreaks of anthrax occurred in heroin users in the United Kingdom, Denmark, France, and Germany.

Clinical Features

Cutaneous anthrax develops when spores enter minor, often unnoticed, breaks in the skin of a mammal. Typical sites are exposed surfaces of the hands, legs, and face (Fig. 52-4). In the hospitable environment, the spores are activated; they revert to rods and begin producing toxins. A dermal papule, often resembling an arthropod bite reaction, develops over several days and soon evolves into a painless edematous ulcer with a central black eschar. One to several lesions may appear, depending on the manner of inoculation. There may be regional lymphadenitis, malaise, and fever. Individual lesions often look pustular, leading to the phrase "malignant pustule." Nevertheless, they contain no pus. In fact, histologic examination of cutaneous anthrax shows edema and necrosis with no inflammatory infiltrate. This is because anthrax is a toxin-mediated disease, an important point because antibiotic treatment of anthrax kills the bacteria but does not alter the course of already-produced toxins.

Diagnosis

Dermatologists played a pivotal role in the diagnosis of anthrax in the letter-borne anthrax incidents of autumn 2001. The acute onset of a painless edematous noduloulcerative lesion with a black eschar should invoke the clinical diagnosis of cutaneous anthrax. Other entities to consider are listed in Table 52-6. The CDC requests that practitioners notify local or state health departments before attempting a laboratory diagnosis of cutaneous anthrax. The American Academy of Dermatology's *Cutaneous Anthrax Management Algorithm* leads one through the proper steps to swab exudates for Gram stain

TABLE 52-6 • Differential Diagnosis for Cutaneous Anthrax

Differential Diagnosis of Eschar and Ulceration

Cutaneous anthrax	Cutaneous diphtheria
Brown recluse spider bite	Orf/Milker nodule
Coumadin necrosis	Plague
Cutaneous leishmaniasis	Rat bite fever
Cutaneous tuberculosis	Pyoderma gangrenosum
Ecthyma gangrenosum	Staphylococcal ecthyma (especially due to methicillin-resistant *S. aureus*)
Glanders	Streptococcal ecthyma
Heparin necrosis	Tropical ulcer
	Tularemia
Antiphospholipid antibody syndrome ulcers	
Opportunistic fungal infections (e.g., due to aspergillosis or mucormycosis)	
Scrub typhus, tick typhus, and rickettsialpox	

Differential Diagnosis for Ulceroglandular Syndromes

Cat scratch disease	Plague
Chancroid	Staphylococcal
Glanders	Streptococcal adenitis
Herpes simplex infection	Syphilis
Lymphogranuloma venereum	Tuberculous adenitis
Melioidosis	Tularemia

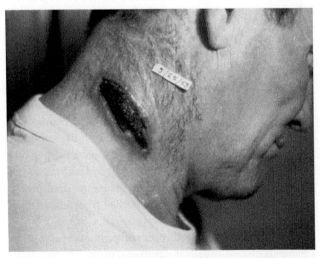

FIGURE 52-4: Lesion of cutaneous anthrax on the neck. Note the central black eschar surrounded by a red rim. The word anthrax derives from the Greek term for burning coal, anthracis. (Courtesy of the Public Health Image Library of the Centers for Disease Control and Prevention.)

and culture, to obtain biopsy specimens for histopathology and immunohistochemical staining, and to draw blood samples for culture and serology.

Patients with inhalational anthrax often present with a flulike illness that rapidly progresses into a severe illness. Inhalational anthrax can be confirmed by examination, culture, or PCR of blood or aspirated pleural fluid. A distinctive radiographic feature of inhalational disease is a widened mediastinum without evidence of a primary pulmonary disorder such as pneumonia.

Treatment

Naturally occurring cutaneous anthrax is susceptible to penicillin and doxycycline, but weaponized anthrax may have been engineered to be resistant to these antibiotics. Therefore, a fluoroquinolone such as ciprofloxacin is recommended for initial treatment of confirmed or suspected anthrax, even in pregnant women and children in whom this class of antibiotic is rarely administered. Once drug sensitivities have been established, the patient may be switched to another antibiotic as clinically indicated. As mentioned, antibiotics kill activated *B. anthracis* rods but do not reverse the effects of toxins that have been produced. Surgical alteration of the cutaneous lesions may exacerbate the injury and therefore is not recommended unless antibiotics are started concurrently. Untreated cutaneous anthrax has a 20% fatality rate. For systemic anthrax, antitoxin, such as raxibacumab or anthrax immunoglobulin, is added to antibiotic therapy.

Although cutaneous anthrax is usually an uncomplicated and readily treatable infection, public health ramifications warrant hospitalization. Standard universal precautions are appropriate, but specific measures against secondary respiratory transmission are unnecessary. Unlike smallpox, anthrax cannot be transmitted from person to person; it is acquired only via exposure to spores, not to the activated bacilli found in people with clinical disease.

Prophylaxis

Anthrax vaccine absorbed (AVA) is the FDA-approved vaccine in the United States and is used regularly by veterinarians, laboratory workers, and animal handlers. The US military uses this vaccine to prevent combat-related exposure to aerosolized anthrax spores, although this remains controversial. The vaccine is administered at 0, 2, and 4 weeks and 6, 12, and 18 months with yearly boosters. If an outbreak were to arise, this complex schedule would cause difficulties in maintaining supplies and vaccinating the public. Research in creating a better vaccine is underway.

BOTULISM

Although a bioterrorism attack involving botulism has never occurred, it is considered an ideal bioweapon. Aerosolization of botulinum toxin would be the most likely method of release in a bioterrorism attack, but other methods such as intentional injection of the toxin by adding it to injectable medications, food-borne botulism by adding it to a food source, and water contamination could also pose a threat.

Botulism occurs when a neurotoxin from *Clostridium botulinum* is absorbed through mucosal membranes or via a wound. *Clostridia* are anaerobic, gram-positive bacilli that form extremely hardy spores. They are found in soil, salt and freshwater sediments, and in the gastrointestinal tract of many animals. There are six clinical syndromes of botulism that include food-borne, infant, wound, adult intestinal toxemia, inhalational, and iatrogenic.

Clinical Features

This section focuses on the clinical features of *wound botulism* as this is most relevant to the dermatologist. This would not be the primary syndrome in a bioterrorist attack, but it is likely that aerosolized botulinum toxin would infect open wounds. In a nonbioterrorist setting, wound botulism is sometimes seen among intravenous drug users who use a technique of injecting black tar heroin subcutaneously called

"skin popping." In an incidence reported by the CDC, the "black tar heroin" (a brown-to-black-colored form of crudely processed heroin commonly from Mexico) is probably contaminated with spores when the heroin is "cut" with dirt or boot polish. Through tissue necrosis and the formation of an abscess, an anaerobic environment is created where *Clostridia* can thrive. As a bioweapon, contamination of wounds with the neurotoxin could also lead to the same result. As with the other syndromes, cranial nerve dysfunction and symmetric descending paralysis ensue.

Diagnosis

The standard method of diagnosis is the mouse bioassay. This method is slow, labor-intensive, and uses live animals. Other options available are real-time PCR (a good option for wound botulism), rapid mass spectrometry (equal sensitivity to the mouse assay), and ELISA testing (a fast screening technique that is less sensitive).

Treatment

Treatment is mostly supportive, and patients should be monitored for respiratory failure. Antitoxin should be given to prevent progression of paralysis. For wound botulism, debridement and antibiotics are recommended to prevent polymicrobial infection.

Vaccine

A vaccine for laboratory personnel in contact with *C. botulinum* had been available from 1965 to 2011, but was discontinued due to decreased immunogenicity of certain toxin serotypes and increase in adverse local reactions.

TULAREMIA

Like botulism, there is no recorded use of tularemia in a bioterrorist attack. Even then, the United States maintained it as a biologic weapon until 1970, and other countries have maintained it as well. If tularemia were to be used as a biologic weapon, aerosol release would be the most probable method leading to an outbreak of pleuropneumonitis, but there would likely be some instances of cutaneous manifestations as aerosolized bacteria might enter broken skin or mucocutaneous surfaces. This cutaneous clinical presentation is described here.

Tularemia is caused by *Francisella tularensis*, an aerobic, intracellular, gram-negative coccobacillus that does not form spores, but instead survives for weeks in water, soil, hay, animal hides, and carcasses. Although tularemia is often called rabbit or deerfly fever because of historically common routes of transmission, the most common vectors today are ticks. Contact with blood or tissues from infected animals, ingestion of contaminated water or meat, and inhalation of aerosols may also transmit the infection. Although tularemia is most often associated with rabbits, other small animals including squirrels, beavers, and rodents are also reservoirs for the disease.

Clinical Features

Tularemia is characterized by seven clinical syndromes including ulceroglandular, glandular, oculoglandular, oropharyngeal, typhoidal, pneumonic, and septic syndromes. Ulceroglandular tularemia is the most common presentation in nature and is the most relevant presentation to the dermatologist. A tender or pruritic papule marks the site of inoculation (most commonly on an exposed extremity) approximately 2 to 5 days after cutaneous exposure. This papule will enlarge to form a sharply demarcated ulcer with a yellowish exudate (Fig. 52-5). Eventually, it develops a necrotic base and may form a black eschar. Regional lymphadenopathy is also present. Ulcers may persist for months and heal leaving a scar.

In addition to the ulceroglandular form itself, "tularemids" are secondary skin eruptions that may appear on the face or extremities in any of the seven clinical forms of tularemia. They can range from papular or macular to petechial, vesicular, or pustular and generally emerge in the second week. Erythema nodosum, erythema multiforme, and Sweet syndrome have also been described as nonspecific secondary manifestations.

Diagnosis

Serology is the most frequent method of diagnosis, although other methods are available. Other methods include fluorescent-labeled antibodies for microscopic examination of tissues or smears; culture of tissue, blood, exudates, and sputum samples; histologic examination of tissue; and PCR. Histology would show a neutrophilic infiltrate early in the disease and a granulomatous response later.

Treatment and Postexposure Prophylaxis

The CDC offers different recommendations for individual cases or mass casualty settings. In isolated cases, streptomycin or gentamicin is recommended for adults, children, and pregnant women. In the setting of a mass casualty, doxycycline

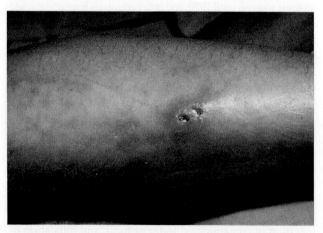

FIGURE 52-5: This sharply demarcated tularemia ulcer formed from a pruritic papule at the site of inoculation. It may evolve into a black eschar. (Courtesy of the James H. Graham, MD, and Gloria F. Graham, MD, Dermatopathology Library.)

and ciprofloxacin are recommended for both treatment and postexposure prophylaxis. Prophylactic treatment for close contacts and isolation precautions are not necessary as there is no person-to-person transmission.

Vaccine

There is no longer an available tularemia vaccine because of concerns about vaccine stability, attenuation, and production. Research is currently being conducted to develop new vaccines.

PLAGUE

It is estimated that 200 million deaths throughout the course of history have been attributed to plague. Because of its high mortality and the panic associated with outbreaks of the disease, it is of great concern as a bioweapon. During World War II, Japanese army units used plague-infected fleas as bioweapons against civilian Chinese populations. Even in the United States, there has been an average of seven new cases and one death per year over the past 10 years.

Plague is caused by *Yersinia pestis*, belonging to the Enterobacteriaceae family, a gram-negative coccobacillus usually transmitted by flea bite or through inadvertent percutaneous inoculation after handling an infected animal. The three forms of the disease are bubonic, pneumonic, and primary septicemic plague.

If the bacterium were used as a bioweapon today, it would most likely be used in an aerosolized form leading to primary pneumonic plague. This manifestation of the disease is rare in the United States and should raise suspicion of bioterrorism.

Clinical Features

Historically, bubonic plague is the most common form. It begins as a skin pustule at the inoculation site and progresses to local or regional lymphadenitis. The swollen, tender lymph nodes are referred to as buboes. The disease may then spread through the lymphatic system. Necrosis of the involved nodes may result in septicemia or secondary yersinial pneumonia. In the pneumonic and septicemic forms, patients may develop cyanosis, petechiae, purpura, ecchymoses, and acral gangrene, also known as "Black Death."

Diagnosis

Culture and staining of bubo aspirate, cerebrospinal fluid, blood, or sputum is the standard method of diagnosis. Direct microscopy of the bubo aspirate, direct immunofluorescence assay, serology, and PCR are also possible. Rapid diagnostic tests have been developed that detect F1 antigen of *Y. pestis* within 15 minutes.

Treatment

It is recommended to isolate any patient with suspected plague for at least 72 hours. Antibiotics should be started immediately upon suspicion of this diagnosis. The CDC recommends the use of IM injection of streptomycin, but owing to limited availability, gentamicin is usually used. In a mass causality setting, oral doxycycline is the treatment of choice. Ciprofloxacin may also be used orally.

Prophylaxis

If a plague outbreak were to occur, patients with symptoms, such as fever, should receive antibiotics immediately. Those in close contact with infected individuals, but without symptoms, are recommended to take a 7-day course of doxycycline as postexposure prophylaxis. The plague vaccine was discontinued in 1999, but research is in progress to develop a new vaccine.

VIRAL HEMORRHAGIC FEVERS

The CDC classifies viral hemorrhagic fevers as "a group of illnesses that are caused by several distinct families of viruses." More than 25 viruses from four families (Filoviridae, Flaviviridae, Bunyaviridae, and Arenaviridae) can cause viral hemorrhagic fevers. The Marburg, Ebola, Lassa, Junin, and Marchupo viruses are of special note because the former Soviet Union had weaponized these viruses. In August 2014, the WHO declared the West Africa Ebola outbreak a Public Health Emergency of International Concern. As of the update of this chapter, there have been 28,454 reported cases and 11,297 deaths worldwide, with the vast majority occurring in Sierra Leone, Liberia, and Guinea. Our discussion will mainly focus on two filoviruses—Ebola and Marburg.

Clinical Features

Viral hemorrhagic fever is a multiorgan system syndrome generally leading to hematologic collapse and is characterized by acute onset of high fever associated with malaise, fatigue, dizziness, weakness, myalgia, diarrhea, and headache. Bleeding under the skin, from internal organs, or from body orifices is also common. Hemorrhagic signs such as petechiae, epistaxis, hematemesis, puncture site bleeding, and bleeding gums manifest themselves in most infected individuals. Progression to DIC is also possible.

Other cutaneous signs commonly may arise. A nonpruritic morbilliform eruption may appear approximately 5 days after a filovirus infection. Generally, the eruption is located on the extremities or trunk and begins in patches that later coalesce and desquamate. Burning and paresthesias may also be associated with the disease whether or not an eruption is apparent.

Diagnosis

Evaluating patients with viral hemorrhagic fevers can be hazardous for health care personnel because collected tissues and fluids can easily transmit the infection. Ebola is diagnosed through culturing the virus, RT-PCR, antigen-capture ELISA, and IgM ELISA. In the 1995 Ebola outbreak in Kikwit, Congo/Zaire, skin biopsies were taken postmortem from infected individuals, and immunohistochemical staining detected the Ebola virus with the same accuracy as the ELISA method.

Treatment

Strict infection control measures, aggressive fluid and electrolyte repletion, and additional supportive care are the only treatments for viral hemorrhagic fevers. There are currently no recommendations for postexposure prophylaxis interventions. In Junin hemorrhagic fever, convalescent serum with specific antibodies has successfully treated this infection. Ribavirin has been effective in treating some individuals with Lassa fever. Neither has been effective with filoviruses. Vaccines are available for yellow fever and Argentine hemorrhagic fever.

The recent Ebola epidemic has accelerated the conduction of trials for antiviral therapies and vaccine development. Phase I/II randomized controlled trials for ZMapp—a cocktail of three monoclonal antibodies targeting Ebola virus surface glycoprotein given to two Americans who survived the Ebola virus—began in February 2015 in Liberia. Although one surviving American did receive TKM-Ebola small interfering RNAs that bind viral messenger RNA sequences, phase II clinical trials only lasted 4 months as no clinical benefit was demonstrated. Favipiravir, an RNA-dependent RNA polymerase inhibitor originally developed in Japan to treat influenza, shows promise in clinical trials for managing Ebola virus in patients with low to moderate viral counts. Convalescent whole blood and plasma transfusion from Ebola survivors are undergoing phase II/III trials; results are expected to be positive. The virus may remain undetected in sequestered body sites such as the eye and testes.

In September 2014, the WHO determined two vaccines as the most developed and initiated safety studies: the recombinant vesicular stomatitis virus-Zaire Ebolavirus (rVSV-ZEBOV) and the chimpanzee-derived adenovirus-Zaire Ebolavirus (cAd3-ZEBOV) vaccines. Both have an Ebola virus gene inserted into a viral vector. Interim analysis of the rVSV-ZEBOV vaccine indicated it was safe and highly effective in preventing disease. The WHO has since then identified two more candidate vaccines being developed by Johnson & Johnson and Novovax. All four vaccines are currently in various clinical trial phases and show encouraging initial results.

Suggested Readings

Arora, S. Cutaneous reactions in nuclear, biological, and chemical warfare. *Indian J Dermatol Venereol Leprol.* 2005;71:80–86.

Bossi P, Tegnell A, Baka A, et al. Bichat guidelines for the clinical management of anthrax and bioterrorism-related anthrax. *Euro Surveill.* 2004;9(12):E3–E4.

Carucci JA, McGovern TW, Norton SA, et al. Cutaneous anthrax management algorithm. *J Am Acad Dermatol.* 2002;47:766–769.

Centers for Disease Control and Prevention. Bioterrorism. http://emergency.cdc.gov/bioterrorism/

Cieslak TJ, Christopher GW, Ottolini MG. Biological warfare and the skin II: viruses. *Clin Dermatol.* 2002;20(4):355–364.

Cieslak TJ, Talbot TB, Hartstein BH. Biological warfare and the skin I: bacteria and toxins. *Clin Dermatol.* 2002;20(4):346–354.

Cronquist SD. Tularemia: the disease and the weapon. *Dermatol Clin.* 2004;22:313–320.

Dellavalle RP, Heilig LF, Francis SO, et al. What dermatologists do not know about smallpox vaccination: results from a worldwide electronic survey. *J Invest Dermatol.* 2006;126(5):986–989.

Dennis D, Inglesby T, Henderson D et al. Tularemia as a biological weapon: medical and public health management. *JAMA*. 2001;285(21):2763–2773.

Fenner F, Henderson DA, Arita I, et al. *Smallpox and its Eradication*. Geneva: World Health Organization; 1988.

Feldmann H, Geisbert TW. Ebola haemorrhagic fever. *Lancet*. 2011;377(9768):849–862.

Guarner J, Shieh WJ, Greer PW, et al. Immunohistochemical detection of *Yersinia pestis* in formalin-fixed, paraffin-embedded tissue. *Am J Clin Pathol*. 2002;117(2):205–209.

Henghold WB. Other biologic toxin bioweapons: ricin, staphylococcal enterotoxin B, and trichothecene mycotoxins. *Dermatol Clin*. 2004;22:257–262.

Jacobs MK. The history of biologic warfare and bioterrorism. *Dermatol Clin*. 2004;22:231–246.

Lupi O, Madkan V, Tyring SK. Tropical dermatology: bacterial tropical diseases. *J Am Acad Dermatol*. 2006;54:559–578.

Marks JD. Medical aspects of biologic toxins. *Anesthesiol Clin North America*. 2004;22(3):509–532.

McGovern TW, Christopher GW, Eitzen EM. Cutaneous manifestations of biological warfare and related threat agents. *Arch Dermatol*. 1999;135:311–322.

Meffert JJ. Biological warfare from a dermatologic perspective. *Curr Allergy Asthma Rep*. 2003;3:304–310.

Noeller, TP. Biological and chemical terrorism: recognition and management. *Cleve Clin J Med*. 2001;68:1001–1016.

Nuovo GJ, Plaza JA, Magro C. Rapid diagnosis of smallpox infection and differentiation from its mimics. *Diagn Mol Pathol*. 2003;12(2):103–107.

Reissman DB, Whitney EA, Taylor TH Jr, et al. One-year health assessment of adult survivors of Bacillus anthracis infection. *JAMA*. 2004;291:1994–1998.

Prentice MB, Rahalison L. Plague. *Lancet*. 2007;369(9568):1196–1207.

Salvaggio MR, Baddley JW. Other viral bioweapons: Ebola and Marburg hemorrhagic fever. *Dermatol Clin*. 2004;22:291–302.

Seward JF, Galil K, Damon I, et al. Development and experience with an algorithm to evaluate suspected smallpox cases in the United States, 2002–2004. *Clin Infect Dis*. 2004;39:1477–1483.

Slifka MK, Hanifin JM. Smallpox: the basics. *Dermatol Clin*. 2004;22:263–274.

Villar RG, Elliot SP, Davenport, KM. Botulism: the many faces of botulinum toxin and its potential for bioterrorism. *Infect Dis Clin North Am*. 2006;20:313–327.

Wenner KA, Kenner JR. Anthrax. *Dermatol Clin*. 2004;22:247–256.

World Health Organization. Ebola outbreak 2014-2015. http://www.who.int/csr/disease/ebola/en/

Wollenberg A, Engler R. Smallpox, vaccination and adverse reactions to smallpox vaccine. *Curr Opin Allergy Clin Immunol*. 2004;4(4):271–275.

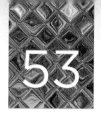

53

Dermatoses of Pregnancy

Jeff K. Shornick MD, MHA and Mackenzie C. Asel, MD

The pregnant woman is subject to the entire repertoire of the dermatologist's trade. Skin changes during pregnancy may be physiologic, unrelated to the pregnancy itself, or characteristic of a specific dermatosis of pregnancy. The rashes specific to pregnancy have been classified into four main categories: pemphigoid gestationis (PG), polymorphic eruption of pregnancy (PEP), atopic eruption of pregnancy (AEP), and cholestasis of pregnancy (CP).

TERMINOLOGY

The generally accepted current classification of skin diseases specific to pregnancy is listed in Table 53-1.

PEMPHIGOID GESTATIONIS

PG is the prototype of rashes specific to pregnancy. It is almost always associated with pregnancy. There are, however, multiple reports of PG in association with choriocarcinoma or trophoblastic tumors in women. There are no reports of a PG-like disease in association with choriocarcinoma in men. Thus, PG appears to be exclusively associated with the presence of placentally derived tissue.

Although the least common pregnancy-related dermatosis (occurring in approximately 1:50,000 pregnancies), PG is the most clearly defined. It remains idiopathic, although it is invariably associated with pregnancy (or trophoblastic tissue), carries a genetic predisposition, and is immunologically mediated.

Presentation and Characteristics

Clinical Appearance

- First onset may occur during any pregnancy, generally during the second or third trimester. Explosive onset in the immediate postpartum period can occur in up to 25% of cases.
- Clinical lesions vary from intensely pruritic urticarial plaques to pemphigoid-like tense blisters (Fig. 53-1). One often sees rapid evolution from the urticarial phase to clustered or arcuate tense blisters. Patients with only urticarial lesions and no further progression have been reported.
- Intense, relentless pruritus is invariable.

Distribution

Onset occurs in the periumbilical area in 50% of the patients but may also first appear on the palms, soles, or extremities. Facial involvement is rare, and mucosal involvement is nearly nonexistent.

TABLE 53-1 • Classification of Dermatoses of Pregnancy	
Classification	**Synonyms or Variants**
Pemphigoid gestationis	Herpes gestationis Gestational pemphigoid
Polymorphic eruption of pregnancy	Pruritic urticarial papules and plaques of pregnancy (PUPPP)
Atopic eruption of pregnancy	Prurigo of pregnancy Pruritic folliculitis of pregnancy Eczema of pregnancy
Cholestasis of pregnancy 1. Prurigo gravidarum 2. Jaundice of pregnancy	Obstetric cholestasis

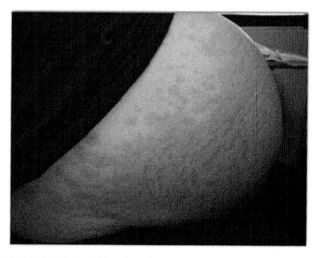

FIGURE 53-1: Urticarial plaques and tense bullae on the thighs of a patient with herpes gestationis.

Course

- Exacerbation at delivery occurs in approximately 75% of patients and may be remarkable.

- PG generally recurs during subsequent pregnancies, although "skip pregnancies" have been reported. There is a tendency for disease to develop earlier in multiparous women. Subsequent flares associated with menstruation or oral contraceptives are reported.

- Spontaneous resolution over weeks to months following delivery is the rule, although case reports of protracted disease are available.

- There is no increased maternal risk in PG.

- Newborns may be affected up to 10% of the time, presumably through passive transfer of the PG IgG. Lesions in newborns are typically mild and self-limited. Positive direct immunofluorescence in circumcision skin from neonates without clinically apparent disease has been reported.

- There is an increased risk of premature delivery (32% before 38 weeks, 16% before 36 weeks), small-for-gestational-age, and low birth weight associated with PG. Earlier onset of symptoms and the presence of blisters are associated with increased risk of adverse outcomes.

Laboratory Findings

- Routine laboratory results are normal. Mild peripheral eosinophilia may occur but is not clearly clinically relevant.

- Histopathology classically shows a subepidermal blister with eosinophils. Eosinophils are often lined up along the dermal–epidermal border.

- Direct immunofluorescence showing complement, with or without IgG deposited in a smooth, linear band along the dermal–epidermal junction, remains the diagnostic sine qua non, occurring in essentially 100% of cases. Split specimens show staining on the epidermal fragment. Indirect immunofluorescence reveals an IgG1 capable of avid complement activation. Titers of the PG antibody are low and historically have not correlated with the extent or severity of skin involvement. Immunoblotting and enzyme-linked immunoassays (NC16A ELISA) have emerged as sensitive tests in PG. More data are needed to determine how well titers correlate with disease activity.

Cause

- The PG antigen is a subcomponent of collagen XVII, a transmembrane glycoprotein with its N-terminal end embedded within the intracellular component of the hemidesmosome and its C-terminal component located extracellularly. The extracellular portion contains 15 collagenous domains interspersed by 16 noncollagenous domains. Antibodies from patients with bullous pemphigoid, mucous membrane pemphigoid, lichen planus pemphigoides, and linear IgA disease all react to specific antigens along the extracellular component of collagen XVII. The 16th noncollagenous A domain (NC16A) lies immediately adjacent to the basal cell membrane and is the target in PG. NC16A is also known as BP180 and BPAg2.

- Pathophysiologically, the PG antibody fixes to the BMZ, triggering complement activation via the classical complement pathway. Chemoattraction and degranulation of eosinophils follow. It is the release of proteolytic enzymes from eosinophilic granules, which appears to dissolve the bond between epidermis and dermis.

- Up to 80% of PG patients carry HLA-DR3, approximately 50% have HLA-DR4, and 40% to 50% have the simultaneous presence of both. HLA-DR3 shows linkage disequilibrium with the C4 null allele, and a corresponding increase in the C4 null allele has also been reported. However, neither HLA-DR3 nor HLA-DR4 is requisite for the development of PG, and there is no obvious correlation between the presence of specific HLA antigen(s) and the extent or severity of disease.

- All patients demonstrate anti-HLA antibodies. Whether this represents phenomenon or epiphenomenon remains to be seen, but because the placenta is the only source of disparate HLA antigens, their strikingly high incidence implies the universal presence of placental compromise.

- Special stains of PG placenta have suggested a primary immunologic reaction in the villous stroma of chorionic villi. Ultrastructural analysis shows detachment of basement membranes and less developed hemidesmosomes. These findings support the suggestion that PG is a primary disease of placental tissue, with secondary involvement of the skin. This hypothesis is attractive from many viewpoints, but remains to be proven.

- Ultrasound of placenta is normal, even in places where ultrastructural findings are not. It seems likely that ultrasound is too insensitive to detect placental insufficiency in PG.

- Antithyroid antibodies are increased; although their clinical relevance is unclear, the majority of patients are clinically euthyroid. On the other hand, the risk of autoimmune thyroid disease, especially Grave's disease, is clearly increased in those with a history of PG (affecting about 10% of patients).

Differential Diagnosis

The primary differential in PG is between PEP and a wide variety of diseases unrelated to pregnancy. Urticaria and arthropod bites can be difficult to differentiate. Immunofluorescence or ELISA is the key to differentiating PG, but both tests are hardly reasonable in all cases of pruritic rashes during pregnancy. Typically, the relentless progression of unbearable itch associated with urticarial lesions, rapidly progressing to tense blisters, helps distinguish PG from other clinical differentials.

Treatment

- PG is sufficiently rare that treatment guidelines are driven by expert opinion.

- Because PG is not associated with significant maternal or fetal risk and because it tends to remit spontaneously postpartum, it is imperative not to create significant risk from therapy.

- Topical steroids and antihistamines are rarely of benefit.

- Systemic steroids (prednisolone 0.25 to 0.5 mg/kg/day or prednisone 0.5 to 1 mg/kg/day) remain the cornerstone of therapy. Many patients improve during the latter part of pregnancy, only to flare at the time of delivery. Because profound flares at delivery are common, one should be prepared to initiate or increase steroids during the immediate postpartum period.

- There has been no clear evidence that PG is associated with increased fetal morbidity or mortality (other than premature birth), although that impression remains from a review of individual case reports.

- There is no evidence that systemic steroids decrease the risk of premature delivery.

- Alternative therapies, including the use of rituximab, intravenous immunoglobulin, and others for recalcitrant disease are presented in case reports.

POLYMORPHIC ERUPTION OF PREGNANCY

> ### SAUER'S NOTES
>
> PUPPP (pruritic urticarial papules and plaques of pregnancy) is now referred to as PEP (polymorphic eruption of pregnancy).

Polymorphic eruption of pregnancy (PEP, formerly called pruritic urticarial papules and plaques of pregnancy or PUPPP) is estimated to occur in 1:130 to 1:300 pregnancies. It is idiopathic, defined clinically, has negative immunofluorescence, and tends not to recur during subsequent gestations.

Presentation and Characteristics

Clinical Appearance

- Most cases (75% to 85%) occur in primiparous women, but first onset after multiple pregnancies has been reported.

- There is an abrupt onset of intensely itchy urticarial or papular lesions, often within abdominal striae during the last trimester of pregnancy (Fig. 53-2) or immediate postpartum period. Rapid spread to the trunk and extremities is characteristic.

- Fine vesicles are present in up to 40% of cases, but there are no tense blisters.

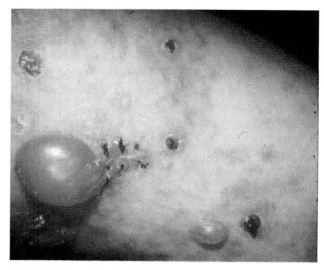

FIGURE 53-2: Urticarial plaques and blisters over the abdomen in the striae of a woman with PEP.

Distribution

There is a curious tendency for lesions to develop first within abdominal striae, although this is certainly not universal. The face and mucosal surfaces are almost always spared.

Course

- Spontaneous resolution within days of delivery is the rule.

- Generally does not recur during subsequent gestations.

- No maternal risks or complications are noted, except for an increased incidence of excessive weight gain and fetal twinning.

Laboratory Findings

- Laboratory investigations are normal.

- Histopathology is nonspecific. An admixture of a variable number of eosinophils scattered in the dermis may or may not be present.

- Direct and indirect immunofluorescence is negative.

- An increase in activated T cells within dermal infiltrates has led to speculation that PEP may be a consequence of a delayed T cell hypersensitivity to skin antigens.

- HLA typing shows no disease associations.

Differential Diagnosis

Because no definitive marker exists for PEP, the diagnosis is clinical and made by exclusion. As with PG, the differential is typically between incidental hives, viral exanthems, and PG. Immunofluorescence or ELISA for BP180 or NC16A, although not indicated in all cases, is the key to distinguishing PG.

Treatment

Potent topical steroids and antihistamines may provide symptomatic support. Systemic steroids are quite helpful, although not always necessary.

ATOPIC ERUPTION OF PREGNANCY

AEP is a disease complex encompassing prurigo of pregnancy, pruritic folliculitis of pregnancy, and eczema in pregnancy (which used to be categorized separately) and collectively represents the most common skin problem in pregnancy. Confusion persists regarding entities reported without histopathology or routine laboratory investigations and prior to the advent of immunofluorescence. Most authors now refer to this group as atopic eruption of pregnancy.

Presentation and Characteristics

Clinical Appearance

- Patients tend to present earlier in pregnancy than with other pregnancy-related dermatoses, often in the first or second trimester.
- Skin changes include eczematous lesions, erythematous papules, and prurigo nodules. There may be pustules, but not blisters. Lesions may or may not be follicular. For many, this rash represents their first manifestation of atopic skin changes, whereas others have an exacerbation of known atopic dermatitis.

Distribution

Any part of the body may be involved, although mucosal surfaces are spared.

Course

- Generally self-limited, symptoms resolve over weeks to months postpartum.
- No fetal or maternal risks have been reported.
- Recurrence during subsequent pregnancies is variable.

Laboratory Findings

- Liver function tests (by definition) are normal. Total IgE may be elevated.
- Histopathology is typically nonspecific. Whether inflammation tends to be follicular or not depends on whether poorly described variants are included in this group.
- Immunofluorescence is characteristically negative.

Differential Diagnosis

By definition, laboratory investigations and immunofluorescence are noncontributory. With no defining marker and only a nonspecific clinical pattern to unite reported variants, there is little guidance to separate AEP from diseases coincident to pregnancy.

Treatment

Treatment is symptomatic; no morbidity or mortality has been associated with this group.

CHOLESTASIS OF PREGNANCY

> **SAUER'S NOTES**
>
> For cholestasis of pregnancy, drug eruptions and hepatitis must be ruled out. Early treatment with vitamin K, ursodeoxycholic acid, or possibly early delivery can prevent fetal damage.

Jaundice occurs in approximately 1 in every 1,500 pregnancies. CP is the second most common cause of gestational jaundice, viral hepatitis being more common. CP accounts for approximately 20% of cases of obstetric jaundice, although the frequency varies both geographically and seasonally.

The incidence of CP varies in different racial groups. It seems to be the highest in Chile-Bolivia (6% to 27%), China (2.3% to 6%), and Sweden (1% to 1.5%) and lowest among blacks. CP occurs in approximately 1:1,000 pregnancies in the United States. The defining features of CP are as follows:

- Generalized pruritus, with or without jaundice, with no history of exposure to hepatitis or hepatotoxic drugs
- The absence of primary lesions
- Elevated serum bile acids (BA), with or without elevated transaminases
- Rapid disappearance of signs and symptoms following pregnancy

There is, however, a broad spectrum of clinical presentations.

CP is not really a primary dermatosis of pregnancy because the defining feature is pruritus associated with cholestasis; there is no primary dermatologic lesion.

Presentation and Characteristics

Clinical Appearance

- Typically presents during the last trimester of otherwise uneventful pregnancies. Onset as early as 7 weeks has been reported.
- Increased incidence of twin pregnancies.
- Intense, generalized pruritus, worse at night and often worst on the palms and soles.
- Skin findings are all secondary.

Distribution

Symptoms are typically most severe on the trunk, palms, and soles.

Course

- Symptoms may wax and wane, with or without changes in liver function tests.
- Up to 50% of patients develop signs of hepatitis including dark urine, light-colored stools, or jaundice—usually within 4 weeks of presentation.

- Recurrences during subsequent gestations occur in 45% to 70% of cases. Recurrences may also occur with the use of oral contraceptives.

- Failure of pruritus to stop within days of delivery or the persistence of elevated liver function tests suggest underlying hepatic or primary biliary disease.

- If intrahepatic cholestasis lasts for weeks, vitamin K absorption may be impaired, leading to a prolonged prothrombin time. Without exogenous vitamin K, fetal prothrombin activity may lead to an increased incidence of intracranial hemorrhage. The prothrombin time should be monitored and intramuscular vitamin K administered as necessary.

- Meconium staining and premature labor occurs in 20% to 60% of cases. An increase in fetal distress is clear. Whether and by how much fetal mortality is increased is disputed.

- Fetal risk appears to be correlated with onset before 28 weeks and with serum BA >40 mmol/L.

- Most authors argue for increased fetal monitoring after 30 weeks, with delivery upon signs of meconium staining or fetal stress. There is growing consensus for delivery at 36 weeks to reduce fetal risks.

- There appears to be a tendency for these women to develop cholelithiasis or gallbladder disease later in life.

Laboratory Findings

- Elevated BA, with or without elevated transaminases, currently defines the disease.

- In those without jaundice, elevated BA may be the only identifiable laboratory abnormality. Conjugated (direct) bilirubin is increased, but rarely above 2 to 5 mg/dL. Alkaline phosphatase, gamma-glutamyl transferase (GGT), and cholesterol are unreliable during pregnancy, and aspartate transaminase (AST) rarely exceeds four times normal, even in those with CP.

- Hepatic ultrasonography is normal. Liver biopsy is not indicated.

Cause

- CP is characterized by impaired transport of BA from hepatic cells into the gallbladder. Increased intracellular BA leads to hepatic injury and leakage of BA into the blood.

- CP remains multifactorial. Defects in at least six canalicular transporter genes have been documented, and multiple environmental risk factors have been identified (hepatitis C, winter onset, low serum selenium, low serum vitamin D, multiple gestations, >35 years at onset).

Differential Diagnosis

Increased BA is the sine qua non and is typically 3 to 100 times normal.

Treatment

- Ursodeoxycholic acid (500 to 2,000 mg/day) is the treatment of choice. It improves pruritus, normalizes liver enzymes, decreases the risk of premature birth, improves fetal outcome, and reduces utilization of the neonatal ICU.

- Antihistamines and bland topicals are helpful to reduce pruritus.

Suggested Readings

Ambros-Rudolph CM, Mullegger RR, Vaughan-Jones SA, et al. The specific dermatoses of pregnancy revisited and reclassified: results of a retrospective two-center study on 505 pregnant patients. *J Am Acad Dermatol.* 2006;54(3):395–404.

Floreani A, Gervasi MT. New insights on intrahapatic cholestasis of pregnancy. *Clin Liver Dis.* 2016;20(1):177–189.

54

Nutritional and Metabolic Diseases and the Skin

Yetunde M. Olumide, MD

Nutrition will always play an important role in the maintenance and protection of the skin. As more is being discovered about the foods we eat and more attention is being paid to different vitamins and minerals, we will undoubtedly find out more important information regarding nutrition and its role in skin maintenance as well as skin disease. Moreover, problems associated with developing countries are becoming more important as more people continue to migrate to the United States from abroad. Because of the increasing elderly population in the United States, adequate nutritional intake among the elderly will continue to be a very important subject for clinicians to be attentive to. Diet is many times inadequate in elderly populations and does not contain enough variety to provide elderly patients with all of the nutrients that they need. Also, as Americans have enjoyed an excess of food in recent times, one of our biggest problems is obesity and the health-related issues it creates for them. The skin is not immune to these problems. We will also discuss how different metabolic diseases can have profound effects on the skin.

The skin does not function as an isolated organ of the human body. Nutritional and metabolic diseases are manifested on the skin in two ways: (1) *primary* impact on the skin as an end organ and (2) skin manifestations *secondary* to involvement of internal organs. In arriving at an accurate diagnosis, it is not only important to know the *primary* manifestations of the diseases on the skin, it is also critical to be aware of potential end organs that may be affected by each disease and how these may manifest as *symptoms* and *signs* discernible through the history of disease given by the patient. Therefore, *awareness* of the spectrum of potential organ involvement in each disease and *listening* to the patient's symptoms are just as crucial as the physical examination of the skin.

VITAMIN DEFICIENCIES

> ### SAUER'S NOTES
>
> Immigration and the ease of travel have brought dietary deficiencies of the third world to be a diagnosis to consider in all the world.

Vitamin A Deficiency

Presentation and Characteristics

Vitamin A deficiency (VAD) is mainly a disease limited to developing countries. One of the first signs of deficiency is night blindness, and it is the leading cause of blindness in developing countries.

The most striking characteristic of the skin associated with vitamin A deficiency is phrynoderma (Fig. 54-1A and B). It is marked by follicular hyperkeratosis with spinous papules at the end of hair follicles. It is symmetrically distributed and often initially located at the extensor surfaces of the thighs, forearms, elbows, knees, buttocks, and back. Mostly, this hyperkeratosis causes the patient's skin to appear like toad skin and sometimes occurs on a background of dry and rough skin that may feel like sandpaper or nutmeg grater. The worst cases often plague children of preschool age. Other signs of deficiency include keratomalacia, pruritus, broken fingernails, and keratinization of mucous membranes.

Treatment

Oral forms of supplementation of vitamin A are effective for lowering the risk of morbidity. Some countries where VAD is a public health problem address its elimination by including vitamin A supplements available in capsule form with National Immunization days (NIDs) for polio eradication or measles. In addition, the delivery of vitamin A supplements, during integrated child health events such as child health days, have helped ensure high coverage of vitamin A supplementation in a large number of lesser-developed countries. Vitamin A capsules cost about US $0.02. The capsules are easy to handle; they do not need to be stored in a refrigerator or vaccine carrier. When the correct dosage is given, vitamin A is safe and has no negative effect on seroconversion rates for oral polio vaccine or measles vaccine. Because NIDs provide only one dose per year, NIDs-linked vitamin A distribution must be complemented by other dose programs to maintain vitamin A in children. Maternal high supplementation benefits both mother and breast-fed infant. High-dose vitamin A supplementation of the lactating mother in the first month postpartum can provide the breast-fed infant with an appropriate amount of vitamin A through breast milk. However, high-dose supplementation

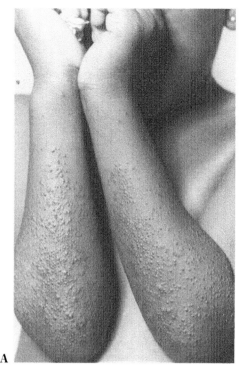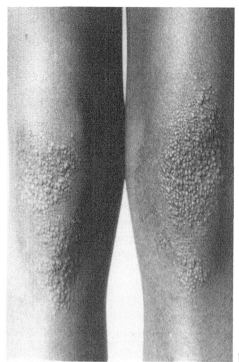

A   B

FIGURE 54-1: **A and B:** Phrynoderma. This is a classic cutaneous manifestation of vitamin A deficiency.

of pregnant women should be avoided because it can cause miscarriage and birth defects. Food fortification is also useful for improving VAD. Vitamin A fortification of fat-based foods, for example, margarine, oil, and milk, are ideal food vehicles for vitamin A delivery. Dietary diversification can also control VAD. Nutritional state can be improved with liver and fish oils, palm oil, carrots, sweet potatoes, leafy green vegetables, dark fruits, orange and yellow vegetables, tomato products, some vegetable oils, fortified foods such as cereal, and a variety of meats such as liver, chicken, beef and eggs. Skin lesions recover impressively with Retin-A cream.

Prevention

It is also extremely important not to take more than the recommended daily allowance (RDA) of Vitamin A, because the amount over and above the RDA is one of the narrowest of all vitamins and minerals. Especially with recent emphasis on vitamins and β-carotene as anticancer agents, accidental chronic overdose (through oral supplementation) is a possible problem. Excessive ingestion of carotenoids (which can cause carotenodermia—discussed in the next section) is nontoxic and does not cause hypervitaminosis A because the conversion of carotene to vitamin A is too slow.

Hypervitaminosis A (Vitamin A Excess)

Presentation and Characteristics

Hypervitaminosis A or vitamin A toxicity may be acute or chronic. Acute toxicity occurs after consuming large amounts of vitamin A over a short period of time, typically within a few hours or days. Chronic toxicity occurs when large amounts of vitamin A build up in the body over a long period of time as in those consuming daily mega doses of vitamin A. In adults, as little as 25,000 IU/day may lead to toxicity, especially in persons with hepatic compromise and dialysis patients on synthetic retinoid.

Symptoms include visual changes, bone pain, and skin changes. Most cases of chronic hypervitaminosis A have been reported in children. There is loss of hair and coarseness of the remaining hair, loss of eyebrows, exfoliative cheilitis, generalized exfoliation and pigmentation of the skin, and clubbing of the fingers. Moderate widespread itching may occur. In infants and children, symptoms may also include softening of the skull bone and bulging of the fontanel, double vision, bulging eyeballs, inability to gain weight, and coma. In adults, the early signs are dryness of the lips and anorexia; these may be followed by joint and bone pains, follicular hyperkeratosis, itchy or branny desquamation of the skin, fissures of the corners of the mouth and nostrils, dryness and loss of scalp hair and eyebrows, and cracked finger nails, fatigue, myalgia, depression, anorexia, headache (from pseudotumor cerebri), strabismus and weight loss commonly occur.

Treatment

The most effective way to treat hypervitaminosis A is to stop taking high-dose vitamin A supplements. Most people will make a full recovery within a few weeks. Complications, such as liver or kidney damage, must be treated independently.

Prevention

People can get most of the vitamin A the body needs from a healthy diet alone. Dietary sources of vitamin A are given in the section of vitamin A deficiency.

Carotenemia

Definition

Carotenemia or carotenaemia (xanthaemia) is the presence of the orange pigment carotene in blood from excessive intake of carrots or other vegetables containing the pigment, resulting in increased serum carotenoids. Carotenoids are lipid-soluble compounds that include α- and β-carotene, β-cryptoxanthin, lycopene, lutein, and zeaxanthin. Carotenoids contribute to normal-appearing human skin color and are a significant component of physiologic ultraviolet photoprotection.

Presentation and Characteristics

Carotenemia is a benign skin condition most often seen in light-skinned patients who have ingested large amounts of foods rich in Vitamin A precursors. Carotenemia commonly occurs in vegetarians and young children. This causes a yellow discoloration of the skin excluding the eyes and oral mucosa. It is important to distinguish this condition from more serious conditions such as jaundice. Carotenemia does not cause selective orange discoloration of the conjunctival membranes over the sclera, and this is unusually easy to distinguish from the yellowing of the skin and conjunctiva caused by bile pigments in states of jaundice. In dark-skinned individuals, the palms and soles may have yellow discoloration, but not the rest of the body. This condition more commonly occurs in children with liver disease, hypothyroidism, or diabetes mellitus. Anorexia nervosa (AN) and renal diseases, for example nephrotic syndrome, may be associated with carotenemia unassociated with the ingestion of carotene. Mothers may induce carotenemia by giving their infants large amounts of carrots in commercial infant food preparation.

An excess of carotenoids, being eliminated via sweat, may cause a marked orange discoloration of the outermost skin layer. This benign and reversible condition, which is most easily observed in light-skinned people, is known as **carotenosis** or **carotenoderma.** Carotenoderma is deliberately caused by β-carotenoid treatment of certain photosensitive dermatitides that discolor the skin. These high doses of β-carotene have been found to be harmless in studies, although being cosmetically displeasing to some.

Treatment

Because carotenemia is a benign condition, it can be treated with dietary modification alone.

Prevention

A lower or more moderate carotene diet will prevent recurrence.

Vitamin B$_2$ (Riboflavin) Deficiency

Presentation and Characteristics

Riboflavin deficiency (also called ariboflavinosis) results in *stomatitis* including red tongue with sore throat, chapped and fissured lips (cheilosis), and inflammation of the corners of the mouth (*angular stomatitis*/perlèche) as shown in **Figure 54-2**. A seborrhea-like follicular keratosis may also be observed. It

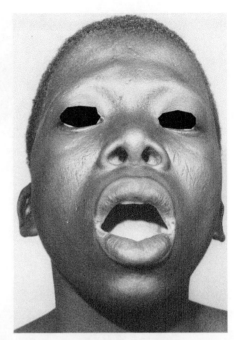

FIGURE 54-2: Angular stomatitis (perlèche). This may be found in Vitamin B$_2$ (Riboflavin) deficiency.

can be generalized, but the areas of the face, chest, abdominal wall, extremities, and the genital areas are most severely and consistently affected. The genital area can show redness with a fine, powdery desquamation. On the face, the roughness can resemble shark skin. There may be oily scaly skin rashes on the scrotum, vulva, philtrum of the lips, or the nasolabial folds. The affected patient is often pale from normochromic normocytic anemia.

Treatment

Treatment consists of taking riboflavin 6 to 30 mg PO q.d. until symptoms resolve.

Prevention

Prevention involves eating foods high in riboflavin, such as milk, cheese, yogurt, meat, and vegetables (especially spinach, asparagus, and broccoli).

Vitamin B$_3$ (Niacin, Nicotinic Acid) Deficiency

Presentation and Characteristics

Symptoms of niacin deficiency depend on whether it is mild or severe deficiency. Symptoms of mild niacin deficiency include indigestion, fatigue, aphthous ulcers (cancer sores), vomiting, and depression. Severe deficiency is called *pellagra*, and this causes symptoms related to the skin (*dermatitis*), digestive system (*diarrhea*), and nervous system (*dementia*, "the three Ds"). There is sometimes a fourth D referred to because, if left untreated for an extended period of time, *death* can result. These symptoms related to skin, digestive system, and nervous system include thick, scaly pigmented rash on sun-exposed areas of the skin, swollen mouth and bright red tongue, vomiting and diarrhea, headache, apathy, fatigue, depression, disorientation, and memory loss. The dermatitis is a symmetrical photodermatitis, affecting sun-exposed areas (Fig. 54-3A and B), areas of friction, or areas of pressure. The patient may report a burning sensation or pain early on. The initial erythema can also subside and darken to a brown color and become brittle, rough, hyperkeratotic, or scaly over time. Almost all patients will have involvement of the dorsal hands. The rash begins in the neck and appears as a broad symmetric hyperpigmented scaly and erythematous collar that has the appearance of a scarf tied around the neck, which then tapers downward, hence the common name "Cassal's necklace" (Fig. 54-3B). The skin rash heals centrifugally with a line of demarcation remaining actively inflamed after the center of the lesion has desquamated.

Treatment

Treatment is supplementation with niacinamide either orally or IV. The usual oral dosage is 0.5 g daily, and the usual dosage of an injection is 50 to 100 mg b.i.d. for a period of 3 months. Skin lesions can be covered with emollients, and because sun protection is important during the recovery phase, sunscreen should be applied to all exposed body areas. Because most patients with pellagra also suffer from other vitamins deficiencies, treating the patient with high-protein diet rich in B-vitamins is also necessary to restore the patient to health. Long-term addition of milk, eggs, and meat is many times necessary to help with recovery. Also, the addition of peanuts, green leafy vegetables, whole or enriched grains, brewer's dry yeast, and meats can enhance niacin uptake in the acute phase of recovery.

Prevention

Niacin deficiency is rare in Western society. It mainly affects societies whose main dietary intake is maize (which has low tryptophan content) and millet or sorghum (both of which interfere with tryptophan metabolism owing to their high leucine content). Because most of their diet was maize, the Native Americans discovered that they could prevent pellagra

by adding lime (an alkaline) that makes niacin more available. It is hypothesized that pellagra is caused not only by niacin deficiency but also due to lack of either tryptophan or one of the vitamin cofactors. Tryptophan is one of the amino acids that makes up proteins. The liver can convert tryptophan from high-protein foods like meats and milk into niacin. However, pellagra does sometimes affect chronic alcoholics, or patients with gastrointestinal disorders or patients with severe psychiatric disturbances in more developed societies like the United States. The best way to prevent pellagra is to have a diet with adequate calories and protein.

Vitamin B_6 Deficiency

Presentation and Characteristics

As far as the skin is concerned, a deficiency can paint a similar clinical picture as pellagra because B_6 is needed by the body to produce its own B_3 vitamin. Although extremely rare, the skin is one of the first organs to show signs of B_6 deficiency and can include nails that are uneven (transverse ridging), scaly facial eruptions resembling seborrheic dermatitis, painful, edematous glossitis, angular cheilitis, and generalized stomatitis. Multiple skin disorders including eczema, acne, and seborrheic dermatitis have been associated with B_6 deficiency.

Treatment

Pyridoxine 50 to 100 mg PO q.d. is usually sufficient for adults.

Prevention

Vitamin B_6 is actually present in most foods; so deficiency is quite rare. As with most vitamin deficiencies, make sure the patient takes in a variety of foods especially poultry, fish, liver, eggs, meat, vegetables, and grains. For patients taking pyridoxine-inactivating drugs such as anticonvulsants, cycloserine, hydralazine, corticosteroids, and penicillamine, the use of pyridoxine in the amount of 50 to 100 mg PO q.d. is recommended. For patients taking isoniazide, a dose of 30 to 50 mg of pyridoxine q.d. is advised.

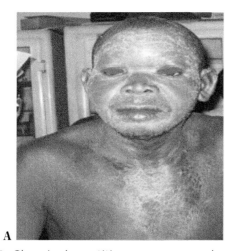
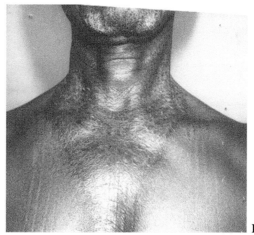

FIGURE 54-3: Chronic dermatitis on sun-exposed areas. **A:** Face and V-area of the upper chest. **B:** "Cassal's necklace" in pellagra. These may be found in vitamin B_3 (Niacin) deficiency.

Vitamin B₁₂ Deficiency

Presentation and Characteristics

Vitamin B_{12} deficiency leads to anemia and neurologic dysfunction. Significant anemia leads to weakness, fatigue, light-headedness, rapid heartbeat, rapid breathing, and pallor of the mucous membranes (e.g., sclera and mouth) and the skin, palms and soles. Glossitis, hyperpigmentation, and canities are the main dermatologic manifestations. The patient may also present with hyperpigmentation of the skin (especially over the dorsum of the hands [Fig. 54-4A] and feet with a concentration over the interphalangeal joints and terminal phalanges). Stomatitis with a bright red atrophic tongue and angular cheilitis (perlèche) are often features of long-standing vitamin B_{12} deficiency (Fig. 54-4B). Vitamin B_{12} deficiency may cause easy bruising or bleeding, including bleeding gums. It may also manifest as angular cheilitis (perlèche) and glossopyrosis (burning mouth syndrome) that can later result in a focal or diffuse smooth painful glossitis. Vitamin B_{12} deficiency may be associated with vitiligo and hair changes. Premature gray hair may occur paradoxically. Megaloblastic anemia is present. Weakness, paresthesias, numbness, ataxia, and other neurologic findings occur. If the deficiency is not corrected, nerve cell damage can result, and this may manifest as tingling or numbness of the fingers and toes, difficulty walking, mood changes, depression, memory loss, disorientation, and, in severe cases, dementia.

Treatment

Treatments can vary, but both IM and oral routes are acceptable. IM administration usually involves initial loading doses followed by monthly maintenance doses. One dose of 1,000 μg q.d. $\times$ 2 weeks followed by a maintenance dose of 1,000 μg q 1 to 3 months is one example. Oral supplementation is usually 1,000 to 2,000 μg PO q.d. $\times$ 8 weeks with a maintenance therapy of 1,000 μg q.d. for life.

Prevention

Because B_{12} is present only in animal foods and cannot be synthesized by the body, a proper diet including fish, meat, poultry, eggs, milk, and milk products is necessary to prevent deficiency. For vegetarians, fortified cereals help prevent deficiency. Rare causes of vitamin B_{12} deficiency including fish tapeworm (*Diphyllobothrium latum*) infection in which the parasite uses luminal vitamin B_{12}, pancreatic insufficiency (with failure to inactivate competing cobalamin-binding protein), and severe Crohn disease, causing sufficient destruction of the ileum to impair vitamin B_{12} absorption, should be investigated and appropriately treated.

Biotin (Vitamin H) Deficiency

Presentation and Characteristics

Classically in neonates, it presents as a universal alopecia with an extensive bran-like erythematous desquamation that is more pronounced in intertriginous areas. Within 3 to 5 weeks of deficient biotin intake, the patient will clinically exhibit seborrheic dermatitis, dry skin, and hair thinning that can progress to total scalp or even universal alopecia over several months. Other associated signs include: fine and brittle hair without abnormalities of the shaft, fungal infections (especially with *Candida albicans*), and rashes including periorificial dermatitis with mild, scaly erythema and crusted erosions. Some patients also exhibit keratoconjunctivitis or blepharitis.

Treatment

Treatment with 10 to 20 mg PO q.d. is normally adequate, although quantities up to 40 mg have been used and tolerated by patients.

Prevention

Prevention depends on the cause, and there are a variety of causes for biotin deficiency. Metabolic causes (biotinidase deficiency or holocarboxylase/multiple carboxylase deficiency) cannot be prevented by diet. For deficiencies caused by anticonvulsants, a switch to another anticonvulsant medication that does not interfere with absorption must be made, or the patients should be supplemented with biotin. For prolonged antibiotic therapy as the cause, the patient should receive biotin supplementation as well if antibiotic therapy must be continued. Otherwise, discontinuation of antibiotic therapy is advised. Patients should also be advised not to consume large amounts of raw eggs or raw egg whites because they both contain avidin. Avidin in large amounts can bind biotin

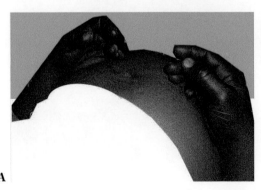
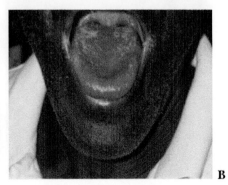

FIGURE 54-4: A: Diffuse hyperpigmentation of the hands in vitamin B_{12} deficiency. (A, Courtesy by Dr Bola Ogunbiyi.) **B:** Stomatitis with atrophic glossitis and angular cheilitis (perlèche) in vitamin B_{12} deficiency.

and prevent absorption in the intestine. A dietary deficiency is quite rare, but foods high in biotin include most vegetables, some fruits, chicken, eggs, and milk.

Vitamin C Deficiency (Scurvy)

Presentation and Characteristics

Scurvy is a disease resulting from a deficiency of vitamin C. Scurvy often presents initially with fatigue. Early symptoms are malaise and lethargy. An even earlier symptom may be a pain in a section of the gums, which interferes with digestion. As the disease progresses, the patients develop shortness of breath, and bone and muscle pains (myalgias). Other symptoms include skin changes with roughness, easy bruising and petechiae, gum disease, loosening of teeth, poor wound healing, and emotional changes (which may appear before any physical changes). The patient may look pale, feel depressed, and be partially immobilized.

The most distinctive skin finding in scurvy is follicular hyperkeratosis with coiled, corkscrew hairs growing out of the follicles on the upper arms, back, buttocks, and lower extremities. Woody edema and petechiae of the legs may develop (Fig. 54-5A). The spots are most abundant on the thighs and legs. Later, patients can get hemorrhagic petechiae in a perifollicular location (Fig. 54-5B) and ecchymoses, spongy bluish-purple gingivae that may become massively swollen, bleeding of gums, and, in extreme cases, bleeding of all mucous membranes. As scurvy advances, there can be open, suppurating wounds, loss of teeth, yellow skin, fever, neuropathy, and finally death from bleeding. Dry mouth and dry eyes similar to Sjögren syndrome may occur. In the late stages, jaundice, generalized edema, oliguria, neuropathy, fever, convulsions, and eventually death are frequently seen.

Treatment

Treatment is vitamin C 300 to 1,000 mg preferably divided into doses of 100 mg throughout the day for at least 1 week and then 400 mg/day until complete recovery.

Prevention

Prevention of scurvy can be accomplished merely by providing a moderate amount of fruits and vegetables in the diet. Foods exceptionally high in vitamin C include bell peppers, brussel sprouts, papaya, broccoli, oranges, strawberries, cantaloupe, kiwifruit, cauliflower, and kale.

IRON DEFICIENCY (SIDEROPENIA OR HYPOFERREMIA)

Presentation and Characteristics

Symptoms of iron deficiency can occur even before the condition has progressed to iron deficiency anemia. Before anemia occurs, the medical condition of iron deficiency

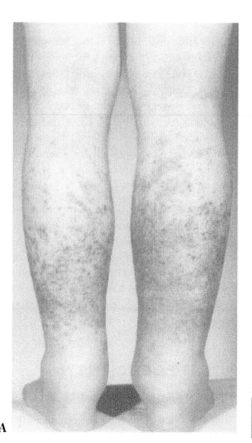
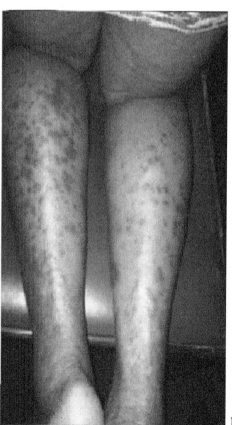

FIGURE 54-5: **A:** Woody edema and petechiae of the legs. This may be found in vitamin C deficiency (scurvy). **B:** Scurvy. Perifollicular hemorrhage and follicular hyperkeratosis.

without anemia is called latent iron deficiency (LID) or iron deficiency erythropoiesis (IDE). Symptoms of iron deficiency are not unique to iron deficiency (i.e., not pathognomonic). Symptoms of iron deficiency include dizziness, pallor, hair loss, twitches, irritability, weakness, pica, pagophagia, restless legs syndrome, and impaired immune function. In Plummer–Vinson syndrome, there is painful atrophy of the mucous membrane covering the tongue, the pharynx, and the esophagus. Some of the skin signs of iron deficiency include pruritus, brittle nails, nails with vertical stripes, koilonychias (spoon-shaped nails), angular stomatitis, a smooth and swollen tongue that can develop a burning sensation, dryness of the throat and mouth, brittle and dry hair, possible increased hair shedding, and pale skin if the patient is anemic.

Treatment

Before commencing treatment, there should be definitive diagnosis of the underlying cause for iron deficiency. This is particularly the case in older patients, who are most susceptible to *colorectal cancer* and the gastrointestinal bleeding it often causes. In adults, 60% of patients with iron deficiency anemia may have underlying gastrointestinal disorders leading to chronic blood loss. It is likely that the cause of the iron deficiency will need treatment as well. In the tropics, hookworm disease is a notable cause of iron deficiency anemia, and this must be treated. Upon diagnosis, the condition can be treated with *iron supplements*. Inflammatory bowel disease (IBD), *dialysis*, or gastrointestinal (GI) bleeding from chronic aspirin use can also result in iron deficiency. Examples of oral iron that are often used are *ferrous sulfate*, *ferrous gluconate*, or amino acid chelate tablets. Blood transfusion is sometimes used to treat iron deficiency with hemodynamic instability.

Prevention

Mild iron deficiency can be prevented or corrected by eating iron-rich foods and by cooking in an iron skillet. Iron from different foods is absorbed and processed differently by the body; for instance, iron in meat (heme iron source) is more easily absorbed than iron in grains and vegetables ("non-heme" iron source). Because iron from plant sources is less easily absorbed than the heme-bound iron of animal sources, vegetarians and vegans should have a higher total daily iron intake than those who eat meat, fish, or poultry. Legumes and dark-green leafy vegetables like broccoli, kale, and oriental greens are especially good sources of iron for vegetarians and vegans. Richest foods in *heme iron* are clam, livers of pork, lamb and beef, lamb kidney, cooked oyster, cuttlefish, octopus, mussel, and beef heart. Richest foods in *non-heme iron* are soybeans, raw yellow beans, lentils, soybean kernels, roasted sesame seeds, spirulina, candied ginger root, and spinach. However, spinach and Swiss chard contain oxalates, which bind iron making it almost entirely unavailable for absorption. Oral iron supplementation is sometimes recommended during periods of increased requirement such as lactation or pregnancy. In the tropics, prevention of intestinal hookworm disease is an important way to prevent iron deficiency anemia. Therefore,

improved sanitation, provision of adequate disposal of human excrements, and not walking about barefooted particularly in farmlands are critical preventive measures against iron deficiency anemia.

IRON OVERLOAD (IRON EXCESS, HEMOCHROMATOSIS)

Definition

Iron overload indicates accumulation of iron in the body from any cause. The most important causes are hereditary hemochromatosis (HHC), a genetic disorder, and transfusional iron overload, which can result from repeated blood transfusions (e.g., patients with sickle cell disease or thalassemia). Hemosiderosis is hemochromatosis caused by excessive blood transfusions, that is, hemosiderosis is a form of secondary hemochromatosis.

Presentation and Characteristics

Organs commonly affected by hemochromatosis are liver, heart, and endocrine organs. The classic triad of hemochromatosis is hyperpigmentation, cirrhosis, and diabetes mellitus. Skin hyperpigmentation is one of the earliest signs of the disease and is therefore very important for the physician to recognize. It is most pronounced on sun-exposed areas, especially the face.

Treatment

Therapeutic phlebotomy is the treatment of choice, and skin hyperpigmentation is often substantially alleviated. For patients not able to tolerate therapeutic phlebotomy due to extreme anemia, Desferal (Deferoxamine) is used to chelate the excess iron. Two newer iron-chelating drugs that are licensed for use in patients receiving regular blood transfusions to treat hemoglobinopathies such as sickle cell disease and thalassemia (and thus develop iron overload) are deferasirox and deferiprone.

Prevention

Hereditary hemochromatosis cannot be prevented. Secondary hemochromatosis can be caused by several factors such as diet, anemia, chronic liver disease, blood transfusion, iron intake, and long-term kidney dialysis. Prevention depends on the factor that caused the disease. Blood transfusions should be sparingly used in hemoglobinopathies in the absence of hemodynamic instability. Oral iron tablets are preferred in chronic iron deficiency anemia.

FOLATE DEFICIENCY

Presentation and Characteristics

Signs of folate deficiency are often subtle. Anemia is a late finding in folate deficiency.

Loss of appetite and *weight loss* can occur. Additional signs are *weakness*, sore tongue, *headaches*, heart *palpitations*, *irritability*, and *behavioral disorders*. In adults, *anemia* (macrocytic, *megaloblastic anemia*) can be a sign of advanced folate deficiency. In infants and children, folate deficiency can slow growth rate. Women with folate deficiency who become *pregnant* are more likely to give birth to *low-birth-weight premature* infants, and infants with *neural tube defects*. Although best known for causing megaloblastic anemia that slowly progresses over months and delays maturation of granulocytes and megakaryocytes, pure folate deficiency has also been known to cause hyperpigmentation of the skin and mucous membranes similar to that which is seen in B$_{12}$ deficiency. Hyperpigmentation is accentuated particularly on the dorsal surfaces of the fingers, toes, as well as in the creases of the palms and soles of patients. The pathogenesis is unknown, but it does clear with appropriate treatment.

Treatment

Treatment consists of oral or IV folic acid supplements on a short-term basis until anemia resolves, and a diet rich in green leafy vegetables and citrus fruits. In cases of intestinal malabsorption, lifelong replacement therapy may be necessary.

Prevention

Prevention involves a high intake of folate-rich foods especially in high-risk patients (i.e., pregnant women, the elderly, celiac patients, cancer patients, alcoholics). For the general population, eating a well-balanced diet and including foods high in folate such as green leafy vegetables, liver, beans, certain fruits (especially oranges and satsumas), brewer's yeast, and fortified breads and cereals is recommended. When cooking, use of steaming or of a food steamer can help keep more folate content in the cooked foods, thus helping to prevent folate deficiency.

ZINC DEFICIENCY

Presentation and Characteristics

Acrodermatitis enteropathica, which is an autosomal recessive disorder affecting the intestinal absorption of zinc, clinically presents as the triad of diarrhea, alopecia, and a periorificial and acral rash (Fig. 54-6A and B). Clinically, it presents in infants that become photophobic and develop a vesiculobullous dermatitis on the hands, feet, periorificial areas, and many times quite drastically in the diaper area 4 to 6 weeks after weaning. Conjunctivitis and blepharitis may also be seen. Acute zinc deficiency from dietary insufficiency will show the same clinical picture with eczematous eruptions of the hands, feet, and anogenital areas. Flat, grayish, bullous lesions surrounded by red-brown erythema will cover the finger flexural creases and palms. Hair growth is slow, with thinning of scalp hair that can lead to alopecia totalis. Zinc deficiency may manifest as acne, eczema, xerosis (dry, scaling skin), seborrheic dermatitis, and paronychia. There may also be impaired wound healing. In the mouth, zinc deficiency can manifest as nonspecific oral ulceration, stomatitis, or white tongue coating. Rarely, it can cause angular cheilitis and burning mouth syndrome. Severe zinc deficiency may disturb the sense of smell and taste. In chronic cases, lesions are seen on the areas subject to repeated pressure or friction such as the elbows, knees, and knuckles. These lesions are well demarcated, thickened, and brownish, and may develop lichenification and scaling. Nails show Beau lines (deep transverse depressions). This condition has been associated with total parenteral nutrition (TPN) and cystic fibrosis.

Treatment

Oral zinc in a dose of 2 mg/kg for acrodermatitis enteropathica can resolve clinical manifestations within 2 weeks. However, the infant should remain on oral zinc supplementation therapy for

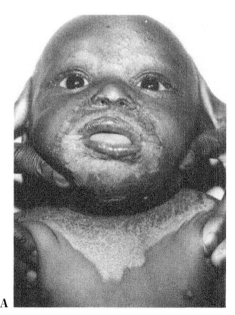
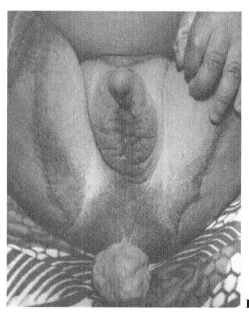

A   **B**

FIGURE 54-6: **A and B:** Acrodermatitis enteropathica. This is found in autosomal recessive zinc deficiency.

life. For dietary zinc deficiency, increasing intake of foods rich in zinc content is suitable for mild deficiency. For a more severe zinc deficiency, zinc picolinate or zinc gluconate can be taken orally, and dosing will vary depending on the severity of the deficiency.

Prevention

Eating a well-rounded diet and including foods that are high in zinc is the best means of prevention. Foods high in zinc include veal liver, red meats, sesame seeds, pumpkin seeds, yogurt, green peas, shrimp, and green leafy vegetables.

COPPER EXCESS (WILSON DISEASE)

Presentation and Characteristics

Wilson disease or hepatolenticular degeneration is an autosomal recessive genetic disorder in which copper accumulates in tissues; this manifests as neurologic or psychiatric symptoms and liver disease. Skin pigmentation and a bluish discoloration at the base of the fingernails (azure lunulae) have been described in patients with Wilson disease.

Treatment

Treatment with copper chelators such as penicillamine, trientine, and zinc acetate is the best therapy to prevent a fatal outcome in these patients.

Prevention

Genetic counseling is recommended for persons with a family history of Wilson disease.

SELENIUM DEFICIENCY

Presentation and Characteristics

Selenium deficiency is relatively rare in healthy, well-nourished individuals. It can occur in patients with severely compromised intestinal function, those undergoing total parenteral nutrition, those who have had gastrointestinal bypass surgery, and also in persons of advanced age. It has also been associated with cholesterol-lowering drugs (e.g., statins). Selenium is also necessary for the conversion of the thyroid hormone thyroxine (T_4) into its more active counterpart, triiodothyronine, and as such a deficiency can cause symptoms of hypothyroidism.

Although best known for causing cardiomyopathy, selenium has been documented in at least one case to cause xerosis, erythematous scaly papules and plaques on the cheeks, hips, thighs, and popliteal areas as well as erosions in the diaper area, and short, thin, light-colored hair.

Treatment

Supplementation with sodium selenite is reported to resolve symptoms. One study found that Brazil nuts alone were just as efficacious as sodium selenite in raising selenium levels in patients with selenium deficiency.

Prevention

Eating a balanced diet and including selenium-rich foods is the best prevention. Foods high in selenium include Brazil nuts, tuna, salmon, shrimp, mushrooms, and halibut.

PROTEIN-ENERGY MALNUTRITION

Definition

Protein-energy malnutrition (PEM) or protein-calorie malnutrition refers to a form of malnutrition in which there is inadequate calorie or protein intake. They include

- *Kwashiorkor* (protein malnutrition predominant)
- *Marasmus* (deficiency in calorie intake)
- *Marasmic kwashiorkor* (marked protein deficiency and marked calorie insufficiency signs present, sometimes referred to as the most severe form of malnutrition).

Kwashiorkor

Presentation and characteristics

The defining sign of kwashiorkor in a malnourished child is pitting edema (swelling of the ankles and feet). Other signs include a distended abdomen, an enlarged liver with fatty infiltrates, thinning hair, loss of teeth, skin depigmentation, and dermatitis. Children with kwashiorkor often develop irritability and anorexia. Victims of kwashiorkor fail to produce antibodies following vaccination against diseases, including diphtheria and typhoid. Generally, the disease can be treated by adding protein to the diet; however, it can have a long-term impact on a child's physical and mental development, and in severe cases may lead to death.

Skin changes are characteristic and progress over a few days. The definition of kwashiorkor is a total body weight of 60% to 80% of the expected weight according to age and height (body mass index [BMI]) with either edema or hypoalbuminemia. The child with Kwashiorkor looks wretched with flaky dermatitis, bloated face, and prominent parotid glands (Fig. 54-7A). The patient will classically have a diffuse, fine reddish-brown scale resembling "flaky paint." Frequently, erosions on areas of friction and vesicles or bullae also occur. Areas of hypo- and hyperpigmentation are also common along with lightening of the hair and "flag sign," which is alternating areas of lighter and darker hair pigmentation. This reflects inconsistent states of nutritional intake in the patient. Mostly, the edema can mask the underlying muscle and subcutaneous tissue atrophy, hence the importance of detecting the cutaneous signs of the disease. Temporal recession and hair loss from the back of the head can occur, likely secondary to pressure when the child lies down. In some cases, loss of hair can be extreme. Hair can also become softer and finer and appear unruly. The eyelashes can undergo the same change, having a so-called "broomstick appearance." Nail plates are thin and soft and may be fissured or ridged. Atrophy of the papillae on the tongue, angular stomatitis, xerophthalmia, and

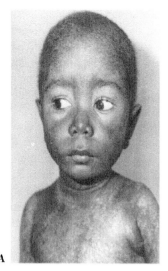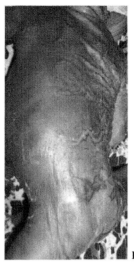

FIGURE 54-7: **A:** Kwashiorkor. The miserable face and dermatitis in a patient. **B:** "Cracked enamel paint skin" in kwashiorkor.

cheilosis can also occur. Depigmentation of hair causes it to be reddish-yellow to white. Curly hair often becomes straightened. Skin changes are characteristic and progress over a few days. The skin becomes dark and dry, and then splits open when stretched (Fig. 54-7B), revealing pale areas between the cracks (also known as "crazy pavement dermatosis" or "enamel paint skin"). This feature is seen especially over pressure areas. In contrast to pellagra, these changes seldom occur on sun-exposed skin. Kwashiorkor typically presents with a failure to thrive, edema, moon facies, a swollen abdomen (potbelly), and a fatty liver. Other nutritional deficiencies often coexist such as vitamin C deficiency, anemia, and niacin deficiency. The poor nutritional state of the patients puts them at increased risk for calciphylaxis, which can ultimately produce ischemia and necrosis of skin.

Treatment

Treatment is similar for both kwashiorkor and marasmus with the goal of therapy to restore the patient's normal body composition and nutritional state. In severe marasmus or kwashiorkor, there are two phases of treatment. The first involves correcting fluid and electrolyte imbalances, treating infections with antibiotics that specifically do not interfere with protein synthesis, and addressing any other related medical problems. The second phase involves slowly replenishing the essential nutrients to prevent taxing the patient's weakened system. Tube feedings can be implemented for certain patients if needed; however, oral refeeding is preferred. If diagnosed on time, both marasmus and kwashiorkor can be treated with complete resolution of symptoms, with the exception of retarded growth and development in more severe cases.

Prevention

The most important prevention strategy for improving nutritional education among communities who are prone to both of these types of protein-energy undernutrition (PEU) is public health measures and reduction of poverty. There is also a form of secondary PEU that can be caused by multiple factors including drugs that interfere with macronutrient absorption; other disorders that affect GI function such as enteritis, enteropathy, and pancreatic insufficiency; wasting disorders such as AIDS, cancer, and renal failure; and any conditions that increase metabolic demands such as infections, hyperthyroidism, pheochromocytoma, burns, or other critical illnesses.

Marasmus

Presentation and Characteristics

Marasmus may have no cutaneous findings. However, inconsistent skin findings include fine, brittle hair, alopecia, impaired growth, and fissuring of the nails. Occasionally, marked growth of lanugo is noted. Most of the times, kwashiorkor and marasmus coexist. Marasmus is caused by a lack of protein and calories. Edema is absent in marasmus. Usually, signs of vitamin A deficiency exist owing to a lack of carrier protein and zinc deficiency. Loss of skin elasticity, failure to develop body fat, muscle wastage, loss of muscle tone, mental dullness, and growth arrest are usually present. In cases of marasmus, the skin is dry, wrinkled, and loose because of marked loss of subcutaneous fat. The "monkey facies," caused by loss of the buccal fat pad, is characteristic. In contrast to kwashiorkor, there is no edema or dermatosis, but the skin is pale and lacks luster. The buttocks are completely flat with gross wasting of the trunk and extremities (Fig. 54-8). The hair can be sparse with a reddish tinge. In adults, there may be prominent follicular hyperkeratosis.

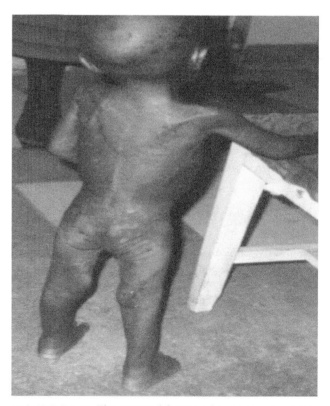

FIGURE 54-8: The wasted figure of a marasmic child.

Treatment

See Kwashiorkor section.

Prevention

See Kwashiorkor section.

EATING DISORDERS

Definition

Eating disorders are *mental disorders* defined by abnormal eating habits that negatively affect a person's *physical* or *mental* health. They include *binge eating disorder* in which people eat a large amount in a short period of time, *anorexia nervosa* in which people eat very little and thus have a low *body weight*, *bulimia nervosa* in which people eat a lot and then try to rid themselves of the food, *pica* in which people eat nonfood items, *rumination disorder* in which people *regurgitate* food, *avoidant/restrictive food intake disorder* in which people have a lack of interest in food, and a group of *other specified feeding or eating disorders*. Anxiety disorders, *depression*, and *substance abuse* are common among people with eating disorders. These disorders do not include *obesity*.

Dermatologic changes in anorexia nervosa (AN) and bulimia nervosa (BN) may be the first signs that an eating disorder is present. Therefore, it is extremely important for the physician to understand the cutaneous signs of eating disorders. Mostly, these two eating disorders coexist, and it has been estimated that approximately 50% of AN patients also practice bulimia.

Bulimia Nervosa

Presentation and Characteristics

BN, also known simply as *bulimia*, is a disorder characterized by binge eating and purging, as well as excessive evaluation of one's self-worth in terms of body weight or shape.

Acne is usually mild or moderate and is common in both BN and AN. Clinically, the patient will usually be of normal or above normal weight. The most classic signs include hypertrichosis, Russell sign (scarring on knuckles or back of hand due to self-induced vomiting), perimylolysis (decalcification of teeth due to gastric acid exposure from chronic vomiting), and self-induced dermatitis. Isolated signs are not predictive of a patient having an eating disorder, but any cluster of or combination of multiple signs in any patient who has a distorted perception of body weight can justify clinical suspicion of an eating disorder. Other signs include enlargement of the submandibular and parotid glands, which indicates frequent

vomiting. Xerosis with mild hyperpigmentation, also called "dirty skin," is another frequent sign, but it is more common in patients with a longer duration of the disease. Occasionally, drug eruptions from laxatives, diuretics, herbal remedies, or diet pills can be seen. Signs from drug consumption can sometimes be specific and include finger clubbing due to senna, photosensitivity due to thiazide diuretics, urticaria due to phenolphthalein, and fixed drug eruption from laxatives. Purpura, edema, and subconjunctival hemorrhage are also quite common in cases of BN. Limb coldness and compulsive washing are also concomitant signs. Acne is usually mild or moderate and is common in both BN and AN. The lesions are more often localized on the face and back and are frequently excoriated. However, because acne has such a high incidence among adolescents, it is difficult to make a distinction between those who developed acne previous to and those who developed acne during the period of the eating disorder. Moreover, interestingly acne can be a risk factor for anorexia in psychologically vulnerable patients who may choose dieting to control their acne. Carotenemia can be found in both AN and BN, but it is more common in BN because of ingestion of carotene-rich vegetables. Acrocyanosis, although uncommon, may occur and is more prevalent among the severely ill patients. Livedo reticularis and, more rarely, acute cutaneous ischemia may also develop. There may be dry mucous membranes, xerosis, and, less frequently, xerophthalmia. In some cases, caries, dental enamel erosions, and tooth abscess can be seen as a result of self-induced vomiting.

Treatment

Depending on the severity of the disease and the patient's nutritional state, the patient may need to be hospitalized for a period of time. However, most cases of bulimia can be treated outside the hospital. Psychotherapy is very helpful in most cases. Also, most of the times, antidepressants are of help in these patients specifically Prozac, which is the only FDA-approved drug for treatment of bulimia. Consulting a dietitian is very helpful.

Prevention

Although there is no true way to prevent bulimia, early detection especially by a pediatrician or a dermatologist can help prevent the disease from progressing, and this may be the most important way in which physicians can help patients with this disease. Questions about eating habits and satisfaction with appearance can sometimes help reveal valuable clinical clues in suspect age groups and certain patient populations.

Anorexia Nervosa

Presentation and Characteristics

AN, often referred to simply as anorexia, is an eating disorder characterized by a low weight, fear of gaining weight, a strong desire to be thin, and food restriction.

Xerosis, lanugo hair (a soft, downy body hair that grows in patients as a result of the body trying to insulate itself owing to loss of body fat), and telogen effluvium are common skin manifestations in AN. Pruritus, hypercarotenemia, edema, acrocyanosis, nail dystrophy, and angular stomatitis are occasionally associated with anorexia, whereas scurvy and pellagra are rarer. Also, erythema ab igne, self-phlebotomy, dermatitis artefacta, and trichotillomania are usually found in these patients. Perniosis (a rare vasculitis from prolonged exposure to cold conditions) and pompholyx have also been reported in some cases. Other general skin signs associated with the starvation and malnutrition associated with AN are interdigital intertrigo, seborrheic dermatitis, follicular hyperkeratosis, striae distensae, gingivitis, depapillated tongue, aphthae, alopecia, opaque hair, pili torti, onychoschizia, and nail fragility. Raynaud phenomenon following the onset of AN has also been reported.

Treatment

Depending on the severity of the disease, the patient may need to be hospitalized in order to correct abnormalities such as electrolyte imbalances, dehydration, or psychiatric problems. There are many day programs or residential programs as well as clinics dedicated just to eating disorders that are helpful in the treatment of AN. Similar to bulimia, a multidisciplinary approach involving dietitians, psychologists, medical personnel, and possibly psychiatric medications (even though there are no FDA-approved drugs for anorexia) can be helpful. Psychiatric drugs can usually help patients deal with anxiety or depression that may be concomitant. One of the most difficult aspects of the disease is convincing patients that they need treatment. Those who do seek treatment have a tough time preventing relapse, and periodic appointments with medical personnel especially during times of stress can be extremely helpful.

Prevention

Just like bulimia, there is no true way to prevent the disease. The best prevention may be detecting the disease early on so that it does not progress into full-blown anorexia. Asking patients about their eating habits and satisfaction with appearance are good screening questions.

Alcohol Abuse

Presentation and Characteristics

During acute alcohol ingestion, flushing is the most common skin manifestation affecting about half of Asians, 80% Native Americans, and about a quarter of Caucasians. Chronic drinkers who have cirrhosis exhibit the cutaneous manifestations of spider angiomas, palmar erythema, jaundice, petechiae, salivary gland hypertrophy, and Dupuytren contracture. Even in the absence of cirrhosis, about 18% of chronic alcoholics have palmar erythema and spider angiomas. Dupuytren contracture is also quite common even in the absence of cirrhosis. Hypoalbuminemia from cirrhosis can lead to edema and ascites. Dilated superficial veins over the abdomen (caput medusae) can be a good clinical clue that a patient has portal hypertension. The following diseases are also listed as occurring more frequently in alcoholics: lichen planus, spontaneous skin necrosis, disseminated superficial

porokeratosis, necrolytic migratory erythema (without glucagonoma), reactive angioendotheliomatosis, and arteriovenous malformations. Alcohol has also been found to induce and aggravate the disease of rosacea. "Breakouts" of pustular and granulomatous lesions can appear after consumption of even small amounts of alcohol, although they are more common after drinking bouts. Telangiectasias in the central portion of the face tend to develop with greater frequency and severity in rosacea patients who drink heavily.

Excessive alcohol consumption is also the most common factor associated with development of porphyria cutanea tarda. Alcohol appears to unmask an underlying inherited defect in the enzyme uroporphyrinogen decarboxylase.

Alcohol also tends to precipitate hemochromatosis owing to its facilitation of the absorption of iron. A pigmented erythema on the lower extremities has been reported to be present in up to 40% of alcoholics below 60 years of age. Alcohol can interfere with the absorption, digestion, and metabolism of vitamins and other nutrients. Even in alcoholics who are not malnourished, vitamin deficiencies are common. Vitamins B and C are the most common vitamins to be deficient in chronic alcoholics. An alcoholic lingual syndrome that consists of a thickened tongue with atrophic mucosa, "lacquer" edges, and an often brown covering has been reported in late-stage alcoholics. Chronic alcoholics also tend to look older and have a "dull expression." Clinically, the facial skin can look corrugated, wrinkled, and flabby with a lack of elasticity.

Treatment

Treatment depends on whether the patient is alcohol-dependent or not. If the patient is dependent on alcohol, then abstinence must be a part of treatment. Cognitive behavioral therapy is often used to help patients deal with the disorder. Several medications have been approved for treatment, including antabuse, campral, and naltrexone. Alcoholics Anonymous is a voluntary, international self-help organization founded in 1935 that uses a 12-step program to assist alcoholics in achieving and maintaining sobriety and is the single most effective therapy.

AN, BN, and alcoholism are pernicious problems throughout the world. Early detection is recognized as an important aspect of therapy. Skin signs can help provide early diagnosis and appropriate referral of these patients.

Prevention

Knowing and recognizing a family history and early intervention are the best ways to prevent alcohol use or abuse from progressing to alcoholism.

ESSENTIAL FATTY ACID DEFICIENCY

Definition

Essential fatty acids (EFAs) are fatty acids that humans must ingest because the body requires them for good health but cannot synthesize them. Only two fatty acids are known to be essential for humans: α-linolenic acid (an ω-3 fatty acid) and linoleic acid (an ω-6 fatty acid).

Presentation and Characteristics

There are several different skin manifestations that are associated with essential fatty acid deficiencies (EFADs). These were discovered by studying patients on long-term parenteral nutrition that did not contain adequate amounts of EFAs, by a study on infant formulas that contained varying amounts of linoleic acid (ω-6), and by studying different case reports in the literature. Through these studies, it has been found that EFAD can lead to hemorrhagic dermatitis, skin atrophy, generalized scaly dermatitis that can resemble congenital ichthyosis, dry skin, keratosis pilaris, edema, scalp dermatitis, alopecia, depigmentation of hair, and hemorrhagic folliculitis. The patient's history will involve either long-term total parenteral nutrition devoid of ω-3 (linolenic acid) or ω-6 (linoleic acid) fatty acids or infant formula devoid of either of these two EFAs. However, most infant formula companies have now added these EFAs to their formulas.

Treatment

Earlier it was thought that topical application of linoleic acid (safflower or sunflower) oil could reverse signs/symptoms of EFAD; however, more recent reports in the literature have shown that topical application of these oils was unable to reverse symptoms. Treatment with dietary EFAs or Intralipid (parenteral lipid) is the treatment of choice.

Prevention

Prevention involves fortifying all parenteral nutrition therapies with parenteral lipid as well as ensuring that infant formula contains adequate amounts of EFAs. Good sources of ω-3s include walnuts, wheat germ oil, flaxseed oil/canola oil, fish liver oils/fish eggs, human milk, organ meats, and seafood/fatty fish like albacore tuna, mackerel, salmon and sardines. Good sources of ω-6s include corn oil, peanut oil, cottonseed oil, soybean oil, and many other plant oils.

METABOLIC DISORDERS

Diabetes Mellitus

Definitions

Diabetes mellitus (DM) occurs because of a lack of insulin or resistance to its action. It is diagnosed by measuring fasting or random blood-glucose concentration (and occasionally by oral glucose tolerance test).

Presentation and Characteristics

Skin diseases that have been described in DM may be either pathognomonic of DM or just associated with DM because they are nonspecific but only seen in greater frequency in diabetics. For example, candidal paronychia (Fig. 54-9A and B), multiple granuloma annulare (Fig. 54-10), and necrobiosis lipoidica diabeticorum (Fig. 54-11A and B) are not pathognomonic but only seen in greater frequency in diabetics. However, the diabetic foot syndrome–ulcer and Charcot foot (Fig. 54-12A and B), scleredema adultorum (Fig. 54-13), diabetic dermopathy (shin spots), and diabetic bullae are pathognomonic of DM. Diabetic foot ulcers are caused by arterial insufficiency (ischemic) ulcer and sensory neuropathic ulcers. Neurogenic arthropathy (Charcot joint) is joint destruction resulting from loss or diminution of proprioception, pain, and temperature perception. Although traditionally associated with tabes dorsalis, it is more frequently seen in diabetic neuropathy and leprosy.

Treatment of DM

The prescribing of drug therapy for DM should be undertaken in a specialist center. Although patients with type 2 diabetes may be controlled on diet alone, many also require oral antidiabetic drugs or insulin (or both) to maintain satisfactory control. In overweight individuals, type 2 diabetes may be prevented by losing weight and increasing physical activity; use of the antiobesity drug orlistat may be considered in obese patients. Treatment of all forms of DM should be aimed at alleviating symptoms and minimizing the risk of long-term complications; tight control of DM is essential. DM is a strong risk factor for

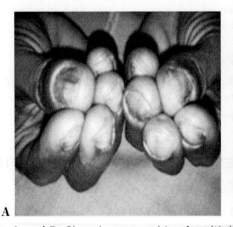
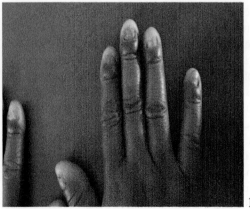

A   **B**

FIGURE 54-9: **A and B:** Chronic paronychia of multiple nails. This can be found in long-standing, poorly controlled diabetes mellitus. (Courtesy by Dr. Ayesha Akinkugbe)

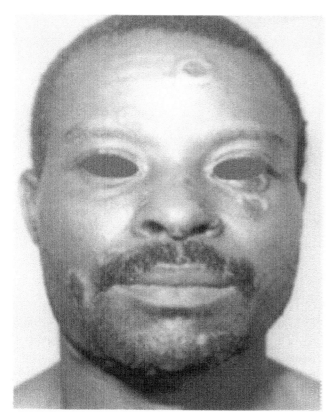

FIGURE 54-10: Granuloma annulare. Multiple lesions may be seen in diabetes mellitus.

cardiovascular disease. Other risk factors for cardiovascular disease such as smoking, obesity, and hyperlipidemia should be addressed. Cardiovascular risk in patients with DM can be further reduced by the use of an angiotensin converting enzyme (ACE) inhibitor, low-dose aspirin, and a lipid-regulating drug.

Prevention of DM Complications

Optimal glycemic control in both type 1 DM and type 2 DM reduces, in the long term, the risk of microvascular complications including retinopathy, development of proteinuria, and to some extent neuropathy. A measure of the total glycosylated (or glycated) hemoglobin (HbA_1) or a specific fraction (HbA_{1c}) provides a good indication of glycemic control over the previous 2 to 3 months. Overall, it is ideal to aim for an HbA_{1c} concentration of 48 to 59 mmol/mol or less.

Diabetics are usually advised to take care of their feet with the attention they give the face! Meticulous hygiene of the feet and the inner lining of the boots should be maintained to prevent infection. Diabetics should not walk about barefooted. Minor traumas from pedicuring instruments or splinter injury usually fester into the diabetic foot syndrome, more so because a neuropathic foot is insensitive. Treatment is directed against the primary disease; mechanical devices are used to assist in weight-bearing and prevention of further trauma. The shoes should not be tight fitting or made of hard fabrics. Well-padded low-heeled boots with appropriate depth with width are recommended. In some instances, amputation becomes unavoidable.

OBESITY

Please see chapter on obesity (Chapter 47).

METABOLIC SYNDROME X

Definition

Metabolic syndrome is a clustering of at least three of five of the following medical conditions: abdominal (central) obesity, elevated blood pressure, elevated fasting plasma glucose,

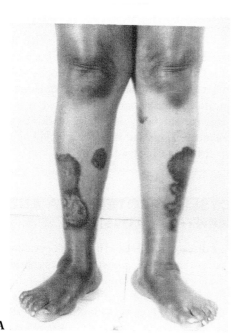
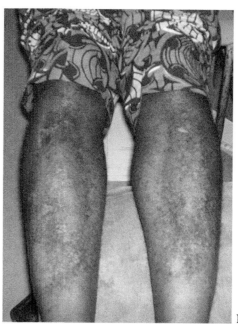

FIGURE 54-11: **A and B:** Necrobiosis lipoidica diabeticorum on the classical site, the shins. (B- Courtesy by Dr Sola Ayanlowo)

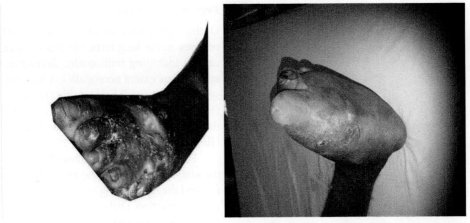

FIGURE 54-12: A: Diabetic foot ulcer. **B:** Charcot foot in diabetes mellitus. (A and B- Courtesy by Dr Olufemi Fasanmade)

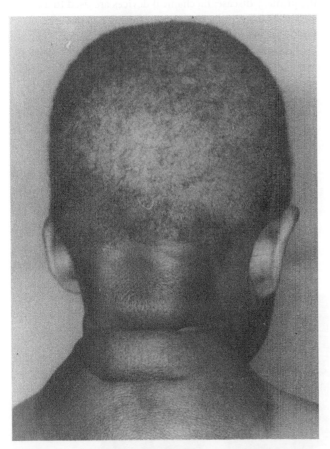

FIGURE 54-13: Scleredema adultorum. Woody induration and thickening of the skin on the upper back and neck in a diabetic man.

high serum triglycerides, and low high-density lipoprotein (HDL) levels.

Metabolic syndrome is also known as *metabolic syndrome X, cardiometabolic syndrome, syndrome X, insulin resistant syndrome, Reaven syndrome* (named after Gerald Reaven), and *CHAOS* (in Australia). CHAOS is an acronym for Coronary artery disease, Hypertension, Atherosclerosis, Obesity, and Stroke.

Presentation and Characteristics

The main sign of metabolic syndrome is *central obesity* (also known as visceral, male-pattern or apple-shaped adiposity), overweight with adipose tissue accumulation particularly around the waist and trunk. Other signs of metabolic syndrome include high blood pressure, decreased fasting serum HDL cholesterol, elevated fasting serum triglyceride level (VLDL triglyceride), impaired fasting glucose, insulin resistance, or prediabetes. Associated conditions include hyperuricemia, fatty liver (especially in concurrent obesity) progressing to nonalcoholic fatty liver disease, polycystic ovarian syndrome (in women), erectile dysfunction (in men), and acanthosis nigricans.

The most significant skin finding is psoriasis. This affects such a large number of patients (3% to 5% of the population) that recognition of this association is very important and often underrecognized.

Multiple skin tags, especially more than 30, can also be associated with the metabolic syndrome.

Some authors have suggested that lichen planus and metabolic syndrome are associated, but more data are needed.

The most recent criteria proposed by the American Heart Association and the National Heart, Lung, and Blood Institute published in 2005 are listed in Table 54-1. Because most patients with metabolic syndrome tend to be obese, cutaneous signs and symptoms would be the same as those described in Chapter 43.

DYSLIPOPROTEINEMIA AND XANTHOMATOSIS

The diseases represented by dyslipoproteinemias and xanthomatoses are diverse, numerous, and of considerable importance because of their relationship to vascular disease. The skin is a particularly valuable index for the diagnosis of dyslipoproteinemias and for following the effects of treatment. Xanthomas are lipid deposits in skin and subcutaneous tissues.

Secondary hyperlipoproteinemia may be found in obstructive liver disease, hematopoietic diseases such as myelomas,

TABLE 54-1 • Criteria for Clinical Diagnosis of Metabolic Syndrome

Measure (Any Three of Five Constitute Diagnosis of Metabolic Syndrome)	Categorical Cutpoints
Elevated waist circumference[a]	≥102 cm (≥40 in) in men
	≥88 cm (≥35 in) in women
Elevated triglycerides	≥150 mg/dL (1.7 mmol/L)
	or
	On drug treatment for elevated triglycerides!
Reduced HDL-C	<40 mg/dL (1.03 mmol/L) in men
	<50 mg/dL (1.3 mmol/L) in women
	or
	On drug treatment for reduced HDL-C!
Elevated blood pressure	≥130 mm Hg systolic blood pressure
	or
	≥85 mm Hg diastolic blood pressure
	or
	On antihypertensive drug treatment in a patient with a history of hypertension
Elevated fasting glucose	≥100 mg/dL
	or
	On drug treatment for elevated glucose

[a] To measure waist circumference, locate top of right iliac crest. Place a measuring tape in a horizontal plane around abdomen at level of iliac crest. Before reading tape measure, ensure that the tape is snug but does not compress the skin and is parallel to the floor. Measurement is made at the end of a normal expiration.

Waldenström macroglobulinemia and occasionally lymphoma, xanthoma diabeticorum, chronic renal failure, myxedema, pancreatitis, and medication-induced hyperlipoproteinemia (e.g., oral prednisone, oral retinoids, indomethacin, highly active antiretroviral therapy [HAART] and olanzapine). There is also normolipoproteinemic xanthomatoses in which serum cholesterol and lipoproteins are normal, yet secondary lipid deposition in the skin occurs.

Classification of Lipoproteins

In clinical medicine as well as in biomedical research, the lipoproteins are usually classified on the basis of their electrophoretic mobility and hydrated density. Frederickson classified **primary** hyperlipoproteinemias into six types on the basis of electrophoretic pattern as follows:

Type I: Excess chylomicrons
Type IIa: Excess β-lipoprotein
Type IIb: Excess β-lipoprotein with slightly elevated VLDLs
Type III: Increased intermediate-density (remnant) lipoprotein
Type IV: Increased pre β-lipoprotein
Type V: Increased pre β-lipoproteins and chylomicrons

Presentation and Characteristics

The type of defect in patients with severe hypertriglyceridemia is suggested by the *age* of onset of the chylomicronemia syndrome. Patients with signs and symptoms before puberty nearly always have *genetic* defects in triglyceride metabolism involving lipoprotein lipase activity. Xanthomas associated with the dyslipoproteinemias are frequently classified as *eruptive* (Fig. 54-14), *tuberous* (Fig. 54-15A and B), *planar*, or *tendinous*.

The characteristic xanthoma accompanying the chylomicronemia syndrome is the *eruptive* xanthoma. These are usually asymptomatic, discrete papules 5 to 6 mm in size, with an yellowish brown center and red halo. They appear in crops over the entire body. Occasionally, eruptive xanthomas may become confluent and associated with tuberous xanthomas. These hybrid lesions have been termed *tuboeruptive xanthomas*.

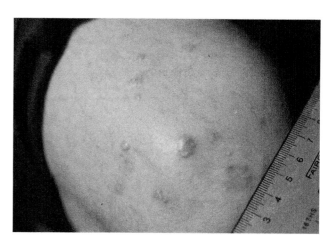

FIGURE 54-14: Eruptive xanthoma over the knee with scattered yellow nodules.

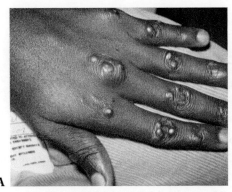
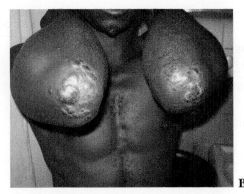

FIGURE 54-15: **A and B:** A patient with tuberous xanthomas on the back of the hands and elbows. These are usually associated with dysbetalipoproteinemia. (Courtesy by Dr. Sola Ayanlowo)

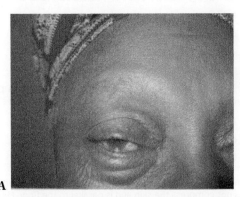
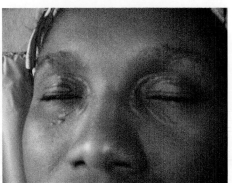

FIGURE 54-16: **A and B:** Xanthelasma palpebrarum. This can be found in familial hypercholesterolemia or normolipemic women. (B, Courtesy by Dr. Debo Oresanya)

Type III hyperlipoproteinemia have virtually pathognomonic *planar* xanthomas on the palmar creases of their hands and tuberous xanthomas on the elbows, knees, and buttocks.

Clinical manifestations of hyperbetalipoproteinemia in a patient with heterozygous familial hypercholesterolemia are arcus juvenilis (a grayish white ring in the cornea owing to accumulation of lipid droplets), xanthelasma, and tendon xanthomas. Xanthelasma palpebrarum (Fig. 54-16A and B) is the most common type of xanthoma. It occurs on the eyelids and is characterized by soft yellowish brown/orange oblong plaques, usually near the inner canthi, frequently symmetrical with a tendency to be coalescent, progressive, and permanent. The disorder is encountered chiefly in middle-aged women who have hepatic or biliary disorders. Xanthelasma may be found in familial hypercholesterolemia; however, the majority of the patients are normolipemic.

Cerebrotendinous xanthomatosis (CTX) is a rare autosomal recessive disease characterized by the accumulation of cholestanol (5,6-dihydroxycholesterol) in plasma lipoproteins and tissues. The cardinal manifestations of CTX include xanthomas, cataracts, severe neurologic deficiencies, mental retardation, dementia, and cardiovascular disease. The xanthomas may be widespread and most commonly occur in tendons, brain, and lungs. Death usually occurs between the fourth and sixth decades and usually results from severe neurologic deficiencies with pseudobulbar paralysis or acute myocardial infarction.

Suggested Readings

Attia E. Anorexia nervosa: current status and future directions. *Annu Rev Med.* 2010;61(1):425–435.

Combs GF Jr. *The Vitamins: Fundamental Aspects in Nutrition and Health.* San Diego: Elsevier, Inc; 2008.

Heath ML, Sidbury R. Cutaneous manifestations of nutritional deficiency. *Curr Opin Pediatr.* 2006;18(4):417–422.

Hunt A, Harrington D, Robinson S. Vitamin B12 deficiency *BMJ.* 2014;349:g5226.

James WD, Berger TG, et al. *Andrews' Diseases of the Skin: Clinical Dermatology.* Philadelphia: Saunders Elsevier, 2006.

Kaur J. A Comprehensive review on metabolic syndrome. *Cardiol Res Pract.* 2014;943162. doi:10.1155/2014/943162.PMC 3966331.

McLaren DS. Skin in protein energy malnutrition [Review]. *Arch Dermatol.* 1987;123(12):1674–1676a.

Olumide YM. Nutritional dermatoses in Nigeria. *Int J Dermatol.* 1995;34(1):11–16.

Oumeish OY, Oumeish I. Nutritional skin problems in children. *Clin Dermatol.* 2003;21(4):260–263.

Sanchez MR. Alcohol, social behavior disorders, and their cutaneous manifestations. *Clin Dermatol.* 1999;17(4):479–489.

Strumia R. Bulimia and anorexia nervosa: cutaneous manifestations. *J Cosmet Dermatol.* 2002;1(1):30–34.

Strumia R. Dermatologic signs in patients with eating disorders. *Am J Clin Dermatol.* 2005;6(3):165–173.

The British National Formulary (BNF) 66. Accessed September, 2013 to March, 2014.

Tyler I, Wiseman MC, Crawford RI, et al. Cutaneous manifestations of eating disorders. *J Cutan Med Surg.* 2002;6(4):345–353.

Vitamin A Deficiency and Supplementation. UNICEF Data. Accessed April 07, 2015. http://data.unicef.org/nutrition/vitamin-a.html.

WHO Vitamin A deficiency/Micronutrient deficiencies. Accessed March 03, 2008.

Where to Look for More Information About a Skin Disease

John C. Hall, MD

"Doctor, I saw a patient yesterday who was diagnosed as having epidermolysis bullosa. I understand this is quite a rare condition. Where can I find the latest information on this subject?" This is the type of question frequently asked of a teaching dermatologist. A computer gives you references, and some databases provide information about a dermatosis. However, assuming that these are not readily available, there are other sources.

PRINT RESOURCES

First, the inquiring physician or student should check out the Dictionary–Index of this book. Even for rare conditions, there is at least a definition of the disease. The Suggested Readings at the end of each chapter can also point one in the right direction for books or papers on a given subject.

Second, there are several comprehensive general texts on dermatology that include rare diseases. The following are suggested.

- Arndt KA, LeBoit DE, Robinson JK, et al. *Cutaneous Medicine and Surgery*. Philadelphia: WB Saunders; 1995.
- Bolognia JL, Jorizzo LJ, Rapini, RP. *Dermatology*. 3rd ed. Elsevier. e-Edition available; 2012.
- Burgdorf WHC, Plewig G, Wolff H, et al. *Braun-Falco's Dermatology*. New York, NY: Springer; 2008.
- Burns T, Breathnach S, Cox N, et al. *Rook's Textbook of Dermatology*. 8th ed. Oxford: Wiley-Blackwell (an imprint of John Wiley & Sons Ltd); 2010.
- Cerroni L, Gatter K, Helmut K. *Skin Lymphoma: The Illustrated Guide*. 3rd ed. United Kingdom: Wiley-Blackwell (an imprint of John Wiley & Sons Ltd); 2009.
- Dellavalle RP. Internet dermatology resources. *J Am Acad Dermatol*. 2013;68:1039.

- Demis DJ, Dahl M, Smith EB, et al. *Clinical Dermatology*. Vol 4. Philadelphia: JB Lippincott (revised annually).
- White GM, Cox NH. *Diseases of the Skin: A Color Atlas and Text*. 2nd ed. St Louis: C. V. Mosby; 2005.
- Edwards L. *Genital Dermatology Atlas*. Hagerstown, MD: Lippincott Williams and Wilkins; 2004.
- Goodheart HP, Gonzalez ME. *Goodheart's Photoguide to Common Pediatric and Adult Skin Disorders: Diagnosis and Management*. 4th ed. Philadelphia: Wolters Kluwer; 2016.
- Habif TP. *Clinical Dermatology: Expert Consult – Online and Print, A Color Guide to Diagnosis and Therapy*. 5th ed. Edinburgh: Elsevier Health Sciences; 2009.
- Jablonski, NG. *Skin: A Natural History*. Berkeley: University of California Press; 2006.
- Lebwohl MG, Heymann WR, Berth-Jones J. *Treatment of Skin Disease: Comprehensive Therapeutic Strategies*. Philadelphia, PA: Elsevier Saunders; 2013.
- Litt JZ. *Litt's Drug Eruption Reference Manual Including Drug Interactions*. 22nd ed. New York: United States: Informa Healthcare; 2016.
- Neill SM, Lewis FM. *Ridley's the Vulva*. 3rd ed. Hoboken: Wiley-Blackwell (an imprint of John Wiley & Sons Ltd); 2009.
- Odum RB, James WD, Berger TG. *Andrew's Diseases of the Skin: Clinical Dermatology*. 10th ed. Philadelphia: WB Saunders; 2006.
- Trozak D. *Dermatology Guide for Primary Care: An Illustrated Guide*. Totowa, NJ: Humana Press; 2006.
- White GM, Cox NH. *Diseases of the Skin*. St. Louis: Mosby; 2005.
- Wolff K, Goldsmith LA, Katz SI, et al. *Fitzpatrick's Dermatology in General Medicine*. 7th ed. New York, NY: McGraw-Hill. Available as e-Edition.

ONLINE RESOURCES

The National Library of Medicine, 8,600 Rockville Pike, Bethesda, MD 20014 (www.nlm.nih.gov), has very good information on different medical sites. Other useful websites include the following:

- A.B. Ackerman's Atlas Online at www.derm101.com
- *Advances in Dermatology* Video Program
- *American Academy of Dermatology* at www.aad.org
- British Association of Dermatologists (clinical practice guidelines) at www.bad.org.uk
- Dermatologic Clinics at www.derm.theclinics.com
- Dermatology Slide Atlas at www.med.unc.edu/derm /atlas/welcome.htm
- *Evidence-Based Dermatology* at http://ebderm.org
- *Internet Journal of Dermatology* at www.ispub.com
- The *Journal of American Academy of Dermatology* at www.eblue.org
- Medical Dermatology at www.labordedermatology.com
- National Organization for Rare Disorders at http:// www.rarediseases.org/
  - Orlow SJ, Strober BE, Hale EK. *Advances in Dermatology Video Program*. http://cmeinfo.com/634. Accessed July 28, 2016.
- Skin Cancer Foundation at www.skincancer.org
  - Testing, E., & Systems, A. (2004). *Board review study questions*. Retrieved July 28, 2016, from http:// dermatologyinreview.com/galderma
- University of Iowa, Dermatology Dictionary Derm-PathTutor at www.tray.dermatology.uiowa.edu/home

The following journals are highly pertinent and are available online:

- *Acta Dermato-Venereologica,* 6 issues per year. Published by Taylor & Francis Group.
- *American Journal of Clinical Dermatology,* 6 issues a year. Published by Adis International.
- *American Journal of Contact Dermatitis,* published by W.B. Saunders. Although this journal is no longer published, you can continue to view the contents of this website and order reprints from 2002 and earlier.

- *American Journal of Dermatopathology,* 6 issues a year. Official journal of the International Society of Dermatopathology.
- *Archives of Dermatology,* a monthly journal published by the American Medical Association, Chicago. It is indexed in both the June and December issues.
- *British Journal of Dermatology,* published monthly by Blackwell Synergy.
- *Clinics in Dermatology,* 6 issues a year. Published by Elsevier.
- *Cutis,* a monthly magazine for the general practitioner, published by Reed Medical Publishers.
- *Dermatologic Surgery,* a journal published by Blackwell Synergy.
- *Dermatologic Therapy,* published by Blackwell Synergy.
- *Dermatology Online Journal,* Senior editor Barbara Burrall, M.D., published by Arthur C. Huntley.
- *Internet Journal of Dermatology,* Editor-in-chief Madeleine Duvic, M.D.
- *Journal of the American Academy of Dermatology,* a monthly journal published by the American Academy of Dermatology.
- *Journal of Cutaneous Pathology,* 10 issues a year. Official publication of the American Society of Dermatopathology. Published by Blackwell Synergy.
- *Journal of Dermatological Treatment,* 6 issues a year. Published by Taylor & Francis Group.
- *Journal of Drugs in Dermatology,* official publication of the International Society for Dermatologic Surgery.
- *Journal of Investigative Dermatology,* a monthly journal published on behalf of the Society for Investigative Dermatology by Blackwell Publishing.
- *Journal Watch Dermatology,* from the publishers of The New England Journal of Medicine, the Massachusetts Medical Society. It is published biweekly on the web and monthly in print.
- *Pediatric Dermatology,* published bimonthly by Blackwell Synergy.
- *Practical Reviews in Dermatology*, Johns Hopkins School of Medicine, Oakstone Publishing. Updated monthly and available online.

Dictionary-Index

Introduction The purpose of the dictionary portion of this index is to define and classify some of the rarer dermatologic terms not covered in the text. Some very rare or unimportant terms have purposely been omitted, but undoubtedly some terms that are *not* rare and *are* important have also been omitted. Just as a picture is worth a thousand words, so the most easily seen of all organs, is described in thousands of words. This leaves the specialty of dermatology as the specialty of unlimited description. Most of the histopathologic terms have been defined. Suggestions or corrections from the reader will be appreciated.

A

Acantholytic dermatosis, transient (Grover's disease) (TAD). Characterized by intensely pruritic, small, firm, reddish-brown, papules mainly on the upper torso, aggravated by sweating. Seen predominantly in white, older men. Histologically, there is acantholysis of the epidermis. There is also a persistent form that is called persistent acantholytic dermatosis (PAD). It has been associated with bone marrow transplantation, underlying malignancy, chronic renal failure, radiation therapy, AIDS and excessive heat, sweating or occlusion. Also with eczema, asteatosis, allergic contact dermatitis and non-specific irritation.

Acanthosis nigricans, 452t

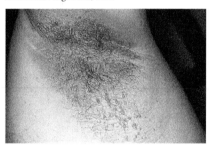

Pseudoacanthosis nigricans of the axilla.

Acne, 8, 25, 43, 180–186, 180f–182f, 186f
    conglobata, 180
    fulminans, 180
    hidradenitis suppurativa, 242
    instruction sheet, 183–185
    inversa, 180
    neonatal, 491, 491t
    rosacea, 186–188, 187f
    scars of, 180, 185–186, 186f
    treatment of, 182, 185–186

Acne keloidalis nuchae. Seen mainly in African American men (ten times more common in dark skinned people than Caucasians). It causes up to 0.5% of all dermatology cases in African Americans. Usually in the occipital scalp and posterior neck. Papules and pustules form hairline keloidal papules and plaques that can be tender, disfiguring and result in scaring alopecia. Topical or intralesional steroids, long term antibiotics, and in severe cases surgery is used for treatment. A prolonged course of Accutane has also been used by some authors., 396

Acne mechanica, 460t, 463

Acne necrotica miliaris, 235t, 238

Acne varioliformis. A chronic inflammatory disorder in adults on the scalp, the forehead, the nose and the cheeks, and rarely the trunk, characterized by the presence of papulopustular lesions that heal within a few days, leaving a smallpox-like scar. Recurrent outbreaks can continue for months and years.

Acquired brachial cutaneous dyschromatosis (ABCD). Usually bilateral, usually female, Caucasian, middle-aged patients with asymptomatic, common, acquired geographic gray brown patches interspersed with hypopigmented macules on dorsal forearms. It is not associated with estrogens but may be associated with angiotensin converting enzyme inhibitors.

Acquired ichthyosis, 456, 457f

Acquired immunodeficiency syndrome (AIDS), 37, 310. *See also* Human immunodeficiency virus

Acquired perforating disease (APD). Intensely pruritic papular eruption that may be hyperkeratotic or form a crater, which tends to koebnerize. Usually on the trunk and extremities and skin biopsy will help confirm the diagnosis. Associated with renal failure, diabetes mellitus, hepatitis, hyperparathyroidism, hypothyroidism, AIDs, atopic dermatitis, herpes zoster, scabies, and as a paraneoplastic disorder, 460. Perforating folliculitis may be the same disease.

Acquired progressive kinking, 398

Acral erythema. Intense redness of palms and soles with dysesthesia and occasionally blisters. Associated with anticancer chemotherapy. Most commonly capecitabine, cytarabine, doxorubicin, 5-flurouracel, and taxanes, 99t

Acral lentiginous melanoma, 357, 357f

Acrochordons (skin tags), 320t, 321t. *See also* Fibromas, pedunculated

Acrocyanosis. Characterized by constant coldness and bluish discoloration of the fingers and the toes, which is more intense in cold weather and on dependence by dangling the legs over a chair or bed. Seen more often in women., 571t

Acrodermatitis chronica atrophicans. A chronic, biphasic disease seen most commonly in western Europe. The first phase begins with an erythematous patch on an extremity, which, in weeks or months, develops the second phase of skin atrophy. The cause is believed to be a mixed infection with group B arboviruses, transmitted by the wood tick *Ixodes ricinus*. It is a penicillin-sensitive bacterium or spirochete. Can be a chronic late stage of Lyme disease., 261, 458

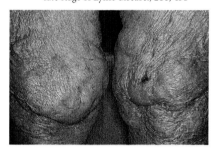

Acrodermatitis chronica atrophicans on the legs.

Acrodermatitis continua of Hallopeau, 404, 404f

Acrodermatitis enteropathica. Condition of zinc deficiency manifested by inflammatory periorificial and acral dermatitis, alopecia, and diarrhea. When zinc was added to pediatric formulas and to hyperalimentation regiments it became rare. Autosomal recessive., 593

Acrodermatitis, papular, of childhood. *See* Gianotti-Crosti syndrome

Acrodynia. Mercury poisoning usually in infants. Itching, painful swelling, pink, cold, clammy hands and feet with hemorrhagic puncta. Stomatitis and loss of teeth occur. Greater than 0.001 mg per liter mercury is found in the urine.

Acrokeratoelastoidosis. Different size, symmetric, horny, glossy translucent papules on the knuckles, thenar eminences, hypothenar eminences, dorsa and sides of the fingers and margins of the hands. May also involve the tibia, anterior ankles, malleoli, Achilles tendon, dorsal feet, and dorsal toes.

Page numbers followed by "b" indicate box; those followed by "f" indicate figure; those followed by "t" indicate table.

Acrokeratosis, paraneoplastic (Bazex's syndrome). A specific sign of cancer of the upper respiratory and upper digestive tracts characterized by plum-colored acral skin lesions, paronychia, nail dysplasias, and keratoderma, 452t

Acrokeratosis verruciformis of Hopf. A rare disease affecting the dorsa of the hands and the feet characterized by flat warty papules. Probably hereditary. Differentiate from *flat warts* and from *epidermodysplasia verruciformis.*

Acromegaly. Hyperpituitary condition causing gross thickening of the skin with characteristic facies, enlarged hands, feet, digits, hyperhidrosis, hypertrichosis, and hyperpigmentation., 385, 410, 416

Acropustulosis of infancy. Tiny pustules or vesicles on the distal extremities that occurwithin the first year of life and are intensely pruritic. Spontaneous resolution usually occurs within the first 2 or 3 years of life. This is frequently seen as a post scabies syndrome, 495t, 496

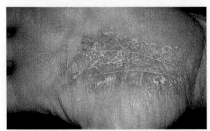

Acropustulosis.

Acropustulosis. Refers to pustular diseases of the palms as soles such as pustular psoriasis of the palms and soles(pustular posriaiasis of barber, dermatitis repens, infantile acropustulosis, and acrodermatitis continua of Hallapeau.

Actinic dermatitis, chronic (Actinic reticuloid). Persistent erythema of the face, hands, and other exposed areas. CD8+ cells infiltrate the skin due to sensitivity to UVA, UVB and even visible light. Especially in elderly men it is associated with increased contact allergies. Strict UVA, UVB and visible light protection isdifficult but beneficial. May become generalized and difficult clinically and histologically to tell from cutaneous T-cell lymphoma (mycosis fungoides). Contact dermatitis is a common association., 472, 472f

Actinic granuloma. *See* Annular elastotic giant cell granuloma

Actinic keratosis, 320t, 321t, 322t, 329f, 328–331, 530,531t

Actinic prurigo. *See* Prurigo, actinic

Actinomycosis, 235t, 252

Acute hemorrhagic edema (Finkelstein disease, AHE). Benign cutaneous leukocytoclastic vasculitis in children under two years ofage. Polycyclic plaques with a dark necrotic center in a medallion, target orcockade configuration sparing thetrunk. Resolves in 1 to 2 weeks without sequelae and can be postinfectious., 536, 537f

Adams-Oliver syndrome. A congenital absence of skin and as aplasia cutis congenita usually involves scalp vertex and terminal transverse limb defects. Autosomal dominant and can be associated with extensive lethal anomalies of internal organs including central nervous system, cardio, pulmonary, gastrointestinal, and genitourinary.

Addison's disease, 442, 454

Adenoma sebaceum (Pringle's disease), 339, 462,463f

Adhesion disorders, 480, 480t, 482f

Adiposis dolorosa (Dercum's disease). A lipoma-like disorder characterized by irregular and painful deposits of fat in the subcutaneous tissue of the trunk and limbs, more common in women than in men.

AESOP syndrome- characterized by regional lymphadenopathy with erythematous skin patch or plaque, chest overlying solitary bone plasmacytoma although there maybe some evidence it can overly other tumors also.

Africa tick bite fever. Occurs in clusters of patients especially in South Africa in game hunters and tourists visiting endemic areas such as the eastern Caribbean. Five to seven days after a bite is the abrupt onset of fever, nausea, headache, myalgias and neck pain. The bites are often multiple and consist of a black, hemorrhagic eschar surrounded by a red halo and tender regional lymphadenopathy. Life threatening complications are rare and doxycycline 100 mgs twice a day for 7days is the treatment of choice. It is caused by the bite of the Amblyomma tick., 262, 262f

Aicardi-Goutières syndrome. Itchy, red, swelling of the fingers, toes, earlobes that mimics chilblains. The hands and feet are puffy and cold. This is accompanied by intracranial calcifications and numerous neurologic complications.

AIDS. *See* Acquired immunodeficiency syndrome

Ainhum. Essentially a tropical disease of blacks that results in the amputation of a toe or toes because of constricting bands.

Albinism, 491t, 491

Albright's hereditary osteodystrophy. Multiple areas of cutaneous ossification, skeletal abnormalities, abnormalities of the parathyroid gland, mental retardation, and shortening of the metacarpal bones.

Albright's syndrome. Large hyperpigmented macules, precocious puberty in females, and polyostotic fibrous dysplasia. The macules have a jagged border like the coastof Maine, unlike café-au-lait macules that usually have a smooth, or coast of California, border, 484

Alkaptonuria. *See* Ochronosis

Allergic granulomatosis (Churg-Strauss syndrome). The combination of transitory pulmonary infiltrations of Loeffler's syndrome, asthma, blood eosinophilia, and nodular purpuric or erythema multiforme-like skin lesions. Target organs beside skin and lung include kidney, upperrespiratory tract, and central nervous system. Diverse cutaneous manifestations probably the commonest manifestation of which is non-thrombocytopenic palpable

purpura. In fewer than 1/3 there is a positive p-ANCA, 157

Alopecia. From the Greek *alopekia,* meaning "hair loss." 99t, 387–396, 387t, 388t

androgenetic pattern, 388

areata, 37, 73, 387t, 388–393, 392f

central centrifugal cicatricial, 426

cicatricial, 394–396

cicatrisata, 238

congenital triangular alopecia. Probably under reported, idiopathic, triangular-shaped temporal area of hair loss. Present at birth or in the first year of life that can be bilateral. (*See* Congenital triangular alopecia)., 393

drugs causing, 391t

frontal fibrosing, cicatricial frontoparietal alopecia mainly in postmenopausal women associated with nonscarring alopecia of the eyebrows., 394, 395f

lipedematous. Rare nonscarring permanent hair loss seen mainly in older black women. Diffuse and mainly on the vertex with a thickened boggy scalp. On lateral radiographic exam the scalp is twice as thick due to increased thickness of subcutaneous fat. On biopsy the hair shaft is replaced by lamellar fibroplasias and hairs cannot grow more than 2 cm and break easily (*See* lipedematous alopecia).

lymphocytic cicatricial, 394

male-pattern, 517

moth eaten scalp, 254

neutrophilic cicatricial, 387

nonscarring diffuse, 388–390

nonscarring patchy, 391–394

scarring, 394–396

syphilis related, 394

Alopecia neoplastica. Infiltrated metastatic cancer to the scalp causing loss of hair. Breast cancer is often the underlying malignancy., 515

Alpha-1-antitrypsin deficiency. *See* Panniculitis, alpha-1-antitrypsin deficiency.

Alternariosis. Plant pathogens that rarely cause human cutaneous infection in patients that are immunocompromised. It can be caused by primary innoculation or endogenous spread after inhalation. Solitary or grouped papules, plaques or macules mainly on the lower extremities. Staining of tissue and culture are needed for diagnosis and medical as well as surgical therapy is often indicated.

Amebiasis, 552, 552f

Amyloidosis.

cutaneous amyloidosis is a rare condition that can be suspected clinically but should be proven by histologic examination. Amyloid is a protein-carbohydrate complex, which on histologic section assumes a diagnostic stain when treated with certain chemicals. Several biochemical varieties have been delineated. Amyloidosis can be systemic or localized.

localized amyloidosis (lichen amyloidosis). The skin only is involved. Clinically, this dermatosis appears as a patch of lichenified papules seen most commonly on the anterior tibial area of the legs. These pruritic lesions can be differentiated from lichen simplex chronicus or hypertrophic lichen planus by biopsy. Some authors feel the amyloid deposits are due to keratinocyte breakdown products caused by scratching and lichen amyloidosis is, therefore, a variant of lichen simplex chronicus.

primary systemic amyloidosis. This peculiar and serious form of amyloidosis commonly involves the skin along with the tongue, the heart, and the musculature of the viscera. The skin lesions appear as transparent-looking, yellowish papules or nodules, which are occasionally hemorrhagic. Commonly (40%) "pinch purpura" which is ecchymosis due to minor trauma. This is often seen on the eyelids. This form is familial., 418

secondary amyloidosis. Secondary amyloid deposits are very rare in the skin but are less rare in the liver, the spleen, and the kidney, where they occur as a result of certain chronic infectious diseases, and in association with multiple myeloma., 249

Androgenetic pattern hair loss, 389

Anetoderma. *See* Atrophies of the skin, macular atrophy

Angioedema, acquired. May be associated with urticaria (*See* Chap 12), other illnesses especially B-cell lymphoproliferative disease (AAE-I) or an autoantibody directed against the C1 inhibitor molecule (AAE-II), 100t

Angioedema, hereditary. Rare autosomal dominant form of angioedema that maybe associated with respiratory and gastrointestinal symptoms. Low level ordysfunctional inhibitor of the first component of complement is the cause., 208

Angioendotheliomatosis, malignant (intravascular large cell lymphoma). Usually fatal B cell intravascular lymphoma in the skin (lower dermal and subcutaneous blood vessels) and central nervous system. Erythematous telangiectatic plaques or nodules especially on the lower extremities. There is a reactive form of this disease, which is now described under a new name intralymphatic histiocytosis. It shows a benign intravascular histiocytic cell proliferation. There is a third variant that is associated with ischemia from arterial occlusion and arthrosclerosis. It is called a diffuse dermal angiomatosis.

Angioendotheliomatosis, reactive. A rare vasculoproliferation of the skin that has also been referred to diffuse dermal angiomatous. Consists of violaceous and occasionally ulcerated plaques which maybe painful and occur most commonly on the lower extremities. Most common comorbidity is sclerosis but it has been reported post-op at the site of a surgical procedure. Local and

systemic corticosteroids and isotrention have been tried but revascularization if possible is the best therapy., 371, 597

Angiofibromas. Asymptomatic skin-colored or pinkish-brown asymptomatic telangiectatic papules usually symmetrically scattered over the central face. When multiple they have been considered pathognomonic for tuberous sclerosis but have been reported with multiple endocrine neoplasia type 1 (MEN1), 462, 463f

Angiohistiocytoma, multinucleated cell. Uncommon tumor with fibrohistiocytic differentiation of vascular proliferation. That is benign may spontaneously regress and appears as solitary or multiple red purple papules especially on the extremities of healthy middle-aged and elderly woman. Diagnosis made by histopathologic examination. *See* Multinucleate cell angiohistiocytoma

Angioleiomyoma. Rare, usually acral, solitary, asymptomatic, subcutaneous, 1 to 4 cm nodule. To be differentiated from angiomyolipoma, which is usually renal and associated with tuberous sclerosis.

Angiolipoleiomyoma (angiomyolipoma). Well-circumscribed, asymptomatic, subcutaneous, rare tumor associated with renal disease and rarely extracutaneous sites may occur especially in the kidney., 463

Angioimmunoblastic lymphadenopathy with dysproteinemia. Fever, night sweats, hepatosplenomegaly and generalized lymphadenopathy. Fifty percent with skin findings that are most often a transient morbilliform eruption. Plaques, purpura, and urticarial lesions also occur. It is a subtype of T-cell lymphoma, which maybe primary or, according to some authors, triggered by a drug allergy orviralinfection.

Angiokeratomas, 334
  Fabry's form, 334
  Fordyce form, 334
  Mibelli's form, 334

Angiolymphoid hyperplasia with eosinophilia (Kimura's disease). A rare benign condition, usually seen on the face, characterized by a solitary or, less frequently, multiple dermal or subcutaneous nodules. There isa blood eosinophilia and there are eosinophils in the histologic infiltrate. Some consider Kimura's disease to be the systemic form only with deeper, larger lesions. When you biopsy be prepared tostop some often impressive bleeding. It has been associated with human herpes virus 8., 321t

Angioma serpiginosum. Characterized by multiple telangiectases, which may start from acongenital vascular nevus but often arisespontaneously. This rare vascular condition is to be differentiated from *Schamberg's disease, Majocchi's disease,* and*pigmented purpuric dermatitis of Gougerot and Blum.*

Angioma, targetoid hemosiderotic. Solitary benign tumor in adults on the trunk or extremities. Violaceous papule with an ecchymotic evanescent ring. It may be caused by trauma.

Angioma, tufted. *See* Tufted angioma (Progressive capillary hemangioma or Nakagawa's angioblastoma). Rare vascular tumor usually on the trunk, slow growing with a tendency to resolve. Usually develops within the first year of life but not present at birth. One third are tender and form dusky reddish-blue subcutaneous plaques or nodules that may be annular with depression resembling a "doughnut." Surrounding skin may be hyperhidrotic or have increased vellus hairs. It can be associated with Kasabach-Merritt syndrome.

Angiomatous, diffuse dermal. *See* Angioednotheliomatosis, reactive

Angiomyxoma (aggressive angiomyxoma). Locally aggressive tumor seen most commonly in the anogenital and pelvic of women in their reproductive age especially in the third decade. It has been described in men in the groin, scrotum, pelvis, and along the spermatic cord. It mimics a bartholin cyst, an MRI may help tell the extent of tumor before removal and recurrence rate is approximately 30%.

Angiosarcoma. Malignancy of vascular tissue usually seen on the face and scalp of elderly male patients, or at the site of chronic lymphedema when it is referred to as Stewart-Treves syndrome. Exertion, an increase in ambient temperature or a tilting of the head below the heart for 5 to 10seconds (head-tilt maneuver) can accentuate redness on the face and aid in early diagnosis., 371

Anhidrosis. The partial or complete absence of sweating, seen in ichthyosis, extensive psoriasis, scleroderma, prickly heat, vitamin A deficiency, one form of ectodermal dysplasia, and other diseases. Partial anhidrosis is producedby many antiperspirants., 464

Anhidrotic asthenia, tropical. Described in theSouth Pacific and in the desert in World War II. Soldiers showed increased sweating of the neck and face and anhidrosis (lack of sweating) below the neck. It was accompanied by weakness, headaches, and subjective warmth and was considered a chronic phase of prickly heat.

Anhidrotic ectodermal dysplasia, 8

Annular atrophic plaques of the face (Christianson's disease). Rare sclerotic annular plaques mainly on the face. Chronic, progressive, recalcitrant to treatment with unknown cause. May be a variant of scleroderma.

Annular elastotic giant cell granuloma (Actinic granuloma). Rare, in fair complexion, middle-aged or older patients. Asymptomatic (rarely intense pruritus) large (20-25 cm) plaques on the trunks and upper extremities. Chronic but may spontaneously remit after years. It may occur with alcoholic liver disease, diabetes, temporal arteritis, and sun bed radiation exposure. May be a variant of granuloma annulare on sun damaged skin.

Annular lichenoid dermatitis of youth. Persistent erythematous macules and papules that are round with a reddish-brown border and hypopigmented centrally especially in the groin and flanks. Phototherapy, topical corticosteroids and systemic corticosteroids were effective but relapse recurred after therapy withdrawal. Histopathology is characteristic.

Anonychia. Absence of all or part of one or several nails. Congenital in diseases such as Apert's syndrome, cartilage-hair dysplasia syndrome, dyskeratosis congenital, Ellis-van Creveld syndrome, nail-patella syndrome, Goltz syndrome, progeria, hypohydrotic ectodermal dysplasia, incontinentia pigmenti, Turner's syndrome, trisomy 13, and trisomy 18. Acquired in diseases such as lichen planus, Stevens-Johnson syndrome, epidermolysis bullosa, and trauma. It can also be seen in a simplex form associated with digital, hand or foot abnormalities.

Anthralin. A proprietary name for dihydroxy-anthranol, which is a strong reducing agent useful in the treatment of chronic cases of psoriasis. Its action is similar to that of chrysarobin. It causes troublesome staining and can be irritating. Short contact anthralin therapy (SCAT) is less irritating., 36, 392

Anthrax. A primary chancre-type disease caused by *Bacillus anthracis,* occurring in persons who work with the hides and the hair of infected sheep, horses, or cattle. A pulmonary form is known. It has the potential for use as a bioterrorist agent, 543–544, 543f, 570t, 575–577, 576f, 576t

Antimalarial agents. Dermatologically active agents include quinacrine (Atabrine), chloroquine (Aralen), and hydroxychloroquine (Plaquenil). Their mode of action is unknown, but these agents are used in the treatment of chronic discoid lupus erythematosus, lymphocytic infiltrate of Jessner, lichen planus, polymorphous light eruption and others. Eye exams by an ophthalmologist should be done at 6 to 12 month intervals to check for retinal damage except with quinacrine. Liver enzyme elevation should also be monitored.

Antiphospholipid antibody syndrome. Hypercoagulable state related to the presence of lupus anticoagulant and anticardiolipin antibodies. Cutaneous necrosis, vasculitis, thrombophlebitis, and ecchymoses occur. Recurrent inflammatory vascular thrombosis of veins and arteries can occur throughout the body and treatment is based on anticoagulation. Recurrent fetal loss and thrombocytopenia can also occur., 576

Antisynthetase syndrome. Antibodies are produced against histidyl-transfer ribonucleic acid synthetase (Jo-1). Mechanic's hands is the characteristic skin sign of the disease which can also have involvement of skeletal muscle, lungs, heart, liver and kidneys.

Apert syndrome. Craniosynostosis, symmetric severe syndactyly and numerous abnormalities of the skin, skeleton, brain and visceral organs. Skin signs include resistant acne, hyperhidrosis, interrupted eyebrows, excessive forehead wrinkling, lateral plantar hyperkeratosis, skin dimpling overjoints, and oculocutaneous hypopigmentation.

Aphthous stomatitis, 416–417, 416f

Aphthous ulcers. *See* Canker sores

Aplasia cutis congenita. Rare condition showing absence of skin at the time of birth. It presents with ulcerations, especially on the scalp that heal with scars.

Apocrine adenomas, 340, 340f

Apocrine epitheliomas, 340, 340f

Aquagenic syringeal acrokeratoderma. Rare symmetric palmar, hyperpigmented plaques and papules that become more prominent on exposure to water.

Aquagenic wrinkling of the palms (aquagenic syringeal acrokeratoderma, aquagenic palmoplantar acrokeratoderma, transient reactive papulotransluscent acrokeratoderma, aquagenic keratoderma). Rapidly forming, transient, edematous, white plaques on the palms after exposure to water (hand in bucket sign) that may be asymptomatic, pruritic or burning. Associated with cystic fibrosis, atopy, and hyperhidrosis. Immersion of the hands in water for 3 minutes in homozygous patients and 7 minutes in heterozygous patients shows translucent papules and marked wrinkling in palms.

Arachnidism, 555–557, 556f

Argyll Robertson pupils. Small irregular pupils that fail to react to light but react to accommodation. This is a late manifestation of neurosyphilis, particularly tabes dorsalis., 459

Argyria, 443

Arsenic. Inorganic arsenic preparation include Fowler's solution and Asiatic pills and were used in the treatment of resistant cases of psoriasis. Can cause arsenical pigmentation, actinic keratoses, Bowen's disease, squamous cell carcinoma, and underlying malignancies (especially lung and bladder). Other sources are well water and industrial sources such as pesticides, sheep dips, metal ores, and fabric dyes. Organic arsenic agents include neoarsphenamine and Mapharsen, used formerly in the treatment of syphilis., 57, 90t, 93t

Arsenical keratosis, 330, 331–332

Arteritis, temporal (giant cell arteritis). Inflammation of the cranial arteries most commonly the temporal artery that may show overlying swelling, erythema, tenderness and pain in the temporal scalp. Blindness may occur due to involvement of the retinal artery. Blindness may be prevented with systemic corticosteroids., 174

Arthus phenomenon. Characterized by local anaphylaxis in a site that has been injected repeatedly with a foreign protein.

Ash-leaf macule, 443, 463

Ashy dermatosis. Also known as erythema dyschromicum perstans. An uncommon pigmentary disorder characterized by ash-colored macules that slowly increase in size and number. The border may be erythematous. Could be a variant of *erythema perstans*. It is more common in nativesof Central and South America., 378

Asymmetric periflexural exanthem of childhood (APEC). *See* Unilateral laterothoracic exanthem

Ataxia-telangiectasia(Louis-Barr syndrome). Clinically shows oculocutaneous telangiectasia, progressive cerebellar ataxia, recurrent sinopulmonary infections, increased incidence of malignancy, x-ray hypersensitivity, and autosomal recessive inheritance., 162, 488t

Athlete's nodules. Benign, symmetric, asymptomatic, firm, flesh-colored, intradermal, 0.5 to 4.0 cm nodules that are sports-related and acquired. Most often over knuckles, knees pretibial area or dorsal aspect of the feet or any areas of chronic friction depending on the activity. Different terms used are knuckle pads (marble players, boxers) on dorsal fingers, surfer's nodules or knots (surfers) on dorsal feet and running shoe nodules or Nike nodules (joggers) on the dorsal aspect of the feet. Morphologically and histologically similar to collagenomas. Treatment is cessation of trauma, high-potency topical corticosteroids, intralesional corticosteroids, and excision. There is the potential for scarring, keloid formation, and recurrence.

Atopic dermatitis, 136, 461, 471t, 499–500, 500f

Atrophie blanche, 37, 158, 513

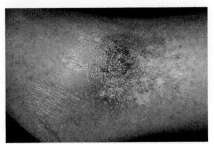

Atrophie blanche on the ankle.

Atrophies of the skin
Acquired atrophies
Inflammatory
Acrodermatitis chronica atrophicans. A rare idiopathic atrophy in older adults, particularly women, characterized by the presence of thickened skin at the onset, with ulnar bands on the forearm, changing into atrophy of the legs below the knee and of the forearms. In the early stages this is to be differentiated from scleroderma. High doses of penicillin may be effective. It may be a late stage of Lyme disease especially noted in Europe., 261, 458
Atrophie blanche (segmental hyalinizing vasculopathy). A form of cutaneous atrophy characterized by porcelain-white scar-like plaques with a border of telangiectasis and hyperpigmentation that cover large areas of the legs and the ankles, mainly of middle-aged or

older women. May ulcerate and biopsy shows a vasculopathy. Treatment is with anticoagulants., 37, 158

Atrophoderma, idiopathic, of Pasini and Pierini. Similar to morphea (localized scleroderma) but without induration. The round or irregular depressed atrophic areas are asymptomatic and appear mainly on the trunk of young females.

Folliculitis ulerythematosa reticulata. A very rare reticulated atrophic condition localized to the cheeks of the face; seen mainly in young adults.

Hemiatrophy. May be localized to one side of the face or may cover the entire half of the body. Vascular and neurogenic etiologies have been proposed, but most cases appear to be a form of *localized scleroderma.*

Lichen sclerosus et atrophicus (kraurosis vulvae, kraurosis penis, and balanitis xerotica obliterans{penis}). An uncommon atrophic process, mainly of women, which begins as a small whitish lesion that contains a central hyperkeratotic pinpoint-sized dell. These 0.5-cm or less whitish macules commonly coalesce to form whitish atrophic plaques. The most common localizations are on the neck, shoulders, arms, axillae, vulva, and perineum. Many consider kraurosis vulvae, kraurosis penis, and balanitis xerotica obliterans(penis) to be variants of this condition. Can be very pruritic and 5% risk of associated squamous cell carcinoma when occurring in adult female genitalia., 420, 539

Macular atrophy (Anetoderma of Jadassohn). A very rare condition characterized by the appearance of circumscribed reddish macules that develop an atrophic center that progresses toward the edge of the lesion, seen mainly on the extremities. May be seen after acne, varicella, syphilis, pilomatrichoma, and other inflammatory skin diseases. There is a primary form that may be associated with systemic lupus erythematosus, vitiligo, alopecia areata, hypothyroidism associated with antithyroid antibodies, and primary Addison disease.

Poikiloderma atrophicans vasculare (Jacobi). This rare atrophic process of adults is characterized by the development of patches of telangiectasis, atrophy, and mottled pigmentation on any area of the body. This resembles chronic radiodermatitis clinically and may be associated with dermatomyositis, lupus erythematosis or scleroderma. May precede the development of a lymphoma and some generalized cases are already mycosis fungoides (cutaneous T-cell lymphoma{CTCL})., 26

Secondary atrophy. From inflammatory diseases such as syphilis, chronic discoid lupus erythematosus, leprosy, tuberculosis, scleroderma, etc.

Ulerythema ophryogenes. A rare atrophic dermatitis that affects the outer part of the eyebrows, resulting in redness, scaling, and permanent loss of the involved hair.

Noninflammatory

Linear atrophy, striae albicantes or *distensae stretch marks.* On the abdomen, thighs, and breasts associated with pregnancy, Cushing's disease, obesity, systemic and topical corticosteroids, adolescence, abuse of androgens, idiopathic, and rapid weight gain.

Macular atrophy (anetoderma of Schweninger-Buzzi). Characterized by the presence of small, oval, whitish depressions or slightly elevated papules, which can be pressed back into the underlying tissue. Associated with antiphospholipid antibodies and thrombotic events.

Secondary atrophy. From sunlight, x-radiation, injury, and nerve diseases. Senile atrophy. Often associated with senile pruritus, senile purpura, and winter itch in the elderly., 332

Congenital atrophies. Associated with other congenital ectodermal defects.

Atrophoderma of Moulin. Hyperpigmented, linear atrophoderma which follows lines of Blaschko beginning during childhood or adolescence

Atypical cutaneous lymphoproliferative disorder (ACLD). Widespread, pruritic papules and plaques, often hyperpigmented (rarely hypopigmented) seen in the later stages of HIV infection. The pathology mimics cutaneous T-cell lymphoma (CTCL) but is usually composed of CD8 (+) cells and only rarely progresses to true CTCL.

Auspitz's sign, 189

Autoeczematous dermatitis, 157, 245

Autoeczematization. *See* Id reaction

Autoerythrocyte sensitization syndrome (Gardner-Diamond syndrome, psychogenic purpura). Bizarre, tender ecchymotic lesions mainly in young females. May be associated with psychological disturbance. Skin lesions reproduced with intradermal injection of whole blood or red blood cell fractions.

Autoimmune bullous disease, 115–116

Autoimmune polyendocrinopathy-candidiasis-ectodermal dystrophy syndrome (APECED). Multiple endocrinopathies in association with chronic mucocutaneous candidiasis. Up to one third have keratitis. The endocrinopathies can develop after childhood. It is due to the AIRE (autoimmune regulatory) gene autosomal recessive defect.

B

Baboon syndrome, 100t. *See* Chapter 9 under Dermatoses and Drugs That Cause Them

Bacterial infection, 524–525, 525, 543–546, 545f

Balanitis, fusospirochetal, 419

Balanitis circumscripta plasmacellularis (balanitis of Zoon). Erythematous papules and plaques on the glans penis in uncircumcised males that is benign and that may resolve after circumcision. A similar condition in females is called *vulvitis circumscripta plasmacellularis.* It has a characteristic histopathology on biopsy.

Balanitis xerotica obliterans, 419

Bamboo hairs. *See* Netherton's syndrome (trichorrhexis invaginata).

Bannayan-Riley-Ruvalcaba syndrome. Also called Riley-Smith, Bannayan-Zonana, or Ruvalcaba-Mybre-Smith syndrome. Rare autosomal dominant with macrocephaly, genital melanotic macules and hamartomatous intestinal polyposis is the classic triad. Numerous other skin, eye, musculoskeletal and nervous system abnormalities are reported.

Bannayan-Zonana syndrome. Macrocephaly, hypotonia, developmental delay, hamartomas such as intestinal polyposis, lipomas and vascular malformations. Pigmented penile macules are common.

Bartonellosis, 543, 543f

Bart's syndrome. Congenital localized absence of skin (CLAS) of the lower extremities, skin and/or mucous membrane blistering, and nail absence and/or deformity. Probably a form of dominant dystrophic epidermolysis bullosa.

Basal cell carcinoma, 346–350, 347f, 470, 530

Basal cell nevus syndrome. A rare hereditary affliction characterized primarily by multiple genetically determined basal cell carcinomas, cysts of the jaws, peculiar pits of the hands and the feet, calcification of the falx cerebri, and developmental anomalies of the ribs, the spine, and the skull, 488t

Battle's sign- ecchymosis around the mastoid process indicating an epidermal hematoma. This sign suggests significant trauma to the skull often with temporal bone fracture from head trauma even if the history is obscure.

Bazex's syndrome. *See* Acrokeratosis, paraneoplastic

Bazin's disease. *See* Erythema induratum.

Beckwith-Wiedemann syndrome. Consists most prominently of EMG (exophthalmos-macroglossia-gigantism). Many other characteristics including renal malformations and embryonal tumors with 20% mortality. To be differentiated from Proteus syndrome and CLOVE syndrome.

Behçet's syndrome, 155, 417

Bejel. The name given to syphilis as it occurs among Arabs, 544, 545

Benign lymphangiomatous papules (BLP). Seen most often following radiation therapy after surgery for breast malignancy but also more rarely following radiation for ovarian endometrioma and other cancers. Clinically showing one or more fleshy colored papules or vesicles located near the area of previous radiation so with breast cancer most often anterior chest wall or axillary folds. Usually asymptomatic and not necessarily accompanied by lymphedema. Although considered benign close clinical follow-up is indicated because some people feel there is a spectrum from BLP to atypical vascular lesions and then progression to angiosarcoma

Benign vulvar melanosis. *See* Vulvar benign

Berloque dermatitis. Similar to the *melanosis of Riehl* and can result from contact with toilet waters containing oil ofbergamot or other essential oils, followed by exposure to sunlight, causing a dermatitis that appears to drip down the neck, like a pendant (berloque)., 442, 442f

Bier spots. Small irregular white macules seen in a dependent or externally compressed limb. They disappear upon elevating the limb or relieving the compression and are felt to be due to microvessel vasoconstriction due to lack of oxygen. Not a sign of significant vascular disease.

Bilharziasis, 554

Bindi leucoderma. Hypopigmentation caused by BTBP (para-tertiary butylphenol) present in high concentration in the glue used by women from Japan, Holland, Russia, and the United Kingdom who tend to wear their religious patch around the clock. The depigmentation may be permanent.

Biologic false-positive reaction, 251

Bioterrorism, cutaneous signs of, 569–579, 570t, 573f, 575f, 576t, 578f

Biotinidase deficiency. Seen in children with partial or complete alopecia, rash, and infection. The rash is periorificial around the mouth, eyes, nose and back. It is eczematous, desquamating and mimics seborrhea. Neurologic manifestations include hypotonia, lethargy, seizures, developmental delay and depression (adults). Oral biotin treats the condition and prevents hearing and vision loss seen in up to 50% of untreated patients., 590

Birthmarks, 491–494, 491t, 492f–494f

Birt-Hogg Dube syndrome. Multiple fibrofolliculomas which are benign, hard papules, 1-3 mm, flesh-colored, common, hair follicle derived tumors especially on the nose, earlobes, forehead, and temples associated with pulmonary cysts, spontaneous pneumothorax, renal tumors, and adenomas of the colon.

Bites

Insect bite reactions may be exaggerated in HIV+ patients and in certain malignancies such as chronic lymphocytic leukemia, acute lymphoblastic leukemia and acute monocytic leukemia, mantle cell lymphoma, large cell lymphoma and myelofibrosis. Many patients do not recall a bite and in some cases this may represent an insect bite-like reaction., 153, 162

Björnstad syndrome. Pili torti with congenital deafness in a variable hereditary pattern., 396t, 398

Black dermographism, 443

Black dot ringworm. Tinea of the hair caused by *Trichophyton tonsurans*. These endothrix fungi do not produce fluorescent hairs under the Wood's light and usually occur in children where broken short hairs are seen ("black dot tinea"), 296

Black heel (talon noir). Black asymptomatic macules on the posterior or lateral aspect of the heel in the area where the skin is thickly keratinized. Related to trauma in such sports as tennis and basketball., 563

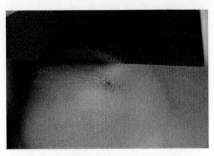

Heel exhibiting black heel (talon noir)in a tennis player.

Black palm (tache noir). Similar to black heel but on the palms of golfers, gymnasts, mountain climbers, tennis players, and weight lifters., 563

Black tongue, 418, 419f

Blackheads, 8, 17

Blaschko's lines. A cutaneous pattern of distribution followed by many skin disorders described in 1901 by Alfred Blaschko. The origin of these lines is not known, may be embryologic. Some of the diseases that can follow Blaschko's lines are lichen striatus, epidermal nevi, linear psoriasis, linear morphea, and linear cutaneous lupus erythematosus., 483, 484, 484f

Blastic plasmacytoid dendritic cell neoplasm (Blastic NK-Cell Lymphomas). Rare hematologic neoplasm with almost always skin involvement but has a poor prognosis even though cytostatic therapy may be initially effective. Rapid systemic dissemination occurs with skin involvement including purpura, bone marrow, lymph node, and other tissues. Purple papules and tumors occur between 0.5 to 6mm and may show dark purplish discoloration and necrosis but without ulceration. Skin lesions were widespread and diagnosis is ultimately made by histopathological examination.

Blastomycosis

North American, 299, 300f

South American (*See* paracoccidioidmycosis)

Blastomycosis-like pyoderma. Seen mainly inimmunosuppressed patients at sites ofinjuries, tattoos, venous stasis and foreign body reactions. Verrucous plaques studded with pustules usually culture staph aureus and biopsy shows neutrophilic abscesses with pseudoepitheliomatous hyperplasia.

Blau syndrome. Rare autosomal dominant disorder usually in childhood with iritis, granulomatous arthritis, and a skin rash. Tiny generalized red dots reveal granulomas on biopsy and usually spontaneously resolve., 152

Bleomycin sulfate injection, 96t

Blister beetle dermatitis. Beetles of the family *Meloidae* contain cantharidin, which on contact with the skin causes the formation of a tense, itching, burning bulla. *See* Paederus dermatitis

Blistering distal dactylitis. Painful, tense blister on a red base over the anterior fat pad of one (due to Group A, beta-hemolytic streptococci) or two (due to staphylococci aureus) fingers usually between 2 and 16 years of age usually without systemic symptoms. Responds to antibiotics.

Bloom's syndrome, 488t

Blue nevus, 336

Blue rubber-bleb nevus syndrome (BEAN syndrome). Rare distinctive gastrointestinal and cutaneous vascular malformations. Gastrointestinal bleeding may occur and rarely other organs are involved. Usually present at birth or early infancy with soft compressible asymptomatic red to blue tumors. Occasionally painful or with overlying hyperhidrosis. Blue macular or pinpoint blue-black areas may be seen. Deeper subcutaneous tumors without overlying skin changes are especially associated with gastrointestinal disease. Disease often progressive and may be associated with other tumors.

Bockhart's impetigo. A very superficial bacterial infection of the hair follicle.

Body odor, 8. *See also* Bromhidrosis

Bohn's nodules (gingival cysts). Innocuous, resolving (weeks to months) white papules in 50 to 80% of newborns on vestibular or lingual surfaces of the alveolar ridge or the palate.

Bolognia's sign. Eccentric foci of hyperpigmentation on clinical examination of pigmented tumor or with dermoscopy which indicates the need for a biopsy to rule out a malignant melanoma.

Bolster sign. Slightly painful red swollen proximal nail folds seen in candida paronychia.

Borreliosis. *See* Lyme disease

Botox. *See* Botulinum toxin

Botryomycosis. Rare, chronic, granulomatous, abscess with granules mimicking actinomycosis but actually due to bacterial masses most often caused by staphylococcus aureus and pseudomonas aeruginosa among many others., 547

Botulinum toxin (BT), 45, 46f

Botulism, 570t

Bowel-associated dermatoarthritis syndrome. Seen in 20% of small bowel bypass patients and occasionally in inflammatory bowel disease. Intermittent neutrophilic pustules in crops with arthritis and increased cryoglobulins.

Bowen's disease, 338f

Brachio-oculo-facial syndrome. Rare disorder caused by malformation of brachial arches. Malformed lip, nose, and ears result. Also lacrimal duct obstruction, brachial cleft sinus, linear neck scars, microphthalmia, auricular and lip pits, cysts of the scalp, high arched palate dental anomalies, cardiac anomalies, and renal anomalies have also been reported.

Brachioradial pruritus. Localized idiopathic, pruritus on the outer upper arms mainly over the elbow area. Sun exposure may be a causative factor.

Branchio-oto-renal syndrome (Melnick-Fraser syndrome). Preauricular pits, renal and ureteral anomalies, hearing loss, and branchial cleft cysts.

Brenner sign. *See* in patients who have a melanoma of a developed erythematous patches and plaques at the site of the melanoma or distant from the primary melanocytic lesion.

Brittle nail syndrome. Affects 20% of the population with women having double the incidence of men. Consists of onychoschezia (lamellar transverse splitting of the distal nail plate) and onychorrhexis (longitudinal nail plate thickening or ridging). Due to dryness and, although difficult to treat, may respond to 2.5 mgs biotin orally each day or topical 50% urea (Kerastik)., 409–410, 409f

Bromhidrosis. The odor of the body that is associated with sweating, commonly called "B.O." Freshly secreted sweat has no odor, but an odor develops when the sweat becomes contaminated with bacteria. Methods used to decrease sweat are curative, 8

Bromoderma. A dermatosis, usually pustular-like, due to the ingestion of bromides. *See also* Drug eruptions

Bronze diabetes. *See* Hemochromatosis

Brooke-Spiegler syndrome. Autosomal dominant association of trichoepitheliomas (usually on the face) and cylindromas (usually on the scalp). Other tumors (especially eccrine spiroadenomas) may also occur.

Brucellosis. The human infection of undulant fever is infrequently accompanied by a nondescript skin eruption. However, after delivering an infected cow, a high percentage of veterinarians experience an itching, red, macular, papular, or pustular dermatitis on the contaminated arms and hands that lasts for a few days to 3 weeks without systemic illness., 571t

Brunauer-Fohs-Siemens syndrome. Keratosis palmoplantaris striate type 1, which is caused by desmoglein 1 abnormalities.

Bubble hair, 397

Buerger's disease, 156

Bullous congenital ichthyosiform erythroderma,477t

Bullous disease of childhood, 495, 495t

Bullous impetigo, 216

Bullous pemphigoid, 37, 219–220

Bullous pyoderma, 452t

Burn
    sun, 496t, 502
    thermal, 496t, 502
    turf, 560t, 561

Burning mouth syndrome. Common, chronic, painful oral mucosae seen mainly in postmenopausal women with no apparent abnormalities visible., 590, 593

Burning tongue, 418

Burrow's solution. A solution of aluminum acetate that in its original formula contained lead. A lead-free Burrow's solution for wet dressings can be made by adding Domeboro tablets or powder to water to make a 1:20 or 1:10 solution

Burton's line- A bluish line around the gums due to lead poisoning. This can be seen at recycling plants such as plants that recycle batteries.

Buschke-Löwenstein. Virally induced giant condyloma of the penis that may progress to invasive squamous cell carcinoma. It is considered a subtype of verrucous carcinoma. *See* Verrucous carcinoma

Buschke-Ollendorf syndrome. A syndrome consisting of connective tissue nevi and osteopoikilosis of the hands, feet, pelvis, and long bones.

Bywaters Lesions. Tiny, painless, proximal nailfold blood clots that can occur on theends of digits where they are painful. Most closely associated with rheumatoid arthritis.

C

CADASIL syndrome (cerebral autosomal dominant arteriopathy with subcortical infarcts and leukoencephalopathy). Familial arteriopathy with migraines, strokes and early onset multi-infarct dementia. Skin biopsy of normal skin with electron microscopy can be diagnostic.

Café-au-lait spots, 320t, 322t

Calcifying epithelioma, 342, 342f

Calcinosis, idiopathic scrotal very common form of idiopathic calcinosis cutis. Serum calcium is normal and surgically removal is optional

Calcinosis cutis, 460

Calcinosis. *Localized calcinosis* can occur in many tumors of the skin and following chronic inflammatory lesions, such as severe acne. *Metabolic calcinosis* may or may not be associated with an excess of blood calcium and is divided into universal calcinosis and circumscribed calcinosis.

Calciphylaxis. Sudden onset cutaneous necrosis and gangrene due to blood vessel and tissue calcification in association with hyperparathyroidism, longterm renal dialysis, renal transplantation, and rarely AIDS or autoimmune disease. Usually fatal(parenteral sodium thiosulfate infusions may be lifesaving) and almost always with marked renal disease, 460

Callus. A hyperkeratotic plaque of the skin dueto chronic pressure and friction, 561,561f

Cancer. *See* Tumors

Candidal intertrigo, 246, 301, 302f

Candidal paronychia, 301

Candidal vulvovaginitis, 303, 304

Candidiasis, 294, 301–305, 302f, 303f, 304f, 491t, 491, 492f

Canker sores (aphthous ulcers), 416, 416f

Capillary hemangiomas, 505

Carbuncle, 235t, 241, 241f

Carcinoid syndrome. A potentially malignant tumor of the argentaffin chromaffin cells of the appendix or the ileum. Some of these tumors or their metastases produce large amounts of serotonin (5-hydroxytryptamine), which causes transient flushing of the skin accompanied by weakness, nausea, abdominal pain, diarrhea, and sweating. The redness usually begins on the head and the neck and then extends down on the body. These episodes last from several minutes to a few hours. Repeated attacks of the erythema lead to the formation of permanent telangiectasias and a diffuse reddish purple hue to the skin. The diagnosis can be made by the finding of over 25 mg of 5-hydroxyindoleacetic acid in a 24-hour urine sample, 452t

Carcinoma en cuirasse. Thickened indurated plaque over large areas of the thorax which may have a peau d'orange appearance that is seen most often with metastatic breast cancer.

Carcinoma erysipelatoides. Rare cutaneous metastasis usually from breast cancer with erythema, tenderness, increased temperature, spreading border and often eventually vesiculation. Unlike erysipelas, which it resembles, there is no systemic toxicity.

Carcinoma, primary cutaneous adenoid cystic. Rare appendageal tumor mainly face, head, and neck associated with favorable survival that can occur on other sites besides the skin including salivary glands, breast, lung, external auditory canal. It is controversial but there is some suggestion it is associated with internal cancers. These underlying malignancies are of the lymph and erythropoietic type.

Carcinoma, verrucous. *See* Verrucous carcinoma

Carcinosarcoma. Rare malignant neoplasm with both epithelial (usually basal cell cancer) and mesencyhmal (usually sarcoma) components. Especially head and neck or older men and may be aggressive with metastasis.

Cardio-facio-cutaneous syndrome. Ectodermal defects especially hair (wooly, friable hair and alopecia), skin lesions in 95% (especially follicular keratin plugging resembling keratosis pilaris), typical facial dysmorphism, cardiac defects, psychomotor retardation and growth failure. Probable autosomal dominant and associated with increased parental age.

Caripito itch is caused by swarms of migrating moths seen in subtropical regions of China and Venezuela near the port of Caripito.

Carney Complex. Myxomas (heart, skin, breast), spotty pigmentation (lentigines, blue nevi), endocrinopathies (Cushing's syndrome, acromegaly, sexual precocity) and schwannomas.

Carotenemia. Buildup of carotene or similar yellow-orange pigment in the blood and keratin layer of the skin. Stains skin a characteristic yellow. Harmless condition due to eating large amounts of foods such as carrots and tomatoes (lycopenemia due to similar pigment called lycopene). It can be seen in hypothyroidism., 588

Carrion's disease, 543

Caseation necrosis. Histologically, this is a form of tissue death with loss of structural detail leaving pale eosinophilic, amorphous, finely granular material. It is seen especially in tuberculosis, syphilis, granuloma annulare, and beryllium granuloma.

Caterpillar dermatitis (erucism). An irritating chemical is released when the hairs of some species of caterpillars penetrate the skin. The onset of irritation is quite immediate. Red macular lesions, then urticarial papules, and occasionally vesicles develop in areas exposed. Mild lesions can be gone

mental deficiency, cyanotic acral edema and characteristic facial features.

Collagen vascular diseases, 463, 464f

Collagenomas. Rare, benign connective tissue nevi (hamartomas) that can be familial, part of tuberous sclerosis as a shagren patch, associated with other various abnormalities, or acquired (eruptive collagenomas).

Collodion baby, 478t

Colloid milium. There are four types of this disease. The juvenile form is rare and apparently disappears around puberty. Clinically on the face and dorsum of the hands, one sees cream-colored or yellowish 1- or 2-mm firm papules. The second type is the adult or acquired form, which is apparently related to the exposure of the skin to the sun and petroleum products. The clinical picture resembles the juvenile form. The third type is nodular colloid degeneration which is one or several larger (up to 5 cm) nodules felt to be related to sun exposure on the face, trunk, and scalp. A fourth type shows pigmented "caviar-like" papules in secondary ochronosis due to chronic topical hydroquinone use., 321t

Coma bullae. Drug induced (especially barbiturates), hypoglycemic or central nervous system induced coma can produce bullae, erythema, violaceous plaques, necrosis or erosions usually, but not exclusively, on pressure sites.

Comedones, 17

Complex regional pain syndrome (Reflex sympathetic dystrophy). A syndrome that results from an injury (50% or greater after a bone fracture especially a Colles' fracture) usually on a limb. Severe pain is not limited to simple peripheral nerve and is disproportionate to the inciting event. Skin findings include edema, hyperhidrosis or anhidrosis, pallor, erythema, coolness and nail dystrophy. Diagnosis is difficult and treatment is of limited success., 186

Compound nevus, 334, 335f

Computer calluses. Trauma induced skin thickening occurs with chronic use of computers such as computer palm, mouse (finger and mousing callus on wrist over the pisiform prominence when wrist has friction with table.)

Condyloma acuminata (venereal warts). Genital viral warts. When types 16, 18 (as well as other subtypes) involved is a precursor of cervical cancer (common), penile cancer (rare) and anal cancer (most common in gay HIV patients). Usually sexually transmitted., 351f

Condylomata lata, 254, 257f

Confluent and reticulated papillomatosis of Gougerot-Carteaud. Pruritic, pigmented, truncal papules especially between the breasts and umbilicus. May become verrucous, erythematous, and reticulated.

Congenital ectodermal defect, 510

Congenital ichthyosiform erythroderma, 477t, 478f. *See also* Ichthyosis

Congenital melanocytic nevus, 491t, 492, 493f

Congenital reticular ichthyosiform erythroderma (CRIE).

Congenital triangular alopecia (Brauer nevus, temporally limited alopecia). Very rare permanent triangular patches on one or both frontotemporal scalp regions beginning at 3 to 5 years of age., 393

Congo red test. An intravenous test used to diagnose generalized amyloidosis. An intradermal skin test using Congo red solution will stain localized amyloid nodules red.

Connective tissue nevus (*See* collagenomas). Hamartomas of connective tissue present as 1) familial cutaneous collagenomas 2) Shagren patch of tuberous sclerosis 3) eruptive collagenomas and 4) isolated collagenomas.

Conradi Hunermann disease, 477t, 479f

Contact dermatitis, 9, 15, 22f, 23, 77–81, 77f–80f, 216, 512

Contraction, 56

Corn. A small, sharply circumscribed, often painful hyperkeratotic lesion that may be either hard with a central horny core or soft, as commonly seen between the toes. Underlying bone protuberances are causative (can be very painful). No tiny clotted capillaries as in warts. Normal skin markings are preserved.

Corticosteroids, 25, 34t, 35, 441

drug eruptions from abuse of

Corynebacterium jeikeium. Normal commensal organism but it is a skin colonizer in up to 50% of hospitalized patients and can be a cause of sepsis in neutropenic patients. In the skin of patients who are septic it is manifest by hemorrhagic or erythematous papular eruption. Histopathology is septic emboli with or without mild inflammation. Skin lesions are indicative of a high mortality.

Cosmeceuticals, 73–76

Cosmetics, 22f, 66–76

Costello syndrome. Formally considered a variant of Noonan syndrome and synonymous with cardiafaciocutaneous syndrome. It can be separated on clinical and genetic findings. Approximately 50% of patients will have verrucous papules with a characteristic histopathology that occurs on the abdomen, face, axillae, knees elbows, vocal cords, face and anus between 2 and 15 years old. The neck, hands and feet have loose redundant skin. Other skin markers include vascular birth marks, acanthosis nigricans, pigmented acral nevi, hyperpigmentation, hyperkeratosis, thin deep set nails, thick eyebrows, and sparse curlyscalp hair. Mental retardation with a sociable personality as well ascardiac abnormalities, musculoskeletal abnormalities, abnormal facies, and increased risk of malignant tumors.

Cowden's disease. Autosomal dominant diseaseassociated with multiple trichilemmomas of the face and multiple papules of the oral mucosa, causing a cobblestone appearance, as well as visceral malignancies, especially cancer of the breast in females, 386t. Other benign conditions in this syndrome include angiomas, multiple subcutaneous lipomas, scrotal tongue, hyperkeratotic papules back of hands (but not on feet) resembling flat

warts, palmoplantaris keratotic punctata, and flat-topped lichenoid papules or papillomas the central face., 488t

Coxsackievirus infections, 275

Crabs. *See* Pediculosis

Creeping eruption, 37

CREST syndrome (Calcinosis cutis, Raynaud's phenomenon, Esophageal dysfunction, Sclerodactyly, Telangiectasias), 447, 449t

Crohn's disease. An inflammatory granulomatous disease of the bowel. Cutaneous manifestations include pyoderma gangrenosum, exfoliative dermatitis, erythema multiforme, Stevens-Johnson syndrome, urticaria, herpes zoster, palmar erythema, cutaneous (metastatic) Crohn's disease, and necrotizing vasculitis., 244

Crouzon's disease. Autosomal dominant (but often spontaneous) craniofacial dystrophy with exophthalmos, craniosynostosis, maxillary hypoplasia, orbitostenosis, hooked nose, and acanthosis nigricans.

Crowe's sign, 462, 484

Cryoglobulinemia. Purpura, livedo reticularis, and ulcers, especially on the lower extremities caused by a complex of proteins that precipitate on cooling in vitro. It can be primary or associated with underlying cancer, collagen vascular diseases, infection, and thromboembolic disease. Hepatitis C may be associated and interferon alpha may be therapeutic. Cryoglobulinemia type 1 is monoclonal with IgG and associated with increased coagulation. Cryoglobulinemia types 2 and 3 are mixed cryoglobulins with IgA or IgM associated with rheumatoid factor and are the 2 types of cryoglobulinemia that cause vasculitis., 163f, 165t, 174, 457

Cryopyrin-associated periodic syndrome. Rare hereditary auto inflammatory disease with 3 prototypes: Familial Cold Autoinflammatory Syndrome, Muckle-Wells syndrome, Neonatal onset multisystem inflammatory disease., 152

Cryotherapy, 469

Cryptococcosis (torulosis). A worldwide disease caused by a yeast-like fungus, *Cryptococcus neoformans*. It characteristically invades the central nervous system via the respiratory tract. Variable skin lesions are uncommon., 281

Crystal storing histiocytosis. Phagocytosis of immunoglobulin crystals of the kappa chain in organs throughout the body which rarely includes the skin. Infiltrated skin colored or erythematous plaques can precede an underlying cancer which is most often multiple myeloma but can be an immunocytoma, amyloidosis or a clofazimine drug induced reaction. Diagnosis is made by biopsy with characteristic histology findings.

CTCL. *See* Cutaneous T-cell lymphoma

Cullen's sign. Bruising around the umbilicus seen in acute hemorrhagic pancreatitis, ectopic pregnancy or blunt trauma and is due to retroperitoneal bleeding.

Cushingoid appearance, 24

Cushing's syndrome, 452t, 454

Cutaneous horn, 18, 328

Cutaneous T-cell lymphoma (CTCL), 146, 375–378, 435t

Diffuse dermal angiomatosis. Cutaneous reactive angiomatosis associated with arteriosclerotic vascular disease, diabetes, and smoking. Seen most often on the lower extremities and may respond to revascularization procedures. Clinically the lesions vary from a solitary erythematous patch to an indurated plaque surrounded by a dusky redness., 449t

Digital myxoid cyst, 413

Digital papular calcific elastosis. Acquired marginal, papular, acrokeratoderma on the radial side of the index finger, first interdigital space, and ulnar side of the thumb. It may be related to manual labor and/or sun exposure.

Digitocutaneous dysplasia. Rare, X-linked dominant, congenital, multiple, digital fibromas. Atrophic plaques, dental abnormalities, dysmorphic features, and bone anomalies.

Dimorphic leprosy, 249, 251f

Diphtheria, cutaneous. The skin ulcer due to *Corynebacterium diphtheriae* has a characteristic rolled firm border and a grayish membrane that progresses to a black eschar with surrounding inflammation, vesicles, and anesthesia., 18, 576t

DIRA (Deficient interleukin 1 receptor antagonist). *See* in children most patients have symptoms from birth to the first two weeks of age including bone pain, deformity, rash that can span from a few pustules to extensive pustules that cover most of the patient's body. Successful treatment has been accomplished with anakinra. It is familial felt to be an inherited mutation in the IL-1RN gene that encodes a protein known as interleukin-1 receptor antagonist. Some people think a clinical phenotype of DIRA is acrodermatitis continua of hallopeau.

Direct immunofluorescence, 217

Dissecting cellulitis of the scalp. *See* Perifolliculitis capitis abscedens et suffodiens

Disseminate recurrent infundibulofolliculitis. Recurrent and disseminate goosebump type follicular rash that is wide spread mildly itchy slightly pink with a brown pigmented edge especially over torso, neck, and arms. Histopathology is fairly characteristic.(DIRF).

Disseminated infundibulofolliculitis. Most often seen in black patients; consists of perifollicular, asymptomatic, flesh-colored papules, most often occurring on the trunk and proximal extremities.

DITRA (deficiency of the interleukin-36 receptor antagonist). This inherited syndrome has similar manifestations to DIRA but has lack of bone involvement. It does have a mucocutaneous pustulosis and can present at any age it also appears to respond to anakinra as does DIRA.

Dock 8 (Dedicator of cytokinesis 8). It's a variant of hyperimmunoglobulin E syndrome. Shares some of the characteristics of Job's syndrome including elevated IgE, dermatitis, recurrent sinopulmonary infections, and cutaneous staphylococcal abscesses. However, it also has recalcitrant wide spread cutaneous viral infections, asthma, food, and environmental allergies as well as the absence of newborn rash and coarse fascies. High rates malignancy are seen in DOCK8 deficiency vs Job's syndrome. Job's syndrome is also called autosomal dominant hyper-IgE syndrome., 352

Dorfman-Chanrin syndrome. Clinical appearance similar to congenital icthyosiform erythroderma. Lipid vacuoles in the skin and throughout other organs. Cataracts, myopathy, sensory-neural deafness, and growth retardation may also be present.

Dowling-Degos disease. Usually beginning in the 4th decade of life are flexural hyperpigmented macules. Autosomal dominant, rare and may present in childhood. Other findings include perioral pitted scars and comedone-like lesions over the neck and back.

Drug eruptions, 95–121, 95t–104t, 105f, 106f, 107f, 108f, 110f, 111, 499, 596

Drug reaction, granulomatous interstitial. Rare drug reaction with characteristic histology that mimics interstitial granuloma annularae. Infiltrative plaques on medial thighs and inner arms is the classic presentation. It can occur weeks to months after drug exposure and take weeks to months to resolve.

Duhring's disease, 222, 455. *See also* Dermatitis herpetiformis

Dyschromatosis, brachial acquired cutaneous. *See* Acquired brachial cutaneous dyschromatosis

Dyshidrosis (pompholyx). A syndrome characterized by pinhead-sized, very pruritic blisters on the palms of the hands, fingers, and feet. Some authors think stress can play a causative role. If the cause is known, this term should not be used. Considered by many to be a subtype of atopic eczema., 22f, 97t, 292

Dyskeratosis, benign. A histopathologic finding of faulty keratinization of individual epidermal cells with formation of corp ronds and corp grains. Seen in Darier's disease and occasionally in familial benign chronic pemphigus.

Dyskeratosis congenita. With pigmentation, dystrophia unguis, and leukokeratosis oris, this is a rare syndrome characterized by a reticulated pigmentation, particularly of the neck, dystrophy of the nails, and a leukoplakia condition of the oral mucosa. Increased sweating and thickening of the palms and soles may occur, 488t

Dyskeratosis, malignant. A histopathologic finding in Bowen's disease and also in squamous cell carcinoma and actinic keratosis in which premature and atypical keratinization of individual cells is seen.

Dysplastic nevus syndrome, 334

Dystrophia unguium mediana canaliformis, 408

E

Ebola, 570t

EBV. *See* Epstein-Barr virus

Ecchymoses, 160. *See also* Purpura

Eccrine angiomatous hamartoma. Rare, benign, painful hyperhidrotic proliferation of eccrine tissue with vascular stroma. Present at birth or early childhood. Surgical excision may be required due to severity of pain.

Eccrine epithelioma, 340f, 342

Eccrine glands, 6

Eccrine hidradenitis. *See* Palmoplantar eccrine hidradenitis

Eccrine poroma, 342, 342f

Eccrine spiradenoma, 342, 342f

Eccrine squamous syringometaplasia. Clinically and etiologically similar to neutrophilic eccrine hidradenitis but with different specific histopathology. Painful erythematous plaques or macules seen especially on the groin, axilla, palms and soles in bone marrow transplant patients due to high dose chemotherapy.

Eccrine syringofibroadenoma (ESFA), 340

Echovirus exanthem, 277

Ecthyma, 235t, 237, 237f

Ecthyma gangrenosum. Rapidly developing painful necrotic escharotic gangrenous plaques usually in the intertriginous areas. Seen in patients with sepsis that is usually due to pseudomonas., 169, 576t

Ectodermal dysplasias, 487, 487f

Ectodermal dysplasia-skin fragility syndrome. Rare genodermatosis caused by defective plakophilin, which is a component of desmosomes. Generalized red skin at birth becomes fragile. Progressive plantar keratoderma, nail dystrophy and alopecia are also a part of this syndrome.

Ectodermosis erosiva pluriorificialis. A synonym for Stevens-Johnson syndrome.

Eczema

atopic. *See* Atopic eczema

craquelé. A French term for cracked appearing skin, especially seen on the legs when skin is very dry.

infantile, 21f, 82

nummular, 20f, 23, 83, 83f, 102t

winter, 23

Eczema etiology, there is curious association with decreased atopic dermatitis risk with exposure to dogs and farm animals at a young age, early daycare, increased contact with non-pathogenic microbes and increased microbial burden, consumption of unpasteurized farm milk, and antenatal helminth infection. An equally curious association is between viral infections and frequent antibiotic use. The risk of smoking causes an increased risk of cutaneous squamous cell cancer but not basal cell cancer.

Eczematous eruption, 100t

Eczematous lesions, 496t, 499–501, 500f–501f

Ehlers-Danlos syndrome, 485

Ehrlichiosis, 252

Elasticity disorders, 485–486

Elastoderma. Acquired, localized laxity of the skin. Dense aggregates of eosinophilic material are present in the dermis.

Elastofibroma dorsi. Rare benign firm subcapsular tumor in elderly women that may be necessary to remove due to pain and difficulty in movement. Abduction of the arms may be necessary to see this subcutaneous tumor with freely movable normal underlying tissue.

Elastosis perforans serpiginosa. A rare asymptomatic disease in which keratotic papules occur in a circinate arrangement around a slightly atrophic patch, usually on the neck. May be seen in association with scleroderma, renal disease, Ehlers-Danlos syndrome, osteogenesis imperfecta, Marfan's syndrome, Rothmund-Thompson syndrome, acrogeria, and especially Down's syndrome., 35, 485

Electrocautery, 53

Electrocoagulation, 53

Elephantiasis nostras verrucosa. Nonfilarial gross enlargement of a body region (usually a limb) due to recurrent streptococcal lymphangitis resulting in dermal woody fibrosis and epidermal papillomatosis and hyperkeratosis causing a dramatically enlarged, firm deformity. Treatment is difficult with compression dressings and long term antibiotics most often used., 243

ELISA (Enzyme-linked immunosorbent assay), 577

EM. See Erythema multiforme

Embolic nodules. Emboli can come from a left atrial myxoma, fat from bone marrow after bone trauma, or from arteriosclerotic plaques with or without vascular surgical procedures, appear as distal, papular, hemorrhagic, sometimes painful areas in the distribution of the vessel involved, 157

Emollients, 29, 31, 69, 62–73, 82, 141, 142

Encephalocraniocutaneous lipomatosis (ECCL). Unilateral lipomas of the face and scalp associated with cerebral and ophthalmologic malformation on the ipsilateral side. Sporadic and very rare in newborns.

Endometriosis. The presence of extracutaneous endometrial tissue. Rarely found in skin usually in abdominal scars related to pelvic surgery (especially caesarean sections). Tumoral nodules are painful and bleed during menstrual cycles and if primary usually occur near the umbilicus.

Entamoeba histolytica, 552

Entire cytopathic human orphan. See ECHO

Eosinophillic annulare erythema. Rare benign annulare erythema and tissue eosinophilia. It is chronic and relapsing and often eventually heals spontaneously. Has rapid response to systemic steroids and is been associated with autoimmune thyroid disease, chronic borreliosis, renal carcinoma, chronic gastritis, diabetes mellitus, and chronic hepatitis C as well as chronic kidney disease. Has rapid response rare lesions seen most often in infancy. It consists of annulare erythema and recurrent appearance of erythematous annulare plaques. It is not associated with any underlying conditions and usually resolves over months to years. The histology is quite characteristic with perivascular deep and superficial lymphocytes and abundant eosinophils.

Eosinophilic cellulitis (Well's syndrome). Characterized by the sudden onset of pruritic, red, infiltrated, urticaria-like patches, which persist for 3 to 4 weeks and can recur. Characteristic histopathology with an infiltrate of eosinophils and "flame figures."

Eosinophilic fasciitis (Shulman's syndrome). Acute onset of induration, tenderness, swelling, and erythema of one or more extremities resulting in sclerodermatous skin changes. Believed by some to be a variant of scleroderma with a diagnosis confirmed by deep biopsy into the fascia showing significant inflammation with eosinophils., 449t

Eosinophilic polymorphic pruritic eruption associated with radiation (EPPER). Excoriated papules, wheals, and vesicles with eosinophilic infiltrate, generalized pruritus and is seen in association with radiation therapy mainly for cervical cancer. It sparesthe palms, soles, and mucous membranes.

Eosinophilic ulcer of the oral mucosa. Uncommon, self-limited ulcer that may be initiated by trauma. Histopathology is usually characteristic. One third are painful and the commonest location of the ulcer is the tongue, buccal mucosa, and lip.

Epidermal nevus. Usually benign overgrowth of epidermal tissue. Can develop into squamous cell carcinoma. Rarely associated with underlying bone, central nervous system, eye or kidney abnormalities (epidermal nevus syndrome), 491t, 493, 493f

Epidermal nevus, inflammatory linear verrucous (ILVEN). Rare verrucous usually unilateral, acquired disorder along Blaschko's lines. Appears during the first few months of life and is pruritic and inflammatory.

Epidermodysplasia verruciformis. A rare, apparently hereditary disease manifested by papulosquamous and warty lesions present at birth with no site of predilection. The prognosis for life is poor because of the eventual development of squamous cell carcinomas from the lesions. Numerous human papilloma viruses (HPV) have been found. HPV types 5 & 8 are especially associated with malignant transformation. Caused by a unique mutation in EVER1 and EVER2 genes. Strict sun protection is indicated to prevent malignant transformation., 279

Epidermolysis bullosa, 216–217, 480, 480t, 482f, 490, 491f, 491t

Epidermolysis bullosa acquisita, 217

Epidermolysis bullosa nevi. Acquired, melanocytic nevi that have so far proven to be benign. Can occur at sitesof previous blisters with a scalloped edge to match the blister border. Clinically the lesions are often large with clinical and dermatoscopic criteria of malignant melanoma. Junctional and dystrophic epidermolysis bullosa are the most commonly associated, 22.

Epidermolysis bullosa pruriginosa. Form of dystrophic epidermolysis bullosa associated with pruritis and hypertrophic, lichenified nodules and plaques.

Epidermophytid. A dermatophytid due to Epidermophyton dermatophyte infection. See also Id reaction

Epidermophytosis. A fungus infection due to Epidermophyton dermatophyte infection.

Epiloia. A triad of mental deficiency, epilepsy, and adenoma sebaceum. See Adenoma sebaceum; Tuberous sclerosis

Epithelioma, 332, 338, 340, 340f, 341f
  apocrine, 340
  calcifying, 342
  cuniculatum. See Verrucous carcinoma
  eccrine, 342
  hair, 342

Epstien's pearls. Small, white, benign, gingival papules on the midline of the palate or junction between the soft and hard palate of an infant's mouth. Common, innocuous benign gingival cysts that usually improves with age.

Epstein-Barr virus (EBV), 282, 374

e-PTFE implants. See Expanded polytetrafluoroethylene facial implants

Epulis. This term refers to any growth involving the gums. Giant epulis is a solitary neoplasm or granuloma arising from the periosteum of the jawbone in the gingival area., 418

Erosio interdigitalis blastomycetica. Erosion and whitish maceration signifying a candidal and gram(-) bacterial infection of the webs between the fingers or toes., 520

Erosive adenomatosis of the nipple. Benign neoplastic conditions usually seen in middle-aged women that mimic Paget's disease clinically and adenocarcinoma histologically. Mastectomies have been unnecessarily done for this condition.

Erosive pustular dermatosis of the scalp. Usually on the scalp of bald men (occasionally on the legs) tiny pustules form on the forehead, temples and scalp that erode and form thick yellowish-brown crusts which when removed show pustular exudates which often cultures staph aureus. It occurs on severely sun- damaged skin and may be after an episode of shingles, trauma or skin cancer surgery. It heals with scars and sometimes increased balding. Treatment is with potassium permanganate or dilute vinegar soaks and oral anti-staph antibiotics. Potent topical corticosteroids and long term minocycline over months have also been advocated. It can be difficult to diagnose skin cancer or actinic keratoses in the crusted areas., 387t, 394

Eruptive melanocytic nevi. Simultaneous abrupt onset of numerous nevi acquired after immunosuppression and bullous eruption. There is increased concern about melanoma in these patients. Seen at blister sites in epidermolysis bullosa, toxic epidermal necrolysis, Stevens-Johnson syndrome, erythema multiforme, and blisters induced by mustard gas. May be idiopathic or associated with HIV, Addison's disease, renal transplantation, PUVA therapy cyclosporine A therapy idiopathic, alpha-melanocyte stimulating hormone, seizures, and underlying malignancy.

Eruptive pseudoangiomatosis. They are benign spontaneously regressing angioma like papules that are erythematous surrounded by a pale halo. Biopsy is distinctive with

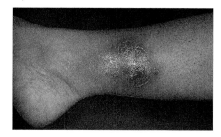

Erythema induratum.

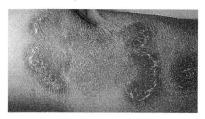

A. Erythema perstans on the elbow (*Drs. H. Shair and L. Grayson*).

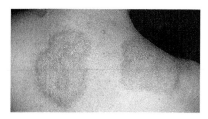

B. Erythema perstans on the back.

F

Proliferative fasciitis is a similar condition that can be differentiated by histology.

Fat autograft muscle injection (FAMI), 45–47, 47f

Fat necrosis of the newborn. Rare indurated, well demarcated subcutaneous nodules and plaques over the arms, legs, cheeks, buttocks or trunk within the first few weeks of life. Usually occurs following a complicated pregnancy and may be associated with hypercalcemia. Usually resolves without sequela.

Fat necrosis, subcutaneous. *See* Subcutaneous fat necrosis

Fat necrosis, subcutaneous, with pancreatic disease. Histologic picture is quite characteristic.

Fatal granulomatous disease of childhood. A very rare, X-linked disease of mainly males characterized by eczematous lesions in infancy with progressive chronic granulomatous bacterial infections.

Favre-Racouchot syndrome. The term for multiple comedones on the high cheek and temple areas in older persons due to chronic sun exposure, 510

Felty syndrome. Triad of arthritis, leucopenia and splenomegaly. Increased leg ulcers (22%), rheumatoid nodules (76%), and mortality (25%) related to increased infections with sepsis.

Fetal alcohol syndrome. Approximately 40% of newborns of alcoholic mothers develop mental retardation, skeletal abnormalities, and cardiac abnormalities. The cutaneous markers are hemangiomas, hypertrichosis, and nail dysplasias with thinning.

Fiberglass dermatitis. Irritant contact dermatitis with itching papules, erythema, vesicles, desquamation, and excoriations. Dorsal hands, fingers and forearms present mainly in workers using reinforcement filling in printed circuit boards. One of the commonest occupational dermatoses.

Fibroelastolytic papulosis. A rare condition with asymptomatic or mildly pruritic whitish-yellow papules that may coalesce into cobblestone-type plaques predilection for women over 40 and seen most often on the neck, supraclavicular area but can occur on face, trunk, and intertriginous skin. Biopsy is characterized by decreased or absent elastic fibers in the papillary and mid-reticular dermis. Probably previous diagnoses of white fibrous papulosis of the neck and pseudoxanthoma elasticum-like papillary dermal elastolysis are really the same disease.

Fibrokeratoma, acquired digital. Tumor occurring in adults on fingers or toes; mimics a rudimentary supernumerary digit but without nerve tissue., 322t

Fibroma, recurrent infantile digital. Fibrous nodules that occur at birth or sometimes during childhood on the fingers and toes; may spontaneously involute and then recur., 322t

Fibromas, pedunculated, 325–326, 325f

Fibrosarcoma, 332

Fibrosis, postirradiation. Gradual onset of dermal atrophy, fibrosis and telangiectasia at a radiation site. Worse with an increase in radiation dose.

Fibroxanthoma, atypical. Relatively uncommon, malignant (metastasis is rare), raised nodular lesion that occurs most often on the head and neck at chronically sun-exposed or irradiated sites. Treated with Mohs surgery to attempt to avoid frequent local recurrence., 321t, 532

Filariasis, 553

Filiform hyperkeratosis. Thin whitish multiple hyperkeratotic and asymptomatic monomorphic projections that are about 1-2mm in size and when present on the palms and soles maybe associated with underlying malignancy and can also be present on the trunk.

Filoviruses, 570t

Finger pebbles (Huntley's papules). Fine asymptomatic flesh colored grouped micropapules on the dorsum of the fingers associated with diabetes mellitus.

Finkelstein disease. *See* Acute hemorrhagic edema

Fish-Odor syndrome (trimethylaminuria). Rare metabolic disease with malodor of the body similar to that of decaying fish. Serious psychosocial problems relate to the malodor. Free urinary trimethylamine should be checked both on a normal and restricted diet. Dietary restriction of choline containing foods such as eggs, peas, beans, marine fish, liver and kidney should be tried. Large quantities of milk, brussel sprouts, and vegetables of the Brassica family should be avoided. Other therapeutic modalities include lactulose, metronidazole, neomycin sulfate, activated charcoal, and copper chlorophyllin.

Flagellate erythema. Uncommon rash with a pattern of linear streaks erythematous or hyperpigmented looking as if the skin has been whipped. Can be caused most characteristically by bleomycin treatment (one to several months after administration), peplomycin (bleomycin derivative), docetaxel, dermatomyositis, adult-onset Still's disease, and shiitake mushroom ingestion.

Flea bites, 210, 556, 557f

Flow cytometry, 13

Flukes. *See* Trematodes dermatosis

Fluorinated corticosteroids, 36

Fluoroscopy-induced chronic radiation injury. Acquired vascular, morphea-like or ulcerated area seen at the site of usually multiple fluoroscopic procedures that is seen over the scapula, back or lateral trunk below the axilla.

Foams, 35

Focal dermal hypoplasia (Goltz syndrome). X linked dominant syndrome showing cribriform atrophy with an increase or decrease in pigment often along Blaschko lines. Eye, skeletal, teeth, nail, and soft tissue abnormalities may occur.

Focal epithelial hyperplasia. Benign condition possibly caused by HPV 13 or 22 consisting of asymptomatic, multiple, mucosal papules especially in young females especially in Native Americans, Eskimos (where it is more common in adults) and South Africans. Seen on the inner upper and lower lips, buccal mucosa, and tongue with a variable course lasting a few months to years. Important to differentiate from condyloma to avoid implications of sexual transmission and abuse. Ablative therapy such as laser, cryotherapy, and surgical excision have been used with variable results.

Follicular plugs, 18

Folliculitis, 235t, 238–240, 239f

   decalvans, 235t, 238

   deep, 235t, 238

   scalp, 235t, 238–240, 239f

   superficial, 235t, 238

   treatment of, 238, 240

Folliculitis, eosinophilic pustular. Recurrent extremely pruritic crops of sterile pustules. Has a characteristic histologic appearance and is seen most often in association with HIV positive patients. There is an adult variant and an infancy variant not associated with immunosuppression.

Folliculitis, hot tub. A bacterial folliculitis with inflammatory nodules caused by *Pseudomonas aeruginosa* in people exposed to poorly chlorinated hot tubs, jacuzzis, whirlpools, and swimming pools., 239f

Folliculitis, perforating, of the nose. A folliculitis of the stiff hairs of the nasal mucocutaneous junction that penetrates deeply through to the external nasal skin. Unless the basic pathology is understood and corrected by plucking the involved stiff hair, the condition cannot be cured. The external papule can simulate a skin cancer.

Fordyce's disease, 339, 417

Foreign body granuloma., 202. *See also* Granuloma, foreign body

Forme fruste, 25

Formaldehyde, 71

Formulary, 28–35, 34t

Foshay test. A 48-hour intradermal test that, if positive, indicates that the person has or has had *tularemia.*

Fordyce disease, Necrotizing infundibular crystalline, waxy papules mainly on head and neck especially on forehead and sometimes the back. Yeast and gram-positive cocci have identified and may respond to topical or systemic antimycotic treatment. Histologically they are folliculocentric filamentous birefringent crystalline deposits.

Fox-Fordyce disease. A rare, intensely pruritic, chronic papular dermatosis of the axillae and the pubic area in women. The intense itching is due to the closure of the apocrine gland pore with rupture of the duct and escape of the apocrine sweat into the surrounding epidermis. Treatment is difficult., 18

Frambesia. *See* Yaws

Freckles, 336, 344, 509f

Frey's syndrome. Auriculotemporal nerve syndrome where gustatory stimuli cause facial flushing or sweating in the distribution of the auriculotemporal nerve. Usually due to trauma to the parotid gland in adults.

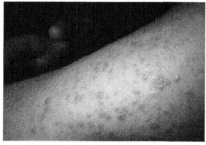

Gianotti-Crosti Syndrome of the upper outer arm

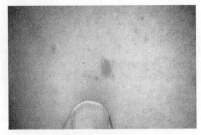

A. Acute GVHD mimicking lichenplanus.

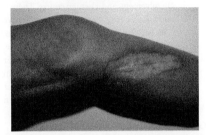

B. Chronic GVHD mimickingscleroderma

Graham-Little Syndrome (Piccardi-Lassueur-Graham-Little Syndrome). Multifocal cicatricial scalp alopecia, non-scarring alopecia of the axillae and/or groin, and keratotic perifollicular papules.

Grain itch. Due to a mite, *Pediculoides ventricosus,* that lives on insects that attack wheat and corn. This mite can attack humans working with the infested grain and cause a markedly pruritic papular, and papulovesicular eruption.

Granular cell schwannoma, 343

Granular cell tumor. *See* granular cell schwannoma

Granular parakeratosis. Especially in women in 5th and 6th decades and intertriginous areas with reddish brown and often asymptomatic papules that coalesce into macerated plaques. Mimics Hailey-Hailey disease and reported to clear with topical tretinoin.

Granuloma
  epithelioid, 202
  foreign body. A granulomatous reaction seen in the dermis due to the introduction, usually by trauma, of certain agents such as lipids, petrolatum, paraffin, indelible pencil, silica and silicates (talc), suture, hair, and zirconium from certain deodorants, 202
  histiocytic, 202
  mixed inflammatory, 202
  necrobiotic, 202
  silica, 204
  swimming pool, 545, 545f. *See also* Swimming pool granuloma

Granuloma annulare, 37, 204–205, 204f, 495t, 496, 498f

Granuloma faciale. Typically occurs as brownish papules or plaques, multiple or single, usually on the face, in middle-aged or older persons (usually men). Asymptomatic, benign, often recalcitrant to therapy and probably represents a form of localized vasculitis. Dapsone, intralesional corticosteroids, and cryosurgery are sometimes beneficial.

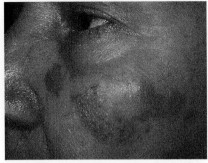

Granuloma faciale (*Dr. J. DeSpain*).

Granuloma gluteale infantum. Purplish, pink nodules in the diaper area in infants or in women wearing garments for incontinence. May be related to prolonged use of fluorinated topical corticosteroid preparations or to candidiasis.

Granuloma inguinale, 235t, 247, 247f

Granuloma, lethal midline. *See* Lethal midline granuloma

Granuloma pyogenicum, 336, 343, 343f

Granulomatosis
  allergic. *See* Allergic granulomatosis
  lymphomatoid. *See* Lymphomatoid granulomatosis

Granulomatous cheilitis. *See* Cheilitis, granulomatous

Granulomatous dermatitis (interstitial granulomatous dermatitis with arthritis). Most often in middle aged women with rheumatoid arthritis. Burning, symmetric, erythematous to violaceous nodules or plaques or linear cords ("rope sign") especially axillae, trunk and inner thighs. Biopsy is needed to make correct diagnosis. Topical corticosteroids, dapsone, and hydroxychloroquine have all been used as effective therapy.

Granulomatous disease of childhood, chronic. An X-linked recessive disorder of leukocyte function characterized by indolent infections of the skin, as well as lymph nodes, lungs, liver, spleen, bone, and bone marrow. 60%–70% of cases have cutaneous disease. Diagnostic pigmented lipid macrophages, found in skin and visceral granuloma.

Granulomatous slack skin syndrome. *See* Slack Skin syndrome

Granulomatous vasculitis, 165t

Grey-Turner's sign. Bruising of the flanks usually seen in acute hemorrhagic pancreatitis due to retroperitoneal bleeding.

Griscelli syndrome. Variable immunodeficiency associated with partial albinism. Characteristic histology of hair and skin is seen.

Grover's disease. *See* Acantholytic dermatosis, transient

Guttate psoriasis, 499, 499f

GVHD. *See* Graft-*versus*-host disease

H

Habit tic deformity, 407, 408f

Hair collar sign. A circle of elongated hyperpigmented hair around a congenital nodule seen in infants with cephalocele, meningocele, hypertrophic brain tissue, membranous aplasia cutis, andcongenital dermatofibrosarcoma protuberans.

Hairy leukoplakia of tongue, 418

Halitosis, 418

Hallermann-Streiff syndrome. Usually mutational, rare, craniofacial dysostoses with bird-like facies, facial telangiectasias, face, and scalp atrophy, alopecia (characteristically along suture lines), skeletal and ocular abnormalities.

Halo nevus, 334, 335f

Hamartoma, congenital smooth muscle. Rare, usually present at birth, hyperpigmented or skin-colored, benign, patch or plaque.

Hamartomas, 462

Hand-foot-and-mouth disease, 418

Hand foot syndrome. *See* Acral erythema

Hanifin/Rajka criteria, 78t

Harlequin fetus, 477t, 495f

Hamartoma syndrome, generalized basaloid follicular. Multiple tan papules that usually present in childhood especially face, scalp, neck, and trunk. Rare, autosomal dominant and can be associated with milia, comedones, and acrochordons. Hypertrichosis, hypohidrosis, and palmoplantar pits are also part of the syndrome. Autoimmune disorders such as myasthenia gravis, alopecia universalis, systemic lupus erythematosus, and antiphospholipid antibodies have been rarely associated. Solitary tumors are not hereditary.

Haverhill Fever. *See* Rat bite fever

Hay-Wells syndrome. Autosomal dominant syndrome with ankyloblepharon, ectodermal dysplasia, and/or cleft lip or cleft palate.

Heck disease. *See* focal epithelial hyperplasia.

Helminthic dermatoses (Roundworms), 210, 552, 553f

Hemangioendothelioma, Kaposi-form, 368, 369. *See* Kaposiform hemangioendothelioma

Hemangioendothelioma, retiform. Rare low-grade angiosarcoma that really metastasizes but frequently recurs. Non-descript clinical lesion but with a characteristic histology.

Hemangioma, 333, 333f, 343
  angiokeratoma, 334
  as birthmarks, 334
  capillary, 321t
  senile, 336
  spider, 333f, 333
  spindle cell. Benign subcutaneous and dermal, firm, red-blue nodules that occur mainly in children and young adults especially on the distal extremities. Satellite nodules develop in the same anatomical region. Histology is diagnostic., 369
  superficial, 330
  targetoid hemosiderotic. Simple benign acquired brown to violaceous papulonodule with pale ring surrounded by a ring of ecchymosis. May be due to trauma and resolves spontaneously. Characteristic histology.
  treatment of, 333–334
  varix, 334
  venous lake, 334
  verrucous, congenital hyperkeratotic, usually unilateral, bluish nodules associated with deep vascular tumors involving skin and subcutaneous tumors. On

Hot foot syndrome. Painful, tender nodules on plantar, weight bearing sites caused bypseudomonas exposure from walking in hot tubs or wading pools. Usually self-limited in 2 weeks but may require systemic fluoroquinolones.

Hound dog appearance, 485

Housewives' hand dermatitis, 80

HPV. *See* Human papillomavirus

HSV-1. *See* Herpes simplex virus 1

HSV-2. *See* Herpes simplex virus 2

HTLV-1 (Human T-cell lymphotropic virus, type 1). Virus associated with human T-cell leukemia lymphoma syndrome and tropical spastic paresis. Endemic in Japan, Caribbean base, South and Central America and southeastern USA. Less than 4% of seropositive patients have overt disease. 0.025% of USA blood donors are seropositive. Latent period may be up to 30 years, 541–542

Human immunodeficiency virus (HIV), 278–284, 279f–284f310–311, 458

Human papillomavirus (HPV), 278–279

Hunter's syndrome. Rare x-linked recessive mucopolysaccharidosis characterized by short stature, stiff joints, claw-like hands, deafness, hepatosplenomegaly, cardiomegaly, unusual facies, and symmetrical ivory-white papulo-nodules that form reticular ridges overthe upper trunk and proximal extremities.

Hutchinson's sign. Extension of pigment onto the lateral and proximal nail fold from a subungual melanoma. Also in herpes simplex where involvement of the nasal tip indicates involvement of thenasociliary branch of the ophthalmic nerve and warrants careful monitoring of the eye for consequent sequalae., 412

Hutchinson's teeth. Changes in the teeth of patients with congenital syphilis characterized especially by narrowing of the upper incisors with a central depression of the cutting edge, 460

Hutchinson's triad. The occurrence in patients with congenital syphilis of ocular keratitis, deafness, and dental defects., 460

Hyalinosis cutis et mucosae. *See* Lipoid proteinosis

Hyaluronic acid, injectable, 47

Hydroa aestivale. This rare recurrent vesicular dermatosis occurs in the summer on the exposed areas of the body. It is more common in young males and usually disappears at the age of puberty. The erythema, urticaria-like lesions, vesicles, and crusted lesions develop following sun exposure andare aggravated by continued exposure. When the vesicle shows a central depression, as in a vaccination, the eruption is called *Hydroa vacciniforme.*

Hydroa vacciniforme. *See* Hydroa aestivale. A severe form of hydroa vacciniforme has been associated with non-Hodgkin's lymphoma. Ebstein-bar virus has been suggested as possibly the causative agent.

Hydrocortisone, 36

α-hydroxy acids, 74

β-hydroxy acids, 74

Hypereosinophilic syndrome. Eosinophilia of 1.5 × 10 cells/L for at least 6 months with systemic involvement without any other identifiable cause of eosinophilia. Urticaria, angioedema, erythematous papules, and nodules are the commonest cutaneous manifestations.

Hyperhidrosis of the palms. Increased sweating of the palms can be a challenging therapeutic problem. Drysol, Drionic, and botulism injections all have their advocates and transthoracic sympathectomy has been used but can cause concomitant morbidity. Subcutaneous suction curettage after tumescent anesthetic distention or excision of sweat glands are more permanent surgical therapies. Usually improves with age., 455

Hyperhidrosis. Primary (idiopathic) form usually involves the palms, soles, and axillae. Social and psychological problems can be significant. Certain-Dri and Drysol are aluminum chloride preparations that can be helpful. Iontophoresis (Drionic) with tap water has been used. Botulism toxin has been tried with some success but it needs to be repeated and is painful. Anticholinergic (probanthine, oxybutinin) drugs can be taken orally but have other side effects. Beta blockers have been used and are occasionally helpful. Sympathectomy is not always helpful and is fraught with numerous complications. Underlying illnesses that need to be considered are lymphoma (night sweats) and other underlying malignancies, infectious etiologies, and hyperthyroidism. Usually improves with age., 287, 455

Hyper-IgE syndrome. Autosomal dominant with "cold" staphylococcal abscesses of the skin, atopic dermatitis, lung infection with pneumatoceles, increased serum IgE, defective granulocyte chemotaxis, osteoporosis, retained teeth, prominent forehead, broad nasal bridge, and rough facial skin with prominent pores., 140

Hyper-IgM immunodeficiency syndrome (HIM). Rare x-linked recessive with increased IgM and IgD and decreased IgA, IgG and IgE. Recurrent pyogenic infections treated with intravenous gamma globulins, and recalcitrant severe oral ulcers, and recalcitrant widespread warts are part of the syndrome.

Hyperimmunoglobulin D syndrome. Laboratory diagnosis depends on at least 2 vitamin D levels greater than 100mg/ml at least 1 month apart. Normal levels of vitamin D have been reported also. It is autosomal recessive with 50% of patients of Dutch ancestry. Mutations occur in the mevalonate kinase (MVK) gene. The first attack is often prior to 1 year of age and lasts 3 to 7 days with a 4 to 8 week asymptomatic period. The attack consists of fever, polymorphic (especially macules) erythematous skin with vasculitis on biopsy, tender cervical lymphadenopathy abdominal pain, 50% splenomegaly, and sometimes aphthous oral or vaginal ulcers.

Hyperkeratosis follicularis en cutem penetrans (Kyrle's disease). A rare, usually nonpruritic eruption, worse on the extremities, of discrete papules with a central keratotic plug. Deeper erythematous papules can leave atrophic scars.

Hyperkeratosis lenticularis perstans (Flegel's disease). Rare disease with tiny keratotic papules usually on the lower extremities in middle aged persons. May have a red halo, and removal leaves pinpoint bleeding site. Can involve oral mucosa.

Hyperpigmentation, 25, 101t, 157, 483–485, 484f

Hypertrichosis, 101t, 384

Hypertrichosis, nevoid. Congenital disorder that is uncommon consisting of terminal hair growth in a localized area and maybe along Blaschko's line. Maybe in a mosaic or segmental pattern and associated with ocular, muscular, as well as other anomalies. A twin spot may appear.

Hypertrichosis lanuginosa acquisita, 452t

Hypertrophic scar, 333

Hypokeratosis (circumscribed acral hypokeratosis). Idiopathic, well-circumscribed, acquired, solitary, asymptomatic, depressed areas with a raised border on the palms and rarely the soles especially on the hypothenar and thenar prominences. Probably a reaction pattern to various stimuli such as human papilloma virus or trauma.

Hypomelanosis of Ito, 443, 483

Hypopigmentation, 25, 429, 481–483, 482f–483f

Hypoplasia, focal dermal (Goltz syndrome). Rare syndrome usually seen in females with linear hypoplastic skin lesions and vertical striations of long bones. Digit and eye abnormalities also occur.

I

Ice pack burn. This can be caused by over 20 minutes exposure to an ice pack causing well demarcated areas that instead of on re-warming causing a pins and needles sensation, the area becomes painful, more red swollen and can leave permanent paresthesias or hyperpigmentation. Gradual warming is the treatment of choice.

Ichthyoses, 476, 477t–478t, 478f

Ichthyosiform erythroderma, 478f, 494

Ichthyosis, 491, 495f

Ichthyosis bullosa of Siemens. Very rare autosomal dominant blistering eruption made worse by warm weather and friction but without scaring or atrophy. May present with erythroderma but less commonly than in bullous congenital ichthyosiform erythroderma which is a more severe disease. Histopathology is helpful as well as electron microscopy.

Ichthyosis vulgaris, 477t

Ichthyosis with confetti. This is a distinct congenital ichthyosiform erythroderma with evolving white spots. A variant of this is the MAUIE syndrome that also includes micropinnae, squamous cell cancers, and ectropion.

Id reaction (autoeczematous reaction). This phenomenon is characterized by an erythematous, vesicular, or eczematous eruption that occurs in disseminated parts of the skin. Most commonly id reactions are seen to follow inflammatory fungal infections of the feet, stasis dermatitis with or without venous ulcers, inflammatory fungus infections of the scalp (kerion), and severe contact dermatitis of the hands, 212. *See also* Dermatophytid; Epidermophytid; Trichophytid; Candidid refers to various organisms involved in the etiology., 78, 83

Idiopathic eruptive macular pigmentation (IEMP). Usually seen in children and adolescents and consists of non-confluent asymptomatic macules that are brownish over the trunk neck proximal aspect of the extremities, absence of preceding inflammation, no history of drug exposure, histology showing basal cell layer hyperpigmentation and prominent dermal melanophages without basal cell layer damage, and normal mast cell count. Tends to resolve spontaneously but may occasionally be persistent.

Idiopathic guttate hypomelanosis (annular depigmented macules). Small macular, whitish, sharply marginated, approximately 0.5-cm lesions found on sun-exposed extremities, mainly the legs, but never on the face. Related to excessive sun exposure in genetically predisposed persons. Therapy is not necessary or effective., 444f

Idiopathic recurrent palmoplantar hidradenitis. Tender multiple red nodules on the palms and soles that occurs in children and spontaneously involutes in 2-21 days without sequelae. May be related to heat or trauma and has a characteristic histopathology when biopsied.

Idiopathic thrombocytopenic purpura, 495t, 499

IFAP. Ichthyosis follicularis, atrichia, and photophobia. Occurring as a rare congenital disordered inherited as X- linked with full manifestations in male patients and milder manifestations with a blaschko linear pattern in female carriers.

IgA pemphigus, 221

IgG4-related skin disease. Autoimmune disease that can affect almost any area of the body even though skin involvement is rare it is manifested by non-specific skin papules, plaques, and nodules that have a psuedolymphomatous appearance. Patients tend to have IgG4 or IgG ratio that is elevated in tissue.

Immediate pigment darkening, 467

Immersion foot. *See* Frostbite

Immersion syndrome (trench foot) and seefrost bite. Immersion of the foot or hand in temperatures from 10 degrees centigrade to 0 degrees centigrade or 50 degrees Fahrenheit to 32 degrees Fahrenheit for prolonged periods. Signs of immersion foot, trench foot, or trench hand are blisters swelling, redness, skin hot to the touch, and bleeding. First phase there is cold without pain and a weak pulse, second phase the limb feels hot and has shooting pains, third phase the skin is pale but maybe bluish discoloration on nail beds and the pulse is weak. Treat by drying, slow re-warming, dry bulky dressing, elevation, and do not rupture the blisters.

Immunofluorescence, 12

Immunohistology, 12, 13f

Impetigo, 235–237, 235t, 236f, 495t, 496560t, 564–565

Impetigo herpetiformis, 218

Incontinentia pigmenti, 218, 442, 484, 485f, 495, 495t, 497f

Indirect immunofluorescence, 219, 219t

Industrial dermatoses, 78

Infantile pedal papules. Relatively common, usually asymptomatic, flesh-colored papules and tumors seen on the medial aspect of the feet in infants. It occasionally extends onto the heels. Most common at 1 year of age and disappear at 2 to 3 years of age. Benign and require no therapy.

Infectious eczematoid dermatitis, 235t, 244–246, 245f

Infectious mononucleosis. Uncommon cutaneous involvement which is relatively nonspecific but a distinct cutaneous ampicillin rash occurs within one week of beginning therapy and the incidences in 80-100% of people with active infectious mononucleosis. It has been reported with other antibiotics including amoxicillin, methicillin, erythromycin, levofloxacin, tetracycline, and cephalexin. Ampicillin can be given after infectious mononucleosis has resolved without any adverse side effects., 274

Inflammatory bowel disease, 455, 456f

Insect bites. *See* Bites

Intensed pulsed light (IPL), 43–44, 43f, 44f

Iododerma. A dermatosis due to the ingestion ofiodides, usually of a pustular nature.

IPL. *See* Intensed pulsed light

Isorlphic response, reverse. *See*Renbok phenomenon

Isotopic response (wolf's isotopic response) is recurrence of a disease at the site of healed lesion of some unrelated disease most commonly reported with herpes zoster, herpes simplex, and varicella being the original illness and the subsequent conditions reported have been tuberculosis, vasculated granuloma, Bowen's disease,squamous cell cancer, actinic keratosis, sarcoid, tinea, angiosarcoma, leukemia cutis, kaposi's sarcoma metastases, lymphoma, granuloma annulare, and furuncles. Can occur as a nonisotopic response where a nonrelated skin disease has healed and a new skin disease spares that site.

Itch, 6. *See also* Pruritus; Scabies
swimmer's, 210, 554
Winter, 23, 212, 512, 512f

Itch-scratch cycle, 232

J

Jacquet's diaper dermatitis. Granulomatous erosive, diaper dermatitis in school age children with chronic urinary and/or fecal incontinence. May mimic condyloma acuminatum., 501f

Janeway nodes. Palmar-plantar, fingers and plantar toes with painless, irregular, hemorrhagic, nonblanchable papules seen with acute bacterial endocarditis.

Jarisch-Herxheimer reaction. *See* Herxheimer reaction

Jellyfish, 554

Jessner's syndrome (lymphocytic infiltrate of Jessner). Benign lymphocytic infiltrationof the skin, mainly of the face,resembling deep chronic discoid lupus erythematosus.

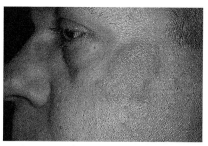

Jessner's benign lymphocytic infiltration of the skin.

Job's syndrome (HIES). Hyperimmunoglobulin E, recurrent infections. Rare, congenital.

Jogger's nipples. Painful erosions of nipples in runners, especially braless females, and when hard, irritating clothing is worn, 560t, 562

Jogger's toe. Subungual hematoma and hyperkeratosis in runners due to repeated trauma due to front of the toe box of the shoe. Tight lacing, high and long toe box, and nail trimming straight and close may all be helpful., 563

Junctional Epidermolysis Bullosa-Pyloric Atresia syndrome. Rare autosomal recessive with atresia of the gastric antrum or pylorus and bullous disease of the skin and oral mucosa.

Junctional nevus, 334, 335f

Jüngling's disease. *Osteitis fibrosa cystica* of the small long bones, particularly of the fingers, due to sarcoidosis.

Juvenile xanthogranuloma, 495t, 498

Juxta-articular nodes. Syphilitic gummatous tumors occurring in the corium or subcutaneous layer of the skin in the region of the joints.

K

Kaposiform hemangioendothelioma. Usually seen on the trunk and develops at birth or in neonates in the first few months of life with approximately 25% mortality rate due to tumor infiltration or Kasabach-Merritt syndrome. Destructive bone changes are not uncommon. Treatment is for as other infantile hemangiomas. Trans-catheter embolization and surgical excision may be required., 368, 368f

Kaposi's sarcoma, 282, 282f, 343, 344f

Kasabach-Merritt syndrome. Rare syndrome ofthrombocytopenia, bleeding and petechiae and association with rapidlyenlarging, tufted angioma orKaposiform hemangioendothelioma.

Kassowitz-Diday's law. The observation that successive children of a syphilitic mother will become progressively less infected with syphilis or not be infected at all.

Kawasaki disease, 38. *See also* Mucocutaneous lymph node syndrome

Kawasaki's syndrome, 38, 453

Keloid, 17, 17f, 24f, 41f, 333, 333f, 429–431, 430f

treatment of. Intralesional corticosteroids, 585-nm pulsed dye laser, 30 second liquid nitrogen cryosurgery and silicon gel sheets for 12 to 24 hours each day for at least 2months., 333

Keratinization disorders, 476–480, 477t–478t, 478f–479f

Keratoacanthoma, 338, 350f

Keratoacanthoma centrifugum marginatum. Arare variant of keratoacanthoma that shows progressive peripheral growth with coincident central healing.

Keratoconjunctivitis sicca, 419

Keratoderma blennorrhagicum. A rare chronic inflammatory dermatosis with horny pustular crusted lesions mainly on thepalms and the soles; occurs in conjunction with gonorrheal infection of the genital tract and Reiter's syndrome.

Keratoderma climacterium. Circumscribed hyperkeratotic lesions of the palms and the soles of women of the menopausal age. These lesions resemble psoriasis, and the majority of cases are considered to be this disease.

Keratoderma, epidermolytic palmoplantar (EPPK of Vörner). Diffuse, yellowish, hyperkeratotic, thickening of the palms and soles. Familiar or sporadic and has a characteristic shape and erythematous line of demarcation. May be hyperhidrotic and rarely with blisters. Autosomal dominant variant called Unna-Thost has a slightly different histopathology.

Keratolytics, 29

Keratoplastic agents, 29

Keratoses, stucco. Discrete, flat, keratotic papules, "stuck on" to the skin in elderly persons especially over legs, ankles, and tops of the feet. They can be removed by scratching without causing bleeding. Probably a type of seborrheic keratoses., 323

Keratosis, 99t
actinic, 25, 320t, 321t, 322t, 328–331, 530, 531t
arsenical, 330, 331, 338

Keratosis follicularis spinulosa decalvans. Rare familial disease with diffuse keratosis pilaris, scarring scalp alopecia, photophobia, facial erythema, and palmoplantar keratoderma.

Keratosis Ichthyosis and Deafness. *See* KID syndrome

Keratosis lichenoides chronica. Rare, chronic, progressive, violaceous, lichenoid papules arranged in linear plaques. May be a variant of lichen planus.

Keratosis pilaris rubra. Variant of keratosis pilaris with accompanying redness over the face, extensor upper arms, extensor thighs and buttocks. No atrophy or hyperpigmentation. Seen mainly in children before puberty.

Keratosis pilaris, 495t, 496

KID syndrome. Keratitis, ichthyosis and deafness in a congenital syndrome affecting ectodermal tissue.

Kikuchi-Fujimoto disease (histiocytic subacute necrotizing lymphadenitis with granulocytic infiltration). Painless lymphadenopathy (mainly cervical), leukopenia, fever, myalgias, sore throat, increased LDH, seen more commonly in women with a mean age of 30 years. 40% have cutaneous lesions that may be exudative erythema, facial rash or erythematous papules, plaques or nodules. Histology examination is diagnostic.

Kimura's disease. *See* Angiolymphoid hyperplasia with eosinophilia

Kindler syndrome. A rare condition presenting simultaneous manifestations of both poikiloderma congenitale and epidermolysis bullosa. The four major features are acral blisters, poikiloderma, atrophy, and photosensitivity.

Kissing bug, 552

Klippel-Trenaunay-Parkes-Weber syndrome. Hemihypertrophy of arm or leg associated with varicosities and nevus flammeus (or hemangioma) with an arteriovenous malformation.

Knuckle pads. Nodules over metacarpal phalangeal and interphalangeal joints. It may be associated with trauma, Dupuytren contracture, camptodactyly, induratio penis plastica, acrokeratoelastoidosis, degenerative collagenous plaques of the hands or Touraine's hereditary polyfibromatosis (knuckle pad disease).

Koebner phenomena, reverse. *See* Renbok pheneomenon

Koebner phenomenon. The ability of the skin to react to trauma by the production of lesions of a previously existing skin disease. This phenomenon occurs in patients with skin diseases such as psoriasis, lichen planus, flat warts (pseudokoebnerization), and lichen nitidus, 190, 197f, 440

KOH preparation, 10

Koplik's spots, 418

Kwashiorkor. Severe dietary protein deficiency seen mainly in poorly developed countries but also in developed countries in infants with protein poor diets (rice milk diets in infants). Diffuse "flaky paint" dermatitis with desquemation as well as stunted growth, decreased stamina, vomiting, diarrhea, anorexia, edema, steatosis, anemia and increased susceptibility to infection. Coma, stupor and fatalities can occur related to infection., 594–595, 595f

Kyrle's disease. *See* Hyperkeratosis follicularis en cutem penetrans

L

Labial melanotic macule (solitary labial lentigo). Pigmented macules (often singular) on the lower lip (most common), tongue or intraoral mucosa. Biopsy shows a lentigo.

LAMB syndrome. **L**entigines, **a**trial myxoma, **m**ucocutaneous myxomas, and **b**lue nevi.

Lamellar ichthyosis, 477t

Langerhans cell, 4

Lanugo hair, 383

Larva migrans, 552, 553f

Lasers, 40–44, 41f–44f
carbon dioxide, 40–41, 41f
neodymium:yttrium aluminum garnet (Nd:Yag), 41, 42f
pulsed dye, 41, 42f
Q-switched, 41, 42f

Lassar's paste. Zinc oxide paste (U.S.P.) containing 25% zinc oxide, 25% starch, and 50% petrolatum.

Latrodectism, 555

Laugier-Hunziker syndrome. Rare disorder of numerous pigmented macules mainly on the lower lip, hand, palate, and tips of the fingers. No underlying gastrointestinal polyposis. Occur in 3rd to 5th decade and may also be seen on the nails (may be a linear band), soles, abdomen, neck, thorax, floor of the mouth, gums, and the labial commissures., 410

Leiden (Factor V) mutation. Commonest blood abnormality associated with thrombosis, increased venous thrombosis, thromboembolism, and venous leg ulcerations,. Associated with an increased thrombosis in pregnant women and women on oral contraceptives as well., 158t

Leiner's disease. A generalized exfoliative erythroderma seen in newborns. Thought to be a severe form of seborrheic dermatitis. Diarrhea and a failure to thrive are seen.

Leiomyoma, 344

Leiomyosarcoma, 344

Leishmaniasis, 550–551, 551f

Lentigines. PUVA-induced. Stellate or star-like brown macules on the buttocks, groin, penis, trunk but spares the palms, soles, gluteal cleft and axillae. May persist up to 2 years after PUVA therapy., 344, 453
tanning bed lentigines. Acral brown macules especially on the legs, arms, neck and chest. May occur abruptly or after prolonged tanning-bed exposure.
generalized lentigines without systemic abnormalities. Eruptive, generalized lentigines occurring abruptly over weeks to years without systemic abnormalities.

Lentiginosis, partial unilateral. Segmental multiple lentigines arising on normal skin. Usually not associated with underlying illness. Begins at childhood and slowly spreads in a wave over months to years.

Lentigo maligna melanoma, 321t, 357

Leonine facies, 25

LEOPARD syndrome. **L**entigines (multiple), **E**lectrocardiographic abnormalities, **O**cular hypertelorism, **P**ulmonary stenosis, **A**bnormalities of genitalia, **R**etardation of growth, **D**eafness and osseous deformities, 453

Lepidopterism. Cutaneous and occasionally mucocutaneous manifestations most often in central and south America from Mexico to Argentina also some tropical regions of China due to a pine caterpillar. The commonest manifestation is on exposed areas forming a papular urticarial eruption with intense itching which can last up to a year. Mucosal lesions including corneal ulcers and even blindness can be associated with anaphylaxis and other systemic symptoms. Removal of urticating hairs by individual removal of hairs with forceps under magnification or adhesive tape removal is recommended. Systemic corticosteroids may be necessary.

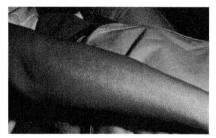

White monotonous papules on the fore arm in lichen nitidis

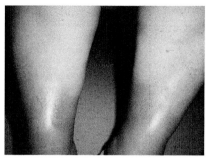

Lipodermatosclerosis of the lower extremities with wine bottle deformity

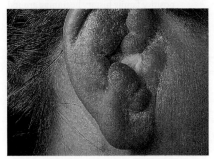

Lymphedema (elephantiasis nostras)of the ear (*Dr. M. Feldaker*).

M

involves the genitourinary tract but can involve the skin in mainly the perineal areas. Michaelis-Gutmann bodies are electron dense intracytoplasmic laminations seen in macrophages.

Malherbe's tumor

Mantoux. *See* Tuberculin tine test

Marshall's syndrome. Pediatric Sweet's syndrome (acute neutrophilic dermatosis) and cutis laxa due to loss of dermal elastic tissue. Associated with Alpha-1 antitrypsin deficiency.

McCune-Albright syndrome. Sexual precocity with polyostotic fibrous dysplasia, café-au-lait spots, pituitary adenomas, adrenal hypercorticolism, hyperthyroidism, and osteomalacia, 484, 484f

McKusick syndrome (cartilage hair hypoplasia). Autosomal recessive with short stature, short limbs, hair abnormalities and immunodeficiency associated with an increased risk of infections and malignancy (especially leukemia and non-Hodgkin's lymphoma)

Mechanic's hands. Hyperkeratotic, lichenified, fissured dermatitis over radial sides of the hands and inner edge of the feet. Similar to calloused hands seen in manual laborers. Most closely associated with antisynthetase syndrome but can also be seen in polymyositis, systemic lupus erythematosus, systemic scleroderma, and overlap syndromes.

Mediterranean Fever, Familial. Autosomal recessive syndrome of recurrent febrile episodes of peritonitis, pleuritis, and joint synovitis. Erysipelas-like skin lesions occur most commonly but bullae, pyoderma, panniculitis, and vasculitis may be seen. Predominantly in Arabic, Turkish, Armenian, and Sephardic Jewish people., 152

Melanoacanthoma a very hyperpigmented seborrhea keratosis that can mimic a malignant melanoma. Histological exam it is a seborrhea keratosis and is always benign., 323

Melanoacanthoma, oral. An oral melanoacanthoma is not a variant of seborrhea keratosis. It is rare and histologically consists of dendritic melanocytes. It could elevated, black, multifocal, and in some cases pain and itching is reported, on the buccal mucosa followed by the palette and lips. Biopsy maybe necessary to rule out a malignant melanoma, no therapy is needed. Some lesions regress spontaneously after biopsy. If it is symptomatic it can be excised.

Melanocytosis, familial genetic. Diffuse brown hyperpigmentation with raindrop hypopigmentation caused by failure of melanocytes to deliver melanin to the surrounding keratinocytes. Probably autosomal dominant with characteristic histopathology.

  signet ring type. Only about 5% of melanoma show this progressive enlargement pigmented erythematous plaque and the cells have a distinct nucleus which is pushed to one side of the cell giving it a "signet ring" morphology.

Melanoma, animal-type. A rare type of melanoma which mimics that of the equine melanocytic disease seen in gray horses. It is associated with a more indolent course but can metastasize and histology is characteristic with large hyperpigmented cells in the dermis and lack of epidermal and junctional component as well as infrequent atypia and infrequent mitosis. Clinically it shows a blue/black voluminous nodule with irregular borders.

Melanonychia. Longitudinal, hyperpigmentation of nailbeds in lines along the long axis due to a normal variant in darkly pigmented patients, PUVA therapy, infliximab, neoplasm, HIV, chemotherapy, and antimalarials. Transverse, hyperpigmentation in transverse lines across nails due to radiation therapy, infliximab, zidovudine, antimalarials, chemotherapy, fungal disease, malignant melanoma, and benign nevi., 410, 410f

Melanosis, Becker's (Becker's nevus). Large localized mottled hypermelanotic noncongenital, and hypertrichotic patches, located especially on the upper back; not associated with underlying structural abnormalities and without cancer potential., 322t

Melanosis, vulvar benign. Intense pigmented macules that maybe irregular and mimic malignant melanoma on the vulva, histologically the lesion is benign and no treatment is necessary.

Melanosis of Riehl. A brownish pigmentation of the skin on the sun-exposed areas of the body that have come into contact with certain tars.

Melanotic macule. *See* Genital melanotic macule; Labial melanotic macule

Melanotic macule of the nail unit. The commonest cause of a pigmented longitudinal streak of the nail plate. Caused by an increase in melanin production by the melanocytes of the nail matrix. It must be biopsied especially in fair skinned patients to rule out a malignant melanoma.

Melasma. *See* Chloasma

Melioidosis. An infectious disease of rodents andhumans with abscesses and pustules ofthe skin and other organs, similar to glanders., 571t, 576t

Melkersson-Rosenthal syndrome. Idiopathic facial swelling, facial nerve palsy, and lingua plicata (fissured tongue, scrotal tongue)., 419

Menkes' Kinky Hair syndrome. Impaired metabolism of copper (serum Cu below 25% of normal), x-linked, hair shaft abnormalities (pili torti, monilethrix), stretchable skin (especially over the hands), central nervous system abnormalities, and failure to thrive.

Merkel cell cancer. Highly malignant (approximately 33 % mortality at 3 years), rare, reddish, dome-shaped tumor of neuroendocrine origin, usually seen on the face. As many as 90% have 3 or more of the AEIOU (asymptomatic/ lack of tenderness, expanding rapidly, immune suppression, older than 50 years, ultraviolet exposed site on a fair complexion patient) criteria., 4, 338, 510

Metabolic syndrome. Polycystic ovaries, insulin resistance, hirsutism, acanthosis nigricans, obesity, skin tags, acne, abnormalities of periods often with amenorrhea. Also associated with increased triglycerides and LDL cholesterol. some studies show an increase in psoriasis and androgenetic alopecia in male and female patients., 385, 599

Meyerson's nevus. An eczematous halo clinically and histologically described in benign nevocellular nevi, atypical nevi, and congenital nevi.

Meyerson's phenomenon. Transient, eczematous dermatitis around nevi, seborrheic keratoses, basal cell carcinomas, squamous cell carcinomas, and dermatofibroma associated with the appearance of these tumors. Affects healthy individuals, is rare, and has no proven etiology. The tumors stop forming after the inflammation dissipates. Seborrheic keratoses may decrease in number., 323

Microcystic adnexal carcinoma. Locally aggressive adnexal malignancy. Often recurs after radiation or surgery. Mainly affects the central face with a slow growing cystic papule or plaque that infiltrates deeply into surrounding structures. It is a difficult clinical diagnosis since it is so nonspecific. Often with sensory changes such as numbness, tenderness or paresthesias. Characteristic pathology., 342

Microscopic polyangiitis. A microscopic form of MPO-ANCA-positive vasculitis now separated from classic polyarteritis nodosa. There is an absence of immunoglobulin and complement localization in vessels. There is often a severe progressive course with necrotizing and crescentic glomerulonephritis and pulmonary capillaritis. Approximately

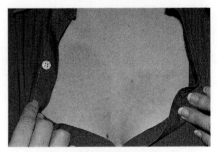

Reticular erythematous mucinosis (REM).

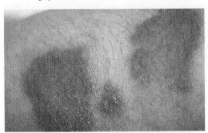

Neutrophilic acute febrile dermatosis (Sweet's syndrome) (*Dr. J. DeSpain*).

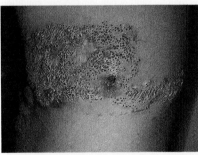

Nevus comedonicus on the abdomen.

progresses to extensive, grotesque, ulcerative, destructive, gangrenous, vegetative growth with destruction of underlying tissue. The children are often shunned by their society. There is a 70 to 90% death rate. It is polymicrobic due mainly to fusobacterium necrophorum and *Prevotella intermedia*. Debridement especially early in its course and systemic penicillin and metronidazole are therapies of choice., 418

Nonbullous congenital ichthyosiform erythroderma, 477t, 478f

Nonthrombocytopenic purpura, 160

Nontropical pyomyositis. Similar to tropical pyomyositis but in temperate climates in debilitated elderly patients in association with diabetes mellitus, HIV infection, connective tissue disease, and underlying malignancy.

North American blastomycosis(blastomycsis), 299, 300f

Notalgia paresthetica, 151. *See also* Pruritic hereditary localized patch on the back. Rarely a sign of a sensory neuropathy.

Nummular eczema, 20f, 23, 83, 83f, 102t, 246

O

Obliterans, arteriosclerosis. A degenerative change mainly in the arteries of the extremities; most commonly seen in elderly men. Leg ulcers and gangrene can result from these vascular changes., 244

Obliterans, thromboangiitis. *Buerger's disease* is an obliterative disease of the arteries and the veins that occurs almost exclusively in young men. It mainly involves the extremities and produces tissue ischemia, ulcers, and gangrene. Cigarette smoking is a usual co-factor., 244

Obstetric cholestasis, 581t

Occipital Horn syndrome, 485

Occlusive dressing therapy, 148

Ochronosis. A rare hereditary metabolic disorder characterized by a brownish or blackish pigmentation of cartilages, ligaments, tendons, and intima of the large blood vessels due to the deposit of a polymer of homogentisic acid. The urine in ochronosis turns black, particularly in the presence of alkali; hence the term *alkaptonuria*. *See also* pigmentary disorders. There is an exogenous form at the site of chronic topical hydroquinone application (*See* Chapter 9), 102t

Ointments, 27, 29, 32–35, 34t

Oleomas. Subcutaneous granulomas due to injection of sesame seed oil used for tissue augmentation or as a slow release substance for anabolic steroids. Usually in bodybuilders.

Olmsted's syndrome. Very rare; consists of congenital keratoderma of the palms andsoles, onychodystrophy, constriction ofdigits, and periorificial keratoses. Can beconfused with acrodermatitis enteropathica.

Omenn's syndrome. Combined immunodeficiency. Rare, congenital. A type of severe combined immunodeficiency with lymphocytosis and leukocytosis with eosinophilia. Often

fatal in childhood with a chronic skin eruption mimicking severe seborrhea, lymphadenopathy, hepatosplenomegaly, recurrent infections, fever, and failure to thrive. Humoral and cellular immunity are both defective, 501

Onchocerciasis, 554

Onycho-. A prefix from the Greek *onyx* meaning "nail."

Onychocryptosis, 406–407, 407f

Onychomadesis. Possibly a severe form of beau's lines with spontaneous separation of the nail plate from the nail bed from proximal to distal and causing complete shedding of the nail. Numerous drugs, fungal therapy, renal failure, infection, Kawasaki disease,male autosomal dominant inheritance type, multiple other severe systemic diseases have been associated with this condition., 102t, 118f

Onychomatricoma. Benign tumor of the nail matrix which causes transverse curvature of the nail plate longitudinal, longitudinal yellowish discoloration, and splinter hemorrhages. Removal of the nail plate reveals a stinger-like fibrokeratogenous projection., 410

Onychomycosis, 401–403, 402f, 403f

Ophiasis. Snake-like form of alopecia areata around the edges of the scalp. May be especially recalcitrant to therapy., 392

Optic atrophy. Atrophy of the optic nerve due to syphilitic involvement of the central nervous system of the tabetic type. Blindness is the end result.

Oral facial granulomatosis. Swelling of the facial or oral tissues with biopsy showing non-caseating granulomatous inflammation. This classification includes Melkersson- Rosenthal syndrome, Miescher chronic granulomatous cheilitis and the localized facial forms of Crohn's disease and sarcoidosis.

Oral florid papillomatosis. *See* Verrucous carcinoma

Orf. A viral infection characterized by a vesicular and pustular eruption of the mouth and the lips of lambs. Sheep herders and veterinarians become inoculated on the hand and develop a primary-chancre type lesion., 18

Oriental sore, 551

Osler's disease, 343

Osler's nodes. *See* Nodes, Osler's.

Osler-Weber-Rendu disease (Hereditary hemorrhagic telangiectasia). Begins in puberty. Progressive telangiectasias on the lips, tongue, palate, nasal mucosa, palms, soles, fingers, nail beds, and throughout the gastrointestinal tract. Pulmonary and intracranial A-V malformations may occur. Epistaxis and bleeding from internal organs is problematic in this autosomal disease,162

Osmidrosis. Malodorous apocrine gland sweating usually in an axillary location related to overgrowth of bacteria.

Osteoma cutis, 344

Ostomy skin care. *See* Stomas

Oxalosis of the skin. Most patients present at an early age with recurrent urolithiasis and renal failure but skin manifestations may be present such as livedo reticularis, acrocyanosis, purpura, gangrene, and ulcerations. Biopsy will show oxalate

deposition with in the lumen vessels shows oxalate crystals under polarization. This disease should be in the differential diagnosis of calciphylaxis and nephrogenic systemic fibrosis since all these patients can present with renal failure and similar cutaneous findings. Secondary disease can be caused by chronic hemodialysis, ileal resection, repeated oral antibiotic use, ascorbic acid excessive intake, pyridoxine deficiency, and various intestinal diseases.

P

Pachonychia congenita, 486, 486f

Pachydermodactyly. Rare benign fibromatosis causing fusiform swelling of multiple fingers over the proximal interphalangeal joints or proximal phalanges. Etiology is uncertain but minor trauma in OCD and in other obsessive compulsive behaviors and other psychiatric conditions is hypothesized. Rare form of digital fibrosis that is painful symmetric swelling around the proximal interphalangeal joints of the hand is associated with poultry processing workers, Dupuytren's contracture, Asperger's syndrome, carpal tunnel syndrome, and tuberous sclerosis.

Pachydermoperiostosis (Touraine-Solente-Golé syndrome and primary hypertrophic osteoarthropathy). Pachydermia,hypertrophic osteoarthropathy, and finger clubbing are part of this rare genetic syndrome. Associated with polyarthritis, cutis verticis gyrata, seborrheic dermatitis, acne, bilateral blepharoptosis, and hyperhidrosis.

Pachyonychia congenita. A rare autosomal dominant condition with thickening of the palms and soles, thickening of the oral mucosa, and hyperkeratosis of the distal nail bed with accumulation of subungual debris., 486, 486f

Paederus dermatitis (Blister beetle dermatitis), 482, 483f. Irritant contact dermatitis seen in the tropics caused by rove beetles (genus Paederus) being crushed on the skin and releasing the vesicant pederin. The result is the sudden onset of a burning vesiculopustular plaque on a red base. Ocular involvement can occur when the toxin is transferred by the patient's fingers., 556–557, 558f

Paget's disease, 338, 452t, 515

Palisaded neutrophilic and granulomatous dermatitis. Benign inflammatory dermatosis that has a distinctive histopathological changes. Consists of recurrent crops of expanding annulare and gyrate plaques usually on the head, neck, torso, and proximal extremities. It is associated with connective tissue diseases and lymphoproliferative disorders

Palmar-Plantar Erythrodysesthesia. *See* Acral erythema.

Palmar-plantar keratoderma, 479, 479f

Palmoplantar eccrine hidradenitis (PEH). Painful, erythematosus palmoplantar nodules in children with resolution after several days of bedrest. On biopsy, inflammation of neutrophils occur in and around eccrine glands and their ducts.

localized cicatricial (Brunsting-Perry). In elderly patients, recurrent blisters are seen, most commonly of the head and neck. Histology and immunofluorescence are similar to cicatricial mucosal pemphigoid, but there is no mucous membrane involvement in this form. Heals with scarring.

Pemphigoid, anti-p200. Rare subepidermal blistering disease with blisters, vesicles, erosion, and urticarial plaques that resembles both bullous pemphigoid and the inflammatory variant of epidermolysis bullosa acquisita. Treatment is with systemic corticosteroids plus or minus dapsone, doxycycline, azathioprine, or cyclosporine.

Pemphigoid gestationis. *See* Herpes gestationis

Pemphigoid nodularis. Uncommon variant of pemphigoid with prurigo nodularis-like nodules with or without blisters. Histopathology of prurigo nodularis but the direct immunofluorescence is compatible with bullous pemphigoid.

Pemphigus
Penile horn. Thick, dry, keratinized epithelium overlying a previously existing lesion on the glans of the penis. Usually preceded by chronic preputial inflammation and long-standing phimosis in individuals who undergo adult circumcision. The underlying tumor can be benign epidermal hyperplasia, warts, keratoacanthoma and, up to 1/3, with a squamous cell carcinoma.

Perforating skin disorders. Several dermatoses exhibit epidermal perforation as a histologic feature. Many represent transepithelial elimination. Four diseases are essential perforating disorders: elastosis perforans serpiginosa, reactive perforating collagenosis, perforating folliculitis, and Kyrle's disease.

Perianal streptococcal dermatitis. Sharply demarcated painful erythema usually in children that may lead to pain, painful defecation, pruritus, tenesmus, constipation, rectal bleeding, and anal discharge. Usually Group A beta hemolytic streptococci (rarely staphylococcus aureus) is causative.

Perianal pyrimidiform protrusion (*See* perianal protrusion, infantile). Exophytic flesh colored to pink soft tissue swelling along the median rafe in the genital area in children especially females. Associated with diarrhea or constipation and may resolve when gastrointestinal normalcy is restored. May be confused with condyloma accuminata.

Perifolliculitis capitis abscedens et suffodiens. (dissecting cellulitis of the scalp). Draining dissecting pustular sinuses and abscesses in the scalp. Part of the follicular occlusion triad that also includes cystic acne and hidradenitis suppurativa.,

Perineal erythema. *See* recurrent toxin-mediated perineal erythema.

Perineal protrusion, infantile (*See* pyradimal pyrimidoform profusion). A pyradimal soft-tissue protrusion with a tongue-like lip and velvety surface located in the midline just anterior to the anus in neonates. It can be genetic, functional after diarrhea, constipation or other irritation or associated with lichen sclerosis et atrophicus. It usually resolves with time and therapy of any underlying condition with rarely a need for surgical intervention.

Periodic fever, aphthous stomatis, pharyngitis, and adenitis (PFAPA). It is the most common cause of periodic fever syndrome in children. Recurring episodes every 2-6 weeks that last for approximately 3-6 days with fever, aphthous stomatis and/or genital ulcers, palmoplantar macules or purpura and erythema, pharyngitis cervical, lymphadenitis and other symptoms of malaise with headache arthritis nausea, vomiting , and enlargement of the spleen. Occurs predominately in the first 5 years of life.,

Perioral dermatitis. Common and mainly seen in women with pinhead sized papules and pustules and some accompanying desquamative erythema. Often with a perioral halo meeting the lips only at the corners of the mouth. First improves with topical corticosteroids and then worsens with topical corticosteroids. Improves within 2 to 4 weeks of oral tetracycline or erythromycin. Topical clindamycin and erythromycin as well as topical metronidazole have been used with some success. Rarely occurs around the eyes, nares and even perirectal so some authors feel it should be called periorificial dermatitis. There is a more chronic granulomatous form,

Pernio. *See* Chilblain; Frostbite

PHACES syndrome. Large facial hemangiomas especially in female infants associated with posterior fossa brain abnormalities (most often Dandy-Walker type malformations). Other anomalies are ocular, cardiac, and vertebral maldevelopment.

Phacomatosis pigmentokeratotica. Rare syndrome with simultaneous occurrence of organoid epidermal nevus and speckled lentigines nevus.

Phacomatosis pigmentovascularis. Rare syndrome of simultaneous occurrence of nevus flammeus and pigmented nevus, nevus pigmentosas, mongolian spot, nevus spilus, nevus verrucosus or nevus anemicus.

PIBIDS. Photosensitivity, ichthyosis, brittle hair (trichothyrodystrophy), intellectual impairment, delayed development, and short stature.

Piedra. The word is Spanish for stone and refers to a fungal infection of the hair shaft forming gritty adherent nodules. Black piedra is caused by Piedraia hortae and appears mainly on scalp hairs in tropical countries as dark hard nodules. White piedra is caused by Trichosporun beigelii and other Trichosporum species and appears as whitenodules on scalp hair in tropical andtemperate regions. The disease mimicsthe nits of pediculosis capitis but can be distinguished by KOH examination of the hair shafts. Treatment is accomplished by antifungal azole shampoos and oral agents.

Piezogenic papules. Herniation of fat into the dermis that are painful or asymptomatic seen only on standing on the lateral or medial heel. 2–5 mm and flesh colored.

Pigmentation, idiopathic eruptive macular. Spontaneously regressing (months to years), idiopathic, asymptomatic, brown, confluent macules. No previous inflammation, no drug association, on the trunk, neck and proximal extremities in children and adolescents. Basal cell layer hyperpigmentation and prominent dermal melanocytes and no increase in mast cells on skin microscopy.

Pilomatrix carcinoma. A rare malignancy derived from follicular matrix cells with high rates of recurrence and metastasizes. Most common in white men and usually on the head and neck in older patients which indicated possible actinic-induced transformation. MOHS microsurgery is probably the treatment choice.

Pilonidal sinus. Cavity lined by epithelial or granulation tissue often containing hair. Usually sacrococcygeal but can occur in other hair-bearing areas. It can be occupational in the interdigital areas of the hands of barbers, milkers, sheep shearers and dog groomers. Treatment is surgical and control of secondary bacterial or fungal infection., 180

Pincer nails. Transverse curling of the nail along its longitudinal axis. It may arise as a developmental abnormality but may be acquired due to subungual exostosis, osteoarthritis, onychomycosis, traumatic acroosteolysis, epidermal cysts, and psoriasis. It is painful and may require nail surgery. *See under* chapter on nails, 406, 406f

Pink disease. *See* Acrodynia

Pinta, 544, 545f

Pitted keratolysis, 287, 560t, 565

Pityriasiform. Used in naming many skin diseases to describe fine, tiny scale.

Pityriasis alba, 427, 427f. *See* Pityriasis simplex faciei

Pityriasis amiantacea. A distinct morphologic entity characterized by masses of sticky, silvery, overlapping scales adherent to the hairs and scalp. When the thick patch of scales is removed, the underlying scalp is red and oozing and often has a foul odor. The underlying cause can be tinea, pyoderma, neurodermatitis erosive pustular dermatosis of the scalp, or psoriasis.

Pityriasis lichenoides chronica (Juliusberg). A form of guttate parapsoriasis. *See* Parapsoriasis.

Pityriasis lichenoides et varioliformis acuta (Mucha-Habermann). An acute disease that appears as a reddish macular generalized eruption that may have mild constitutional signs including fever and malaise. Vesicles may develop and also papulonecrotic lesions. This disease gradually disappears in several months. Histologically, it is characterized by a vasculitis that differentiates it from the parapsoriasis group of diseases. It may improve with UVB therapy or oral antibiotics (tetracycline, erythromycin). There is a febrile ulceronecrotic form that can involve the liver and gastrointestinal tract and be fatal. Methotrexate, dapsone and systemic corticosteroids may be life-saving, Some authors think pityriasis lichenoides chronica is a chronic form of this disease., 26

Pityriasis rosea, 19f, 23, 92t, 194–196, 194f–195f, 197, 201, 496t, 499

Pityriasis rubra pilaris. Papulosquamous psoriasiform eruption that often begins in the scalp and progresses to an erythroderma with islands of normal skin. Keratoderma of the palms and soles ("keratotic sandal") is common. Clinically mimics psoriasis and histological examination may help in differentiation. It has a bimodal distribution in the first and fifth decades. Retinoids and methotrexate are the mainstays of therapy which is not always satisfactory., 170t, 227, 227f

Pityriasis rotunda. Rare asymptomatic well defined round scaly area that may have increased or decrease pigment, usually found in the trunk, buttock or extremities. May well be an acquired form of ichthyosis but may possible

also be a paraneoplastic condition. Type 1 tends to be more increased in pigment in black and Asian patients where systemic malignancy may be as high as 30%, this also includes malignant transformation of the lesion. Type 2 is more common in white patients has hypopigmentation and not associated with systemic disease and is more apt to be familial.

Pityriasis simplex faciei (pityriasis alba). A common disorder of children seen predominantly in the winter as a well-localized, scaly, hypopigmented, oval patch on the cheeks, upper outer arms, and upper outer legs. The end result is hypopigmentation of the area, but the normal pigment returns when the eruption clears up (usually in the summer, however, an initial tan may make it temporarily more prominent). We believe this condition to be a mild form of atopic eczema., 139, 427, 427f, 558

Plague, 570t

Plantar fibromatosis (Ledderhose disease). The equivalent of Dupuytren's contracture (palmar fibromatosis) except it occurs on the plantar surface of the foot. Abnormal fibrous tissue replaces the plantar aponeurosis. Contractures are rare but there are slowly growing, sometimes painful, flesh-colored, fixed nodules especially on the central or medial sole of the foot. It can be bilateral and, if painful, intralesional corticosteroids or surgery for more aggressive disease is indicated. Recurrence is common.

Plasma cell mucositis. It is commonly and first described on the glans penis but also seen on the vulva, oral mucosa, and perirectal tissue, it is a chronic idiopathic inflammatory condition usually asymptomatic and most commonly occurs middle-aged and older. It is usually bright reddish-pink and well demarcated and the etiology is unknown. Histopathology examination is necessary to help rule out extramammary paget's disease, metastatic cancer, basal cell carcinoma, and other adenocarcinomas.

Plasmacytoma. Rare cutaneous B-cell lymphoma. Erythematous papules and plaques. Death from disseminated disease occurs in a minority of patients.

Plica polonica. Rare disorder where scalp hair shafts become irreversibly entangled into a matt of malodorous encrusted, sticky, moist mass. Predisposng factors include pediculosis capitis, pyoderma, poor hygiene, and deficient hair care. Removal of the plait of hair is necessary for therapeutic improvement. Some ethnic groups consider it a sign of health and recommend it to be left in place ("polish plat," "Rasfarian hair style,").

Plummer-Vinson syndrome. A syndrome characterized by dysphagia, glossitis, hypochromic anemia, and spoon nails in middle-aged women. The associated dryness and atrophy of the mucous membranes of the throat may lead to leukoplakia and squamous cell carcinoma, 592

Podoconiosis (non-filarial endemic elephantiasis of the lower legs). Asymmetric, bilateral elephantiasis nostras of the lower extremities seen in the highlands of Africa, Central and South America, and Indonesia due to walking barefoot on volcanic soil where small amounts of silica are absorbed through the feet and obstruct the lymphatics.

POEMS syndrome.(**P**olyneuropathy,**O**rganomegaly,**E**ndocrinopathy,**M**-protein, and **S**kin changes). Cherry-type and subcutaneous hemangiomas, hyperpigmentation, and hypertrichosis are reported in this syndrome. Glomeruloid hemangioma may be quite specific.

Poikiloderma, 26, 450t

Poikiloderma atrophicans vasculare (Jacobi), 26. *See* Atrophies of the skin

Poikiloderma congenitale. A rare syndrome characterized by telangiectasis, pigmentation, defective teeth, and bone cysts; may be similar to dyskeratosis congenita.

Poikiloderma of Civatte, 43, 442, 510, 510f

Poison ivy dermatitis, 9, 78f, 80–81

Poison weed dermatitis, 244

Poliosis. Localized loss of hair pigment. It has been associated with vitiligo, regrowth of hair in alopecia areata, piebaldism, tuberous sclerosis, malignant melanoma, intradermal nevi, congenital pigmented nevi, halo nevi, and Waardenburg syndrome.

Polyarteritis nodosa, 165t. *See* Periarteritis nodosa

Polychondritis, relapsing. Inflammation of cartilage most often involving the auricle of the ear but that may also involve inflammation of the eye, joints, nose, and most significantly heart valves or upper respiratory tract. The ear will demonstrate recurrent attacks of redness, pain, and swelling. Some authors have noticed a tense, fixed, urticarial papule and plaque eruption that is annulare on the trunk and mainly in males and it can occur months to years before the polychondritis., 37

Polycystic ovary syndrome (Stein-Leventhal). Amenorrhea and large polycystic ovaries, hirsutism (2/3), obesity (1/2) and insulin resistant hyperinsulinemia. Great variations in this syndrome make diagnosis and classification difficult., 385, 521

Polyfibromatosis. Rare syndrome with multiple cutaneous fibrotic conditions (Dupuytren's contracture, keloids, Peyronie's disease, plantar fibromatosis).

Polymorphic eruption of pregnancy. *See* Pruritic urticarial papules and plaques of pregnancy

Polymorphous light eruption, 471t, 471f, 471, 496t, 502

Pool toes. Erythematous, tender areas seen from friction against the cement bottom of pools at the beginning of swimming season. Treat by wearing protective footwear, avoiding contact with the bottom of the pool or be observed since protective calluses usually form with time.

Porokeratosis. Begins as a small, slightly elevated, wart-like papule that slowly enlarges, leaving an atrophic center with a keratotic, ridge-like border (coronoid lamellae). The small individual lesions may coalesce, this is the Mibelli type, and squamous cell cancers can arise (1-2% especially if very hyperkeratotic) in these tumors. A disseminated form (disseminated superficial actinic porokeratosis of Chernowski,DSAP) develops in middle-aged persons on sun-exposed limbs. Three other types are linear porokeratosis, porokeratosis punctuate palmaris et plantaris, and porokeratosis palmaris plantaris et disseminate. Histopathology may be characteristic., 320t, 330

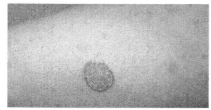

Porokeratosis of the leg.

Potassium permanganate. An oxidizing antiseptic usually used as a wet dressing in the concentration of 1:10,000., 221
Prausnitz-Küstner reaction. A demonstration of passive sensitization of the skin of a nonsensitive person. This is accomplished by the intradermal injection of serum from a sensitive patient into the skin of a nonsensitive person. After 24 to 48 hours, the allergen to be tested is injected intracutaneously into the previously injected site on the nonsensitive person's skin. Passive transfer of the sensitivity is manifested by the formation of a wheal.
Prayer marks. Lichenification and hyperpigmentation seen mainly in Muslims over bony prominences that experience repeated, extended pressure during times of prayer.
Precalcaneal congenital fibrolipomatosus (podalic papules, bilateral congenital fatty heel pads). Congenital, bilateral nonpulsatile, nontender, soft, skin color, elastic nodules between 0.5 and 1.5cm. Covered with normal epidermis, they are unattached to underlying tissue and do not transilluminate. Usually no therapy is necessary but surgery has been done if there is impairment of function.
Progeria. Extremely rare autosomal dominant mutation condition. Noticed early in life with characteristics of the elderly but no mental changes. Most patients die between 10 and 15 years of age. A factor may be a defect of hyaluronic acid.
Progressive hemifacial atrophy See Parry-Romberg Syndrome
Progressive symmetric erythrokeratodermia. SeeErythrokeratodermia progressive symmetrica

Prolidase deficiency. Rare hereditary syndrome affecting protein degradation. Resistant skin ulcers of the lower extremities are the commonest and most troublesome finding. Scar formation, xerosis, telangiectasias, purpura, poliosis, telangiectasias, and erythematous rash are among many other manifestations.
Proliferating trichilemmal cysts (proliferating pilar tumor). Locally aggressively, rapidly growing, scalp (90% of time) tumors usually in women. Rare malignant transformation., 321t
Protein kinase inhibitors. Anitcancer agents that are selective inhibitors of signal transduction molecules. Research in dermatology is being done for possible treatment for melanoma, nonmelanoma skin cancer, dermatofibrosarcoma protuberans, Merkel cell carcinoma, Kaposi's sarcoma, and systemic mastocytosis. Tyrosine kinase inhibitors are the commonest but threonine and serine can also be inhibited as well as combinations of all three(dual treatment). Histidine kinases inhibitors are also in development.
Proteus syndrome. Sporadic, progressive, congenital, rare condition which includes hemihypertrophy, epidermal nevi, macrodactyly, scoliosis, exostoses, and a variety of benign hamartomatous skin and sift tissue tumors. Elephant man (John Hermick) exhibited this syndrome even though some authors incorrectly diagnosed neurofibromatosis.
Protothecosis. Very rare chronic cutaneous infections with a nonpigmented algae (usually Prototheca wickerhamii) having protean clinical manifestations. Usually found in immunocompromised patients and the organism can be found in trees, lakes, rivers, sewage treatment plants, soil, and household garbage.
Protozoal dermatoses, 210, 550-552, 551f
Prurigo. This term is used more commonly in Europe. It lacks a precise definition but implies itchy bumps.
  actinic. A chronic photodermatitis seen in native Americans and Hispanics.
  pregnancy with, 581t, 584
Prurigo nodularis. A rare chronic dermatosis, usually of middle-aged women, consisting of discrete nodular pruritic excoriated papules and tumors scattered over the arms and the legs. This can be a warning sign of anemia, liver disease, renal disease, underlying cancer, and human immunodeficiency virus infection., 240
Prurigo pigmentosa. Rare inflammatory pruritic papules mainly over the upper trunk healing with netlike hyperpigmentation. Pathology is nonspecific. Reportedly mainly in the Japanese literature. A rare distinctive inflammatory disease with recurrent pruritic pink macules, papules, and papulous vesicles that resolve with a reticulate increase in pigment. Reported mainly in Japan but they are suggesting it may be under diagnosed.

Pruritic hereditary localized patch on the back (notalgia paresthetica). A rather common, benign problem manifested by a single patch of approximately 4 to 8 cm, usually lichenified, on the back. Frequently, the person rubs the area on the door jam orsimilar scratching post. May be slightlyhyperpigmented. Can rarely be associated with impingement on a spinal nerve., 151
Pruritic papular eruption. Papular, chronic, symmetrical, pruritic eruption in HIV (+) patients without other identifiable cause of pruritus. Common in HIV (+) patients and often seen early in the infection.
Pruritic urticarial papules and plaques of pregnancy (PUPPP syndrome). Most common gestational dermatoses (1 in 200 pregnancies) especially in the third trimester with first pregnancy and more common with twins. Very pruritic papules and plaques beginning in stretch marks on the abdomen (usually spares the periumbilical area) then spreads to the extremities. No perinatal risk to the mother or neonate. Treat with topical or occasionally systemic corticosteroids, 581t, 583
Pseudochancre redux. A late, gummatous, syphilitic inflammation occurring at the site of the original chancre.
Pseudocyst of auricle. Asymptomatic, noninflammatory swelling of the antihelix of the ear, seen mainly in middle-aged men. Treatment consists of draining the viscous (olive oil-like) sterile, clear to serosanguineous fluid. Minor trauma may play a role in etiology.
Pseudoepitheliomatous hyperplasia, 300
Pseudoepitheliomatosus, keratotic and micaceous balanitis. Large, well-demarcated, thick, solitary, micaceous, hyperkeratotic plaque with phimosis and hyperkeratotic foreskin. Indolent, chronic, relapsing, and may occur with a squamous cell carcinoma.

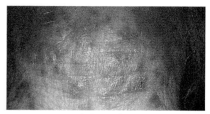

Pseudolymphoma of Spiegler-Fendt.

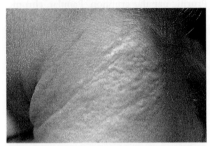
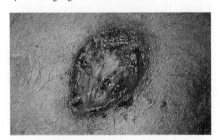

facies and mental retardation. Also pulmonary stenosis, keloid formation, large foramen magnum, and vertebral and sternal abnormalities.

Runner's rump. Increase pigment of the superior intergluteal cleft that results from ecchymosis in long distance runners. Due to rubbing of buttocks together.

Ruvalcaba-Myhre syndrome. Mental deficiency, colonic polyps, angiolipomas and macrocephaly associated with penile hyperpigmented areas, and café au lait spots.

S

Salicylic acid (beta hydroxy acid). Locally, this agent acts as a keratoplastic chemical in strengths up to 3% and as a keratolytic in strengths over 3%. Its greatest use is in the treatment of chronic fungus infection of the feet and lichenified patches seen with psoriasis or neurodermatitis. It macerates and peels off the thickened horny layer of the skin when used in the stronger strengths. In a 40% plaster in can be used for plantar warts, 36

Salmon patch, 491t, 493, 493f

San Joaquin valley fever. See Coccidioidomycosis

SAPHO syndrome, Synovitis, acne, pustulosis, hyperostosis, and osteitis

Sarcoid, Darier-Roussy. A deep subcutaneous form of sarcoid resembling erythema induratum.

Sarcoidosis, 38, 203–204, 204f, 461, 461f

Scabies, 17, 210–212, 211f, 312–314, 313f, 514, 554, 555f

Scarlet fever, 235t, 246

Schamberg's disease, 160

Schick test. An intradermal test using diphtheria toxin that, if positive as shown by the development of an erythematous wheal, indicates that the person lacks immunity for diphtheria.

Schilder's disease, 442

Schistosomiasis, 554

Schnitzler syndrome. Rare and probably underrecognized chronic urticarial rash and monoclonal IgM (seldom IgG) antibody. Also with disabling bone pain, fever, hyperostosis, and elevated sedimentation rate. Up to 15% of patients may develop lymphoproliferative disorders in 20 years.

Schultz-Charlton reaction. A blanching reaction seen when the scarlet fever antitoxin or convalescent serum is injected intradermally into a bright red area of the scarlet fever rash. Neutralization of the streptococcal toxin causes the blanching.

Scleredema. A self-limited rare disease characterized by benign but spreading induration and swelling of the skin and the subcutaneous tissues. It usually follows an acute infection. It resembles scleroderma but usually involutes in 3 to 12 months. May be associated with diabetes. Deep skin biopsy should allow differentiation of scleroderma from scleredema.

Sclerema neonatorum. Diffuse wax-like cutaneous and subcutaneous hardening in the first few weeks of life. 50%-75% mortality and seen in debilitated infants with sepsis, dehydration, congenital heart disease, respiratory stress

or diarrhea. Symmetrical, nonpitting, rock-hard, yellow-white, cadaver-like, cold skin develops. Twenty-five percent of mothers have been ill. No proven therapy.

Scleroderma, 162, 442, 447, 448f, 449t, 464, 464f

Scleromyxedema. Rare syndrome with plaques and lichenoid papules especially on the trunk and upper extremities associated with sclerodactyly, Raynaud's phenomenon, myopathy, neurologic defects, restrictive lung disease, esophageal dysmotility, and monoclonal gammopathy. Need skin biopsy to differentiate from scleroderma. Papular mucinosis and lichen myxedematosus are interchangeable terms. Infiltrates may be dramatic enough to cause a leonine facies., 449t

Sclerotherapy. An injection technique to rid patients of varicosities and occasionally also for hemangiomas., 134

Scurvy., 416, 591

Seabather's eruption, 554, 554f

Sebaceous adenoma, 339

Sebaceous hyperplasia, 339, 339f

Sebaceous nevus, 339, 339f

Seborrheic dermatitis, 19f, 23, 148, 177–180, 178f–179f, 187, 283, 390t, 423, 424f, 471t, 496t, 500, 500f

Seborrheic keratoses, 323–325, 323t, 324f, 510, 511f

Seborrhiasis. A name for an entity that clinically appears as a cross between seborrhea and psoriasis. Sebopsoriasis is a similar term.

Sebum, 7

Senear-Usher syndrome. Another term for pemphigus erythematosus.

Senile keratoses, 336

Senile pruritis, 146

Senile purpura, 160, 507

Servelle-Martorell syndrome (angio-osteohypotrophic syndrome). Venous (and rarely arterial) malformations associated with skeletal abnormalities. Venous ectasia and anuerysmal deformities can result in monstrous deformities and be confused with Klippel-Trenaunay-Weber syndrome.

Seven-year itch. See Scabies

Severe combined immunodeficiency, 501

Sézary syndrome, 227, 337t, 345

Shampoos, 30, 67, 179, 214

Shiitake dermatitis. Skin eruption of flagellate lesions due to eating raw or half-cooked shiitake which are mushrooms that contain a toxin called lentinan. This occurs mainly in Japan but can occur elsewhere as these mushrooms are cultivated worldwide .

Sicca syndrome. Xerostomia (dry mouth) and xerophthalmia (dry eyes, also called keratoconjunctivitis sicca) usually associated with Sjögren's syndrome.

Sign of Leser-Trélat, 452t, 515

Siliconoma. Subcutaneous granulomas seen as foreign body reactions to silicone injection.

Simmond's disease. Also known as hypophyseal cachexia, this disease is characterized by emaciation, amenorrhea, hypogenitalism, hypoglycemia, hypotension, and generalized pigmentation. The disease is due to necrosis of the pituitary, usually due to postpartum hemorrhage into the gland.

Sinus pericranii. Nodule on the scalp (usually frontal) that represents a communication with an intracranial dural sinus through dilated diploic veins. Clinically it presents as a flesh colored tortuous "hair of snakes" or bluish-red nodule. Usually in childhood or young adults with the most common symptoms of vertigo, headache or localized pain. Lesions dissipate on pressure or standing up. Hemorrhage, infection or emboli are potentially fatal complications which warrant neurosurgical consultation and appropriate imaging studies.

Sister Mary Joseph's nodule. Firm indurated nodule of the umbilicus indicating metastatic carcinoma., 515

Sixth disease. Another term for roseola infantum.

Sjögren-Larsson syndrome, 478t

Sjögren's syndrome, 419

Skin grafting, 159, 441

Skin tags, 325–326, 519. See also Fibromas, pedunculated

Slack Skin syndrome (granulomatous slack skin syndrome). Rare cutaneous T-cell lymphoma characterized by wrinkled pendulous erythematous folds of skin. Granulomatous inflammation and phagocytosis of elastic stroma as well as atypical lymphocytes are seen on histopathology. Especially in young males., 337t, 373

SLE. See Systemic lupus erythematosus

Smallpox, 569–574, 573f, 573t, 574t, 575f

Smith-Lemli-Opitz syndrome. Autosomal recessive with deficient 7-dehydrocholesterol reductase with resultant low cholesterol. Multiple malformations and development delays occur and the skin manifestation is photosensitivity which may be severe.

Smooth muscle hamartoma, congenital. See Hamartoma

Sneddon's syndrome. Livedo reticularis associated with slowly progressive multisystem medium and small vessel occlusion and vasculitis. Central nervous system often involved.

Soaks, 29

Soaps, 29

Sodoku. See Rat bite fever

Solar elastosis, 468

Solar urticaria, 471t, 472, 472f

Solenonychia. An acquired, longitudinal tubular deformity of a nail plate. Probably synonymous with median nail dystrophy.

Sparing phenomena, This where an unrelated skin disease spares the site of an already existing disease.

Spherulocytosis (myospherulosis). In Western countries, this benign, cystic mass usually affects the nose, paranasal sinuses and middle ear after surgery or topical treatment with greasy bases such as antibiotic ointments. In Africa, it usually precedes trauma with subcutaneous nodules developing on the limbs and buttocks. Hemorrhage in tissue with a high lipid content results in spherules which are clumps of red blood cells that start a foreign body reaction. Fat necrosis may ensue. "Brown bodies of Perls" represent extracellular hemosiderin.

microorganisms (Baccilus fusiformis) and spirochetes (Treponema vincenti). May reach the muscle and periosteum. Treatment is tetracycline and metronidazole., 576t

Troisier's Sign. An enlarged lymph node (Virchow's node) in the supraclavicular fossa due to metastasis from an abdominal malignancy. The spread of the cancer occurs via the thoracic duct.

Trousseau's syndrome. *See* Thrombophlebitis, superficial migratory

T.R.U.E. Test (Glaxo), 9

Trypanosomiasis, 551

Tuberculin tine test (Mantoux), 9

Tuberculoid leprosy, 249, 250f

Tuberculosis of the skin, 38, 235t, 248–251, 249t, 250f–251f

Tuberous sclerosis, 339, 462–463, 462f, 483f

Tufted angioma. Rare skin and subcutaneous slowly growing benign tumors that will occasionally self-involute. Often painful, tender and with hyperhidrosis and can develop the Kasabach-Merritt syndrome. They are dull, red, brown-red or purple patches or plaques that usually present prior to 5 years of age, may be multifocal and can develop in port-wine stains. *See* Angioma, tufted

Tularemia. The most common form is the ulceroglandular form with its primary chancre-type lesion and regional and generalized lymphadenopathy. Caused by *Pasteurella tularensis*. Other forms are oculoglandular, glandular, and typhoidal, 570t

Tumor necrosis factor receptor associated autoinflammatory syndrome (TRAPS) Rare Autosomal dominant disease with symptoms that include fever, pain in the joints, abdominal muscles, skin, and eye disease. The skin involvement includes migratory patches, erysipelas like erythema, edematous plaques, urticaria, and periorbital edema with or without conjunctivitis, 152

Tumors, 15, 16f, 320–345

Tungiasis. Caused by skin penetration of the pregnant female of the Tunga penetrans flea. A white to yellow-gray, papulonodule with a brown-black central tip forms as the flea begins to produce eggs and enlarges up to 1 cm by a phenomenon called physiogastry. Seen in Central and South America, sub-Saharan Africa and central Asia. Treatment is surgical excision., 556

Turf burn, 560t, 561

Twenty-nail dystrophy, 496t, 502

Tyrosinemia Type II (*See* Richer-Hanhart syndrome) (keratosis palmoplantar circumscriptus). Rare autosomal recessive syndrome of bilateral hyperkeratosis of the palms and soles (Richer-Hanhart syndrome) and (if tyrosine and phenylalanine are not restricted from the diet) mental retardation. Due to hepatic deficiency of hepatic tyrosine aminotransferase (TAT).

Tzanck smear. Cells scraped with a 15 Bard Parker blade from the floor of fresh bullae of pemphigus. These cells are altered epithelial cells, rounded, and devoid of intercellular attachments. Similar multinuclear giant cells seen in herpes simplex and herpes zoster. Smear is left to dry and stained with Giemsa for one minute and examined after drying under high magnification after applying a drop of emersion oil and coverslip., 267, 307, 308f

U

Ulcerative colitis, 455, 456f

Ulcerative lichen planus of the sole. Rare variant of lichen planus especially in females often accompanied by loss of toenails and scarring alopecia in addition to chronic, painful, progressive, ulcerations of the soles with histopathology indicative of lichen planus which may be present on other areas of the skin as well.

Ulcers, 17
chiclero, 551
decubitus, 244
infected, 235t, 244
mal perforans, 18
nonhealing leg, 158t
phagedenic, 244
pyodermic, 158
stasis, 157–160

Ulerythema ophryogenes. *See* Atrophies of the skin

Ultraviolet light, 466–475, 467t, 469f, 471t, 472f–475f, 474t

Uncombable hair syndrome ("Cheveux incoiffables," pili canaliculi, pili canaliculi et trianguli). Congenital, slowly growing, frizzy, scalp hair that is fragile and difficult to brush or comb. Rarely associated with ectodermal dysplasia. Electron microscopy may show a longitudinal groove (may also be seen on light microscopy) and a triangular, kidney bean or oval shape, 398, 398f, 486t

Unilateral laterothoracic exanthem (ULE). Also called asymmetric periflexural exanthem of childhood (APEC). Maculopapular or eczematous unilateral exanthem of childhood (mean age of onset 24 months) mean duration exanthem 5–6 weeks with regional lymphadenopathy. Probable viral origin. Spreads from the axilla and has an increased incidence in females (2:1). Unique eccrine lymphocytic infiltrate on biopsy.

Unilateral nevoid telangiectasia. Usually acquired but occasionally congenital Blaschkoid or dermatomal confluent telangiectasias acquired more common in women, congenital more common in men. May be associated with higher levels of estrogen such as pregnancy, puberty, and hormone therapy. There has also been an association with hyperthyroidism, chronic liver disease, alcoholic cirrhosis, and viral infections., 162

Urea. 29, 31, 69, 71, 76, 86t, 141, 145, 159, 179, 182, 398, 406, 409, 529

Uremic pruritus. A difficult problem of extreme pruritis associated with renal failure. May be helped by ultraviolet radiation, cholestyramine, oral charcoal, or lidocaine infusions. Consult the literature for cautions on different therapeutic interventions.

Urticaria, 38, 104t, 105–106, 105f, 152–154, 162, 206–209, 336, 472
physical, 560t

Urticaria-adrenergic. 1-5mm reddish macules or papules with a very characteristic pale halo around the edge occurring within 10-15 minutes after emotional upset. If severe the plaques maybe quite large. The lesions can be replicated by intradermal injection of noradrenaline but not acetylcholine. There is also associated increase plasma noradrenaline and adrenaline.

Urticaria pigmentosa, 336, 495t, 498, 498f

Uta, 551

V

Vaccinia. Generalized viral exanthema seen as a rare complication of smallpox vaccine. It usually resolves after a benign course. A generalized maculopapular eruption which often vesiculates and becomes umbilicated in a febrile moderately ill patient., 574, 575f

Van der Woude syndrome. Rare autosomal dominant with symmetric congenital lower lip pits that may have a salivary discharge. May be associated with hypodontia, bifid uvula, syngnathia, symblepharon, ankyloblepharon, polythelia, megacolon, auricular septal defect, congenital heart disease, syndactyly, equinovarus foot deformity, and sternal abnormalities.

Varicella. *See* Chickenpox

Varicella-zoster virus (VZV), 266–268, 267f, 279, 514–515, 514f

Varicelliform, 26

Varioliformis, 26

Varix. *See* Venous Lake

Vascular steal syndrome. In hemodialysis patients with arteriovenous fistulas, distal to the fistula a hernia can result in pain at rest, coolness, numbness, paresthesias, cyanosis, loss of distal pulses, muscle atrophy of the thenar muscles, paralysis, and gangrene of the digits and hand. Treatment is prompt surgical shunt ligation. Symptoms can develop from 1 week to 1 month after the fistula has been created.

Vasculitis, 162, 163f, 165t, 495t, 499
Giant cell arteritis, 165t
granulomatous, 165t
leukocytoclastic, 165t
polyarteritis nodosa, 165t
rheumatic, 165t
urticarial, especially in young female and associated with systemic lupus erythematosus, Sjögren's syndrome, IgM paraproteinemia, (Schitzler's syndrome), infection (hepatitis B and C, and mononucleosis), serum sickness, and drug allergies. Clinically mimics urticaria but lasts greater than 24 hours, often painful, resolves with purpura and hyperpigmentation and shows leukocytoclastic vasculitis on biopsy. Associated with decreased complement